COMPANION CD

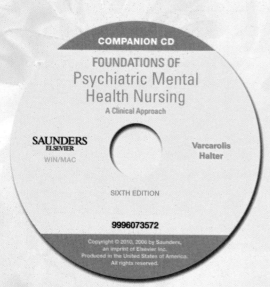

Your Companion CD for *Foundations of Psychiatric Mental Health Nursing* contains the following study aids to help you prepare for class tests as well as the NCLEX® Examination.

TEST-TAKING STRATEGIES

Learn to deconstruct and think critically about psychiatric mental health nursing test questions with the **Test-Taking Strategies** tutorial. This self-paced presentation (1) explains the various types of test questions you are likely to encounter on exams, (2) provides examples and techniques for answering them, and (3) offers general tips for testing success.

REVIEW QUESTIONS

Once you have the strategies for how to approach psychiatric mental health nursing test questions … practice, practice, practice! The **Review Questions** give you practice where you need it: you can mix and match questions across all chapters of the book and determine the total number of questions in each session. Each question includes the answer, a detailed rationale, the appropriate test-taking strategy, and relevant step of the nursing process (if applicable).

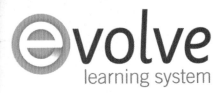

learning system

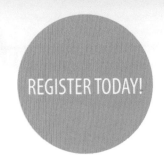

REGISTER TODAY!

To access your Evolve Resources, visit:

http://evolve.elsevier.com/Varcarolis/foundations

Evolve® Student Resources for Varcarolis and Halter: *Foundations of Psychiatric Mental Health Nursing,* 6th edition, include:

- **Audio Chapter Summaries,** available for online streaming or download, recap key points and important concepts from each chapter

- **Audio Glossary & Flashcards** highlight 150 psychiatric mental health nursing terms with definitions, audio pronunciations, and printable flashcards

- **Case Studies and Nursing Care Plans** supplement those in the textbook

- **Chapter Review Answers and Rationales** provide answers, rationales, cognitive level, NCLEX® Client Needs category, and step of the nursing process (if applicable) for the Chapter Review questions at the end of each chapter

- **Concept Map Creator** walks you through the process of creating individualized concept maps

- **Critical Thinking Answer Guidelines** provide possible outcomes for the Critical Thinking questions at the end of each chapter

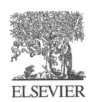

ELSEVIER

FOUNDATIONS OF
Psychiatric Mental Health Nursing

A Clinical Approach

SIXTH EDITION

Elizabeth M. Varcarolis, RN, MA
Professor Emeritus
Formerly Deputy Chairperson, Department of Nursing
Borough of Manhattan Community College
Associate Fellow
Albert Ellis Institute for Rational Emotional Behavioral
    Therapy (REBT)
New York, New York

Margaret Jordan Halter, PhD, PMHCNS-BC
Associate Professor
College of Nursing
University of Akron
Akron, Ohio

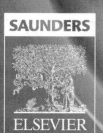

SAUNDERS

ELSEVIER

SAUNDERS
ELSEVIER

3251 Riverport Lane
St. Louis, Missouri 63043

FOUNDATIONS OF PSYCHIATRIC MENTAL
HEALTH NURSING: A CLINICAL APPROACH, SIXTH EDITION

ISBN: 978-1-4160-6667-5

Notice

Foundations of psychiatric mental health nursing : a clinical approach. --6th ed./[edited by] Elizabeth M. Varcarolis, Margaret J. Halter.
　　p. ; cm.
　Rev. ed. of: Foundations of psychiatric mental health nursing / [by] Elizabeth M. Varcarolis, Verna Benner Carson, Nancy Christine Shoemaker. 5th ed. 2006.
　Includes bibliographical references and index.
　ISBN 978-1-4160-6667-5 (hardback : alk. paper) 1. Psychiatric nursing. I. Varcarolis, Elizabeth M. II. Halter, Margaret J. (Margaret Jordan) III. Varcarolis, Elizabeth M. Foundations of psychiatric mental health nursing.
　[DNLM: 1. Mental Disorders--nursing. 2. Psychiatric Nursing. WY 160 F771 2010]
　RC440.F58 2010
　616.89'0231--dc22

　　　　　　　　　　　2009029783

Vice President and Publisher: Tom Wilhelm
Managing Editor: Jill Ferguson
Developmental Editor: Tiffany Trautwein
Publishing Services Manager: Anne Altepeter
Project Manager: Cindy Thoms
Senior Book Designer: Amy Buxton

Printed in the United States of America

Last digit is the print number: 9 8 7 6 5 4 3 2

DEDICATION

I want to give thanks to my husband, Paul, for all of the years he supported me through five revisions of *Foundations* with love and patience.

To Margaret Halter, who I am thrilled and grateful will be carrying this text onward with extensive expertise in the field of psychiatric nursing and genuine care for humanity in her heart. Good luck always, Ms. Peggy.

Betsy Varcarolis

To my girls, Emily, Elissa, and Monica, and their girls, Vivienne and Kiran. The world is a better and brighter place with you in it.

Fear gu aois, is bean gu bàs.

To my friend and mentor, Betsy. Thank you for your unwavering trust, support, and friendship. Your work has shaped two decades of psychiatric nursing knowledge, the way that nurses provide care, and how nurses think about the people for whom they provide care. With every best wish for you,

Peggy Halter

ACKNOWLEDGMENTS

The sixth edition of *Foundations* was based upon years of work and the contributions of countless experts whose voices continue to come through in a rich and personable way. Special thanks to returning chapter contributors—your knowledge and passion will continue to influence psychiatric nursing. These veteran contributors were joined by a new team of writers whose expertise was both recognized and sought. It has truly been a joy working with each of you. Thanks for the countless hours you spent researching, writing, and rewriting!

A huge debt of gratitude goes to the many educators and clinicians who reviewed the manuscript and offered valuable suggestions, ideas, opinions, and criticisms. All were welcomed and greatly helped refine and strengthen the individual chapters. Many thanks to contributors of past editions, whose influence on the text continues to be evident: Carrol Alvarez, Susan Caverly, Helene (Kay) Charron, Kathleen Smith DiJulio, Sally K. Holzapfel, Gloria Kuhlman, Catherine M. Lala, Francesca Profiri, Julius Trubowitz, and Thomas Wenzka.

Throughout this project, a number of people at Elsevier provided superb editorial and publishing services. Thanks to Tom Wilhelm, vice president and publisher. It is clear why Elsevier has entrusted much to him—he is a sparkling star. Any conversation with Tom is guaranteed to be informative, candid, and entertaining. Sincere thanks go to other valuable Elsevier players: Cindy Thoms, our gracious project manager; Amy Buxton, a talented and creative designer; and Brian Dennison, senior developmental editor, who was instrumental in coordinating and setting the stage for the sixth edition.

Special appreciation goes to Jill Ferguson, managing editor, and Tiffany Trautwein, developmental editor. During weekly conference calls we brainstormed, pored over countless details, and developed timelines. Their professionalism and support were invaluable. From five hundred miles away, these two women became part of my extended family. Thank you, Jill and Tiffany—we did it!

And finally, thanks to my nuclear family and to my friends for your patience and support throughout this revision.

Peggy Halter

CONTRIBUTORS

Lois Angelo, APRN, BC
Assistant Professor of Nursing
Massachusetts College of Pharmacy and Health
  Sciences
Boston, Massachusetts
Instructor's Manual

Timothy Kevin Blake, RN, MSN
Associate Professor of Nursing
Ohio University Zanesville
Zanesville, Ohio
Critical Thinking Answer Guidelines

Leslie A. Briscoe, PMHNP-BC
Psychiatric Nurse Practitioner
U.S. Veterans Affairs Department
Cleveland, Ohio
Chapter 29 Psychosocial Needs of the Older Adult

Penny S. Brooke, APRN, MS, JD
Professor and Director of Outreach
College of Nursing
University of Utah
Salt Lake City, Utah
Chapter 7 Legal and Ethical Guidelines for Safe Practice

Teresa S. Burckhalter, MSN, RN, BC
Nursing Instructor
Technical College of the Lowcountry
Beaufort, South Carolina
Test-Taking Strategies
Test Bank

Claudia A. Cihlar, PhD, PMHCNS-BC
Coordinator of Behavioral Health Services
Center for Psychiatry
Akron General Medical Center
Akron, Ohio
Chapter 19 Personality Disorders

Avni Cirpili, RN, MSN
Chief Nursing Officer
Department of Psychiatry
Ohio State University Harding Hospital
Columbus, Ohio
*Chapter 4 Psychiatric Mental Health Nursing in
  Acute Care Settings*
*Chapter 5 Psychiatric Mental Health Nursing in
  Community Settings*

Alison M. Colbert, PhD, APRN, BC
Assistant Professor
Duquesne University
Pittsburgh, Pennsylvania
Chapter 33 Forensic Psychiatric Nursing

Joe Councill III, RN, MSN
Assistant Professor
Clarkson College
Omaha, Nebraska
Chapter 18 Addictive Disorders

Carissa R. Enright, RN, MSN, PMHNP-BC
Associate Clinical Professor
Texas Woman's University
Psychiatric Consult Liaison
Presbyterian Hospital of Dallas
Dallas, Texas
Chapter 16 Eating Disorders

Elizabeth Hite Erwin, PhD, APRN, BC
Assistant Professor
University of Virginia School of Nursing
Charlottesville, Virginia
Chapter 28 Disorders of Children and Adolescents

Christine Heifner Graor, PhD, PMHCNS-BC
Assistant Professor
College of Nursing
University of Akron
Akron, Ohio
Chapter 23 Crisis and Disaster

Faye J. Grund, PMHNP-BC
President and Associate Professor
MedCentral College of Nursing
Board Member of NAMI Richland County
Mansfield, Ohio
Chapter 22 Somatoform, Factitious, and Dissociative Disorders

Mary A. Gutierrez, PharmD, BCPP
Professor of Clinical Pharmacy and Psychiatry
Department of Pharmacotherapy and
  Outcome Science
School of Pharmacy
Loma Linda University
Loma Linda, California
*Chapter 3 Biological Basis for Understanding
  Psychotropic Drugs*

Edward A. Herzog, RN, BSN, MSN, APN
Lecturer
College of Nursing
Kent State University
Kent, Ohio
Chapter 15 Schizophrenia
Chapter 30 Serious Mental Illness
Chapter Review Questions
Test Bank

Mallie Kozy, PhD, PMHCNS-BC
Associate Professor
Associate Chair for Undergraduate Curriculum
School of Nursing, Lourdes College
Sylvania, Ohio
Chapter 13 Depressive Disorders

Kathy Kramer-Howe, MA, MSN, LCSW
Bereavement Team Leader
Hospice of the Valley
Phoenix, Arizona
Chapter 32 Care for the Dying and for Those Who Grieve

Karyn I. Morgan, RN, MSN, CNS
Instructor
University of Akron College of Nursing
Clinical Nurse Specialist
Intensive Outpatient Psychiatry
Summa Health System
Akron, Ohio
Chapter 34 Therapeutic Groups

Lorann Murphy, MSN, PMHCNS-BC
Clinical Nurse Specialist
Lutheran Hospital
Cleveland, Ohio
Chapter 25 Anger, Aggression, and Violence

Cherie R. Rebar, MSN, MBA, RN, FNP, ND, PhD(c)
Associate Professor
Kettering College of Medical Arts
Chair, Associate of Science Nursing Program
Dayton, Ohio
Chapter Review Questions
Companion CD Review Questions

Judi Sateren, MS, RN
Associate Professor
St. Olaf College
Northfield, Minnesota
Chapter 26 Child, Older Adult, and Intimate Partner Abuse

L. Kathleen Sekula, PhD, APRN-BC
Associate Professor and Director
Forensic Graduate Nursing Programs
Duquesne University
Pittsburgh, Pennsylvania
Chapter 33 Forensic Psychiatric Nursing

Kathleen Slyh, RN, MSN
Nursing Instructor
Technical College of the Lowcountry
Beaufort, South Carolina
PowerPoint® Presentations

Jane Stein-Parbury, RN, BSN, MEd, PhD, FRCNA
Professor of Mental Health Nursing
Faculty of Nursing, Midwifery and Health
University of Technology
Director, Area Professorial Mental Health
    Nursing Unit
South East Sydney Area Health Service
Sydney, Australia
Chapter 17 Cognitive Disorders

Sylvia Stevens, APRN, MS, BC
Professor of Nursing
Montgomery College
Silver Spring, Maryland
Psychotherapy Private Practice
Washington, District of Columbia
Chapter 35 Family Interventions

Margaret Trussler, ANP-BC
Instructor
University of Massachusetts
Nurse Practitioner
Sleep Health Centers
Worcester, Massachusetts
Chapter 20 Sleep Disorders

Roberta Waite, EdD, RN, PMHCNS-BC
Assistant Professor
College of Nursing and Health Professions
Drexel University
Philadelphia, Pennsylvania
*Chapter 31 Psychological Needs of Patients with Medical
    Conditions*

M. Selena Yearwood, EdD, MSN, RN-BC
Professor
Chamberlain College of Nursing
Phoenix, Arizona
Chapter 24 Suicide

Rothlyn P. Zahourek, PhD, PMHCNS-BC, AHN-BC
Private Holistic Psychotherapy
Consultation and Education Practice
Belchertown, Massachusetts
Chapter 36 Integrative Care

Rick Zoucha, PhD, APRN-BC, CTN
Associate Professor
College of Nursing
Duquesne University
Pittsburgh, Pennsylvania
Chapter 6 Cultural Implications for Psychiatric Mental Health Nursing

REVIEWERS

Nancy Buccola, RN, APRN, MSN, CNS
Assistant Professor of Clinical Nursing
Louisiana State University
New Orleans, Louisiana

Mary Ann Camann, PhD, APRN, BC
Associate Professor of Nursing
Kennesaw State University
Kennesaw, Georgia

Sherry D. Chin, RN, MSN
Clinical Instructor of Nursing
Montgomery College
Takoma Park, Maryland

Nancy A. Craig-Williams, MS, RN, PhD(c)
Professor of Nursing
Greenfield Community College
Greenfield, Massachusetts

Nancy R. Cyr, DHSc, RN
Assistant Professor of Nursing
North Georgia College and State University
Dahlonega, Georgia

Chyllia Dixon, LMT, RPP, CHt
Banner Nurse Fellow/Student Nurse
Maricopa Community College District
    Nursing Program
GateWay Community College
Phoenix, Arizona

Dianna H. Douglas, DNS, APRN-CNS
Professor of Nursing
Louisiana State University
New Orleans, Louisiana

Eleanor Falkingham, RN, MSN, CNE
Assistant Professor of Nursing
University of South Dakota
Watertown, South Dakota

Debra A. Gottel, MHS, RN
Instructor of Nursing
University of South Florida
Tampa, Florida

Mary Paulette Humphries, RN, MA, MS
Nursing Lecturer
Indiana University East
Richmond, Indiana

Ann C. Keely, RN, MN, APRN-BC, LMFT
Assistant Professor of Nursing
Georgia Baptist College of Nursing
Mercer University
Atlanta, Georgia

Deborah Kindy, PhD, RN
Professor of Nursing
Sonoma State University
Rohnert Park, California

Barbara Wolfe Magenheim, EdD, MSN, BSN, RN, CNE
Nursing Faculty
Chandler-Gilbert Community College
Chandler, Arizona

Marina Martinez-Kratz, RN, BSN, MS
Professor of Nursing
Jackson Community College
Jackson, Michigan

Mary L. Spath, RN, CNS, PhD(c), CNE
Associate Professor of Nursing
University of St. Francis
Fort Wayne, Indiana

Jeanne Venhaus Stein, DNP, MSN, RN, CNS
Assistant Professor of Nursing
California State University, Long Beach
Long Beach, California

Linda Turchin, MSN, RN, CNE
Assistant Professor of Nursing
Fairmont State University
Fairmont, West Virginia

Kim Webb, RN, MN
Nursing Chair
Northern Oklahoma College
Tonkawa, Oklahoma

Stephanie Lenz Windle, MSN, RN
Nursing Instructor
Merritt College
Oakland, California

TO THE INSTRUCTOR

The role of the health care provider continues to become more challenging as our health care system is compromised by increasing federal cuts, lack of trained personnel, and the dictates of health maintenance organizations (HMOs) and behavioral health maintenance organizations (BHMOs). We nurses and our patients are from increasingly diverse cultural and religious backgrounds, bringing with us a wide spectrum of beliefs and practices. An in-depth consideration and understanding of cultural, religious/spiritual, and social practices is paramount in the administration of appropriate and effective nursing care and is emphasized throughout this text.

We are living in an age of fast-paced research in neurobiology, genetics, and psychopharmacology, as well as research to find the most effective evidence-based approaches for patients and their families. Legal issues and ethical dilemmas faced by the health care system are magnified accordingly. Given these myriad challenges, knowing how best to teach our students and serve our patients can seem overwhelming. With contributions from several knowledgeable and experienced nurse educators, our goal is to bring to you the most current and comprehensive trends and evidence-based practices in psychiatric mental health nursing.

CONTENT NEW TO THIS EDITION

The following topics are at the forefront of nursing practice and, as such, considered in detail in this sixth edition:

- Issues involving mental health parity and other current legislations (Chapter 4)
- Disaster preparedness (Chapter 5)
- Emphasis on the fact that we are all "from another culture" to encourage cultural awareness (Chapter 6)
- Neurotransmitter and immune stress responses, stress-inducing events and stress-reducing techniques, self-assessment of the nurse's stress level, and mindfulness (Chapter 11)
- Evidence-based practices and an enhanced emphasis on health promotion, resiliency, and recovery in disorders chapters (Unit 4)
- Depression screenings in children, adolescents, and older adults; vagus nerve stimulation; and additional subtypes of depression under consideration for the *DSM-IV* (Chapter 13)
- Nursing interventions for injury prevention (Chapter 17)

- Emphasis throughout the text on recovery versus rehabilitation, victimization, social isolation and loneliness, unemployment and poverty, involuntary treatment, incarceration, wellness and recovery action plans, interventions to promote adherence to treatment, and more
- Chapter 20, Sleep Disorders, recognizing the increased prevalence and implications of sleep disturbances with a focus on their relationship to psychiatric illness and the nurse's role in assessment and management
- Chapter 21, Sexual Dysfunction and Sexual Disorders, introducing the complex issue of sexual behavior and providing the knowledge of normal and abnormal sexuality necessary to conduct a sexual assessment, identify deviations from normal sexual behavior, recognize nursing implications, and formulate interventions

Refer to the To the Student section of this introduction on pages x-xi for examples of thoroughly updated **familiar features with a fresh perspective**, including Evidence-Based Practice boxes, Integrative Therapy boxes, Considering Culture boxes, Key Points to Remember, Assessment Guidelines, and Vignettes, among others.

ORGANIZATION OF THE TEXT

Chapters are grouped in units to emphasize the clinical perspective and facilitate location of information. All clinical chapters are organized in a clear, logical, and consistent format with the nursing process as the strong, visible framework. The basic outline for clinical chapters is:

- **Clinical Picture**—Identifies disorders that fall under the umbrella of the general chapter name. Presents an overview of the disorder(s) and includes *DSM-IV-TR* criteria as appropriate.
- **Epidemiology**—Helps the student to understand the extent of the problem and characteristics of those who would more likely be affected. This section provides information related to prevalence, lifetime incidence, age of onset, and gender differences.
- **Comorbidity**—Describes the most commonly associated comorbid conditions. Knowing that comorbid disorders are often part of the clinical picture of specific disorders helps students as well as clinicians understand how to better assess and treat their patients.

- **Etiology**—Provides current views of causation along with formerly held theories. It is based on the biopsychosocial triad and includes biological, psychological, and environmental factors.
- **Assessment:**
  - **General Assessment**—Appropriate assessment for a specific disorder, including assessment tools and rating scales. The rating scales included help to highlight important areas in the assessment of a variety of behaviors or mental conditions. Because many of the answers are subjective in nature, experienced clinicians use these tools as a guide when planning care, in addition to their knowledge of their patients.
  - **Self-Assessment**—Discusses the nurse's thoughts and feelings that may need to be addressed to enhance self-growth and provide the best possible and most appropriate care to the patient.
  - **Assessment Guidelines**—Summary of specific areas to assess by disorder.
- **Diagnosis**—NANDA International–approved nursing diagnoses are used in all nursing process sections, and *DSM-IV-TR* (2000) taxonomy and criteria are used throughout.
- **Outcomes Identification**—NIC classifications for interventions and NOC classifications for outcomes are introduced in Chapter 8 and used throughout the text when appropriate.
- **Planning**
- **Implementation**—Interventions follow the Standards of Practice and Professional Performance set by the *Psychiatric-Mental Health Nursing: Scope and Standards of Practice* (2007) developed collaboratively by the American Nurses Association, American Psychiatric Nurses Association, and International Society of Psychiatric–Mental Health Nurses. These standards are incorporated throughout the chapters and are listed on the inside back cover for easy reference.
- **Evaluation**

TEACHING AND LEARNING RESOURCES

For Instructors

All instructor resources are easily accessible on **Evolve** (http://evolve.elsevier.com/Varcarolis/foundations). The **Instructor's Manual** includes an expansive Introduction with course preparation guidelines and teaching tips, Objectives and Key Terms from each chapter, annotated Chapter Outlines, Thoughts About Teaching the Topic, and Concept Maps. **PowerPoint®** **Presentations** offer approximately 750 slides for in-class lectures. **Audience Response Questions,** 2 to 5 multiple-answer questions embedded within each chapter's PowerPoint® presentation, stimulate class discussion and assess student understanding of key concepts. The **Test Bank** has more than 1800 test items, complete with the correct answer, rationale, cognitive level of each question, corresponding step of the nursing process, appropriate NCLEX® Client Needs label, and text page reference(s).

For Students

Students will find a wealth of valuable learning resources on their free **Companion CD** (bound with the textbook) and on **Evolve**. The Evolve Resources page in the front of the book gives login instructions and a description of each resource. Reminders also appear in each chapter to help readers along the way.

We are grateful to educators who send suggestions and provide feedback and hope this sixth edition continues to help students learn and appreciate the scope of psychiatric mental health nursing practice.

Peggy Halter and Betsy Varcarolis

TO THE STUDENT

Psychiatric mental health nursing challenges us to understand the complexities of human behavior. In the chapters that follow, you will learn about people with psychiatric disorders and how to provide them with quality nursing care. As you read, keep in mind these special features.

READING AND REVIEW TOOLS

1 **Key Terms and Concepts** and **2** **Objectives** introduce the chapter topics and provide a concise overview of the material discussed.

Key Points to Remember listed at the end of each chapter reinforce essential information.

Critical Thinking activities at the end of each chapter are scenario-based critical thinking problems for practice in applying what you have learned. **Answer guidelines** can be found on the Evolve website.

Multiple choice **Chapter Review** questions at the end of each chapter help you review the chapter material and study for exams. **Answers** are located in the back of your book, and **rationales** and textbook **page references** are available on the Evolve website.

ADDITIONAL LEARNING RESOURCES

The **Companion CD** included in your textbook contains **Test-Taking Strategies** for psychiatric mental health nursing and more than 300 **Review Questions** to help you prepare for the NCLEX® Examination.

3 Your free **Evolve Resources** at **http://evolve.elsevier. com/Varcarolis/foundations** offer more helpful study aids, such as Audio Chapter Summaries, an Audio Glossary & Flashcards, additional Case Studies and Nursing Care Plans, and a Concept Map Creator.

CHAPTER FEATURES

4 **Vignettes** describe the unique circumstances surrounding individual patients with psychiatric disorders.

5 **Self-Assessment** sections discuss the nurse's thoughts and feelings that may need to be addressed to enhance self-growth and provide the best possible and most appropriate care to the patient.

6 **Assessment Guidelines** at the end of each Assessment section in the clinical chapters provide summary points for patient assessment.

7 **Evidence-Based Practice** boxes demonstrate how current research findings affect psychiatric mental health nursing practice and standards of care.

8 **Guidelines for Communication** boxes provide tips for communicating therapeutically with patients and their families.

Considering Culture boxes reinforce the importance of providing culturally competent care.

Drug Treatment tables present the latest information on medications used to treat psychiatric disorders.

Integrative Therapy boxes discuss significant nursing considerations for complementary and alternative therapies and examine relevant study findings.

9 **Patient and Family Teaching** boxes underscore the nurse's role in helping patients and families understand psychiatric disorders, treatments, complications, and medication side effects, among other important issues.

Case Studies and Nursing Care Plans present individualized histories of patients with specific psychiatric disorders following the steps of the nursing process. Interventions with rationales and evaluation statements are presented for each patient goal.

A Nurse Speaks narratives, which introduce select units, provide personal stories of individual nurses in various practice settings. **A Patient Speaks** narratives, written in the patient's own words, describe how psychiatric disorders affect them, their families, and their caregivers.

CHAPTER 14

Bipolar Disorders

Margaret Jordan Halter and Elizabeth M. Varcarolis

1 **Key Terms and Concepts**

acute phase, 288
anticonvulsant drugs, 294
bipolar I disorder, 281
bipolar II disorder, 281
clang associations, 287
continuation phase, 288
cyclothymia, 281
flight of ideas, 286
grandiosity, 287
hypomania, 281
lithium carbonate, 292
maintenance phase, 288
mania, 281
mood stabilizers, 299
rapid cycling, 281
seclusion protocol, 297

2 **Objectives**

1. Assess a patient experiencing mania for (a) mood, (b) behavior, and (c) thought processes, and be alert to possible dysfunction.
2. Formulate three nursing diagnoses appropriate for a patient with mania, and include supporting data.
3. Explain the rationales behind five methods of communication that may be used with a patient experiencing mania.
4. Teach a classmate at least four expected side effects of lithium therapy.
5. Distinguish between signs of early and severe lithium toxicity.
6. Write a medication care plan specifying five areas of patient teaching regarding lithium carbonate.
7. Compare and contrast basic clinical conditions that may respond better to anticonvulsant therapy with those that may respond better to lithium therapy.
8. Evaluate specific indications for the use of seclusion for a patient experiencing mania.
9. Defend the use of electroconvulsive therapy for a patient in specific situations.
10. Review at least three of the items presented in the patient and family teaching plan (see Box 14-2) with a patient with bipolar disorder.
11. Distinguish the focus of treatment for a person in the acute manic phase from the focus of treatment for a person in the continuation or maintenance phase.

3 evolve Visit the Evolve website for an **Audio Glossary & Flashcards, Concept Map Creator,** and additional resources related to the content in this chapter: **http://evolve.elsevier.com/Varcarolis/foundations**

Once commonly known as *manic-depression,* bipolar disorder is a chronic, recurrent illness that must be carefully managed throughout a person's life. Bipolar disorder frequently goes unrecognized, and people suffer for an average of 6 years before receiving a proper diagnosis and treatment (Wang et al., 2005). Bipolar disorder is marked by shifts in mood, energy, and ability to function. The course of the illness is variable, and symptoms range from severe mania—an exaggerated euphoria or irritability—to severe depression (Figure 14-1). Periods of normal functioning may alternate with periods of illness (highs, lows, or a combination of both). However, many individuals continue to experience chronic interpersonal or occupational difficulties even during remission. The mortality rate for bipolar disorder is severe; 25% to 60% of individuals with bipolar disorder will make a suicide attempt at least once in their lifetime, and nearly 20% of all deaths among this population are from suicide (Tondo & Baldessarini et al., 2006).

280

226 Unit 4 Psychobiological Disorders

7 **EVIDENCE-BASED PRACTICE**

Teenage Pregnancy and the Trauma of Giving Birth

Anderson, C., & McGuiness, T. M. (2008). Do teenage mothers experience childbirth as traumatic? *Journal of Psychosocial Nursing and Mental Health Services, 46*(4), 21–24.

Problem

Despite the fact that hundreds of thousands of teenagers give birth every year in the United States, little is known about the psychological impact it has on these girls. Although giving birth can be a stressor at any age, teenagers often lack social support and resources for coping. Adverse psychological consequences can have a profoundly negative impact on both the mother's level of health and that of her infant.

Purpose of Study

The purpose of this study was to assess for posttraumatic stress (PTS) and postpartum depression (PPD) in teenage mothers.

Methods

For this pilot (initial) study, 28 teenage mothers were interviewed by telephone 9 months after childbirth. They were between the ages of 15 and 19 and included 13 Latina, 8 African Americans, and 6 Caucasians. The participants were asked to rate their perception of childbirth, respond to questions assessing for PTS, and respond to questions assessing for PPD.

Key Findings

- Most of the mothers rated their experience with childbirth at a midway point between *awful* and *great.*
- Fourteen of the participants were afraid of losing control during labor, and 13 believed that they would die in childbirth.
- Scores from a third of the participants indicated PTS as the result of childbirth experiences.
- Scores from more than half the participants indicated the presence of mild to severe depression.

Implications for Nursing Practice

Some teenage mothers are vulnerable to PTS and PPD because of lack of social support, low self-esteem, chaotic/harsh upbringing, and family conflict. Carefully assessing the patient's history for risk factors can be the first step in minimizing these vulnerabilities. Educational programs in which girls are provided with information related to the process of labor and delivery, pain management methods, and what to expect postpartum can reduce fear and possibly reduce psychiatric complications.

Psychiatric mental health nurses care for adolescent girls who have been abused or sexually assaulted, have eating disorders, and/or abuse alcohol and drugs. Understanding the additional stress childbirth may bring about should be considered when assessing and intervening with teenagers who have given birth. Collaboration between maternal-child health nurses and psychiatric mental health nurses could provide the ideal support for pregnant teenagers and teenagers who have given birth.

Behavioral theories suggest that anxiety is a learned response to specific environmental stimuli (classical conditioning). An example of classical conditioning is a boy who experiences anxiety when his abusive mother enters the room and then generalizes this anxiety as a response to all women (Sadock & Sadock, 2008). The social learning model suggests that anxiety is learned through the modeling of parents or peers. For example, a mother who is fearful of thunder and lightning and hides in closets during storms may transmit her anxiety to her children, who continue to adopt her behavior into adult life. Such individuals can unlearn this behavior by observing others who react normally to a storm by lighting candles and telling stories.

Cognitive theorists believe that anxiety disorders are caused by distortions in an individual's thoughts and perceptions. Because individuals with such distortions may believe that any mistake will have catastrophic results, they experience acute anxiety.

Cultural Considerations

Reliable data on the incidence of anxiety disorders are sparse, but sociocultural variation in symptoms of anxiety disorders has been noted. In some cultures, individuals express anxiety through somatic symptoms, whereas in other cultures, cognitive symptoms predominate. Panic attacks in Latin Americans and Northern Europeans often involve sensations of choking, smothering, numbness, or tingling, as well as fear of dying. In other cultural groups, panic attacks involve fear of magic or witchcraft. Social phobias in Japanese and Korean cultures may relate to beliefs that the individual's blushing, eye contact, or body odor is offensive to others (APA, 2000).

The *DSM-IV-TR* (APA, 2000) notes cultural aspects of each psychiatric disorder to alert the clinician to cultural contexts that must be considered before making a psychiatric diagnosis. The Considering Culture box discusses factors relevant to one anxiety disorder (ataque de nervios) primarily experienced by people from Hispanic cultures. Also review Chapter 6 for more discussion of cultural issues.

384 Unit 4 Psychobiological Disorders

are confusing, and he does not know what they are doing there, anyway. Sometimes he tries to walk away from the terrifying feelings and the strangers. He tries to find something he has lost long ago…if he could only remember what it is. ■

Stage 4: Late Alzheimer's Disease

Late in AD, the following symptoms may occur: **agraphia** (inability to read or write), **hyperorality** (the need to taste, chew, and put everything in one's mouth), blunting of emotions, visual agnosia (loss of ability to recognize familiar objects), and **hypermetamorphosis** (manifested by touching of everything in sight). At this stage, the ability to talk, and eventually the ability to walk, is lost. End-stage AD is characterized by stupor and coma. Death frequently is secondary to infection or choking.

4 VIGNETTE

Mrs. Collins and the children keep Mr. Collins at home until his outbursts become frightening. Once he is lost for 2 days after he somehow unlocks the front door. Finally Mrs. Collins admits her husband to a Veterans Administration (VA) hospital. When his wife comes to visit, Mr. Collins sometimes cries, but he never talks. He is usually restrained in his chair during her visits. The staff explain to her that although Mr. Collins can still walk, he keeps getting into other people's beds and scaring them. They explain that perhaps he wants comfort and misses human touch. They encourage her visits, even though Mr. Collins does not seem to recognize her. He does respond to music. His wife brings a radio, and when she plays the country and western music he has always loved, Mr. Collins nods and claps his hands.

Mrs. Collins is torn between guilt and love, anger and despair. She is confused and depressed. She is going through the painful process of mourning the loss of the man she has loved and shared a life with for 34 years. Three months after his admission to the VA hospital, and 8 years after the incident of the crossed wires at the telephone company, Mr. Collins chokes on some food, develops pneumonia, and dies. ■

5 **Self-Assessment**

Working with cognitively impaired people in any setting should make us aware of the tremendous responsibility placed on caregivers. The behavioral problems these patients may display can cause tremendous stress for professionals and family caregivers alike. Caring for people who are unable to communicate and have lost the ability to relate and respond to others is extremely difficult, especially for student nurses or nurses who do not understand dementia or AD.

Nurses working in facilities for residents who are cognitively impaired (e.g., nursing homes and extended care facilities) need special education and skills. Education must include information about the process of the disease and effective interventions, as well as knowledge regarding antipsychotic drugs. Support and educational opportunities should be readily available, not just to nurses but also to nurse aides, who are often directly responsible for administering basic care.

Because stress is a common occurrence when working with persons with cognitive impairments, staff need to be proactive in minimizing its effects, which can be facilitated by:

- Having a realistic understanding of the disease so that expectations for the person are realistic.
- Establishing realistic outcomes for the person and recognizing when they are achieved. These outcomes may be as minor as *patient feeds self with spoon,* yet remember that even the smallest achievement can be a significant accomplishment for the impaired individual.
- Maintaining good self-care. As nurses, we need to protect ourselves from the negative effects of stress by obtaining adequate sleep and rest, eating a nutritious diet, exercising, engaging in relaxing activities, and addressing our own emotional and spiritual needs.

Assessment Guidelines Dementia 6

1. Evaluate the person's current level of cognitive and daily functioning.
2. Identify any threats to the person's safety and security and arrange their reduction.
3. Evaluate the safety of the person's home environment (e.g., with regard to wandering, eating inedible objects, falling, engaging in provocative behaviors toward others).
4. Review the medications (including, herbs, complementary agents) the patient is currently taking.
5. Interview family to gain a complete picture of the person's background and personality.
6. Explore how well the family is prepared for and informed about the progress of the person's dementia, depending on cause (if known).
7. Discuss with the family members how they are coping with the patient and their main issues at this time.
8. Review the resources available to the family. Ask family members to describe the help they receive from other family members, friends, and community resources. Determine if caregivers are aware of community support groups and resources.
9. Identify the needs of the family for teaching and guidance (e.g., how to manage catastrophic reactions, lability of mood, aggressive behaviors, and nocturnal delirium and increased confusion and agitation at night [sundowning]).

324 Unit 4 Psychobiological Disorders

8 **BOX 15-4 Guidelines for Communication with Patients Experiencing Delusions**

- To build trust, be open, honest, and reliable.
- Respond to suspicions in a matter-of-fact, empathic, supportive, and calm manner.
- Ask the patient to describe the delusions. Example: "Tell me more about someone trying to hurt you."
- Avoid debating the delusional content, but interject doubt where appropriate. Example: "It seems like it would be hard for that petite girl to hurt you."
- Focus on the feelings that underlie or flow from the delusions. Example: "You seem to wish you could be more powerful," or "It must feel frightening to think others want to hurt you."
- Once it is understood and addressed, do not dwell further on the delusion. Instead, focus on more reality-based topics. If the patient obsesses about delusions, set firm limits on the amount of time you will talk about them, and explain your reason.
- Observe for events that trigger delusions. If possible, help the patient find ways to reduce or manage them.
- Validate if part of the delusion is real. Example: "Yes, there was a man at the nurse's station, but I did not hear him talk about you."

Data from Farhall, J., Greenwood, K. M., & Jackson, H. J. (2007). Coping with hallucinated voices in schizophrenia. A review of self-initiated strategies and therapeutic interventions. *Clinical Psychology Review, 27,* 476–493.

BOX 15-5 Patient and Family Teaching: Coping with Auditory Hallucinations or Delusions 9

Distraction

- Listening to music
- Reading (aloud may help more)
- Counting backwards from 100
- Watching television

Interaction

- Looking at others—do they seem to be hearing/fearing what you are? If not, ignore the voices/thoughts.
- Talking with another person

Activity

- Walking
- Cleaning the house
- Having a relaxing bath
- Playing the guitar or singing
- Going to the gym (or anyplace you enjoy being, where others will be present)

Talking to Yourself

- Telling the voices or thoughts to go away
- Telling yourself that the voices and thoughts are a symptom and not real
- Telling yourself that no matter what you hear, voices can be safely ignored

Social Action

- Talking to a trusted friend or member of the family
- Calling a help line or going to a drop-in center
- Visiting a favorite place or a comfortable public place

Physical Action

- Taking extra medication when ordered (call your prescriber)
- Going for a walk or doing other exercise
- Using breathing exercises and other relaxation methods

Data from Farhall, J., Greenwood, K. M., & Jackson, H. J. (2007). Coping with hallucinated voices in schizophrenia: A review of self-initiated strategies and therapeutic interventions. *Clinical Psychology Review, 27,* 476-493; and Jenner, J. A., Neinhuis, F. J., van de Willige, G., & Wiersma, D. (2006). "Hitting" voices of schizophrenia patients may lastingly reduce persistent auditory hallucinations and their burden: 18-month outcome of a randomized controlled trial. *Canadian Journal of Psychiatry, 51*(3), 169–177.

on delusional thoughts. The more time the patient spends engaged in activities or with people, the more opportunities there are to receive feedback about and become comfortable with reality.

Work with the patient to find out which coping strategies succeed and how the patient can make the best use of them. Box 15-4 lists techniques for communicating with patients experiencing delusions, and Box 15-5 presents patient and family teaching topics for coping with hallucinations and delusions.

Associative Looseness

Associative looseness often mirrors the patient's autistic thoughts and reflects poorly organized thinking. An increase in associative looseness often indicates that the patient is feeling increased anxiety or overwhelmed by internal and external stimuli. The patient's ramblings may also produce confusion and frustration in the nurse. The following guidelines are useful for intervention with a patient whose speech is confused and disorganized:

- Do *not* pretend you understand the patient's words or meaning when you don't; tell the patient you are having difficulty understanding.
- Place the difficulty in understanding on yourself, *not* on the patient. Example: "I'm having trouble following what you are saying," *not* "You're not making any sense."
- Look for recurring topics and *themes* in the patient's communications, and *tie these to events*

DETAILED CONTENTS

A NURSE SPEAKS

Fifty years ago psychiatry was practiced in an environment vastly different from the one in which it is practiced today. Most patients were treated in large state hospitals, which were like small towns with their own stores, restaurants, churches, farms, power plants, carpentry shops, and buildings housing thousands of patients and staff. There were buildings for admission and for treatment, infirmaries, chronic quiet units, and chronic disturbed units.

As nursing students, we were taught to care for patients who were receiving sedation, insulin shock, electric shock, malaria therapy, continuous hydrotherapy, wet packs, supraorbital lobotomies, physical restraints, and seclusion. All of these treatments were designed to make the patients more amenable to psychotherapy, to calm them, or for the safety of themselves or others. The disturbed wards were usually noisy and very active places in which patients acted out their psychoses both physically and vocally. Care for these patients was mostly custodial and involved keeping them clean, fed, safe, and calm.

I distinctly remember one patient who was almost continuously kept in seclusion because of his bizarre and aggressive behavior. He would not keep his clothes on, could not safely use eating utensils, and roared like a lion. Because of his behavior, he was frequently referred to as the Lion Man. Keeping him clean and fed was a major project for the staff and always required several people. It was a frustrating experience because we all wanted to help him and see him behave in a more acceptable manner.

During the Korean War, I was away in the Air Force for four years. For three years I was a part of a system that treated young men for psychiatric problems by using many of the same modalities that were used in the state hospitals. The treatment there was somewhat more successful than that provided in the state hospitals because most of the men's visible signs of psychoses were of recent origin, having been caused by the stress of basic training or the stress of being in battle.

During my fourth year in the Air Force, psychotropic drugs were introduced. We began to use them cautiously on our patients, with very limited success. As the doctors became more familiar with the drugs and increased the dosages, we saw much improved behavior in most patients. Gradually no patients were being put into packs, and the hydrotherapy room was seldom used.

After being discharged from the Air Force, I returned to the hospital in which I had trained. As I went to the different buildings, I was surprised to see that here too there had been a decrease in the use of the old treatment modalities. Patients for the most part appeared much calmer; no patients were in seclusion all of the time, not even the Lion Man.

One day, while I was walking on the grounds with one of the charge attendants, he asked me if I knew who a patient sitting on a bench talking with another patient was. I said, "No. Who is he?" "That is the guy we used to call the Lion Man." What a change! The attendant told me that they had given him Thorazine and that within one week he was out of seclusion and keeping his clothes on. Gradually he began to socialize with staff and other patients. Within one month he was playing checkers, and within one year he was granted ground privileges.

John A. Payne

John Payne died in April 2001 after a long illness.

CHAPTER **1**

Mental Health and Mental Illness

Margaret Jordan Halter

Key Terms and Concepts

advanced practice registered nurse–psychiatric
   mental health (APRN-PMH), 19
basic level registered nurse, 18
clinical epidemiology, 11
comorbid condition, 11
Diagnostic and Statistical Manual of Mental
   Disorders, fourth edition, text revision
   (DSM-IV-TR), 5
electronic health care, 20
epidemiology, 10
evidence-based practice, 18
incidence, 10

mental health, 3
mental health continuum, 4
mental illness, 4
Nursing Interventions Classification (NIC), 17
Nursing Outcomes Classification (NOC), 17
phenomena of concern, 17
prevalence, 10
psychiatric mental health nursing, 17
psychiatry's definition of mental health, 3
registered nurse–psychiatric mental health
   (RN-PMH), 18
resilience, 5

Objectives

1. Describe the continuum of mental health and mental illness.
2. Explore the role of resilience in the prevention of and recovery from mental illness, and consider your own resilience in response to stress.
3. Identify how culture influences our view of mental illnesses and behaviors associated with them.
4. Discuss the nature/nurture origins of psychiatric disorders.
5. Summarize the social influences of mental health care in the United States.

6. Explain how epidemiological studies can improve medical and nursing care.
7. Identify how the *DSM-IV-TR* multiaxial system can influence a clinician to consider a broad range of information before making a diagnosis.
8. Describe the specialty of psychiatric mental health nursing, and list three phenomena of concern.
9. Compare and contrast a *DSM-IV-TR* medical diagnosis with a nursing diagnosis.
10. Discuss future challenges and opportunities for mental health care in the United States.

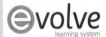 Visit the Evolve website for an **Audio Glossary & Flashcards, Concept Map Creator,** and additional resources related to the content in this chapter: **http://evolve.elsevier.com/Varcarolis/foundations**

If you are a fan of vintage films, you may have witnessed a scene similar to the following: A doctor, wearing a lab coat and an expression of deep concern, enters a hospital waiting room and delivers the bad news to an obviously distraught gentleman who is seated there. The doctor says, "I'm afraid your wife has suffered a nervous breakdown." From that point on, the woman's condition is only vaguely hinted at. The husband dutifully visits her at a gated asylum where the staff regards him with sad expressions. He may find his wife confined to her bed, or standing by the window and staring vacantly into the middle distance, or sitting motionless in the hospital garden. The viewer can only speculate about the nature of the problem but assumes she has had an emotional collapse.

CONTINUUM OF MENTAL HEALTH AND MENTAL ILLNESS

We have come a long way in acknowledging psychiatric disorders and increasing our understanding of them since the days of "nervous breakdowns." In fact, the World Health Organization (WHO) (2007) maintains that a person cannot be considered healthy without taking into account mental health, as well as physical health. The WHO defines mental health as a state of well-being in which each individual is able to realize his or her own potential, cope with the normal stresses of life, work productively and fruitfully, and make a contribution to the community. Mental health provides people with the capacity for rational thinking, communication skills, learning, emotional growth, resilience, and self-esteem (U.S. Department of Health and Human Services [USDHHS], 1999). Some of the attributes of mentally healthy people are presented in Figure 1-1.

Psychiatry's definition of mental health evolves over time. It is a definition shaped by the prevailing culture and societal values, and it reflects changes in cultural norms, society's expectations, political climates, and even reimbursement criteria by third-party payers. In the past, the term *mental illness* was applied to behaviors considered "strange" and "different"—behaviors that occurred infrequently and

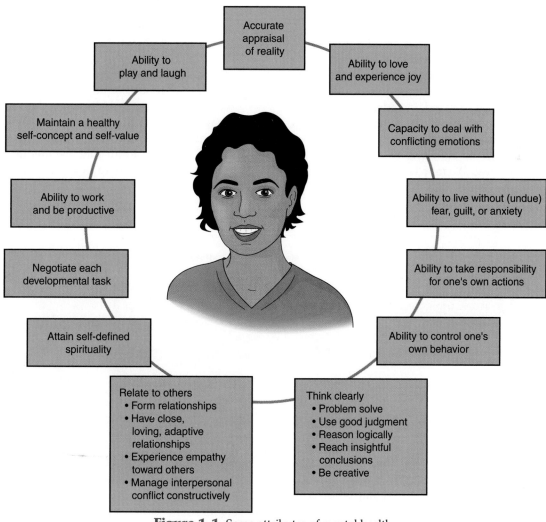

Figure 1-1 Some attributes of mental health.

deviated from an established norm. Such criteria are inadequate because they suggest that mental health is based on conformity. But there is a further problem in viewing people whose behavior is "strange" or "different" as mentally ill. If such definitions were used, nonconformists and independent thinkers like Abraham Lincoln, Mahatma Gandhi, and Socrates would be judged mentally ill. And although the sacrifices of a Mother Teresa or the dedication of Martin Luther King Jr. are uncommon, virtually none of us would consider these much-admired behaviors to be signs of mental illness.

Mental illness is considered to be a clinically significant behavioral or psychological syndrome marked by the patient's distress, disability, or the risk of suffering disability or loss of freedom (APA, 2000). *Mental illness* refers to all mental disorders with definable diagnoses. Thinking may be impaired—as in Alzheimer's disease; mood may be affected—as in major depression; and behavioral alterations may be apparent—as in schizophrenia; or the patient may display some combination of the three.

You may be wondering if there is some middle ground between mental health and mental illness. After all, it is a rare person who does not have doubts as to his or her sanity at one time or another. The answer is a definite *yes*, there is a middle ground; in fact, mental health and mental illness can be conceptualized as points along a **mental health continuum** (Figure 1-2).

Well-being is characterized by adequate to high-level functioning in response to routine stress and resultant anxiety or distress. Nearly all of us experience emotional problems or concerns or occasions when we are not at our best. We may feel lousy temporarily, but signs and symptoms are not of sufficient duration or intensity to warrant a psychiatric diagnosis. We may spend a day or two in a gray cloud of self-doubt and recrimination over a failed exam, a sleepless night filled with worry and obsessing about normally trivial concerns, or months of genuine sadness and mourning after the death of a loved one. During those times, we are fully or vaguely aware that we are not functioning optimally. However, these problems or concerns may be alleviated by time, exercise, a balanced diet, rest, talking with others, mental reframing, or even early intervention and treatment. It is not until we experience marked distress or suffer from impairment or inability to function in our everyday lives that the line is crossed into mental illness.

People who have experienced mental illness can testify to the existence of changes in functioning. The following comments of a 40-year-old woman illustrate the continuum between illness and health as her condition ranged from (1) deep depression to (2) mania to (3) health:

1. It was horror and hell. I was at the bottom of the deepest and darkest pit there ever was. I was worthless and unforgivable. I was as good as—no, worse than—dead.
2. I was incredibly alive. I could sense and feel everything. I was sure I could do anything, accomplish any task, create whatever I wanted, if only other people wouldn't get in my way.
3. Yes, I am sometimes sad and sometimes happy and excited, but nothing as extreme as before. I am much calmer. I realize now that, when I was manic, it was a pressure-cooker feeling. When I am happy now, or loving, it is more peaceful and real. I have to admit that I sometimes miss the intensity—the sense of power and creativity—of those manic times. I never miss anything about

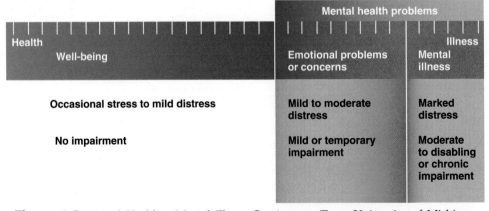

Figure 1-2 Mental Health – Mental Illness Continuum. (From University of Michigan, "Understanding U." [2007]. *What is mental health?* <http://www.hr.umich.edu/mhealthy/programs/mental_emotional/understandingu/learn/mental_health.html> Accessed 30.07.08.)

the depressed times, but of course the power and the creativity never bore fruit. Now I do get things done, some of the time, like most people. And people treat me much better now. I guess I must seem more real to them. I certainly seem more real to me (Altrocchi, 1980).

Contributing Factors

Many factors can affect the severity and progression of a mental illness, as well as the mental health of a person who does not have a mental illness (Figure 1-3). If possible, these influences need to be evaluated and factored into an individual's plan of care. In fact, the *Diagnostic and Statistical Manual of Mental Disorders, fourth edition, text revision (DSM-IV-TR)*, a two-inch thick manual that classifies more than 300 mental disorders, states that there is evidence suggesting that the symptoms and causes of a number of disorders are influenced by cultural and ethnic

factors (APA, 2000). The *DSM-IV-TR* is discussed in further detail later in this chapter.

Resilience

Researchers, clinicians, and consumers are all interested in actively facilitating mental health and reducing mental illness. A characteristic of mental health, increasingly being promoted and essential to the recovery process, is **resilience**. Resilience is closely associated with the process of adapting and helps people facing tragedies, loss, trauma, and severe stress (APA, 2004). Disasters, such as the attack on the World Trade towers in 2001 and the devastation of Hurricane Katrina in 2005, in which people pulled together to help one another and carried on despite horrendous loss, illustrate resilience. Being resilient does not mean being unaffected by stressors. It means that rather than falling victim to negative emotions, resilient people recognize the feelings, readily deal with them, and learn from the experience.

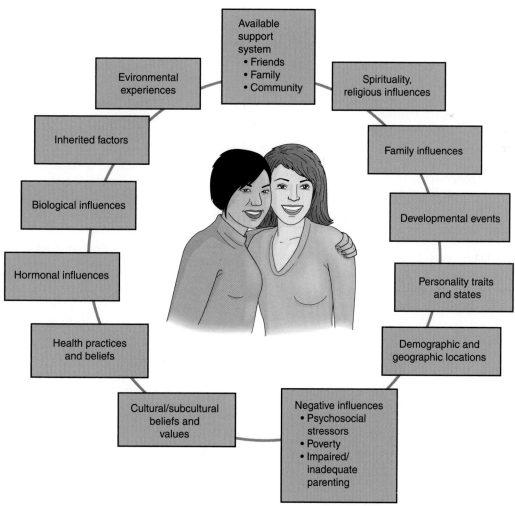

Figure 1-3 Influences that can have an impact on an individual's mental health.

The promotion of resilience has implications for improving not only individual responses to stress and mental illness but also the level of happiness and well-being of the general population (Cloninger, 2006). Accessing and developing this trait assists people to bounce back from painful experiences and difficult events. It is characterized by optimism, a sense of mastery, and competence. It is not an unusual quality but one that is possessed by regular, everyday people and can be enhanced in almost everyone.

Research demonstrates that early experiences in mastering difficult or stressful situations enhance the prefrontal cortex's resiliency in coping with difficult situations later. According to Amat and colleagues (2006), when rats were exposed to uncontrollable stresses, their brains turned off mood-regulating cells, and they developed a syndrome much like major depression. However, rats that were first given the chance to control a stressful situation were better able to respond to subsequent stress for up to a week following the success. In fact, when the successful rats were faced with uncontrollable stress, their brain cells responded as if they were in control.

People who are resilient are effective at regulating their emotions and not falling victim to negative, self-defeating thoughts. You can get an idea of how good you are at regulating your emotions by taking the Resilience Factor Test in Box 1-1.

Culture

There is no standard measure for mental health, in part because it is culturally defined and is based on interpretations of what effective functioning is according to societal norms (WHO, 2007). One approach to differentiating mental health from mental illness is to consider what a particular culture regards as acceptable or unacceptable. In this view, the mentally ill are those who violate social norms and thus threaten (or make anxious) those observing them. For example, traditional Japanese may consider suicide to be an act of honor, and Middle Eastern "suicide bombers" are considered holy warriors or martyrs. Contrast these viewpoints with Western culture, where people who attempt or complete suicides are nearly always considered mentally ill.

Throughout history, people have interpreted health or sickness according to their own current views. A striking example of how cultural change influences the interpretation of mental illness is an old definition of *hysteria*. According to Webster's Dictionary (Porter, 1913), hysteria was "A nervous affection, occurring almost exclusively in women, in which the emotional and reflex excitability is exaggerated, and the will power correspondingly diminished, so that the patient loses control over the emotions, becomes the victim of imaginary sensations, and often falls into paroxysm or fits." Treatment for this condition often involved

---

BOX 1-1 The Resilience Factor Test

Use the following scale to rate each item listed below:
1 = Not true of me
2 = Sometimes true
3 = Moderately true
4 = Usually true
5 = Very true

1. Even if I plan ahead for a discussion with my spouse, my boss, or my child, I still find myself acting emotionally.
2. I am unable to harness positive emotions to help me focus on a task.
3. I can control the way I feel when adversity strikes.
4. I get carried away by my feelings.
5. I am good at identifying what I am thinking and how it affects my mood.
6. If someone does something that upsets me, I am able to wait until an appropriate time when I have calmed down to discuss it.
7. My emotions affect my ability to focus on what I need to get done at home, school, or work.
8. When I discuss a hot topic with a colleague or family member, I am able to keep my emotions in check.

Add your score on the following items:
3 _____
5 _____
6 _____
8 _____

Add your score on the following items:
1 _____
2 _____
4 _____
7 _____

Positive total = _____   Negative total = _____

Positive total minus negative total = _____

A score higher than 13 is rated as above average in emotional regulation.

A score between 6 and 13 is inconclusive.

A score lower than 6 is rated as below average in emotional regulation.

If your emotional regulation is below average, you may need to master some calming skills.

Here are a few tips:
- When anxiety strikes, your breathing may become shallow and quick. You can help control the anxiety by controlling your breathing. Inhale slowly through your nose, breathing deeply from your belly, not your chest.
- Stress will make your body tight and stiff. Again, you can counter the effects of stress on the body and brain if you relax your muscles.
- Try positive imagery; create an image that is relaxing, such as visualizing yourself on a secluded beach.
- Resilience is within your reach.

From Reivich, K., & Shatte, A. (2003). *The resilience factor: 7 essential skills for overcoming life's inevitable obstacles.* New York: Broadway Books.

sexual outlets for afflicted women, whose condition was thought to be the result of sexual deprivation. According to some authors, this diagnosis fell into disuse as women's rights improved, the family atmosphere became less restrictive, and societal tolerance of sexual practices increased.

Cultures differ in not only their views regarding mental illness but also the types of behavior categorized as mental illness. **Culture-bound syndromes** seem to occur in specific sociocultural contexts and are easily recognized by people in those cultures (Sadock & Sadock, 2008). For example, one syndrome recognized in parts of Southeast Asia is **running amok**, in which a person (usually a male) runs around engaging in furious, almost indiscriminate violent behavior. **Pibloktoq**, an uncontrollable desire to tear off one's clothing and expose oneself to severe winter weather, is a recognized psychological disorder in parts of Greenland, Alaska, and the Arctic regions of Canada. In the United States, **anorexia nervosa** (see Chapter 16) is recognized as a psychobiological disorder that entails voluntary starvation. The disorder is well known in Europe, North America, and Australia but unheard of in many other parts of the world.

What is to be made of the fact that certain disorders occur in some cultures but are absent in others? One interpretation is that the conditions necessary for causing a particular disorder occur in some places but are absent in other places. Another interpretation is that people learn certain kinds of abnormal behavior by imitation. However, the fact that some disorders may be culturally determined does not prove that all mental illnesses are so determined. The best evidence suggests that schizophrenia (see Chapter 15) and bipolar disorders (see Chapter 14) are found throughout the world. The symptom patterns of schizophrenia have been observed among indigenous Greenlanders and West African villagers, as well as in Western culture.

Perceptions of Mental Health and Mental Illness

Mental Illness versus Physical Illness

People commonly make a distinction between mental illnesses and physical illnesses. It is an odd distinction, considering that *mental* refers to the brain, the most complex and sophisticated part of the body, the organ responsible for the higher thought processes that set us apart from other creatures. Surely the workings of the brain—the synaptic connections, the areas of functioning, the spinal innervations and connections—are *physical*. One problem with this distinction is that it implies that psychiatric disorders are "all in the head" and therefore under personal control and indistinguishable from a choice to indulge in bad behavior. Although some physical disorders, such as a broken

arm from skiing or lung cancer from smoking, are blamed on the victim, the majority of physical illnesses are considered to be beyond personal responsibility.

Perhaps the origin of this distinction between mental and physical illness lies in the religious and philosophical tradition of explaining the unexplainable by assigning a mystical or spiritual origin to cognitive processes and emotional activities. Despite many advances in understanding, mental illnesses continue to be viewed differently from illnesses that originate in other parts of the body.

Consider that people with epilepsy were once thought to be possessed by demons, under the attack of gods, or cursed; they were subjected to horrible "cures" and treatments. Today, most people would say that epilepsy is a disorder of the mind and not under personal control, because we can *see* epilepsy on brain scans as areas of overactivity and excitably. But there are no specific biological tests to diagnose most psychiatric disorders—no cranium culture for depression and no MRI for obsessive-compulsive disorder (OCD). However, researchers are convinced that the root of most mental disorders lies in intercellular abnormalities, and we can now see clear signs of altered brain function in several mental disorders, including schizophrenia, OCD, stress disorders, and depression.

Nature versus Nurture

For students, one of the most intriguing aspects of learning about mental illnesses is understanding their origins. Although for centuries people believed that extremely unusual behaviors were due to demonic forces, in the late 1800s, the mental health pendulum swung briefly to a biological focus with the "germ theory of diseases." Germ theory explained mental illness in the same way other illnesses were being described—that is, they were caused by a specific agent in the environment (Morgan, McKenzie, & Fearon, 2008). This theory was abandoned rather quickly, since clinicians and researchers could not identify single causative factors for mental illnesses; there was no "mania germ" that could be viewed under a microscope and subsequently treated.

Although ineffective biological treatments for mental illness continued to be explored, over the next half century, psychological theories dominated and focused on the science of the mind and behavior. These theories explained the origin of mental illness as faulty psychological processes that could be corrected by increasing personal insight and understanding. For example, a patient experiencing depression and apathy might be assisted to explore feelings left over from childhood, when his attempts at independence were harshly discouraged by overly protective parents.

This psychological focus was challenged in 1952 when chlorpromazine (Thorazine) was found to have a calming effect on agitated, out-of-control patients.

Imagine what this must have been like for clinicians who had resorted to every biological treatment imaginable, including wet wraps, insulin shock therapy, and psychosurgery (in which holes were drilled in the head of a patient and probes inserted in the brain) in a futile attempt to change behavior. Many began to believe that if psychiatric problems respond to medications that alter intercellular components, then there must be a disruption of intercellular components to begin with. At this point, the pendulum made steady and sure progress to a biological explanation of psychiatric problems and disorders.

Currently, the **diathesis-stress model**—in which diathesis represents biological predisposition, and stress represents environmental stress or trauma—is the most accepted explanation for mental illness. This nature-*plus*-nurture argument asserts that most psychiatric disorders result from a combination of genetic vulnerability and negative environmental stressors. While one person may develop major depression largely as the result of an inherited and biological vulnerability that alters brain chemistry, another person with little vulnerability may develop depression from changes in brain chemistry caused by the insults of a stressful environment.

Social Influences on Mental Health Care

Consumer Movement and Mental Health Recovery

In the latter part of the 20th century, tremendous energy was expended on putting the notion of equality into widespread practice in the United States. Treating people fairly and extinguishing labels became focuses of the culture. In regard to mental illness, decades of institutionalization had created political and social concerns that gave rise to a mental health movement similar to women's rights movements, civil rights movements, disabilities rights movements, and gay rights movements. Groups of people with mental illnesses—or **mental health consumers**—began to advocate for their rights and the rights of others with mental illness and to fight stigma, discrimination, and forced treatment.

In 1979, a nationwide advocacy group, the National Alliance on Mental Illness (NAMI), was formed by people with mental illnesses and their families. In the 1980s, individuals in the consumer movement, now organized by NAMI, began to resist the traditional arrangement of mental health care providers who dictated care and treatment of the patient. This "paternalistic" relationship was not just demoralizing; it also implied that patients were not competent to make their own decisions. Consumers rebelled and demanded increased involvement in decisions concerning their treatment.

The consumer movement also promoted the notion of **recovery**, which was both a new and an old idea in mental health. On one hand, it represents a concept that has been around a long time: that some people—even those with the most serious illnesses, such as schizophrenia—recover. One such recovery was depicted in the movie "A Beautiful Mind," wherein a brilliant mathematician, John Nash, seems to have emerged from a continuous cycle of devastating psychotic relapses to a state of stabilization and recovery (Howard, 2001). On the other hand, a newer conceptualization of recovery evolved into a consumer-focused process "in which people are able to live, work, learn, and participate fully in their communities" (U.S. Department of Health and Human Services, 2003).

According to the Substance Abuse and Mental Health Services Administration (SAMHSA) (2005), there are 10 fundamental components of the recovery process:

1. **Self-directed:** Consumers lead, control, exercise choice over, and determine their own path of recovery.
2. **Individual- and person-centered:** Recovery is based on unique strengths and resiliencies, as well as needs, preferences, experiences (including past trauma), and cultural backgrounds.
3. **Empowering:** Consumers have the authority to choose from a range of options, participate in all decisions that will affect their lives, and be educated and supported in so doing.
4. **Holistic:** Recovery encompasses an individual's whole life, including mind, body, spirit, and community.
5. **Nonlinear:** Recovery is based on continual growth, occasional setbacks, and learning from experience.
6. **Strengths-based:** Recovery is focused on valuing and building on the multiple capacities, resiliencies, talents, coping abilities, and inherent worth of individuals.
7. **Peer-supported:** Consumers encourage and engage each other in recovery and provide a sense of belonging, supportive relationships, valued roles, and community.
8. **Respect:** Community, systems, and societal acceptance and appreciation of consumers—including protecting their rights and eliminating discrimination and stigma—are crucial in achieving recovery.
9. **Responsibility:** Consumers have a personal responsibility for their own self-care and recovery, for understanding and giving meaning to their experiences, and for identifying coping strategies and healing processes to promote their own wellness.
10. **Hope:** Recovery provides the essential motivating message of a better future: that people can and do overcome the barriers and obstacles that confront them. Hope is the catalyst of the recovery process.

VIGNETTE

Jeff is a mental health consumer who has schizophrenia. Involvement in a recovery support group has changed his view of himself, and he has taken the lead role in his own recovery: "See, nobody knows your body better than you do, and some, maybe some mental health providers or doctors, think, 'Hey, I am the professional, you're the person seeing me, I know what's best for you.' But technically, it isn't true. They only provide you with the tools to get better. They can't crawl inside you and see how you are." ■

Decade of the Brain

In 1990, President George H. W. Bush designated the last decade of the 1900s as the Decade of the Brain. The overriding goal of this designation was to make legislators and the general public aware of the advances that had been made in neuroscience and brain research. This U.S. initiative stimulated a worldwide growth of scientific research (Tandon, 2000). Among the advances and progress made during the Decade of the Brain were:

- Understanding the genetic basis of embryonic and fetal neural development
- Mapping genes involved in neurological illness, including mutations associated with Parkinson's disease, Alzheimer's disease, and epilepsy
- Discovering that the brain uses a relatively small number of neurotransmitters but has a vast assortment of neurotransmitter receptors
- Uncovering the role of cytokines (proteins involved in the immune response) in such brain disorders as depression
- Refining neuroimaging techniques, such as positron emission tomography (PET) scans, magnetic resonance imaging (MRI), magneto encephalography, and event-related electroencephalography (EEG), which have improved our understanding of normal brain functioning, as well as areas of difference in pathological states
- Bringing together computer modeling and laboratory research, which resulted in the new discipline of computational neuroscience.

Surgeon General's Report on Mental Health

The first Surgeon General's report on the topic of mental health was published in 1999 (USDHHS, 1999). This landmark document was based on an extensive review of the scientific literature in consultation with mental health providers and consumers. The two most important messages from this report were that (1) mental health is fundamental to overall health, and (2) there are effective treatments for mental health. The report is reader-friendly and a good introduction to mental health and illness. You can review the

report at http://www.surgeongeneral.gov/library/mentalhealth/home.html.

Human Genome Project

The Human Genome Project was a 13-year project that lasted from 1990–2003 and was completed on the 50th anniversary of the discovery of the DNA double helix. The project has strengthened biological and genetic explanations for psychiatric conditions (Cohen, 2000). The goals of the project (U.S. Department of Energy, 2008) were to:

- **Identify** the approximately 20,000 to 25,000 genes in human DNA.
- **Determine** the sequences of the 3 billion chemical base pairs that make up human DNA.
- **Store** this information in databases.
- **Improve** tools for data analysis.
- **Address** the ethical, legal, and social issues that may arise from the project.

Although researchers have begun to identify strong genetic links to mental illness (as you will see in the chapters on clinical disorders); it will be some time before we understand the exact nature of genetic influences on mental illness. What we do know is that most psychiatric disorders are the result of multiple mutated or defective genes, each of which in combination may contribute to the disorder.

President's New Freedom Commission on Mental Health

In 2003, the President's New Freedom Commission on Mental Health released its recommendations for mental health care in America. This was the first commission since First Lady Rosalyn Carter's (wife of President Jimmy Carter) in 1978. The report noted that the system of delivering mental health care in America was "in a shambles." It called for a streamlined system with a less fragmented delivery of care. It advocated early diagnosis and treatment, a new expectation for principles of recovery, and increased assistance in helping people find housing and work. Box 1-2 describes the goals necessary for such a transformation of mental health care in the United States.

Institute of Medicine

The "Improving the Quality of Health Care for Mental and Substance-Use Conditions: Quality Chasm Series" was released in 2005 by the Institute of Medicine (IOM). It highlights the effective treatments for mental illness and at the same time addresses the huge gap between the best care and the worst. It focuses on such issues as the problem of coerced (forced) treatment, a system that treats mental health issues separately from physical health problems, and lack of quality control. This report (IOM, 2006, p. 7) makes strong, sound recommendations for treating mental illness—from the standpoint of both providers and financial

BOX 1-2 Goals for a Transformed Mental Health System in the United States

Goal 1

Americans understand that mental health is essential to overall health.

Goal 2

Mental health care is consumer- and family-driven.

Goal 3

Disparities in mental health services are eliminated.

Goal 4

Early mental health screening, assessment, and referral to services are common practice.

Goal 5

Excellent mental health care is delivered, and research is accelerated.

Goal 6

Technology is used to access mental health care and information.

Data from U.S. Department of Health and Human Services, President's New Freedom Commission on Mental Health. (2003). *Achieving the promise: Transforming mental health care in America.* USDHHS Publication No. SMA-03–3832. <http://www.mentalhealthcommission.gov/reports/finalreport/fullreport-02.htm>

reimbursers of care—and stipulates that to have high-quality mental health care (or any health care), the system must aim to be:

- **Safe:** The provided care should not add further injury (e.g., nosocomial infections).
- **Effective:** Services should be based on scientific knowledge, and services with little benefit should be reduced or abandoned.
- **Patient-centered:** Care should be given in an atmosphere of respect and responsiveness, and the patient's values (rather than our own) should guide care.
- **Timely:** Delays in care should be reduced.
- **Efficient:** Waste of supplies, ideas, and energy should be avoided.
- **Equitable:** Care resources should be distributed fairly, regardless of individual circumstances.

Mental Health Parity Act

Imagine insurance companies singling out a group of disorders such as cardiac diseases and then requiring higher co-pays and specifying the number of times patients could be reimbursed for treatment in their lives. People would be outraged by such discrimination, yet this is exactly what happens with psychiatric

disorders. While this saves money for insurers, costs are shifted to taxpayers, and many people suffer needlessly. Advocates have fought to remedy reimbursement inequities for years. In response to this problem, the Mental Health Parity Act of 1996 was signed into law. *Parity* refers to equality, and this legislation required insurers that provide mental health coverage to offer annual and lifetime benefits at the same level provided for medical/surgical coverage. Unfortunately, by the year 2000, the Government Accounting Office found that although 86% of health plans complied with the 1996 law, 87% of those plans actually imposed new limits on mental health coverage.

The Wellstone-Domenici Parity Act built on the 1996 legislation. It was enacted into law on October 3, 2008 for group health plans with more than 50 employees. While mental health coverage is still not mandated under any plan, the new law requires that any plan providing mental health coverage must do so in the same manner as medical/surgical coverage. Equal coverage includes deductibles, copayments, coinsurance, and out-of-pocket expenses as well as treatment limitations (e.g., frequency of treatment and number/frequency of visits).

EPIDEMIOLOGY OF MENTAL DISORDERS

Epidemiology, as it applies to psychiatric mental health, is the quantitative study of the distribution of mental disorders in human populations. Once the distribution of mental disorders has been determined quantitatively, epidemiologists can identify high-risk groups and high-risk factors associated with illness onset, duration, and recurrence. The further study of risk factors for mental illness may then lead to important clues about the etiology of various mental disorders.

Two different but related words used in epidemiology are **incidence** and **prevalence**. *Incidence* refers to the *number of new cases* of mental disorders in a healthy population within a given period of time—for example, the number of New York City adolescents who were diagnosed with major depression between 2000 and 2010. *Prevalence* describes the *total number of cases*, new and existing, in a given population during a specific period of time, regardless of when they became ill (e.g., the number of adolescents who screen positive for major depression in New York City schools between 2000 and 2010). Each level of investigation supplies information that can be used to improve clinical practice and plan public health policies.

The National Institute of Mental Health (NIMH) (2001) provides a summary of statistics describing the prevalence of mental disorders in the United States. Annually, according to this summary, an estimated 21.1% of Americans aged 18 and older—about one in five adults—suffer from a diagnosable mental disorder. When this percentage is applied to the 1998 U.S. Census residential population estimate, the figure translates into 44.3 million people. In addition, mental disorders—specifically major depression, schizophrenia, bipolar disorder, and obsessive-compulsive disorder—comprise 4 of the 10 leading causes of disability in the United States, as well as in other developed countries. Many individuals have more than one mental disorder at a time; this is known as having a **comorbid condition**.

Some disorders may have a high incidence but a low prevalence, and vice versa. A disease with a short duration, such as the common cold, tends to have a high incidence (many new cases in a given year) and a low prevalence (not many people suffering from a cold

at any given time). Conversely a chronic disease such as diabetes will have a low incidence, because after the first year (or whatever time increment is being used), the person will be dropped from the list of new cases. Lifetime risk data, or the risk that one will develop a disease in the course of a lifetime, will be higher than both incidence and prevalence. According to Kessler and colleagues (2005), about 50% of all Americans will meet criteria for a psychiatric disorder in a lifetime. Table 1-1 shows the prevalence of some psychiatric disorders in the United States.

Clinical epidemiology is a broad field that addresses what happens after people with illnesses are seen by providers of clinical care. Studies use traditional epidemiological methods and are conducted in groups usually defined by the illness or symptoms or by diagnostic

TABLE 1-1 Twelve-Month Prevalence of Psychiatric Disorders in the United States

Disorder	Prevalence Over 12 Months (%)	Estimated No. of People Affected by Disorder in United States	Comments
Schizophrenia	1.1	2.4 million	Affects men and women equally May appear earlier in men than in women
Major depressive disorder	6.7	14.8 million	Leading cause of disability in United States and established economies worldwide Nearly twice as many women (6.5%) as men (3.3%) suffer from major depressive disorder every year
Bipolar affective disorder	2.6	5.7 million	Affects men and women equally
Generalized anxiety disorder	3.1	6.8 million	Can begin across life cycle; risk is highest between childhood and middle age
Panic disorder	2.7	6 million	Typically develops in adolescence or early adulthood About 1 in 3 people with panic disorder develops agoraphobia
Obsessive-compulsive disorder	1	2.2 million	First symptoms begin in childhood or adolescence
Posttraumatic stress disorder (PTSD)	3.5	7.7 million	Can develop at any time About 30% of Vietnam veterans experienced PTSD after the war; percentage high among first responders to 9/11/01 U.S. terrorist attacks
Social phobia	6.8	15 million	Typically begins in childhood or adolescence
Agoraphobia	.08	1.8 million	Begins in young adulthood
Specific phobia	8.7	19.2 million	Begins in childhood
Alzheimer's disease	10 (65 years+) 50 (85 years+)	4.5 million	Rare, inherited forms can strike in the 30s-40s

Data from National Institute of Mental Health. (2008). *The numbers count: Mental disorders in America* <http://www.nimh.nih.gov/health/publications/the-numbers-count-mental-disorders-in-america/index/shtml>Accessed 19.03.09.

procedures or treatments given for the illness or symptoms. Clinical epidemiology includes the following:

- Studies of the natural history of an illness
- Studies of diagnostic screening tests
- Observational and experimental studies of interventions used to treat people with the illness or symptoms

Results of epidemiological studies are now routinely included in the *DSM-IV-TR* to describe the frequency of mental disorders. Analysis of such studies can reveal the frequency with which psychological symptoms appear together with physical illness. For example, epidemiological studies demonstrate that depression is a significant risk factor for death in people with cardiovascular disease and premature death in people with breast cancer.

CLASSIFICATION OF MENTAL DISORDERS

Nursing care, as opposed to medical care, is care based on responses to illness. We nurses do not treat major depression per se; we treat the problems associated with depression, such as insomnia or hopelessness. We care for people by providing effective nursing care, using the nursing process as a guide. If we believe that human beings have biological, psychological, social, and spiritual components and needs, then we believe in *holistic* nursing and know that our work as nurses is to assess and plan for the whole individual under our care. Nurses and physicians are two parts of a multidisciplinary team that, when well coordinated, can provide optimal care for the biological, psychological, social, and spiritual needs of patients.

To carry out their diverse professional responsibilities, educators, clinicians, and researchers need clear and accurate guidelines for identifying and categorizing mental illness. For clinicians in particular, such guidelines help in planning and evaluating their patients' treatment. A necessary element for categorization is agreement regarding which behaviors constitute a mental illness. At present, there are two major classification systems: the *DSM-IV-TR* and the *International Classification of Disease, tenth version (ICD-10)* (WHO, 2007). Both are important in terms of planning for patient care and determining reimbursement for services rendered. We will discuss both the *DSM-IV-TR* and the *ICD-10*, although more attention will be devoted to the *DSM-IV-TR* because it is the dominant mode of understanding and diagnosing mental illness in the United States and the framework for describing psychiatric disorders in this text. Psychiatric nurses often function as members of a multidisciplinary treatment team, and professional language must be consistent.

The *DSM-IV-TR*

The *DSM-IV-TR* conceptualizes each of the mental disorders as a clinically significant behavioral or psychological syndrome or pattern that occurs in an individual and is associated with present **distress** (e.g., a painful symptom), **disability** (i.e., impairment in one or more important areas of functioning), or with a significantly increased risk of suffering death, pain, disability, or an important loss of freedom (APA, 2000). This syndrome or pattern must not be merely an expected and transient response to a particular event, such as the death of a loved one. Whatever its original causes, the behavior must currently be considered a manifestation of a behavioral, psychological, or biological dysfunction to be classified as a mental disorder. Deviant behavior (e.g., political, religious, or sexual) and conflicts between the individual and society are not considered mental disorders per se, but if the deviance or conflict is a symptom of dysfunction in the individual, then it may be considered a symptom of the illness.

A common misconception is that a classification of mental disorders classifies *people*, when actually the *DSM-IV-TR* classifies *disorders* people have. For this reason, the *DSM-IV-TR* (and this textbook) avoids the use of expressions such as "a schizophrenic" or "an alcoholic" and instead uses the more accurate terms "an individual with schizophrenia" or "an individual with alcohol dependence." Since the third edition of the *DSM* appeared in 1980, the criteria for classification of mental disorders have been sufficiently detailed for clinical, teaching, and research purposes. As an example, Box 1-3 shows the specific criteria provided by the *DSM-IV-TR* for the diagnosis of generalized anxiety disorder.

The *DSM-IV-TR* in Culturally Diverse Populations

Special efforts have been made in the *DSM-IV-TR* to incorporate an awareness that the manual is used in culturally diverse populations in the United States and internationally. Clinicians evaluate individuals from numerous ethnic groups and cultural backgrounds (including many who are recent immigrants). Diagnostic assessment can be especially challenging when a clinician from one ethnic or cultural group uses the *DSM-IV-TR* classification to evaluate an individual from a different ethnic or cultural group. For example, among certain cultural groups, particular religious practices or beliefs (e.g., hearing or seeing a deceased relative during bereavement) may be misdiagnosed as manifestations of a psychotic disorder; furthermore, a syndrome often takes different superficial forms in different cultures. Also, people from minority or migrant populations may have good reason to be distrustful, and it should not be assumed that these patients are suffering from paranoia or paranoid schizophrenia.

The *DSM-IV-TR* includes information specifically related to culture in three areas:

1. A discussion of cultural variations for each of the clinical disorders
2. A description of culture-bound syndromes

BOX 1-3 *DSM-IV-TR* Criteria for Generalized Anxiety Disorder

A. Excessive anxiety and worry (apprehensive expectation), occurring more days than not for at least 6 months, about a number of events or activities (such as work or school performance).
B. The person finds it difficult to control the worry.
C. The anxiety and worry are associated with three (or more) of the following six symptoms (with at least some symptoms present for more days than not for the past 6 months). Note: Only one item is required in children.
  (1) Restlessness or feeling keyed up or on edge
  (2) Being easily fatigued
  (3) Difficulty concentrating or mind going blank
  (4) Irritability
  (5) Muscle tension
  (6) Sleep disturbance (difficulty falling or staying asleep; or restless, unsatisfying sleep)
D. The focus of the anxiety and worry is not confined to features of an Axis I disorder, for example, the anxiety or worry is not about having a panic attack (as in panic disorder), being embarrassed in public (as in social phobia), being contaminated (as in obsessive-compulsive disorder), being away from home or close relatives (as in separation anxiety disorder), gaining weight (as in anorexia nervosa), having multiple physical complaints (as in somatization disorder), or having a serious illness (as in hypochondriasis), and the anxiety and worry do not occur exclusively during posttraumatic stress disorder.
E. The anxiety, worry, or physical symptoms cause significant distress or impairment in social, occupational, or other important areas of functioning.
F. The disturbance is not due to the direct physiologic effects of a substance (e.g., a drug of abuse, a medication) or a general medical condition (e.g., hyperthyroidism) and does not occur exclusively during a mood disorder, a psychotic disorder, or a pervasive developmental disorder.

From American Psychiatric Association. (2000). *Diagnostic and statistical manual of disorders* (4th ed., text rev.). Washington, DC: Author.

TABLE 1-2 *DSM-IV-TR* Multiaxial System of Evaluation

Axis	Category	Example
I	Clinical disorders Other conditions that may be a focus of clinical attention	Major depressive disorder
II	Personality disorders Mental retardation	Dependent personality disorder
III	General medical conditions	Diabetes
IV	Psychosocial and environmental problems	Divorce 3 months previously
V	Global Assessment of Functioning	31 years old and unable to work or respond to family and friends

Data from American Psychiatric Association. (2000). *Diagnostic and statistical manual of mental disorders* (4th ed., text rev.). Washington, DC: Author.

Axis I refers to the collection of signs and symptoms that together constitute a particular disorder (e.g., schizophrenia) or a condition that may be a focus of treatment. There are 16 major categories of disorders:

1. Disorders usually first diagnosed in infancy, childhood, or adolescence
2. Delirium, dementia, and amnestic and other cognitive disorders
3. Mental disorders due to a general medical condition
4. Substance-related disorders
5. Schizophrenia and other psychotic disorders
6. Mood disorders
7. Anxiety disorders
8. Somatoform disorders (i.e., disorders with somatic symptoms)
9. Factitious disorders (i.e., disorders involving "faking")
10. Dissociative disorders (e.g., multiple personality disorder)
11. Sexual and gender identity disorders
12. Eating disorders
13. Sleep disorders
14. Impulse control disorders not elsewhere classified
15. Adjustment disorders
16. Other conditions that may be a focus of clinical attention

Axis II refers to personality disorders (see Chapter 19) and mental retardation (see Chapter 28). Thus axes I and II constitute the classification of abnormal behavior. Axes I and II were separated to ensure that the possible presence of a long-term disturbance is considered

3. An outline designed to assist the clinician in evaluating and reporting the impact of the individual's cultural context

Chapter 6 of this text offers a detailed discussion of the differing ways people view the world and presents a review of discrete cultural syndromes.

The *DSM-IV-TR* Multiaxial System

The *DSM-IV-TR* axis system, by requiring judgments to be made on each of five axes, forces the diagnostician to consider a broad range of information (Table 1-2).

when attention is being directed to another, current, problem. For example, a heroin addict would be diagnosed on axis I as having a substance-related disorder; this patient might also have a longstanding antisocial personality disorder, which would be noted on axis II. The main personality disorders are:

1. Obsessive-compulsive
2. Narcissistic
3. Histrionic
4. Paranoid
5. Borderline
6. Dependent
7. Schizoid
8. Anxious/Avoidant
9. Schizotypal
10. Antisocial

Although the remaining three axes are not needed to make the actual diagnosis, their inclusion in the *DSM-IV-TR* indicates the recognition that factors other than a person's symptoms should be considered in an assessment. On axis III, the clinician indicates any general medical conditions believed to be relevant to the mental disorder in question. In some individuals, a physical disorder (e.g., a neurological dysfunction) may be the cause of the abnormal behavior, whereas in others, it may be an important factor in the individual's overall condition (e.g., diabetes in a child with a conduct disorder).

Axis IV is for reporting psychosocial and environmental problems that may affect the diagnosis, treatment, and prognosis of a mental disorder. These may include occupational problems, educational problems, economic problems, interpersonal difficulties with family members, and a variety of problems in other life areas. Often a psychosocial assessment will uncover these (see Chapter 8).

Finally, axis V, called *Global Assessment of Functioning* (GAF), gives an indication of the person's best level of psychological, social, and occupational functioning during the preceding year, rated on a scale of 1 to 100 (where 1 indicates persistent danger of severely hurting oneself or others, and 100 indicates superior functioning in a variety of activities at the time of the evaluation, as well as the highest level of functioning for at least a few months during the past year). Box 1-4 presents the GAF Scale. Table 1-3 illustrates how the multiaxial system of classification might be applied to a hypothetical case. As a clinical exercise, you may want to try to rate yourself on this scale.

The *ICD-10*

In an increasingly global society, it is important to view the United States' diagnosis and treatment of mental illness as part of a bigger picture. An international standard for diagnostic classification for all diseases is the *ICD-10* (WHO, 2007), a document that helps identify epidemiological trends among populations in an effort

to report and manage the global burden of disease. Although more frequently revised, the *ICD* has been published alongside the *DSM-IV-TR*, and psychiatric diagnoses in each text correspond with one another. United States government reimbursement has traditionally been based on *ICD* codes. Clinical descriptions of mental and behavioral disorders are divided into 10 disease classifications:

1. Organic—including symptomatic—mental disorders
2. Mental and behavioral disorders due to psychoactive substance use
3. Schizophrenia, schizotypal, and delusional disorders
4. Mood (affective) disorders
5. Neurotic, stress-related, and somatoform disorders
6. Behavioral syndromes associated with physiological disturbances and physical factors
7. Disorders of adult personality and behavior
8. Mental retardation
9. Disorders of psychological development
10. Behavioral and emotional disorders with onset usually occurring in childhood and adolescence

PSYCHIATRIC MENTAL HEALTH NURSING

In all clinical settings, nurses work with people who are going through crises, including physical, psychological, mental, and spiritual distress. You will encounter patients who are experiencing feelings of hopelessness, helplessness, anxiety, anger, low self-esteem, or confusion. You will meet people who are withdrawn, suspicious, elated, depressed, hostile, manipulative, suicidal, intoxicated, or withdrawing from a substance. Many of you have already come across people who are going through difficult times in their lives. You may have handled these situations skillfully, but at other times you may have wished you had additional skills and knowledge. Basic psychosocial nursing concepts will become central to your practice of nursing and increase your competency as a practitioner in all clinical settings. Whatever setting you choose to work in, you will have the opportunity to improve the lives of people who are experiencing mental illness as an additional challenge to their health care needs.

Your experience in the psychiatric nursing rotation can help you gain insight into yourself and greatly increase your insight into the experiences of others. This part of your nursing education can also give you guidelines and the opportunity to learn new skills for dealing with a variety of challenging behaviors. The following sections of this chapter present a brief overview of what professional psychiatric nurses do, their scope of practice, their role in managed care, and the challenges and evolving roles for the future health care environment.

BOX 1-4 **Global Assessment of Functioning (GAF) Scale**

Consider psychological, social, and occupational functioning on a hypothetical continuum of mental health-mental illness. Do not include impairment in functioning that is a result of physical (or environmental) limitations. *Note:* Use intermediate codes when appropriate (e.g., 45, 68, 72).

Code

100
↓
91
Superior functioning in a wide range of activities, life's problems never seem to get out of hand, is sought out by others because of his or her many positive qualities. No symptoms.

90
↓
81
Absent or minimal symptoms (e.g., mild anxiety before an exam), **good functioning in all areas, interested and involved in a wide range of activities, socially effective, generally satisfied with life, no more than everyday problems or concerns** (e.g., an occasional argument with family members).

80
↓
71
If symptoms are present, they are transient and expected reactions to psychosocial stressors (e.g., difficulty concentrating after family argument); **no more than slight impairment in social, occupational, or school functioning** (e.g., temporarily falling behind in schoolwork).

70
↓
61
Some mild symptoms (e.g., depressed mood and mild insomnia) **OR some difficulty in social, occupational, or school functioning** (e.g., occasional truancy, or theft within the household), **but generally functioning pretty well, has some meaningful interpersonal relationships.**

60
↓
51
Moderate symptoms (e.g., flat affect and circumstantial speech, occasional panic attacks) **OR moderate difficulty in social, occupational, or school functioning** (e.g., few friends, conflicts with peers or co-workers).

50
↓
41
Serious symptoms (e.g., suicidal ideation, severe obsessional rituals, frequent shoplifting) **OR any serious impairment in social, occupational, or school functioning** (e.g., no friends, unable to keep a job).

40
↓
31
Some impairment in reality testing or communication (e.g., speech is at times illogical, obscure, or irrelevant) **OR major impairment in several areas, such as work or school, family relations, judgment, thinking, or mood** (e.g., depressed man avoids friends, neglects family, and is unable to work; child frequently beats up younger children, is defiant at home, and is failing at school).

30
↓
21
Behavior is considerably influenced by delusions or hallucinations OR serious impairment in communication or judgment (e.g., sometimes incoherent, acts grossly inappropriately, suicidal preoccupation) **OR inability to function in almost all areas** (e.g., stays in bed all day; no job, home, or friends).

20
↓
11
Some danger of hurting self or others (e.g., suicide attempts without clear expectation of death; frequently violent; manic excitement) **OR occasionally fails to maintain minimal personal hygiene** (e.g., smears feces) **OR gross impairment in communication** (e.g., largely incoherent or mute).

10
↓
1
Persistent danger of severely hurting self or others (e.g., recurrent violence) **OR persistent inability to maintain minimal personal hygiene OR serious suicidal act with clear expectation of death.**

0
Inadequate information.

From American Psychiatric Association. (2000). *Diagnostic and statistical manual of mental disorders* (4th ed., text rev.). Washington, DC: Author, 34.

The rating of overall psychological functioning on a scale of 0 to 100 was operationalized by Luborsky (1962) in the Health-Sickness Rating Scale. Spitzer and colleagues developed a revision of the Health-Sickness Rating Scale called the *Global Assessment Scale* (GAS) (Endicott et al., 1976). A modified version of the GAS was included in the *Diagnostic and Statistical Manual of Mental Disorders,* third edition, revised (APA, 1987) as the Global Assessment of Functioning Scale.

This rating scale highlights important areas in the assessment of functioning. Because many of the judgments are subjective, experienced clinicians use this tool as a guide when planning care and draw on their knowledge of their patients.

What Is Psychiatric Mental Health Nursing?

Psychiatric mental health nursing, a core mental health profession, employs a purposeful use of self as its art and a wide range of nursing, psychosocial, and neurobiological theories and research evidence as its science (American Psychiatric Nurses Association, et al., 2007). Psychiatric mental health nurses work with people throughout the lifespan: children, adolescents, adults, and the elderly. Psychiatric mental health nurses assist healthy people who are in crisis or who

TABLE 1-3 Clinical Example Demonstrating *DSM-IV-TR* Axes

DSM-IV-TR Axis	Disorder	Clinical Example
I	Schizophrenic disorder, paranoid	For the past 9 months, Michael, a 33-year-old sales representative, has suffered delusions of grandeur and persecution. Believing himself to be a genius, he became convinced that another salesman in his firm was trying to kill him because the other man could not tolerate Michael's superiority. In the past 2 weeks, Michael has become certain that this other man has had a pale green gas pumped into his office through the air-conditioning ducts, but there is no objective evidence of such gas or any other malfunctioning of the air-conditioning system.
II	Paranoid traits, no personality disorder	Michael has always tended to be suspicious and distrustful of people. He looks constantly for evidence that others are trying to get the better of him or to harm him, and his manner is guarded. He has trouble relaxing, and others see him as cold and unemotional. He has no close friends and is considered a loner. He was extremely jealous of his wife, from whom he is now separated, and often accused her, falsely, of having affairs with other men.
III	Colitis	Michael sees a flare-up of his colitis (inflammation of the colon) as evidence that the salesman is poisoning him, even though Michael has had the same symptoms many times before.
IV	Psychosocial and environmental problems a. Marital separation b. Loss of work responsibility Rated severe	Michael left his wife 10 months ago. Two months ago, the president of Michael's firm reassigned one of Michael's important accounts to the salesman Michael now suspects of hostile intent. Michael thinks this was maneuvered by the other salesman, but in fact, the president acted because the quality of Michael's work was deteriorating. His work had slowed visibly, and co-workers complained that they could not perform their work properly when he was present.
V	Highest level of adaptive functioning in last year (GAF) Serious symptoms 45-50 Rated moderate to serious	Michael's functioning was adequate until he separated from his wife. At that point, he began to withdraw further from friends and acquaintances. He appeared to concentrate more on his job but actually spent his time checking and rechecking his work. When the firm's president reassigned his major account, Michael's work deteriorated further, and Michael began to air some of his suspicions about the partner who took over the account. When his colitis flared up 2 weeks ago, he requested an appointment with the president and accused the partner openly. Michael was fired.

GAF, Global Assessment of Functioning.
Adapted from Altrocchi, J. (1980). *Abnormal behavior*. New York: Harcourt Brace Jovanovich; American Psychiatric Association. (2000). *Diagnostic and statistical manual of mental disorders* (4th ed., text rev.). Washington, DC: Author.

are experiencing life problems, as well as those with long-term mental illness. Their patients may include people with dual diagnoses (a mental disorder and a coexisting substance disorder), homeless persons and families, forensic patients (people in jail), individuals who have survived abusive situations, and people in crisis. Psychiatric mental health nurses work with individuals, couples, families, and groups in every nursing setting. They work with patients in hospitals, in their homes, in halfway houses, in shelters, in clinics, in storefronts, on the street—virtually everywhere.

The specific activities of the psychiatric mental health nurse are defined by the *Psychiatric-Mental Health Nursing: Scope and Standards of Practice*. This publication—jointly written in 2007 by the American

Nurses Association (ANA), the American Psychiatric Nurses Association (APNA), and the International Society of Psychiatric-Mental Health Nurses (ISPN)—defines the focus of psychiatric mental health nursing as "promoting mental health through the assessment, diagnosis, and treatment of human responses to mental health problems and psychiatric disorders" (p. 14). The psychiatric mental health nurse uses the same nursing process you have already learned to assess and diagnose patients' illnesses; identify outcomes; and plan, implement, and evaluate nursing care. Box 1-5 describes phenomena of concern for psychiatric mental health nurses.

BOX 1-5 Phenomena of Concern for Psychiatric-Mental Health Nurses

Phenomena of concern for psychiatric-mental health nurses include:

- Promotion of optimal mental and physical health and well-being and prevention of mental illness.
- Impaired ability to function related to psychiatric, emotional, and physiological distress.
- Alterations in thinking, perceiving, and communicating due to psychiatric disorders or mental health problems.
- Behaviors and mental states that indicate potential danger to self or others.
- Emotional stress related to illness, pain, disability, and loss.
- Symptom management, side effects, or toxicities associated with self-administered drugs, psycho-pharmacological intervention, and other treatment modalities.
- The barriers to treatment efficacy and recovery posed by alcohol and substance abuse and dependence.
- Self-concept and body image changes, developmental issues, life process changes, and end-of-life issues.
- Physical symptoms that occur along with altered psychological status.
- Psychological symptoms that occur along with altered physiological status.
- Interpersonal, organizational, sociocultural, spiritual, or environmental circumstances or events which have an effect on the mental and emotional well-being of the individual and family or community.
- Elements of recovery, including the ability to maintain housing, employment, and social support, that help individuals re-engage in seeking meaningful lives.
- Societal factors such as violence, poverty, and substance abuse.

From American Psychiatric Nurses Association, International Society of Psychiatric-Mental Health Nurses, & American Nurses Association. (2007). *Psychiatric-mental health nursing: Scope and standards of practice.* Silver Spring, MD: NurseBooks.org.

Classification of Nursing Diagnoses, Outcomes, and Interventions

To provide the most appropriate and scientifically sound care, the psychiatric mental health nurse uses standardized classification systems developed by professional nursing groups. The *Nursing Diagnoses: Definitions and Classification 2009–2011* of the North American Nursing Diagnosis Association International (NANDA-I) (2009) provides 201 standardized diagnoses, more than 40% of which are related to psychosocial care. These diagnoses provide a common language to aid in the selection of nursing interventions and ultimately lead to outcome achievement.

DSM-IV-TR and NANDA-I–Approved Nursing Diagnoses

Psychiatric mental health nursing includes the diagnosis and treatment of human responses to actual or potential mental health problems. A nursing diagnosis is "a clinical judgment about individual, family, or community responses to actual or potential health problems/life processes" (NANDA-I, 2009–2011, p. 419). While the *DSM-IV-TR* is used to diagnose a psychiatric disorder, a well-defined nursing diagnosis provides the framework for identifying appropriate nursing interventions for dealing with the patient's reaction to the disorder. Those reactions might include confusion, low self-esteem, impaired ability to function in job or family situations, and so on.

Part 2 lists the NANDA-I–approved nursing diagnoses and the 13 individual domains offer suggestions for potential nursing diagnoses for the behaviors and phenomena often encountered in association with specific disorders. A more thorough discussion of nursing diagnoses in psychosocial nursing can be found in Chapter 8.

Nursing Outcomes Classification (NOC)

The *Nursing Outcomes Classification (NOC)* is one reference that provides "a comprehensive list of standardized outcomes, definitions, and measures to describe client outcomes influenced by nursing practice" (Moorhead et al., 2008, p. 15). Outcomes are organized into seven domains: functional health, physiological health, psychosocial health, health knowledge and behavior, perceived health, family health, and community health. The psychosocial health domain includes four classes: psychological well-being, psychosocial adaptation, self-control, and social interaction.

Nursing Interventions Classification (NIC)

The *Nursing Interventions Classification (NIC)* is another tool used to standardize, define, and measure nursing care. Bulechek and colleagues (2008) define a nursing intervention as "any treatment, based upon clinical judgment and knowledge, that a nurse performs to enhance patient/client outcomes" (p. xxi), including direct and indirect care through a series of nursing activities. There are seven domains: basic physiological, complex physiological, behavioral, safety, family, health system, and community. Two domains relate specifically to psychiatric nursing: behavioral—including communication, coping, and education—and safety, covering crisis and risk management.

Evidence-Based Practice

The three nursing diagnosis classification systems mentioned have been extensively researched by nurses across a variety of treatment settings. They form a foundation for the novice or experienced nurse to provide evidence-based practice; that is, care based on the "collection, interpretation and integration of valid, important, and applicable patient-reported, clinician-observed, and research-derived evidence" (APNA et al., 2007, p. 66). In the chapters that follow, you will see examples of applying these classifications to specific patients in Vignettes and Case Studies, along with brief descriptions of other relevant research in the Evidence-Based Practice boxes.

Levels of Psychiatric Mental Health Clinical Nursing Practice

Psychiatric mental health nurses are registered nurses educated in nursing and licensed to practice in their individual states. Psychiatric nurses are qualified to practice at two levels, basic and advanced, depending on educational preparation. Table 1-4 describes basic and advanced psychiatric nursing interventions.

Basic Level

The term basic level registered nurse refers to professionals who have completed a nursing program, passed the state licensure examination, and is qualified to work in most any general or specialty area. The registered nurse–psychiatric mental health (RN-PMH) is a nursing graduate who possesses a diploma, associate degree, or baccalaureate degree and chooses to work in the specialty of psychiatric mental health nursing. An RN with a Bachelor of Science degree in nursing (BSN) may take a basic certification examination sponsored by the American Nurses Credentialing

TABLE 1-4 Basic Level and Advanced Practice Psychiatric Mental Health Nursing Interventions	
Basic Level Intervention	**Description**
Coordination of care	Coordinates implementation of the nursing care plan and documents coordination of care.
Health teaching and health maintenance	Individualized anticipatory guidance to prevent or reduce mental illness or enhance mental health (e.g., community screenings, parenting classes, stress management)
Milieu therapy	Provides, structures, and maintains a safe and therapeutic environment in collaboration with patients, families, and other health care clinicians
Pharmacological, biological, and integrative therapies	Applies current knowledge to assessing patient's response to medication, provides medication teaching, and communicates observations to other members of the health care team
Advanced Practice Intervention	**Description**
All of the above plus:	
Medication prescription and treatment	Prescription of psychotropic medications, with appropriate use of diagnostic tests; hospital admitting privileges
Psychotherapy	Individual, couple, group, or family therapy, using evidence-based therapeutic frameworks and the nurse-patient relationship
Consultation	Sharing of clinical expertise with nurses or those in other disciplines to enhance their treatment of patients or address systems issues

Data from American Psychiatric Nurses Association, International Society of Psychiatric-Mental Health Nurses, & American Nurses Association. (2007). *Psychiatric-mental health nursing: Scope and standards of practice.* Silver Spring, MD: NurseBooks.org.

Center (the credentialing arm of the American Nurses Association) to demonstrate clinical competence in psychiatric mental health nursing. Certification gives nurses a sense of mastery and accomplishment, identifies them as competent clinicians, and may be required by employers in some states for reimbursement purposes. At the basic level, nurses work in various supervised settings and perform multiple roles such as staff nurse, case manager, home care nurse, and so on. Nearly 4% of all registered nurses work in a psychiatric setting (USDHHS, 2004).

Advanced Practice

The advanced practice registered nurse–psychiatric mental health (APRN-PMH) is a licensed RN with a Master of Science in Nursing (MSN) or Doctor of Nursing Practice (DNP) in psychiatric nursing. This DNP is not to be confused with a doctoral degree in nursing (PhD), which is a research degree. Certification is an additional requirement and is obtained through the American Nurses Credentialing Center. Four examinations are currently available, including two for psychiatric nurse practitioners (NPs) and two for clinical nurse specialists (CNSs):

1. Adult Psychiatric and Mental Health Nurse Practitioner–Board Certified (PMHNP-BC)
2. Adult/Family Psychiatric and Mental Health Nurse Practitioner–Board Certified (PMHNP-BC)
3. Clinical Nurse Specialist in Adult Psychiatric and Mental Health–Board Certified (PMHCNS-BC)
4. Clinical Nurse Specialist in Child/Adolescent Psychiatric and Mental Health–Board Certified (PMHCNS-BC)

The APRN-PMH may function autonomously and is eligible for specialty privileges. Some advanced practice nurses continue their education to the doctoral (PhD) level. Nearly 10% of advanced practice nurses are educated and credentialed in psychiatric mental health nursing (USDHHS, 2004).

Future Challenges and Roles for Psychiatric Mental Health Nurses

Psychiatric mental health nurses at both the basic and advanced practice level continue to be in great demand. As with any specialty area in hospital settings, psychiatric nurses are caring for more acutely ill patients. In the 1980s, it was common for patients who were depressed and suicidal to have insurance coverage for about 2 weeks. Now patients are lucky to be covered for 3 days, if they are covered at all. This means that nurses need to be more skillful and be prepared to discharge patients for whom the benefit of their care will not always be evident.

Challenges in educating students who possess the skills to eventually become psychiatric mental health nurses are related to this level of acute care, as well as to dwindling inpatient populations. Clinical rotations in general medical centers are becoming less available and faculty are fortunate to secure rotations in state psychiatric hospitals and veterans administration facilities. Community psychiatric settings also provide students with valuable experience, but the logistics of placing and supervising students in multiple sites has required creativity on the part of nursing educators. Some schools have established integrated rotations that allow students to work outside the psychiatric setting with patients who have mental health issues—for example, caring for a person with depression on an orthopedic floor.

As community-based care becomes dominant in the clinical setting, psychiatric mental health nurses will need to enhance their **case management** skills. Case management is an integral part of psychiatric home care for the elderly, in-home services for children and adolescents, and long-term treatment for the chronically mentally ill.

Nurse-run clinics are becoming increasingly common. **Community nursing centers** serve low-income and uninsured people, as long as they can secure funding. In this model, psychiatric mental health nurses work with primary care nurses to provide comprehensive care, usually funded by scarce grants from academic centers. These centers use a nontraditional approach of combining primary care and health promotion interventions. Advanced practice psychiatric nurses have also been extremely successful in setting up private practices where they provide both psychotherapy and medication management.

Three significant trends that will affect the future of psychiatric nursing in the United States include the aging population, increasing cultural diversity, and expanding technology. As the number of older adults grows, the prevalence of Alzheimer's disease and other dementias requiring skilled nursing care in inpatient settings is likely to increase. Healthier older adults will need more services at home, in retirement communities, or in assisted living facilities. For more information on the needs of older adults, refer to Chapters 17, 26, and 29.

Cultural diversity is steadily increasing in the United States. The United States Census Bureau (2008) projects that between 2010 and 2050; the percentage of white Americans will decrease from almost 80% to less than 74%. Percentages of Hispanics (who may be of any race) are projected to nearly double in numbers during those years, from 16% of the population to over 30%. Psychiatric mental health nurses will need to increase their **cultural competence**, that is, their sensitivity to different cultural views regarding health, illness, and response to treatment.

Science, Technology, and Electronic Health Care

Genetic mapping from the Human Genome Project has resulted in a steady stream of research discoveries concerning genetic markers implicated in a variety of psychiatric illnesses. This information could be helpful in identifying at-risk individuals and in targeting medications specific to certain genetic variants and profiles. However, the legal and ethical implications of responsibly using this technology are staggering. Questions arise, such as: Would you want to know you were at risk for a psychiatric illness like bipolar disorder? Who should have access to this information—your primary care provider, insurer, future spouse, a lawyer in a child-custody battle? "Who will regulate genetic testing centers to protect privacy and prevent 21st-century problems like identity theft and fraud?" Despite these concerns, the next decade holds great promise in the diagnosis and treatment of psychiatric disorders, and nurses will be central as educators and caregivers.

Scientific advances through research and technology are certain to shape psychiatric mental health nursing practice. Magnetic resonance imaging research, in addition to comparing healthy people to people diagnosed with mental illness, is now focusing on development of preclinical profiles of children and adolescents. The hope of this type of research is to identify people at risk for developing mental illness, which allows earlier interventions to try to decrease impairment.

Electronic health care services provided from a distance are gaining wide acceptance. In the early days of the Internet, consumers were cautioned against the questionable wisdom of seeking advice through an unregulated medium. However, the Internet has transformed the way we approach our health care needs. It is used liberally by young and old alike, and men in particular seem to feel more comfortable researching online than seeking care in person (Ybarra & Suman, 2006). The Internet has empowered people to advocate for themselves and explore health problems and options related to treatment.

Telepsychiatry via microphones and/or web cams is being promoted by the American Psychiatric Association (2008) as an effective way to reach underserved populations and those who are homebound. This method allows for assessment and diagnosis, medication management, and even group therapy. Psychiatric nurses may become more active in developing websites for mental health education, screening, or support, especially to reach geographically isolated areas. Many health agencies hire nurses to staff help lines or hotlines, and provision of these cost-effective services will likely increase, with more need for bilingual resources.

Advocacy and Legislative Involvement

The role of the psychiatric mental health nurse as **patient advocate** will continue to evolve. Nurses advocate for the psychiatric patient through direct care and indirect community action. In all treatment settings, the nurse has the responsibility to communicate to the patient and uphold patients' rights. Chapter 7 offers an in-depth discussion of ethics and patient rights.

As a patient advocate, the nurse reports incidents of abuse or neglect to the appropriate authorities for immediate action. The nurse also upholds patient confidentiality, which is becoming more challenging as the use of computerized patient records increases. Another form of nursing advocacy is supporting the patient's right to make decisions regarding treatment. Within managed care, situations in which the patient disagrees with the treatment approved continue to arise. Nurses can teach patients about the appeal process—including internal appeal procedures for the managed behavioral health care organization (MBHO)—as well as procedures for appeal to the external review bodies available in most states (Sabin, Granoff, & Daniels, 2003).

On an indirect level, the nurse may choose to be active in consumer mental health groups (such as NAMI) and state and local mental health associations to reduce the **stigma** of mental illness and to support consumers of mental health care. The nurse can also be vigilant about reviewing local and national legislation affecting health care to identify potential detrimental effects on the mentally ill. Especially during times of fiscal crisis, lawmakers are inclined to decrease or eliminate funding for vulnerable populations who do not have a strong political voice.

The APNA (2008) is investing greater energy in influencing politicians, lawmakers, and the public, and its efforts to positively affect the care of people with psychiatric disorders is ongoing. As the 24-hours-a-day, 7-days-a-week caregivers and members of the largest group of health care professionals, nurses are in the enviable position of being expert advocates for individuals with mental illness. We have the potential to exert tremendous influence in the legislative arena.

When commissions and task forces are developed, however, nurses are not usually the first group to be considered to provide input and expertise for national, state, and local decision-makers. In fact, nursing presence is often absent at the policy-making table. Consider the President's New Freedom Commission on Mental Health (USDHHS, 2003) which included psychiatrists (medical doctors), psychologists (PhDs), academics, and policy makers—but no nurses. It is difficult to understand how the largest contingent of mental health care providers in the United States could be excluded from a group that would determine the future of mental health care.

It is in the best interest of consumers of mental health care that all members of the collaborative health care team, including nurses, be involved in decisions and legislation that will affect their care. Current political issues that need monitoring and support include mental health parity, discriminatory media portrayal, standardized language and practices, and advanced practice issues, such as prescriptive authority over Schedule II drugs and government reimbursement.

At the 2003 NAMI National Convention, one presenter thoughtfully summarized his knowledge gained from a 45-year career in mental health care as follows:

> Mental health services look very different now than they did a half century ago. The good news is that we know more, have better treatment tools, and provide useful services to more people. The bad news is that many signs of neglect remain, particularly for the most poor and most disenfranchised individuals. As the history of mental illness attests, a decent mental health system depends as much on the interest and compassion of the larger public as it does on the concerned professionals who make mental health their work, and this area requires improvement (Mechanic, 2003, p. 1232).

KEY POINTS TO REMEMBER

- Mental health and mental illness are not either/or propositions, but end points on a continuum.
- Resilience is a personal characteristic that helps to promote adaptation to stressful circumstances. This is a trait that can be promoted and improved to strengthen responses to stress.
- Culture influences behavior, and symptoms may reflect a person's cultural patterns or beliefs. Symptoms must be understood in terms of a person's cultural background.
- The United States mental health care system has been influenced by scientific shifts in thinking, broad-reaching reports, and legislative initiatives.
- The consumer and recovery movement shifted the focus of mental health care from something done *to* patients to something consumers *choose*.
- The study of epidemiology can help identify high-risk groups and behaviors, which can lead to a better understanding of the causes of some disorders. Incidence provides us with the number of new cases in a given period of time. Prevalence rates help us to identify the proportion of a population experiencing a specific mental disorder at a given time.
- Comorbid conditions are those disorders that occur at the same time as another condition. For example, a person with schizophrenia may also have comorbid diabetes, depression, and hypertension.
- The five axes of the *DSM-IV-TR* make it possible for clinicians to make a more holistic and realistic assessment of their patients and thus allow for more comprehensive and appropriate interventions.
- Psychiatric mental health nurses work with a broad population of patients in diverse settings to promote optimal mental health. They may be prepared as basic level nurse generalists, or they may gain additional training and function as advanced practice nurses.
- Due to social, cultural, scientific, and political factors, the future holds many challenges and possibilities for the psychiatric mental health nurse.

CRITICAL THINKING

1. Brian, a 19-year-old college sophomore with a grade point average of 3.4, is brought to the emergency department after a suicide attempt. He has been extremely depressed since the death of his girlfriend 5 months previously when the car he was driving crashed. His parents are devastated. They believe taking one's own life prevents a person from going to heaven. Brian has epilepsy and has had more seizures since the auto accident. He says he should be punished for his carelessness and does not care what happens to him. He has not been to school or shown up for his part-time job tutoring children in reading.
   A. What might be a possible *DSM-IV-TR* diagnosis for axis I? What information should be included on axis III? What should be included on axis IV? What score (range) might you give to Brian on the GAF Scale?
   B. Before you plan your care, what are some other factors you would like to assess regarding aspects of Brian's overall health and other influences that can affect his mental health?
   C. Do you think that an antidepressant could help Brian's grieving process? Why or why not? What additional care do you think Brian needs?
   D. Formulate at least two potential nursing diagnoses for Brian.
   E. Would Brian's parents' religious beliefs factor into your plan of care? If so, how?

2. In a small study group, share experiences you have had with others from unfamiliar cultural, ethnic, religious, or racial backgrounds, and identify two positive learning experiences from these encounters.

3. Consider what it would be like working with a group of healthy women preparing for parenthood versus working with a group of depressed women in a mental health clinic. What do you feel are the advantages and disadvantages of working with each group?

4. Would you feel comfortable referring a family member to a mental health clinician? What factors make you feel that way?

5. How do basic and advanced practice psychiatric mental health nurses work together to provide the highest quality of care?

6. Would you consider joining a professional group or advocacy group that promotes mental health? Why or why not?

CHAPTER REVIEW

1. Resilience, the capacity to rebound from stressors via adaptive coping, is associated with positive mental health. Your friend has just been laid off from his job. Which of the following responses on your part would most likely contribute to enhanced resilience?
   1. Using your connections to set up an interview with your employer
   2. Connecting him with a friend of the family who owns his own business
   3. Supporting him in arranging, preparing for, and completing multiple interviews
   4. Helping him to understand that the layoff resulted from troubles in the economy and is not his fault

2. Which of the following situations best supports the stress-diathesis model of mental illness development?
   1. The rate of suicide increases during times of national disaster and despair.
   2. Four of five siblings in the Jones family develop bipolar disorder by the age of 30.
   3. A man with no prior mental health problems experiences sadness after his divorce.
   4. A man develops schizophrenia, but his identical twin remains free of mental illness.

3. Identify all of the following statements about mental illness which are correct:
   1. In any given year, about 20% of adults experience a mental disorder.
   2. Mental health is best represented as a continuum of levels of functioning.
   3. Mental disorders and diagnoses occur very consistently across cultures.
   4. Most serious mental illnesses are psychological rather than biological in nature.
   5. The President's New Freedom Commission highlighted significant gaps in care.
   6. "Parity" refers to relating to mentally ill persons the same as to the non–mentally ill.

4. Which of the following disorders would be included on Axis I of the *DSM IV-TR*?
   1. Major depression, dementia, and alcoholism
   2. Diabetes type I or II, Parkinson's disease, and seizure disorders
   3. Narcissistic, borderline, and paranoid personality disorders
   4. Mental retardation and psychosocial stressors such as divorce

5. Which of the following actions represent the primary focus of psychiatric nursing for a basic-level registered nurse?
   1. Determining a patient's diagnosis according to the *DSM-IV-TR*
   2. Ordering diagnostic tests such as EEGs or CT or MRI scans
   3. Identifying how a patient is coping with a symptom such as hallucinations
   4. Guiding a patient to learn and use a variety of stress-management techniques
   5. Helping a patient without transportation find a way to his treatment appointments
   6. Collecting petition signatures seeking the removal of stigmatizing images on television

---

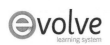 Visit the Evolve website for an **Audio Chapter Summary, Chapter Review Answers & Rationales, Critical Thinking Answer Guidelines,** and additional resources related to the content in this chapter: **http://evolve.elsevier.com/Varcarolis/foundations**

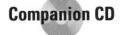 Use the Companion CD to prepare for tests and the NCLEX® Examination with **Test-Taking Strategies** for psychiatric mental health nursing and hundreds of **Review Questions**.

References

Altrocchi, J. (1980). *Abnormal behavior.* New York: Harcourt Brace Jovanovich.

Amat, J., Paul, E., Zarza, C., Watkins, L. R., & Maier, S. F. (2006). Previous experience with behavioral control over stress blocks the behavioral and dorsal raphe activating effects of later uncontrollable stress: Role of the ventral medial prefrontal cortex. *Journal of Neuroscience, 26,* 13,264–13,272.

American Psychiatric Association. (2008). Topic 4: Telepsychiatry. Retrieved March 10, 2009 from http://www.psych.org/ Departments/HSF/underservedclearinghouse/Linked documents/telepsychiatry.aspx

American Psychiatric Nurses Association. (2008). *Institute for mental health advocacy.* Retrieved June 24, 2008 from http://www.apna.org/i4a/pages/index.cfm?pageid=3637

American Psychiatric Nurses Association, International Society of Psychiatric-Mental Health Nurses, & American Nurses Association. (2007). *Psychiatric-mental health nursing: Scope and standards of practice.* Silver Spring, MD: NurseBooks.org.

American Psychiatric Association. (2000). *Diagnostic and statistical manual of mental disorders (DSM-IV-TR)* (4th ed., text rev.). Washington, DC: Author.

American Psychological Association. (2004). *The road to resilience*. Retrieved June 25, 2008 from http://apahelpcenter.org/featuredtopics/feature.php?id=6

Bulechek, G. M., Butcher, H. K., & Dochterman, J. M. (Eds.). (2008). *Nursing interventions classification (NIC)* (5th ed.). St. Louis: Mosby.

Cloninger, C. R. (2006). The science of well-being: An integrated approach to mental health and its disorders. *World Psychiatry, 5*(2), 71–76.

Cohen, J. I. (2000). Stress and mental health: A biobehavioral perspective. *Issues in Mental Health Nursing, 21*, 185–202.

Endicott, J., Spitzer, R. L., Fleiss, J. L., & Cohen, J. (1976). The global assessment scale: A procedure for measuring overall severity of psychiatric disturbance. *Archives of General Psychiatry, 33*, 766–771.

Howard, R. (Director). (2001). *A beautiful mind* [motion picture]. United States: Universal Pictures.

Institute of Medicine. (2006). *Improving the quality of health care for mental and substance-use conditions: Quality chasm series*. Washington DC: National Academies Press.

Kessler, R. C., Berglund, P., Demler, O., Jin, R., & Walters, E. E. (2005). Lifetime prevalence and age-of-onset distributions of *DSM-IV* disorders in the national comorbidity survey replication. *Archives of General Psychiatry, 62*, 593–602.

Mechanic, D. (2003). Improving mental health services: Some lessons from the past. *Psychiatric Services, 54*(9), 1227–1232.

Moorhead, S., Johnson, M., Maas, M., & Swanson, E. (Eds.). (2008). *Nursing outcomes classification (NOC)* (3rd ed.). St. Louis: Mosby.

Morgan, C., McKenzie, K., & Fearon, P. (2008). *Society and psychosis*. Cambridge: London.

National Institute of Mental Health. (2008; updated Feb 2009). *The numbers count: Mental disorders in America*. Retrieved March 19, 2009, from <http://www.nimh.nih.gov/health/publications/the-numbers-count-mental-disorders-in-america/index/shtml>

North American Nursing Diagnosis Association International (NANDA-I). (2009). *NANDA nursing diagnoses: Definitions and classification 2009–2011*. Oxford, United Kingdom. Author.

Peplau, H. E. (1952). *Interpersonal relations in nursing: A conceptual frame of reference for psychodynamic nursing*. New York: Putnam.

Porter, N. (Ed.) (1913). Webster's revised unabridged dictionary. Boston, MA: Merriam.

Sabin, J., Granoff, K., & Daniels, N. (2003). Strengthening the consumer voice in managed care: VI. Initial lessons from independent external review. *Psychiatric Services, 54*(1), 24–25.

Sadock, B. J., & Sadock, V. A. (2008). *Kaplan and Sadock's concise textbook of clinical psychiatry* (3rd ed.). Philadelphia: Lippincott Williams & Wilkins.

Substance Abuse and Mental Health Services Administration. (2005). *Promoting self-determination for individuals with psychiatric disabilities through self-directed service*. Retrieved March 10, 2009 from http://mentalhealth.samhsa.gov/publications/allpubs/NMH05-0192/default.asp

Tandon, P. N. (2000). The decade of the brain: A brief review. *Neurology India, 48*(3), 199–207.

U.S. Census Bureau. (2008). *An older and more diverse nation by midcentury*. Retrieved March 10, 2009 from http://www.census.gov/Press-Release/www/releases/archives/population/012496.html

U.S. Department of Energy. (2008). *The human genome project information*. Retrieved September 18, 2008 from http://www.ornl.gov/sci/techresources/Human_Genome/home.shtml

U.S. Department of Health and Human Services, Health Resources and Services Administration. (2004). *The registered nurse population: Findings from the 2004 national sample survey of registered nurses*. Retrieved June 25, 2008 from http://bhpr.hrsa.gov/healthworkforce/rnsurvey04/

U.S. Department of Health and Human Services, President's New Freedom Commission on Mental Health. (2003). *Achieving the promise: Transforming mental health care in America*. USDHHS Publication No. SMA-03–3832 <http://www.mentalhealthcommission.gov/reports/finalreport/fullreport-02.htm>

U.S. Department of Health and Human Services, U.S. Public Health Service. (1999). *Mental health: A report of the Surgeon General*. Washington, DC: U.S. Government Printing Office.

World Health Organization. (2007). *Mental health: A state of well-being*. Retrieved June 13, 2008 from http://www.who.int/features/factfiles/mental_health/en/index.html

World Health Organization. (2007). *International statistical classification of diseases and related health problems* (10th rev.) (ICD-10). Geneva: Author.

Ybarra, M., & Suman, M. (2006). Reasons, assessments, and actions taken: Sex and age differences in uses of Internet health information. *Health Education Research, 23*, 512–521.

CHAPTER 2

Relevant Theories and Therapies for Nursing Practice

Margaret Jordan Halter and Verna Benner Carson

Key Terms and Concepts

Objectives

1. Evaluate the premises behind the various therapeutic models discussed in this chapter.
2. Describe the evolution of therapies for psychiatric disorders.
3. Identify ways each theorist contributes to the nurse's ability to assess a patient's behaviors.
4. Drawing on clinical experience, provide the following:
   a. An example of how a patient's irrational beliefs influenced behavior.
   b. An example of countertransference in your relationship with a patient.
   c. An example of the use of behavior modification with a patient.
5. Identify Peplau's framework for the nurse-patient relationship.
6. Choose the therapeutic model that would be most useful for a particular patient or patient problem.

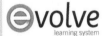
Visit the Evolve website for an **Audio Glossary & Flashcards, Concept Map Creator,** and additional resources related to the content in this chapter: **http://evolve.elsevier.com/Varcarolis/foundations**

Every professional discipline, from math and science to philosophy and psychology, bases its work and beliefs on theories. Most of these theories can best be described as explanations, hypotheses, or hunches, rather than testable facts. For students, the word theory may conjure up some dry, conceptual images vaguely recalling the physicists' theory of relativity or the geologists' plate tectonics. However, compared to most other theories, psychological theories are filled with familiar concepts, since terms from psychological theories have filtered their way into parts of mainstream thinking and speech. We all recognize advertisements that use the behaviorist ploy of linking a gorgeous, seductive woman to the family-style utilitarian minivan. And who has not attributed language mistakes to subconscious motivation? As the fictional king greets his queen, "Good morning, my beheaded...I mean my beloved!" we comprehend the Freudian slip.

Dealing with other people is one of the most universally anxiety-provoking activities we face, and psychological theories provide us with plausible explanations for perplexing behavior. Maybe the guy at the front desk who never greets you in the morning does not really despise you; maybe he has an inferiority complex because his mother was cold and his father was absent from the home. In much the same way, our patients challenge us to understand stories that are complex and always unique. We do well to have a broad base of knowledge about personality development, human needs, the ingredients of mental health, contributing factors to mental illness, and the importance of relationships.

This chapter will provide you with snapshot views of some of the most influential psychological theories. It will also provide an overview of the treatment, or **therapy**, they inspired and the contributions they have made to our practice of psychiatric mental health nursing. We begin our theoretical journey with a look at Sigmund Freud, often referred to as the "father of psychoanalysis." We travel on to Erik Erickson and Harry Stack Sullivan, who initially were devotees of Freud but found Freudian theory lacking and so took a divergent path. We will then focus on the theory of the "mother of psychiatric nursing," Hildegard Peplau, then Abraham Maslow, our representative theorist from the humanistic approach to psychiatry. We continue on with a look at Ivan Pavlov, John B. Watson, and B. F. Skinner as representatives of the behaviorist approach. As we near the final leg of this trip, we will explore the two dominant approaches to treating psychiatric illness, cognitive-behavioral therapy and biological therapies. Each of these theoretical approaches and therapies are evaluated for relevance to psychiatric mental health nursing. Let's begin our expedition!

PSYCHOANALYTIC THEORIES AND THERAPIES

Sigmund Freud's Psychoanalytic Theory

Sigmund Freud (1856-1939), an Austrian neurologist, revolutionized thinking about mental health disorders with his groundbreaking theory of personality structure, levels of awareness, anxiety, the role of defense mechanisms, and the stages of psychosexual development. Originally, he was searching for biological treatments for psychological disturbances and even experimented with using cocaine as medication. He soon abandoned the physiological approach and focused on psychological treatments. Freud came to believe that the vast majority of mental disorders were due to unresolved issues that originated in childhood. He arrived at this conclusion through his experiences treating people with hysteria—individuals who were suffering physical symptoms despite the absence of an apparent physiological cause.

As part of his treatment, Freud initially used hypnosis, but this provided mixed therapeutic results.

He then changed his approach to talk therapy, known as the *cathartic method*. Today we refer to catharsis as "getting things off our chests." Talk therapy evolved to include "free association," which requires full and honest disclosure of thoughts and feelings as they come to mind. Freud (1961, 1969) concluded that talking about difficult emotional issues had the potential to heal the wounds causing mental illness. Viewing the success of these therapeutic approaches led Freud to construct his psychoanalytic theory.

Levels of Awareness

Through the use of talk therapy and free association, Freud came to believe that there were three levels of psychological awareness in operation. He offered a topographic theory of how the mind functions—a description, if you will, of the landscape of the mind. He used the image of an iceberg to describe these levels of awareness (Figure 2-1).

Conscious. Freud described the conscious part of the mind as the tip of the iceberg. It contains all the material a person is aware of at any one time, including perceptions, memories, thoughts, fantasies, and feelings.

Preconscious. Just below the surface of awareness is the preconscious, which contains material that can be retrieved rather easily through conscious effort.

Unconscious. The unconscious includes all repressed memories, passions, and unacceptable urges lying deep below the surface. It is believed that the memories and emotions associated with trauma are often "placed" in the unconscious because the individual finds it too painful to deal with them. The unconscious exerts a powerful yet unseen effect on the conscious thoughts and feelings of the individual. The individual is usually unable to retrieve unconscious material without the assistance of a trained therapist; however, with this assistance, unconscious material can be brought into conscious awareness.

Personality Structure

Freud (1960) delineated three major and distinct but interactive systems of the personality: the id, the ego, and the superego.

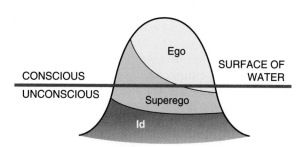

Figure 2-1 The mind as an iceberg.

Id. At birth we are all id. The **id** is the source of all drives, instincts, reflexes, needs, genetic inheritance, and capacity to respond, as well as all the wishes that motivate us. The id cannot tolerate frustration and seeks to discharge tension and return to a more comfortable level of energy. The id lacks the ability to problem solve; it is not logical and operates according to the pleasure principle. A hungry, screaming infant is the perfect example of id.

Ego. The **ego** develops because the needs, wishes, and demands of the id cannot be satisfactorily met through primary processes and reflex action. The ego, which emerges in the fourth or fifth month of life, is the problem solver and reality tester. It is able to differentiate subjective experiences, memory images, and objective reality and attempts to negotiate a solution with the outside world. The ego follows the reality principle, which says to the id, "You have to delay gratification for right now," and then sets a course of action. For example, a hungry man feels tension arising from the id. His ego allows him not only to think about his hunger but to plan where he can eat and to seek that destination. This process is known as *reality testing*, because the individual is factoring in reality to implement a plan to decrease tension.

Superego. The **superego**, the last portion of the personality to develop, represents the moral component of personality. The superego consists of the conscience (all the "should nots" internalized from parents) and the ego ideal (all the "shoulds" internalized from parents). The superego represents the ideal rather than the real; it seeks perfection, as opposed to seeking pleasure or engaging reason.

In a mature and well-adjusted individual, the three systems of the personality—the id, the ego, and the superego—work together as a team under the administrative leadership of the ego. If the id is too powerful, the person will lack control over impulses; if the superego is too powerful, the person may be self-critical and suffer from feelings of inferiority.

Defense Mechanisms and Anxiety

Freud (1969) believed that anxiety is an inevitable part of living. The environment in which we live presents dangers and insecurities, threats and satisfactions. It can produce pain and increase tension or produce pleasure and decrease tension. The ego develops defenses, or **defense mechanisms**, to ward off anxiety by preventing conscious awareness of threatening feelings.

Defense mechanisms share two common features: (1) they all (except suppression) operate on an unconscious level, and we are not aware of their operation; and (2) they deny, falsify, or distort reality to make it less threatening. Although we cannot survive without defense mechanisms, it is possible for our defense mechanisms to distort reality to such a degree that we experience difficulty with healthy adjustment and personal growth. Chapter 12 offers further discussions of defense mechanisms.

Psychosexual Stages of Development

Freud believed that human development proceeds through five stages from infancy to adulthood. His main focus, however, was on events that occur during the first 5 years of life. From Freud's perspective, experiences during the early stages determine an individual's lifetime adjustment patterns and personality traits. In fact, Freud thought that personality was formed by the time the child entered school and that subsequent growth consisted of elaborating on this basic structure. Freud's psychosexual stages of development are presented in Table 2-1.

Implications for Psychiatric Mental Health Nursing

Freud's theory has relevance to psychiatric mental health nursing practice at many junctures. First, the theory offers a comprehensive explanation of complex human processes and suggests that the formation of a patient's personality is influenced by many diverse sources rooted in past events. Freud's theory of the unconscious is particularly valuable as a baseline for considering the complexity of human behavior. By considering conscious and unconscious influences, a nurse can identify and begin to think about the root causes of patient suffering. Freud emphasized the importance of individual talk sessions characterized by attentive listening, with a focus on underlying themes as an important tool of healing in psychiatric care.

Classical Psychoanalysis

Classical psychoanalysis, as developed by Sigmund Freud, is seldom used today. Freud's premise that all mental illness is caused by early intrapsychic conflict is no longer widely thought to be valid, and such therapy requires an unrealistically lengthy period of treatment, making it prohibitively expensive for most. However, there are two concepts from classic psychoanalysis that are important for all psychiatric nurses to know: transference and countertransference (Freud, 1969).

Transference develops when the patient experiences feelings toward the nurse or therapist that were originally held toward significant others in his or her life. When transference occurs, these feelings become available for exploration with the patient. Such exploration helps the patient to better understand certain feelings and behaviors. **Countertransference** is the health care worker's unconscious, personal response to the patient. For instance, if the patient reminds you of someone you do not like, you may unconsciously react as if the patient were that individual.

TABLE 2-1 Freud's Psychosexual Stages of Development

Stage (Age)	Source of Satisfaction	Primary Conflict	Tasks	Desired Outcomes	Other Possible Personality Traits
Oral (0-1 yr)	Mouth (sucking, biting, chewing)	Weaning	Mastery of gratification of oral needs; beginning of ego development (4-5 mo)	Development of trust in the environment, with the realization that needs can be met	Fixation at the oral stage is associated with passivity, gullibility, and dependence; the use of sarcasm; and the development of orally focused habits (e.g., smoking, nail-biting).
Anal (1-3 yr)	Anal region (expulsion and retention of feces)	Toilet training	Beginning of development of a sense of control over instinctual drives; ability to delay immediate gratification to gain a future goal	Control over impulses	Fixation at the anal stage is associated with anal retentiveness (stinginess, rigid thought patterns, obsessive-compulsive disorder) or anal-expulsive character (messiness, destructiveness, cruelty).
Phallic (oedipal) (3-6 yr)	Genitals (masturbation)	Oedipus and Electra	Sexual identity with parent of same sex; beginning of super-ego development	Identification with parent of the same sex	Lack of successful resolution may result in difficulties with sexual identity and difficulties with authority figures.
Latency (6-12 yr)	—	—	Growth of ego functions (social, intellectual, mechanical) and the ability to care about and relate to others outside the home (peers of the same sex)	The development of skills needed to cope with the environment	Fixations can result in difficulty identifying with others and in developing social skills, leading to a sense of inadequacy and inferiority.
Genital (12 yr and beyond)	Genitals (sexual intercourse)	—	Development of satisfying sexual and emotional relationships with members of the opposite sex; emancipation from parents—planning of life goals and development of a strong sense of personal identity	The ability to be creative and find pleasure in love and work	Inability to negotiate this stage could result in difficulties in becoming emotionally and financially independent, lack of strong personal identity and future goals, and inability to form satisfying intimate relationships.

Data from Gleitman, H. (1981). *Psychology*. New York: W. W. Norton.

Countertransference underscores the importance of maintaining self-awareness and seeking supervisory guidance as therapeutic relationships progress. Chapter 19 talks more about countertransference and the nurse-patient relationship.

Psychodynamic Therapy

Psychodynamic therapy follows the psychoanalytic model by using many of the tools of psychoanalysis, such as free association, dream analysis, transference, and countertransference. However, the therapist has increased involvement and interacts with the patient more freely than in traditional psychoanalysis. Also, the therapy is oriented more to the here and now and makes less of an attempt to reconstruct the developmental origins of conflicts (Dewan, et al., 2008). Psychodynamic therapy tends to last longer than other common therapeutic modalities and may extend for more than 20 sessions.

The best candidates for brief psychotherapy are relatively healthy and well-functioning individuals, sometimes referred to as the "worried well," who have a clearly circumscribed area of difficulty and are intelligent, psychologically minded, and well motivated for change. Patients with psychosis, severe depression, borderline personality disorders, and severe character disorders often are not appropriate candidates for this type of treatment. Supportive therapies, which are within the scope of practice of the basic level psychiatric nurse, are useful for these patients. A variety of supportive therapies are described in chapters concerning specific disorders (see Chapters 12 to 22).

At the start of treatment, the patient and therapist agree on what the focus will be and concentrate their work on that focus. Sessions are held weekly, and the total number of sessions to be held is determined at the outset of therapy. There is a rapid, back-and-forth pattern between patient and therapist, with both participating actively. The therapist intervenes constantly to keep the therapy on track, either by redirecting the patient's attention or by interpreting deviations from the focus to the patient.

Brief therapies share the following common elements:

- Assessment tends to be rapid and early.
- Clear expectations are established for time-limited therapy with improvement demonstrated within a small number of sessions.
- Goals are concrete and focus on improving the patient's worst symptoms, improving coping skills, and helping the patient understand what is going on in his or her life.
- Interpretations are directed toward present life circumstances and patient behavior rather than toward the historical significance of feelings.
- There is a general understanding that psychotherapy does not cure but that it can help troubled individuals learn to better deal with life's inevitable stressors.

Erik Erikson's Ego Theory

Erik Erikson (1902-1994), an American psychoanalyst, was also a follower of Freud. However, Erikson (1963) believed that Freudian theory was restrictive and negative in its approach. He also stressed that an individual's development is influenced by more than the limited mother-child-father triangle and that culture and society exert significant influence on personality. According to Erikson, personality was not set in stone at age 5, as Freud suggested, but continued to develop throughout the lifespan.

Erikson described development as occurring in eight predetermined and consecutive life stages (psychosocial crises), each of which consists of two possible outcomes (e.g., industry vs. inferiority). The successful or unsuccessful completion of each stage will affect the individual's progression to the next (Table 2-2). For example, Erikson's crisis of industry versus inferiority occurs from the ages of 7 to 12. During this stage, the child's task is to gain a sense of personal abilities and competence and expand relationships beyond the immediate family to include peers. The attainment of this task (industry) brings with it the virtue of confidence. The child who fails to navigate this stage successfully is unable to gain a mastery of age-appropriate tasks, cannot make a connection with peers, and will feel like a failure (inferiority).

Implications for Psychiatric Mental Health Nursing

Nurses use Erikson's developmental model as an important part of patient assessment. Analysis of behavior patterns using Erikson's framework can identify age-appropriate or arrested development of normal interpersonal skills. A developmental framework helps the nurse know what types of interventions are most likely to be effective. For example, children in Erikson's initiative-versus-guilt stage of development respond best if they actively participate and ask questions. Older adults respond to a life review strategy that focuses on the integrity of their life as a tapestry of experience. In the therapeutic encounter, individual responsibility and the capacity for improving one's functioning are addressed. Treatment approaches and interventions can be tailored to the patient's developmental level.

INTERPERSONAL THEORIES AND THERAPIES

Harry Stack Sullivan's Interpersonal Theory

Harry Stack Sullivan (1892-1949), an American-born psychiatrist, initially approached patients from a Freudian framework, but he became frustrated by dealing with what he considered unseen and private mental processes within the individual. He turned his attention to interpersonal processes that could be observed in a social framework. Sullivan (1953) defined *personality* as behavior that can be observed within interpersonal relationships. This premise led to the development of his interpersonal theory.

TABLE 2-2 Erikson's Eight Stages of Development

Approximate Age	Developmental Task	Psychosocial Crisis	Successful Resolution of Crisis	Unsuccessful Resolution of Crisis
Infancy (0-1½ yr)	Forming attachment to mother, which lays foundations for later trust in others	Trust vs. mistrust	Sound basis for relating to other people; trust in people; faith and hope about environment and future "I'm confident that my son will arrange for me to stay with his family until I'm able to live on my own again."	General difficulties relating to people effectively; suspicion; trust-fear conflict; fear of future "I can't trust anyone; no one has ever been there when I needed them."
Early childhood (1½-3 yr)	Gaining some basic control of self and environment (e.g., toilet training, exploration)	Autonomy vs. shame and doubt	Sense of self-control and adequacy; will power "I'm sure that with the proper diet and exercise program, I can achieve my target weight."	Independence/fear conflict; severe feelings of self-doubt "I could never lose the weight they want me to, so why even try?"
Late childhood (3-6 yr)	Becoming purposeful and directive	Initiative vs. guilt	Ability to initiate one's own activities; sense of purpose "I like to help mom by setting the table for dinner."	Aggression/fear conflict; sense of inadequacy or guilt "I know it's wrong, but I wanted the candy, so I took it."
School age (6-12 yr)	Developing social, physical, and school skills	Industry vs. inferiority	Competence; ability to work "I'm getting really good at swimming since I've been taking lessons."	Sense of inferiority; difficulty learning and working "I can't read as well as the others in my class; I'm just dumb."
Adolescence (12-20 yr)	Making transition from childhood to adulthood; developing sense of identity	Identity vs. role confusion	Sense of personal identity; fidelity "I'm homosexual, and I'm OK with that."	Confusion about who one is; submersion of identity in relationships or group memberships "I belong to the gang because without them, I'm nothing."
Early adulthood (20-35 yr)	Establishing intimate bonds of love and friendship	Intimacy vs. isolation	Ability to love deeply and commit oneself "My husband has been my best friend for 25 years."	Emotional isolation; egocentricity "It's nearly impossible to find a man who is worth marrying."
Middle adulthood (35-65 yr)	Fulfilling life goals that involve family, career, and society; developing concerns that embrace future generations	Generativity vs. self-absorption	Ability to give and to care for others "I've arranged for a 6-month leave of absence to stay with my mother, now that her illness is terminal."	Self-absorption; inability to grow as a person "I've lived with this scar on my face for 3 years; it's worse than having cancer."
Later years (65 yr to death)	Looking back over one's life and accepting its meaning	Integrity vs. despair	Sense of integrity and fulfillment; willingness to face death; wisdom "I've led a happy, productive life, and I'm ready to die."	Dissatisfaction with life; denial of or despair over prospect of death "I'm not ready to die; the doctors are wrong, you'll see they are wrong."

Data from Erikson, E. H. (1963). *Childhood and society.* New York: W. W. Norton; and Altrocchi, J. (1980). *Abnormal psychology* (p. 196). New York: Harcourt Brace Jovanovich.

According to Sullivan, the purpose of all behavior is to get needs met through interpersonal interactions and to decrease or avoid anxiety. He defined *anxiety* as any painful feeling or emotion that arises from social insecurity or prevents biological needs from being satisfied. Sullivan coined the term *security operations* to describe measures the individual employs to reduce anxiety and enhance security. Collectively, all of the security operations an individual uses to defend against anxiety and ensure self-esteem make up the *self-system*.

There are many parallels between Sullivan's notion of security operations and Freud's concept of defense mechanisms. Both are processes of which we are unaware, and both are ways in which we reduce anxiety. However, Freud's defense mechanism of repression is an intrapsychic activity, whereas Sullivan's security operations are interpersonal relationship activities that can be observed.

Implications for Psychiatric Mental Health Nursing

Sullivan's theory is the foundation for Hildegard Peplau's nursing theory of interpersonal relationships that we examine later in this chapter. Sullivan believed that therapy should educate patients and assist them in gaining personal insight. Sullivan first used the term *participant observer*, which underscores that professional helpers cannot be isolated from the therapeutic situation if they are to be effective. Sullivan would insist that the nurse interact with the patient as an authentic human being. Mutuality, respect for the patient, unconditional acceptance, and empathy, which are considered essential aspects of modern therapeutic relationships, were important aspects of Sullivan's theory of interpersonal therapy.

Sullivan also demonstrated that a psychotherapeutic environment, characterized by an accepting atmosphere that provided numerous opportunities for practicing interpersonal skills and developing relationships, is an invaluable treatment tool. Group psychotherapy, family therapy, and educational and skill training programs, as well as unstructured periods, can be incorporated into the design of a psychotherapeutic environment to facilitate healthy interactions. This method is used today in virtually all residential and day hospital settings.

Interpersonal Psychotherapy

Interpersonal psychotherapy is an effective short-term therapy derived from the school of psychiatry that originated with Adolph Meyer and Harry Stack Sullivan. The assumption is that psychiatric disorders are influenced by interpersonal interactions and the social context. The goal of interpersonal psychotherapy is to reduce or eliminate psychiatric symptoms (particularly depression) by improving interpersonal functioning and satisfaction with social relationships (Sadock & Sadock, 2008). Interpersonal psychotherapy has proved successful in the treatment of depression. Treatment is predicated on the notion that disturbances in important interpersonal relationships (or a deficit in one's capacity to form those relationships) can play a role in initiating or maintaining clinical depression. In interpersonal psychotherapy, the therapist identifies the nature of the problem to be resolved and then selects strategies consistent with that problem area. Four types of problem areas have been identified (Hollon & Engelhardt, 1997):

1. **Grief**—complicated bereavement following the death or loss of a loved one
2. **Role disputes**—conflicts with a significant other
3. **Role transition**—problematic change in life status or social or vocational role
4. **Interpersonal deficit**—an inability to initiate or sustain close relationships

Hildegard Peplau's Theory of Interpersonal Relationships in Nursing

Hildegard Peplau (1909-1999) (Figure 2-2), influenced by the work of Sullivan and learning theory, developed the first systematic theoretical framework for psychiatric nursing in her groundbreaking book *Interpersonal Relations in Nursing* (1952). Peplau not only established

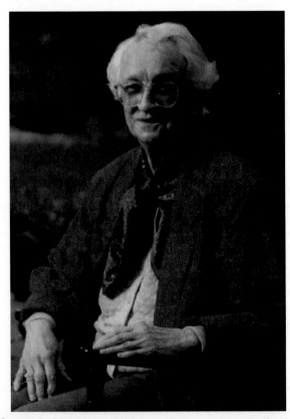

Figure 2-2 Hildegard Peplau. (Courtesy Anne Peplau.)

the foundation for the professional practice of psychiatric nursing but also continued to enrich psychiatric nursing theory and work for the advancement of nursing practice throughout her career.

Peplau was the first nurse to identify psychiatric mental health nursing both as an essential element of general nursing and as a specialty area that embraces specific governing principles. She was also the first nurse theorist to describe the nurse-patient relationship as the foundation of nursing practice (Forchuk, 1991). In shifting the focus from what nurses do *to* patients to what nurses do *with* patients, Peplau (1989) engineered a major paradigm shift from a model focused on medical treatments to an interpersonal relational model of nursing practice.

She viewed nursing as an educative instrument designed to help individuals and communities use their capacities in living more productively (Peplau, 1987). Her theory is mainly concerned with the processes by which the nurse helps patients make positive changes in their health care status and well-being. She believed that illness offered a unique opportunity for experiential learning, personal growth, and improved coping strategies and that psychiatric nurses play a unique role in facilitating this growth (Peplau, 1982a, 1982b).

Peplau identified stages of the nurse-patient relationship (see Chapter 9) and also used the technique of process recording to help her students hone their communication and relationship skills (see Table 10-4). The skills of the psychiatric nurse include observation, interpretation, and intervention. The nurse observes and listens to the patient, developing impressions about the meaning of the patient's situation. By employing this process, the nurse is able to view the patient as a unique individual. The nurse's inferences are then validated with the patient for accuracy.

Peplau proposed an approach in which nurses are both participants and observers in therapeutic conversations. She believed it was essential for nurses to observe the behavior not only of the patient but also of themselves. This self-awareness on the part of the nurse is essential in keeping the focus on the patient, as well as keeping the social and personal needs of the nurse out of the nurse-patient conversation.

Peplau spent a lifetime illuminating the science and art of professional nursing practice, and her work has had a profound effect on the nursing profession, nursing science, and the clinical practice of psychiatric nursing (Haber, 2000). The *art* component of nursing consists of the care, compassion, and advocacy nurses provide to enhance patient comfort and well-being. The *science* component of nursing involves the application of knowledge to understand a broad range of human problems and psychosocial phenomena, intervening to relieve patients' suffering and promote growth (Haber, 2000). In her works, Peplau (1995) constantly reminds nurses to "care for the person as well as the illness" and "think exclusively of patients as persons."

Implications for Psychiatric Mental Health Nursing

Perhaps Peplau's most universal contribution to the everyday practice of psychiatric mental health nursing is her application of Sullivan's theory of anxiety to nursing practice. She described the effects of different levels of anxiety (mild, moderate, severe, and panic) on perception and learning. She promoted interventions to lower anxiety, with the aim of improving patients' abilities to think and function at more satisfactory levels. More on the application of Peplau's theory of anxiety and interventions is presented in Chapter 12.

Table 2-3 lists selected nursing theorists and summarizes their major contributions and the impact of these contributions on psychiatric mental health nursing.

BEHAVIORAL THEORIES AND THERAPIES

Behavioral theories also developed as a protest response to Freud's assumption that a person's destiny was carved in stone at a very early age. Behaviorists have no concern with inner conflicts but argue that personality simply consists of learned behaviors. Consequently, personality becomes synonymous with behavior—if behavior changes, so does the personality.

The development of behavioral models began in the 19th century as a result of Ivan Pavlov's laboratory work with dogs. It continued into the 20th century with John B. Watson's application of these models to shape behavior and B.F. Skinner's research on rat behavior. These behavioral theorists developed systematic learning principles that could be applied to humans. Behavioral models emphasize the ways in which observable behavioral responses are learned and can be modified in a particular environment. Pavlov's, Watson's, and Skinner's models focus on the belief that behavior can be influenced through a process referred to as *conditioning*. Conditioning involves pairing a behavior with a condition that reinforces or diminishes the behavior's occurrence.

Ivan Pavlov's Classical Conditioning Theory

Ivan Pavlov (1849-1936) was a Russian physiologist. He won a Nobel Prize for his outstanding contributions to the physiology of digestion, which he studied through his well-known experiments with dogs. In incidental observation of the dogs, Pavlov noticed that the dogs were able to anticipate when food would be forthcoming and would begin to salivate even before actually tasting the meat. Pavlov labeled this process *psychic secretion*.

TABLE 2-3 Selected Nursing Theorists, Their Major Contributions, and Their Impact on Psychiatric Mental Health Nursing

Nursing Theorist	Focus of Theory	Contribution to Psychiatric Mental Health Nursing
Patricia Benner	"Caring" as foundation for nursing	Benner encourages nurses to provide caring and comforting interventions. She emphasizes the importance of the nurse-patient relationship and the importance of teaching and coaching the patient and bearing witness to suffering as the patient deals with illness.
Dorothea Orem	Goal of self-care as integral to the practice of nursing	Orem emphasizes the role of the nurse in promoting self-care activities of the patient; this has relevance to the seriously and persistently mentally ill patient.
Sister Callista Roy	Continual need for people to adapt physically, psychologically, and socially	Roy emphasizes the role of nursing in assisting patients to adapt so they can cope more effectively with changes.
Betty Neuman	Impact of internal and external stressors on the equilibrium of the system	Neuman emphasizes the role of nursing in assisting patients to discover and use stress-reducing strategies.
Joyce Travelbee	Meaning in the nurse-patient relationship and the importance of communication	Travelbee emphasizes the role of nursing in affirming the suffering of the patient and being able to alleviate that suffering through communication skills used appropriately through the stages of the nurse-patient relationship.

Data from Benner, P., & Wrubel, J. (1989). *The primacy of caring: Stress and coping in health and illness.* Menlo Park, CA: Addison-Wesley; Leddy, S., & Pepper, J. M. (1993). *Conceptual bases of professional nursing* (3rd ed., pp. 174–175). Philadelphia: Lippincott; Neuman, B., & Young, R. (1972). A model for teaching total-person approach to patient problems. *Nursing Research, 21,* 264–269; Orem, D. E. (1995). *Nursing: Concepts of practice* (5th ed.). New York: McGraw-Hill; Roy, C., & Andrews, H. A. (1991). *The Roy adaptation model: The definitive statement.* Norwalk, CT: Appleton & Lange; and Travelbee, J. (1961). *Intervention in psychiatric nursing.* Philadelphia: F. A. Davis.

He hypothesized that the psychic component was a learned association between two events: the presence of the experimental apparatus and the serving of meat.

Pavlov formalized his observations of behaviors in dogs in a theory of classical conditioning. Pavlov (1928) found that when a neutral stimulus (a bell) was repeatedly paired with another stimulus (food that triggered salivation), eventually the sound of the bell alone could elicit salivation in the dogs. An example of this response in humans would be an individual who became very ill as a child after eating spoiled coleslaw at a picnic and later in life feels nauseated whenever he smells coleslaw. It is important to recognize that classical conditioned responses are *involuntary*—not under conscious personal control—and are not spontaneous choices.

John B. Watson's Behaviorism Theory

John B. Watson (1878-1958) was an American psychologist who rejected the unconscious motivation of psychoanalysis as being too subjective. He developed the school of thought referred to as *behaviorism*, which he believed was more objective or measurable. Watson contended that personality traits and responses—adaptive and maladaptive—were socially learned through classical conditioning (Watson, 1919). In a famous (but terrible) experiment, Watson stood behind Little Albert, a 9-month-old who liked animals, and made a loud noise with a hammer every time the infant reached for a white rat. After this experiment, Little Albert became terrified at the sight of white fur or hair, even in the absence of a loud noise. Watson concluded that behavior could be molded by controlling the environment and that anyone could be trained to be anything, from a beggar man to a merchant.

B.F. Skinner's Operant Conditioning Theory

B.F. Skinner (1904-1990) represented the second wave of behavioral theorists. Skinner (1987) researched operant conditioning, in which *voluntary* behaviors are learned through consequences, and behavioral responses are elicited through reinforcement, which causes a behavior to occur *more* frequently. A consequence can be a positive reinforcement, such as receiving a reward (getting a 3.8 GPA after studying hard all semester), or a **negative reinforcement**, such as the removal of an objectionable or aversive stimulus (walking freely through a park once the vicious dog is picked up by the dogcatcher).

Other techniques can cause behaviors to occur *less* frequently. One technique is an unpleasant consequence, or **punishment**. Driving too fast may result in a speeding ticket, which—in mature and healthy individuals—decreases the chances that speeding will occur. Absence of reinforcement, or **extinction**, also decreases behavior by withholding a reward that has become habitual. If a person tells a joke and no one laughs, for example, the person is less apt to tell jokes because his joke-telling behavior is not being reinforced. Teachers employ this strategy in the classroom when they ignore acting-out behavior that had previously been rewarded by more attention.

Figure 2-3 illustrates the differences between classical conditioning (in which an involuntary reaction is caused by a stimulus) and operant conditioning (in which voluntary behavior is learned through reinforcement).

Implications for Psychiatric Mental Health Nursing

Skinner's behavioral model provides a concrete method for modifying or replacing behaviors. Behavior management and modification programs based on his principles have proven to be successful in altering targeted behaviors. *Programmed learning* and *token economies* represent extensions of Skinner's thoughts on learning. Behavioral methods are particularly effective with children, adolescents, and individuals with many forms of chronic mental illness.

Behavioral Therapy

Behavioral therapy is based on the assumption that changes in maladaptive behavior can occur without insight into the underlying cause. This approach works best when it is directed at specific problems and the goals are well defined. Behavioral therapy is effective in treating people with phobias, alcoholism, schizophrenia, and many other conditions. Four types of behavioral therapy

are discussed here: modeling, operant conditioning, systematic desensitization, and aversion therapy.

Modeling

In modeling, the therapist provides a role model for specific identified behaviors, and the patient learns through imitation. The therapist may do the modeling, provide another person to model the behaviors, or present a video for the purpose. Bandura and Colleagues (1969) were able to help people reduce their phobias about nonpoisonous snakes by having them first view close-ups of filmed encounters between people and snakes that resulted in successful outcomes, and then view live encounters between people and snakes that also had successful outcomes. In a similar fashion, some behavioral therapists use role playing in the consulting room. They demonstrate patterns of behaving that might prove more effective than those usually engaged in, and then have the patients practice these new behaviors. For example, a student who does not know how to ask a professor for an extension on a term paper would watch the therapist portray a potentially effective way of making the request. The clinician would then help the student practice the new skill in a similar role-playing situation.

Operant Conditioning

Operant conditioning is the basis for behavior modification and uses positive reinforcement to increase desired behaviors. For example, when desired goals are achieved or behaviors are performed, patients might be rewarded with tokens. These tokens can be exchanged for food, small luxuries, or privileges. This reward system is known as a *token economy*.

Operant conditioning has been useful in improving the verbal behaviors of mute, autistic, and developmentally disabled children. In patients with severe and persistent mental illness, behavior modification has helped increase levels of self-care, social behavior, group participation, and more. You may find this a useful technique as you proceed through your clinical rotations.

We all use positive reinforcement in our everyday lives, whether we are aware of it or not. A familiar case in point is the mother who takes her preschooler along to the grocery store, and the child starts acting out, demanding candy, nagging, crying, and yelling. Here are examples of three ways the child's behavior can be reinforced:

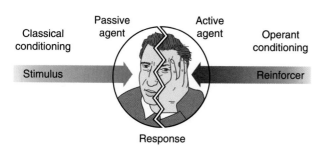

Passive agent — Active agent

Classical conditioning ← Stimulus | Operant conditioning ← Reinforcer

Response

Figure 2-3 Classical versus operant conditioning. (From Carson, V. B. [2000]. *Mental health nursing: The nurse-patient journey* [2nd ed., p. 121]. Philadelphia: Saunders.)

Action	Result
1. The mother gives the child the candy.	The child continues to use this behavior. This is positive reinforcement of negative behavior.
2. The mother scolds the child.	Acting out may continue, because the child gets what he really wants—attention. This positively rewards negative behavior.

Action	Result
3. The mother ignores the acting out but gives attention to the child when he is acting appropriately.	The child gets a positive reward for appropriate behavior.

Systematic Desensitization

Systematic desensitization is another form of behavior modification therapy that involves the development of behavioral tasks customized to the patient's specific fears; these tasks are presented to the patient while using learned relaxation techniques. The process involves four steps:

1. The patient's fear is broken down into its components by exploring the particular stimulus cues to which the patient reacts. For example, certain situations may precipitate a phobic reaction, whereas others do not. Crowds at parties may be problematic, whereas similar numbers of people in other settings do not cause the same distress.
2. The patient is incrementally exposed to the fear. For example, a patient who has a fear of flying is introduced to short periods of visual presentations of flying—first with still pictures, then with videos, and finally in a busy airport. The situations are confronted while the patient is in a relaxed state. Gradually, over a period of time, exposure is increased until anxiety about or fear of the object or situation has ceased.
3. The patient is instructed in how to design a hierarchy of fears. For fear of flying, a patient might develop a set of statements representing the stages of a flight, order the statements from the most fearful to the least fearful, and use relaxation techniques to reach a state of relaxation as they progress through the list.
4. The patient practices these techniques every day.

Aversion Therapy

Today, aversion therapy (which is akin to punishment) is used widely to treat behaviors such as alcoholism, sexual deviation, shoplifting, hallucinations, violent and aggressive behavior, and self-mutilation. Aversion therapy is sometimes the treatment of choice when other less drastic measures have failed to produce the desired effects. The following are three paradigms for using aversive techniques:

1. Pairing of a maladaptive behavior with a noxious stimulus (e.g., pairing the sight and smell of alcohol with electric shock), so that anxiety or fear becomes associated with the once-pleasurable stimulus
2. Punishment (e.g., punishment applied after the patient has had an alcoholic drink)
3. Avoidance training (e.g., patient avoids punishment by pushing a glass of alcohol away within a certain time limit)

Simple examples of extinguishing undesirable behavior through aversion therapy include painting foul-tasting substances on the fingernails of nail biters or the thumbs of thumb suckers. Other examples of aversive stimuli are chemicals that induce nausea and vomiting, noxious odors, unpleasant verbal stimuli (e.g., descriptions of disturbing scenes), costs or fines in a token economy, and denial of positive reinforcement (e.g., isolation).

Before initiating any aversive protocol, the therapist, treatment team, or society *must* answer the following questions:

- Is this therapy in the best interest of the patient?
- Does its use violate the patient's rights?
- Is it in the best interest of society?

If aversion therapy is chosen as the most appropriate treatment, ongoing supervision, support, and evaluation of those administering it must occur.

Biofeedback

Biofeedback is also a form of behavioral therapy and is successfully used today, especially for controlling the body's physiological response to stress and anxiety. Biofeedback is discussed in detail in Chapter 11.

COGNITIVE THEORIES AND THERAPIES

While behaviorists focused on increasing, decreasing, or eliminating measurable behaviors, little attention was paid to the thoughts, or cognitions, that were involved in these behaviors. Rather than thinking of people as passive recipients of environmental conditioning, cognitive theorists proposed that there is a dynamic interplay between individuals and the environment. These theorists believe that thoughts come before feelings and actions, and thoughts about the world and our place in it are based on our own unique perspectives, which may or may not be based on reality. Two of the most influential theorists and their therapies are presented here.

Rational-Emotive Behavior Therapy

Rational-Emotive Behavior Therapy (REBT) was developed by Albert Ellis (1913-2007) in 1955. The aim of REBT is to eradicate core irrational beliefs by helping people recognize thoughts that are not accurate, sensible, or useful. These thoughts tend to take the form of shoulds (e.g., "I should always be polite."), oughts (e.g., "I ought to consistently win my tennis games."), and musts (e.g., "I must be thin."). Ellis described negative thinking as a simple A-B-C process. *A* stands for the activating event, *B* stands for beliefs about the event, and *C* stands for emotional consequence as a result of the event.

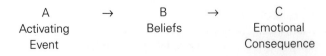

A	→	B	→	C
Activating Event		Beliefs		Emotional Consequence

Perception influences all thoughts, which in turn influence our behaviors. It often boils down to the simple notion of perceiving the glass as half full or half empty. For example, imagine you have just received an invitation to a birthday party (activating event). You think, "I hate parties. Now I have to hang out with people who don't like me, instead of watching my favorite television shows. They probably just invited me to get a gift." (Beliefs) You will probably be miserable (emotional consequence) if you go. On the other hand, you may think, "I love parties (activating event)! This will be a great chance to meet new people, and it will be fun to shop for the perfect gift." (Beliefs) You could have a delightful time (emotional consequence).

Although Ellis (Figure 2-4) admits that the role of past experiences is instrumental in our current beliefs, the focus of rational-emotive behavior therapy is on present attitudes, painful feelings, and dysfunctional behaviors. If our beliefs are negative and self-deprecating, we are more susceptible to depression and anxiety. Ellis noted that while we cannot change the past, we can change the way we are now. He was pragmatic in his approach to mental illness and colorful in his therapeutic advice. "It's too [darn] bad you panic, but you don't die from it! Get them over the panic about panic, you may find the panic disappears" (Ellis, 2000).

Cognitive-Behavioral Therapy (CBT)

Aaron T. Beck (see Figure 2-4), another follower of Sigmund Freud, originally trained in psychoanalysis but is regarded as a Neo-Freudian. When he attempted to study depression from a psychoanalytic perspective, he became convinced that people with depression generally had stereotypical patterns of negative and self-critical thinking that seemed to distort their ability to think and process information. Cognitive-behavioral therapy (CBT) is based on both cognitive psychology and behavioral theory. It is a commonly employed, effective, and well-researched therapeutic tool.

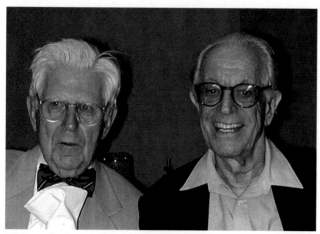

Figure 2-4   Aaron Beck and Albert Ellis. (Courtesy Fenichel, 2000.)

Beck's method (Beck et al., 1979), the basis for CBT, is an active, directive, time-limited, structured approach used to treat a variety of psychiatric disorders (e.g., depression, anxiety, phobias, and pain problems). It is based on the underlying theoretical principle that how people feel and behave is largely determined by the way they think about the world and their place in it (Beck, 1967). Their cognitions (verbal or pictorial events in their stream of consciousness) are based on attitudes or assumptions developed from previous experiences. These cognitions may be fairly accurate, or they may be distorted.

According to Beck, we all have *schemata* or unique assumptions about ourselves, others, and the world around us. For example, if a person has the schema (singular of schemata) "The only person I can trust is myself," they will have expectations that everyone else has questionable motives, will lie, and will eventually hurt them. Other negative schemata include incompetence, abandonment, evilness, and vulnerability. We are typically not aware of such cognitive biases, but recognizing them as beliefs and attitudes based on distortions and misconceptions will help make it apparent when dysfunctional schemas underlie our thinking.

Rapid, unthinking responses based on schemas are known as **automatic thoughts**. These responses are particularly intense and frequent in psychiatric disorders such as depression and anxiety. Often automatic thoughts, or **cognitive distortions**, are irrational and lead to false assumptions and misinterpretations. For example, if a person interprets all experiences in terms of whether he or she is competent and adequate, thinking may be dominated by the cognitive distortion, "Unless I do everything perfectly, I'm a failure." Consequently, the person reacts to situations in terms of adequacy, even when these situations are unrelated to whether he or she is personally competent. Table 2-4 describes common cognitive distortions.

The therapeutic techniques of the cognitive therapist are designed to identify, reality test, and correct distorted conceptualizations and the dysfunctional beliefs underlying them. In other words, the cognitive therapist helps patients to change the way they think and thereby reduce symptoms. Patients are taught to challenge their own negative thinking and substitute it with positive, rational thoughts. They are taught to recognize when thinking is based on distortions and misconceptions. Homework assignments play an important role in CBT. A particularly useful technique is the use of a four-column format to record the precipitating event or situation, the resulting automatic thought, the proceeding feeling(s) and behavior(s), and finally, a challenge to the negative thoughts, based on rational evidence and thinking. The following is an example of the type of analysis done by a patient receiving CBT.

TABLE 2-4 Common Cognitive Distortions

Distortion	Definition	Example
All-or-nothing thinking	Thinking in black and white, reducing complex outcomes into absolutes	Although Marcia earned the second highest score in the state's cheerleading competition, she consistently referred to herself as "a loser."
Overgeneralization	Using a bad outcome (or a few bad outcomes) as evidence that nothing will ever go right again	Marty had a minor traffic accident. She refuses to drive and says, "I shouldn't be allowed on the road." When asked why, she answers, "I'm a horrible driver; I could have killed someone!"
Labeling	A form of overgeneralization where a characteristic or event becomes definitive and results in an overly harsh label for self or others	"Because I failed the advanced statistics exam, I am a failure. I might as well give up. I may as well quit and look for an easier major."
Mental filter	Focusing on a negative detail or bad event and allowing it to taint everything else	Anne's boss evaluated her work as exemplary and gave her a few suggestions for improvement. She obsessed about the suggestions and ignored the rest.
Disqualifying the positive	Maintaining a negative view by rejecting information that supports a positive view as being irrelevant, inaccurate, or accidental	"I've just been offered the job I've always wanted. No one else must have applied."
Jumping to conclusions	Making a negative interpretation despite the fact that there is little or no supporting evidence	"My fiancé, Juan, didn't call me for 3 hours, which just proves he doesn't love me anymore."
a. Mind-reading	Inferring negative thoughts, responses, and motives of others	"The grocery store clerk was grouchy and barely made eye contact, so I must have done something wrong."
b. Fortune-telling error	Assuming a negative outcome is inevitable	"I'll ask her out, but I know she won't have a good time."
Magnification or minimization	Exaggerating the importance of something (such as a personal failure or the success of others) or reducing the importance of something (such as a personal success or the failure of others)	"I'm alone on a Saturday night because no one likes me. When other people are alone, it's because they want to be."
a. Catastrophizing	Catastrophizing is an extreme form of magnification in which the very worst is assumed to be a probable outcome.	"If I don't make a good impression on the boss at the company picnic, she will fire me."
Emotional reasoning	Drawing a conclusion based on an emotional state	"I'm nervous about the exam. I must not be prepared. If I were, I wouldn't be afraid."
"Should" and "must" statements	Rigid self-directives that presume an unrealistic amount of control over external events	"My patient is worse today. I should give better care so she will get better."
Personalization	Assuming responsibility for an external event or situation that was likely outside personal control.	"I'm sorry your party wasn't more fun. It's probably because I was there."

Data from Burns, D.D. (1989). *The feeling good handbook*. New York: William Morrow.

A 24-year-old nurse recently discharged from the hospital for severe depression presented this record (Beck et al., 1979):

Event	Feeling	Cognitions	Other Possible Interpretations
While at a party, Jim asked me, "How are you feeling?" shortly after I was discharged from the hospital.	Anxious	Jim thinks I am a basket case. I must really look bad for him to be concerned.	He really cares about me. He noticed that I look better than before I went into the hospital and wants to know if I feel better too.

Box 2-1 presents an example of cognitive-behavioral therapy, and Table 2-5 compares and contrasts psychodynamic, interpersonal, cognitive-behavioral, and behavioral therapies.

Implications for Psychiatric Mental Health Nursing

Recognizing the interplay between events, negative thinking, and negative responses can be beneficial from both a patient-care standpoint and a personal one. As a supportive therapeutic measure, helping the patient identify negative thought patterns is a worthwhile intervention. Workbooks are available to aid in the process of identifying cognitive distortions.

Personal benefits from this cognitive approach could help the nurse understand her/his own response to a variety of difficult situations. One example

---

BOX 2-1 Example of Cognitive-Behavioral Therapy

The patient was an attractive woman in her early 20s. Her depression of 18 months' duration was precipitated by her boyfriend's leaving her. She had numerous automatic thoughts that she was ugly and undesirable. These automatic thoughts were handled in the following manner:

Therapist: Other than your subjective opinion, what evidence do you have that you are ugly?

Patient: Well, my sister always said I was ugly.

Therapist: Was she always right in these matters?

Patient: No. Actually, she had her own reasons for telling me this. But the real reason I know I'm ugly is that men don't ask me out. If I weren't ugly, I'd be dating now.

Therapist: That is a possible reason why you're not dating. But there's an alternative explanation. You told me that you work in an office by yourself all day and spend your nights alone at home. It doesn't seem like you're giving yourself opportunities to meet men.

Patient: I can see what you're saying, but still, if I weren't ugly, men would ask me out.

Therapist: I suggest we run an experiment: that is, for you to become more socially active, stop turning down invitations to parties and social events, and see what happens.

After the patient became more active and had more opportunities to meet men, she started to date. At this point, she no longer believed she was ugly.

Therapy then focused on her basic assumption that one's worth is determined by one's appearance. She readily agreed this didn't make sense. She also saw the falseness of the assumption that one must be beautiful to attract men or be loved. This discussion led to her basic assumption that she could not be happy without love (or

attention from men). The latter part of treatment focused on helping her to change this belief.

Therapist: On what do you base this belief that you can't be happy without a man?

Patient: I was really depressed for a year and a half when I didn't have a man in my life.

Therapist: Is there another reason why you were depressed?

Patient: As we discussed, I was looking at everything in a distorted way. But I still don't know if I could be happy if no one was interested in me.

Therapist: I don't know either. Is there a way we could find out?

Patient: Well, as an experiment I could not go out on dates for a while and see how I feel.

Therapist: I think that's a good idea. Although it has its flaws, the experimental method is still the best way currently available to discover the facts. You're fortunate in being able to run this type of experiment. Now, for the first time in your adult life you aren't attached to a man. If you find you can be happy without a man, this will greatly strengthen you and also make your future relationships all the better.

In this case, the patient was able to stick to a "cold turkey" regimen. After a brief period of dysphoria, she was delighted to find that her well-being was not dependent on another person.

There were similarities between these two interventions. In both, the distorted conclusion or assumption was delineated, and the patient was asked for evidence to support it. An experiment to gather data was also suggested in both instances. However, to achieve the results, a contrasting version of the same experimental situation was required.

From Beck, A. T, Rush, A. J., Shaw, B. F., & Emery, G. (1979). *Cognitive therapy of depression.* New York: Guilford Press.

TABLE 2-5 Comparison of Psychodynamic, Interpersonal, Cognitive-Behavioral, and Behavioral Therapies

	Psychodynamic Therapy	Interpersonal Therapy	Cognitive-Behavioral Therapy	Behavioral Therapy
Treatment focus	Unresolved past relationships and core conflicts	Current interpersonal relationships and social supports	Thoughts and cognitions	Learned maladaptive behavior
Therapist role	Significant other Transference object	Problem solver	Active, directive, challenging	Active, directive teacher
Primary disorders treated	Anxiety Depression Personality disorders	Depression	Depression Anxiety/panic Eating disorders	Posttraumatic stress disorder Obsessive compulsive disorder Panic disorder
Length of therapy	20 + sessions	Short term (12-20 sessions)	Short term (5-20 sessions)	Varies, typically fewer than 10 sessions
Technique	Therapeutic alliance Free association Understanding transference Challenging defense mechanisms	Facilitate new patterns of communication and expectations for relationships	Evaluating thoughts and behaviors Modifying dysfunctional thoughts and behaviors	Relaxation Thought stopping Self-reassurance Seeking social support

Data from Dewan, M. J., Steenbarger, B. N., & Greenberg, R. P. (2008). Brief psychotherapies. In R. E. Hales, S. C. Yudofsky, & G. O. Gabbard (Eds.), *Textbook of psychiatry* (5th ed., pp. 1155–1170). Washington, DC: American Psychiatric Publishing.

might be the anxiety that some students feel regarding the psychiatric nursing clinical rotation. Students may overgeneralize ("All psychiatric patients are dangerous.") or personalize ("My patient doesn't seem to be better; I'm probably not doing him any good.") the situation. The key to effectively using this approach in clinical situations is to challenge the negative thoughts not based on facts, and then replace them with more realistic appraisals.

HUMANISTIC THEORIES

In the 1950s, humanistic theories arose as a protest against both the behavioral and psychoanalytic schools, which were thought to be pessimistic, deterministic, and dehumanizing. Humanistic theories focus on human potential and free will to choose life patterns that are supportive of personal growth. Humanistic frameworks emphasize a person's capacity for self-actualization. This approach focuses on understanding the patient's perspective as she or he subjectively experiences it. There are a number of humanistic theorists. Our journey will stop to explore Abraham Maslow and his theory of self-actualization.

Abraham Maslow's Humanistic Psychology Theory

Abraham Maslow (1908-1970), considered the father of humanistic psychology, introduced the concept of a "self-actualized personality" associated with high productivity and enjoyment of life (Maslow, 1963, 1968). He criticized psychology for focusing too intently on humanity's frailties and not enough on its strengths. Maslow contended that the focus of psychology must go beyond experiences of hate, pain, misery, guilt, and conflict to include love, compassion, happiness, exhilaration, and well-being.

Hierarchy of Needs

Maslow conceptualized human motivation as a hierarchy of dynamic processes or needs that are critical for the development of all humans. Central to his theory is the assumption that humans are active rather than passive participants in life, striving for self-actualization. Maslow (1968) focused on human need fulfillment, which he categorized into six incremental stages; beginning with physiological survival needs and ending with self-transcendent needs (Figure 2-5). The hierarchy of needs is conceptualized as a pyramid, with the strongest, most fundamental

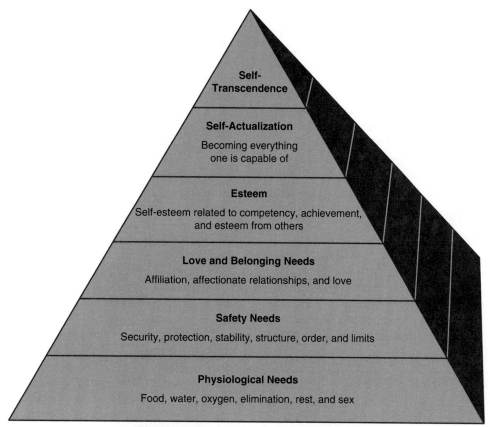

Figure 2-5 Maslow's hierarchy of needs.

needs placed on the lower levels. The higher levels—the more distinctly human needs—occupy the top sections of the pyramid. When lower-level needs are met, higher needs are able to emerge.

- *Physiological needs.* The most basic needs are the physiological drives—needing food, oxygen, water, sleep, sex, and a constant body temperature. If all needs were deprived, this level would take priority over the rest.
- *Safety needs.* Once physiological needs are met, safety needs emerge. They include security, protection, freedom from fear/anxiety/chaos, and the need for law, order, and limits. Adults in a stable society usually feel safe, but they may feel threatened by debt, job insecurity, or lack of insurance. It is during times of crisis, such as war, disasters, assaults, and social breakdown, that safety needs really take precedence. Children, who are more vulnerable and dependent, respond far more readily and intensely to safety threats.
- *Belongingness and love needs.* People have a need for intimate relationships, love, affection, and belonging and will seek to overcome feelings of aloneness and alienation. Maslow stresses the importance of having a family and a home and being part of identifiable groups.

- *Esteem needs.* People need to have a high self-regard and have it reflected to them from others. If self-esteem needs are met, we feel confident, valued, and valuable. When self-esteem is compromised, we feel inferior, worthless, and helpless.
- *Self-actualization.* We are preset to strive to be everything we are capable of becoming. Maslow said, "What a man *can* be, he *must* be." What we are capable of becoming is highly individual—an artist must paint, a writer must write, and a healer must heal. The drive to satisfy this need is felt as a sort of restlessness, a sense that something is missing. It is up to each person to choose a path that will bring about inner peace and fulfillment.

Although Maslow's early work included only five levels of needs, he later took into account two additional factors: (1) cognitive needs (the desire to know and understand) and (2) the aesthetic needs (Maslow, 1970). He describes the acquisition of knowledge (our first priority) and the need to understand (our second priority) as being hard-wired and essential; he identified the aesthetic need for beauty and symmetry as universal. How else, after all, do we explain the impulse to straighten a crooked picture?

Maslow based his theory on the results of clinical investigations of people who represented self-actualized individuals who moved in the direction of achieving and reaching their highest potentials. Among those Maslow chose to investigate were historical figures such as Abraham Lincoln, Thomas Jefferson, Harriet Tubman, Walt Whitman, Beethoven, William James, and Franklin D. Roosevelt, as well as others like Albert Einstein, Eleanor Roosevelt, and Albert Schweitzer, who were living at the time they were studied. This investigation led Maslow (1963, 1970) to identify some basic personality characteristics that distinguish self-actualizing people from those who might be called "ordinary" (Box 2-2).

Implications for Psychiatric Mental Health Nursing

The value of Maslow's model in nursing practice is two-fold. First, an emphasis on human potential and the patient's strengths is key to successful nurse-patient relationships. Second, the model helps establish what is most important in the sequencing of nursing actions in the nurse-patient relationship. For example, to collect

---

BOX 2-2 Some Characteristics of Self-Actualized Persons

- Accurate perception of reality. Not defensive in their perceptions of the world.
- Acceptance of themselves, others, and nature.
- Spontaneity, simplicity, and naturalness. Self-actualized individuals (SAs) do not live programmed lives.
- Problem-centered rather than self-centered orientation. Possibly the most important characteristic. SAs have a sense of a mission to which they dedicate their lives.
- Enjoyment of privacy and detachment. Pleasure in being alone; ability to reflect on events.
- Freshness of appreciation. SAs don't take life for granted.
- Mystical or peak experiences. A peak experience is a moment of intense ecstasy, similar to a religious or mystical experience, during which the self is transcended. More recently, Mihaly Csikszentmihalyi developed the term *flow experience* to describe times when people become so totally involved in what they are doing that they lose all sense of time and awareness of self.
- Active social interest.
- An unhostile sense of humor.
- Democratic character structure. SAs display little racial, religious, or social prejudice.
- Creativity, especially in managing their lives.
- Resistance to conformity (enculturation). SAs are autonomous, independent, and self-sufficient.

From Maslow, A. H. (1970). *Motivation and personality.* New York: Harper & Row.

---

any but the most essential information when a patient is struggling with drug withdrawal is inappropriate. Following Maslow's model as a way of prioritizing actions, the nurse meets the patient's physiological need for stable vital signs and pain relief before collecting general information for a nursing database.

BIOLOGICAL THEORIES AND THERAPIES

The Advent of Psychopharmacology

In 1950, a French drug firm synthesized chlorpromazine—a powerful antipsychotic medication—and psychiatry experienced a revolution. The advent of psychopharmacology presented a direct challenge to psychodynamic approaches to mental illness. The dramatic experience of observing patients freed from the bondage of psychosis and mania by powerful drugs such as chlorpromazine and lithium left witnesses convinced of the critical role of the brain in psychiatric illness. In fact, President George H. W. Bush declared the 1990s the Decade of the Brain, and vast amounts of research monies and effort were directed at study of the structure and functions of the brain.

Since the discovery of chlorpromazine, many other medications have proven effective in controlling psychosis, mania, depression, and anxiety. These medications greatly reduce the need for hospitalization and dramatically improve the lives of people suffering with serious psychiatric difficulties. Today we know that psychoactive medications exert differential effects on different neurotransmitters and help restore brain function, allowing patients with mental illness to continue living productive lives with greater satisfaction and far less emotional pain.

The Biological Model

A biological model of mental illness focuses on neurological, chemical, biological, and genetic issues and seeks to understand how the body and brain interact to create emotions, memories, and perceptual experiences. A biological perspective views abnormal behavior as part of a disease process or a defect and seeks to stop or alter it. The biological model locates the illness or disease in the body—usually in the limbic system of the brain and the synapse receptor sites of the central nervous system—and targets the site of the illness using physical interventions such as drugs, diet, or surgery.

The recognition that psychiatric illnesses are as physical in origin as diabetes and coronary heart disease serves to decrease the stigma surrounding them. Just as someone with diabetes or heart disease cannot be held responsible for their illness, patients with schizophrenia or bipolar affective disorder are no more to blame. It often happens that one of the most helpful things we can tell those whose lives are affected by psychiatric illness is that they are not responsible or to blame.

Implications for Psychiatric Mental Health Nursing

Historically, psychiatric mental health nurses always have attended to the physical needs of psychiatric patients. Nurses administer medications; monitor sleep, activity, nutrition, hydration, elimination, and other functions; and prepare patients for somatic therapies, such as electroconvulsive therapy. They have continued to do so with the advancement of the biological model, which has not altered the basic nursing strategies: focusing on the qualities of a therapeutic relationship, understanding the patient's perspective, and communicating in a way that facilitates the patient's recovery.

One of the risks in adopting a biological model to the exclusion of all other theoretical perspectives is that such a theory ignores the myriad other influences, including social, environmental, cultural, economic, spiritual, and educational factors that play a role in the development and treatment of mental illness.

ADDITIONAL THERAPIES

Milieu Therapy

In 1948, Bruno Bettelheim coined the term milieu therapy to describe his use of the total environment to treat disturbed children. Bettelheim created a comfortable, secure environment (or milieu) in which psychotic children were helped to form a new world. Staff members were trained to provide 24-hour support and understanding for each child on an individual basis. In 1953, Maxwell Jones in Great Britain wrote the book *The Therapeutic Community*. This book both laid the groundwork for the milieu therapy movement in the United States and defined the nurse's role in this therapy.

Milieu is sometimes a difficult concept to grasp. It is an all-inclusive term that recognizes the people, setting, structure, and emotional climate as all important to healing. Milieu therapy takes naturally occurring events in the environment and uses them as rich learning opportunities for patients. There are certain basic characteristics of milieu therapy, regardless of whether the setting involves treatment of psychotic children, patients in a psychiatric hospital, drug abusers in a residential treatment center, or psychiatric patients in a day hospital. Milieu therapy, or a therapeutic community, has as its locus a living, learning, or working environment. Such therapy may be based on any number of therapeutic modalities, from structured behavioral therapy to spontaneous, humanistic-oriented approaches.

Implications for Psychiatric Mental Health Nursing

Milieu therapy is a basic intervention in nursing practice. Nurses are constantly involved in the assessment and provision of safe and effective milieus for their patients. Common examples include providing a safe environment for the suicidal patient or a patient with a cognitive disorder (e.g., Alzheimer's disease), referring abused women to safe houses, and advocating for children suspected of being abused in their home environments.

You will be introduced to other therapeutic approaches later in the book. Crisis intervention (see Chapter 23) is an approach you will find useful, not only in psychiatric mental health nursing but also in other nursing specialties. Group therapy (see Chapter 34) and family interventions (see Chapter 35), which are appropriate for the basic level practitioner, will also be discussed.

Table 2-6 lists additional theorists whose contributions influence psychiatric mental health nursing.

TABLE 2-6 Additional Theorists Whose Contributions Influence Psychiatric Mental Health Nursing			
Theorist	**School of Thought**	**Major Contributions**	**Relevance to Psychiatric Mental Health Nursing**
Carl Rogers	Humanism	Developed a person-centered model of psychotherapy. Emphasized the concepts of: Congruence—authenticity of the therapist in dealings with the patient Unconditional acceptance and positive regard—climate in the therapeutic relationship that facilitates change. Empathetic understanding—therapist's ability to apprehend the feelings and experiences of the patient as if these things were happening to the therapist.	Encourages nurses to view each patient as unique. Emphasizes attitudes of unconditional positive regard, empathetic understanding, and genuineness that are essential to the nurse-patient relationship. *Example:* The nurse asks the patient, "What can I do to help you regain control over your anxiety?"

Continued

TABLE 2-6 Additional Theorists Whose Contributions Influence Psychiatric Mental Health Nursing—cont'd

Theorist	School of Thought	Major Contributions	Relevance to Psychiatric Mental Health Nursing
Jean Piaget	Cognitive development	Identified stages of cognitive development, including sensorimotor (0-2 yr); preoperational (2-7 yr); concrete operational (7-11 yr); and formal operational (11 yr-adulthood). These describe how cognitive development proceeds from reflex activity to application of logical solutions to all types of problems.	Provides a broad base for cognitive interventions, especially with patients with negative self-views. *Example:* The nurse shows an 8-year-old all the equipment needed to start an IV when discussing the fact that he will need one prior to surgery.
Lawrence Kohlberg	Moral development	Posited a six-stage theory of moral development.	Provides nurses with a framework for evaluating moral decisions.
Albert Ellis	Existentialism	Developed approach of rational emotive behavioral therapy that is active and cognitively oriented; confrontation used to force patients to assume responsibility for behavior; patients are encouraged to accept themselves as they are and are taught to take risks and try out new behaviors.	Encourages nurses to focus on "here-and-now" issues and to help the patient live fully in the present and look forward to the future. *Example:* The nurse encourages the patient to vacation with her family even though she will be wheelchair bound until her leg fracture heals
Albert Bandura	Social learning theory	Responsible for concepts of modeling and self-efficacy: person's belief or expectation that he or she has the capacity to affect a desired outcome through his or her own efforts.	Includes cognitive functioning with environmental factors, which provides nurses with a comprehensive view of how people learn. *Example:* The nurse helps the teenage patient identify three negative outcomes of tobacco use
Viktor Frankl	Existentialism	Developed "logotherapy," a form of support offered to help people find their sense of self-respect. Logotherapy is a future-oriented therapy focused on one's need to find meaning and value in living as one's most important life task.	Focuses nurse beyond mere behaviors to understanding the meaning of these behaviors to the patient's sense of life meaning. *Example:* The nurse listens attentively as the patient describes what it's been like since her daughter died.

Data from Bandura, A. (1977). *Social learning theory.* Englewood Cliffs, NJ: Prentice-Hall; Bernard, M. E., & Wolfe, J. L. (Eds.). (1993). *The RET resource book for practitioners.* New York: Institute for Rational-Emotive Therapy; Ellis, A. (1989). *Inside rational emotive therapy.* San Diego, CA: Academic Press; Frankl, V. (1969). *The will to meaning.* Cleveland, OH: New American Library; Kohlberg, L. (1986). A current statement on some theoretical issues. In S. Modgil & C. Modgil (Eds.), *Lawrence Kohlberg.* Philadelphia: Palmer; and Rogers, C. R. (1961). *On becoming a person.* Boston: Houghton Mifflin.

KEY POINTS TO REMEMBER

- Sigmund Freud advanced the first theory of personality development.
- Freud articulated levels of awareness (unconscious, preconscious, conscious) and demonstrated the influence of our unconscious behavior on everyday life, as evidenced by the use of defense mechanisms.
- Freud identified three psychological processes of personality (id, ego, superego) and described how they operate and develop.
- Freud articulated one of the first modern developmental theories of personality, based on five psychosexual stages.

- Various psychoanalytic therapies have been used over the years. Currently a short-term, time-limited version of psychotherapy is common.
- Erik Erikson expanded on Freud's developmental stages to include middle age through old age. Erikson called his stages *psychosocial stages* and emphasized the social aspect of personality development.
- Harry Stack Sullivan proposed the interpersonal theory of personality development, which focuses on interpersonal processes that can be observed in a social framework.
- Hildegard Peplau, a nursing theorist, developed an interpersonal theoretical framework that has become the foundation of psychiatric mental health nursing practice.

- Abraham Maslow, the founder of humanistic psychology, offered the theory of self-actualization and human motivation that is basic to all nursing education today.
- Cognitive-behavioral therapy is the most commonly used, accepted, and empirically validated psychotherapeutic approach.
- A biological model of mental illness and treatment dominates care for psychiatric disorders.
- Milieu therapy is a philosophy of care in which all parts of the environment are considered to be therapeutic opportunities for growth and healing. The milieu includes the people (patients and staff), setting, structure, and emotional climate.

CRITICAL THINKING

1. Consider the theorists and theories discussed in this chapter. The following questions address how they may impact your nursing practice.
   A. How do Freud's concepts of the conscious, preconscious, and unconscious affect your understanding of patients' behaviors?
   B. Do you believe that Erikson's psychosocial stages represent a sound basis for identifying disruptions in stages of development in your patients? Support your position with a clinical example.
   C. What are the implications of Sullivan's focus on the importance of interpersonal relationships for your interactions with patients?
   D. Peplau believed that nurses must exercise self-awareness within the nurse-patient relationship. Describe situations in your student experience in which this self-awareness played a vital role in your relationship(s) with patient(s).
   E. Identify someone you believe to be self-actualized. What characteristics does this person have that support your assessment?
   F. How do/will you make use of Maslow's hierarchy of needs in your nursing practice?
   G. What do you think about the behaviorist point of view that a change in behavior results in a change in thinking? Can you give an example of this in your own life?

2. Which of the therapies described in this chapter do you think are/will be the most helpful to you in your nursing practice? Explain your choice.

CHAPTER REVIEW

1. The nurse is working with a patient who lacks the ability to problem solve and seeks ways to self-satisfy without regard for others. The nurse understands that which system of the patient's personality is most pronounced?
   1. Id
   2. Ego
   3. Conscience (superego)
   4. Ego ideal (superego)

2. Which behavior, seen in a 30-year-old patient, would alert the nurse to the fact that the patient is not in his appropriate developmental stage according to Erikson?
   1. States he is happily married
   2. Frequently requests to call his brother "just to check in"
   3. Looks forward to visits from a co-worker
   4. Says "I'm still trying to find myself."

3. A patient has difficulty sitting still and listening to others during group therapy. The therapist plans to use operant conditioning as a form of behavioral modification to assist the patient. Which action would the nurse expect to see in group therapy?
   1. The therapist will act as a role model for the patient by sitting still and listening.
   2. The patient will receive a token from the therapist for each session in which she sits still and listens.
   3. The patient will be required to sit in solitude for 30 minutes after each session in which she does not sit still or listen.
   4. The therapist will ask that the patient sit still and listen for only 2 minutes at a time to begin and will increase the time incrementally until the patient can sit and listen 10 minutes at a time.

4. The nurse is planning care for a patient with anxiety who will be admitted to the unit shortly. Which nursing action is most important?
   1. Consider ways to assist the patient to feel valued during his stay on the unit.
   2. Choose a roommate for the patient so that a friendship can develop.
   3. Identify a room where the patient will have comfortable surroundings, and order a balanced meal plan.
   4. Plan methods of decreasing stimuli that could cause heightened anxiety in the patient.

5. An experienced nurse is monitoring a new nurse. Which action of the new nurse would cause the experienced nurse to intervene?
   1. Considering ways to decrease suicide risk of a suicidal patient
   2. Referring an abused patient to a shelter
   3. Providing a safe environment for a patient with Alzheimer's disease
   4. Asking a patient to justify her behaviors

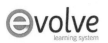 Visit the Evolve website for an **Audio Chapter Summary, Chapter Review Answers & Rationales, Critical Thinking Answer Guidelines,** and additional resources related to the content in this chapter: **http://evolve.elsevier.com/Varcarolis/foundations**

Companion CD   Use the Companion CD to prepare for tests and the NCLEX® Examination with **Test-Taking Strategies** for psychiatric mental health nursing and hundreds of **Review Questions.**

References

Bandura, A., Blahard, E.B., & Ritter, B. (1969). Relative efficacy of desensitization and modeling approaches for inducing behavioral, affective, and attitudinal changes, *Journal of Personality and Social Psychology*, 13(3), 173–99.

Beck, A. T. (1967). *Depression: Clinical, experimental and theoretical aspects*. New York: Harper & Row.

Beck, A. T., Rush, A. J., Shaw, B. F., & Emery, G. (1979). *Cognitive therapy of depression*. New York: Guilford.

Dewan, M. J., Steenbarger, B. N., & Greenberg, R. P. (2008). In R. E. Hales, S. C. Yudofsky, & G. O. Gabbard (Eds.), *Textbook of psychiatry* (pp. 1155–1170). Washington, DC: American Psychiatric Publishing.

Ellis, A. (2000, August). *On therapy: A dialogue with Aaron T. Beck and Albert Ellis*. Discussion at the American Psychological Association's 108th Convention, Washington, DC.

Erikson, E. H. (1963). *Childhood and society*. New York: Norton.

Forchuk, C. (1991). A comparison of the works of Peplau and Orlando. *Archives of Psychiatric Nursing*, 5(1), 38–45.

Freud, S. (1960). *The ego and the id* (J. Strachey, Trans.). New York: Norton.

Freud, S. (1961). *The interpretation of dreams* (J. Strachey, Ed. & Trans.). New York: Scientific Editions.

Freud, S. (1969). *An outline of psychoanalysis* (J. Strachey, Trans.). New York: W. W. Norton.

Haber, J. (2000). Hildegard E. Peplau: The psychiatric nursing legacy of a legend. *Journal of the American Psychiatric Nurses Association*, 6(2), 56–62.

Hollon, S. D., & Engelhardt, N. (1997). Review of psychosocial treatment of mood disorders. In D. L. Dunner (Ed.), *Current psychiatric therapy II*. Philadelphia: Saunders.

Maslow, A. H. (1963). Self-actualizing people. In G. B. Levitas (Ed.), *The world of psychology* (Vol. 2). New York: Braziller.

Maslow, A. H. (1968). *Toward a psychology of being*. Princeton, NJ: Van Nostrand.

Maslow, A. H. (1970). *Motivation and personality* (2nd ed.). New York: Harper & Row.

Pavlov, I. (1928). *Lectures on conditioned reflexes* (W. H. Grant, Ed. & Trans.). New York: International Publishers.

Peplau, H. E. (1952). *Interpersonal relations in nursing: A conceptual frame of reference for psychodynamic nursing*. New York: Putnam.

Peplau, H. E. (1982a). Therapeutic concepts. In S. A. Smoyak & S. Rouslin (Eds.), *A collection of classics in psychiatric nursing literature* (pp. 91–108). Thorofare, NJ: Slack.

Peplau, H. E. (1982b). Interpersonal techniques: The crux of psychiatric nursing. In S. A. Smoyak & S. Rouslin (Eds.), *A collection of classics in psychiatric nursing literature* (pp. 276–281). Thorofare, NJ: Slack.

Peplau, H. E. (1987). Interpersonal constructs for nursing practice. *Nursing Education Today*, 7, 201–208.

Peplau, H. E. (1989). Future directions in psychiatric nursing from the perspective of history. *Journal of Psychosocial Nursing*, 27(2), 18–28.

Peplau, H. E. (1995). Another look at schizophrenia from a nursing standpoint. In C. A. Anderson (Ed.), *Psychiatric nursing 1946–94: The state of the art*. St. Louis, Mosby.

Sadock, B. J., & Sadock, V. A. (2008). *Concise textbook of clinical psychiatry* (3rd ed.). Philadelphia: Lippincott, Williams & Wilkins.

Skinner, B. F. (1987). Whatever happened to psychology as the science of behavior? *American Psychologist*, 42, 780–786.

Sullivan, H. S. (1953). *The interpersonal theory of psychiatry*. New York: W. W. Norton.

Watson, J. B. (1919). *Psychology from the standpoint of a behaviorist*. Philadelphia: Lippincott.

CHAPTER 3

Biological Basis for Understanding Psychotropic Drugs

Mary A. Gutierrez and John Raynor

Key Terms and Concepts

antagonists, 68
antianxiety (anxiolytic) drugs, 59
anticholinesterase drugs, 71
atypical antipsychotics, 69
circadian rhythms, 48
conventional antipsychotics, 68
hypnotic, 61
limbic system, 53
lithium, 66
monoamine oxidase inhibitors (MAOIs), 65
mood stabilizer, 66

neurons, 49
neurotransmitter, 49
pharmacodynamics, 59
pharmacokinetics, 59
receptors, 46
reticular activating system (RAS), 53
reuptake, 51
selective serotonin reuptake inhibitors (SSRIs), 64
synapse, 49
therapeutic index, 67
tricyclic antidepressants, 64

Objectives

1. Identify at least eight functions of the brain and the way these functions can be altered by psychotropic drugs.
2. Describe how a neurotransmitter functions as a neuromessenger.
3. Draw the three major areas of the brain and identify at least three functions of each.
4. Explain how specific brain functions are altered in certain mental disorders (e.g., depression, anxiety, schizophrenia).
5. Describe how the use of imaging techniques can be helpful for understanding mental illness.
6. Develop a teaching plan that includes side effects from dopamine blockage, such as motor abnormalities.
7. Describe the result of blockage of the muscarinic receptors and the α_1 adrenergic receptors by the standard neuroleptic drugs.

8. Identify the main neurotransmitters affected by the following psychotropic drugs and their subgroups:
   a. Antianxiety agents
   b. Sedative-hypnotic agents
   c. Antidepressants
   d. Mood stabilizers
   e. Antipsychotic agents
   f. Anticholinesterase drugs
9. Discuss special dietary and drug restrictions in a teaching plan for a patient taking a monoamine oxidase inhibitor.
10. Identify specific cautions you might incorporate into your medication teaching plan with regard to:
    a. Herbal medicine
    b. Pharmacogenetics (i.e., variations in effects and therapeutic actions of medications among different ethnic groups)

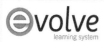

Visit the Evolve website for an **Audio Glossary & Flashcards, Concept Map Creator,** and additional resources related to the content in this chapter: **http://evolve.elsevier.com/Varcarolis/foundations**

Whether conscious or unconscious, all mental activity has its locus in the brain. This implies that a primary goal of psychiatry is to understand both normal and abnormal mental processes in terms of brain function. Ultimately, we would like to be able to apply this understanding to the treatment of mental disease and the alleviation of mental suffering. Approached in relation to brain function, psychiatric problems are explained and treated in the same way as any other biological problems.

Implied in the biological approach to psychiatric illness is the idea that although the origin of a psychiatric illness may be related to any number of factors (e.g., genetics, neurodevelopmental factors, drugs, infection, psychosocial experience), there will eventually be an alteration in cerebral function that accounts for the disturbances in the patient's behavior and mental experiences. These physiological alterations are the targets of the psychotropic drugs used to treat mental disease. From a holistic point of view, mental disorders then have neurobiopsychological components that support the efficacy of treating these disorders both pharmacologically and with appropriate psychotherapy.

Reversal of these alterations is the goal of the use of psychotropic drugs in the treatment of mental illnesses. During recent years there has been an explosion of information in this area. Earlier theories, such as the dopamine theory of schizophrenia and the monoamine theory of depression, are currently seen as overly simplistic because a large number of other neurotransmitters, hormones, and coregulators are now thought to play important and complex roles. The importance of receptor subtypes and the role of these receptors in normal physiology, pathology, and pharmacology are also receiving increasing attention.

The goal of this chapter is to relate psychiatric disturbances and the psychotropic drugs used to treat them to normal brain structure and function. We first look at the normal functions of the brain and how they are carried out from an anatomical and physiological perspective. We then review current theories of the neuropsychological basis of various types of emotional and physiological dysfunctions. These theories focus primarily on neurotransmitters and their receptors. Finally, we attempt to relate both the beneficial and the untoward effects of psychiatric drugs to their interaction with various neurotransmitter-receptor systems.

Although the modern era of the treatment of mental illness with psychotropic drugs extends back almost half a century, a full understanding of how these drugs improve the symptoms of these illnesses continues to elude investigators. The focus of research is on neurotransmitters—their release from presynaptic cells and their actions on postsynaptic cells—and how psychotropic drugs interact with the physiology of these substances. In recent years, many subtypes of receptors for the various neurotransmitters have been discovered, and long-term changes induced in postsynaptic cells have taken on increased significance. This information is becoming increasingly important for nurses to understand. Such an understanding is particularly crucial for advanced practice psychiatric mental health nurses, who in many states have the authority to write prescriptions.

Included in this chapter is an overview of the major drugs used to treat mental disorders and an explanation of how they work. Additional and detailed information regarding adverse and toxic effects, dosage, nursing implications, and teaching tools is presented in the appropriate clinical chapters (see Chapters 12 to 22).

Despite new information known about the complex brain functions and neurotransmitters, there is still much to be clarified in understanding the complex ways in which the brain carries out its normal functions, is altered during disease, and is improved by pharmacological intervention. After reading this chapter, you should have a neurobiological framework into which you can place existing, as well as future, information about mental illness and its treatment.

STRUCTURE AND FUNCTION OF THE BRAIN

Functions and Activities of the Brain

Regulating behavior and carrying out mental processes are important, but far from the only, responsibilities of the brain. Box 3-1 summarizes some of the major functions and activities of the brain. Because all these brain functions are carried out by similar mechanisms (interactions of neurons) and often in similar locations, it is not surprising that mental disturbances are often associated with alterations in other brain functions and that the drugs used to treat mental disturbances can also interfere with other activities of the brain.

BOX 3-1 Functions of the Brain

- Monitor changes in the external world
- Monitor the composition of body fluids
- Regulate the contractions of skeletal muscles
- Regulate the internal organs
- Initiate and regulate the basic drives: hunger, thirst, sex, aggressive self-protection
- Mediate conscious sensation
- Store and retrieve memories
- Regulate mood (affect) and emotions
- Think and perform intellectual functions
- Regulate the sleep cycle
- Produce and interpret language
- Process visual and auditory data

Maintenance of Homeostasis

The brain serves as the coordinator and director of the body's response to both internal and external changes. Appropriate responses require a constant monitoring of the environment, interpretation and integration of the incoming information, and control over the appropriate organs of response. The goal of these responses is to maintain homeostasis and thus to maintain life.

Information about the external world is relayed from various sense organs to the brain by the peripheral nerves. This information, which is at first received as gross sensation (light, sound, touch), must ultimately be interpreted (a picture, a train whistle, a hand on the back). Interestingly, a component of major psychiatric disturbance (e.g., schizophrenia) is an alteration of sensory experience. Thus the patient may experience a sensation that does not originate in the external world. For example, people with schizophrenia may hear voices talking to them (auditory hallucination).

The brain not only monitors the external world but also keeps a close watch on internal functions. Information about blood pressure, body temperature, blood gases, and the chemical composition of the body fluids is continuously received by the brain, signaling it to direct the appropriate responses required to maintain homeostasis.

To respond to external changes, the brain has control over the skeletal muscles. This control involves the ability not only to initiate contraction (e.g., to contract the biceps and flex the arm) but also to fine-tune and coordinate contraction so a person can, for example, guide the fingers to the correct keys on a piano. Unfortunately, both psychiatric disease and the treatment of psychiatric disease with psychotropic drugs are associated with movement disturbances.

It is important to remember that the skeletal muscles controlled by the brain include the diaphragm—essential for breathing—and the muscles of the throat, tongue, and mouth—essential for speech. Thus drugs that affect brain function can stimulate or depress respiration or lead to slurred speech.

Adjustments to changes within the body require that the brain exert control over the various internal organs. For example, if blood pressure drops, the brain must direct the heart to pump more blood and the smooth muscles of the arterioles to constrict. This increase in cardiac output and vasoconstriction allows the body to return blood pressure to its normal level.

Regulation of the Autonomic Nervous System and Hormones

The autonomic nervous system and the endocrine system serve as the communication links between the brain and the cardiac muscle, smooth muscle, and glands of which the internal organs are composed (Figure 3-1). If the brain needs to stimulate the heart, it must activate the sympathetic nerves to the sinoatrial node and the ventricular myocardium. If the brain needs to bring about vasoconstriction, it must activate the sympathetic nerves to the smooth muscles of the arterioles.

The linkage between the brain and the internal organs that allows for the maintenance of homeostasis may also serve to translate mental disturbances, such as anxiety, into alterations of internal function. For example, anxiety in some people can cause activation of parasympathetic nerves to the digestive tract, leading to hypermotility and diarrhea. Likewise, anxiety can activate the sympathetic nerves to the arterioles, leading to vasoconstriction and hypertension.

The brain also exerts influence over the internal organs by regulating hormonal secretions of the pituitary gland, which in turn regulates other glands. A specific area of the brain, the hypothalamus, secretes hormones called *releasing factors*. These hormones act on the pituitary gland to stimulate or inhibit the synthesis and release of pituitary hormones. Once in the general circulation, they influence various internal activities. An example of this linkage is the release of gonadotropin-releasing hormone by the hypothalamus at the time of puberty. This hormone stimulates the release of two gonadotropins—follicle-stimulating hormone and luteinizing hormone—by the pituitary gland, which consequently activate the ovaries or testes. This linkage may explain why anxiety or depression in some women may lead to disturbances of the menstrual cycle.

The relationship between the brain, the pituitary gland, and the adrenal glands is particularly important in normal and abnormal mental function. Specifically, the hypothalamus secretes **corticotropin-releasing hormone (CRH)** which stimulates the pituitary to release corticotropin, which in turn stimulates the cortex of each adrenal gland to secrete the hormone cortisol. This system is activated as part of the normal response to a variety of mental and physical stresses. Among many other actions, all three hormones—CRH, corticotropin, and cortisol—influence the functions of the nerve cells of the brain. There is considerable evidence that in both anxiety and depression, this system is overactive and does not respond properly to negative feedback.

Control of Biological Drives and Behavior

To understand the neurobiological basis of mental disease and its treatment, it is helpful to distinguish between the various types of brain activity that serve as the basis of mental experience and behavior. An understanding of these activities shows where to look for disturbed function and what to hope for in treatment. The brain, for example, is responsible for the basic drives such as sex and hunger that play a strong role in molding behavior. Disturbances of

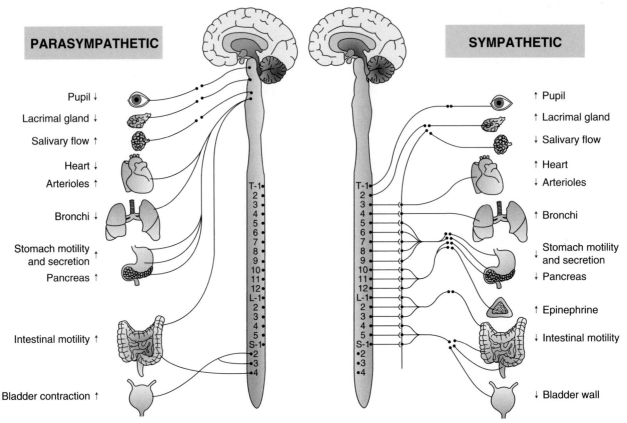

Figure 3-1 The autonomic nervous system has two divisions: the sympathetic and parasympathetic. The sympathetic division is dominant in stress situations such as fear and anger—known as the *fight-or-flight response*.

these drives (e.g., overeating or undereating, loss of sexual interest) can be an indication of an underlying psychiatric disorder such as depression.

Cycle of Sleep and Wakefulness. The entire cycle of sleep and wakefulness, as well as the intensity of alertness while the person is awake, are regulated and coordinated by various regions of the brain. Although we do not fully understand the true homeostatic function of sleep, we know that it is essential for both physiological and psychological well-being. Assessment of sleep patterns is part of what is required to determine a psychiatric diagnosis.

Unfortunately, many of the drugs used to treat psychiatric problems interfere with the normal regulation of sleep and alertness. Drugs with a sedative-hypnotic effect can blunt the degree to which a person feels alert and focused and can cause drowsiness. The sedative-hypnotic effect requires caution in using these drugs while engaging in activities that require a great deal of attention, such as driving a car or operating machinery. One way of minimizing the danger is to take such drugs at night just before bedtime.

Circadian Rhythms. The cycle of sleep and wakefulness is only one aspect of circadian rhythms, the fluctuation of various physiological and behavioral

parameters over a 24-hour cycle. Other variations include changes in body temperature, secretion of hormones such as corticotropin and cortisol, and secretion of neurotransmitters such as norepinephrine and **serotonin**. Both norepinephrine and serotonin are thought to be involved in mood, and daily fluctuations of mood may be related in part to circadian variations in these neurotransmitters. There is evidence that the circadian rhythm of neurotransmitter secretion is altered in psychiatric disorders, particularly in those that involve mood.

Conscious Mental Activity

All aspects of conscious mental experience and sense of self originate from the neurophysiological activity of the brain. Conscious mental activity can be a basic, meandering, stream-of-consciousness flow among thoughts of future responsibilities, memories, fantasy, and so on. Conscious mental activity can also be much more complex when it is applied to problem solving and the interpretation of the external world. Both the random stream of consciousness and the complex problem solving and interpretation of the environment can become distorted in psychiatric illness. Thus a person with schizophrenia may have chaotic and incoherent speech and thought patterns (a jumble of unrelated words known as **word salad**; unconnected phrases and topics known as **looseness of association**) and delusional interpretations of personal interactions, such as beliefs about people or events that are not supported by data or reality.

Memory

An extremely important component of mental activity is memory, the ability to retain and recall past experience. From both an anatomical and a physiological perspective, there is thought to be a major difference in the processing of short- and long-term memory. This can be seen dramatically in some forms of cognitive mental disorders such as dementia, in which a person has no recall of the events of the previous 8 minutes, but may have vivid recall of events that occurred decades earlier.

Social Skills

An important and often neglected aspect of brain functioning involves the social skills that make interpersonal relationships possible. In almost all types of mental illness, from mild anxiety to severe schizophrenia, difficulties in interpersonal relationships are important parts of the disorder, and improvements in these relationships are important gauges of progress. The connection between brain activity and social behavior is an area of intense research and is believed to be influenced by a combination of genetic make-up and individual experience. There is evidence that positive reward-based experiential learning and negative avoidance learning may involve different areas of the brain.

Cellular Composition of the Brain

The brain is composed of approximately 100 billion neurons, nerve cells that conduct electrical impulses, as well as other types of cells that surround the neurons. Most functions of the brain, from regulation of blood pressure to the conscious sense of self, are thought to result from the actions of individual neurons and the interconnections between them. Although neurons come in a great variety of shapes and sizes, all carry out the same three types of physiological actions: (1) they respond to stimuli, (2) they conduct electrical impulses, and (3) they release chemicals called *neurotransmitters*.

An essential feature of neurons is their ability to conduct an electrical impulse from one end of the cell to the other. This electrical impulse consists of a change in membrane permeability that first allows the inward flow of sodium ions and then the outward flow of potassium ions. The inward flow of sodium ions changes the polarity of the membrane from positive on the outside to positive on the inside. Movement of potassium ions out of the cell returns the positive charge to the outside of the cell. Because these electrical charges are self-propagating, a change at one end of the cell is conducted along the membrane until it reaches the other end (Figure 3-2). The functional significance of this propagation is that the electrical impulse serves as a means of communication between one part of the body and another.

Once an electrical impulse reaches the end of a neuron, a neurotransmitter is released. A neurotransmitter is a chemical substance that functions as a neuromessenger. Neurotransmitters are released from the axon terminal at the **presynaptic** neuron on excitation. This neurotransmitter then diffuses across a space, or synapse, to an adjacent **postsynaptic** neuron, where it attaches to receptors on the neuron's surface. It is this interaction from one neuron to another by way of a neurotransmitter and receptor that allows the activity of one neuron to influence the activity of other neurons. Depending on the chemical structure of the neurotransmitter and the specific type of receptor to which it attaches, the postsynaptic cell will be rendered either more or less likely to initiate an electrical impulse. It is the interaction between neurotransmitter and receptor that is a major target of the drugs used to treat psychiatric disease. Table 3-1 lists important neurotransmitters

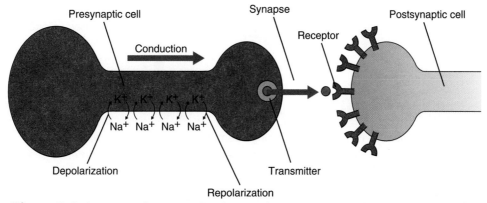

Figure 3-2 Activities of neurons. Conduction along a neuron involves the inward movement of sodium ions (Na⁺) followed by the outward movement of potassium ions (K⁺). When the current reaches the end of the cell, a neurotransmitter is released. The neurotransmitter crosses the synapse and attaches to a receptor on the postsynaptic cell. The attachment of neurotransmitter to receptor either stimulates or inhibits the postsynaptic cell.

TABLE 3-1 Transmitters and Receptors

Transmitters	Receptors	Effects/Comments	Association with Mental Health
MONOAMINES			

Dopamine (DA)	D_1, D_2, D_3, D_4, D_5	Involved in fine muscle movement
		Involved in integration of emotions and thoughts
		Involved in decision making
		Stimulates hypothalamus to release hormones (sex, thyroid, adrenal)
			Decrease:
			  Parkinson's disease
			  Depression
			Increase:
			  Schizophrenia
			  Mania

Norepinephrine (NE) (noradrenaline)	α_1, α_2, β_1, β_2	Level in brain affects mood
		Attention and arousal
		Stimulates sympathetic branch of autonomic nervous system for "fight or flight" in response to stress
			Decrease:
			  Depression
			Increase:
			  Mania
			  Anxiety states
			  Schizophrenia

Serotonin (5-HT)	5-HT_1, 5-HT_2, 5-HT_3, 5-HT_4	Plays a role in sleep regulation, hunger, mood states, and pain perception
		Hormonal activity
		Plays a role in aggression and sexual behavior
			Decrease:
			  Depression
			Increase:
			  Anxiety states

Histamine	H_1, H_2	Involved in alertness
		Involved in inflammatory response
		Stimulates gastric secretion
			Decrease:
			  Sedation
			  Weight gain

AMINO ACIDS			

Gamma-aminobutyric acid (GABA)	$GABA_A$, $GABA_B$	Plays a role in inhibition; reduces aggression, excitation, and anxiety
		May play a role in pain perception
		Anticonvulsant and muscle-relaxing properties
		May impair cognition and psychomotor functioning
			Decrease:
			  Anxiety disorders
			  Schizophrenia
			  Mania
			  Huntington's disease
			Increase:
			  Reduction of anxiety

Glutamate	NMDA, AMPA	Is excitatory
		AMPA plays a role in learning and memory
			Decrease (NMDA):
			  Psychosis
			Increase (NMDA):
			  Prolonged increased state can be neurotoxic
			  Neurodegeneration in Alzheimer's disease
			Increase (AMPA):
			  Improvement of cognitive performance in behavioral tasks

CHOLINERGICS			

Acetylcholine (ACh)	Nicotinic, muscarinic (M_1, M_2, M_3)	Plays a role in learning, memory
		Regulates mood: mania, sexual aggression
		Affects sexual and aggressive behavior
		Stimulates parasympathetic nervous system
			Decrease:
			  Alzheimer's disease
			  Huntington's disease
			  Parkinson's disease
			Increase:
			  Depression

TABLE 3-1 Transmitters and Receptors—cont'd			
Transmitters	**Receptors**	**Effects/Comments**	**Association with Mental Health**
PEPTIDES (NEUROMODULATORS)			
Substance P (SP)	SP	Centrally active SP antagonist has antidepressant and antianxiety effects in depression Promotes and reinforces memory Enhances sensitivity to pain receptors to activate	Involved in regulation of mood and anxiety Role in pain management
Somatostatin (SRIF)	SRIF	Altered levels associated with cognitive disease	*Decrease:* 　Alzheimer's disease 　Decreased levels of SRIF in spinal fluid of some depressed patients *Increase:* 　Huntington's disease
Neurotensin (NT)	NT	Endogenous antipsychotic-like properties	Decreased levels in spinal fluid of schizophrenic patients

AMPA, α-Amino-3-hydroxy-5-methyl-4-isoxazolepropionic acid; *NMDA*, N-methyl-ᴅ-aspartate.

and the types of receptors to which they attach. Also listed are the mental disorders associated with an increase or decrease in these neurotransmitters.

After attaching to a receptor and exerting its influence on the postsynaptic cell, the neurotransmitter separates from the receptor and is destroyed. The process of neurotransmitter destruction is described in Box 3-2. There are two basic mechanisms by which neurotransmitters are destroyed. Some neurotransmitters (e.g., acetylcholine) are destroyed by specific enzymes at the postsynaptic cell. The enzyme that destroys **acetylcholine** is called **acetylcholinesterase**. Other neurotransmitters (e.g., norepinephrine) are taken back into the presynaptic cell from which they were originally released by a process called cellular reuptake. Upon their return to these cells, the neurotransmitters are either reused or destroyed by intracellular enzymes. In the case of the monoamine neurotransmitters (e.g., norepinephrine, **dopamine**, serotonin), the destructive enzyme is called **monoamine oxidase (MAO)**.

As a means of regulating the concentration of neurotransmitters at the **postsynaptic receptors**, many neurotransmitters exert a feedback inhibition of their own release. This is accomplished by the attachment of neurotransmitters to **presynaptic receptors** at the synapse, which act to inhibit the further release of neurotransmitters.

The concept of a neuron releasing a specific neurotransmitter that stimulates or inhibits a postsynaptic membrane receptor and acts through negative feedback on a presynaptic receptor is an accurate but far from complete picture of the interaction between nerve cells. Researchers have found that in many cases, neurons release more than one chemical at the same time. Neurotransmitters such as norepinephrine or **acetylcholine**—which have immediate effects on postsynaptic membranes—are often joined by larger molecules, neuropeptides, that may initiate long-term changes in the postsynaptic cells. These changes may involve basic cell functions, such as genetic expression, and lead to modifications of cell shape and responsiveness to stimuli. Ultimately, this means that the action of one neuron on another affects not only the immediate response of that neuron but also its sensitivity to future influence. The long-term implications of this for neural development, normal and abnormal mental health, and the treatment of psychiatric disease are being investigated.

The communication between neurons at a synapse is not unidirectional. **Neurotrophic factors** are proteins and even simple gases, such as carbon monoxide and nitrous oxide that are released by postsynaptic cells and influence the growth, shape, and activity of presynaptic cells. These factors are thought to be particularly important during the development of the fetal brain, guiding the growing brain to form the proper neuronal connections. However, it is now apparent that the brain retains anatomical plasticity throughout life and that internal and external influences can alter the synaptic network of the brain. The role of altered genetic expression or environmental trauma in the action of these factors and the negative and positive consequences of these changes on mental function and psychiatric disease is an area of much research.

The development and responsiveness of neurons is dependent not only on chemicals released by other neurons but also on chemicals brought to the

BOX 3-2 Destruction of Neurotransmitters

A full explanation of the various ways psychotropic drugs alter neuronal activity requires a brief review of the manner in which neurotransmitters are destroyed after attaching to the receptors. To avoid continuous and prolonged action on the postsynaptic cell, the neurotransmitter is released shortly after attaching to the postsynaptic receptor. Once released, the neurotransmitter is destroyed in one of two ways.

One way is the immediate inactivation of the neurotransmitter at the postsynaptic membrane. An example of this method of destruction is the action of the enzyme acetylcholinesterase on the neurotransmitter acetylcholine. Acetylcholinesterase is present at the postsynaptic membrane and destroys acetylcholine shortly after it attaches to nicotinic or muscarinic receptors on the postsynaptic cell.

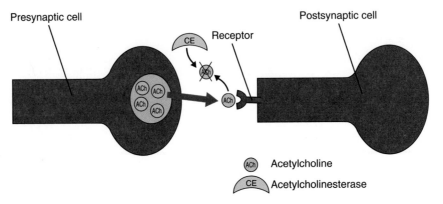

A *second* method of neurotransmitter inactivation is a little more complex. After interacting with the postsynaptic receptor, the neurotransmitter is released and taken back into the presynaptic cell, the cell from which it was released. This process, referred to as the *reuptake of neurotransmitter*, is a common target for drug action. Once inside the presynaptic cell, the neurotransmitter is either recycled or inactivated by an enzyme within the cell. The monoamine neurotransmitters norepinephrine, dopamine, and serotonin are all inactivated in this manner by the enzyme monoamine oxidase.

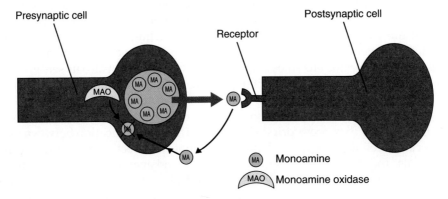

Looking at this second method, you might naturally ask what prevents the enzyme from destroying the neurotransmitter before its release. The answer is that before release, the neurotransmitter is stored within a membrane and is thus protected from the degradative enzyme. After release and reuptake, the neurotransmitter is either destroyed by the enzyme or reenters the membrane to be used again.

neurons by the blood, particularly the **steroid hormones**. Estrogen, testosterone, and cortisol can bind to neurons, where they can cause short- and long-term changes in neuronal activity. A clear example of this is seen in the psychosis that can sometimes result from the hypersecretion of cortisol in Cushing's disease or from the use of prednisone in high doses to treat chronic inflammatory disease.

Organization of the Brain

Brainstem

The central core of the brainstem regulates the internal organs and is responsible for such vital functions as the regulation of blood gases and the maintenance of blood pressure. The hypothalamus, a small area in the ventral superior portion of the brainstem, plays a vital role in such basic drives as hunger, thirst, and sex. It also serves as a crucial psychosomatic link between higher brain activities, such as thought and emotion, and the functioning of the internal organs. The brainstem also serves as an initial processing center for sensory information that is then sent on to the cerebral cortex. Through projections of the **reticular activating system (RAS)**, the brainstem regulates the entire cycle of sleep and wakefulness and the ability of the cerebrum to carry out conscious mental activity.

Other ascending pathways, referred to as *mesolimbic* and *mesocortical pathways,* seem to play a strong role in modulating the emotional value of sensory material. These pathways project to those areas of the cerebrum collectively known as the **limbic system** which play a crucial role in emotional status and psychological function. They use norepinephrine, serotonin, and dopamine as their neurotransmitters. Much attention has been paid to the role of these pathways in normal and abnormal mental activity. For example, it is

thought that the release of dopamine from the *ventral tegmental pathway* plays a role in psychological reward and drug addiction. The neurotransmitters released by these neurons are major targets of the drugs used to treat psychiatric disease.

Cerebellum

Located posteriorly to the brainstem, the cerebellum (Figure 3-3) is primarily involved in the regulation of skeletal muscle coordination and contraction and the maintenance of equilibrium. It plays a crucial role in coordinating contractions so that movement is accomplished in a smooth and directed manner.

Cerebrum

The human brainstem and cerebellum are similar in both structure and function to these same structures in other mammals. The development of a much larger and more elaborate cerebrum is what distinguishes human beings from the rest of the animal kingdom.

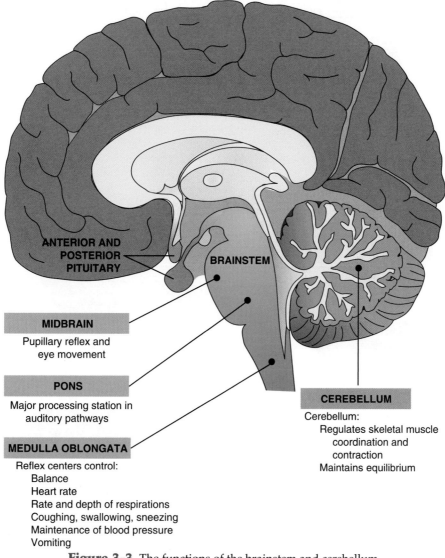

Figure 3-3 The functions of the brainstem and cerebellum.

The cerebrum, situated on top of and surrounding the brainstem, is responsible for mental activities and a conscious sense of being. The cerebrum is responsible for our conscious perception of the external world and our own body, emotional status, memory, and control of skeletal muscles that allow willful direction of movement. It is also responsible for language and the ability to communicate.

The cerebrum consists of surface and deep areas of integrating gray matter (the cerebral cortex and basal ganglia) and the connecting tracts of white matter that link these areas with each other and the rest of the nervous system. The cerebral cortex, which forms the outer layer of the brain, is responsible for conscious sensation and the initiation of movement. Specific areas of the cortex are responsible for specific sensations: the parietal cortex for touch, the temporal cortex for sound, the occipital cortex for vision, and so on. The initiation of skeletal muscle contraction is controlled by a specific area of the frontal cortex. All areas of the cortex are interconnected to enable an appropriate picture of the world to be formed and, if necessary, linked to a proper response (Figure 3-4).

Specialized areas of the cerebral cortex are responsible for language in both its sensory and motor aspects.

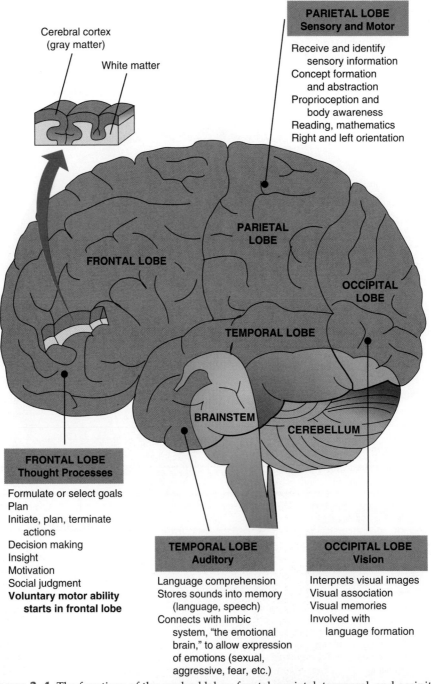

Cerebral cortex
(gray matter)

White matter

PARIETAL LOBE
Sensory and Motor

Receive and identify
    sensory information
Concept formation
    and abstraction
Proprioception and
    body awareness
Reading, mathematics
Right and left orientation

PARIETAL LOBE

FRONTAL LOBE

OCCIPITAL LOBE

TEMPORAL LOBE

BRAINSTEM

CEREBELLUM

FRONTAL LOBE
Thought Processes

Formulate or select goals
Plan
Initiate, plan, terminate
    actions
Decision making
Insight
Motivation
Social judgment
Voluntary motor ability
    starts in frontal lobe

TEMPORAL LOBE
Auditory

Language comprehension
Stores sounds into memory
    (language, speech)
Connects with limbic
    system, "the emotional
    brain," to allow expression
    of emotions (sexual,
    aggressive, fear, etc.)

OCCIPITAL LOBE
Vision

Interprets visual images
Visual association
Visual memories
Involved with
    language formation

Figure 3-4 The functions of the cerebral lobes: frontal, parietal, temporal, and occipital.

Sensory language functions include the ability to read, understand spoken language, and know the names of objects perceived by the senses. Motor functions involve the physical ability to use muscles properly for speech and writing. In both neurological and psychological dysfunction, the use of language may become compromised or distorted. The change in linguistic ability may be a factor in determining a diagnosis.

In addition to the gray matter forming the surface of the cerebrum, there are pockets of integrating gray matter deep within the cerebrum. Some of these, the basal ganglia, are involved in the regulation of movement. Others, the **amygdala** and **hippocampus**, are involved in emotions, learning, memory, and basic drives. Significantly, there is an overlap of these various areas both anatomically and in the types of neurotransmitters employed. One consequence is that drugs used to treat emotional disturbances may cause movement disorders, and drugs used to treat movement disorders may cause emotional changes.

Visualizing the Brain

A variety of noninvasive imaging techniques is used to visualize brain structure, functions, and metabolic activity. Table 3-2 identifies some common brain imaging techniques and preliminary findings as they relate to psychiatry. There are basically two types of neuroimaging techniques: structural and functional. **Structural imaging techniques** (e.g., computed

TABLE 3-2 Common Brain Imaging Techniques			
Technique	Description	Uses	Psychiatric Relevance and Preliminary Findings
STRUCTURAL: SHOW GROSS ANATOMICAL DETAILS OF BRAIN STRUCTURES			
Computed tomography (CT)	Series of x-ray images are taken of the brain, and computer analysis produces "slices," providing a precise 3D-like reconstruction of each segment	Can detect: Lesions Abrasions Areas of infarct Aneurysm	Schizophrenia: Cortical atrophy Third ventricle enlargement Cognitive disorders: Abnormalities
Magnetic resonance imaging (MRI)	Magnetic field is applied to the brain; nuclei of hydrogen atoms absorb and emit radio waves that are analyzed by computer, providing 3D visualization of the brain's structure in sectional images	Can detect: Brain edema Ischemia Infection Neoplasm Trauma	Schizophrenia: Enlarged ventricles Reduction in temporal lobe and prefrontal lobe
Functional magnetic resonance imaging (fMRI)	Functional imaging approach that avoids exposure to ionizing radiation	(See MRI)	(See MRI)
FUNCTIONAL: SHOW SOME ACTIVITY OF THE BRAIN			
Positron-emission tomography (PET)	Radioactive substance (tracer) injected, travels to the brain, and shows up as bright spots on the scan; data collected by detectors are relayed to a computer, which produces images of the activity and 3D visualization of CNS	Can detect: Oxygen utilization Glucose metabolism Blood flow Neurotransmitter/ receptor interaction	Schizophrenia: Increased D_2, D_3 receptors in caudate nucleus Abnormalities in limbic system Mood disorders: Abnormalities in temporal lobes Adult ADHD: Decreased utilization of glucose
Single photon emission computed tomography (SPECT)	Similar to PET but uses radionuclides that emit gamma-radiation (photons); measures various aspects of brain functioning and provides images of multiple layers of the CNS (as does PET)	Can detect: Circulation of cerebrospinal fluid Similar functions to PET	(See PET)

ADHD, Attention deficit hyperactivity disorder; *CNS,* central nervous system; *3D,* three-dimensional.

tomography [CT] and magnetic resonance imaging [MRI]) identify gross anatomical changes in the brain. **Functional imaging techniques** (e.g., positron emission tomography [PET] and single photon emission computed tomography [SPECT]) reveal physiological activity in the brain, as described in Table 3-2.

PET scans are particularly useful in identifying physiological and biochemical changes as they occur in living tissue. Usually a radioactive "tag" is used to trace compounds such as glucose. In the brain, glucose use is related to functional activity in certain areas. For example, in patients with schizophrenia, PET scans may show a decreased use of glucose in the frontal lobes of untreated individuals. Figure 3-5 shows lower brain activity in the frontal lobe of a twin diagnosed with schizophrenia than in the asymptomatic twin. The area affected in the frontal cortex of the twin with schizophrenia is an area associated with reasoning skills, which are greatly impaired in people with schizophrenia. Scans such as these suggest a location in the frontal cortex as the site of functional impairment in people with schizophrenia.

In people with obsessive-compulsive disorder (OCD), PET scans show that brain metabolism is increased in certain areas of the frontal cortex. Figure 3-6 shows increased brain metabolism in an individual with OCD compared with a control, suggesting altered brain function in people with OCD.

PET scans of individuals with depression show decreased brain activity in the prefrontal cortex. Figure 3-7 shows the results of a PET scan taken after a form of radioactively tagged glucose was used as a tracer to visualize brain activity. The patient with depression shows reduced brain activity compared with a control. Finally, Figure 3-8 shows three views of a PET scan of the brain of a patient with Alzheimer's disease.

Modern imaging techniques have also become important tools in assessing molecular changes in mental disease and marking the receptor sites of drug action. From a psychiatric perspective, we would like to be able to understand where in the brain the various components of psychological activity take place and what types of neurotransmitters and receptors underlie this activity physiologically. Currently our understanding of both of these questions is far from complete. However, it is thought that the limbic system—a group of structures that includes parts of the frontal cortex, the basal ganglia, and the brainstem—is a major locus of psychological activity.

Within these areas, the monoamine neurotransmitters (norepinephrine, dopamine, and serotonin), the amino acid neurotransmitters (glutamate and

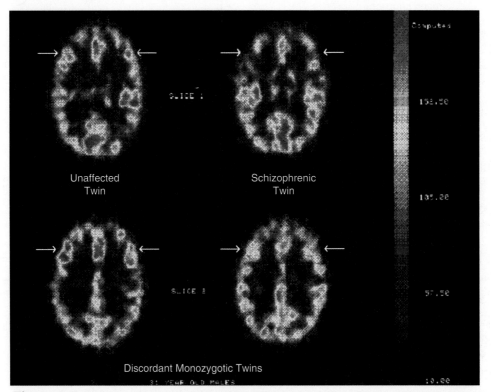

Figure 3-5 Positron emission tomographic (PET) scans of blood flow in identical twins, one of whom has schizophrenia, illustrate that individuals with this illness have reduced brain activity in the frontal lobes when asked to perform a reasoning task that requires activation of this area. Patients with schizophrenia perform poorly on the task. This suggests a site of functional impairment in schizophrenia. (From Karen Berman, MD, courtesy of National Institute of Mental Health, Clinical Brain Disorders Branch.)

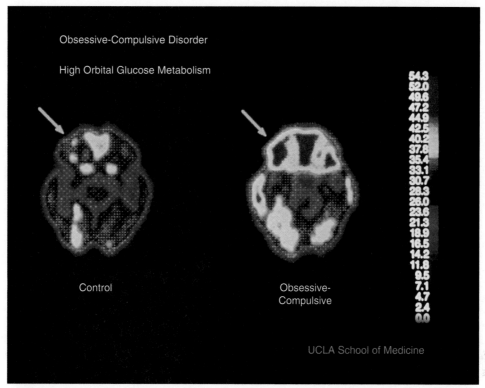

Figure 3-6 Positron emission tomographic (PET) scans show increased brain metabolism *(brighter colors)*, particularly in the frontal cortex, in a patient with obsessive-compulsive disorder (OCD), compared with a control. This suggests altered brain function in OCD. (From Lewis Baxter, MD, University of Alabama, courtesy National Institute of Mental Health.)

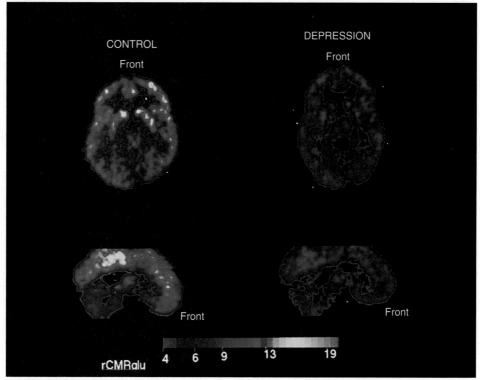

Figure 3-7 Positron emission tomographic (PET) scans of a patient with depression *(right)* and a person without depression *(left)* reveal reduced brain activity *(darker colors)* in depression, especially in the prefrontal cortex. A form of radioactively tagged glucose was used as a tracer to visualize levels of brain activity. (From Mark George, MD, courtesy National Institute of Mental Health, Biological Psychiatry Branch.)

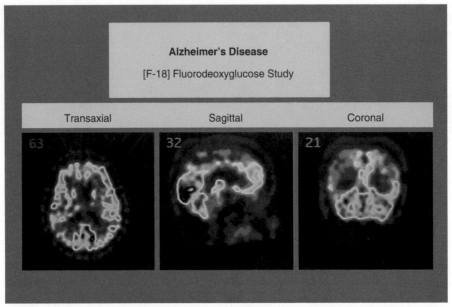

Figure 3-8 Positron emission tomographic (PET) scan of a patient with Alzheimer's disease demonstrates a classic pattern for areas of hypometabolism in the temporal and parietal regions of the brain. Areas of reduced metabolism (*dark blue and black regions*) are very noticeable in the sagittal and coronal views. (Courtesy PET Imaging Center, Department of Radiology, University of Iowa Hospitals and Clinics, Iowa City.)

gamma-aminobutyric acid [GABA]), and the neuropeptides (CRH and endorphin), as well as acetylcholine, play a major role. Alterations in these areas appear to form the basis of psychiatric disease and are the target for pharmacological treatment.

Disturbances of Mental Function

Most occurrences of mental dysfunction are of unknown origin. Among known causes are drugs (e.g., lysergic acid diethylamide [LSD]), long-term use of prednisone, excess levels of hormones (e.g., thyroxine, cortisol), infection (e.g., encephalitis, acquired immunodeficiency syndrome [AIDS]), and physical trauma. Even when the cause is known, however, the link between the causative factor and the mental dysfunction is far from understood.

There is often a genetic predisposition for psychiatric disorders. The incidence of both thought and mood disorders is higher in relatives of people with these diseases than in the general population. There is also a strong concordance among identical twins, even when they are raised apart. *Concordance* refers to how often one twin will be affected by the same illness as the other. Psychosocial stress, either in the family of origin or in contacts with society at large, increases the likelihood of mental problems, as does physical disease. Genetics and environment interact in complex ways so that some people are better able to cope with stress than others.

Researchers ultimately want to be able to understand mental dysfunction in terms of altered activity of neurons in specific areas of the brain. The hope is that such an understanding will lead to better treatments and possible prevention of mental disorders. Current interest is focused on certain neurotransmitters and their receptors—particularly in the limbic system, which links the frontal cortex, basal ganglia, and upper brainstem. As mentioned earlier, the neurotransmitters that have been most consistently linked to mental activity are norepinephrine, dopamine, serotonin, GABA, and glutamate.

Although the underlying physiology is complex, it is thought that a deficiency of norepinephrine or serotonin (or both) may serve as the biological basis of depression. Figure 3-9 shows that an insufficient degree of transmission may be due to a deficient release of neurotransmitters by the presynaptic cell or to a loss of the ability of postsynaptic receptors to respond to the neurotransmitters. Changes in neurotransmitter release and receptor response can be both a cause and a consequence of intracellular changes in the neurons involved. Thought disorders such as schizophrenia are associated physiologically with excess transmission of the neurotransmitter dopamine, among other changes. As illustrated in Figure 3-10, this may be due to either an excess release of neurotransmitter or an increase in receptor responsiveness.

The neurotransmitter **gamma-aminobutyric acid (GABA)** seems to play a role in modulating neuronal

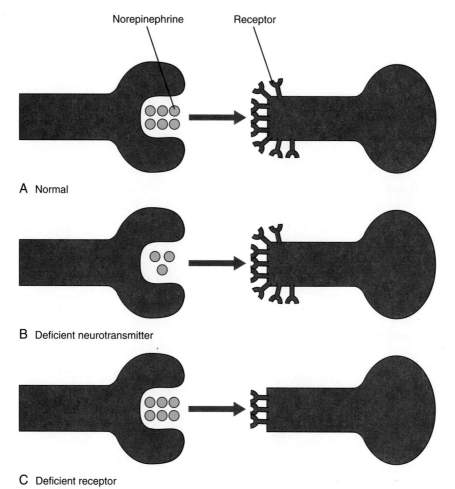

Figure 3-9 Normal transmission of neurotransmitters (**A**). Deficiency in transmission may be due to deficient release of neurotransmitter, as shown in **B**, or to a reduction in receptors, as shown in **C**.

excitability and anxiety. Not surprisingly, many **antianxiety (anxiolytic) drugs** act by increasing the effectiveness of this neurotransmitter. This is accomplished primarily by increasing receptor responsiveness.

It is important to keep in mind that the various areas of the brain are interconnected structurally and functionally by a vast network of neurons. This network serves to integrate the many and varied activities of the brain. A limited number of neurotransmitters are used in the brain, and thus a particular neurotransmitter is often used by different neurons to carry out quite different activities. For example, dopamine is used by neurons involved in not only thought processes but also the regulation of movement. Alterations in neurotransmitter activity due to a mental disturbance or to the drugs used to treat the disturbance can affect more than one area of brain activity. In other words, alterations in mental status, whether arising from disease or from medication, are often accompanied by changes in basic drives, sleep patterns, body movement, and autonomic functions.

MECHANISMS OF ACTION OF PSYCHOTROPIC DRUGS

When studying drugs, it is important to keep in mind the concepts of pharmacodynamics and pharmacokinetics. **Pharmacodynamics** refers to the biochemical and physiological effects of drugs on the body, which include the mechanisms of drug action and its effect. **Pharmacokinetics** refers to the actions of the body on the drug. How is the drug absorbed into the blood? How is it transformed in the liver? How is it distributed in the body? How is it excreted by the kidney? Pharmacokinetics determines the blood level of a drug and is used to guide the dosage schedule. It is also used to determine the type and amount of drug used in cases of liver and kidney disease.

The processes of pharmacokinetics and pharmacodynamics play an extensive role in how genetic factors give rise to interindividual and cross-ethnic variations in drug response (Lin, et al., 2003). The Considering Culture box discusses how the area of pharmacogenetics may influence the way health care providers tailor their prescriptions for patients.

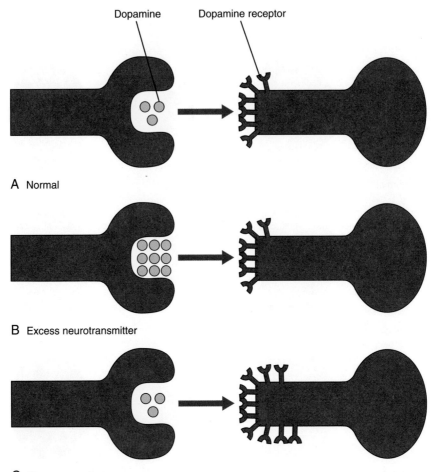

Dopamine   Dopamine receptor

A Normal

B Excess neurotransmitter

C Excess receptors

Figure 3-10 Causes of excess transmission of neurotransmitters. Excess transmission may be due to excess release of neurotransmitter, as shown in **B**, or to excess responsiveness of receptors, as shown in **C**.

CONSIDERING CULTURE

Pharmacogenetics

Pharmacogenetics explains how genetic variation leads to clinical differences in drug response of different individuals and ethnic groups. Variation of drug metabolism via the CYP450 enzymes leads to significant differences in psychotropic drug concentrations between those who metabolize drugs poorly and those who metabolize drugs extensively. Metabolism of many psychotropic drugs (e.g., risperidone) involves the CYP450 2D6 enzymes. Poor metabolizers of these enzymes (about 5% to 10% of Caucasians) may experience more side effects from higher drug levels. About 20% to 30% of Asian subgroups are poor metabolizers of CYP450 2C19 enzymes and have reduced clearance of many of the psychotropic drugs, compared to Caucasians (Bertilsson, 2007).

Many factors influence adherence with the medical regimen in all groups of people, but individuals from some ethnic and cultural groups have even greater adherence issues for a variety of reasons. For example, cultural and ethnic beliefs surrounding mental illness, attitudes toward the mental health system, and the cultural practices of an ethnic group all impact greatly a patient's degree of engagement with and adherence to the medical regimen. This topic is discussed more fully in Chapter 6.

Bertilsson, L. (2007). Metabolism of antidepressant and neuroleptic drugs by cytochrome P450s: Clinical and interethnic aspects. *Clinical pharmacology and therapeutics, 82,* 606–609.

Many drugs are transformed by the liver into active metabolites—chemicals which themselves have pharmacological actions. This knowledge is used by researchers in designing new drugs that make use of the body's own mechanisms to activate a chemical for pharmacological use.

An ideal psychiatric drug would relieve the mental disturbance of the patient without inducing additional cerebral (mental) or somatic (physical) effects. Unfortunately, in psychopharmacology—as in most areas of pharmacology—there are no drugs that are both fully effective and free of undesired side effects. Researchers are working toward developing medications that target the symptoms while producing no or few side effects.

Because all activities of the brain involve actions of neurons, neurotransmitters, and receptors, these are the targets of pharmacological intervention. Most psychotropic drugs act by either increasing or decreasing the activity of certain neurotransmitter-receptor systems. It is generally agreed that different neurotransmitter-receptor systems are dysfunctional in persons with different psychiatric conditions. These differences offer more specific targets for drug action. In fact, much of what is known about the relationship between specific neurotransmitters and specific disturbances has been derived from knowledge of the pharmacology of the drugs used to treat these conditions. For example, most agents that were effective in reducing the delusions and hallucinations of schizophrenia blocked the D_2 dopamine receptors. It was concluded that delusions and hallucinations result from overactivity of dopamine at these receptors.

Antianxiety and Hypnotic Drugs

Gamma-aminobutyric acid is the major **inhibitory** (calming) neurotransmitter in the central nervous system (CNS). There are three major types of GABA receptors: $GABA_A$, $GABA_B$, and $GABA_C$ receptors. The various subtypes of $GABA_A$ receptors are the targets of benzodiazepines, barbiturates, and alcohol. Drugs that enhance $GABA_A$ receptors exert a sedative-hypnotic action on brain function. The most commonly used antianxiety agents are the benzodiazepines and more recently the antidepressants (selective serotonin reuptake inhibitors and selective norepinephrine reuptake inhibitors).

Benzodiazepines

Benzodiazepines **potentiate**, or promote, the activity of GABA by binding to a specific receptor on the $GABA_A$

receptor complex. This binding results in increased frequency of chloride channel opening, causing membrane hyperpolarization, which inhibits cellular excitation. If cellular excitation is decreased, the result is a calming effect. Figure 3-11 shows that benzodiazepines, such as diazepam (Valium), clonazepam (Klonopin), and alprazolam (Xanax), bind to $GABA_A$ receptors with different alpha subunits. Alpha-2 subunits may be the most important for decreasing anxiety.

Since benzodiazepines are nonselective for $GABA_A$ receptors with different alpha subunits, all can cause sedation at higher therapeutic doses. There are five benzodiazepines approved by the U.S. Food and Drug Administration (FDA) for treatment of insomnia—flurazepam (Dalmane), temazepam (Restoril), triazolam (Halcion), estazolam (Prosom), and quazepam (Doral)—with a predominantly **hypnotic** (sleep-inducing) effect. Other Benzodiazepines, such as lorazepam (Ativan) and alprazolam (Xanax), reduce anxiety without being as **soporific** (sleep producing) at lower therapeutic doses.

The fact that the benzodiazepines potentiate the ability of GABA to inhibit neurons probably accounts for their efficacy as anticonvulsants and for their ability to reduce the neuronal overexcitement of alcohol withdrawal. When used alone, even at high dosages, these drugs rarely inhibit the brain to the degree that respiratory depression, coma, and death result. However, when combined with other central nervous system (CNS) depressants, such as alcohol, opiates, or tricyclic antidepressants (TCAs), the inhibitory actions of the benzodiazepines can lead to life-threatening CNS depression.

Any drug that inhibits electrical activity in the brain can interfere with motor ability, attention, and judgment. A patient taking benzodiazepines must be cautioned about engaging in activities that could be dangerous if reflexes and attention are impaired, including specialized activities such as working in construction and more common activities such as driving a car. In older adults, the use of benzodiazepines may contribute to falls and broken bones. Ataxia is a common side effect secondary to the abundance of GABA receptors in the cerebellum.

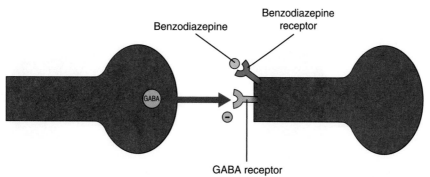

Figure 3-11 Action of the benzodiazepines. Drugs in this group attach to receptors adjacent to the receptors for the neurotransmitter gamma-aminobutyric acid (GABA). Drug attachment to these receptors strengthens the inhibitory effects of GABA. In the absence of GABA, there is no inhibitory effect of benzodiazepines.

Short-Acting Sedative-Hypnotic Sleep Agents

A newer class of hypnotics, termed the "Z-hypnotics," includes zolpidem (Ambien), zaleplon (Sonata), and eszopiclone (Lunesta). They have sedative effects without the antianxiety, anticonvulsant, or muscle relaxant effects of benzodiazepines, and they demonstrate selectivity for $GABA_A$ receptors containing alpha-1 subunits (Sanger, 2004). The drugs' affinity to alpha-1 subunits has the potential for amnesiac and ataxic (unsteadiness) side effects, and the onset of action is faster than that of most benzodiazepines. It is important to inform patients taking non-benzodiazepine hypnotic agents about the quick onset and advise them to take the drug when they are ready to go to sleep.

Most of these drugs have short half-lives, which determine the duration of action. Eszopiclone has the longest duration of action (an average of 7 to 8 hours of sleep per therapeutic dose); the half-lives of zolpidem and zaleplon are much shorter. Eszopiclone also has the unique side effect of an unpleasant taste upon awakening. Although tolerance and dependence are reportedly less than with benzodiazepines, all of the benzodiazepines and Z-hypnotics are categorized as schedule C-IV by the U.S. Drug Enforcement Administration (DEA).

Melatonin Receptor Agonists

Melatonin is a hormone that is only excreted at night as part of the normal circadian rhythm. Ramelteon (Rozerem), the latest FDA-approved hypnotic agent, is a melatonin receptor agonist and acts much the same way as endogenous (naturally occurring) melatonin. It has a high selectivity and potency at the melotonin-1 receptor site—thought to regulate sleepiness—and at the melotonin-2 receptor site—thought to regulate circadian rhythms. This is the only hypnotic medication approved for the treatment of insomnia that is not classified as a scheduled substance, or one having abuse potential, by the DEA. Side effects include headache and dizziness. Although most of the hypnotics are indicated for short-term use, the two newest hypnotics on the U.S. market, eszopiclone and ramelteon, are not restricted to short-term use on the package labeling. Long-term use of ramelteon above therapeutic doses can lead to increased prolactin and associated side effects (e.g., sexual dysfunction) (Due & Fitzgerald, 2006).

Buspirone

Buspirone (BuSpar) is a drug that reduces anxiety without having strong sedative-hypnotic properties. Because this agent does not leave the patient sleepy or sluggish, it is often much better tolerated than the benzodiazepines. It is not a CNS depressant and thus does not have as great a danger of interaction with other CNS depressants such as alcohol. Also, there is not the potential for addiction that exists with benzodiazepines.

Although at present the mechanism of action of buspirone is not clearly understood, one possibility is illustrated in Figure 3-12. Buspirone seems to act as a partial serotonin agonist. it also has a moderate affinity for dopamine-2 receptors. Side effects include headache, dizziness, light-headedness, nausea, and insomnia.

Refer to Chapter 12 on anxiety disorders for a discussion of the adverse reactions, dosages, nursing implications, and patient and family teaching for the antianxiety drugs.

Treating Anxiety Disorders with Antidepressants

The symptoms, neurotransmitters, and circuits associated with anxiety disorders overlap extensively with those of depressive disorders (see Chapter 13), and many antidepressants have proven to be effective

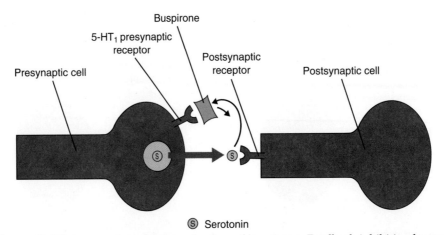

Figure 3-12 Proposed mechanism of action of buspirone. Feedback inhibition by serotonin is blocked, leading to increased release of serotonin by the presynaptic cell. *5-HT₁*, Serotonin.

treatments for anxiety disorders (Stahl, 2008). Selective serotonin reuptake inhibitors (SSRIs) are often used to treat OCD, social anxiety disorder (SAD), generalized anxiety disorder (GAD), panic disorder (PD), and post-traumatic stress disorder (PTSD). Venlafaxine (Effexor XR), is used to treat GAD, SAD, and PD. Duloxetine (Cymbalta) has recently received FDA approval for GAD.

Antidepressant Drugs

Our understanding of the neurophysiological basis of mood disorders is far from complete. However, a great deal of evidence seems to indicate that the neurotransmitters norepinephrine and serotonin play a major role in regulating mood. It is thought that a transmission deficiency of one or both of these monoamines within the limbic system underlies depression. One piece of evidence is that all of the drugs that show efficacy in the treatment of depression increase the synaptic level of one or both of these neurotransmitters. Figure 3-13 identifies the side effects of specific neurotransmitters being blocked or activated. Figure 3-14 illustrates the normal release, reuptake, and destruction of the monoamine neurotransmitters. A grasp of this underlying physiology is essential for understanding the

mechanisms by which the antidepressant drugs are thought to act.

Three hypotheses of antidepressants' mechanism of action:

1. The *monoamine hypothesis of depression* suggests there is a deficiency in one or more of the three neurotransmitters—serotonin, norepinephrine, or dopamine. The theory is that increasing these neurotransmitters alleviates depression.
2. The *monoamine receptor hypothesis of depression* suggests that low levels of neurotransmitters cause postsynaptic receptors to be up-regulated (increased in sensitivity or number). Increasing neurotransmitters by antidepressants results in down-regulation (desensitization) of key neurotransmitter receptors (Stahl, 2008). Delayed length of time for down-regulation may answer the question of why it takes so long for antidepressants to work, especially if they rapidly increase neurotransmitters.
3. Another hypothesis for the mechanism of antidepressant drugs is that they increase production of neurotrophic factors with prolonged use of antidepressants. These factors regulate the survival of neurons and enhance the sprouting of axons to form new synaptic connections (Stahl 2008).

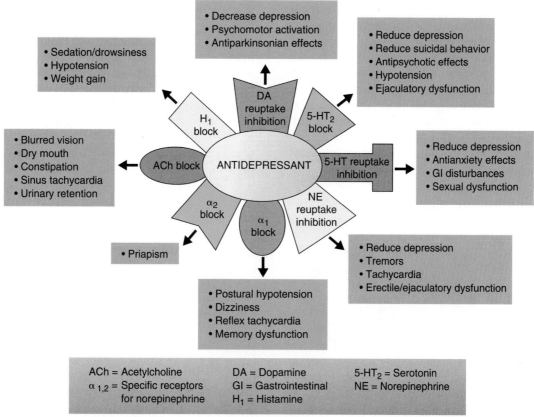

Figure 3-13 Possible effects of receptor binding of the antidepressant medications.

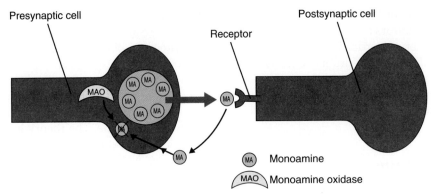

Figure 3-14 Normal release, reuptake, and destruction of the monoamine neurotransmitters.

Tricyclic Antidepressants

Tricyclic and heterocyclic antidepressants were widely used prior to the development of SSRIs. TCAs are no longer considered first-line treatment for depression, since they have more side effects, take longer to reach an optimal dose, and are far more lethal in overdose. The tricyclic antidepressants (TCAs) are thought to act primarily by blocking the reuptake of norepinephrine for the secondary amines (e.g., nortriptyline [Pamelor]) and both norepinephrine and serotonin for the tertiary amines (e.g., amitriptyline [Elavil], imipramine [Tofranil]). As shown in Figure 3-15, this blockage prevents norepinephrine from coming into contact with its degrading enzyme, MAO, and thus increases the level of norepinephrine at the synapse. Similarly, the tertiary TCAs block the reuptake and destruction of serotonin and increase the synaptic level of this neurotransmitter. Visit the Evolve website for a more thorough discussion of how tricyclic antidepressants work.

To varying degrees, many of the tricyclic drugs also block the muscarinic receptors that normally bind acetylcholine. This blockage leads to typical anticholinergic effects, such as blurred vision, dry mouth, tachycardia, urinary retention, and constipation. These adverse effects can be troubling to patients and limit their adherence with the regimen.

Depending on the individual drug, these agents can also block histamine-1 receptors in the brain. Blockage of these receptors by any drug causes sedation and drowsiness, an unwelcome side effect in daily use (see Figure 3-13). People taking the TCAs often have adherence issues because of their adverse reactions. TCA overdose can be fatal, secondary to cardiac conduction disturbances from excessive sodium channel blockade.

Selective Serotonin Reuptake Inhibitors

As the name implies, the selective serotonin reuptake inhibitors (SSRIs), such as fluoxetine (Prozac), sertraline (Zoloft), paroxetine (Paxil), citalopram (Celexa), escitalopram (Lexapro), and fluvoxamine (Luvox), preferentially block the reuptake and thus the destruction of serotonin. SSRIs as a group have less ability to block the muscarinic and histamine-1 receptors than do the TCAs. As a result of their more selective action, they seem to show comparable efficacy without eliciting the anticholinergic and sedating side effects that limit patient adherence. However, SSRIs have other side effects resulting from stimulation of a variety of serotonin receptors. Stimulation of various serotonin receptors may inhibit the spinal reflexes of orgasm, lead to apathy and low libido, and may cause

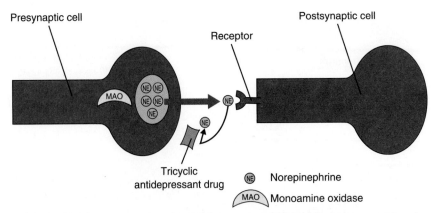

Figure 3-15 How the tricyclic antidepressants (TCAs) block the reuptake of norepinephrine.

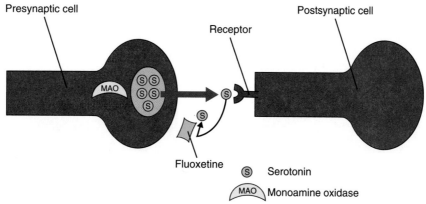

Figure 3-16 How the selective serotonin reuptake inhibitors (SSRIs) work.

nausea or vomiting (Stahl, 2008) (Figure 3-16). Visit the Evolve website for a more detailed explanation of how the SSRIs work.

Serotonin-Norepinephrine Reuptake Inhibitors

Serotonin-norepinephrine reuptake inhibitors (SNRIs) are medications that increase both serotonin and norepinephrine. Venlafaxine (Effexor) is more of a serotonergic agent at lower therapeutic doses, but norepinephrine reuptake blockade occurs at higher doses, leading to the dual SNRI action. Hypertension, induced in about 5% of patients, is a dose-dependent effect based on norepinephrine reuptake blockade. Doses higher than 150 mg/day can increase diastolic blood pressure about 7 to 10 mm Hg.

Duloxetine (Cymbalta) is an SNRI indicated for both depression and diabetic peripheral neuropathy. Like the TCAs, many of the SNRIs also have therapeutic effects on neuropathic pain. The common underlying mechanism of neuropathic pain is nerve injury or dysfunction. The mechanism by which TCAs and SNRIs reduce neuropathic pain is through activation of the descending norepinephrine and serotonin pathways to the spinal cord, thereby limiting pain signals ascending to the brain.

Serotonin-Norepinephrine Disinhibitors

The class of drugs described as **serotonin norepinephrine disinhibitors (SNDIs)** is represented by only one drug, mirtazapine (Remeron), which increases norepinephrine and serotonin transmission by antagonizing (blocking) presynaptic alpha-2 noradrenergic receptors. Mirtazapine offers both antianxiety and antidepressant effects, with minimal sexual dysfunction secondary to serotonin blockade. This antidepressant is particularly suited for the patient with nausea, because it is an antiemetic via serotonin blockade. The most common side effects are sedation and weight gain (Stahl, 2008).

Monoamine Oxidase Inhibitors

Monoamine oxidase inhibitors (MAOIs) are a group of antidepressant drugs that illustrate the principle that drugs can have a desired and beneficial effect in the brain, while at the same time having possibly dangerous effects elsewhere in the body. To understand the action of these drugs, keep in mind the following definitions:

- **Monoamines:** a type of organic compound; includes the neurotransmitters norepinephrine, epinephrine, dopamine, and serotonin, as well as many different food substances and drugs
- **Monoamine oxidase (MAO):** an enzyme that destroys monoamines
- **Monoamine oxidase inhibitors (MAOIs):** drugs that prevent the destruction of monoamines by inhibiting the action of MAO

The monoamine neurotransmitters, as well as any monoamine food substance or drug, are degraded (destroyed) by the enzyme MAO, which is located in neurons and in the liver. Antidepressant drugs such as phenelzine (Nardil), tranylcypromine (Parnate), selegiline (EMSAM) are MAOIs that act by inhibiting the enzyme and interfering with the destruction of the monoamine neurotransmitters. This in turn increases the synaptic level of the neurotransmitters and makes possible the antidepressant effects of these drugs (Figure 3-17). Visit the Evolve website for a more comprehensive explanation of how MAOIs work.

The use of MAO-inhibiting drugs is complicated by the fact that MAO is also present in the liver and is responsible for degrading monoamine substances that enter the body via food or drugs. Of particular importance is the monoamine tyramine, which is present in many food substances: aged cheeses, pickled or smoked fish, and wine. Tyramine poses a threat of hypertensive crisis because it can produce significant vasoconstriction—and thus an elevation in blood pressure—if allowed to circulate freely in the blood. Normally this does not happen, because tyramine is

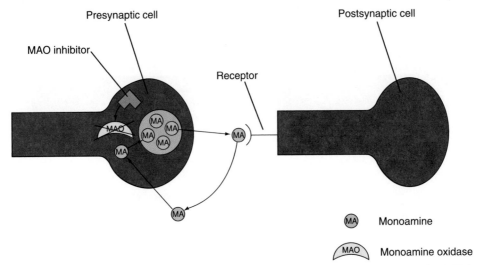

Figure 3-17 Blocking of monoamine oxidase (MAO) by inhibiting agents (MAOIs), which prevents the breakdown of monoamine by MAO.

destroyed by MAO as it passes through the liver before entering the general blood circulation. However, in the presence of MAOIs, tyramine is not destroyed by the liver and can cause serious, even life-threatening, hypertensive crisis.

A substantial number of drugs are chemically monoamines. The dosages of these drugs are determined by the rate at which they are destroyed by MAO in the liver. In a patient taking MAOIs, the blood level of monoamine drugs can reach high levels and cause serious toxicity. Thus MAOIs are contraindicated with concurrent use of any other antidepressants and sympathomimetic drugs. Concurrent use with some over-the-counter products with sympathomimetic properties (e.g., oral decongestants) should be avoided.

Because of the dangers that result from inhibition of hepatic MAO, patients taking MAOIs must be given a list of foods high in tyramine and drugs that must be avoided. Chapter 13 discusses the treatment of depression and contains a list of forbidden foods and foods to be eaten in moderation, along with nursing measures and instructions for patient teaching.

Other Antidepressants

Bupropion is an effective antidepressant (Wellbutrin) that is also used for smoking cessation (Zyban). It seems to act as a dopamine-norepinephrine reuptake inhibitor and also inhibits nicotinic acetylcholine receptors to reduce the addictive action of nicotine. Since bupropion has no serotonin action, it does not cause sexual side effects. Side effects include insomnia, tremor, anorexia, and weight loss. Bupropion is contraindicated in patients with a seizure disorder, in patients with a current or prior diagnosis of bulimia or anorexia nervosa, and in patients undergoing abrupt discontinuation of alcohol or sedatives (including benzodiazepines), owing to the additive seizure risk.

Trazodone is not a first choice for antidepressant treatment, but it is often given along with another agent because sedation, one of the common side effects, helps with insomnia. Its antidepressant effects are only seen at high therapeutic doses. The common side effects are sedation and orthostasis. Trazodone's sedative effect is from potent histamine-1 blockade; orthostasis is from α_1 adrenergic blockade. Its potent α_1 blockade with minimal anticholinergic effects can lead to another rare side effect: priapism (painful prolonged penile erection).

Mood Stabilizers

Lithium

Although the efficacy of lithium (Eskalith, Lithobid) as a mood stabilizer in patients with bipolar (manic-depressive) disorder has been established for many years, its mechanism of action is still far from understood. As a positively charged ion, similar in structure to sodium and potassium, lithium may well act by affecting electrical conductivity in neurons.

As discussed earlier, an electrical impulse consists of the inward, depolarizing flow of sodium followed by an outward, repolarizing flow of potassium. These electrical charges are propagated along the neuron; if they are initiated at one end of the neuron, they will pass to the other end. Once they reach the end of a neuron, a neurotransmitter is released.

It may be that an overexcitement of neurons in the brain underlies bipolar disorder and that lithium interacts in some complex way with sodium and potassium at the cell membrane to stabilize electrical activity. Also, lithium may reduce the excitatory neurotransmitter **glutamate** and exert an antimanic effect. The other proposed mechanisms by which lithium works to regulate mood include the noncompetitive inhibition of the enzyme **inositol monophosphatase**. Inhibition of serotonin autoreceptors by lithium is more related to the agent's antidepressant effects than its antimanic effects (Shaldubina et al., 2001).

While we do not know exactly how lithium works, we are certain that its influence on electrical conductivity results in adverse effects and toxicity. By altering electrical conductivity, lithium represents a potential threat to all body functions regulated by electrical currents. Foremost among these functions is cardiac contraction; lithium can induce, although not commonly, sinus bradycardia. Extreme alteration of cerebral conductivity with overdose can lead to convulsions. Alteration in nerve and muscle conduction can commonly lead to tremor at therapeutic doses or more extreme motor dysfunction with overdose.

The fact that sodium and potassium play a strong role in regulating fluid balance and the distribution of fluid in various body compartments explains the disturbances in fluid balance that can be caused by lithium. These include polyuria (the output of large volumes of urine) and edema (the accumulation of fluid in the interstitial space). Long-term use of lithium can cause hypothyroidism in some patients by interfering with iodine molecules and affecting formation of and conversion to the active form of thyroid hormone, triiodothyronine (T3). In addition, hyponatremia can increase the risk of lithium toxicity, because increased renal reabsorption of sodium leads to increased reabsorption of lithium as well.

Primarily because of its effects on electrical conductivity, lithium has a low therapeutic index. The therapeutic index represents the ratio of the lethal dose to the effective dose and is a measure of overall drug safety in regards to the possibility of overdose or toxicity. It can be expressed as therapeutic index = median lethal dose/median effective dose. A *low therapeutic index* means that the blood level of a drug that can cause death is not far above the blood level required for drug effectiveness. This mandates that the blood level of lithium be monitored on a regular basis to be sure the drug is not accumulating and rising to dangerous levels. Table 3-3 lists some of the adverse and toxic effects of lithium. Chapter 14 considers lithium treatment in more depth and discusses specific dose-related adverse and toxic effects, nursing implications, and the patient teaching plan.

TABLE 3-3 Adverse/Toxic Effects of Lithium

System	Adverse/Toxic Effects
Nervous and muscular	Tremor, ataxia, confusion, convulsions
Digestive	Nausea, vomiting, diarrhea
Cardiac	Arrhythmias
Fluid and electrolyte	Polyuria, polydipsia, edema
Endocrine	Goiter and hypothyroidism

Anticonvulsant Drugs

Valproate (available as divalproex sodium [Depakote] and valproic acid [Depakene]), carbamazepine (Tegretol), and lamotrigine (Lamictal) have demonstrated efficacy in the treatment of bipolar disorders (APA, 2008). Their anticonvulsant properties derive from the alteration of electrical conductivity in membranes; in particular, they reduce the firing rate of very-high-frequency neurons in the brain. It is possible that this membrane-stabilizing effect accounts for the ability of these drugs to reduce the mood swings that occur in patients with bipolar disorders. Other proposed mechanisms as mood stabilizers are glutamate antagonists and GABA agonists.

Valproate

Valproate (Depakote, Depakene) is structurally different from other anticonvulsants and psychiatric drugs that show efficacy in the treatment of bipolar disorder. Divalproex is recommended for mixed episodes and has been found useful for rapid cycling. Common side effects include tremor, weight gain, and sedation. Occasional serious side effects are thrombocytopenia, pancreatitis, hepatic failure, and birth defects. Baseline levels are measured for liver function indicators and complete blood count (CBC) before an individual is started on this medication, and measurements are repeated periodically. In addition, the therapeutic blood level of the drug is monitored.

Carbamazepine

Carbamazepine (Tegretol) is useful in preventing mania and during episodes of acute mania. It reduces the firing rate of overexcited neurons by reducing the activity of sodium channels. Common side effects include anticholinergic side effects (e.g., dry mouth, constipation, urinary retention, blurred vision), orthostasis, sedation, and ataxia. Rash may occur in 10% of patients (Sadock & Sadock, 2008). Recommended baseline laboratory work includes liver function tests, CBC, electrocardiogram, and electrolyte levels. Blood levels are monitored to avoid toxicity (>12 mcg/mL), but there are no established therapeutic blood levels for carbamazepine in the treatment of bipolar disorder.

Lamotrigine

Lamotrigine (Lamictal) is approved by the FDA for maintenance therapy of bipolar disorder, but it is not effective in acute mania (Preston et al., 2005). Lamotrigine works well in treating the depression of bipolar disorder, with less incidence of switching the patient into mania than antidepressants. It modulates the release of glutamate and aspartate. Patients should promptly report any rashes, which could be a sign of life-threatening Stevens-Johnson syndrome. This can be minimized by slow titration to therapeutic doses.

Other Anticonvulsants

Other anticonvulsants used as mood stabilizers are gabapentin (Neurontin), topiramate (Topamax), and oxcarbazepine (Trileptal). None of them have FDA approval as mood stabilizers, and studies have not provided strong support for their use as primary treatments for bipolar disorder. Antipsychotic medications and antianxiety medications, such as clonazepam (Klonopin), are used for their calming effects during mania. Chapter 14 offers a more detailed discussion of these medications.

Antipsychotic Drugs

Conventional Antipsychotics

First-generation antipsychotic drugs, or conventional antipsychotics (also called *typical* or *standard*), are strong antagonists at the D_2 dopamine receptors. By binding to these receptors and blocking the attachment of dopamine, they reduce dopaminergic transmission. It has been postulated that an overactivity of the dopamine system in certain areas of the mesolimbic system may be responsible for at least some of the symptoms of schizophrenia; thus blockage of dopamine may reduce these symptoms. This is thought to be particularly true of the "positive" symptoms of schizophrenia, such as delusions (e.g., paranoid and grandiose ideas) and hallucinations (e.g., hearing or seeing things not present in reality). Chapter 15 presents a more detailed discussion of schizophrenia and its symptoms.

These drugs are also antagonists, to varying degrees, of the muscarinic receptors for acetylcholine, α_1 adrenergic receptors for norepinephrine, and histamine-1 receptors. Although it is unclear if this antagonism plays a role in the beneficial effects of the drugs, it is certain that antagonism is responsible for some of their major side effects (see Chapter 15). Visit the Evolve website for a more detailed description of how these drugs block not only dopamine but also muscarinic receptors for acetylcholine and α_1 adrenergic receptors for norepinephrine.

Figure 3-18 illustrates the proposed mechanism of action of the conventional antipsychotics, which include the phenothiazines, thioxanthenes, butyrophenones, and pharmacologically related agents. As summarized in Figure 3-19, many of the untoward side effects of these drugs can be understood as a logical extension of their receptor-blocking activity. Because dopamine in the basal ganglia plays a major role in the regulation of movement, it is not surprising that dopamine blockage can lead to motor abnormalities (extrapyramidal side effects) such as parkinsonism, akinesia, akathisia, dyskinesia, and tardive dyskinesia.

Nurses and physicians often monitor patients for evidence of involuntary movements after administration of the conventional antipsychotic agents. One popular scale is called the *Abnormal Involuntary Movement Scale (AIMS)*. Chapter 15 provides an example AIMS and a discussion of the clinical use of antipsychotic drugs, side effects, specific nursing interventions, and patient teaching strategies.

An important physiological function of dopamine is that it acts as the hypothalamic factor that inhibits the release of prolactin from the anterior pituitary gland, so blockage of dopamine transmission can lead to increased pituitary secretion of prolactin. In women, this hyperprolactinemia can result in amenorrhea (absence of the menses) or galactorrhea (breast milk flow); in men, it can lead to gynecomastia (development of the male mammary glands).

Acetylcholine is the neurotransmitter released by the postganglionic neurons of the parasympathetic nervous system. Through its attachment to muscarinic receptors on internal organs, it serves to help regulate internal function. Blockage of the muscarinic receptors by phenothiazines and a wide variety of other psychiatric drugs can lead to a constellation of untoward effects, which are predictable based on knowledge of the normal physiology of the parasympathetic nervous system. These side effects usually involve blurred

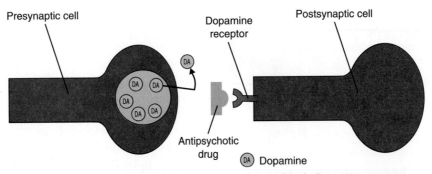

Figure 3-18 How the conventional antipsychotics block dopamine receptors.

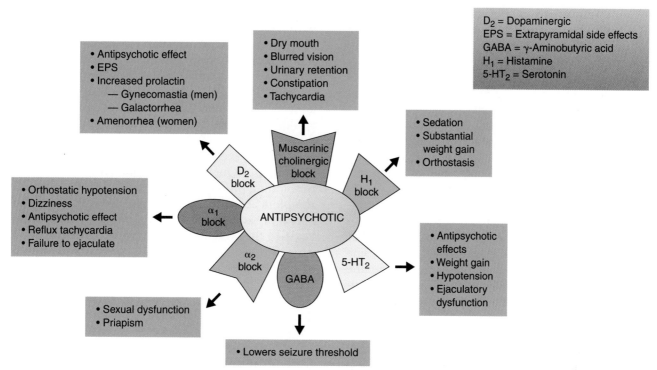

Figure 3-19 Adverse effects of receptor blockage of antipsychotic agents. (From Varcarolis, E. [2004]. *Manual of psychiatric nursing care plans* [2nd ed.]. St. Louis: Elsevier.)

vision, dry mouth, constipation, and urinary hesitancy. These drugs can also impair memory, since acetylcholine is important for memory function.

In addition to blocking dopamine and muscarinic receptors, many of the conventional antipsychotic drugs act as antagonists at the α_1 adrenergic receptors for norepinephrine. These receptors are found on smooth muscle cells that contract in response to norepinephrine from sympathetic nerves. For example, the ability of sympathetic nerves to constrict blood vessels is dependent on the attachment of norepinephrine to α_1 adrenergic receptors. Blockage of these receptors can bring about vasodilation and a consequent drop in blood pressure. Vasoconstriction mediated by the sympathetic nervous system is essential for maintaining normal blood pressure when the body is in the upright position; blockage of the α_1 adrenergic receptors can lead to orthostatic hypotension.

The α_1 adrenergic receptors are also found on the vas deferens and are responsible for the propulsive contractions leading to ejaculation. Blockage of these receptors can lead to a failure to ejaculate. Potent α_1 adrenergic antagonists with little anticholinergic effects, such as trazodone, can lead to priapism, secondary to the inability for detumescence (subsidence of erection).

Finally, many of these conventional antipsychotic agents, as well as a variety of other psychiatric drugs, block the histamine-1 receptors for histamine. The two most significant side effects of blocking these receptors are sedation and substantial weight gain. The sedation may be beneficial in severely agitated patients. Nonadherence to the medication regimen is a significant issue because of these troublesome side effects, and the atypical antipsychotic agents have consequently become the drugs of choice.

Atypical Antipsychotics

The second generation of antipsychotic drugs includes the **atypical antipsychotics**, which produce fewer extrapyramidal side effects (EPS) and target both the negative and positive symptoms of schizophrenia (see Chapter 15). These newer agents are often chosen as first-line treatment over the conventional antipsychotics because of their lower risk of EPS. However, five of the seven available atypical antipsychotics can increase the risk of metabolic syndrome, with increased weight, blood glucose, and triglycerides. The simultaneous blockade of 5-HT_{2C} and histamine-1 receptors is associated with weight gain due to increased appetite stimulation via the hypothalamic eating centers. Strong antimuscarinic properties at the M3 receptor on the pancreatic beta cells can cause insulin resistance, leading to hyperglycemia. The receptor responsible for elevated triglycerides is currently unknown (Stahl, 2008). Clozapine and olanzapine have the highest risk of causing metabolic syndrome; aripiprazole and ziprasidone have the lowest risk.

The atypical antipsychotics are predominantly dopamine and serotonin antagonists (blockers). The blockade at the mesolimbic dopamine pathway is thought to decrease psychosis, similar to the mechanism by which the conventional antipsychotics work. Decreasing dopamine can reduce psychosis but cause adverse effects elsewhere such as the movement side effects of EPS, the worsening of cognitive and negative symptoms, and an increase in the hormone prolactin, leading to gynecomastia, galactorrhea, amenorrhea, and low libido (Stahl, 2008).

Clozapine. Clozapine (Clozaril), the first of the atypicals, is an antipsychotic drug that is relatively free of the motor side effects of the phenothiazines and other atypical antipsychotics. It is thought that clozapine preferentially blocks the dopamine receptors in the mesolimbic system, rather than those in the nigrostriatal area. This allows it to exert an antipsychotic action without leading to difficulties with EPS.

Although people who take clozapine are more likely to adhere to their medication regimen than those who are taking other atypical antipsychotics, it can cause a potentially fatal side effect in up to 0.8% of patients (McEvoy et al., 2006). Clozapine has the potential to suppress bone marrow and induce agranulocytosis. Because any deficiency in white blood cells renders a person prone to serious infection, regular measurement of white blood cell count is required. Typically the count is measured weekly for the first 6 months, every other week for the next 6 months, and monthly thereafter. However, new research indicates that it is medically justifiable to discontinue blood counts after 6 months if a knowledgeable patient does not want them, especially if adherence is jeopardized (Schulte, 2006).

Clozapine has the potential for inducing convulsions, a dose-related side effect, in 3.5% of patients. Caution should be used with other drugs that can increase the concentration of clozapine. There is also a potential for myocarditis that should be monitored, but the most common side effects of clozapine are drowsiness and sedation (39%), hypersalivation (31%), weight gain (31%), reflex tachycardia (25%), constipation (14%), and dizziness (19%) (Novartis, 2009).

Risperidone. Risperidone (Risperdal) has a very low potential for inducing agranulocytosis or convulsions. However, high therapeutic dosages (>6 mg/day) may lead to motor difficulties. It has the highest risk of EPS among the atypical antipsychotics and may increase prolactin, which may lead to sexual dysfunction. Risperidone can cause orthostatic hypotension that can lead to falls, which are a serious problem among older adults. Weight gain, sedation, and sexual dysfunction are adverse effects that may affect adherence

with the medication regimen and should be discussed with patients. It is notable that risperidone is the first atypical antipsychotic available as a long-acting injection. Risperdal Consta, administered every two weeks, provides an alternative to the depot form of conventional antipsychotics. A rare but serious side effect is an increased risk of cerebrovascular accidents in older adults with dementia who are being treated for agitation (Lee et al., 2004).

Quetiapine. Quetiapine (Seroquel) has a broad receptor-binding profile. Its strong blockage of histamine-1 receptors accounts for the high sedation. The combination of histamine-1 and serotonin receptor blockage leads to the weight gain associated with use of this drug and also to a moderate risk for metabolic syndrome. It causes moderate blockage of α_1 adrenergic receptors and associated orthostasis. Quetiapine has a low risk for EPS or prolactin elevation from low D_2 dopamine binding due to rapid dissociation at these receptors.

Other Atypical Antipsychotics. Other atypical antipsychotics include olanzapine (Zyprexa), ziprasidone (Geodon), aripiprazole (Abilify), and paliperidone (Invega).

- **Olanzapine** is similar to clozapine in chemical structure. Side effects include sedation, weight gain, hyperglycemia with new-onset type 2 diabetes, and higher risk for metabolic syndrome.
- **Ziprasidone** is a serotonin-norepinephrine reuptake inhibitor. The main side effects are dizziness and moderate sedation. Ziprasidone is contraindicated in patients with a known history of QT interval prolongation, recent acute myocardial infarction, or uncompensated heart failure.
- **Aripiprazole** is a unique atypical antipsychotic known as a *dopamine system stabilizer*. In areas of the brain with excess dopamine, it lowers the dopamine level by acting as a receptor antagonist; however, in regions with low dopamine, it stimulates receptors to raise the dopamine level. It has little sedation and weight gain. Side effects include insomnia and akathisia.
- **Paliperidone**, the newest antipsychotic in the United States, is the major active metabolite of risperidone. It has similar side effects, such as EPS and prolactin elevation. Its side effects are orthostasis and sedation. The Osmotic Release Oral System (OROS) provides consistent 24-hour release of medication, leading to minimal peaks and troughs in plasma concentrations.

Chapter 15 discusses the conventional and atypical antipsychotic drugs in detail, including the indications for use, adverse reactions, nursing implications, and patient and family teaching.

Drug Treatment for Attention Deficit Hyperactivity Disorder

Children and adults with attention deficit hyperactivity disorder (ADHD) show symptoms of short attention span, impulsivity, and overactivity. Paradoxically, the mainstay of treatment for this condition in children—and increasingly in adults—is the administration of psychostimulant drugs. Both methylphenidate (Ritalin) and dextroamphetamines such as Adderall seem to show efficacy in these conditions. They are sympathomimetic amines and have been shown to function as direct and indirect agonists at adrenergic receptor sites. Psychostimulants act directly at the postsynaptic receptor, mimicking the effects of norepinephrine or dopamine. They block the reuptake of norepinephrine and dopamine into the presynaptic neuron and increase the release of these monoamines into the extraneuronal space. How this translates into clinical efficacy is far from understood, but it is thought that the monoamines may inhibit an overactive part of the limbic system.

Among many concerns with the use of these drugs are the side effects of agitation, exacerbation of psychotic thought processes, hypertension, and long-term growth suppression, as well as their potential for abuse. One nonstimulant medication available for the treatment of ADHD is atomoxetine hydrochloride (Strattera), a norepinephrine reuptake inhibitor approved for use in children 6 years and older. Common side effects include decreased appetite and weight loss, fatigue, and dizziness. Refer to Chapter 28 for more on these agents.

Drug Treatment for Alzheimer's Disease

The insidious and progressive loss of memory and other higher brain functions brought about by Alzheimer's disease is a great individual, family, and social tragedy. Because the disease seems to involve progressive structural degeneration of the brain, there are two major pharmacological directions in its treatment. The first is to attempt to prevent or slow the structural degeneration. Although actively pursued, this approach has been unsuccessful so far. The second is to attempt to maintain normal brain function for as long as possible.

Much of the memory loss in this disease has been attributed to dysfunction of neurons that secrete acetylcholine. Tacrine and donepezil are **anticholinesterase drugs** (also called *cholinesterase inhibitors*) that show some efficacy in slowing the rate of memory loss and in some patients may even improve memory. The drugs work by interfering with the action of acetylcholinesterase. Inactivation of this enzyme leads to less destruction of the neurotransmitter acetylcholine and therefore a higher concentration at the synapse. There are five agents FDA-approved for the treatment of Alzheimer's disease in the United States, four of which are acetylcholinesterase inhibitors: tacrine (Cognex), donepezil (Aricept), galantamine (Reminyl), and rivastigmine (Exelon). Among the acetylcholinesterase inhibitors, tacrine is no longer used extensively because of the risk of hepatic toxicity in some patients.

The fifth agent approved by the FDA for treatment of Alzheimer's disease is memantine (Namenda), a noncompetitive *N*-methyl-D-aspartate (NMDA) receptor antagonist. The glutamatergic neurotransmitter system plays an important role in memory formation. Amyloid plaques in the brain can lead to glutamatergic dysfunction and excess glutamate. When glutamate binds to NMDA receptors, calcium flows freely from the cell; overexposure to calcium results in cell degeneration. Memantine fills the NMDA receptor sites and reduces the degeneration. Memantine was shown to be effective in the treatment of moderate to severe Alzheimer's disease.

Refer to Chapter 17 for a more detailed discussion of these drugs, as well as their nursing considerations and patient and family teaching.

Herbal Treatments

The growing interest in medicinal herbs is driven by a variety of factors. Many people believe that herbal treatments are safer because they are "natural" or that they may have fewer side effects than more costly traditional medications.

Herbal treatments have been researched in efforts to understand their mechanisms of action. They have also been studied in clinical trials to determine their safety and efficacy. This is especially true of kava kava and St. John's wort (Sarris, 2007). Some medicinal herbs have been found to be nontherapeutic and others even deadly if taken over long periods of time or in combination with other chemical substances and prescription drugs (Preston et al., 2005). The risk of bleeding may be increased in patients taking ginkgo biloba and warfarin, and kava kava may increase the risk of hepatotoxicity at doses over 240 mg/day.

Among the major concerns of health care professionals are the potential long-term effects of some herbal agents (nerve, kidney, and liver damage) and the possibility of adverse chemical reactions when herbal agents are taken in conjunction with other substances, including conventional medications.

St. John's wort can have serious interactions with a number of conventional medications. Taking St. John's wort with other serotonergic agents (e.g., SSRIs, triptans) can cause serotonin syndrome. It may also reduce the effectiveness of other medications by increasing their rate of metabolism and reducing blood levels of these medications. St. John's wort is a cytochrome P450 (CYP450) 3A4 enzyme inducer. Patients taking CYP450 3A4 metabolized medications (e.g., oral contraceptives, digoxin, theophylline, some immunosuppressives) concurrently with St. John's wort may experience increased metabolism and subtherapeutic drug levels (Alpert, 2008).

Another key concern regarding the use of alternative herbs and nutrients is the quality of herbal supplements on the market. Many brands are of poor quality, have dosing inconsistencies, or are of questionable purity or stability. This is partly because herbal preparations are sold as dietary supplements rather than drugs; thus they avoid regulation under the FDA's Federal Food, Drug, and Cosmetic Act. Health care professionals, and especially nurses, need to stay current, using unbiased sources of product information and passing this information on to patients taking alternative agents (Brown, et al., 2003). Independent evaluation of many brands with updates can be found at www.consumerlab.com or www.supplementwatch.com. Recalls and warnings to stop use of certain brands are available at www.fda.gov/medwatch (Brown, et al., 2003).

It is important that nurses and other health care professionals explore the patient's use of herbal supplements in a nonjudgmental manner by asking, "What over-the-counter medications or herbs do you take to help your symptoms? Do they help? How much are you taking? How long have you been taking them?" Individuals taking medications or other supplements should be made aware of drug/substance interactions and product safety. Such discussion should be part of the initial and ongoing interviews with patients. Chapter 36 covers complementary and integrative therapies in more detail.

KEY POINTS TO REMEMBER

- All actions of the brain—sensory, motor, and intellectual—are carried out physiologically through the interactions of nerve cells. These interactions involve impulse conduction, neurotransmitter release, and receptor response. Alterations in these basic processes can lead to mental disturbances and physical manifestations.

- In particular, it seems that excess activity of dopamine is involved in the thought disturbances of schizophrenia, and deficiencies of norepinephrine, serotonin, or both underlie depression and anxiety. Insufficient activity of GABA also plays a role in anxiety.

- Pharmacological treatment of mental disturbances is directed at the suspected neurotransmitter-receptor problem. Antipsychotic drugs decrease dopamine, antidepressant drugs increase synaptic levels of norepinephrine and/or serotonin, and antianxiety drugs increase

the effectiveness of GABA or increase 5-HT and/or norepinephrine.

- Because the immediate target activity of a drug can result in many downstream alterations in neuronal activity, drugs with a variety of chemical actions may show efficacy in treating the same clinical condition. Thus newer drugs with novel mechanisms of action are being used in the treatment of schizophrenia, depression, and anxiety.

- Unfortunately, agents used to treat mental disease can cause various undesired effects. Prominent among these can be sedation or excitement, motor disturbances, muscarinic blockage, α antagonism, sexual dysfunction, and weight gain. There is a continuing effort to develop new drugs that are effective, safe, and well tolerated.

CRITICAL THINKING

1. No matter where you practice nursing, individuals under your care will be taking psychotropic drugs. Consider the importance of understanding normal brain structure and function as they relate to mental disturbances and psychotropic drugs by addressing the following questions:

   A. How can you use the knowledge of normal brain function (control of peripheral nerves, skeletal muscles, the autonomic nervous system, hormones, and circadian rhythms) to better understand how a patient can be affected by psychotropic drugs or psychiatric illness?

   B. What information from the various brain imaging techniques can you use to understand and treat patients with mental disorders and provide support to their families? How might you use that information for patient and family teaching?

2. Based on your understanding of symptoms that may occur when the following neurotransmitters are altered, what specific information would you include in medication teaching?

   A. Dopamine D_2 (as with use of antipsychotic drugs)

   B. Blockage of muscarinic receptors (as with use of phenothiazines and other drugs)

   C. α_1 Receptors (as with use of phenothiazines and other drugs)

   D. Histamine (as with use of phenothiazines and other drugs)

   E. Monoamine oxidase (MAO) (as with use of a monoamine oxidase inhibitor [MAOI])

   F. Gamma-aminobutyric acid (GABA) (as with use of benzodiazepines)

   G. Serotonin (as with the use of selective serotonin reuptake inhibitors [SSRIs] and other drugs)

   H. Norepinephrine (as with the use of selective norepinephrine reuptake inhibitors [SNRIs])

CHAPTER REVIEW

1. The nurse is assessing a new patient. Which patient statement would the nurse attribute to a neurobiological basis of mental disease?
   1. "I like to eat all day long."
   2. "I sleep 7 hours nightly."
   3. "I have a number of close friends."
   4. "I enjoy solving word puzzles."

2. The physician has written orders for four patients. Which medication order would the nurse question?
   1. BuSpar, take in the morning
   2. Restoril, take at bedtime
   3. Ambien, take early in the morning
   4. Rozerem, take at bedtime

3. Which patient statement would require the nurse to provide further teaching?
   1. "I should report any unusual bleeding when I take gingko biloba."
   2. "I should not take St. John's Wort with Zoloft."
   3. "Herbal treatments are safe because they are made with all-natural ingredients."
   4. "I will tell my doctor that I am taking an herbal supplement."

4. The nurse is caring for a patient who is taking lithium. Which adverse effect would the nurse anticipate?
   1. Oliguria
   2. Confusion
   3. Constipation
   4. Hyperthyroidism

5. The nurse understands that norepinephrine is involved with the stimulation of which bodily process?
   1. The "fight-or-flight" response to stress
   2. The hypothalamus to release hormones
   3. Involvement in the inflammatory response
   4. The parasympathetic nervous system

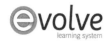

Visit the Evolve website for an **Audio Chapter Summary, Chapter Review Answers & Rationales, Critical Thinking Answer Guidelines,** and additional resources related to the content in this chapter: **http://evolve.elsevier.com/Varcarolis/foundations**

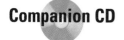

Use the Companion CD to prepare for tests and the NCLEX® Examination with **Test-Taking Strategies** for psychiatric mental health nursing and hundreds of **Review Questions.**

References

Alpert, J. E. (2008). Drug-drug interactions in psychopharmacology. In T. A. Stern, J. F. Rosenbaum, M. Fava, J. Biederman, & S. L. Rauch (Eds.), *Comprehensive clinical psychiatry* (pp. 687–704). Philadelphia: Elsevier.

American Psychiatric Association. (2008). *Practice guidelines for the treatment of patients with bipolar disorder* (2nd ed.). Retrieved July 18, 2008 from www.psychiatryonline.com/popup.aspx?aID=50099&print=yes

Brown, R., Gerbarg, P. L., & Muskin, P. R. (2003). Complementary and alternative treatment in psychiatry. In A. Tashman, J. Kay, & J. A. Lieberman (Eds.), *Psychiatry* (2nd ed.). London: Wiley.

Lee, P. E., Gill, S. S., Freedman, M., Bronskill, S. E., Hillmer, M. P., Rochon, P. A. (2004). Atypical antipsychotic drugs in the treatment of behavioural and psychological symptoms of dementia: Systematic review. *British Medical Journal*, 329, 75. Retrieved from: http://bmj.bmjjournals.com/cgi/content/full/329/7457/75.

Lin, K. M., Smith, M. W., & Lin, M. T. (2003). Psychopharmacology. In A. Tashman, J. Kay, & J. A. Lieberman (Eds.), *Psychiatry* (2nd ed.). London: Wiley.

McEvoy, J. P., Lieberman, J. A., Stroup, T. S., Davis, S. M., Meltzer, H. Y., Rosenheck, et al, for the CATIE Investigators. (2006). Effectiveness of clozapine versus olanzapine, quetiapine, and risperidone in patients with chronic schizophrenia who did not respond to prior atypical antipsychotic treatment. *American Journal of Psychiatry*, 163, 600–610.

Novartis. (2009). Clozaril prescribing information. Retrieved March 10, 2009 from http://www.pharma.us.novartis.com/product/pi/pdf/clozaril.pdf

Preston, J. D., O'Neal, J. H., & Talaga, M. C. (2005). *Handbook of clinical psychopharmacology for therapists* (3rd ed.). Oakland, CA: New Harbinger.

Sadock, B. J., & Sadock, V. A. (2008). *Concise textbook of clinical psychiatry* (3rd ed.). Philadelphia: Lippincott, Williams & Wilkins.

Sanger, D. J. (2004). The pharmacology and mechanisms of action of new generation, non-benzodiazepine hypnotic agents. *CNS Drugs, 18*(Suppl. 1), 9–15.

Sarris, J. (2007). Herbal medicines in the treatment of psychiatric disorders: A systematic review. *Phytotherapy Research, 21,* 703–716.

Schulte, F. J. (2006). Risk of clozapine-associated agranulocytosis and mandatory white blood cell monitoring. *The Annals of Pharmacotherapy, 40,* 683–688.

Shaldubina, A., Adam, G., & Belmaker, R. H. (2001). The mechanism of lithium action: state of the art, ten years later. *Progress in Neuropsychopharmacology and Biological Psychiatry, 25,* 855–866.

Stahl, S. W. (2008). *Stahl's Essential Psychopharmacology* (3rd ed.). New York: Cambridge University Press.

U.S. Food and Drug Administration. (2004). *Antidepressant use in children, adolescents, and adults.* Updated May 2, 2007. Retrieved July 29, 2008 from http://www.fda.gov/cder/drug/antidepressants/

Foundations for Practice

A NURSE SPEAKS

As a psychiatric mental health home care nurse, I took care of an older adult patient named Lucy who was diagnosed with major depression. Lucy resided in an assisted living facility (ALF). Initially, I administered the Geriatric Depression Scale and the Mini-Mental State Exam. These assessments demonstrated that Lucy was seriously depressed and appeared to be suffering with dementia as well. I focused my interventions on depression as well as dementia.

Lucy seemed to be responding to my nursing care until one night at about 10 PM, when one of the staff members called me to report that Lucy was crying and screaming. I provided suggestions to calm Lucy. This same scenario repeated itself the next two nights. On the third night I decided to visit the ALF. I arrived to find Lucy cowering in a corner, crying, wringing her hands, and incredibly distraught. I saw a nursing assistant pointing her finger and yelling at Lucy to stop crying. This made Lucy more upset. I asked the nursing assistant to tell me what had happened, and she explained that for the last few nights Lucy had come out of her room at about 10 PM asking to see Lou. The nursing assistant said, "Every night I tell her the same thing: Lou is dead. He has been dead for ten years. Stop asking to see him when you know he is dead!"

With that explanation of what had occurred, I asked if I could intervene. I walked over to Lucy, placed my arm around her shoulder, and asked her what was wrong. Through her tears Lucy said to me, "They tell me that Lou is dead. How can that be? He is my husband—wouldn't I know if he were dead? Why would they say something so cruel to me?" I said, "Lucy, Lou is not here. He went out. Let's go back to your room and spend a little time together." Lucy immediately calmed. We walked to Lucy's room, where we each had a cup of tea and played cards until Lucy said, "I'm tired now. I think I'll go to sleep."

I left Lucy's room and gathered the nursing staff together to teach them about memory loss and dementia. I instructed them on the value of the "therapeutic fib"—an intervention that recognizes that when a patient has lost certain memories, the patient can no longer handle reality as we know it—and how much kinder it is for us to enter into the patient's reality, even if it means that we have to fib. The staff actually enjoyed this and provided examples of other resident situations in which telling the truth made things worse.

This incident took place years ago, but I remember it as if it happened yesterday. It confirmed that as a psychiatric mental health home care nurse my focus is certainly the patient but it is also everyone else who is involved in the care of that patient. It also reminded me that sometimes the most effective interventions are also the simplest.

Katherine Vanderhorst

CHAPTER **4**

Psychiatric Mental Health Nursing in Acute Care Settings

Avni Cirpili and Margaret Swisher

Key Terms and Concepts

admission criteria, 78
clinical pathway, 79
codes, 84
elopement, 82
**managed behavioral health care
  organizations (MBHOs),** 77

managed care plans, 77
mental health parity, 77
milieu, 82
multidisciplinary treatment plan, 79
psychiatric case management, 77
psychosocial rehabilitation, 84

Objectives

1. Describe the population served by inpatient psychiatric care.
2. Identify funding options for acute care of psychiatric conditions and legislation related to insurance reimbursement.
3. List the criteria for admission to inpatient care.
4. Discuss the purpose of identifying the rights of hospitalized psychiatric patients.
5. Explain how the multidisciplinary treatment team collaborates to plan and implement care for the hospitalized patient.

6. Explain the importance of monitoring patient safety during hospitalization.
7. Describe the role of the nurse as advocate and provider of care for the patient.
8. Discuss the managerial and coordinating roles of nursing on an inpatient acute care unit.
9. Discuss the process for preparing patients to return to the community for ongoing care.

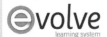 Visit the Evolve website for an **Audio Glossary & Flashcards, Concept Map Creator,** and additional resources related to the content in this chapter: **http://evolve.elsevier.com/Varcarolis/foundations**

Inpatient psychiatric care has undergone significant change over the past quarter century. During the 1980s, inpatient stays were at their peak as private and non-federal general hospital psychiatric units proliferated. However, by the mid-1990s, the number of patient days, psychiatric beds, and psychiatric facilities were dipping sharply. This decline was caused by improvements brought about by managed care, tougher limitations of covered days by insurance plans, and alternatives to inpatient care such as partial hospitalization programs and residential facilities. Lengths of stay decreased from weeks to days.

Hospitalization remains an option for the treatment of patients with mental disorders and emotional crises. In fact, one out of four hospital stays are related to a mental illness and/or substance-abuse diagnosis (Owens et al., 2007). The top five mental health diagnoses treated are mood disorders, substance-related disorders, delirium/dementia, anxiety disorders, and schizophrenia. Admission is commonly reserved for those people who are suicidal, homicidal, or extremely disabled and in need of short-term, acute-care (Simon & Shuman, 2008). Most inpatient treatment today takes place in general hospitals or private psychiatric hospitals. There are also state psychiatric hospitals that exist as a resource for the uninsured and for specialty populations, such as forensic patients referred for evaluation or treatment by the court system.

FUNDING PSYCHIATRIC MENTAL HEALTH CARE

Most U.S. citizens are covered by private insurance that pays varying amounts for mental health care. Standard private insurance policies allow people to choose their own providers and seek treatment and then provide some portion of reimbursement. Managed care plans provide members with a list of health care providers they may visit and then either cover the entire cost or collect co-pays from members. Low-income Medicaid and Medicare recipients may also enroll in managed care plans.

The goal of managed care is to provide coordination of all health services—with an emphasis on preventive care—to control costs. Managed care organizations offer two basic types of health plans. *Health maintenance organizations (HMOs)* provide comprehensive services to members within a defined provider network for a fixed yearly rate and use a primary care physician as the gatekeeper for specialty care. *Preferred provider organizations (PPOs)* give members a choice of providers within a defined network for a fixed co-payment or providers outside the network for a higher co-payment.

Managed behavioral health care organizations (MBHOs) were developed separately, or "carved out," from medical services to provide mental health and substance-abuse treatment. Both private and public (Medicaid) MBHOs monitor psychiatric care through preadmission reviews, continuing treatment authorizations, or retroactive chart reviews.

A program that coordinates services for individual patient care is psychiatric case management. In the inpatient setting, case managers on the hospital team communicate daily or weekly with the patient's insurer and provide the treatment team with guidance regarding the availability of resources. Once the patient returns to the community, multiple levels of intervention are available within case management services, ranging from daily assistance with medications to ongoing resolution of housing and financial issues. Ideally, psychiatric case managers establish enduring relationships with patients, facilitate their involvement in outpatient settings, and access resources, thereby helping to avoid the crises that result in readmission to the acute care hospital.

Mental Health Funding Legislation

Having private insurance is not a guarantee that one will be provided with adequate coverage for mental health care. Insurance companies have skirted coverage by excluding some diagnoses for reimbursement, charging higher co-pays or deductibles, limiting numbers of treatments per year, and placing lifetime caps for mental health care days. In response to this unequal treatment, the U.S. government enacted a mental health parity (equality) law in 1996 that made

it illegal for companies with more than 50 employees to limit annual or lifetime dollar mental health benefits unless they also limited benefits for physical illnesses. While this federal legislation was a good start, problems remained. Insurers and employers got around the law by limiting the number of treatment sessions for psychiatric problems and charging higher co-payments and deductibles.

Mental health advocates and providers pushed for state legislation to shore up the gaps in the federal bill with some success. By 2008, 5 states had adopted parity laws that prohibited exemptions and/or limitations under private insurance plans for mental health and substance-abuse disorders; 7 states had "good" parity laws; 25 states had limited parity laws, and 13 states had no mental health parity laws (National Mental Health Association, 2008).

Finally in 2008, the House and Senate passed landmark legislation that improved mental health and substance coverage for more than a third of Americans (Kaiser Network, 2008). This legislation is called the *Paul Wellstone and Peter Domenici Mental Health and Addiction Equity Act of 2008*. The bill was named for the late Senator Paul Wellstone and Senator Pete Domenici, both long-time advocates for mental health. This new law restricts insurance companies from requiring higher co-payments or imposing higher deductibles for mental health or substance-abuse treatment. If existing state laws are stricter than this federal legislation, the stricter state laws will continue to be upheld.

Uninsured Patients

Since most health insurance is employer-based, and serious mental illness can lead to job loss, many individuals with psychiatric disorders have no coverage. Furthermore, most private insurance plans (along with Medicare) have coverage limits that are more restrictive for treatment of mental illness than other physical illnesses, with annual or lifetime caps on days of care or total expenses.

State systems exist in part as a safety net for the limits in health insurance, and public assistance is available for mental health care and costs of living. Four government assistance programs are Medicare, Medicaid, Social Security, and Veterans Administration benefits. Medicare is a national program that provides benefits to those who are 65 years of age or older and those who have become disabled. In the case of mental illness, benefits are limited, and coverage may be 50% for outpatient mental health care, compared to 80% for non–mental health outpatient care. Medicaid operates under federal guidelines and state regulations and pays mental health care costs for people who have extreme financial need. States vary widely in how they fund mental health care, but all states must provide benefits for inpatient care, physicians' services, and treatment for those under age 21.

Social Security has two federal programs designed to help people with disabilities. Social Security Disability Insurance (SSDI) may be awarded to individuals who have worked a required length of time, have paid into Social Security, and are disabled for 12 months or more. Supplemental Security Income (SSI) provides benefits based on economic need (Social Security Administration [SSA], 2008). More than 60% of children and 50% of adults on SSI have brain disorders (mental illness and/or disability), and the cost of providing disability benefits is projected to escalate rapidly during the next 20 years (Depression and Bipolar Support Alliance, 2006).

For people who have actively served in the armed forces, another federal program that provides comprehensive inpatient and outpatient mental health care is the Veterans Administration (Veterans Administration, 2008). The amount and range of coverage depends on (1) the degree to which the mental health condition is service-related and (2) income criteria.

INPATIENT PSYCHIATRIC MENTAL HEALTH CARE

Entry to Inpatient Care

Although some patients are directly admitted based on a psychiatrist or primary care provider referral, the majority of patients receiving inpatient acute psychiatric care are admitted through the emergency department (ED). The average ED wait time for a patient in need of hospitalization is increasing—in some areas, the wait can be days. Nurses who work on psychiatric units should recognize that patients admitted from the ED may need additional patience and attention. They may have been deprived of medication, treatments, sleep, or proper food.

People with psychiatric symptoms are often isolated and ignored from the outset of their hospitalization. An extreme outcome of excess waiting occurred in 2008. A hospital videotape documents the plight of a 49-year-old woman in a Brooklyn psychiatric hospital who died on the floor of a waiting room and lay there for more than an hour before help was summoned (Hartocollis, 2008).

In the ED, the patient is generally evaluated by an emergency department physician and a social worker who will determine if the patient meets criteria to justify admission. The **admission criteria** to a hospital begin with the premise that the person is suffering from a mental illness, and there is evidence of one or more of the following:

1. Imminent danger of harming self
2. Imminent danger of harming others
3. Unable to care for basic needs, placing individual at imminent risk of harming self

If patients meet the admission criteria, they are then given the option of being admitted on a voluntary basis, which means that they agree with the need for treatment and hospitalization. The vast majority of patient admissions to psychiatric inpatient units are voluntary. If patients do not wish to be hospitalized, but mental health professionals feel that admission is necessary, they can be admitted against their wishes, commonly known as an *involuntary admission.* Involuntarily admitted patients still have rights and can petition the court for release. If the admission is contested, the treating psychiatrist—or in some states the advanced practice registered nurse—must present the case to the court, supporting hospitalization as necessary for the safety of the patient or others and explaining how the patient will benefit from treatment. The court then decides whether or not to continue hospitalization. Chapter 7 discusses legal requirements for admissions, commitment, and discharge procedures in more detail.

VIGNETTE

Shane is a 22-year-old male who was brought to the emergency room by police after expressing thoughts of suicide. He reports having had difficulty sleeping and eating for the past several days and has lost 5 pounds. He is restless and demanding. When approached, he becomes very irritable and threatening to the nurses and physicians, stating that he wants to leave and does not understand why he needs to be here. He states that he was tricked by his mother and brother, who are only trying to have him admitted so they can take his money. He is exhibiting poor judgment, insight, and impulse control. He has been nonadherent with his antipsychotic medication and stopped taking it 3 weeks ago because of side effects.

Shane did not want to be admitted, and despite several attempts by the nursing staff, he continued to refuse hospitalization. The decision was made to involuntarily admit him to the locked psychiatric inpatient unit. On arrival to the inpatient unit, Shane was informed of his rights and the fact that he was involuntarily committed to the unit. ■

Rights of the Hospitalized Patient

Patients admitted to any psychiatric unit retain rights as citizens, which vary from state to state, and are entitled to certain privileges. Laws and regulatory standards require that patients' rights be explained in a timely fashion after an individual has been admitted to the hospital, and that the treatment team must always be aware of these rights. Any infringement by the team during the patient's hospitalization—such as a failure to protect patient safety—must be documented, and actions must be justifiable. All mental health facilities provide a written statement

---

BOX 4-1   Typical Items Included in Hospital Statements of Patients' Rights

- Right to be treated with dignity
- Right to be involved in treatment planning and decisions
- Right to refuse treatment, including medications
- Right to request to leave the hospital, even against medical advice
- Right to be protected against harming oneself or others
- Right to the benefit of the legally prescribed process of an evaluation occurring within a limited period (in most states, 72 hours) in the event of a request for discharge against medical advice that may lead to harm to self or others
- Right to legal counsel
- Right to vote
- Right to communicate privately by telephone and in person
- Right to informed consent
- Right to confidentiality regarding one's disorder and treatment
- Right to choose or refuse visitors
- Right to be informed of research and to refuse to participate
- Right to the least restrictive means of treatment
- Right to send and receive mail and to be present during any inspection of packages received
- Right to keep personal belongings unless they are dangerous
- Right to lodge a complaint through a plainly publicized procedure
- Right to participate in religious worship

---

of patients' rights, often with copies of applicable state laws attached. Box 4-1 provides a sample list of patients' rights, and Chapter 7 offers a more detailed discussion of this issue.

Multidisciplinary Treatment Team

Psychiatric mental health nurses are core members of the multidisciplinary treatment team, a group of professionals and nonprofessionals who work together to provide care (Box 4-2). The full team generally meets within 72 hours of the patient's admission to formulate a full treatment plan. The nurse's role in this process is often to lead the planning meeting. This nursing leadership reflects the holistic nature of nursing, as well as the fact that nursing is the discipline that is represented on the unit at all times. Nurses are in a unique position to contribute valuable information such as continuous assessment findings, the patient's adjustment to the unit, and any health concerns, psychoeducational needs, and deficits in self-care the patient may have.

Ultimately the treatment plan will be the guideline for the patient's care during the hospital stay. It is based on goals for the hospitalization and defines how achievement of the goals will be measured. Input from the patient and family (if available and desirable) is critical in formulating goals. Incorporating the patient's feedback in developing the treatment plan goals increases the likelihood of the success of the outcomes.

Members of each discipline are responsible for gathering data and participating in the planning of care. Newly admitted patients may find this extremely stressful or threatening; team members must consider appropriate timing. The urgency of the need for data should be weighed against the patient's ability to tolerate assessment. Often, assessments made by the intake worker and the nurse provide the basis for initial care. In most settings, the psychiatrist must evaluate the patient and provide orders within a limited timeframe. Medical problems are usually referred to a primary care physician or specialist, who assesses the patient and consults with the unit physicians.

The plan of care reflects a nursing process–based or multidisciplinary path–based approach to care. The latter approach may be in the form of a **multidisciplinary treatment plan** or a **clinical pathway**. Clinical pathways seek to standardize the daily expected outcomes for patients (Rossi, 2003). The team either composes the plan of care or selects the clinical pathway, revising the plan if the patient's progress differs from the expected outcomes. In the managed care environment, it is common for a member of the hospital's case management services, often the social worker, to participate in all treatment planning conferences and daily report meetings to monitor patient progress. The reduction of overt symptoms and development of an adequate outpatient plan signal that discharge is imminent.

VIGNETTE

June is assigned as Shane's primary nurse, and Rachel as his evening shift nurse. June met with the treatment team to plan Shane's care during the hospitalization. The physician's diagnosis was major depression with psychotic features. The major problems the team identified based on reports of the past 2 days and nursing assessments, were safety, paranoia, nonadherence with medications, and hypertension. June identified that the nursing diagnoses were risk for self-directed violence, disturbed thought processes, noncompliance, and deficient knowledge. Along with the treatment team, June identified the nursing education groups that Shane should participate in and recommended that suicide-precaution monitoring should be maintained, owing to Shane's inability to contract for safety. ■

BOX 4-2 Members of the Multidisciplinary Treatment Team

Psychiatric mental health registered nurses: Licensed registered nurses whose focus is on mental health and mental illness and who may or may not be certified in psychiatric mental health nursing. The registered nurse is typically the only 24-hour-a-day, 7-days-a-week professional working in acute care. Among the responsibilities of the registered nurse are diagnosing and treating responses to psychiatric disorders, coordinating care, counseling, giving medication and evaluating responses, and providing education.

Psychiatric mental health advanced practice registered nurses: Licensed registered nurses who are prepared at the master's or doctoral level and hold specialty certification as either clinical nurse specialists or nurse practitioners. These nurses are qualified for clinical functions such as diagnosing psychiatric conditions, prescribing psychotropic medications and integrative therapy, conducting psychotherapy; they are involved in case management, consulting, education, and research.

Social workers: Basic level social workers help the patient prepare a support system that will promote mental health on discharge from the hospital. This includes contacts with day treatment centers, employers, sources of financial aid, and landlords. Licensed clinical social workers undergo training in individual, family, and group therapies, and often are primary care providers.

Counselors: Counselors prepared in disciplines such as psychology, rehabilitation counseling, and addiction counseling may augment the treatment plan by co-leading groups, providing basic supportive counseling, or assisting in psychoeducational and recreational activities.

Psychologists: In keeping with their master's or doctoral degree preparation, psychologists conduct psychological testing, provide consultation for the team, and offer direct services such as specialized individual, family, or marital therapies.

Occupational, recreational, art, music, and dance therapists: Based on their specialist preparation, these therapists assist patients in gaining skills that help them cope more effectively, gain or retain employment, use leisure time to the benefit of their mental health, and express themselves in healthy ways.

Psychiatrists: Depending on their specialty of preparation, psychiatrists may provide in-depth psychotherapy or medication therapy or head a team of mental health providers functioning as a private service based in the community. As physicians, psychiatrists may be employed by the hospital or may hold practice privileges in the facility. Because they have the legal power to prescribe and to write orders, psychiatrists often function as the leaders of the teams managing the care of patients individually assigned to them.

Medical physicians: Medical physicians provide medical diagnosis and treatments on a consultation basis. Occasionally a physician trained as an addiction specialist may play a more direct role on a unit that offers treatment for addictive disease.

Mental health workers: Mental health workers, including nursing assistants, function under the direction and supervision of registered nurses. They provide assistance to patients in meeting basic needs and also help the community to remain supportive, safe, and healthy.

Pharmacists: In view of the intricacies of prescribing, coordinating, and administering combinations of psychotropic and other medications, the consulting pharmacist can offer a valuable safeguard. Physicians and nurses collaborate with the pharmacist regarding new medications, which are proliferating at a steady rate.

Nursing Care

Admission Assessment

Being admitted to a hospital is anxiety-provoking for anyone, and anxiety can be severe for patients admitted to a psychiatric unit. Especially for the first-time patient, admission often summons preconceptions about psychiatric hospitals and the negative stigma associated with them. Patients may experience shame, and families may be reluctant to be forthcoming with pertinent information. Psychiatric mental health nurses can be most effective when they are sensitive to both the patient and family during the traumatizing effect of being hospitalized. In this initial encounter with the patient, psychiatric mental health nurses must try to provide reassurance and hope.

The goal of the admission assessment is to gather information that will enable the treatment team to accurately develop a plan of care, ensure that safety needs are identified and addressed, identify the learning needs of the patient so the appropriate information can be provided, and initiate a therapeutic relationship between the nurse and the patient. Chapter 8 presents a more detailed discussion of how to perform an admission assessment, as well as a mental status

TABLE 4-1   Common Nursing Diagnoses, with Sample Outcomes and Interventions for Patients During Admission to the Acute Care Hospital

Nursing Diagnoses (NANDA International)	Nursing Outcomes Classification (NOC)	Nursing Interventions Classification (NIC)
Risk for other-directed violence: At risk for behaviors in which an individual demonstrates that he or she can be physically, emotionally, and/or sexually harmful to others	*Aggression Self-Control:* Self-restraint of assaultive, combative, or destructive behaviors towards others	*Anger Control Assistance:* Facilitation of the expression of anger in an adaptive, nonviolent manner
Risk for self-directed violence: At risk for behaviors in which an individual demonstrates that he or she can be physically, emotionally, and/or sexually harmful to self	*Suicide Self-Restraint:* Personal actions to refrain from gestures and attempts at killing self	*Behavior Management: Self-Harm:* Assisting the patient to decrease or eliminate self-mutilating or self-abusive behaviors
Disturbed sensory perception (auditory): Change in the amount or patterning of incoming stimuli accompanied by a diminished, exaggerated, distorted, or impaired response to such stimuli	*Communication: Receptive:* Reception and interpretation of verbal and/or nonverbal messages	*Hallucination Management:* Promoting the safety, comfort, and reality orientation of a patient experiencing hallucinations

Data from North American Nursing Diagnosis Association International (2009). *NANDA-I nursing diagnoses: Definitions and classification 2009-2011*. Oxford, United Kingdom: Author.; Moorhead, S., Johnson, M., Maas, M., & Swanson, E. (Eds.). (2008). *Nursing outcomes classification (NOC)* (3rd ed.). St. Louis: Mosby.; and Bulechek, G. M., Butcher, H. K., & Dochterman, J. M. (Eds.). (2008). *Nursing interventions classification (NIC)* (5th ed.). St. Louis: Mosby.

examination. Table 4-1 illustrates common nursing diagnoses, sample nursing interventions, and sample nursing outcomes to guide the nurse in evidence-based practice during a patient's admission for acute psychiatric care.

Ensuring Safety

Safety is one of the most important aspects of care in any inpatient setting. Protecting the patient is essential, but equally important is the safety of the staff and other patients. Safety needs are identified, and individualized interventions begin, on admission. Staff should check all personal property and clothing to prevent any potentially harmful items from being taken onto the unit (e.g., medication, alcohol, sharp objects). Some people are at greater risk of suicide than others, and psychiatric mental health nurses must be skillful in evaluating this risk through questions and observations. Understanding the types of precautions used in the hospital is one of the most important tasks a new staff member or nursing student can learn.

The Joint Commission (TJC), an agency that accredits hospitals, developed National Patient Safety Goals (2009) specific to specialty areas within hospitals to promote improvements in patient safety. Box 4-3 lists safety goals specific to behavioral health care. Centers for Medicare and Medicaid Services (CMMS) have also put more emphasis on patient safety and have iden-

tified several preventable hospital-acquired injuries they will not cover. One example of such an injury is a fracture due to a patient fall. It is likely that other health insurance providers will also begin to limit payment for preventable injuries.

The nurse supervises the unit for overall safety, and one of the most important interventions is tracking patients' whereabouts and activities. These checks are done periodically or continuously, depending upon patients' risk for harming themselves or others. Visitors are another potential safety hazard. Although visitors can contribute to patients' healing through socialization, acceptance, and familiarity, visits may be overwhelming or distressing. Also, visitors may unwittingly or purposefully provide patients with unsafe items; bags and packages should be inspected by unit staff. Sometimes the unsafe items take the form of comfort foods from home or a favorite restaurant and should be monitored because they may be incompatible with diets or medications.

Intimate relationships between patients are generally discouraged or expressly prohibited. There are risks for sexually transmitted diseases, pregnancy, and emotional distress at a time when patients are vulnerable and may lack the capacity for consent.

Aggression and violence may also occur as a result of living in close quarters with reduced outlets for frustration. Psychiatric staff should have specialized

---

BOX 4-3 National Patient Safety Goals in Behavioral Health Care

- Improve the accuracy of patient identification:
  - Use at least two ways to identify patients, such as patient's name and date of birth.
- Improve the effectiveness of communication among caregivers:
  - Read back verbal orders.
  - Create a list of abbreviations and symbols that are not to be used.
  - Promptly report critical tests and critical results.
- Improve the safety of using medications:
  - Create a list of look-alike and sound-alike medications.
- Reduce the risk of health care–associated infections:
  - Use hand cleaning guidelines from the World Health Organization.
  - Record and report death or injury from infection.
- Accurately and completely reconcile medications across the continuum of care:
  - Compare current and newly ordered medications for compatibility.
  - Give a list of medications to the next provider and regular caregiver.
  - Provide a medication list to both the patient and family.
- Encourage patients' active involvement in their own care:
  - Encourage patients and families to report safety concerns.
- Identify safety risks inherent in its patient population:
  - Identify individuals at risk for suicide.

Adapted from The Joint Commission (2009). *Standards improvement initiative.* Retrieved August 1, 2008 from www.jointcommission.org/NR/rdonlyres/BF11F12D-8CE5-442E-B375-CE1E4883FD12/0/BHC_NPSG_Outline.pdf

---

training to minimize hostility while maintaining an atmosphere that promotes healthy and appropriate expression of anger and other feelings. Most units are locked, since some patients are hospitalized involuntarily, and elopement (escape) must be prevented in a way that avoids an atmosphere of imprisonment (see Chapter 7).

One of the most important safety aspects of a psychiatric unit's design is in patient rooms. The rooms are usually less institutional looking than other hospital rooms and tend to resemble hotels. Closets may be equipped with "break-bars" designed to hold a minimal amount of weight, windows are locked, and beds are often platforms rather than mechanical hospital beds that can be dangerous because of their crushing potential. Showers may be in individual rooms or dormitory-style, with one or two per hallway, and have non–weight bearing shower heads.

Physical Health Assessment

The psychiatric mental health nurse is in an excellent position to assess not only mental health but also physical health. Researchers have become increasingly interested in the staggering number of individuals who suffer from combinations of medical and psychiatric illness and recognize the impact the conditions have on one another. For example, depressive symptoms may impair a patient's ability to cope with the added stress of a medical illness and negatively affect follow-up treatment recommendations (Howard et al., 2007).

As discussed previously, access to health care services is problematic for many individuals with psychiatric illnesses. Even if patients with psychiatric disorders have sought health care in the past, medical conditions may have been overlooked or ignored by other health care professionals. Often when patients with preexisting or comorbid conditions seek treatment in the ED for a medical condition, health care providers will downplay or attribute the patient's physical complaints to the psychiatric condition. Patients also report reluctance to seek out health care providers, owing to the stigma they encounter when they reveal they are being treated for a comorbid psychiatric illness. This reluctance to seek treatment not only adversely impacts the patient's quality of life but also contributes to a decreased life expectancy (Miller, et al., 2006).

Milieu Management

Peplau (1989) advocated for the milieu as a therapeutic modality on inpatient units. A well-managed milieu offers patients a sense of security and comfort. Structured aspects of the milieu include activities, unit rules, reality orientation practices, and unit environment. In addition to the structured components of the milieu, Peplau (1989) described other less tangible factors of the milieu, such as the interactions that occur among patients and staff, patients and patients, patients and visitors, and so forth. This is quite different from medical units where patients generally remain in their rooms, often with closed doors, and rarely interact with other patients or the milieu. On psychiatric units, patients are in constant contact with their peers and staff. These interactions help patients engage and can increase the sense of social competence and worth.

The therapeutic milieu can serve as a real-life training ground for learning about the self and practicing communication and coping skills in preparation for a return to the community. Even events that seemingly distract from the program of therapies can be turned into valuable learning opportunities for the members of the milieu. Psychiatric mental health nurses can support the milieu and intervene when necessary. They usually develop an uncanny ability to assess the mood of the unit (e.g., calm, anxious, disengaged, or tense) and predict environmental risk. Nurses observe the dynamics of interactions, reinforce adaptive social skills, and redirect patients during negative interactions. Reports from shift to shift provide information on the emotional climate and level of tension on the unit.

Structured Group Activities

Experienced psychiatric mental health nurses conduct specific, structured activities involving the therapeutic community, special groups, or families on most mental health units. Examples of these activities include morning goal-setting meetings and evening goal-review meetings. Community meetings may be held daily or at other scheduled times of the week. At these meetings, new patients are greeted, and departing patients are given farewells; ideas for unit activities are discussed; community problems or successes are considered; and other business of the therapeutic community is conducted.

Nurses also offer psychoeducational groups for patients and families on topics such as stress management, coping skills, grieving, medication management, and communication skills. Group therapy is a specialized therapy led by a mental health practitioner with advanced training. This therapy addresses communication and sharing, helps patients explore life problems and decrease their isolation and anxiety, and engages patients in the recovery process. Chapter 34 presents a more detailed discussion of therapeutic groups led by nurses.

VIGNETTE

During the evening shift, Rachel observes that Shane is restless and pacing in the hallway. Rachel recalls that when he was admitted, Shane was asked if he had been aggressive in the past. He stated that he had periods of being angry when he felt people were not listening to him or were telling him what to do. Rachel also recalls that Shane said that he has never struck or hit anyone before, and that he usually handles anger by taking a walk around the neighborhood or going to his room.

Rachel asks Shane how things are going. He tells her he is upset because he told the doctor he wanted to be discharged, and the doctor said he was not ready yet. Rachel affirms that this must be frustrating. She suggests that Shane practice some of the relaxation techniques he learned in the coping group today to manage the feelings of anger. Rachel also asks Shane if he would like the medication that has been ordered for feelings of agitation. Shane agrees to a prn medication and to relax in his room until he feels in better control of his anger. Rachel goes back to meet with Shane after 30 minutes. She provides positive feedback about his ability to successfully handle his aggressive feelings. ▪

Documentation

Documentation of patient progress is the responsibility of the entire mental health team. Although communication among team members and coordination of services are the primary goals when choosing a system for charting, practitioners in the inpatient setting must also consider professional standards, legal issues, requirements for reimbursement by insurers, and accreditation by regulatory agencies. Information must also be in a format that is retrievable for quality assurance monitoring, utilization management, peer review, and research. For nursing, the nursing process step of documentation is a guiding concern and is reflected in the different reporting formats commonly found in psychiatric hospitals. Chapter 8 gives an overview of documentation options.

Medication Administration

The safe administration of medications and monitoring their effects is a 24-hour responsibility for the nurse, who is expected to have detailed knowledge of psychoactive medications and the interactions and psychological side effects of other medications. Staff nurse reports regarding the patient's adherence with the medication regimen, the presence or absence of side effects, or changes in the patient's behaviors exert great influence on the physician's or nurse practitioner's medication decisions. For example, feedback about excessive sedation or increased agitation may lead to a decrease or increase in the dosage of an antipsychotic medication.

Psychiatric mental health nurses often have numerous decisions to make about medications that are prescribed to be administered prn (as needed). These decisions must be based on a combination of factors: the patient's wishes, the team's plan, attempts to use alternative methods of coping, and the nurse's judgments regarding timing and the patient's behavior. Documentation for administering each prn medication must include the rationale for its use and the effects.

Medication Adherence. Medication adherence, or compliance, is a common problem for psychiatric patients, often because of side effects. One of the nurse's goals during hospitalization is to assist the patient to learn the importance of medication adherence during and after hospitalization. Educating patients on how to recognize, report, and manage potential side effects can help empower patients and increase treatment success. This approach encourages the patient to seek out the nurse when it is time for medications to be administered and fosters responsibility and involvement in the treatment process.

Pain Management. Just like others in the general population, psychiatric patients often suffer from medical problems that result in pain. Neck, back, and spine problems, arthritis, and migraine headaches are common conditions that result in pain. People with psychiatric conditions are often viewed as being unable to accurately assess their own sensations or are labeled "drug seeking," which results in untreated or undertreated pain. In fact, addressing the issue of pain is so important that The Joint Commission has made pain assessment and pain management a major part of its regulatory evaluation of hospitals.

Beyond humanitarian considerations, pain is a distraction that limits a patient's ability to benefit from hospitalization. A patient in pain is less able to participate in formal activities on the unit and will have greater difficulty focusing on education. Who wants to participate in group therapy when a back injury makes it excruciatingly painful to sit for more than a few minutes? Adequate assessment and treatment of pain within the psychiatric population may actually have a positive impact on the course of mental disorders.

Crisis Management

Medical Crises. Nurses anticipate, prevent, and manage emergencies and crises on the unit. These crises may be of a medical or behavioral nature. Mental health units, whether situated in a general hospital or independent facilities, must be able to stabilize the condition of a patient who experiences a medical crisis. Mental health or addictive disease units that manage detoxification (withdrawal from alcohol or other drugs) must anticipate several common medical crises associated with that process. Mental health units therefore store crash carts containing the emergency medications used to treat shock and cardiorespiratory arrest. Nurses must maintain their cardiopulmonary resuscitation skills and be able to use basic emergency equipment. To be effective and practice at a high level of competency, nurses are advised to attend in-service sessions and workshops designed to teach and maintain skills. Nurses must be able to alert medical support systems quickly and mobilize transportation to the appropriate medical facility.

Behavioral Crises. Behavioral crises can lead to patient violence toward self or others and are usually, but not always, observed to escalate through fairly predictable stages. Crisis prevention and management techniques are practiced by staff in most mental health facilities. Many psychiatric hospitals have special teams made up of nurses, psychiatric aides, and other professionals who respond to psychiatric emergencies called codes. Each member of the team takes part in the team effort to defuse a crisis in its early stages. If preventive measures fail, each member of the team participates in a rapid, organized movement designed to immobilize, medicate, or seclude a patient. The nurse is most often this team's leader, not only organizing the plan but also timing the intervention and managing the concurrent use of prn medications. The nurse can initiate such an intervention in the absence of a physician in most states but must secure a physician's order for restraint or seclusion within a specified time. The nurse also advocates for patients by ensuring that their legal rights are preserved, no matter how difficult their behavior may be for the staff to manage. Refer to Chapters 7 and 25 for further discussions and protocols for use of restraints and seclusion.

Crises on the unit are upsetting and threatening to other patients as well. A designated staff member usually addresses their concerns and feelings. This person removes other patients from the area of crisis and helps them express their fears. Patients may be concerned for their own safety or the welfare of the patient involved in the crisis. They may fear that they too might experience such a loss of control.

Preparation for Discharge to the Community

Discharge planning begins on admission and is continuously modified as required by the patient's condition until the time of discharge. The reduction of overt symptoms and development of an adequate outpatient plan signal that discharge is imminent. As members of the multidisciplinary team, nurses assist patients and their families to prepare for independent or assisted living in the community. Community-based programs provide patients with psychosocial rehabilitation, which moves the mentally ill beyond stabilization toward recovery and a higher quality of life. This is especially important to the concept and practice of managed behavioral health care, which aims to reduce the length and frequency of hospital stays.

Nurses therefore focus on precipitating factors that led to the crisis and hospital admission. Patients are assisted to learn coping skills and behaviors that will help them avert future crises. Psychoeducational groups, individual exploration of options and supports, and on-the-spot instruction (such as during medication administration) offer the patient numerous learning opportunities. Nurses encourage patients to use their everyday experiences on the unit to practice newly learned behavior.

The treatment plan or clinical pathway chosen for the patient should reflect this discharge planning emphasis as early as the day of admission. The patient is expected to begin to progress toward a resolution of acute symptoms, assume personal responsibility, and improve interpersonal functioning. Patients with prolonged mental illness benefit most from a seamless transition to community services. This is facilitated by collaboration with community mental health services and the intensive case management programs available there. Readiness for community reentry should include preparation by members of the patient's support system for their role in enhancing the patient's mental health. Chapter 5 has a more detailed discussion of the nurse's roles in the community setting.

VIGNETTE

Rachel meets with Shane and his mother on the day of discharge to review the aftercare arrangements. Rachel reviews the goals that were established by the treatment team and Shane's own goal for hospitalization. She reviews the accomplishments Shane made during the hospitalization, reinforces the importance of medication adherence, reviews each prescription, highlighting how the medication must be taken each day, and tells Shane when and where the aftercare appointment is scheduled. Rachel answers Shane's and his mother's questions. ■

KEY POINTS TO REMEMBER

- Inpatient care has increasingly become more acute and short-term. Private insurers and a variety of governmental sources fund inpatient psychiatric care.
- Inpatient psychiatric mental health nursing requires strong skills in management, communication, and collaboration.
- The nurse plays a leadership role and also functions as a member of the multidisciplinary treatment team.
- The nurse advocates for the patient and ensures that the patient's rights are protected.
- Monitoring the environment and providing for safety are important components of good inpatient care. Psychiatric mental health nurses are skilled in protecting patients from suicidal impulses and aggressive behavior.
- Basic level nursing interventions include admission, providing a safe environment, psychiatric and physical assessments, milieu management, documentation, medication administration, and preparation for discharge to the community.
- Documentation is an important form of communication to promote consistency in patient care and justify the patient's stay in the hospital.
- Discharge planning begins on the day of admission and requires input from the treatment team and the community mental health provider.

CRITICAL THINKING

1. Imagine that you were asked for your opinion in regards to your patient's ability to make everyday decisions for himself. What sort of things would you consider as you weighed out safety versus autonomy and personal rights?

2. If nurses function as equal members of the multidisciplinary mental health team, what differentiates the nurse from the other members of the team?

3. What effect do managed care plans have on the treatment of patients with mental illness?

4. How might the community be affected when patients with serious mental illness live in group homes? How would you feel about having a group home in your neighborhood?

CHAPTER REVIEW

1. A friend recognizes that his depression has returned and tells you he is suicidal and afraid he will harm himself. He wishes to be hospitalized but does not have health insurance. Which of the following responses best meets his immediate care needs and reflects the options for care a person in his position typically has?
    1. Provide emotional support and encourage him to contact his family to see if they can help him arrange and pay for inpatient care.
    2. Advise him that state hospitals serve persons unable to pay, and immediately accompany him to the nearest state hospital pre-admission evaluation facility.
    3. Help him apply for Medicaid coverage, arrange for him to be monitored by family and friends, and once Medicaid coverage is in place, take him to an emergency room for evaluation.
    4. Assist him to obtain an outpatient counseling appointment at an area community mental health center, and call him frequently to assure he is safe until his appointment occurs.

2. You are about to interview a newly admitted patient on your inpatient mental health unit. This is his first experience with psychiatric treatment. Which of the following interventions would be appropriate for this patient? *Select all that apply.*
    1. Discuss outpatient care options for after discharge.
    2. Anticipate and address possible increased anxiety and shame.
    3. Ensure that the individual understands his rights as a patient on your unit.
    4. Confirm his insurance coverage or other plans for payment of charges.
    5. Assess the patient for physical health needs which may have been overlooked.
    6. Carefully check all clothing and possessions for potentially dangerous items.

3. Which of the following nursing actions is appropriate in maintaining a safe therapeutic inpatient milieu? *Select all that apply.*
   1. Interact frequently with both individuals and groups on the unit.
   2. Ensure that none of the unit fixtures can be used for suicide by hanging.
   3. Initiate and support group interactions via therapeutic groups and activities.
   4. Stock the unit with standard hospital beds and other sturdy hospital furnishings.
   5. Provide and encourage opportunities to practice social and other life skills.
   6. Collaborate with housekeeping to provide a safe, pleasant environment.

4. A patient becomes agitated and hostile, threatening to smash a chair into the nurses station door. Which of the following responses would be most appropriate for the student nurse to take?

1. Maintain a safe distance, and attempt to de-escalate the patient verbally.
2. When the response team arrives, assist in physically restraining the patient.
3. Assist in promptly moving other patients to a safe distance or separate location.
4. Meet with the patient immediately after the crisis to help him process what happened.

5. A student is considering a career in psychiatric nursing. Which of the following statements accurately reflects the role and expectations of psychiatric nurses in acute care settings?
   1. The primary role of the nurse is to monitor the patients from the nurses' station.
   2. Psychiatric patients rarely need medical care, so nurses need fewer medical nursing skills.
   3. The close relationships developed with patients can lead to later romantic relationships.
   4. Psychiatric nursing requires a high degree of interpersonal comfort and therapeutic skill.

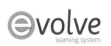

Visit the Evolve website for an **Audio Chapter Summary, Chapter Review Answers & Rationales, Critical Thinking Answer Guidelines,** and additional resources related to the content in this chapter: **http://evolve.elsevier.com/Varcarolis/foundations**

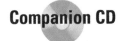

Use the Companion CD to prepare for tests and the NCLEX® Examination with **Test-Taking Strategies** for psychiatric mental health nursing and hundreds of **Review Questions**.

References

Depression and Bipolar Support Alliance. (2006). *The state of depression in America.* Chicago: Author.

Hartocollis, A. (2008 July 2). Video of dying mental patient being ignored spurs changes at Brooklyn Hospital. *New York Times* [online edition]. Retrieved January 23, 2009 from http://www.nytimes.com/2008/07/02/nyregion/02hosp.html

Howard, P., El-Mallakh, P., Rayens, M., & Clark, J. (2007). Comorbid medical illnesses and perceived general health among adult recipients of Medicaid mental health services. *Issues in Mental Health Nursing, 28,* 255–278.

The Joint Commission (2009). *Standards improvement initiative.* Retrieved March 11, 2009 from http://www.jointcommission.org/NR/rdonlyres/BF11F12D-8CE5–442E-B375-CE1E4883FD12/0/BHC_NPSG_Outline.pdf

Kaiser Network. (October 6, 2008). *Administration news: President Bush signs $700b financial bailout bill that includes mental health parity provisions.* Retrieved on October 6, 2008 from http://www.kaisernetwork.org/daily_reports/rep_index.cfm?hint=3&DR_ID=54845

Miller, B., Paschall, C., & Sevenson, D. (2006). Mortality and medical comorbidity among patients with serious mental illness. *Psychiatric Services, 57*(10), 1482–1487.

National Mental Health Association. (2008). *What have states done to ensure insurance parity?* Retrieved July 31, 2008 from http://www.nmha.org/go/parity/states

Owens, P., Myers, M., Elixhauser, A., & Brach, C. (2007). *Care of adults with mental health and substance-abuse disorders in U.S. community hospitals, 2004. HCUP Fact Book No. 10.* AHRQ Publication No. 07-0008, January 2007. Rockville, MD: Agency for Healthcare Research and Quality.

Peplau, H. E. (1989). Interpersonal constructs for nursing practice. In A.W. O'Toole & S. R. Welt (Eds.), *Interpersonal theory in nursing practice: Selected works of Hildegard E. Peplau* (pp. 42–55). New York: Putnam.

Rossi, P. (2003). *Case management in health care* (2nd ed.). Philadelphia: Saunders.

Simon, R. I., & Shuman, D. W. (2008). Psychiatry and the law. In R. E. Hales, S. C. Yudofsky, & G. O. Gabbard (Eds.). *Textbook of psychiatry* (pp. 1555–1959). Arlington, VA: American Psychiatric Publishing.

Social Security Administration. (2008). *Benefits for people with disabilities.* Retrieved January 23, 2009 from http://www.ssa.gov/disability/

Veterans Administration. (2008). *Federal benefits for veterans and dependents.* VA Pamphlet 80-0-01, P94663. Washington, DC: Government Printing Office.

CHAPTER 5

Psychiatric Mental Health Nursing in Community Settings

Avni Cirpili and Nancy Christine Shoemaker

Key Terms and Concepts

assertive community treatment (ACT), 95
barriers to treatment, 97
continuum of psychiatric mental health treatment, 92
decompensation, 92

deinstitutionalization, 88
ethical dilemmas, 97
serious mental illness, 88

Objectives

1. Explain the evolution of the community mental health movement.
2. Identify elements of the nursing assessment that are critically important to the success of community treatment.
3. Explain the role of the nurse as the biopsychosocial care manager in the multidisciplinary team.
4. Discuss the continuum of psychiatric treatment.
5. Describe the role of the community psychiatric mental health nurse in disaster preparedness.

6. Describe the role of the psychiatric nurse in four specific settings: partial hospitalization program, psychiatric home care, assertive community treatment, and community mental health center.
7. Identify two resources to assist the community psychiatric nurse in resolving ethical dilemmas.
8. Discuss barriers to mental health treatment.
9. Examine influences on the future of community psychiatric mental health nursing.

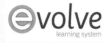 Visit the Evolve website for an **Audio Glossary & Flashcards, Concept Map Creator**, and additional resources related to the content in this chapter: **http://evolve.elsevier.com/Varcarolis/foundations**

Psychiatric mental health nursing in the community began with nurses who specialized in community care who moved about within the community, were comfortable meeting with patients in the home or neighborhood center, were competent to act independently, used professional judgment in unanticipated situations, and possessed knowledge of community resources. The heritage of these nurses can be traced back to European women who cared for the sick at home and American women who organized religious and secular societies during the 1800s to visit the sick in their homes. By 1877, trained nurses worked as public health nurses, visiting the homes of the poor in northeastern cities, and generalist nurses made community visits to rural areas for health promotion and care of the sick (Smith, 1995).

THE EVOLUTION OF PSYCHIATRIC CARE IN THE COMMUNITY

During the 1960s, patients began to leave state hospitals in huge numbers. This was due in part to unprecedented civil rights movements. It is not surprising that the rights of *mental patients* (as they were then called) were part of the focus. Libertarian lawyers called for their freedom, sued states successfully, and forced discharges of patients who later found it extremely difficult to be rehospitalized (Torrey et al., 2007).

Financial pressure on the state system was also a factor in decreasing hospitalization, since inpatients were not eligible for federal assistance, and states were left to pick up the tab. Many hospitals were indeed grossly overcrowded, patients' rights were often disregarded, and seclusion and restraint were overused. Due to the largely custodial nature of inpatient treatment, patients were left with little incentive for growth or participation in their own care.

Finally the introduction of psychotropic drugs, beginning with chlorpromazine (Thorazine), made community living a more realistic option.

In 1963, President John F. Kennedy signed into law the Community Mental Health Centers Act, which stipulated that individuals with mental illness were to be treated in their own communities. The goal of this act was to provide much-needed mental health services while maintaining the individual as an active member of the community in close proximity to families, jobs, and friends. This shifting of patients from hospitals to the community is known as **deinstitutionalization**. Policymakers believed that community care would be more humane and less expensive than hospital-based care.

To provide for formerly institutionalized patients, community mental health centers were formed to serve in catchment areas (specific geographical areas within each state); they often partnered with large state hospitals to assist in aftercare services and crisis management. During the 1960s, several federal entitlement programs were created to assist patients in moving out of institutions and into the community. Programs included Social Security Disability Insurance, Supplemental Security Income, Medicaid, Medicare, housing assistance, and food stamps. The number of public psychiatric beds available in 2005, compared to 1955, was reduced from 340 to 17 per 100,000 in the population (Torrey et al., 2007).

Caring for patients with **serious mental illness** in the community presented many challenges in the early years after deinstitutionalization. At the time, there were few choices for outpatient treatment, usually a community mental health center or therapy in a private office. Government promises to expand funding for community services were not kept, and there were more patients than resources. Many patients with serious mental illness resisted treatment with available providers, and providers began to use scarce resources for the less disabled but more adherent population. Despite these problems, a second wave of deinstitutionalization took place in the 1980s after President Carter's Commission on Mental Health highlighted the needs of this underserved and unserved population.

Currently, optimism for improving lives of people with mental illness has been bolstered by a report from President George W. Bush's New Freedom Commission on Mental Health (U.S. Department of Health and Human Services [UDHHS], 2003), which will provide direction for mental health care in the United States for the next quarter century. The report emphasized that mental illness is not a hopeless life sentence in which people have no control, but rather a condition from which recovery is possible. *Recovery* is described as the ability of the individual to work, live, and participate in the community. It is a journey that provides patients with hope, empowerment, and confidence to take an active role in determining their own treatment paths.

Ideally, recovery would be facilitated by interconnected community agencies that work in harmony to assist consumers of mental health care as they navigate an often confusing system. Realistically, funding has always been an issue in treating people with mental illness, and current economic realities have not done much to improve the situation. Psychiatric mental health nurses may be the answer to transforming an illness-driven and dependency-oriented system into a system that emphasizes recovery and empowerment. Nurses are adept at understanding the system and coordinating care. They "can work between and within systems, connecting services and acting as an important safety net in the event of service gaps" (American Psychiatric Nurses Association [APNA] et al., 2007).

Over the past 30 years—with advances in psychopharmacology and psychosocial treatments—psychiatric care in the community has become more sophisticated, with a continuum of care that provides more settings and options for people with mental illness. The role of the community psychiatric mental health registered nurse has grown to include service provision in a variety of these treatment settings, and nursing roles have developed outside traditional treatment sites.

For example, psychiatric needs are well known in the criminal justice system and the homeless population. The number of individuals suffering from a serious mental illness in the correctional systems is growing, with estimates that approximately 18% of individuals in state prisons suffer from a serious mental illness (Lamb et al., 2007). The community nurse's role is not only to provide care to individuals as they leave the criminal justice system and reenter the community but also to educate police officers and justice staff in how to work with individuals entering the criminal system. The percentage of homeless people with serious mental illness has been estimated to be as high as 15% (Folsom et al., 2005). The challenge to psychiatric mental health nurses is in making contact with these people, who are outside the system but desperately in need of treatment.

To support nurses' interventions, the principles of the public health concept of prevention are useful. *Primary prevention* activities are directed at healthy populations and include providing information and teaching coping skills to reduce stress, with the goal of avoiding mental illness. (A nurse may teach parenting skills in a well-baby clinic.) *Secondary prevention* involves the early detection and treatment of psychiatric symptoms, with the goal of minimizing impairment. (A nurse may conduct screening for depression at a work site.) *Tertiary prevention* involves services that address residual impairments in psychiatric patients in

BOX 5-1 Possible Community Mental Health Practice Sites

Primary Prevention

- Adult and youth recreational centers
- Schools
- Day care centers
- Churches, temples, synagogues, mosques
- Ethnic cultural centers

Secondary Prevention

- Crisis centers
- Shelters (homeless, battered women, adolescents)
- Correctional community facilities
- Youth residential treatment centers
- Partial hospitalization programs
- Chemical dependency programs
- Nursing homes
- Industry/work sites
- Outreach treatment in public places
- Hospices and acquired immunodeficiency syndrome programs
- Assisted living facilities

Tertiary Prevention

- Community mental health centers
- Psychosocial rehabilitation programs

an effort to promote the highest level of community functioning. (A nurse may provide long-term treatment in a clinic.) Box 5-1 presents examples of community practice sites for the psychiatric mental health nurse.

COMMUNITY PSYCHIATRIC MENTAL HEALTH NURSING

Psychiatric mental health nursing in the community setting requires strong problem-solving and clinical skills, cultural competence, flexibility, solid knowledge of community resources, and comfort functioning more autonomously than acute care nurses. Patients need assistance with problems related to individual psychiatric symptoms, family and support systems, and basic living needs, such as housing and financial support. Community treatment hinges on enhancing patient strengths in the same environment daily life is maintained in, which makes individually tailored psychiatric care imperative. Treatment in the community permits patients and those involved in their support to learn new ways of coping with symptoms or situational difficulties. The result can be one of empowerment and self-management for patients and their support systems.

Roles and Functions

As noted in Chapter 1, psychiatric mental health nurses are educated at a variety of levels, including associate, diploma, baccalaureate, master's, and doctoral. Perhaps the most significant distinction among the multiple levels of preparation is the degree to which the nurse acts autonomously and provides consultation to other providers, both inside and outside the particular agency. The nurse practice acts of individual states grant nurses authority to practice, and the Standards of Practice developed by the American Nurses Association—in collaboration with the American Psychiatric Nurses Association and the International Society of Psychiatric-Mental Health Nurses (2007)—also define levels of practice (see Chapter 8). Table 5-1 describes the roles of psychiatric mental health nurses according to level of education.

Biopsychosocial Assessment

Assessment of the biopsychosocial needs and capacities of patients living in the community requires expansion of the general psychiatric mental health nursing assessment (see Chapter 8). To be able to plan and implement effective treatment, the community psychiatric mental health nurse must also develop a comprehensive understanding of the patient's ability to cope with the demands of living in the community. Box 5-2 identifies the areas covered in a biopsychosocial assessment.

Key elements of this assessment are strongly related to the probability that the patient will experience successful outcomes in the community. Problems in any of these areas require immediate attention because they can seriously impair the success of other treatment goals:

- Housing adequacy and stability: If a patient faces daily fears of homelessness, it is not possible to focus on other treatment issues.
- Income and source of income: A patient must have a basic income—whether from an entitlement, a relative, or other sources—to obtain necessary medication and meet daily needs for food and clothing.
- Family and support system: The presence of a family member, friend, or neighbor supports the patient's recovery and gives the nurse a contact person, with the patient's consent.
- Substance abuse history and current use: Often hidden or minimized during hospitalization, substance abuse can be a destructive force, undermining medication effectiveness and interfering with community acceptance and procurement of housing.
- Physical well-being: Factors that increase health risks and decrease life span for individuals with mental illnesses include decreased physical activity, smoking, medication side effects, and lack of routine health exams.

TABLE 5-1   Community Psychiatric Mental Health Nursing Roles Relevant to Educational Preparation

Role	Advanced Practice (MS, PhD)	Basic Practice (Diploma, AA, BS)
Practice	Nurse practitioner or clinical nurse specialist; manage consumer care and prescribe or recommend interventions independently	Provide nursing care for consumer and assist with medication management as prescribed, under direct supervision
Consultation	Consultant to staff about plan of care, to consumer and family about options for care; collaborate with community agencies about service coordination and planning processes	Consult with staff about care planning and work with nurse practitioner or physician to promote health and mental health care; collaborate with staff from other agencies
Administration	Administrative or contract consultant role within mental health agencies or mental health authority	Take leadership role within mental health treatment team
Research and education	Role as educator or researcher within agency or mental health authority	Participate in research at agency or mental health authority; serve as preceptor to undergraduate nursing students

---

BOX 5-2   Elements of a Biopsychosocial Nursing Assessment

- Presenting problem and referring party
- Psychiatric history, including symptoms, treatments, medications, and most recent service utilization
- Health history, including illnesses, treatments, medications, and allergies
- Substance abuse history and current use*
- Family history, including health and mental health disorders and treatments
- Psychosocial history, including:
  ○ Developmental history
  ○ School performance
  ○ Socialization
  ○ Vocational success or difficulty
  ○ Interpersonal skills or deficits
  ○ Income and source of income*
  ○ Housing adequacy and stability*
  ○ Family and support system*
  ○ Level of activity
  ○ Ability to care for needs independently or with assistance
  ○ Religious or spiritual beliefs and practices
- Legal history
- Mental status examination
- Strengths and deficits of the patient
- Cultural beliefs and needs relevant to psychosocial care

*Strongly related to the probability that the patient will experience successful outcomes in the community.

Individual cultural characteristics are also very important to assess. For example, working with a patient who speaks a different language from the nurse requires the nurse to consider the implications of language and cultural background. The use of a translator or cultural consultant from the agency or from the family is essential when the nurse and patient speak different languages (see Chapter 6).

Treatment Goals and Interventions

In the community setting, treatment goals and interventions are negotiated rather than imposed on the patient. To meet a broad range of patient needs, community psychiatric mental health nurses must approach interventions with flexibility and resourcefulness. The complexity of navigating the mental health and social service funding systems is often overwhelming to patients. Not unexpectedly, patient outcomes with regard to mental status and functional level have been found to be more positive and achieved with greater cost effectiveness when the community psychiatric mental health nurse integrates case management into the professional role (Chan et al., 2000).

Differences in characteristics, treatment outcomes, and interventions between inpatient and community settings are outlined in Table 5-2. Note that all of these interventions fall within the practice domain of the basic level registered nurse.

Multidisciplinary Team Member

The concept of using multidisciplinary treatment teams originated with the Community Mental Health Centers Act of 1963. Psychiatric nursing practice was

TABLE 5-2 Characteristics, Treatment Outcomes, and Interventions by Setting

Inpatient Setting	Community Mental Health Setting
CHARACTERISTICS	
Unit locked by staff	Home locked by patient
24-hour supervision	Intermittent supervision
Boundaries determined by staff	Boundaries negotiated with patient
Milieu with food, housekeeping, security services	Patient-controlled environment with self-care, safety risks
TREATMENT OUTCOMES	
Stabilization of symptoms and return to community	Stable or improved level of functioning in community
INTERVENTIONS	
Develop short-term therapeutic relationship.	Establish long-term therapeutic relationship.
Develop comprehensive plan of care, with attention to sociocultural needs of patient.	Develop comprehensive plan of care for patient and support system, with attention to sociocultural needs.
Enforce boundaries by seclusion or restraint as needed.	Negotiate boundaries with patient.
Administer medication.	Encourage adherence with medication regimen.
Monitor nutrition and self-care with assistance as needed.	Teach and support adequate nutrition and self-care with referrals as needed.
Provide health assessment and intervention as needed.	Assist patient in self-assessment, with referrals for health needs in community as needed.
Offer structured socialization activities.	Use creative strategies to refer patient to positive social activities.
Plan for discharge with family/significant other with regard to housing and follow-up treatment.	Communicate regularly with family/support system to assess and improve level of functioning.

identified as one of the core mental health disciplines, along with psychiatry, social work, and psychology. This recognition permitted the allocation of resources to educate psychiatric nurses and emphasized their unique contributions to the team.

In multidisciplinary team meetings, the individual and discipline-specific expertise of each member is recognized. Generally the composition of the team reflects the availability of fiscal and professional resources in the area. Similar to the multidisciplinary team defined in Chapter 4, the community psychiatric team may include psychiatrists, nurses, social workers, psychologists, dual-diagnosis specialists, and mental health workers. Recognition of the ability of nurses to have an equal voice in team treatment planning with other professionals was novel at the time the team approach was implemented in the 1960s. This level of professional performance was later used as a model for other nursing specialties.

The nurse is able to integrate a strong nursing identity into the team perspective. At the basic or advanced practice level, the community psychiatric mental health nurse is in a critical position to link the biopsychosocial and spiritual components relevant to mental health care. The nurse also communicates in a manner that the patient, significant others, and other members of the team can understand. In particular, the management and administration of psychotropic medications have become significant tasks the community nurse is expected to perform.

Biopsychosocial Care Manager

The role of the community psychiatric mental health nurse includes coordinating mental health, physical health, spiritual health, social service, educational service, and vocational realms of care for the mental health patient. The reality of community practice in the new millennium is that few patients seeking treatment have uncomplicated symptoms of a single mental illness. The severity of illness has increased, and it is often accompanied by substance abuse, poverty, and stress. Repeated studies show that people with mental illnesses also have a higher risk for medical disorders than the general population (Robson & Gray, 2007).

The community psychiatric mental health nurse is in an excellent position to assist the team in bridging the gap between the psychiatric and physical needs of the patient. The nurse meets not only with the mental health treatment team but also with the patient's primary care team, serving as the liaison between the two. According to Griswald and colleagues (2005), integrating a nurse case manager to assist patients with primary care needs facilitates greater success with follow-up and adherence with appointments.

The 1980s brought increased emphasis on implementing case management as a core service in treating the patient with serious mental illness. In the private domain, case management, or care management, also found a niche. The intent was to charge case managers with designing individually tailored treatment services for patients and tracking outcomes of care. The new case management included assessing patient needs, developing a plan for service, linking the patient with necessary services, monitoring the effectiveness of services, and advocating for the patient as needed. Newer models have been developed, particularly team concepts, which will be discussed later in this chapter.

Promoting Continuation of Treatment

A significant number of patients treated in the community have problems continuing treatment and following through with prescribed treatments plans, particularly in taking medication. Traditionally these problems have been called *noncompliance*. Many people find this word objectionable, since it implies a medical "paternalism" (i.e., the patient is treated as a child who needs to be told what to do). Deegan and Drake (2006) contend that there are actually two experts involved in the care of people with mental illnesses. One is the healthcare professional—who has advanced skills and training in psychiatric disorders—and the other is the consumer of care—who has intimate knowledge of the disorder and its response to treatment. Shared decision making is the key to improving treatment adherence and success.

To share decision making, a patient must be knowledgeable about the illness and treatment options. Research demonstrates that people with mental illness want more than watered-down and simplistic information. (Imagine a pamphlet entitled, "You and Your Mental Illness.") To fully participate in the treatment plan, patients need current, evidence-based information about their illness and treatment options (Tanenbaum, 2008).

A successful life in the community is more likely when medications are taken as prescribed. Nurses are in a position to help the patient manage medication, recognize side effects, and be aware of interactions among drugs prescribed for physical illness and mental illness. Patient-family education and behavioral strategies, in the context of a therapeutic relationship

with the clinician, have been shown to significantly increase adherence with the medication regimen (Lacro & Glassman, 2004).

Evolving Venues of Practice

Many community psychiatric mental health nurses originally practiced on site at community mental health centers, but practice locations have evolved because of financial, health care, regulatory, cultural, and population changes. Nurses are providing primary mental health care at therapeutic day care centers, schools, partial hospitalization programs, and shelters. In addition to these more traditional environments for care, psychiatric mental health nurses are also entering forensic settings and drug and alcohol treatment centers.

Mobile mental health units have been developed in some service areas. In a growing number of communities, mental health programs are collaborating with other health or community services to provide integrated approaches to treatment. A prime example of this is the growth of dual-diagnosis programming at both mental health and chemical dependency clinics.

Technology contributes to the change of venues for providing community care. Telephone crisis counseling, telephone outreach, and the Internet are being used to enhance access to mental health services. Although face-to-face interaction is still preferred, technology has the potential to improve support, confidence, and health status among mental health consumers (Akesson et al., 2007).

Figure 5-1 presents the **continuum of psychiatric mental health treatment**. Movement along the continuum is fluid, from higher to lower levels of intensity, and changes are not necessarily step by step. Upon discharge from acute hospital care or a 24-hour supervised crisis unit, many patients need intensive services to maintain their initial gains or to "step down" in care. Failure to follow up in outpatient treatment increases the likelihood of rehospitalization and other adverse outcomes (Kruse & Rohland, 2002).

Other patients with a preexisting community treatment team may return directly to their community mental health center or psychosocial rehabilitation program. Homeless patients may be referred to a shelter with linkage to intensive case management or assertive community treatment. Patients with a substantial substance abuse problem may be transferred directly into a residential treatment program (see Chapter 18). It is also notable that patients may pass through the continuum of treatment in the reverse direction; that is, if symptoms do not improve, a lower-intensity service may refer the patient to a higher level of care in an attempt to prevent total **decompensation** (deterioration of mental health) and hospitalization.

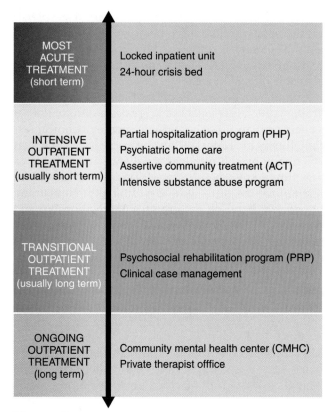

MOST ACUTE TREATMENT (short term)	Locked inpatient unit 24-hour crisis bed
INTENSIVE OUTPATIENT TREATMENT (usually short term)	Partial hospitalization program (PHP) Psychiatric home care Assertive community treatment (ACT) Intensive substance abuse program
TRANSITIONAL OUTPATIENT TREATMENT (usually long term)	Psychosocial rehabilitation program (PRP) Clinical case management
ONGOING OUTPATIENT TREATMENT (long term)	Community mental health center (CMHC) Private therapist offfice

Figure 5-1 The continuum of psychiatric mental health treatment.

COMMUNITY SETTINGS

Four different community psychiatric settings are described in the following sections, with examples of basic-level nursing interventions in each:

- Counseling—assessment interviews, crisis intervention, problem solving in individual, group, or family sessions
- Promotion of self-care activities—fostering grooming, instruction in use of public transportation, budgeting (The nurse may directly assist as necessary in home settings.)
- Psychobiological interventions—medication administration, teaching relaxation techniques, promotion of sound eating and sleep habits
- Health teaching—medication use, illness characteristics, coping skills, relapse prevention
- Case management—communication with family, significant others, and other health care or community resource personnel to coordinate an effective plan of care

Partial Hospitalization Programs

Partial hospitalization programs (PHPs) offer intensive, short-term treatment similar to inpatient care, except that the patient is able to return home each day. Criteria for referral to a PHP include the need for prevention of hospitalization for serious symptoms

or step-down from acute inpatient treatment *and* the presence of a responsible relative or caregiver who can assure the patient's safety (Shoemaker, 2000). Referrals come from inpatient or outpatient providers. Patients receive 5 to 6 hours of treatment daily, and programs operate 5 days a week, with some programs operating on weekends. The average length of stay is approximately 2 to 3 weeks, depending on the program, and the multidisciplinary team consists of at minimum a psychiatrist, RN, and social worker.

The following vignette illustrates a typical day for a psychiatric mental health nurse in a PHP.

VIGNETTE

Michael Sanders is a nurse in a PHP that is part of the only community mental health center in this region, which includes one state hospital and one private inpatient unit. Michael is the nurse member of the multidisciplinary team, and today his schedule is as follows.

8:30-9:00: Michael arrives at the PHP and meets with the team to review the patients expected to arrive in the program today. He prepares to meet with the patients who are scheduled for medication review with the psychiatrist. He also prepares the teaching outline for her medication group.

9:00-10:00: Michael meets with eight patients to teach them how to manage their medication regimen and how to talk with the psychiatrist about any concerns. Throughout the session, Michael assesses each patient's understanding of the prescribed medications and any concerns that have arisen.

10:00-10:30: Michael reviews the cases of three newly admitted patients. He is responsible for reviewing the medical history and confirming the medication list for each. In addition, he has met with the two patients who were instructed to bring their medication with them so that he could directly observe them taking their medications.

10:30-11:30: Michael conducts an intake interview with a newly admitted patient. Ms. Brown is a 50-year-old woman with a history of major depression who was hospitalized for 1 week after a drug overdose following an argument with her boyfriend. Michael completes the standardized interview form, paying extra attention to risk factors for suicide. When asked about substance abuse, Ms. Brown admits that she has been drinking heavily for the past 2 years, including the night she took the drug overdose. When the interview is completed, the patient is referred to the psychiatrist for a diagnostic evaluation.

12:30-2:00: Michael meets with each patient scheduled to meet with the psychiatrist. He reviews the cases with the psychiatrist and ensures that the patients understand any changes in the medication regimens.

2:00-2:30: Michael has a discharge meeting with Mr. Jones, a 48-year-old man with a diagnosis of schizophrenia. He was referred to the PHP by his clinic therapist to prevent hospitalization due to increasing paranoia and agitation. After 2 weeks in the PHP, he has restabilized and recognizes that he must be adherent with his antipsychotic medication regimen. Michael finalizes Mr. Jones's medication teaching and confirms his aftercare appointments with his previous therapist and psychiatrist.

2:30-3:00: To ensure Ms. Brown's safety, Michael meets with her again before she goes home, assessing her suicide risk potential. Michael also shares the preliminary individual treatment plan and begins a discussion of resources for alcohol treatment, including Alcoholics Anonymous.

3:00-4:30: Michael meets with the team for daily rounds. He presents Ms. Brown, and the team develops an individual treatment plan. In this treatment plan, the team notes discharge planning needs for referrals to a community mental health center and alcohol treatment program. As a critical member of the treatment team, Michael reviews the remaining cases and makes needed adjustments to their treatment plans. He completes his notes and discharge summary. He also makes case-management telephone calls to arrange for community referrals, communicate with families, and report to managed behavioral care programs for utilization review. ∎

Psychiatric Home Care

Psychiatric home care was defined by Medicare regulations in 1979 as requiring four elements: (1) homebound status of the patient, (2) presence of a psychiatric diagnosis, (3) need for the skills of a psychiatric registered nurse, and (4) development of a plan of care under orders of a physician. Other payers besides Medicare also authorize home care services.

Homebound refers to the patient's inability to leave home independently to access community mental health care because of physical or mental conditions. Patients are referred to psychiatric home care following an acute inpatient episode—either psychiatric or somatic—or to prevent hospitalization. The psychiatric mental health nurse visits the patient 1 to 3 times per week for approximately 1 to 2 months and usually sees 5 or 6 patients daily. By going to the patient's home, the nurse is better able to address the concerns of access to services and adherence with treatment. With the growing number of older adults being treated in the community for psychiatric and medical issues, the role of psychiatric home care is becoming even more important.

Family members or significant others are closely involved in most cases of psychiatric home care. Because many patients are older than 65, there are usually concurrent somatic illnesses to assess and monitor. The nurse acts as case manager to coordinate all specialists involved in the patient's care (e.g., physical therapist, occupational therapist, and home health aide). The nurse is supervised by an advanced practice registered nurse (APRN) team leader who is always available by telephone.

Boundaries become important in the home setting. Walking into a person's home creates a different set of dynamics than those commonly seen in a clinical setting. It may be important for the nurse to begin a visit informally by chatting about patient family events or accepting refreshments offered. This interaction can be a strain for the nurse who has difficulty maintaining boundaries between the professional relationship and a personal one. However, there is great significance to the therapeutic use of self in such circumstances to establish a level of comfort for the patient and family.

The following vignette illustrates a typical day for a psychiatric mental health registered nurse conducting home care.

VIGNETTE

Monica Castillo is a registered nurse employed by a home care agency in a large rural county. She visits patients in a radius of 50 miles from her home and has daily telephone contact with her supervisor. She stops by the office weekly to drop off paperwork and attends the team meeting once a month. The team includes her team leader, other field nurses, a team psychiatrist consultant, and a social worker. Monica chooses to make her visits from 8:00 AM until 3:30 PM and then completes her documentation at home.

8:00-9:00: Monica's first patient is Mr. Johnson, a 66-year-old man with a diagnosis of major depression after a stroke. He was referred by his primary care physician because of suicidal ideation. Monica has met with Mr. Johnson and his wife 3 times a week for the past 2 weeks. He has contracted for safety and has been adherent in his antidepressant regime. Today she teaches the couple about stress-management techniques. Case-management responsibilities for Mr. Johnson include supervision of the home health aide, who helps him with hygiene, and coordination with the physical and occupational therapists that also treat him.

9:30-11:30: Monica has an intake interview scheduled with Ms. Barker, a 45-year-old single woman with a diagnosis of schizophrenia. Ms. Barker lives with her mother and was referred by an inpatient psychiatrist following an involuntary hospitalization for repeatedly calling 911 with bizarre reports of violence in her backyard. Ms. Barker was nonadherent with her medication plan and appointments prior to being hospitalized. Monica completes the extensive structured intake interview, including the mother's feedback. She teaches them about the new antipsychotic medication Ms. Barker is taking and sets up the weekly medication box. Monica explains that she will visit 2 times a week for the next

2 months. Her case-management role will include assisting Ms. Barker to keep the scheduled appointment and referral to a family support group for the mother.

12:30-1:30: Monica sees Mrs. Graves, a 62-year-old widow diagnosed with major depression after the death of her husband and a move into an assisted living facility. Ms. Graves has diabetes and is wheelchair bound due to an amputation. She was referred by the nurse director of the assisted living facility. Monica has met with her 2 times a week for the past 4 weeks, teaching about depression, grief, medications, and coping skills. Today her focus is on identifying a new social system, including increased contact with long-distance relatives, social activities at the facility, and spiritual support. With input from the director, Monica learns of a grief-counseling group run by a pastoral counselor at the local church and recommends that resource to Mrs. Graves.

2:00-3:00: Monica's last patient for the day is Mr. Cooper, a 55-year-old single man with a diagnosis of panic disorder with agoraphobia. Mr. Cooper lives with his older brother and was referred by his brother's primary care physician after the physician found out that the patient had not been out of the house for 5 years since the death of his mother. Monica has been working with Mr. Cooper for 7 weeks and has decreased visits to once a week. She has taught Mr. Cooper about his illness, medication, and relaxation techniques. He has progressed to being able to walk outside for 15 minutes at a time. Today's plan is to attempt riding in the car with his brother for 10 minutes, in preparation for discharge when he will have to ride for 30 minutes to reach the community mental health center.

Following this visit, Monica returns home to complete documentation, call in a report to her team leader and the physicians, and make other case-management telephone contacts for community referrals. ▪

Assertive Community Treatment

Assertive community treatment (ACT) is an intensive type of case management developed in response to the community-living needs of people with serious, persistent psychiatric symptoms and patterns of repeated hospitalization for services such as emergency room and inpatient care (Minzenberg et al., 2008). Patients are referred to ACT teams by inpatient or outpatient providers because of a pattern of repeated hospitalizations with severe symptoms, along with an inability to participate in traditional treatment. ACT teams work intensively with patients in their homes or in agencies, hospitals, and clinics—whatever settings patients find themselves in. Creative problem solving and interventions are hallmarks of care provided by mobile teams. The ACT concept takes into account that people need support and resources after 5:00 PM; teams are on call 24 hours a day.

ACT teams are multidisciplinary and typically composed of psychiatric mental health registered nurses, social workers, psychologists, APRNs, and psychiatrists. One of these professionals (often the registered nurse) serves as the case manager and may have a case load of 10 patients who require visits 3 to 5 times per week. The nurse is usually supervised by an APRN or psychiatrist. Length of treatment may extend to years until the patient is ready to accept transfer to a more structured site for care.

The following vignette illustrates a typical day for a psychiatric mental health registered nurse on an ACT team.

VIGNETTE

Maria Rodriguez is a nurse who works on an ACT team at a large, inner-city, university medical center. She had 5 years of inpatient experience before joining the ACT team, and she works with two social workers, two psychiatrists, and a mental health worker. She is supervised by an APRN.

8:00-9:00: Maria starts the day at the clinic site with team rounds. Because she was on call over the weekend, she updates the team on three emergency department visits: two patients were able to return home after she met with them and the emergency department physician; one patient was admitted to the hospital because he made threats to his caregiver.

9:30-10:30: Maria's first patient is Mr. Donaldson, a 35-year-old man with a diagnosis of bipolar disorder and alcohol dependence. He lives with his mother and has a history of five hospitalizations with nonadherence to outpatient clinic treatment. Except during his manic episodes, he isolates himself at home or visits a friend in the neighborhood, at whose house he drinks excessively. Today he is due for his biweekly decanoate injection (a long-acting antipsychotic medication). Maria goes first to his house and learns that he is not at home. She speaks with his mother about his recent behavior and an upcoming medical clinic appointment. Then she goes to the friend's house and finds Mr. Donaldson playing cards and drinking a beer. He and his friend are courteous to her, and Mr. Donaldson cooperates in receiving his injection. He listens as Maria repeats teaching about the risks of alcohol consumption. She encourages his attendance at an Alcoholics Anonymous meeting. He reports that he did go to one meeting yesterday. Maria praises him and encourages him and his friend to go again that night.

11:00-1:00: The next patient is Ms. Abbott, a 53-year-old single woman with a diagnosis of schizoaffective disorder and hypertension. She lives alone in a senior-citizen building and has no contact with family. Ms. Abbott was referred by her clinic team because she experienced three hospitalizations for psychotic decompensation over a period of a year, despite receiving monthly decanoate injections. The ACT team is now the payee for her Social Security check. Today Maria has to take Ms. Abbott out to pay her bills and go to her primary care physician for a checkup. Ms. Abbott greets Maria warmly at the door, wearing excessive makeup and inappropriate summer clothing. With gentle encouragement, she agrees to wear warmer clothes. She is reluctant to show Maria her medication box and briefly gets irritable when Maria points out that she has not taken her morning medications. As they stop by the apartment office to pay the rent, Maria talks with the manager briefly. This apartment manager is the team's only contact person and calls the team whenever any of the other residents report that Ms. Abbott is exhibiting unusual behavior. Over the next hour and a half, Maria and Ms. Abbott drive to various stores and Ms. Abbott's somatic appointment.

2:00-4:30: The last patient visit of the day is with Mr. Hunter, a 60-year-old widowed man diagnosed with schizophrenia and cocaine dependence. Mr. Hunter was referred by the emergency department last year after repeated visits due to psychosis and intoxication. Initially he was homeless, but he now lives in a recovery house shelter and has been clean of illegal substances for 6 months. He receives a monthly decanoate injection and is socially isolated in the house. Now that he receives Social Security Disability Insurance, he is seeking an affordable apartment. Maria has made appointments at two apartment buildings. After greeting him, Maria notes that he is wearing the same clothes he had on 2 days earlier, and his hair is uncombed. She suggests that he shower and change his clothes before they go out, and he agrees.

At the end of the day, Maria jots down information she will use to write her progress notes in patients' charts the next day when she returns to the clinic. ▪

Community Mental Health Centers

Community mental health centers were created in the 1960s and have since become the main resource for those who have no access to private mental health care. The range of services available at such centers varies, but generally they provide emergency services, adult services, and children's services. Common treatments include medication administration, individual therapy, psychoeducational and therapy groups, family therapy, and dual-diagnosis treatment. A clinic may also be aligned with a **psychosocial rehabilitation program** that offers a structured day program, vocational services, and residential services. Some community mental health centers have an associated intensive case management service to assist patients in finding housing or obtaining entitlements.

Community mental health centers also utilize multidisciplinary teams. The psychiatric mental health nurse may carry a caseload of 60 patients, each of whom is seen one to four times a month. The basic level nurse

is supervised by an APRN. Patients are referred to the clinic for long-term follow-up by inpatient units or other providers of outpatient care at higher intensity levels. Patients may attend the clinic for years or be discharged when they improve and reach desired goals.

The following vignette illustrates the typical day for a nurse in a community mental health center.

VIGNETTE

Amanda Jordan is a registered nurse at a community mental health center. She is on the adult team and carries a caseload of patients diagnosed with chronic mental illness. She is supervised by an APRN.

8:30-9:00: Upon arriving at the clinic, Amanda receives a voicemail message from Ms. Thompson, who is crying and says she is out of medication. Amanda consults with the psychiatrist and calls Ms. Thompson to arrange for an emergency appointment later that day.

9:00-9:30: Amanda's first patient is Mr. Enright, a 35-year-old man diagnosed with schizophrenia, who has been in treatment at the clinic for 10 years. During their 30-minute counseling session, Mary assesses Mr. Enright for any exacerbation of psychotic symptoms (he has a history of grandiose delusions), eating and sleep habits, and social functioning in the psychosocial rehabilitation program that he attends 5 days a week. Today he presents as stable. Mary gives Mr. Enright his decanoate injection and schedules a return appointment for a month from now, reminding him of his psychiatrist appointment the following week.

10:00-11:00: Amanda co-leads a medication group with a psychiatrist. This group consists of seven patients with chronic schizophrenia who have been attending biweekly group sessions and receiving decanoate injections for the past 5 years. She leads the group discussion, and the psychiatrist writes prescriptions for each patient because most of the members also take oral medication. Today Amanda asks the group to explain relapse prevention to a new member. She teaches significant elements, including adherence with the medication regimen and healthy habits. As group members give examples from their own experiences, she assesses each patient's mental status. At the end of the meeting, she administers injections and gives members appointment cards for the next group session. After the patients leave, she meets with the psychiatrist to evaluate the session and discuss any necessary changes in treatment.

11:00-12:00: Amanda documents progress and medication notes, responds to telephone calls, and prepares for the staff meeting.

12:00-2:00: All adult team staff attends the weekly intake meeting, at which new admissions are discussed and individual treatment plans are written with team input. Amanda presents a patient in intake, reading from the standardized interview form. She also gives nursing input about treatment for the other five newly admitted patients. The new patient she presented is assigned to her, and she plans to call him later in the afternoon to set up a first appointment.

2:00-3:00: Amanda co-leads a dual-diagnosis therapy group with the dual-diagnosis specialist, who is a social worker. The group is made up of seven patients who have concurrent diagnoses of substance abuse and a major psychiatric illness. The leaders take a psychoeducational approach, and today's planned topic is teaching about the physical effects of alcohol on the body. Amanda focuses on risks associated with the interaction between alcohol and medications and answers the members' questions. Because this is an ongoing group, members take a more active role, and discussion may vary according to members' needs instead of following planned topics. After the session, the co-leaders discuss the group dynamics and write progress notes.

3:30-4:00: Amanda meets with Ms. Thompson, who arrives at the clinic tearful and agitated. Ms. Thompson says that she missed her appointment this month because her son died suddenly. Amanda uses crisis intervention skills to assess Ms. Thompson's status (e.g., any risks for her safety related to her history of suicidal ideation). After helping Ms. Thompson clarify a plan to increase support from her family, Amanda notes that insomnia is a new problem. She takes Ms. Thompson to the psychiatrist covering "emergency prescription time" and explains the change in the patient's status. The psychiatrist refills Ms. Thompson's usual antidepressant and adds a medication to aid sleep. Amanda makes an appointment for the patient to return to see her in 1 week instead of the usual 1 month and also schedules her to meet with her assigned psychiatrist that same day.

4:00-4:30: Amanda completes all notes, makes necessary telephone calls to other staff in the psychosocial rehabilitation program who are working with her patients, and phones her new patient to schedule an appointment. ■

DISASTER PREPAREDNESS

In the last decade, we have seen several disasters that have tested community mental health systems across the United States. Educators now believe that all nurses need core competencies in emergency preparedness to be ready for natural and human-created disasters (Edwards et al., 2007). Following a disaster, the immediate goal is to ensure that shelter, food, and first aid are provided. Then the community mental health nurse provides crisis management for victims and volunteers who have arrived to assist in the relief efforts. After the crisis passes, the community psychiatric mental health nurse must find those individuals whose care was disrupted and help them to link back into the system. The nurse administers "psychological first aid" by assisting victims to meet basic needs, listening to

individuals who need to share their stories, directing individuals to agencies that can help, and providing compassion and appropriate hope. After hurricane Katrina, survivors with mental illnesses often went untreated because of disruption of existing services and failure to initiate services (Wang et al., 2008). Chapter 23 offers a more detailed discussion of crisis and disaster.

ETHICAL ISSUES

As community psychiatric mental health nurses assume greater autonomy and accountability for the care they deliver, ethical concerns become a more pressing issue. **Ethical dilemmas** are common in disciplines and specialties that care for the vulnerable and disenfranchised.

Psychiatric mental health nurses have an obligation to develop a model for assessing the ethical implications of their clinical decisions. Each incident requiring ethical assessment is somewhat different, and the individual nurse brings personal insights to each situation. The role of the nurse is to act in the best interests of the patient and of society, to the degree that this is possible.

In most organizations that employ nurses, there is a designated resource for consultation regarding ethical dilemmas. For example, hospitals (with associated outpatient departments) are required by regulatory bodies to have an ethics committee to respond to clinicians' questions. Home care agencies or other independent agencies may have an ethics consultant in the administrative hierarchy of the organization. Professional nursing organizations and even boards of nursing can be used as a resource by the individual practitioner. Refer to Chapter 7 for an in-depth discussion of ethical guidelines for nursing practice.

FUTURE ISSUES

Barriers to Treatment

Despite the current availability and variety of community psychiatric treatments in the United States, many patients in need of services still do not receive them because of various **barriers to treatment**. The National Survey on Drug Use and Health in 2007 estimated that 24.3 million adults had serious psychological distress (U.S. Department of Health and Human Services, 2007). Less than half, however, received treatment in 2007.

The stigma of mental illness has lessened over the past 40 years, in part because mental illnesses are recognized as biologically-based, and many well-known people have come forward to admit that they have received psychiatric treatment. Yet many people still are afraid to admit to a psychiatric diagnosis. Instead, they seek medical care for vague somatic complaints from primary care providers, who too often fail to diagnose anxiety or depressive disorders.

In addition to stigma, there are geographic, financial, and systems factors that impede access to psychiatric care. Mental health services are scarce in some rural areas, and many families cannot afford health insurance even if they are working. The New Freedom Commission on Mental Health (USDHHS, 2003) identified national system and policy problems, including fragmented care for children and adults with serious mental illness, high unemployment and disability among those with serious mental illness, undertreatment of older adults, and lack of national priorities for mental health and suicide prevention. Parity in reimbursement for services provided by community mental health care providers will decrease the gap in insurance coverage between mental health and other health coverage.

Nursing Education

A baccalaureate degree is preferred in more autonomous community settings and will become increasingly in demand as the trend away from hospital-based acute care settings continues. However, educators believe that non-BSN nurses also should be trained to meet the challenges of providing community care. Clinical experiences in community settings are valuable for all nursing students; they increase cultural sensitivity, teaching skills, and an appreciation for strong multidisciplinary teams (Sensenig, 2007).

Community psychiatric mental health nursing is a specialty area in transition. As this specialty area develops, competence-based position descriptions and scope-of-practice guidelines will be vital to ensuring that nurses with diverse levels of education (including licensed practical nurses) are performing appropriate tasks and functions (Kudless, 2007).

Nurses who elect to work with older psychiatric patients with increasingly complex health care needs will be in demand as the population ages. As with other populations and other types of care, there will be pressure to expand the proportion of community-based psychiatric care (Ryan et al., 2006). Community psychiatric mental health nurses may collaborate more with primary health care practitioners to fill the gap in existing community services. This problem is particularly acute in rural areas where psychiatrists are scarce (Hanrahan & Hartley, 2008). Certainly, community psychiatric mental health nurses need to be committed to teaching the public about resources for mental health care for long-term, serious mental illness or for short-term, situational stress.

KEY POINTS TO REMEMBER

- Community psychiatric mental health nursing has historical roots dating to the 1800s and has been significantly influenced by public policies.

- Deinstitutionalization brought promise, as well as problems, for people with chronic, serious mental illness.
- The basic level community psychiatric mental health nurse practices in many traditional and nontraditional sites.
- In the multidisciplinary team, the community psychiatric mental health nurse functions as a biopsychosocial care manager.
- The continuum of psychiatric treatment includes numerous community treatment alternatives with varying degrees of intensity of care.
- The community psychiatric mental health nurse needs access to resources to address ethical dilemmas encountered in clinical situations.
- There are still barriers to mental health care that the community psychiatric mental health nurse may be able to diminish through daily practice.

CRITICAL THINKING

1. You are a nurse working at a local community mental health center. During an assessment of a 45-year-old single, male patient, he reports that he has not been sleeping and that his thoughts seem to be "all tangled up." Although he does not admit directly to being suicidal, he remarks, "I hope that this helps today, because I don't know how much longer I can go on like this."

   He is disheveled and has been sleeping in homeless shelters. He has little contact with his family and becomes agitated when you suggest that it might be helpful to contact them. He reports a recent hospitalization at the local veterans hospital and previous treatment at a dual-diagnosis facility, yet he denies substance abuse. When asked about his physical condition he says that he has tested positive for hepatitis C and is "supposed to take" multiple medications that he cannot name.

   A. List your concerns about this patient in order of priority.
   B. Which of these concerns must be addressed before he leaves the clinic today?
   C. Do you feel there is an immediate need to consult with any other members of the multidisciplinary team today about this patient?
   D. Keeping in mind that the patient must always be an active part of his own care, how will you start to develop trust with the patient to gain his cooperation with the treatment plan?

CHAPTER REVIEW

1. Which of the following factors contribute to the movement of patients out of large state institutions and into community-based mental health treatment? *Select all that apply.*
   1. States desire to save money by moving the patients to the community, where the federal government would pick up more of the cost.
   2. The growing availability of generous mental health insurance coverage gave more patients the ability to seek private care in the community.

3. A system of coordinated and accessible community care was developed by forward-thinking communities and offered more effective treatment.

4. The Community Mental Health Centers Act of 1963 required states to develop and offer care in community-based treatment programs.

5. Patient advocates exposed deficiencies of state hospitals and took legal actions, leading to the identification of a right to treatment in the least restrictive setting.

6. New psychotropic medications controlled symptoms more effectively, allowing many patients to live and receive care in less restrictive settings.

2. You are a community mental health nurse meeting with a patient who has just been discharged from the hospital where he had received his first episode of psychiatric care. Which of the following activities would you expect to undertake in your role as the nurse on the treatment team caring for this patient?
1. Take medications to the patient's home each day and administer them.
2. Solve day-to-day problems for the patient to minimize his exposure to stress.
3. Refer him to counselors or other providers when he indicates a need to talk with someone.
4. Take a ride on the local bus system with the patient to help him learn routes and schedules.

3. A nurse providing in-home mental health care enjoys working with Mr. Jones, an elderly man suffering from depression since the loss of his wife and a recent below-knee amputation that has left him homebound. A fondness develops between the two, with the nurse reminding Mr. Jones of his daughter when she was young, and the patient reminding the nurse of her grandfather. Mr. Jones begins to offer the nurse small statues and other trinkets that had belonged to his wife and seem of little monetary value. She tries to decline, but he persists with each visit and seems hurt when she does not accept the items. Which of the following responses is most appropriate and professional?

1. Agree to accept one, and only one, small token gift to appease the patient.
2. Continue to decline the gifts while helping him find other ways to express his feelings.
3. Consult with her supervisor or designated ethics resource person about what to do next.
4. Identify Mr. Jones's efforts as a boundary violation and request not to be assigned to him.

4. Mr. Johnson has been hospitalized twice in 5 years with a severe, chronic psychiatric disorder. He responds well to inpatient and community treatment and is usually stable, but he also has a history of becoming socially withdrawn and failing to provide for his self-care needs in the months following inpatient care. Hospital staff feel he no longer needs inpatient care but do feel that he needs a higher level of care than the typical periodic outpatient appointments at a community mental health center would provide. He is not homebound, has access to transportation and secure housing, and has a supportive family. Given these circumstances, which of the following programs would the nurse suggest for Mr. Johnson immediately after discharge?
1. Psychiatric home care
2. Partial hospitalization program
3. Assertive Community Treatment
4. Mobile mental health program

5. Mrs. Smith, a patient at the community mental health center, tends to stop taking her medications at intervals, usually leading to decompensation. Which of the following interventions would most likely improve her adherence to her medications?
1. Help Mrs. Smith to understand her illness and share in decisions about her care.
2. Advise Mrs. Smith that if she stops her medications, her doctor will hospitalize her.
3. Arrange for Mrs. Smith to receive daily home care so her use of medications is monitored.
4. Discourage Mrs. Smith from focusing on side effects and other excuses for stopping her pills.

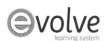

Visit the Evolve website for an **Audio Chapter Summary, Chapter Review Answers & Rationales, Critical Thinking Answer Guidelines,** and additional resources related to the content in this chapter: **http://evolve.elsevier.com/Varcarolis/foundations**

Companion CD   Use the Companion CD to prepare for tests and the NCLEX® Examination with **Test-Taking Strategies** for psychiatric mental health nursing and hundreds of **Review Questions.**

References

Akesson, K. M., Saveman, B. I., & Nilsson, G. (2007). Health care consumers' experiences of information communication technology: A summary of literature. *International Journal of Medical Informatics, 76*, 633–645.

American Psychiatric Nurses Association, International Society of Psychiatric-Mental Health Nurses, & American Nurses Association. (2007). *Psychiatric-mental health nursing: Scope and standards of practice.* Silver Spring, MD: NurseBooks.org.

Chan, S., Mackenzie, A., & Jacobs, P. (2000). Cost-effectiveness analysis of case management versus a routine community care organization for patients with chronic schizophrenia. *Archives of Psychiatric Nursing, 14*(2), 98–104.

Deegan, P. E., & Drake, R. E. (2006). Shared decision making and medication management in the recovery process. *Psychiatric Services, 57*, 1636–1639.

Edwards, D., Williams, L. H., Scott, M. A., & Beatty, J. (2007). When disaster strikes: Maintaining operational readiness. *Nursing Management, 38*(9), 64–66.

Folsom, D. P., Hawthorne, W., Lindamer, L., Gilmer, T., Bailey, A., Golshan, S., et al. (2005). Prevalence and risk factors for homelessness and utilization of mental health services among 10,340 patients with serious mental illness in a large public mental health system. *American Journal of Psychiatry, 162*, 370–376.

Griswald, K., Servoss, T., Leonard, K., Pastore, P., Smith, S., Wagner, C., et al. (2005). Connections to primary care after psychiatric crisis. *Journal of the American Board of Family Practice, 18*(3), 166–172.

Hanrahan, N. P., & Hartley, D. (2008). Employment of advanced-practice psychiatric nurses stem rural mental health workforce shortages. *Psychiatric Services, 59*, 109–111.

Kruse, G. R., & Rohland, B. M. (2002). Factors associated with attendance at a first appointment after discharge from a psychiatric hospital. *Psychiatric Services, 53*, 473–476.

Kudless, M. W. (2007). Competencies and roles of community mental health nurses. *Journal of Psychosocial Nursing, 45*(5), 36–44.

Lacro, J., & Glassman, R. (2004). Medication adherence. *Medscape Psychiatry & Mental Health, 9*(1), 1–4. <http://www.medscape.com>

Lamb, H., Weinberger, L., Marsh, J., & Gross, B. (2007). Treatment prospects for persons with severe mental illness in an urban county jail. *Psychiatric Services, 58*, 782–786.

Minzenberg, M. J., Yoon, J. H. & Carter, C. S. (2008). Schizophrenia. In R. E. Hales, S. C. Yudofsky, & G. O. Gabbard (Eds.), *Textbook of psychiatry* (5th ed., pp. 407–456). Arlington, VA: American Psychiatric Publishing.

Robson, D., & Gray, R. (2007). Serious mental illness and physical health problems: A discussion paper. *International Journal of Nursing Studies, 44*, 457–466.

Ryan, R., Garlick, R., & Happell, B. (2006). Exploring the role of the mental health nurse in community mental health care for the aged. *Issues in Mental Health Nursing, 27*(1), 91–105.

Sensenig, J. A. (2007). Learning through teaching: Empowering students and culturally diverse patients at a community-based nursing care center. *Journal of Nursing Education, 46*, 373–379.

Shoemaker, N. (2000). The continuum of care. In V. B. Carson (Ed.), *Mental health nursing: The nurse-patient journey* (2nd ed., pp. 368–387). Philadelphia: Saunders.

Smith, C. M. (1995). Origins and future of community health nursing. In C. M. Smith & F. A. Maurer (Eds.), *Community health nursing: Theory and practice* (pp. 30–52). Philadelphia: Saunders.

Tanenbaum, S. J. (2008). Consumer perspectives on information and other inputs to decision-making: Implications for evidence-based practice. *Community Mental Health Journal,* 2008 April 10. [Epub ahead of print]. PMID18401710. <http://www.ncbi.nlm.nih.gov/pubmed/18401710>

Torrey, E. F., Entsminger, K., Gellar, J., Stanley, J., & Jaffe, D. J. (2007). *The shortage of public hospitals for mentally ill persons: A report by the Treatment Advocacy Center.* Retrieved January 23, 2009 from http://www.psychlaws.org/Reportbedshortage.htm

U. S. Department of Health and Human Services. (2003). *New freedom commission on mental health. Achieving the promise: Transforming mental health care in America. Final Report* [DHHS Pub. No. SMA–03–3832]. Rockville, MD: Author

U.S. Department of Health and Human Services. (2007). *Results from the 2007 national survey on drug use and health: National findings.* Retrieved September 28, 2008 from http://www.oas.samhsa.gov/nsduh/2k7nsduh/2k7Results.cfm#8.1.1

Wang, P., Gruber, M., Powers, R., Schoenbaum, M., Speier, A., Wells, K., et al. (2008). Disruption of existing mental health treatments and failure to initiate new treatment after hurricane Katrina. *American Journal of Psychiatry, 165*, 34–41.

CHAPTER 6

Cultural Implications for Psychiatric Mental Health Nursing

Rick Zoucha and Mary Curry Narayan

Key Terms and Concepts

acculturation, 111
assimilation, 111
cultural competence, 112
culture, 102
culture-bound syndromes, 109
Eastern tradition, 104
enculturation, 106
ethnicity, 102
ethnocentrism, 106

ethnopharmacology, 110
indigenous culture, 104
minority status, 102
race, 102
refugee, 111
somatization, 109
stereotyping, 113
Western tradition, 103
worldview, 102

Objectives

1. Explain the importance of culturally relevant care in psychiatric mental health nursing practice.
2. Discuss potential problems in applying Western psychological theory to patients of other cultures.
3. Compare and contrast Western nursing beliefs, values, and practices with the beliefs, values, and practices of patients from diverse cultures.

4. Perform culturally sensitive assessments that include risk factors and barriers to quality mental health care that culturally diverse patients frequently encounter.
5. Develop culturally appropriate nursing care plans for patients of diverse cultures.

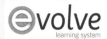 Visit the Evolve website for an **Audio Glossary & Flashcards, Concept Map Creator**, and additional resources related to the content in this chapter: **http://evolve.elsevier.com/Varcarolis/foundations**

According to Mental Health: Culture, Race, and Ethnicity—a 2001 report issued by the U.S. Surgeon General—cultural, racial, and ethnic minorities in America have not had the same access to quality mental health services as white Americans (U.S. Department of Health and Human Services [USDHHS], 2001). This report identifies culturally inappropriate services as one of the reasons minority groups in America do not receive and/or benefit from needed mental health services.

Psychiatric mental health nurses must practice **culturally relevant nursing** if we are to meet the needs of culturally diverse patients. The goal of nursing is to promote health and well-being, and if we are to achieve this goal, mental health providers must strive to provide care that is as congruent as possible with patients' cultural beliefs, values, and practices—keeping in mind that certain cultural practices (e.g., sweat lodges, sun ceremonies, witchcraft) may be impractical, harmful, or even illegal. This kind of **culturally competent care** has been given other names: culturally appropriate care, culturally comfortable care, culturally sensitive care, and culturally congruent care. But whatever the name, *effective* care calls for adapting psychiatric mental health nursing assessments and interventions to each patient's cultural needs and preferences.

This chapter focuses on culture and how it affects the mental health and care of patients with mental illness. In this chapter you will learn about:

- Culture, race, ethnicity, minority status, and how they are related
- Demographic shifts, which make it essential that mental health nurses know how to provide culturally competent care
- The impact of cultural worldviews on mental health nursing
- Variations in cultural beliefs, values, and practices that affect mental health and care of patients with mental health problems
- Barriers to providing quality mental health services to culturally diverse patients
- Culturally diverse populations at increased risk of developing mental illness
- Techniques for providing culturally competent care to diverse populations

CULTURE, RACE, ETHNICITY, AND MINORITY STATUS

The 2001 Surgeon General's report discussed culture, race, and ethnicity in relation to minority groups (USDHHS, 2001). Although the definitions of these terms distinguish them from one another, they are related.

Minority status is connected more with economic and social standing in society than with cultural identity. However, many cultural, racial, and ethnic minority groups are also economically and socially disadvantaged groups.

Culture comprises the shared beliefs, values, and practices that guide a group's members in patterned ways of thinking and acting. Culture can also be viewed as a blueprint for guiding actions that impact care, health, and well-being (Leininger & McFarland, 2006). Culture is more than ethnicity and social norms; it includes religious, geographic, socioeconomic, occupational, ability- or disability-related, and sexual orientation–related beliefs and behaviors. Each group has cultural beliefs, values, and practices that guide its members in ways of thinking and acting. **Cultural norms** help members of the group make sense of the world around them and make decisions about appropriate ways to relate and behave. Because cultural norms prescribe what is "normal" and "abnormal," culture helps develop concepts of mental health and illness.

Ethnic groups have a common heritage and history (**ethnicity**). These groups share a **worldview**, a system for thinking about how the world works and how people should behave in it and in relationship to one another. From this worldview, they develop beliefs, values, and practices that guide members of

the group in how they should think and act in different situations.

Acknowledging the inadequacy of describing minority groups according to a single biological **race**, the U.S. Census Bureau will continue to use the 2000 census combined race-ethnicity categorization system for the 2010 census. Respondents are first asked whether they are of Hispanic, Latino, or Spanish origin; if not, they are asked to further identify their race. Federally defined racial groups will be expanded from six categories in 2000 to sixteen in 2010 (U.S. Census Bureau, 2008a). Respondents who do not identify with any of the predefined categories are encouraged to use blank spaces provided to classify their race (Figure 6-1).

The purpose of categorizing individuals according to racial-ethnic descriptions is to help the government understand the needs of its citizens. The Surgeon General used data from the 2000 census classification system to identify disparities in mental health care along racial-ethnic lines. Recording these classifications also helps to determine when and how the health care needs of these populations are being met.

Despite the benefits, this convention of classifying groups of people can be confusing, confounding, and offensive. Consider the following:

Is Person 1 of Hispanic, Latino, or Spanish origin?
- ☐ No, not of Hispanic, Latino, or Spanish origin
- ☐ Yes, Mexican, Mexican Am., Chicano
- ☐ Yes, Puerto Rican
- ☐ Yes, Cuban
- ☐ Yes, another Hispanic, Latino, or Spanish origin — *Print origin, for example, Argentinean, Columbian, Dominican, Nicaraguan, Salvadoran, Spaniard, and so on.*

A

What is Person 1's race? *Mark ☒ one or more boxes.*
- ☐ White
- ☐ Black, African Am., or Negro
- ☐ American Indian or Alaska Native — *Print name of enrolled or principal tribe.*

- ☐ Asian Indian
- ☐ Chinese
- ☐ Filipino
- ☐ Other Asian — *Print race, for example, Hmong, Laotian, Thai, Pakistani, Cambodian, and so on.*

- ☐ Japanese
- ☐ Korean
- ☐ Vietnamese

- ☐ Native Hawaiian
- ☐ Guamanian or Chamorro
- ☐ Samoan
- ☐ Other Pacific Islander — *Print race, for example, Fijian, Tongan, and so on.*

- ☐ Some other race — *Print race.*

B

Figure 6-1 Race-ethnicity categorizations to be included in the 2010 U.S. Census. **A,** Respondents are first asked if they are of Hispanic, Latino, or Spanish origin. **B,** Respondents are asked to further identify their race.

- Each racial group contains multiple ethnic cultures. There are over 560 Native American and Alaskan tribes and over 40 countries in Asia and the Pacific Islands. The cultural norms of blacks or African Americans whose ancestors were brought to the United States centuries ago as slaves are very different from the norms of those who have recently immigrated from Africa or the Caribbean. Americans of European origin are a diverse group, some of whom have been in the United States for hundreds of years and some of whom are new immigrants.
- The Latino-Hispanic group is a cultural group based on a shared language, but all its members are also members of a racial group or groups (white, black, and/or Native American) and may include Mexican Americans, Puerto Ricans, and Cuban Americans, just to name a few.
- People from the Middle East and the Arabian subcontinent are considered "white" in the classification system.
- Although children of multiracial, multicultural, multiheritage marriages fall into more than one category, their unique identity is not distinguished and sometimes viewed as invisible.

Categorizing people according to a racial-ethnic system carries inherent problems. In psychiatric mental health nursing, we can assess patients further and make better decisions on their behalf if our focus is on *culture* rather than race.

DEMOGRAPHIC SHIFTS IN THE UNITED STATES

In 2006, about one in three Americans was a minority (U.S. Census Bureau, 2007). Hispanics have surpassed African Americans (who make up about 13.4% of the population) as the largest minority group and now constitute about 15% of the population. The United States is 5% Asian and 1.5% Hawaiian or other Pacific Islander.

The U.S. Census Bureau predicts that by the year 2042, no single racial-ethnic group will hold a majority population position, and more than half of Americans will be members of a minority group (Table 6-1). With these changing demographics, every psychiatric mental health nurse will care for culturally diverse patients. We need to know how to provide culturally relevant care and help reduce the problem of mental health disparities among culturally diverse populations.

WORLDVIEWS AND PSYCHIATRIC MENTAL HEALTH NURSING

Nursing theories, psychological theories, and the understanding of mental health and illness used by

TABLE 6-1 Year 2050 Population Projections (Percentage of Total Population)*

	2008	2050
White, non-Hispanic	66	46
Black, non-Hispanic	13	13
Hispanic (of any race)	15	30
Asian	4	8
All other races	3	5

*Population percentages are rounded to the nearest 1%.
Shortly after the year 2050, the white, non-Hispanic population will represent less than 46% of the United States population. The Hispanic and Asian populations are growing at the fastest rates.
Data from U.S. Census Bureau. (August 14, 2008). *U.S. interim projections by age, sex, race, and Hispanic origin.* <http://www.census.gov/population/www/projections/summarytables.html> Accessed 10.09.08.

nurses in the United States have all grown out of a Western philosophical and scientific framework, which is in turn based on Western cultural ideals, beliefs, and values. Because psychiatric mental health nursing is grounded in Western culture, consider how your core assumptions about personality development, emotional expression, ego boundaries, and interpersonal relationships affect your nursing care of any patient.

A long history of Western science and European-American norms for mental health has shaped present-day American beliefs and values about people. Our understanding of how a person relates to the world and to other people are based on Greek, Roman, and Judeo-Christian thought. Other Western scientists and philosophers, such as Descartes (credited with the Western concept of body-mind dualism), have contributed to the Western scientific tradition. Nursing knowledge of psychology, development, and mental health and illness is based on this tradition.

However, a vast number of people throughout the world have very different philosophical histories and traditions from those of Western cultures (Table 6-2). The Eastern cultures of Asia are based on the philosophical thought of Chinese and Indian philosophers and the spiritual traditions of Confucianism, Buddhism, and Taoism. Diverse cultures found among Native Americans, African tribes, Australian and New Zealand aborigines, and tribal peoples on other continents frequently include rich cultural traditions based on deep personal connections to the natural world and the tribe.

In the **Western tradition**, one's identity is found in one's individuality, which inspires the valuing of autonomy, independence, and self-reliance. Mind and

TABLE 6-2 Worldviews

World cultures have grown out of different worldviews and philosophical traditions. Worldview shapes how cultures perceive reality, the person, and the person in relation to the world and to others. Worldview also shapes perceptions about time, health and illness, and rights and obligations in society. The three worldviews compared here are broad categories and generalizations created to contrast some of the themes found in diverse world cultures. They do not necessarily fit any particular cultural group.

Western (Science)	Eastern (Balance)	Indigenous (Harmony)
Roman, Greek, Judeo-Christian; the Enlightenment; Descartes.	Chinese and Indian philosophers: Buddha, Confucius, Lao-tse.	Deep relationship with nature.
The "real" has form and essence; reality tends to be stable.	The "real" is a force or energy; reality is always changing.	The "real" is multidimensional; reality transcends time and space.
Cartesian dualism: body and mind-spirit.	Mind-body-spirit unity.	Mind, body, and spirit are considered so united that there may not be words to indicate them as distinct entities.
Self is starting point for identity.	Family is starting point for identity.	Community is starting point for identity—a person is only an entity in relation to others. The self does not exist except in relation to others. There may be no concept of person or personal ownership.
Time is linear.	Time is circular, flexible.	Time is focused on the present.
Wisdom: preparation for the future.	Wisdom: acceptance of what is.	Wisdom: knowledge of nature.
Disease has a cause (pathogen, toxin, etc.) that creates the effect; disease can be observed and measured.	Disease is caused by a lack of balance in energy forces (e.g., yin-yang, hot-cold); imbalance between daily routine, diet, and constitutional type (Ayurveda).	Disease is caused by a lack of personal, interpersonal, environmental, or spiritual harmony; thoughts and words can shape reality; evil spirits exist.
Ethics of rights and obligations: Based on the individual's right *Value given to:* Right to decide Right to be informed Open communication Truthfulness	*Ethics of care:* Based on promoting positive relationships *Value given to:* Sympathy, compassion, fidelity, discernment Action on behalf of those with whom one has a relationship Persons in need of health care considered to be vulnerable and to require protection from cruel truth	*Ethics of community:* Based on needs of the community *Value given to:* Contribution to community

© 2002, 2004 by Mary Curry Narayan.

body are seen as two separate entities, so different practitioners treat disorders of the body and the mind. Disease is considered to have a specific, measurable, and observable cause, and treatment is aimed at eliminating the cause. Time is seen as linear, always moving forward, and waiting for no one. Success in life is obtained by preparing for the future.

Eastern tradition, however, sees the family as the basis for one's identity, so that family interdependence and group decision making are the norm.

Body-mind-spirit are seen as a single entity; there is no sense of separation between a physical illness and a psychological one (Chan et al., 2006). Time is seen as circular and recurring, as in the belief in reincarnation. One is born into an unchangeable fate, with which one has a duty to comply. For the Chinese, disease is caused by fluctuations in opposing forces—the yin-yang energies.

The term **indigenous culture** refers to those people who have inhabited a country for thousands of years and includes such groups as New Zealand Maoris, Australian aborigines, American natives, and native Hawaiians. These groups place special significance on the place of humans in the natural world and frequently manifest a more dramatic difference from Western views (Cunningham & Stanley, 2003). Frequently, the basis of one's identity is the tribe. There may be no concept of person; instead, a person is an entity only in relation to others. The holism of body-mind-spirit may be so complete that there may be no adequate words in the language to describe them as separate entities. Disease is frequently seen as a lack of harmony of the individual with others or the environment.

Psychiatric mental health nursing theories and methods are themselves part of a cultural tradition and our nursing care is a culturally derived set of interventions designed to promote verbalization of feelings, teach individually focused coping skills, and assist patients with behavioral and emotional self-control—all consistent with Western cultural ideals. When nurses understand that many of the concepts and methods found in psychiatric mental health nursing are based on different assumptions than those of our patients, we have begun the process of becoming *culturally competent*.

CULTURE AND MENTAL HEALTH

Diverse cultures have evolved from the three broad categories of worldview described in the previous section. Cultures develop norms consistent with their worldviews and adapted to their own historical experiences and the influences of the "outside" world. Cultures are not static; they change and adjust, although usually very slowly. Each culture has different patterns of nonverbal communication (Table 6-3), etiquette norms (Box 6-1), beliefs and values that shape the culture

TABLE 6-3 Selected Nonverbal Communication Patterns

People perceive very strong messages from nonverbal communication patterns. However, the same nonverbal communication pattern can mean very different things to different cultures, as this table indicates. This table does not provide an exhaustive list of possible differences.

Nonverbal Communication Pattern	Predominate Patterns in the United States	Patterns Seen in Other Cultures
Eye contact	Eye contact is associated with attentiveness, politeness, respect, honesty, and self-confidence.	Eye contact is avoided as a sign of rudeness, arrogance, challenge, or sexual interest.
Personal space	*Intimate space:* 0-1½ ft *Personal space:* 1½-3 ft In a personal conversation, if a person enters into the intimate space of the other, the person is perceived as aggressive, overbearing, and offensive. If a person stays more distant than expected, the person is perceived as aloof.	Personal space is significantly closer or more distant than in U.S. culture. *Closer*—Middle Eastern, Southern European, and Latin American cultures *Farther*—Asian cultures When closer is the norm, standing very close frequently indicates acceptance of the other.
Touch	Moderate touch indicates personal warmth and conveys caring.	Touch norms vary. *Low-touch cultures*—Touch may be considered an overt sexual gesture capable of "stealing the spirit" of another or taboo between women and men. *High-touch cultures*—People touch one another as frequently as possible (e.g., linking arms when walking or holding a hand or arm when talking).
Facial expressions and gestures	A nod means "yes." Smiling and nodding means "I agree." Thumbs up means "good job." Rolling one's eyes while another is talking is an insult.	Raising eyebrows or rolling the head from side to side means "yes." Smiling and nodding means "I respect you." Thumbs up is an obscene gesture. Pointing one's foot at another is an insult.

BOX 6-1 Norms of Etiquette

People tend to feel offended when their rules for "polite" behavior are violated. However, the rules for polite behavior vary greatly from one culture to another. Unless we are aware of cultural differences in etiquette norms, we could infer rudeness on the part of a patient who is operating from a different set of cultural norms and believes his or her behavior is respectful.

Norms of etiquette that vary across cultures include:

- Whether "promptness" is expected and how important it is to be on time
- How formal one should be in addressing others
- Which people deserve recognition and honor and how respect is shown
- Whether shaking hands and other forms of social touch are appropriate
- Whether or not shoes can be worn in the home
- How much clothing must be worn to be "modest"
- What it means to accept or reject offers of food or drink and other gestures of hospitality
- What importance is given to "small talk" and how long it should continue before "getting down to business"
- Whether communication should be direct and forthright or circuitous and subtle
- What the tone of voice and pace of the conversation should be
- Which topics are considered taboo
- Whether or not the children in the home can be touched and admired

(Table 6-4), and beliefs, values, and practices that influence how the culture understands health and illness (Table 6-5). For instance, in American culture, eye contact is a sign of respectful attention, but in many other cultures, it may be considered arrogant and intrusive. In Western culture, emotional expressiveness is valued, but in many other cultures, it may be a sign of immaturity. In American culture, independence and self-reliance are encouraged, and the family interdependence valued by other cultures may be seen as a symbiotic relationship, or a pathological *enmeshment*.

The culture's worldview, beliefs, values, and practices are transmitted to its members in a process called enculturation. As children, we learn from our parents which behaviors, beliefs, values, and actions are "right" and which are "wrong." The individual is free to make choices, but the culture expects these choices to be made from its acceptable range of options.

Deviance from cultural expectations is considered to be a problem and frequently is defined by the cultural group as "illness." Mental health is often seen as the degree to which a person fulfills the expecta-

tions of the culture. The culture defines which differences are still within the range of normal (mentally healthy) and which are outside the range of normal (mentally ill).

The same thoughts and behaviors considered mentally healthy in one culture can be considered mentally ill in another. For example, many religious traditions view "speaking in tongues" as mentally healthy and a gift from God, whereas a different cultural group might consider this same behavior as psychosis and a sign of mental illness. Considering culture creates challenges for the psychiatric mental health nurse. And even if the nurse and patient agree the patient has a mental health problem, they may advocate very different ways of treating it.

All people are raised to view the world and everything in it through their own cultural lens, and nurses are no exception. We are products of our culture of professional socialization. Nurses may be tempted to think that the only "good care" is the care they have learned to believe in, value, and practice. However, this can lead to ethnocentrism, the universal tendency of humans to think their way of thinking and behaving is the only correct and natural way (Purnell, 2008). Most people are, to a certain degree, ethnocentric; but as nurses, we must examine our assumptions about other cultures to give the best and most culturally competent care possible. Imposing cultural norms on members of other cultural groups is known as **cultural imposition** (Leininger & McFarland, 2006).

BARRIERS TO QUALITY MENTAL HEALTH SERVICES

The first part of this chapter focused on the impact of culture on mental health and illness in a theoretical way. In the following sections, you will learn about some practice issues that nurses are likely to encounter when providing care to culturally diverse patients. You will also learn ways to overcome these barriers.

Communication Barriers

Therapeutic communication is key to the nursing care of patients with mental illness, yet often nurses and patients do not even speak the same language. The USDHHS Office of Minority Health (2007) states that health care organizations must offer and provide language assistance services, including an interpreter, at no cost to each patient with limited English proficiency at all points of contact and in a timely manner during all hours of operation and service. Patients with **limited English proficiency** are those who cannot speak English or do not speak English well enough to meet their communication needs.

TABLE 6-4 Cultural Belief and Value Systems

This table contrasts cultural beliefs and values that are predominant in the United States with those that are common in various other world cultures. Belief and value systems are best viewed as a continuum. The beliefs and values of cultures, and of the individuals within cultures, fall at various points along the continuum.

Predominant Culture Patterns and Concepts in the United States	Patterns and Concepts in Various Other Cultures
Individualism Independence, self-reliance Autonomy, autonomous decision making	Familism Interdependence of family Interconnectedness Family decision making
Egalitarianism—everyone has an equal voice and deserves equal opportunities	Social hierarchy—some deserve more honor or power than others because of their age, gender, occupation, or role in the family; family hierarchies can be patriarchal or matriarchal.
Youth Physical beauty	Age Wisdom
Competition Achievement Materialistic orientation Possessions	Cooperation Relationships Metaphysical orientation Spirituality, nature, relationships
Reason and logic Doing and activity	Meditation and intuition Being and receptivity
Mastery over nature Latest technology	Harmony with nature Natural, traditional ways
Master of one's fate—"I am the master of my destiny." Optimism Internal locus of control: life events and circumstances are the result of one's actions	Fate is one's master—"Fate is responsible for my destiny." Fatalism External locus of control: life events and circumstances are beyond one's own control and rest in the hands of fate, chance, other people, or God
Future orientation—"He who prepares for tomorrow will be successful." Punctuality ("clock time")—"Time waits for no one." "Time flies." "Time is money." Being on time is a sign of courtesy and responsibility.	Present orientation—"Live for today and let tomorrow take care of itself." Past orientation—tradition "People time"—time is flexible, indefinite; "Time starts when the group gathers." "Time walks. *El tiempo anda.*" Being on time can be a sign of compulsiveness and disregard for the people one was with before the appointment time.

© 2000, 2004 by Mary Curry Narayan.

When a professional interpreter is engaged, the interpreter should be matched to the patient as closely as possible in gender, age, social status, and religion. In addition to interpreting the language, the interpreter can alert the nurse to the meaning of nonverbal communication patterns and cultural norms that are relevant to the encounter. In this way, the interpreter acts as a **cultural broker**, interpreting not only the language but also the culture.

Interpreters should not be relatives or friends of the patient. The stigma of mental illness may prevent the openness needed during the encounter. Also, those close to the patient may not have the language skills necessary to meet the demands of interpretation, which is a very complex task. Languages frequently cannot be translated word for word; the literal translations of words in one language can carry many different connotations in the other language, and certain concepts are so culturally linked that an adequate translation is very difficult.

Even people who speak English very well may have difficulty communicating emotional nuances in English; these may be more accessible to patients in their own languages. Idioms and figures of

TABLE 6-5 Cultural Beliefs and Values About Health and Illness

This table contrasts the views typically held by Western nurses and the views about health and illness their patients from diverse cultures may hold.

	Western Biomedical Perspective	Perspective of Various Other Cultures
Health	Absence of disease Ability to function at a high level	Being in a state of balance Being in a state of harmony Ability to perform family roles
Disease causation	Measurable, observable cause that leads to measurable, observable effect Pathogens, mutant cells, toxins, poor diet	Frequently intangible, immeasurable cause Lack of balance (yin and yang) Lack of harmony with environment
Location of disorder	Body Mind	Whole entity: mind, body, and spirit are completely merged Disorder causing disease in the person may be in the family or environment
Decisions about care	Made by patient or holder of power of attorney Goals are autonomy and confidentiality Truth telling required so patient has information to make decisions	Made by the whole family or family head Goals are protection and support of patient Hope should be preserved; patient should be protected from painful truth
Sick role	Sick people should be as independent and self-reliant as possible Self-care is encouraged; one gets better by "getting up and getting going"	Sick people should be as passive as possible Family members should "take care of" and "do for" the sick person Passivity stimulates recovery
Best treatments	Physician-prescribed drugs and treatments Advanced medical technology	Regaining of lost balance or harmony by counteracting negative forces with positive ones and vice versa Treatment by folk healers and traditional remedies
Pain	Stoicism valued Pain described quantitatively Able to pinpoint location of pain In cultures in which negative feelings are not expressed freely, pain is kept as silent as possible: Northern European, Asian, Native American	Pain expressed vocally and dramatically Use of quantitative scales to measure pain is difficult Pain experienced globally In cultures in which emotional expression is encouraged, more dramatic pain expression is expected: Southern European, African, Middle Eastern
Ethics	Based on bioethical principles of autonomy, beneficence, justice, and confidentiality Informed consent requires truthfulness	Based on virtue or community needs Hope should be preserved, painful truth hidden Support and care should be provided Emphasis is on greatest good for the greatest number

© 2002, 2004 by Mary Curry Narayan.

speech can be extremely confusing. For instance, the terms *feeling blue* or *feeling down* may have no meaning at all in the patient's literal understanding of English.

Nonverbal communication patterns may also be influenced by culture. Some Native American cultures use silence to a far greater degree than the dominant culture, and their silence can be mistaken for belligerence or sullenness, when in fact it is a common response to dealing with strangers and is even considered a sign of wisdom. The downcast eyes of an Asian woman may be viewed as a sign of evasiveness, when it is actually a sign of respect. Nonverbal communication patterns must be interpreted from within the patient's cultural perspective, not from the Western medical perspective (Munoz & Luckmann, 2005).

Stigma of Mental Illness

Mental illnesses are highly stigmatized disorders. Many people, in all sectors of society in the United States, associate mental illness with moral weakness. Others express fear of, or bias against, those with mental health problems. However, in many cultural groups, the stigma of mental illness is more severe and prevalent than it generally is in the United States.

In cultural groups that emphasize the interdependence and harmony of the family, mental illness may be perceived as a failure of the family. In such groups, the pressures on both the individual with the mental illness and the family are increased. Not just the individual is perceived as ill, but the whole family—and the illness reflects badly on the character of all family members. Stigma and shame can lead to reluctance to seek help, so members of these cultural groups may enter the mental health care system at an advanced stage, when the family has exhausted its ability to cope with the problem.

Misdiagnosis

Studies indicate that blacks and African Americans, Afro-Caribbeans, and Latino-Hispanic Americans run a significant risk of being misdiagnosed with schizophrenia when the true diagnosis is bipolar disease or an affective disorder (Suite et al., 2007). Why does this happen? One reason for misdiagnosis is the use of culturally inappropriate psychometric instruments and other diagnostic tools. Most available tools have been validated using subjects of European origin. For instance, Kim (2002) states that although there are over 40 validated depression scales, they tend to be "linguistically irrelevant and culturally inappropriate" (p. 110) for some groups, and they fail to identify depression in Koreans. Kim argues that the current scales measure Western ways of expressing depression by focusing on the affective domain, whereas for Koreans, more attention needs to be given to the somatic domain. To rectify this problem, Kim created and validated a depression scale for Korean Americans.

As this inadequacy of diagnostic tools suggests, psychological distress is manifested in different cultures in different ways. In cultures in which the body and mind are seen as one entity, or in cultures in which there is a high degree of stigma associated with mental health problems, people frequently somatize their feelings of psychological distress. In **somatization**, psychological distress is experienced as physical problems. Instead of perceiving the distress as emotional or affective, the psychological distress is perceived in the body. For example, a Cambodian woman may describe feelings of back pain, fatigue, and dizziness and say nothing about feelings of sadness or hopelessness (Henderson et al., 2008).

Somatization is just one example of how psychological distress is manifested, however. Just as we learn from our parents whether the appropriate way to deal with pain is either dramatic expressiveness or stoicism and denial, we learn different ways to manifest and express mental pain and pathology. Because of this, many cross-cultural mental health experts (Marsella, 2003) are skeptical about using the criteria of the *Diagnostic and Statistical Manual of Mental Disorders*, fourth edition, text revision *(DSM-IV-TR)* (American Psychiatric Association [APA], 2000) for diagnosing mental illness in culturally diverse populations, because the criteria are based on studies with predominately white American samples.

The Glossary of Culture-Bound Syndromes, added to the *DSM-IV-TR*, acknowledges the limits of the *DSM-IV*'s ability to capture and name the symptoms and pathology of culturally diverse patients. **Culture-bound syndromes** are sets of signs and symptoms that are common in a limited number of cultures but virtually nonexistent in most other cultural groups (Henderson et al., 2008) (Box 6-2).

Culture-bound illnesses may seem exotic or irrational to American nurses and cannot be understood within a Western medical framework. Symptoms may be shocking, and other-culture explanations regarding causation and treatment may be mystifying. However, these illnesses are frequently well understood by the people within the cultural group. They know the name of the problem, its etiology, its course, and the way it should be treated; frequently when these illnesses are treated in culturally prescribed ways, the remedies are quite effective.

Many culture-bound syndromes have been identified. Some of these syndromes seem to be mental health problems that manifest in somatic ways. *Hwa-byung* and *neurasthenia* have many similarities to depression (Park et al., 2001), but because the somatic complaints are so prominent, and patients frequently deny feelings of sadness or depression, they may not fit the *DSM-IV* diagnostic criteria for depression.

Ataque de nervios and *ghost sickness* (see Box 6-2) belong to another group of culture-bound illnesses characterized by abnormal behaviors people in the culture understand as illness but that are not found in other cultures. These types of illness seem to be culturally acceptable ways for patients to express that they can no longer endure the stressors in their lives. People in the culture understand the patient is ill and provide support using culturally prescribed treatments, which actually relieve the stresses through cultural remedies the patient finds helpful.

Another kind of culture-bound illness seems to be merely a cultural explanation of an illness Western medicine understands as having a biomedical cause. From a Western perspective, the patient may be experiencing depression, anxiety, or posttraumatic stress disorder, but the patient believes he is experiencing the

BOX 6-2 Examples of Culture-Bound Syndromes

Because so many culture-bound syndromes have been identified, they cannot all be described in this chapter. However, the list here includes some of the syndromes the psychiatric mental health nurse might encounter.

Ataque de nervios: Latin American. Characterized by a sudden attack of trembling, palpitations, dyspnea, dizziness, and loss of consciousness. Thought to be caused by an evil spirit and related to intolerable stress. Treated by an *espiritista* (spiritual healer) and by the support of the family and community, who provide aid to the patient and consider the patient to be calling for help in a culturally acceptable way.

Ghost sickness: Navajo. Characterized by "being out of one's mind," dyspnea, weakness, and bad dreams. Thought to be caused by an evil spirit. Treated by overcoming the evil spirit with a stronger spiritual force the healer, a "singer," calls forth through a powerful healing ritual.

Hwa-byung: Korean. Characterized by epigastric pain, anorexia, palpitations, dyspnea, and muscle aches and pains. Thought to be caused by a lack of harmony in the body or in interpersonal relationships. Treated by reestablishing harmony. Some researchers feel that it is closely related to depression.

Neurasthenia: Chinese. Characterized by somatic symptoms of depression (e.g., anorexia, weight loss, fatigue, weakness, trouble concentrating, insomnia), although feelings of sadness or depression are denied. Thought to be related to a lack of yin-yang balance.

Susto: Latin American. Characterized by a broad range of somatic and psychological symptoms. Thought to be related to a traumatic incident or fright that caused the patient's soul to leave the body. Treated by an *espiritista* (spiritual healer).

Wind illness: Chinese, Vietnamese. Characterized by a fear of cold, wind, or drafts. Derived from the belief that yin-yang and hot-cold elements must be in balance in the body or illness occurs. Treated by keeping very warm and avoiding foods, drinks, and herbs that are cold or considered to have a cold quality, as well as "cold" colors, emotions, and activities. Also treated by a variety of means designed to pull the "cold wind" out of the patient, such as by coining (vigorously rubbing a coin over the body) or cupping (applying a heated cup to the skin, creating a vacuum).

do not value the thinness so prized by European and North American cultural groups (Marsella, 2003). Some feel that almost all the descriptions of psychological illness in the *DSM-IV* are culture-bound to Western patients because the *DSM-IV* criteria were developed through studies of Western patients.

When we fail to consider culture in diagnosis and treatment, we are more likely to see culturally normal behavior as "abnormal" instead of merely different. In African American churches, it is common to talk about spiritual experiences in terms such as "I was talking to Jesus this morning." The speaker may have meant he was praying, but the clinician unfamiliar with the culture may misinterpret such a statement as delusional (Neighbors, 2003). If a Vietnamese father says he tried to take the "wind illness" out of his child by vigorously rubbing a coin down her back, the clinician may believe the father is a potential threat to the child.

When there is a cultural mismatch between the clinician and the patient, misdiagnosis and culturally inappropriate treatments frequently result in cultural imposition (Leininger & McFarland, 2006). One might be tempted to think that the only way to solve these problems is to ensure that patients have mental health providers who match the patient's culture. However, another way to solve the problem is to take the time to study the patient's culture, learn the patient's cultural perspective, and adapt your nursing care to meet the patient's cultural needs.

Ethnic Variation in Pharmacodynamics

A third clinical practice issue that presents a barrier to quality mental health services for some groups is genetic variation in drug metabolism. There is a growing realization that many drugs vary in their action and effects along genetic-ethnic lines. What was found true in drug studies primarily performed with subjects of European origin may not be true in ethnically diverse populations. Genetic variations in drug metabolism have been documented for several classifications of drugs, including antidepressants and antipsychotics.

The relatively new field of **ethnopharmacology** investigates the genetic and ethnic variations in drug pharmacokinetics. Many drugs are metabolized at least in part by the more than 20 cytochrome P-450 (CYP) enzymes present in human beings (Henderson et al., 2008). Genetic variations in these enzymes may alter drug metabolism, and these variations tend to be propagated through racial and ethnic populations.

Most antidepressants and antipsychotics are metabolized by CYP enzymes. Some genetic variations result in rapid metabolism, and if medications are metabolized too quickly, serum levels become too low, and therapeutic effects are minimized. Other variations

illness as *susto* or "soul loss" due to an extremely disturbing or frightening experience (Lim, 2006).

Culture-bound illnesses are frequently thought of as being found only in "other" (i.e., non-Western) cultures. However, some authors have pointed out that anorexia nervosa and bulimia seem to be bound to Western culture, apparently because other cultures

may result in poor metabolism. If medications are metabolized too slowly, serum levels become too high, and intolerable side effects are increased.

Awareness that genetic variations in drug metabolism are found in people of all races and ethnicities is growing. Although statistically, people of European origin have more CYP enzymes than those of African and Asian origin, the CYP enzyme is found in people of all ethnicities. So making treatment decisions based on statistical differences among various ethnic groups may increase the odds but does not guarantee an appropriate dosage. The ideal way to determine appropriate dosage is to determine the underlying phenotype of the patient (a capability not yet available in general practice) and treat by phenotype, rather than by current drug dosage charts or ethnicity.

For now, psychiatric mental health nurses need to be aware that there are ethnic variations in drug metabolism. Munoz and Hilgenberg (2005) suggest the following interventions to minimize risk:

- Keep abreast of current findings related to the drugs most likely to bring about adverse responses and effects in people from various ethnic groups.
- Carry out cultural assessments with all patients.
- Carefully monitor and document drug responses, and give the lowest possible safe dose.
- Incorporate cultural context in nursing education for patients and families.

POPULATIONS AT RISK FOR MENTAL ILLNESS AND INADEQUATE CARE

Many people in the United States are subject to experiences that challenge their mental health in ways that members of the majority group do not have to face. Among these challenges are issues related to the experience of being an immigrant and the socioeconomic disadvantages of minority status.

Immigrants

Immigrants face many unknowns. Upon arriving in the United States, they may not speak English, yet need to learn how to navigate new economic, political, legal, educational, transportation, and health care systems. Many who had status and skills in their homeland—jobs as teachers, administrators, or other professional positions—find that because of certification requirements or limited English skills, only menial jobs are open to them. After immigration, family roles may be upset, with wives finding jobs before their husbands. Immigrant families may find the struggle to live successfully in America arduous and wearisome. Long-honored cultural values and traditions, which once provided stability, are challenged by new cultural norms. During the period of adjustment, many immigrants find that the hope they felt on first immigrating turns into anxiety and depression.

Immigrants and their families embark on a process of **acculturation**—learning the beliefs, values, and practices of their new cultural setting—that sometimes takes several generations. Some immigrants adapt to the new culture quickly, absorbing the new worldview, beliefs, values, and practices rapidly until they are more natural than the ones they learned in their homeland (**assimilation**). Others attempt to maintain their traditional cultural ways. Some may become **bicultural**—able to move in and out of their traditional culture and their new culture, depending on where they are and with whom they associate. Some immigrants may suffer **culture shock**, finding the new norms disconcerting or offensive because they contrast so deeply with their traditional beliefs, values, and practices.

Many families find that the children assimilate the new culture at a rapid pace, whereas the elders maintain their traditional cultural beliefs, values, and practices. This sets the stage for intergenerational conflict. The traditional status of elders in a hierarchical family may be challenged by children who are assimilating different values about family. Some children may feel lost between two cultures and unsure of where to place their cultural identity.

Refugees

A **refugee** is a special kind of immigrant. Whereas the immigrant generally values the new culture and wishes to enjoy a change in life circumstances, the refugee has left his or her own homeland to escape intolerable conditions and would have preferred to stay in the culture if that had been possible. Refugees do not perceive entry into the new culture as an active choice and may experience the stress of adjusting as imposed on them against their will. Many refugees from Southeast Asia, Central America, and Africa have been traumatized by war, genocide, torture, starvation, and other catastrophic events. Many have lost family members, a way of life, and a homeland to which they can never return. The degree of trauma and loss they have experienced may make them particularly vulnerable to a variety of psychiatric disorders, including depression and posttraumatic stress disorder (PTSD).

Cultural "Minorities"

Individuals who are considered "minorities" (nonwhites) may be vulnerable to a variety of disadvantages, including poverty and limited opportunities for education and jobs. Cultural minority groups are frequent victims of bias, discrimination, and racism—subtle but pervasive forms of rejection that diminish self-esteem and self-efficacy and leave victims feeling excluded and marginalized.

In the United States, the incidence of various types of mental health disorders among cultural and racial minority groups is similar to that among whites *if* the poor and other vulnerable populations (e.g., homeless, institutionalized, children in foster care, victims of trauma) within the minority groups are excluded. However, if people in these vulnerable populations are included, the incidence of mental health problems among minorities increases. Therefore, the higher incidence of mental health problems is related to poverty not ethnicity (USDHHS, 2001).

People who live in poverty are two to three times more likely to develop mental illness than those who live above the poverty line. In 2007, 8% of non-Hispanic whites lived in poverty; 10% of Asian, 22% of Latino-Hispanic Americans, and 24% of blacks and African Americans live below the poverty line (U.S. Census Bureau, 2008b). Poverty is highly associated with other disadvantages, such as scarce educational and economic opportunities, which in turn are associated with substance abuse and violent crime. People who are poor are subject to a daily struggle for survival, and this takes its toll on mental health.

People from cultural minorities have reported that they perceived bias and experienced culturally uncomfortable care from health care providers, which made them less likely to seek medical services in the future. According to a report issued by the Institute of Medicine, *Unequal Treatment: Confronting Racial and Ethnic Disparities in Healthcare*, bias and discrimination infect the health care system; resulting in further stresses on the mental health of those in minority groups instead of delivering the help they need (Smedley et al., 2003).

CULTURALLY COMPETENT CARE

So far, this chapter has explained why the nursing needs of culturally diverse patient populations are so varied. Mental health and illness are biological, psychological, social, and *cultural* processes. Cultural competence is required of nurses if we are to assist patients in achieving mental health and well-being. But how, exactly, are psychiatric mental health nurses to practice culturally competent care? The remainder of this chapter suggests techniques that answer this question.

The USDHHS Office of Minority Health (2007) defines culturally competent care as attitudes and behaviors that enable a nurse to work effectively *within* the patient's cultural context. Cultural and linguistic competence is a set of congruent behaviors, attitudes, and policies that come together in a system, agency, or among professionals and enable effective work in cross-cultural situations. Cultural competence means that nurses adjust *their* practices to meet their patients' cultural beliefs, practices, needs, and preferences. Having cultural sensitivity or awareness is an essential component of cultural competence. Culturally competent care goes beyond culturally sensitive care by adapting care to the patient's cultural needs and preferences (Narayan, 2006).

Campinha-Bacote (2008) recommends a blueprint for psychiatric mental health nurses in providing culturally effective care: the Process of Cultural Competence in the Delivery of Healthcare Services. In this model, nurses view themselves as *becoming* culturally competent rather than *being* culturally competent. This model suggests that nurses must constantly see themselves as learners throughout their careers—always open to, and learning from, the immense cultural diversity they will see among their patients. The model consists of five constructs that promote the process and journey of cultural competence:

1. Cultural awareness
2. Cultural knowledge
3. Cultural encounters
4. Cultural skill
5. Cultural desire

Cultural Awareness

Through cultural awareness, the nurse recognizes the enormous impact culture makes on what patients' health values and practices are, how and when patients decide they are ill and need care, and what treatments they will seek when illness occurs.

Cultural awareness should inspire us as nurses to first acknowledge ourselves as cultural beings, so close to the norms of our own ethnic and professional cultures that these norms seem "right" (ethnocentrism) and not just "cultural." In accordance with the demands of cultural awareness, nurses must also examine all beliefs, values, and practices to ascertain which ones are cultural and which ones could be universally held (Campinha-Bacote, 2003). Through cultural awareness and cultural humility, we often discover that many of our norms are cultural, few are universal, and that we have an obligation to be open to and respectful of patients' cultural norms.

By practicing cultural awareness, we also examine our cultural assumptions and expectations about what constitutes mental health, a "healthy" self-concept, a "healthy" family, and the "right way" to behave in society. Assumptions and expectations about how people manifest psychological distress must also be examined. The culturally aware nurse questions whether the evidence-based guideline (derived from studies involving primarily subjects of European origin) should be modified to address the cultural aspects of a particular patient's life and illness (Campinha-Bacote, 2002).

A culturally aware nurse recognizes that three cultures are intersecting during any encounter with a patient: the culture of the patient, the culture of the nurse, and the culture of the setting (agency, clinic, hospital) (USDHHS, 2001). As a patient advocate, our job is to negotiate and support the patient's cultural needs and preferences.

Cultural Knowledge

Nurses can enhance their cultural knowledge in various ways. They can attend cultural events and programs, forge friendships with members of diverse cultural groups, and participate in in-service programs at which members of diverse groups talk about their cultural norms. Another way to obtain cultural knowledge is to study print or online resources designed for health care providers.

Cultural knowledge is proactive when it prevents us from assuming that a patient's underlying worldview and values are the same as ours; it alerts us to areas in which there may be cultural differences. Cultural knowledge also helps us understand behaviors that might otherwise be misinterpreted. Cultural knowledge helps us establish rapport, ask the right questions, avoid misunderstandings, and identify cultural variables that may need to be considered when planning nursing care (Narayan, 2002).

Available cultural guides and resources offer valuable information about various ethnic and religious cultures (Campinha-Bacote, 2002), including:

- Worldview, beliefs, and values that permeate the culture
- Nonverbal communication patterns, such as the meaning of eye contact, facial expressions, gestures, and touch
- Etiquette norms, such as the importance of punctuality, the pace of conversation, and the way respect and hospitality are shown
- Family roles and psychosocial norms, such as the way decisions are made and the degree of independence versus interdependence of family members
- Cultural views about mental health and illness, such as the degree of stigma and the nature of the "sick role"
- Patterns related to health and illness, including culture-bound syndromes, ethnopharmacological variations, and folk and herbal treatments frequently used within the culture

Cultural Encounters

Although obtaining cultural knowledge sets a foundation, cultural guides cannot tell us anything about a particular patient. According to Campinha-Bacote (2008), multiple cultural encounters with diverse patients deter nurses from stereotyping. Although generalizations can be made about cultures, stereotyping individuals within the group robs them of the individuality they possess and robs the culture of its diversity.

Stereotyping is the tendency to believe that every member of a group is like all other members. However, multiple cultural encounters enable us to experience the intra-ethnic diversity of cultural groups and come to understand that although there are patterns that characterize a culture, individual members of the culture adhere to the culture's norms in diverse ways.

Each person is a unique blend of the many ethnic, religious, socioeconomic, geographic, educational, and occupational cultures to which he or she belongs. Each person brings a unique personality, life experiences, and creative thought to self-development and makes choices about which cultural norms to adopt or abandon. In the end, each person is a unique individual who never adheres to all (and may not adhere to any) of the norms of his or her culture of origin. The only way to know about the norms of a patient's culture is to ask the patient.

Cultural encounters help nurses develop confidence in cross-cultural interactions. Every nurse is likely to make cultural blunders and will need to recover from cultural mistakes. Cultural encounters help develop our skill at recognizing, avoiding, and reducing the cultural pain that can occur when nursing care causes the patient discomfort or offense by failing to be sensitive to cultural norms (Kavanagh, 2008). Every nurse can learn to recognize signs of cultural pain, such as a patient's discomfort or alienation, and take measures to recover trust and rapport by asking what has caused the offense, apologizing for any lack of sensitivity, and expressing willingness to learn from the patient how care can be provided in a culturally sensitive way.

Cultural Skill

Cultural skill is the ability to perform a cultural assessment in a sensitive way (Campinha-Bacote, 2008). The first step is to ensure that meaningful communication can occur. If the patient is not proficient in English, a professional medical interpreter should be engaged.

Many cultural assessment tools are available (Andrews & Boyle, 2008; Purnell, 2008; Spector, 2004; Giger & Davidhizar, 2003; Narayan, 2003; Leininger, 2002). An appendix of the *DSM-IV-TR* (APA, 2000), Outline for Cultural Formulation, recommends cultural assessment areas. A very useful mental health assessment tool is the classic set of questions proposed by Kleinman and colleagues (1978):

- What do you call this illness? *(diagnosis)*
- When did it start? Why then? *(onset)*
- What do you think caused it? *(etiology)*
- How does the illness work? What does it do to you? *(course)*
- How long will it last? Is it serious? *(prognosis)*

- How have you treated the illness? How do you think it should be treated? *(treatment)*

These questions allow the patient to feel heard and understood. They also help in eliciting culture-bound syndromes. They can be expanded to include questions such as:

- What are the chief problems this illness has caused you?
- What do you fear most about this illness? Do you think it is curable?
- Do you know others who have had this problem? What happened to them? Do you think this will happen to you?

Approaching these questions conversationally is generally more effective than using a direct, formal approach. One indirect technique is to ask the patient what another family member thinks is causing the problem. Instead of saying, "What do you call this illness? When did it start and why?" The nurse can ask, "What does your family think is wrong? Why do they think it started? What do they think you should do about it?" After the patient describes what the family thinks, the nurse can simply ask in a nonjudgmental way if the patient agrees.

Another technique for promoting openness is to make a declaratory statement before asking the questions. For instance, before asking about cultural treatments the patient has tried, the nurse can first say, "Everyone has remedies they find help them when they are ill. Are there any special healers or treatments you have used or that you think might be helpful to you?"

Some areas that deserve special attention during an assessment interview are:

- Ethnicity, religious affiliation, and degree of acculturation to Western medical culture
- Spiritual practices that are important to preserving or regaining health
- Degree of proficiency in speaking and reading English
- Dietary patterns, including foods prescribed for sick people
- Attitudes about pain and experiences with pain in a Western medical setting
- Attitudes about and experience with Western medications
- Cultural remedies such as healers, herbs, and practices the patient may find helpful
- Who the patient considers "family," who should receive health information, and how decisions are made in the family
- Cultural customs the patient feels are essential to preserve and is fearful will be violated in the mental health setting

The purpose of a culturally sensitive assessment is to develop a therapeutic plan that is mutually agreeable, culturally acceptable, and potentially productive of positive outcomes. While gathering assessment data, you should identify cultural patterns that may support or interfere with the patient's health and recovery process. Your professional knowledge can then be used to categorize the patient's cultural norms into three different groups:

1. Those that facilitate the patient's health and recovery, from the Western medical perspective
2. Those that are neither helpful nor harmful, from the Western medical perspective
3. Those that are harmful to the patient's health and well-being, from the Western medical perspective

Leininger and McFarland (2006) suggest a **preservation/maintenance, accommodate/negotiate, repatterning/restructuring framework** for care planning. Using this framework, effective nursing care **preserves** the aspects of the patient's culture that, from a Western perspective, promote health and well-being—such as a strong family support system and traditional values like cooperation and emphasis on relationships.

Cultural values and practices that are neither helpful nor harmful are **accommodated** or may be **negotiated**. You may encourage the patient's use of neutral values and practices, such as folk remedies and healers. By including these culture-specific interventions in the care as complementary interventions, nursing care builds on the patient's own coping and healing systems. For example, Native Americans with substance abuse problems may find tribal healing ceremonies helpful as a complement to the therapeutic program.

Finally, when cultural patterns are determined harmful, the nurse must make attempts to **repattern/restructure** them. For instance, if a patient is taking an herb that interferes with the prescription medication regimen, you will do well to educate and negotiate until a mutually agreeable therapeutic program is developed.

Cultural Desire

The final construct in Campinha-Bacote's cultural competence model for psychiatric mental health nurses (2008) is **cultural desire**. Cultural desire indicates that the nurse is not acting out of a sense of duty but from a sincere and genuine concern for patients' welfare. This concern ideally leads to attempts to truly understand each patient's viewpoint. Nurses exhibit cultural desire through patience, consideration, and empathy. Giving the impression that you are willing to learn from the patient is the hallmark of cultural desire; as opposed to behaving as if you know what is best and are going to impose the "correct" treatment on the patient.

Cultural desire inspires openness and flexibility in applying nursing principles to meet the patient's cultural needs. Although it may be easier to establish a therapeutic relationship with someone who comes from a similar cultural background, cultural desire enables the nurse to achieve good outcomes with culturally diverse patients.

KEY POINTS TO REMEMBER

- Mental health and illness are biological, psychological, social, and cultural phenomena.
- As the diversity of the world and the United States increases, psychiatric mental health nurses will be caring for more and more people of diverse cultural groups.
- Nurses must learn to deliver culturally competent care, meaning culturally sensitive assessments and culturally congruent interventions.
- *Culture* is the shared beliefs, values, and practices of a group that shape their thinking and behavior in patterned ways. Cultural groups share these norms with new members of the group through *enculturation*.
- A group's culture influences its members' worldview, nonverbal communication patterns, etiquette norms, and ways of viewing the person, the family, and the "right" way to think and behave in society.
- The concept of mental health is formed within a culture, and deviance from cultural expectations can be defined as "illness" by other members of the group.
- Psychiatric mental health nursing is based on personality and developmental theories advanced by Europeans and Americans and grounded in Western cultural ideals and values.
- Nurses are as influenced by their own professional and ethnic cultures as patients are by theirs. Nurses must guard against ethnocentric tendencies when caring for patients, because cultural imposition does not promote patient health and well-being.
- Barriers to quality mental health care include communication barriers, ethnic variations in psychotropic drug metabolism, and misdiagnoses caused by culturally inappropriate diagnostic tools.
- Immigrants (especially refugees) and minority groups who suffer from the effects of low socioeconomic status, including poverty and discrimination, are at particular risk for mental illness.
- Cultural competence consists of five constructs: cultural awareness, cultural knowledge, cultural encounters, cultural skill, and cultural desire.
- Through cultural awareness, nurses recognize that they, as well as patients, have cultural beliefs, values, and practices.
- Cultural knowledge is obtained by seeking cultural information from friends, participating in in-service programs, immersing oneself in the culture, or consulting print and online sources.
- Nurses experience intra-ethnic diversity through multiple cultural encounters, which prevents nurses from stereotyping their patients.
- Nurses demonstrate cultural skill by performing culturally sensitive assessment interviews and adapting care to meet patients' cultural needs and preferences.
- Care can be adapted by using the care planning preservation/maintenance, accommodate/negotiate, repatterning/

restructure framework of Leininger & McFarland (2006) when creating the therapeutic plan.
- Cultural desire is a genuine interest in the patient's unique perspective; it enables nurses to provide considerate, flexible, and respectful care to patients of all cultures.

CRITICAL THINKING

1. Describe the cultural factors that have influenced the development of Western psychiatric mental health nursing practice. Contrast these Western influences with the cultural factors that influence patients who come from an Eastern or indigenous culture.

2. What do you think about the claim that mental illness, such as schizophrenia, is a cultural phenomenon and that people are judged to be mentally ill if they do not fit within the social definition of normal? What implications (good or bad) does a diagnosis of a mental illness have?

3. Analyze the effects cultural competence (or incompetence) can have on psychiatric mental health nurses and their patients.

4. How can barriers such as misdiagnosis and communication problems impede competent psychiatric mental health care? What can the members of the health care team do to overcome such barriers?

CHAPTER REVIEW

1. Which patient behavior would alert the nurse to the potential for somatization?
   1. States, "I am so sad that I don't know what to do."
   2. Shows the nurse bottles of medication used to treat anxiety.
   3. Presents with concerns involving back pain, dizziness, and fatigue.
   4. States, "My doctor diagnosed me with bipolar disorder."

2. The nurse is caring for a patient who states that he has "ghost sickness." Which is the appropriate nursing response?
   1. "I have no idea what 'ghost sickness' is."
   2. "How does 'ghost sickness' make you feel?"
   3. "There is not a disorder known as 'ghost sickness.'"
   4. "Why do you believe in evil spirits?"

3. Which nursing actions demonstrate cultural competence? *Select all that apply.*
   1. Planning mealtime around the patient's prayer schedule
   2. Advising a patient to visit with the hospital chaplain
   3. Researching foods that a lacto-ovo-vegetarian patient will eat
   4. Providing time for a patient's spiritual healer to visit
   5. Ordering standard meal trays to be delivered three times daily

4. The nurse is planning care for a patient of the Latin-American culture. Which goal is appropriate?
   1. Patient will visit with spiritual healer once weekly.
   2. Patient will experience rebalance of yin-yang by discharge.
   3. Patient will identify sources that increase "cold wind" within 24 hours of admission.
   4. Patient will contact "singer" to provider healing ritual within 3 days of admission.

5. A nurse is caring for a patient of another culture. Which nursing action is appropriate?
   1. Maintain eye contact at all times.
   2. Assume that personal space is significantly closer than in the United States.
   3. State, "You can beat this diagnosis; you are in control of yourself."
   4. Ask the patient if family should be included in the decision-making process.

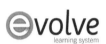

Visit the Evolve website for an **Audio Chapter Summary, Chapter Review Answers & Rationales, Critical Thinking Answer Guidelines,** and additional resources related to the content in this chapter: **http://evolve.elsevier.com/Varcarolis/foundations**

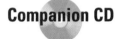

Companion CD Use the Companion CD to prepare for tests and the NCLEX® Examination with **Test-Taking Strategies** for psychiatric mental health nursing and hundreds of **Review Questions.**

References

American Psychiatric Association. (2000). *Diagnostic and statistical manual of mental disorders (DSM-IV-TR)* (4th ed., text rev.). Washington, DC: Author.

Andrews, M., & Boyle, J. (2008). *Transcultural concepts in nursing care* (5th ed.). Philadelphia: Lippincott.

Campinha-Bacote, J. (2002). Cultural competence in psychiatric nursing: Have you asked the right questions? *Journal of the American Psychiatric Nurses Association, 8*(6), 183–187.

Campinha-Bacote, J. (2003). *The process of cultural competence in the delivery of healthcare services* (4th ed.). Cincinnati, OH: Transcultural C.A.R.E. Associates Press.

Campinha-Bacote, J. (2008). Cultural desire: 'caught' or 'taught'? *Contemporary Nurse: Advances in Contemporary Transcultural Nursing, 28*(1-2), 141–148.

Chan, C. L. W., Ng, S. M., Ho, R. T. H., & Chow, Y. M. (2006). East meets West: Applying Eastern spirituality in clinical practice. *Journal of Clinical Nursing, 15,* 822–832.

Cunningham, C., & Stanley, F. (2003). Indigenous by definition, experience, and worldview. *British Medical Journal, 327,* 403–404.

Giger, J. N., & Davidhizar, R. E. (2003). *Transcultural nursing: Assessment and intervention* (3rd ed.). St. Louis: Mosby.

Henderson, D. C., Yeung, A., Fan, X., & Fricchione, G. L. (2008). Culture and psychiatry. In T. A. Stern, J. F. Rosenbaum, M. Fava, J. Biederman, & S. L. Rauch (Eds.), *Comprehensive clinical psychiatry* (pp. 907–916). Philadelphia: Mosby.

Kavanagh, H. K. (2008). Transcultural perspectives in mental health nursing. In M. M. Andrews, & J. S. Boyle (Eds.), *Transcultural concepts in nursing care* (5th ed., pp. 226–260). Philadelphia: Wolters.

Kim, M. (2002). Measuring depression in Korean Americans: Development of the Kim Depression Scale for Korean Americans. *Journal of Transcultural Nursing, 13*(2), 109–117.

Kleinman, A., Eisenberg, L., & Good, B. (1978). Culture, illness and care: Clinical lessons from anthropologic and cross-cultural research. *Annals of Internal Medicine, 88,* 251–258.

Leininger, M. (2002). Culture care assessments for congruent competency practices. In M. Leininger, & M. McFarland (Eds.), *Transcultural nursing: Concepts, theories, research and practice* (3rd ed., pp. 117–144). New York: McGraw-Hill.

Leininger, M., & McFarland, M. (2006). *Culture care diversity & universality: A worldwide nursing theory* (2nd ed.). Sudbury, MA: Jones & Bartlett.

Lim, R. F. (2006). *Clinical manual of cultural psychiatry.* Arlington, VA: American Psychiatric Publishing.

Marsella, A. J. (2003). Cultural aspects of depressive experience and disorders. In W. J. Lonner, D. L. Dinnel, S. A. Hayes, & D. N. Sattler (Eds.), *Online readings in psychology and culture* (Unit 9, Chapter 4). Retrieved November 17, 2004, from Western Washington University, Center for Cross-Cultural Research website: http://www.ac.wwu.edu/culture/Marsella.htm

Munoz, C., & Hilgenberg, C. (2005). Ethnopharmacology. *American Journal of Nursing, 105*(8), 40–48.

Munoz, C., & Luckmann, J. (2005). *Transcultural communication in nursing* (2nd ed.). Clifton Park, NJ: Delmar.

Narayan, M. C. (2002). Six steps to cultural competence: A clinician's guide. *Home Health Care Management and Practice, 14,* 378–386.

Narayan, M. C. (2003). Cultural assessment and care planning. *Home Healthcare Nurse, 21,* 611–618.

Narayan, M. C. (2006). Culturally relevant mental health nursing: A global perspective. In E. M. Varcarolis, V. B. Carson, & N. C. Shoemaker (Eds.), *Foundations of psychiatric mental health nursing* (5th ed., pp. 99–113). Philadelphia: Saunders.

Neighbors, H. (2003, January 22). *The (mis)diagnosis of African Americans implementing DSM criteria in the hospital and the community.* Retrieved April 4, 2004, from University of Michigan Department of Psychiatry, Psychiatry Grand Rounds website: http://www.med.umich.edu/psych/ mlk2003.htm

Office of Minority Health. (2007). *National standards on culturally and linguistically appropriate services.* Washington, DC: U.S. Department of Health and Human Services, Office of Minority Health. Retrieved on January 23, 2009 from http://www.omhrc.gov/templates/browse.aspx?lvl=2&lvlID=15

Park, Y., Kim, H., Kang, H., & Kim, J. (2001). A survey of hwa-byung in middle-age Korean women. *Journal of Transcultural Nursing, 12*(2), 115–122.

Purnell, L. D. (2008). Transcultural diversity and health care. In L. D. Purnell, & B. J. Paulanka (Eds.), *Transcultural health care* (3rd ed.). Philadelphia: Davis.

Smedley, B., Stith, A., & Nelson, A. (2003). *Unequal treatment: Confronting racial and ethnic disparities in healthcare* (Institute of Medicine Report). Washington, DC: National Academy Press.

Spector, R. E. (2004). *Cultural diversity in health and illness* (6th ed.). Upper Saddle River, NJ: Prentice-Hall.

Suite, D. H., LaBril, R., Primm, A., & Harrison-Ross, P. (2007). Beyond misdiagnosis, misunderstanding, and mistrust: Relevance of the historical perspective in the medical and mental health treatment of people of color. *Journal of the National Medical Association*, 99(8), 1–7.

U.S. Census Bureau. (2007, May 18). Minority population tops 100 million. *U.S. Census Bureau News*. Retrieved October 10, 2008 from http://www.census.gov/Press-Release/www/releases/archives/population/010048.html

U.S. Census Bureau. (2008). *Income, poverty, and health insurance coverage in the United States, 2007*. Retrieved on October 11, 2008 from http://www.census.gov/prod/2008pubs/p60–235.pdf

U.S. Census Bureau. (2008). *Questions planned for the 2010 census and American community survey*. Retrieved October 11, 2008 from http://www.census.gov/2010census/pdf/2010ACSnotebook.pdf

U.S. Department of Health and Human Services. (2001). *Mental health: Culture, race, and ethnicity: A supplement to Mental health: A report of the surgeon general*. Rockville, MD: U.S. Department of Health and Human Services, Substance Abuse and Mental Health Services Administration, Center for Mental Health Services.

CHAPTER **7**

Legal and Ethical Guidelines for Safe Practice

Penny S. Brooke

Key Terms and Concepts

assault , 129
battery, 129
bioethics, 119
civil rights, 119
competency, 124
conditional release, 121
confidentiality, 125
duty to protect, 127
duty to warn, 126
ethical dilemma, 119
ethics, 119
false imprisonment, 129
Health Insurance Portability and
 Accountability Act (HIPAA), 126
implied consent, 124
informal admission, 120
informed consent, 123

intentional torts, 129
involuntary admission, 120
involuntary outpatient admission, 121
least restrictive alternative doctrine, 120
long-term involuntary admission, 121
malpractice, 129
negligence, 129
right to privacy, 126
right to refuse treatment, 122
right to treatment, 122
temporary admission, 120
tort, 128
unconditional release, 121
unintentional torts, 129
voluntary admission, 120
writ of habeas corpus, 120

Objectives

1. Compare and contrast the terms *ethics* and *bioethics*, and identify five principles of bioethics.
2. Discuss at least five patient rights, including the patient's right to treatment, right to refuse treatment, and right to informed consent.
3. Identify the steps nurses are advised to take if they suspect negligence or illegal activity on the part of a professional colleague or peer.
4. Apply legal considerations of patient privilege (a) after a patient has died, (b) if the patient tests positive for human immunodeficiency virus, or (c) if the patient's employer states a "need to know."

5. Provide explanations for situations in which health care professionals have a duty to break patient confidentiality.
6. Discuss a patient's civil rights and how they pertain to restraint and seclusion.
7. Develop awareness of the balance between the patient's rights and the rights of society with respect to the following legal concepts relevant in nursing and psychiatric mental health nursing: (a) duty to intervene, (b) documentation, and (c) confidentiality.
8. Identify legal terminology (e.g., torts, negligence, malpractice) applicable to psychiatric nursing and explain the significance of each term.

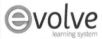 Visit the Evolve website for an **Audio Glossary & Flashcards, Concept Map Creator**, and additional resources related to the content in this chapter: **http://evolve.elsevier.com/Varcarolis/foundations**

This chapter introduces current legal and ethical issues you may encounter in the practice of psychiatric mental health nursing. A fundamental goal of psychiatric care is to strike a balance between the rights of the individual patient and the rights of society at large. This chapter is designed to assist you to understand the implications of ethical or legal issues during the provision of care in a psychiatric setting.

An ethical dilemma results when there is a conflict between two or more courses of action, each carrying favorable and unfavorable consequences. How we respond to these dilemmas is based partly on our own morals (beliefs of right or wrong) and values. Suppose you are caring for a pregnant woman with schizophrenia who wants to carry the baby to term, but whose family insists she get an abortion. To promote fetal safety, her antipsychotic medication will need to be reduced, putting her at risk of exacerbation of the illness. Furthermore, there is a question as to whether she can safely care for the child. If you rely on the ethical principle of autonomy, you may conclude that she has the right to decide. Would other ethical principles be in conflict with autonomy in this case?

At times, your values may be in conflict with the value system of the institution. This situation further complicates the decision-making process and necessitates careful consideration of the patient's desires. For example, you may experience a conflict of values in a setting where older adult patients are routinely tranquilized to a degree you do not feel comfortable with. Whenever one's value system is challenged, increased stress results.

ETHICAL CONCEPTS

Ethics is the study of philosophical beliefs about what is considered right or wrong in a society. The term bioethics is the study of specific ethical questions that arise in health care. The five basic principles of bioethics are:

1. **Beneficence**—the duty to act to benefit or promote the good of others (e.g., spending extra time to help calm an extremely anxious patient).
2. **Autonomy**—respecting the rights of others to make their own decisions (e.g., acknowledging the patient's right to refuse medication promotes autonomy).
3. **Justice**—the duty to distribute resources or care equally, regardless of personal attributes (e.g., an ICU nurse devotes equal attention to someone who has attempted suicide as to someone who suffered a brain aneurysm).
4. **Fidelity** (nonmaleficence)—maintaining loyalty and commitment to the patient and doing no wrong to the patient (e.g., maintaining expertise in nursing skill through nursing education).
5. **Veracity**—one's duty to communicate truthfully (e.g., describing the purpose and side effects of psychotropic medications in a truthful and non-misleading way).

Laws tend to reflect the ethical values of society. It should be noted that although you may feel obligated to follow ethical guidelines, these guidelines should not override laws. For example, if you are aware of a statute or a specific rule or regulation created by the state board of nursing to prohibit a certain action (e.g., restraining patients against their will), and you feel you have an ethical obligation to protect the patient by engaging in such an action (e.g., using restraints), you would be wise to follow the law.

MENTAL HEALTH LAWS

Laws have been enacted to regulate the care and treatment of the mentally ill. Mental health laws—or statutes—vary from state to state; therefore, you are encouraged to review your state's code to better understand the legal climate in which you will be practicing. This can be accomplished by visiting the web page of your state mental health department or by doing an Internet search using the keywords "mental + health + statutes + (your state)."

Many of these laws have undergone major revision since the enactment of the Community Mental Health Centers Act of 1963 under President John F. Kennedy (see Chapter 5). The changes reflect a shift in emphasis from institutional care of the mentally ill to community-based care. Along with this shift in setting has come the more widespread use of psychotropic drugs in the treatment of mental illness—which has enabled many people to integrate more readily into the larger community—and an increasing awareness of the need to provide the mentally ill with humane care that respects their civil rights.

Civil Rights of Persons with Mental Illness

Persons with mental illness are guaranteed the same rights under federal and state laws as any other citizen. Most states specifically prohibit any person from depriving an individual receiving mental health services of his or her civil rights, including but not limited to:

- The right to vote
- The right to civil service ranking
- The right to receive, forfeit, or deny a driver's license
- The right to make purchases and enter contractual relationships (unless the patient has lost legal capacity by being adjudicated incompetent)
- The right to press charges against another person

- The right to humane care and treatment (medical, dental, and psychiatric needs must be met in accordance with the prevailing standards of these professions)
- The right to religious freedom and practice
- The right to social interaction
- The right to exercise and participate in recreational opportunities

Incarcerated persons with mental illness are afforded the same protections.

ADMISSION AND DISCHARGE PROCEDURES

Due Process in Involuntary Admission

The courts have recognized that involuntary admission (see Chapter 4) to a psychiatric inpatient setting is a "massive curtailment of liberty" (*Humphrey v. Cady*, 1972, p. 509) requiring due process protections in the civil commitment procedure. This right derives from the Fifth Amendment of the U.S. Constitution, which states that "no person shall . . . be deprived of life, liberty, or property without due process of law."

The Fourteenth Amendment explicitly prohibits *states* from depriving citizens of life, liberty, and property without due process of law. State civil commitment statutes, if challenged in the courts on constitutional grounds, must afford minimal due process protections to pass the court's scrutiny (*Zinernon v. Burch*, 1990). In most states, a patient can challenge commitments through a writ of habeas corpus, which means a "formal written order" to "free the person." The writ of habeas corpus is the procedural mechanism used to challenge unlawful detention by the government.

The writ of habeas corpus and the least restrictive alternative doctrine are two of the most important concepts applicable to civic commitment cases. The least restrictive alternative doctrine mandates that the least drastic means be taken to achieve a specific purpose. For example, if someone can safely be treated for depression on an outpatient basis, hospitalization would be too restrictive and unnecessarily disruptive.

Admission Procedures

Several types of admissions will be discussed in the following sections, all of which must be based on several fundamental guidelines:

- Neither voluntary nor involuntary admission determines a patient's ability to make informed decisions about their health care.
- A medical standard or justification for admission must exist.
- A well-defined psychiatric problem must be established, based on current illness classifications in the *Diagnostic and Statistical Manual of*

Mental Disorders, fourth edition, text revision *(DSM-IV-TR)* (American Psychiatric Association [APA], 2000).

- The presenting illness should be of such a nature that it causes an immediate crisis situation or that other less restrictive alternatives are inadequate or unavailable.
- There must be a reasonable expectation that the hospitalization and treatment will improve the presenting problems.

You are encouraged to become familiar with the laws in your state and provisions for admissions, discharges, patients' rights, and informed consent.

Informal Admission

Informal admission is one type of voluntary admission that is similar to any general hospital admission in which there is no formal or written application (Sadock& Sadock, 2008). An informal admission is sought by the patient. Under this model, the normal doctor-patient relationship exists, and the patient is free to stay or leave, even against medical advice.

Voluntary Admission

Voluntary admission is sought by the patient or the patient's guardian through a written application to the facility. Voluntarily admitted patients have the right to demand and obtain release; however, few states require voluntarily admitted patients to be notified of the rights associated with their status. In addition, many states require that a patient submit a written release notice to the facility staff, who reevaluate the patient's condition for possible conversion to involuntary admission status according to criteria established by state law.

Temporary Admission

Temporary admission is used (1) for people who are so confused or demented they cannot make decisions on their own or (2) for people who are so ill they need emergency admission. A temporary admission is initiated by a physician, and then the need for hospitalization must be confirmed by a psychiatrist employed by the hospital. The primary purpose of this type of hospitalization is observation, diagnosis, and treatment of those who have mental illness or pose a danger to themselves or others. The length of time and procedures vary markedly from state to state; generally patients can be held no more than 15 days under the temporary procedure.

Involuntary Admission

Involuntary admission is admission to a facility without the patient's consent. Generally, involuntary admission is necessary when a person is in need of psychiatric treatment, presents a danger to self or others, or is unable to meet his or her own basic needs.

Involuntary admission requires that the patient retain freedom from unreasonable bodily restraints, the right to informed consent, and the right to refuse medications, including psychotropic or antipsychotic medications.

Involuntary admission procedures include that a specified number of physicians must certify that a person's mental health status justifies detention and treatment. Close family members are made aware of the hospitalization (if they were not already). Patients have the right of access to legal council and the right to take their case before a judge, who may order a release (Sadock & Sadock, 2008).

Patients can be kept involuntarily hospitalized for 60 days. After that time, their cases are reviewed by a panel of professionals that includes psychiatrists, medical doctors, lawyers, and private citizens. A patient who believes that he is being held without just cause can file a petition for a writ of habeas corpus, which the hospital must immediately submit to the court. The court must then decide if the patient has been denied due process of law.

Forced treatment raises ethical dilemmas regarding autonomy versus paternalism, privacy rights, duty to protect, and right to treatment.

VIGNETTE

Elizabeth is a 50-year-old woman with a long history of admissions to psychiatric hospitals. During previous hospitalizations, she was diagnosed with paranoid schizophrenia. She has refused visits from her case worker and quit taking medication, and her young-adult children have become increasingly concerned about her behavior. When they stop to visit, she is typically unkempt and smells bad, her apartment is filthy and filled with cats, there is no food in the refrigerator except for ketchup and an old container of yogurt, and she is not paying her bills. Elizabeth accuses her children of spying on her and of being in collusion with the government to get at her secrets of mind control and oil-rationing plans. Elizabeth is making vague threats to the local officials, claiming that people who have caused the problems need to be "taken care of." Her daughter contacts her psychiatrist with this information, and a decision is made to begin emergency involuntary admission proceedings. ∎

Long-Term Involuntary Admission. Long-term involuntary admission has as its primary purpose extended care and treatment of the mentally ill. Those who undergo extended involuntary hospitalization are admitted through medical certification, judicial review, or administrative action. Some states do not require a judicial hearing before involuntary long-term admission but often provide the patient with an opportunity for a judicial review after admission procedures. This type

of involuntary hospitalization generally lasts 60 to 180 days, but may also be for an indeterminate period.

Involuntary Outpatient Admission. Involuntary outpatient admission arose in the 1990s, when states began to pass legislation that permitted outpatient admission as an alternative to forced inpatient treatment. This type of admission can be a preventive measure, allowing a court order before the onset of a psychiatric crisis that would result in an inpatient admission. The order for involuntary outpatient admission is usually tied to receipt of goods and services provided by social welfare agencies, including disability benefits and housing. To access these goods and services, the patient is mandated to participate in treatment and may face inpatient admission if he or she fails to participate in treatment (Chan, 2003).

Discharge Procedures

Release from hospitalization depends on the patient's admission status. As previously discussed, voluntarily admitted patients have the right to request and receive release. Some states, however, do provide for conditional release of voluntary patients, which enables the treating physician or administrator to order continued treatment on an outpatient basis if the clinical needs of the patient warrant further care.

Conditional Release

Conditional release usually requires outpatient treatment for a specified period to determine the patient's adherence with medication protocols, ability to meet basic needs, and ability to reintegrate into the community. Generally, a voluntarily admitted patient who is conditionally released can only be involuntarily admitted through the usual methods described above. However, an involuntarily admitted patient who is conditionally released may be reinstitutionalized although the commitment is still in effect without recommencement of formal admission procedures.

Unconditional Release

Unconditional release is the termination of a patient-institution relationship. This release may be court ordered or administratively ordered by the institution's officials. Generally, the administrative officer of an institution has the discretion to discharge patients.

Release Against Medical Advice (AMA)

In some cases, there is a disagreement between the mental health care providers and the patient as to whether continued hospitalization is necessary. In cases where treatment seems beneficial, but there is no compelling reason (e.g., danger to self or others) to seek an involuntary continuance of stay, patients may be released against medical advice.

PATIENTS' RIGHTS UNDER THE LAW

Psychiatric facilities usually provide patients with a written list of basic rights derived from a variety of sources, especially legislation that came out of the 1960s. Since that time, rights have been modified to some degree, but most lists share commonalities described in the following sections.

Right to Treatment

With the enactment of the Hospitalization of the Mentally Ill Act in 1964, the federal statutory right to psychiatric treatment in public hospitals was created. The statute requires that medical and psychiatric care and treatment be provided to all persons admitted to a public hospital.

Although state courts and lower federal courts have decided that there may be a federal constitutional right to treatment, the U.S. Supreme Court has never clearly defined the right to treatment as a constitutional principle. Based on the decisions of a number of early court cases, treatment must meet the following criteria:

- The environment must be humane.
- Staff must be qualified and sufficient to provide adequate treatment.
- The plan of care must be individualized.

The initial cases presenting the psychiatric patient's right to treatment arose in the criminal justice system. An interesting case regarding the right to treatment is *O'Connor v. Donaldson* (1975). The Court held that a "state cannot constitutionally confine a nondangerous individual who is capable of surviving safely in freedom by himself or with the help of willing and responsible family members or friends" (*O'Connor v. Donaldson*, 1975, p. 576). Such court cases provide an interesting history of the evolution and shortcomings of our mental health delivery system.

Right to Refuse Treatment

Just as patients have the undeniable right to receive treatment, they also have the right to refuse it. Patients may withhold consent or withdraw consent at any time. Retraction of consent previously given must be honored, whether it is a verbal or written retraction. However, the mentally ill patient's right to refuse treatment with psychotropic drugs has been debated in the courts, based partly on the issue of mental patients' competency to give or withhold consent to treatment and their status under the civil commitment statutes. Early cases—initiated by state hospital patients—considered medical, legal, and ethical considerations such as basic treatment problems, the doctrine of informed consent, and the bioethical principle of autonomy. Tables 7-1 and 7-2

TABLE 7-1 Right to Refuse Treatment: Evolution of Massachusetts Case Law to Present Law

Case	Court	Decision
Rogers v. Okin, 478 F. Supp. 1342 (D. Mass. 1979)	Federal district court	Ruled that involuntarily hospitalized patients with mental illness are competent and have the right to make treatment decisions. Forcible administration of medication is justified in an emergency if needed to prevent violence and if other alternatives have been ruled out. A guardian may make treatment decisions for an incompetent patient.
Rogers v. Okin, 634 F.2nd 650 (1st Cir. 1980)	Federal court of appeals	Affirmed that involuntarily hospitalized patients with mental illness are competent and have the right to make treatment decisions. The staff has substantial discretion in an emergency. Forcible medication is also justified to prevent the patient's deterioration. A patient's rights must be protected by judicial determination of competency or incompetency.
Mills v. Rogers, 457 U.S. 291 (1982)	U.S. Supreme Court	Set aside the judgment of the court of appeals, with instructions to consider the effect of an intervening state court case.
Rogers v. Commissioner of the Department of Mental Health, 458 N.E.2d 308 (Mass. 1983)	Massachusetts Supreme Judicial Court answering questions certified by federal court of appeals	Ruled that involuntarily hospitalized patients are competent and have the right to make treatment decisions unless they are judicially determined to be incompetent.

TABLE 7-2 Right to Refuse Treatment: Evolution of New Jersey Case Law to Present Law

Case	Court	Decision
Rennie v. Klein, 476 F. Supp. 1292 (D. N.J. 1979)	Federal district court	Ruled that involuntarily hospitalized patients with mental illness have a qualified constitutional right to refuse treatment with antipsychotic drugs. Voluntarily hospitalized patients have an absolute right to refuse treatment with antipsychotic drugs under New Jersey law.
Rennie v. Klein, 653 F.2d 836 (3d Cir. 1981)	Federal court of appeals	Ruled that involuntarily hospitalized patients with mental illness have a constitutional right to refuse antipsychotic drug treatment. The state may override a patient's right when the patient poses a danger to self or others. Due process protections must be complied with before forcible medication of patients in nonemergency situations.
Rennie v. Klein, 454 U.S. 1078 (1982)	U.S. Supreme Court	Set aside the judgment of the court of appeals, with instructions to consider the case in light of the U.S. Supreme Court decision in *Youngberg v. Romeo*.
Rennie v. Klein, 720 F.2d 266 (3d Cir. 1983)	Federal court of appeals	Ruled that involuntarily hospitalized patients with mental illness have the right to refuse treatment with antipsychotic medication. Decisions to forcibly medicate must be based on "accepted professional judgment" and must comply with due process requirements of the New Jersey regulations.

summarize the evolution of two landmark sets of cases regarding the patient's right to refuse treatment.

The notion of refusing treatment becomes especially important if we consider medication to be a "chemical restraint." If it is, then the infringement on a person's liberty is at least equal to that with involuntary admission. The noninstitutionalized, competent patient with mental illness has the right, through substituted judgment, to determine whether to be involuntarily committed or medicated.

Cases involving the right to refuse psychotropic drug treatment are still evolving, and without clear direction from the Supreme Court, there will continue to be different case outcomes in different jurisdictions. The numerous cases involving the right to refuse medication have illustrated the complex and difficult task of translating social policy concerns into a clearly articulated legal standard.

Right to Informed Consent

The principle of **informed consent** is based on a person's right to self-determination, as enunciated in the landmark case of *Canterbury v. Spence* (1972):

The root premise is the concept, fundamental in American jurisprudence, that every human being of adult years and sound mind has a right to determine what shall be done with his own body. . . . True consent to what happens to one's self is the informed exercise of choice, and that entails an opportunity to evaluate knowledgeably the options available and the risks attendant on each. (p. 780)

Proper orders for specific therapies and treatments are required and must be documented in the patient's medical record. Consent for surgery, electroconvulsive treatment, or the use of experimental drugs or procedures must be obtained. In some state institutions, consent is required for each medication addition or change. Patients have the right to refuse participation in experimental treatments or research and the right to voice grievances and recommend changes in policies or services offered by the facility, without fear of punishment or reprisal.

For consent to be effective legally, it must be informed. Generally, the informed consent of the patient must be obtained by the physician or other health professional before a treatment or procedure is performed. Patients must be informed of the following:
- The nature of their problem or condition
- The nature and purpose of a proposed treatment
- The risks and benefits of that treatment
- The alternative treatment options

- The probability that the proposed treatment will be successful
- The risks of not consenting to treatment

It is important that psychiatric mental health nurses know that the presence of psychotic thinking does not mean that the patient is incompetent or incapable of understanding.

Competency is the capacity to understand the consequences of one's decisions. Patients must be considered legally competent until they have been declared incompetent through a legal proceeding. If found incompetent, the patient may be appointed a legal guardian or representative who is legally responsible for giving or refusing consent for the patient, while always considering the patient's wishes.

Guardians are typically selected from among family members. The order of selection is usually (1) spouse, (2) adult children or grandchildren, (3) parents, (4) adult siblings, and (5) adult nieces and nephews. In the event a family member is either unavailable or unwilling to serve as guardian, the court may also appoint a court-trained and approved social worker, representing the county or state, or a member of the community.

Many procedures nurses perform have an element of implied consent attached. For example, if you approach the patient with a medication in hand, and the patient indicates a willingness to receive the medication, implied consent has occurred. It should be noted that many institutions—particularly state psychiatric hospitals—have a requirement to obtain informed consent for every medication given. A general rule for you to follow is that the more intrusive or risky the procedure, the higher the likelihood that informed consent must be obtained. The fact that you may not have a legal duty to be the person to inform the patient of the associated risks and benefits of a particular medical procedure does not excuse you from clarifying the procedure to the patient and ensuring his or her expressed or implied consent.

Rights Regarding Involuntary Admission and Advance Psychiatric Directives

Patients concerned that they may be subject to involuntary admission can prepare an advance psychiatric directive document that will express their treatment choices. The advance directive for mental health decision making should be followed by health care providers when the patient is not competent to make informed decisions. This document can clarify the patient's choice of a surrogate decision maker and instructions about hospital choices, medications, treatment options, provider preferences, and emergency interventions. Identification of persons who are to be notified of the patient's hospitalization and who may have visitation rights is especially helpful, given the privacy demands of the Health Insurance Portability and Accountability Act (HIPAA) (Bazelon, 2003).

Rights Regarding Restraint and Seclusion

As previously mentioned, the use of the least restrictive means of restraint for the shortest duration is always the general rule. Verbal interventions or asking the patient for cooperation are the first approach, and medications are considered if verbal interventions fail. Chemical interventions (i.e., medications) are usually considered less restrictive than physical/mechanical interventions (i.e., restraints and seclusion), but they can have a greater impact on the patient's ability to relate to the environment because medication alters our ability to think and produces other side effects. However, when used judiciously, psychopharmacology is extremely effective and helpful as an alternative to physical methods of restraint.

The history of mechanical restraint and seclusion is marked by abuse, overuse, and even a tendency to use restraint as punishment. This was especially true prior to the 1950s when there were no effective chemical treatments. Legislation has dramatically reduced this problem by mandating strict guidelines. Behavioral restraint and seclusion are authorized as an intervention under the following circumstances:

- When the particular behavior is physically harmful to the patient or a third party
- When alternative or less restrictive measures are insufficient to protect the patient or others from harm
- When a decrease in sensory overstimulation (seclusion only) is needed
- When the patient anticipates that a controlled environment would be helpful and requests seclusion

As indicated earlier, most state laws prohibit the use of unnecessary physical restraint or isolation. The use of seclusion and restraint are permitted under the following circumstances:

- On the written order of a physician
- When orders are confined to specific time-limited periods (e.g., 2 to 4 hours)
- When the patient's condition is reviewed and documented regularly (e.g., every 15 minutes)
- When the original order is extended after review and reauthorization (e.g., every 24 hours) and specifies the type of restraint

Nurses must also know under which circumstances the use of seclusion is contraindicated (Box 7-1).

In an emergency, the nurse may place a patient in seclusion or restraint and obtain a written or verbal order as soon as possible thereafter. With the exception of a patient-initiated request to be placed in seclusion,

---

BOX 7-1 Contraindications to Seclusion

- Extremely unstable medical and psychiatric conditions*
- Delirium or dementia leading to inability to tolerate decreased stimulation*
- Severe suicidal tendencies*
- Severe drug reactions or overdoses or need for close monitoring of drug dosages*
- Desire for punishment of patient or convenience of staff

---

*Unless close supervision and direct observation are provided.
From Simon, R. I. and Shuman, Daniel, W. (2007). *Clinical Manual of psychiatry and law.* Washington, DC: American Psychiatric Publishing, Inc.

---

federal laws require an emergency situation to exist in which an immediate risk of harm to the patient or others can be documented. Although in restraints, the patient must be protected from all sources of harm. The behavior leading to restraint or seclusion and the time the patient is placed in and released from restraint must be documented. The patient in restraint must be assessed at regular and frequent intervals (e.g., every 15 to 30 minutes) for physical needs (e.g., food, hydration, toileting), safety, and comfort; and these observa-tions must also be documented every 15 to 30 minutes. The patient must be removed from restraints when safer and quieter behavior is observed.

Agencies have continued to revise their policies and procedures regarding restraint and seclusion, further limiting these practices after recent changes in laws. Despite deep-held beliefs of efficacy among practi-tioners who have used restraints, most agencies have found no negative impact associated with the reduced use of restraints and seclusion, and alternative meth-ods of therapy and cooperation with the patient have proven successful.

Rights Regarding Confidentiality

Confidentiality of care and treatment is also an important right for all patients, particularly psychiat-ric patients. Any discussion or consultation involving a patient should be conducted discreetly and only with individuals who have a need and a right to know this privileged information.

The American Nurses Association's (ANA's) *Code of Ethics for Nurses* (2001) asserts that it is a duty of the nurse to protect confidential patient information (Box 7-2). Failure to provide this protection may harm the nurse-patient relationship, as well as the patient's well-being. However, the code clarifies that this duty

---

BOX 7-2 Code of Ethics for Nurses

The House of Delegates of the American Nurses Association approved these nine provisions of the *Code of Ethics for Nurses* at its June 30, 2001, meeting in Washington, DC. In July of 2001, the Congress of Nursing Practice and Economics voted to accept the new language of the interpretive statements, resulting in a fully approved revised *Code of Ethics for Nurses with Interpretive Statements*.

1. The nurse, in all professional relationships, practices with compassion and respect for the inherent dignity, worth, and uniqueness of every individual, unrestricted by considerations of social or economic status, personal attributes or the nature of health problems.
2. The nurse's primary commitment is to the patient, whether an individual, family, group, or community.
3. The nurse promotes, advocates for, and strives to protect the health, safety, and rights of the patient.
4. The nurse is responsible and accountable for individual nursing practice and determines the appropriate delegation of tasks consistent with the nurse's obligation to provide optimum patient care.
5. The nurse owes the same duties to self as to others, including the responsibility to preserve integrity and safety, to maintain competence, and to continue personal and professional growth.
6. The nurse participates in establishing, maintaining, and improving health care environments and conditions of employment conducive to the provision of quality health care and consistent with the values of the profession through individual and collective action.
7. The nurse participates in the advancement of the profession through contributions to practice, education, administration, and knowledge development.
8. The nurse collaborates with other health professionals and the public in promoting community, national, and international efforts to meet health needs.
9. The profession of nursing, as represented by associations and their members, is responsible for articulating nursing values, for maintaining the integrity of the profession and its practice, and for shaping social policy.

From American Nurses Association. (2001). *Code of ethics for nurses with interpretive statements.* Washington, DC: American Nurses Publishing.

is not absolute. In some situations, disclosure may be mandated to protect the patient, other persons, or the public health.

Health Insurance Portability and Accountability Act (HIPAA)

The psychiatric patient's right to receive treatment and to have medical records kept confidential is legally protected by the Health Insurance Portability and Accountability Act (HIPAA), which was enacted in 1996. The fundamental principle underlying the ANA code on confidentiality is a person's constitutional right to privacy. Generally, your legal duty to maintain confidentiality is to protect the patient's right to privacy.

The HIPAA Privacy Rule became effective on April 14, 2003. According to this rule, you may not, without the patient's consent, disclose information obtained from the patient or the medical record to anyone except those persons for whom it is necessary for implementation of the patient's treatment plan. HIPAA also gives special protection to notes taken during psychotherapy that are kept separate from the patient's health information (HIPAA, 2003). Discussions about a patient in public places such as elevators and the cafeteria—even if the patient's name is not mentioned—can lead to disclosures of confidential information and liabilities for you and the facility.

For example, without the patient's consent, release of information to a patient's employer about his or her condition is a breach of confidentiality that subjects you to liability for the tort of invasion of privacy, as well as a HIPAA violation. On the other hand, discussion of a patient's history with other staff members to determine a consistent treatment approach is not a breach of confidentiality.

Generally, for a situation to be created in which information is privileged, a patient–health professional relationship must exist, and the information must concern the care and treatment of the patient. The health professional may refuse to disclose information to protect the patient's privacy. However, the right to privacy is the patient's right, and health professionals cannot invoke confidentiality for their own defense or benefit.

Confidentiality After Death

A person's reputation can be damaged even after death. Therefore, it is important that you do not divulge information after a person's death that you would not have been able to share legally before the death. The Dead Man's Statute protects confidential information about people when they are not alive to speak for themselves.

Confidentiality of Professional Communications

A legal privilege of confidentiality is enacted legislatively and exists to protect the confidentiality of professional communications (e.g., nurse-patient [in some states], physician-patient, attorney-patient). The theory behind such privileged communications is that patients will not be comfortable or willing to disclose personal information about themselves if they fear their confidential conversations will be repeated.

In some states in which the legal privilege of confidentiality has not expressly been legislated for nurses, you must respond to a court's inquiries regarding the patient's disclosures, even if this information implicates the patient in a crime. In these states, the confidentiality of communications cannot be guaranteed. If a duty to report exists, you may be required to divulge private information shared by the patient.

Confidentiality and Human Immunodeficiency Virus Status

Some states have enacted mandatory or permissive statutes that direct health care providers to warn a spouse if a partner tests positive for human immunodeficiency virus (HIV). Nurses must understand the laws in their jurisdiction of practice regarding privileged communications and warnings of infectious disease exposure.

Exceptions to the Rule

Duty to Warn and Protect Third Parties. The California Supreme Court, in its 1974 landmark decision *Tarasoff v. Regents of University of California*, ruled that a psychotherapist has a duty to warn a patient's potential victim of potential harm. A university student who was in counseling at the University of California was despondent over being rejected by Tatiana Tarasoff, whom he had once kissed. The psychologist notified police verbally and in writing that the young man might pose a danger to Tarasoff. The police questioned the student, found him to be rational, and secured his promise to stay away from his love interest. The student killed Tarasoff 2 months later.

This case created much controversy and confusion in the psychiatric and medical communities over (1) breach of patient confidentiality and its impact on the therapeutic relationship in psychiatric care, and (2) over the ability of the psychotherapist to predict when a patient is truly dangerous. This trend continues as other jurisdictions have adopted or modified the California rule despite objections from the psychiatric community.

The *Tarasoff* case acknowledged that generally there is no common-law duty to aid third persons. An exception is when special relationships exist, and the court found the patient-therapist relationship sufficient to create a duty of the therapist to aid Ms. Tarasoff, the victim. The duty to protect the intended victim from danger arises when the therapist determines—or, pursuant to professional standards, should have determined—that the patient presents a serious danger to another.

The California Supreme Court held a second hearing in 1976 in the case of *Tarasoff v. Regents of the University of California* (now known as *Tarasoff II*). They delivered a second ruling that broadened the earlier duty to warn. When a therapist determines that a patient presents a serious danger of violence to another, the therapist has the duty to protect that other person. In providing protection, it may be necessary for the therapist to call and warn the intended victim, the victim's family, or the police or to take whatever steps are reasonably necessary under the circumstances.

Most states currently have similar laws regarding the duty to protect third parties of potential life threats. The duty to protect usually includes the following:

- Assessing and predicting the patient's danger of violence toward another
- Identifying the specific persons being threatened
- Taking appropriate action to protect the identified victims

Implications for psychiatric mental health nursing. As this trend toward the therapist's duty to warn third persons of potential harm continues to gain wider acceptance, it is important for students and nurses to understand its implications for nursing practice. Although none of these cases has dealt with nurses, it is fair to assume that in jurisdictions that have adopted the *Tarasoff* doctrine, the duty to warn third persons will be applied to advanced practice psychiatric mental health nurses in private practice who engage in individual therapy. If, however, a staff nurse—who is a member of a team of psychiatrists, psychologists, psychiatric social workers, and other psychiatric nurses— does not report to other members of the team a patient's threats of harm against specified victims or classes of victims, this failure is likely to be considered substandard nursing care.

Failure to communicate and record relevant information from police, relatives, or the patient's old records might also be deemed negligent. Breach of patient-nurse confidentiality should not pose ethical or legal dilemmas for nurses in these situations, because a team approach to the delivery of psychiatric care presumes communication of pertinent information to other staff members to develop a treatment plan in the patient's best interest.

Statutes for Reporting Child and Elder Abuse. All 50 states and the District of Columbia have enacted child abuse reporting statutes. Although these statutes differ from state to state, they generally include a definition of child abuse, a list of persons required or encouraged to report abuse, and the governmental agency designated to receive and investigate the reports. Most statutes include civil penalties for failure to report. Many states specifically require nurses to report cases of suspected abuse. Refer to Box 7-3 for a possible example of how to report abuse.

There is a conflict between federal and state laws with respect to child abuse reporting when the health care professional discovers child abuse or neglect during

---

BOX 7-3 How Does A Nurse Go About Reporting Child Abuse?

Institutions usually have policies for reporting abuse. Often the responsibility goes to social workers who have expertise in these matters and know how to navigate the system. However, if you are caring for a child covered in old and new bruises or who has a broken bone and decaying teeth, and you suspect abuse, it is your legal and ethical responsibility to make a report to your state's child welfare agency. You should also let the child's parents/ guardians know that you are filing the report. Whether the physician or your peers agree with you or not, if you report suspected child abuse in good faith, you will be protected from criminal or civil liability. More importantly, you may save one child from further suffering.

---

the suspected abuser's alcohol or drug treatment. Federal laws and regulations governing confidentiality of patient records, which apply to almost all drug abuse and alcohol treatment providers, prohibit any disclosure without a court order. In this case, federal law supersedes state reporting laws, although compliance with the state law may be maintained under the following circumstances:

- If a court order is obtained, pursuant to the regulations
- If a report can be made without identifying the abuser as a patient in an alcohol or drug treatment program
- If the report is made anonymously (some states, to protect the rights of the accused, do not allow anonymous reporting)

As reported incidents of abuse to other persons in society surface, states may require health professionals to report other kinds of abuse. A growing number of states are enacting **elder abuse reporting statutes**, which require registered nurses and others to report cases of abuse of older adults (those 65 years of age and older). Agencies that receive federal funding (e.g., Medicare or Medicaid) must follow strict guidelines for reporting and preventing elder abuse.

These laws also apply to dependent adults—adults between the ages of 18 and 64 whose physical or mental limitations restrict their ability to carry out normal activities or to protect themselves—when the registered nurse has actual knowledge that the person has been the victim of physical abuse. Under most state laws, a person who is required to report suspected abuse, neglect, or exploitation of a disabled adult and willfully does not do so is guilty of a misdemeanor crime. Most state statutes declare that anyone who makes a report in good faith is immune from civil liability in connection with the report.

You may also report knowledge or reasonable suspicion of mental abuse or suffering. Both dependent adults and elders are protected by the law from purposeful physical or fiduciary neglect or abandonment. **Because state laws vary, students are encouraged to become familiar with the requirements of their states**.

Failure to Protect Patients

Legal issues common in psychiatric mental health nursing relate to the failure to protect the safety of patients (Table 7-3). If a suicidal patient is left alone with the means of self harm, the nurse who has a duty to protect the patient will be held responsible for the resultant injuries. Leaving a suicidal patient alone in a room on the sixth floor with an open window is an example of unreasonable judgment on the part of the nurse. Precautions to prevent harm also must be taken whenever a patient is restrained. Miscommunications and medication errors are common in all areas of nursing, including psychiatric care. Another common area of liability in psychiatry is abuse of the therapist-patient relationship. Issues of sexual misconduct during the

therapeutic relationship have become a source of concern in the psychiatric community. Misdiagnosis is also frequently charged in legal suits.

Tort Law

A **tort** is a civil wrong for which money damages may be collected by the injured party (the plaintiff) from the responsible party (the defendant). The injury can be to person, property, or reputation. Because tort law has general applicability to nursing practice, this section may contain a review of material previously covered elsewhere in your nursing curriculum.

Intentional Torts

Nurses in psychiatric settings may encounter provocative, threatening, or violent behavior that may require the use of restraint or seclusion. However, use of such interventions must be carefully determined and used only in the most extreme situations. As discussed earlier in this chapter, restraint and seclusion historically were used with little regard to patients' rights, and overuse and abuses were common. Stories of patients

TABLE 7-3 Common Liability Issues

Issue	Examples
Patient safety	Failure to notice or take action on suicide risks Failure to use restraints properly or monitor the patient Miscommunication Medication errors Violation of boundaries (e.g., sexual misconduct) Misdiagnosis

Intentional torts
  May carry criminal penalties
  Punitive damages may be awarded
  Not covered by malpractice insurance
	Voluntary acts intended to bring a physical or mental consequence
	Purposeful acts
	Recklessness
	Not obtaining patient consent
	Note: Self-defense or protection of others may serve as a defense to charges
	  of an intentional tort.

Negligence/malpractice	Carelessness Foreseeability of harm
Assault and battery	Person apprehensive (assault) of harmful/offensive touching (battery) Threat to use force (words alone are not enough) with opportunity and ability Treatment without patient's consent
False imprisonment	Intent to confine to a specific area Indefensible use of seclusion or restraints Detention of voluntarily admitted patient, with no agency or legal policies to support detaining

Defamation of character
  Slander (spoken)
  Libel (written)
	Sharing private information with people who aren't directly involved with care
	Confidential documents shared with people who aren't directly involved with care

Supervisory liability (vicarious liability)	Inappropriate delegation of duties Lack of supervision of those supervising

restrained and left to lie in their own excrement or locked in seclusion for days for being annoying have resulted in strict laws. Accordingly, the nurse in the psychiatric setting should understand intentional torts, which are willful or intentional acts that violate another person's rights or property. Some examples of intentional torts include assault, battery, and false imprisonment (see Table 7-3).

Other types of intentional torts may hurt a person's sense of self or their financial status. They are **invasion of privacy** and **defamation of character**. Invasion of privacy in health care has to do with breaking a person's confidences or taking photographs without explicit permission. Defamation of character includes slander (verbal), such as talking about patients on the elevator with others around, and libel (printed), where written information about the patient is shared with people outside the professional setting.

Unintentional Torts

Unintentional torts are unintended acts against another person that produce injury or harm. Negligence is a general tort for which anyone may be found guilty. For example, if you do not shovel the snow from your driveway, and a visitor falls and breaks his hip, you may be charged with negligence. When health care professionals fail to act in accordance with professional standards, or when they fail to foresee consequences that other professionals with similar skills and education should foresee, they can be liable for a tort of professional negligence, or malpractice. Malpractice is an act or omission to act that breaches the duty of due care and results in or is responsible for a person's injuries. The five elements required to prove negligence are (1) duty, (2) breach of duty, (3) cause in fact, (4) proximate cause, and (5) damages. Foreseeability or likelihood of harm is also evaluated.

Duty. When nurses represent themselves as being capable of caring for psychiatric patients and accept employment, a **duty** of care has been assumed. As a nurse, you have the duty to understand the theory and medications used in the specialty care of psychiatric patients. Persons who represent themselves as possessing superior knowledge and skill, such as psychiatric mental health nurse specialists, are held to a higher standard of care in the practice of their profession. The staff nurse who is assigned to a psychiatric unit must be knowledgeable enough to assume a reasonable or safe duty of care for the patients.

Breach of Duty. If you are not capable of providing the standard of care that other nurses would be expected to supply under similar circumstances, you have breached the duty of care. **Breach of duty** is any conduct that exposes the patient to an unreasonable risk of harm, through either commission or omission of acts by the nurse. If you do not have the required education and experience to provide certain interventions, you have breached the duty by neglecting or omitting the provision of necessary care. You can also act in such a way that the patient is harmed and can thus be guilty of negligence through acts of commission.

Cause in Fact, Proximate Cause, and Damages. **Cause in fact** may be evaluated by asking the question, "Except for what the nurse did, would this injury have occurred?" **Proximate cause**, or legal cause, may be evaluated by determining whether there were any intervening actions or persons that were, in fact, the causes of harm to the patient.

Damages include actual damages (e.g., loss of earnings, medical expenses, and property damage), as well as pain and suffering. They also include incidental or consequential damages. For example, giving a patient the wrong medication may have actual damage of a complicated hospital stay, but it also may result in permanent disability which may require such things as special education needs and special accommodations in the home. Furthermore, incidental damages may deprive others of the benefits of the injured person, such as losing a normal relationship with a husband or father.

Forseeability of harm evaluates the likelihood of the outcome under the circumstances. If the average, reasonable person could foresee that injury would result from the action or inaction, then the injury was foreseeable.

Box 7-4 gives a description of a case of false imprisonment, negligence, and malpractice.

DETERMINATION OF A STANDARD OF CARE

Professional standards of practice determined by professional associations differ from the minimal qualifications set forth by state licensure for entry into the profession of nursing because the primary purposes are different. The state's qualifications for practice provide consumer protection by ensuring that all practicing nurses have successfully completed an approved nursing program and passed the national licensing examination. The professional association's primary focus is to elevate the practice of its members by setting standards of excellence. The Standards of Practice and Professional Performance from the *Psychiatric-Mental Health Nursing: Scope and Standards of Practice* (ANA et al., 2007) are provided on the inside back cover of this book.

Nurses are held to a basic standard of care. This standard is based on what other nurses who possess the same degree of skill or knowledge in the same or similar circumstances would do. Psychiatric patients have the right to the standard of care recognized by professional bodies governing nursing, whether they are in a

---

BOX 7-4 False Imprisonment, Negligence, and Malpractice: *Plumadore v. State of New York* (1980)

Mrs. Plumadore was admitted to Saranac Lake General Hospital for a gallbladder condition. Her medical workup revealed emotional problems stemming from marital difficulties, which had resulted in suicide attempts several years before her admission. After a series of consultations and tests, she was advised by the attending surgeon that she was scheduled to have gallbladder surgery later that day. After the surgeon's visit, a consulting psychiatrist who examined her directed her to dress and pack her belongings; he had arranged to have her admitted to a state hospital at Ogdensburg.

Subsequently, two uniformed state troopers handcuffed her and strapped her into the back seat of a patrol car. She was also accompanied by a female hospital employee and was transported to the state hospital. On arrival, the admitting psychiatrist recognized that the referring psychiatrist lacked the requisite authority to order her involuntary admission. He therefore requested that she sign a voluntary admission form, which she refused to do. Despite Mrs. Plumadore's protests regarding her admission to the state hospital, the psychiatrist assigned her to a ward without physical or psychiatric examination and without the opportunity to contact her family or her medical doctor. The record of her admission to the state hospital noted an "informed admission," which is patient-initiated voluntary admission in New York.

The court awarded $40,000 to Mrs. Plumadore for malpractice and false imprisonment on the part of health care professionals, and negligence on the part of the troopers.

---

large, small, rural, or urban facility. Nurses must participate in continuing education courses to stay current with existing standards of care.

Hospital policies and procedures define institutional criteria for care, and these criteria may be introduced in legal proceedings to prove that a nurse met or failed to meet them. The weakness of this method is that the hospital's policy may be substandard. For example, an institution may determine that patients can be kept in seclusion for up to 6 hours, based on the original physician's order, but state licensing laws for institutions might set a limit of 4 hours. **Substandard institutional policies do not absolve the individual nurse of responsibility to practice on the basis of professional standards of nursing care.**

Like hospital policy and procedures, custom can be used as evidence of a standard of care. In the absence of a written policy on the use of restraint, testimony might be offered regarding the customary use of restraint in emergency situations in which the combative, violent,

or confused patient poses a threat of harm to self or others. Using custom to establish a standard of care may result in the same defect as in using hospital policies and procedures: custom may not comply with the laws, recommendations of the accrediting body, or other recognized standards of care. Custom must be carefully and regularly evaluated to ensure that substandard routines have not developed. Substandard customs do not protect you when a psychiatric patient charges that a right has been violated or that harm has been caused by the staff's common practices.

GUIDELINES FOR ENSURING ADHERENCE TO STANDARDS OF CARE

Negligence, Irresponsibility, or Impairment

It is not unusual for a student or practicing nurse to suspect negligence on the part of a peer. In most states, you have a legal duty to report such risks of harm to the patient. It is also important to document the evidence clearly and accurately before making serious accusations against a peer. If you question a physician's or fellow nurse's orders or actions, it is wise to communicate these concerns directly to the person involved. If the risky behavior continues, you have an obligation to communicate these concerns to a supervisor, who should then intervene to ensure that the patient's rights and well-being are protected.

If you suspect a peer of being chemically impaired or of practicing irresponsibly, you have an obligation to protect not only the rights of the peer but also the rights of all patients who could be harmed by this person. If the danger persists after you have reported suspected behavior of concern to a supervisor, you have a duty to report the concern to someone at the next level of authority. It is important to follow the channels of communication in an organization, but it is also important to protect the safety of the patients. If the supervisor's actions or inactions do not rectify the dangerous situation, you have a continuing duty to report the behavior of concern to the appropriate authority, such as the state board of nursing.

A useful reference for nurses is the ANA's *Guidelines on Reporting Incompetent, Unethical or Illegal Practices* (1994).

Unethical or Illegal Practices

The issues become more complex when a professional colleague's conduct (including that of a student nurse) is criminally unlawful. Specific examples include the diversion of drugs from the hospital and sexual misconduct with patients. Increasing media attention and the recognition of substance abuse as an occupational hazard for health professionals have led to the establishment of substance abuse programs for health care workers in many states. These programs provide appropriate treatment for impaired professionals to protect the public from harm and to rehabilitate the professional.

The problem of reporting impaired colleagues—as previously discussed—becomes a difficult one, particularly when no direct harm has occurred to the patient. Concern for professional reputations, damaged careers, and personal privacy has generated a code of silence regarding substance abuse among health professionals.

Several states now require reporting of impaired or incompetent colleagues to the professional licensing boards. In the absence of such a legal mandate, the questions of whether to report and to whom to report become ethical ones. Chapter 18 deals more fully with issues related to the chemically impaired nurse, and you are again urged to use the ANA's *Guidelines on Reporting Incompetent, Unethical or Illegal Practices* (1994).

The duty to intervene includes the duty to report known abusive behavior. Most states have enacted statutes to protect children and older adults from abuse and neglect. Psychiatric mental health nurses working in the community may be required by law to report unsafe relationships they discover.

Duty to Intervene and Duty to Report

The psychiatric mental health nurse has a duty to intervene when the safety or well-being of the patient or another person is obviously at risk. A nurse who knowingly follows an incorrect or possibly harmful order is responsible for any harm that results to the patient. **If you have information that leads you to believe that the physician's orders need to be clarified or changed, it is your duty to intervene and protect the patient.** It is important that you communicate with the physician who has ordered the treatment to explain the concern. If the treating physician does not appear willing to consider your concerns, you should carry out the duty to intervene through other appropriate channels. The following Vignette illustrates two possible outcomes of a nurse intervening in a medication issue.

VIGNETTE

Amanda is a new nurse on the crisis management unit. She completed the hospital and unit orientations 2 weeks ago and has begun to care for patients independently. As she prepares to give her 5:00 PM medications, Amanda notices that Greg Thorn, a 55-year-old man admitted after a suicide attempt, has been given a new order for the antidepressant sertraline (Zoloft). Amanda remembers that Mr. Thorn had been taking phenelzine (Nardil) prior to his admission and seems to recall something unsafe about mixing these two medications. She looks the antidepressants up in her drug guide and realizes that Nardil is a monoamine oxidase inhibitor (MAOI) and that adding this second antidepressant within 2 weeks of discontinuing the Nardil could result in severe side effects and possibly a lethal response.

After clarifying with Mr. Thorn that he had been on Nardil and discussing the issue with another nurse, Amanda realizes she needs to put the medication on hold and contact Mr. Thorn's psychiatrist, Dr. Cruz, by phone. Amanda begins by saying, "I see that Mr. Thorn has been ordered Zoloft. I am looking at his nursing admission assessment, and it says that he had been taking Nardil up until a few days ago. However, I don't see it listed on the medical assessment that was done by the resident."

First Possible Outcome

Dr. Cruz responds, "Thank you for calling that to my attention. When I make my rounds in the morning, I'll decide what to do with his medications. For now, please put a hold on the Zoloft." Amanda clarifies what Dr. Cruz has said, writes the order, and documents what happened in the nurses notes.

Second Possible Outcome

Dr. Cruz responds, "Are you telling me how to do my job? If it wasn't on the medical assessment, then he wasn't taking it. A nurse must have made a mistake—again. I wrote an order for Nardil, give him the Nardil." He hangs up. Amanda documents the exchange, determines that the safest and most appropriate response is to hold the medication for now, and contacts her nursing supervisor. The supervisor supports her decision and follows up with the chief of psychiatry.

You should express concerns to your supervisor so that the supervisor can communicate with the appropriate medical staff. It is also important to follow agency policies and procedures for communicating differences of opinion. If you fail to intervene and the patient is injured, you may be partly liable for the injuries that result because of failure to use safe nursing practice and good professional judgment.

The duty to intervene on the patient's behalf poses legal and ethical dilemmas for nurses in the workplace. Institutions that have a chain-of-command policy or other reporting mechanisms offer some assurance that the proper authorities in the administration are notified. Most patient-care issues regarding physicians' orders or treatments can be settled fairly early in the process by the nurse's discussion of the concerns with the physician. If further intervention by the nurse is required to protect the patient, the next step in the chain of command can be followed. Generally, the nurse then notifies the immediate nursing supervisor, who discusses the problem with the physician and then the chief of staff of a particular service until a resolution is reached. If there is no time to resolve the issue through the normal process because of the life-threatening nature of the situation, the nurse has no choice but to act to protect the patient's life.

The legal concept of **abandonment** may also arise when a nurse does not leave a patient safely back in the hands of another health professional before discontinuing treatment. When the nurse is given an assignment to care for a patient, the nurse must provide the care or ensure that the patient is safely reassigned to another nurse. Abandonment issues arise when accurate, timely, and thorough reporting has not occurred or when follow-through of patient care, on which the patient is relying, has not occurred.

The same principles apply for the psychiatric mental health nurse who is working in a community setting. For example, if a suicidal patient refuses to come to the hospital for treatment, you must take the necessary steps to ensure the patient's safety. These actions may include enlisting the assistance of the law in involuntarily admitting the patient on a temporary basis.

DOCUMENTATION OF CARE

The purposes of the medical record are to provide accurate and complete information about the care and treatment of patients and to give health care personnel a means of communicating with each other, allowing continuity of care. A record's usefulness is determined by evaluating how accurately and completely it portrays the patient's behavioral status at the time it was written. The patient has the right to see the medical record, but it belongs to the institution. The patient must follow appropriate protocol to view his or her records.

For example, if a psychiatric patient describes to a nurse a plan to harm himself or another person, and that nurse fails to document the information—including the need to protect the patient or the identified victim—the information will be lost when the nurse leaves work. If the patient's plan is carried out, the harm caused could be linked directly to the nurse's failure to communicate this important information. Even though documentation takes time away from the patient, the importance of communicating and preserving the nurse's memory through the medical record cannot be overemphasized.

Facility Use of Medical Records

The medical record has many other uses aside from providing information on the course of the patient's care and treatment by health care professionals. A retrospective medical record review can provide valuable information to the facility on the quality of care provided and on ways to improve that care. A facility may conduct reviews for risk management purposes to determine areas of potential liability for the facility and to evaluate methods used to reduce the facility's exposure to liability. For example, documentation of the use of restraints and seclusion for psychiatric patients may be reviewed by risk managers. Accordingly, the medical record may be used to evaluate care for quality assurance or peer review. Utilization review analysts evaluate the medical record to determine appropriate use of hospital and staff resources consistent with reimbursement schedules. Insurance companies and other reimbursement agencies rely on the medical record in determining what payments they will make on the patient's behalf.

Medical Records as Evidence

From a legal perspective, the medical record is a recording of data and opinions made in the normal course of the patient's hospital care. It is deemed to be good evidence because it is presumed to be true, honest, and untainted by memory lapses. Accordingly, the medical record finds its way into a variety of legal cases for a variety of reasons. Some examples of its use include determining (1) the extent of the patient's damages and pain and suffering in personal injury cases, such as when a psychiatric patient attempts suicide while under the protective care of a hospital; (2) the nature and extent of injuries in child abuse or elder abuse cases; (3) the nature and extent of physical or mental disability in disability cases; and (4) the nature and extent of injury and rehabilitative potential in workers' compensation cases.

Medical records may also be used in police investigations, civil conservatorship proceedings, competency hearings, and involuntary admission procedures. In states that mandate mental health legal services or a patients' rights advocacy program, audits may be performed to determine the facility's compliance with state laws or violation of patients' rights. Finally, medical records may be used in professional and hospital negligence cases.

During the initial, or discovery, phase of litigation, the medical record is a pivotal source of information for attorneys in determining whether a cause of action exists in a professional negligence or hospital negligence case. Evidence of the nursing care rendered will be found in what the nurse documented.

Guidelines for Electronic Documentation

Accurate, descriptive, and legible nursing notes serve the best interests of the patient, the nurse, and the institution. Electronic documentation is commonplace and has created new challenges for protecting the confidentiality of the records of psychiatric patients. Institutions must protect against intrusions into the privacy of patient record systems. At the same time, they must provide a method by which information can be shared appropriately. Sensitive information regarding treatment for mental illness can adversely impact patients who are seeking employment, insurance, and credit (Fung & Paynter, 2008).

Concerns for the privacy of patients' records have been addressed by federal laws that provide guidelines for agencies that use electronic documentation. These guidelines include the recommendation that staff be assigned a password for entering patients' records to identify which staff have gained access to confidential patient information. There are penalties, including termination of employment, if a staff member enters a record without authorization for access. Only staff who have a legitimate need to know about the patient are authorized to access a patient's electronic medical record.

It is important to keep your password private and never allow someone else to access a record under your password. You are responsible for all entries into records using your password. The various systems used allow specific time frames within which the nurse must make any necessary corrections if a documentation error is made.

Any documentation method that improves communication between care providers should be encouraged. Courts assume that nurses and physicians read each other's notes on patient progress. Many courts take the attitude that if care is not documented, it did not occur. Your documentation also serves as a valuable memory refresher if the patient sues years after the care is rendered. In providing complete and timely information on the care and treatment of patients, the medical record enhances communication among health professionals. Internal institutional audits of the record can improve the quality of care rendered. Chapter 8 describes common documentation forms and gives examples and the pros and cons of each.

FORENSIC NURSING

The new and evolving specialty of forensic nursing includes the application of nursing principles in a court of law to assist in reaching a decision on a contested issue. The nurse acts as an advocate, educating the court about the science of nursing. Examples of psychiatric mental health forensic nursing may include cases related to patient competency, fitness to stand trial, and involuntary admission or responsibility for a crime. The application of nursing facts are related and applied to the legal facts. Forensic nurses also focus on victims of crime and violence, the collection of evidence, and the provision of health care in prison settings. See Chapter 33 for a complete discussion of forensic nursing.

VIOLENCE IN THE PSYCHIATRIC SETTING

Nurses must protect themselves in both institutional and community settings. Nurses have placed themselves knowingly in the range of danger by agreeing to care for unpredictable patients, and employers typically are not held responsible for employee injuries due to violent patient behavior. It is therefore important for nurses to protect themselves by participating in setting policies that create a safe environment. Good judgment means not placing oneself in a potentially violent situation.

Nurses, as citizens, have the same rights as patients not to be threatened or harmed. Appropriate security support should be readily available to the nurse practicing in an institution. When you work in community settings, you must avoid placing yourself unnecessarily in dangerous environments, especially when alone at night. You should use common sense and enlist the support of local law enforcement officers when needed. A violent patient is not being abandoned if placed safely in the hands of the authorities.

The psychiatric mental health nurse must also be aware of the potential for violence in the community when a patient is discharged following a short-term stay. The duty of the nurse to protect the patient and warn others who may be threatened by the violent patient is discussed earlier in this chapter. The nurse's assessment of the patient's potential for violence must be documented and acted on if there is legitimate concern regarding discharge of a patient who is discussing or exhibiting potentially violent behavior. The psychiatric mental health nurse must communicate his or her observations to the medical staff when discharge decisions are being considered.

KEY POINTS TO REMEMBER

- The states' power to enact laws for public health and safety and for the care of those unable to care for themselves often pits the rights of society against the rights of the individual.
- Psychiatric mental health nurses frequently encounter problems requiring ethical choices.
- The nurse's privilege to practice carries with it the responsibility to practice safely, competently, and in a manner consistent with state and federal laws.
- Knowledge of the law, the ANA's *Code of Ethics for Nurses*, and the Standards of Practice and Professional Performance from the *Psychiatric-Mental Health Nursing: Scope and Standards of Practice* (ANA et al., 2007) are essential for providing safe, effective psychiatric mental health nursing care and will serve as a framework for decision making.

CRITICAL THINKING

1. Joe and Beth are registered nurses who have worked together on the psychiatric unit for two years. Beth confided to Joe that her marital situation has become particularly difficult over the last six months. He expressed concern and shared his observation that she seems to be distracted and not as happy lately. Privately, Joe concludes that this explains why Beth has become so irritable and distracted.

As Joe prepares the medication for the evening shift, he notices that two of his patients' medications are missing; both are bedtime Ativan (lorazepam). When he phones the pharmacy to send up the missing medications, the pharmacist responds, "You people need to watch your carts more carefully because this has become a pattern." Shortly after, another patient complains to Joe that he did not receive his 5 PM Xanax (alprazolam). On the medication administration record Beth has recorded that she has given the drugs. Joe suspects that Beth may be diverting the drugs.

A. What action, if any, should Joe take?

B. Should Joe confront Beth with his suspicions?

C. If Beth admits that she has been diverting the drugs, should Joe's next step be to report Beth to the supervisor or to the board of nursing?

D. When Joe talks to the nursing supervisor, should he identify Beth or should he state his suspicions in general terms?

F. How does the nature of the drugs affect your responses? That is, if the drugs were to treat a 'physical' condition such as hypertension would you be more concerned?

G. What does the nurse practice act in your state mandate regarding reporting the illegal use of drugs by a nurse?

2. Linda has been employed in a psychiatric setting for five years. One day she arrives at work and is informed that the staffing office has requested that a nurse from the psychiatric unit assist the intensive care unit (ICU) staff in caring for an agitated car accident victim with a history of schizophrenia. Linda goes to the ICU and joins a nurse named Corey in providing care for the patient. Eventually, the patient is stabilized, he goes to sleep, and Corey leaves the unit for a break. Since Linda is unfamiliar with the telemetry equipment, she fails to recognize that the patient is having an arrhythmia and the patient experiences a cardiopulmonary arrest. Although he is successfully resuscitated after six minutes, he suffers permanent brain damage.

A. Can Linda legally practice in this situation? (That is, does her RN license permit her to practice in the intensive care unit?)

B. Does the ability to practice legally in an area differ from the ability to practice competently in that area?

C. Did Linda have any legal or ethical grounds to refuse the assignment to the intensive care unit?

D. What are the risks in accepting an assignment in an area of specialty in which you are professionally unprepared to practice?

E. What are the risks in refusing an assignment in an area of specialty in which you are professionally unprepared to practice?

F. Would there have been any way for Linda to minimize the risk of retaliation by the employer had she refused the assignment?

G. What action could Linda have taken to protect the patient and herself when Corey left the unit for a break?

H. If Linda is negligent, is the hospital liable for any harm to the patient caused by her?

3. A 40-year-old man is admitted to the emergency department for a severe nosebleed and has both of his nostrils packed. Because of a history of alcoholism and the possibility for developing delirium tremens (withdrawal), the patient is transferred to the psychiatric unit. His physician orders a private room, restraints, continuous monitoring, and 15 minute checks of vital signs and other indicators. At the next 15 minute check, the nurse discovers that the patient does not have a pulse or respiration. The patient had apparently inhaled the nasal packing and suffocated.

A. Does it sound like the nurse was responsible for the patient's death?

B. Was the order for the restraint appropriate for this type of patient?

C. What factors did you consider in making your determination?

4. Assume that there are no mandatory reporting laws for impaired or incompetent colleagues in the following clinical situation. A 15-year-old boy is admitted to a psychiatric facility voluntarily at the request of his parents because of violent, explosive behavior. This behavior began after his father's recent remarriage after his parents' divorce. In group therapy, he has become incredibly angry in response to a discussion about weekend passes for Mother's Day. "Everyone has abandoned me, no one cares," he screamed. Several weeks later, on the day before his discharge, he convinces his nurse to keep his plan to kill his mother confidential.

Consider the ANA *Code of Ethics for Nurses* on patient confidentiality, the principles of psychiatric nursing, the statutes on privileged communications, and the duty to warn third parties in answering the following questions:

A. Did the nurse use appropriate judgment in promising confidentiality?

B. Does the nurse have a legal duty to warn the patient's mother of her son's threat?

C. Is the duty owed to the patient's father and stepmother?

D. Would a change in the admission status from voluntary to involuntary protect the patient's mother without violating the patient's confidentiality?

E. What nursing action, if any, should the nurse take after the disclosure by the patient?

CHAPTER REVIEW

1. A patient with depression presents with her family in the emergency room. The family feels the patient should be admitted because "she might hurt herself." An assessment indicates moderate depression with no risk factors for suicide other than the depressed mood itself, and the patient denies any intent or thoughts about self-harm. The family agrees that the patient has not done or said anything to suggest that she might be a danger to herself. Which of the following responses is consistent with the concept of "least restrictive alternative" doctrine?
   1. Admit the patient as a temporary inpatient admission.
   2. Persuade the patient to agree to a voluntary inpatient admission.
   3. Admit the patient involuntarily to an inpatient mental health treatment unit.
   4. Arrange for an emergency outpatient counseling appointment the next day.

2. After 15 days, a patient is released from an inpatient treatment unit where he had been committed by a judge for a period of 90 days. Upon discharge, in return for placement in a mental health group home, the patient is required to attend weekly appointments with his case manager and counselor, take all ordered medications, and meet twice monthly with his psychiatrist. He is told that the judge has ordered that the patient be readmitted to the inpatient facility if he fails to follow these requirements. This scenario includes examples of which of the following type(s) of admissions and/or releases? *Select all that apply.*
   1. Involuntary admission
   2. Long-term involuntary admission
   3. Unconditional release
   4. Conditional release
   5. Involuntary outpatient admission

3. An advanced practice nurse wishes to initiate treatment with an antipsychotic medication which, although very likely to benefit the patient, in a small percentage of patients may cause a dangerous side effect. The nurse explains the purpose, expected benefits, and possible risks of the medication. The patient readily signs a form accepting the medication, stating, "These pills will poison the demons inside of me." Although he has been informed of the risk of side effects, he is unable to state what these are and simply reports that he "won't have side effects because I am iron and cannot be killed." Which of the following responses would be most appropriate under these circumstances?
   1. Begin administration of the medications based on his signed permission, because he has legally consented to treatment.
   2. Petition the court to appoint a guardian to substitute for the patient's being unable to comprehend the proposed treatment.

   3. Administer the medications even though consent is unclear, because the patient is clearly psychotic and in need of the medications.
   4. Withhold the medication until the patient is able to identify the benefits and risks of both consenting and refusing consent to the medications.

4. A patient incidentally shares with you that he has difficulty controlling his anger when around children because their play irritates him, leading to resentment and fantasies about attacking them. He has a history of impulsiveness and assault, escalates easily on the unit, and has a poor tolerance for frustration. This weekend he has an overnight pass, which he will spend with his sister and her family. As you meet with the patient and his sister just prior to the pass, the sister mentions that she has missed her brother because he usually helps her watch the children, and she has to work this weekend and needs him to babysit. The patient becomes visibly apprehensive upon hearing this. Which of the following responses would best reflect appropriate nursing practice relative to the conflict this situation presents between safety and the patient's right to confidentiality?
   1. Cancel the pass without explanation to the sister, and reschedule it for a time when babysitting would not be required of the patient.
   2. Suggest that the sister make other arrangements for child care, but withhold the information the patient shared regarding his concerns about harming children.
   3. Speak with the patient about the safety risk involved in babysitting, seeking his permission to share this information and advising against the pass if he declines to share the information.
   4. Meet with the patient's sister, sharing with her the patient's previous disclosure about his anger towards children and the resultant risk that his babysitting would present.

5. Mrs. Smith is admitted for treatment of depression with suicidal ideation triggered by marital discord. She had spoken with staff about her fears that the marriage will end, had indicated that she did not know how she could cope if her marriage ended, and has a history of suicide attempts when the marriage had seemed threatened in the past. Her spouse visits one night and informs Mrs. Smith that he has decided to file for divorce. Staff are aware of the visit and the husband's intentions regarding divorce but take no further action, feeling that the q15-minute suicide checks Mrs. Smith is already on are sufficient. Thirty minutes after the visit ends, staff make rounds and discover Mrs. Smith has hanged herself in her bathroom, using hospital pajamas she had tied together into a rope. Which of the following statements best describes this situation? *Select all that apply.*
   1. The nurses have created liability for themselves and their employer by failing in their duty to protect Mrs. Smith.

2. The nurses have breached their duty to reassess Mrs. Smith for increased suicide risk after her husband's visit.

3. Given Mrs. Smith's history, the nurses should have expected an increased risk of suicide after the husband's announcement.

4. The nurses correctly reasoned that suicides cannot always be prevented and did their best to keep Mrs. Smith safe via the q15-minute checks.

5. The nurses are subject to a tort of professional negligence for failing to prevent the suicide by increasing the suicide precautions in response to Mrs. Smith's increased risk.

6. Had the nurses restricted Mrs. Smith's movements or increased their checks on her, they would have been liable for false imprisonment and invasion of privacy, respectively.

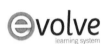

Visit the Evolve website for an **Audio Chapter Summary, Chapter Review Answers & Rationales, Critical Thinking Answer Guidelines,** and additional resources related to the content in this chapter: **http://evolve.elsevier.com/Varcarolis/foundations**

Companion CD Use the Companion CD to prepare for tests and the NCLEX® Examination with **Test-Taking Strategies** for psychiatric mental health nursing and hundreds of **Review Questions**.

References

American Nurses Association. (1994). *Guidelines for reporting incompetent, unethical, and illegal practices.* Kansas City, MO: Author.

American Nurses Association. (2001). *Code of ethics for nurses with interpretive statements.* Washington, DC: American Nurses Publishing. Retrieved November 18, 2004, from the American Nurses Association website: http://www.nursingworld.org/ethics/code/ethicscode150.htm

American Nurses Association, American Psychiatric-Mental Health Nurses Association, & International Society of Psychiatric-Mental Health Nurses. (2007). *Psychiatric mental health nursing: Scope and standards of practice.* Silver Spring, MD: American Nurses Association.

American Psychiatric Association. (2000). *Diagnostic and statistical manual of mental disorders (DSM-IV-TR)* (4th ed., text rev.). Washington, DC: Author.

Bazelon, D. L. (2003). *Advance psychiatric directives.* Washington, DC: Bazelon Center for Mental Health Law.

Canterbury v. Spence, 464 F.2d 722 (D.C. Cir. 1972), quoting *Schloendorf v. Society of N.Y. Hosp.*, 211 N.Y. 125 105 N.E.2d 92, 93 (1914).

Chan, C. (2003, May 13–18). *Mandatory outclient treatment: Issues to consider.* Paper presented at the 153rd annual meeting of the American Psychiatric Association, Chicago, IL.

Fung, M. Y. L., & Paynter, J. (2008). The impact of information technology in healthcare privacy. In P. Duquenoy, C. George, & K. Kimppa (Eds.), *Ethical, legal, and social issues in medical informatics* (pp. 186–227). Hershey, PA: Idea Group.

Health Insurance Portability and Accountability Act, U.S.C.45C.F.R § 164.501 (2003).

Humphrey v. Cady, 405 U.S. 504 (1972).

Illinois v. Russel, 630 N.E.2d 794 (Ill. Sup. Ct. 1994).

O'Connor v. Donaldson, 422 U.S. 563 (1975).

Plumadore v. State of New York, 427 N.Y.S.2d 90 (1980).

Sadock, B. J., & Sadock, V. A. (2008). *Concise textbook of clinical psychiatry* (3rd ed.). Philadelphia: Lippincott, Williams & Wilkins.

Tarasoff v. Regents of University of California, 529 P.2d 553, 118 Cal Rptr 129 (1974).

Tarasoff v. Regents of University of California, 551 P.2d 334, 131 Cal Rptr 14 (1976).

Zinernon v. Burch, 494 U.S. 113, 108 L.Ed.2d 100, 110 S. Ct. 975 (1990).

A NURSE SPEAKS

Communication that conveys knowledge, care, encouragement, and support can lead a psychiatric patient along a path that endorses wellness and well-being. This is termed *therapeutic communication* or *therapeutic relating*. Let me share a story from my own experience that illustrates the power of such communication.

I was working in a psychiatric day treatment program when I met Sue. Sue was brand new to the program. I could see the same confusion and denial in Sue that I so often see in persons newly diagnosed with mental health problems. Sue truly did not believe that she was facing a diagnosis of schizophrenia. She believed she was overly stressed but certainly not mentally ill. If the health care team would just listen to her, believe her, and help her, she could get over this. She described the attacks "they" were making upon her person and her life. "They" followed her, repeated to her segments of conversations she had with her family, invaded the privacy of her home, and harassed her at her job.

As Sue's psychiatric mental health nurse, I perceived that she was experiencing fear, panic, and feelings that her life was totally out of control. I acknowledged the feelings that this frightened woman expressed. I offered Sue support and help as treatment with medications and therapy began. Adjusting to an antipsychotic medication was difficult, especially because Sue really did not think she needed it. After all, she believed that she was just very stressed and talking to someone about it was bound to help.

I provided Sue with some simple explanations about how the antipsychotic medication would work to correct the chemical imbalance that existed in her brain.

I was fully aware that these explanations and ongoing teaching would mean nothing if Sue did not feel that I cared and was sincerely interested in her. Sue needed to feel safe, cared about, and protected at a time when her world was so foreboding.

As medication dulled the delusional thoughts that raced through Sue's mind, I could see her transform into a calmer, more trusting person. Sue's gifts became apparent—she was smart and very creative. I acknowledged these gifts and called them into play. This bolstered Sue's self-confidence, which had been badly battered by the symptoms of the illness.

I was determined to focus on Sue's personal gifts and talents, as well as the evident manifestations of the disease, addressing both as I could. Sue's response to this approach was positive. She began to feel less like a "sick, overwhelmed person." She was encouraged to grasp and hold on to that which had been good and positive in her life before the onset of her illness. I truly believe that reaching out to the well person that Sue could and would become was helpful.

The progress was slow and painstaking. I believed it was worth all of the effort involved. My hope was that Sue would leave treatment stabilized, less stressed, and aware that a nurse she met at the day program believed in her, reached out to her, and walked the road to wellness with her.

Miriam Jacik

CHAPTER 8

The Nursing Process and Standards of Care for Psychiatric Mental Health Nursing

Elizabeth M. Varcarolis

Key Terms and Concepts

evidence-based practice (EBP), 149
health teaching, 150
mental status examination (MSE), 143
milieu therapy, 151
Nursing Interventions Classification (NIC), 149
Nursing Outcomes Classification (NOC), 147

outcome criteria, 147
Psychiatric-Mental Health Nursing: Scope and Standards of Practice, 138
psychosocial assessment, 144
self-care activities, 150

Objectives

1. Compare the different approaches you would consider when performing an assessment with a child, an adolescent, and an older adult.
2. Differentiate between the use of an interpreter and a translator when performing an assessment with a non–English speaking patient.
3. Conduct a mental status examination (MSE).
4. Perform a psychosocial assessment, including brief cultural and spiritual components.
5. Explain three principles a nurse follows in planning actions to reach agreed-upon outcome criteria.

6. Construct a plan of care for a patient with a mental or emotional health problem.
7. Identify three advanced practice psychiatric mental health nursing interventions.
8. Demonstrate basic nursing interventions and evaluation of care following the ANA's Standards of Practice.
9. Compare and contrast *Nursing Interventions Classification (NIC)*, *Nursing Outcomes Classification (NOC)*, and evidence-based practice (EBP).

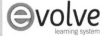 Visit the Evolve website for an **Audio Glossary & Flashcards, Concept Map Creator**, and additional resources related to the content in this chapter: **http://evolve.elsevier.com/Varcarolis/foundations**

The nursing process is a six-step problem-solving approach intended to facilitate and identify appropriate, safe, culturally competent, developmentally relevant, and quality care for individuals, families, groups, or communities. Psychiatric mental health nursing practice bases nursing judgments and behaviors on this accepted theoretical framework (Figure 8-1). Theoretical paradigms such as developmental theory, psychodynamic theory, systems theory, holistic theory, cognitive theory, and biological theory are some examples. Whenever possible, interventions are also supported by scientific theories when we apply evidence-based research to our nursing plans and actions of care (see Chapter 1).

The nursing process is also the foundation of the Standards of Practice as presented in *Psychiatric-*

Mental Health Nursing: Scope and Standards of Practice (ANA et al., 2007), which in turn provide the basis for the:

- Criteria for certification
- Legal definition of nursing, as reflected in many states' nurse practice acts
- National Council of State Boards of Nursing Licensure Examination (NCLEX-RN®)

The following sections describe the Standards of Practice, which "describe a competent level of psychiatric-mental health nursing care as demonstrated by the critical thinking model known as the nursing process (ANA et al., 2007)." The Standards of Practice and Professional Performance are listed on the inside back cover of this book.

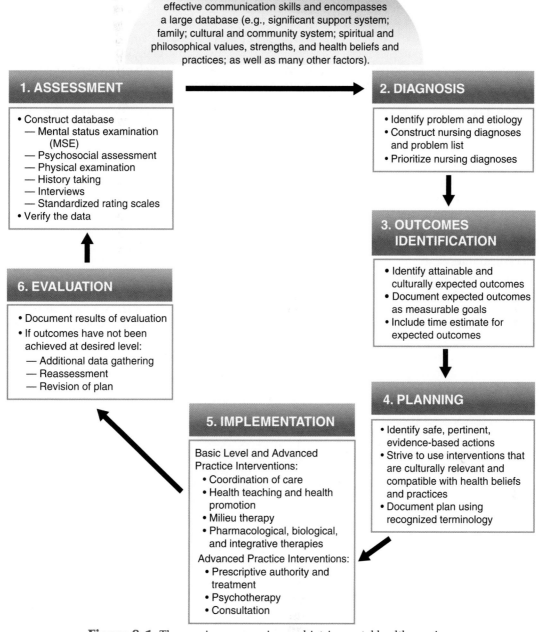

Figure 8-1 The nursing process in psychiatric mental health nursing.

STANDARD 1: ASSESSMENT

A view of the individual as a complex blend of many parts is consistent with nurses' holistic approach to care. Nurses who care for people with physical illnesses ideally maintain a holistic view that involves an awareness of psychological, social, cultural, and spiritual issues. Likewise, nurses who work in the psychiatric mental health field need to assess or have access to past and present medical history, a recent physical examination, and any physical complaints, as well as document any observable physical conditions or behaviors (e.g., unsteady gait, abnormal breathing patterns, wincing as if in pain, doubling over to relieve discomfort).

The assessment process begins with the initial patient encounter and continues throughout the care of the patient. To develop a basis for the plan of care and in preparation for discharge, every patient should have a thorough, formal nursing assessment on entering treatment. Subsequent to the formal assessment, data is collected continually and systematically as the patient's condition changes and—hopefully—improves.

Perhaps the patient came into treatment actively suicidal, and the initial focus of care was on protection from injury; through regular assessment, it may be determined that although suicidal ideation has diminished, negative self-evaluation is still certainly a problem.

Assessments are conducted by a variety of professionals, including nurses, psychiatrists, social workers, dietitians, and other therapists. Virtually all facilities have standardized nursing assessment forms to aid in organization and consistency among reviewers. These forms may be paper or electronic versions, according to the resources and preferences of the institution. The time required for the nursing interview—a standard aspect of the formal nursing assessment—varies, depending on the assessment form and the patient's response pattern (e.g., a patient who is lengthy or rambling, is prone to tangential thought, has memory disturbances, or gives markedly slowed responses). Refer to Chapter 10 for sound guidelines for setting up and conducting a clinical interview.

In emergency situations, immediate intervention is often based on a minimal amount of data. In all situations, however, legal consent must be given by the patient, who must also receive a copy of the Health Insurance Portability and Accountability Act (HIPAA) guidelines. Essentially, the purpose of the HIPAA privacy rule is to ensure that an individual's health information is properly protected, while at the same time allowing health care providers to obtain personal health information for the purpose of providing and promoting high-quality health care (USDHHS, 2003). HIPAA was first enacted in 1996, but compliance was not mandated until April 14, 2003. Chapter 7 has a more detailed discussion of HIPAA. Visit www.hhs.gov/ocr/privacy/hipaa/understanding/index.html for a full overview.

The nurse's *primary source* for data collection is the patient; however, there may be times when it is necessary to supplement or rely completely on another for the assessment information. These *secondary sources* can be invaluable when caring for a patient experiencing psychosis, muteness, agitation, or catatonia. Such secondary sources include members of the family, friends, neighbors, police, health care workers, and medical records.

The best atmosphere in which to conduct an assessment is one of minimal anxiety. Therefore, if an individual becomes upset, defensive, or embarrassed regarding any topic, the topic should be abandoned. The nurse can acknowledge that the subject makes the patient uncomfortable and suggest within the medical record that the topic be discussed when the patient feels more comfortable. It is important that the nurse not probe, pry, or push for information that is difficult for the patient to discuss. However, it should be recognized that increased anxiety about any subject is data in itself. The nurse can note this in the assessment without obtaining any further information.

Age Considerations

Assessment of Children

When assessing children, it is important to gather data from a variety of sources. Although the child is the best source in determining inner feelings and emotions, the caregivers (parents or guardians) often can best describe the behavior, performance, and conduct of the child. Caregivers also are helpful in interpreting the child's words and responses. However, a separate interview is advisable when an older child is reluctant to share information, especially in cases of suspected abuse (Arnold & Boggs, 2007).

Developmental levels should be considered in the evaluation of children. One of the hallmarks of psychiatric disorders in children is the tendency to regress (i.e., return to a previous level of development). Although it is developmentally appropriate for toddlers to suck their thumbs, such a gesture is unusual in an older child.

One study found that children felt more comfortable if their health care provider was the same gender (Bernzweig et al., 1997). Another study indicated that although 60% of parents preferred that their children be cared for by a man, 79% of the children, regardless of gender, requested that a female physician care for them (Waseem & Ryan, 2005). Age-appropriate communication strategies are perhaps the most important factor in establishing successful communication (Arnold & Boggs, 2007).

Assessment of children should be accomplished by a combination of interview and observation. Watching children at play provides important clues to their functioning. From a psychodynamic view, play is a safe area for the child to act out thoughts and emotions and can serve as a safe way in which children can release pent-up emotions—for example, having a child act out their story with the use of anatomically correct dolls or tell a story of their family using a family of dolls. Asking the child to tell a story, draw a picture, or engage in specific therapeutic games can be useful assessment tools when determining critical concerns and painful issues a child may have difficulty expressing. Usually, a clinician with special training in child and adolescent psychiatry works with young children. Chapter 28 presents a more extensive overview of assessing children.

Assessment of Adolescents

Adolescents are especially concerned with confidentiality and may fear that anything they say to the nurse will be repeated to their parents. Lack of confidentiality can become a barrier of care with this population. Adolescents need to know that their records are private; they should receive an explanation as to how information will be shared among the treatment team. Questions related to such topics as substance abuse and sexual abuse demand confidentiality

(Arnold & Boggs, 2007). However, threats of suicide, homicide, sexual abuse, or behaviors that put the patient or others at risk for harm must be shared with other professionals, as well as with the parents. Because identifying risk factors is one of the key objectives when assessing adolescents, it is helpful to use a brief, structured interview technique such as the HEADSSS interview (Box 8-1). Chapter 28 offers more on assessment of adolescents.

Assessment of Older Adults

As we get older, our five senses (taste, touch, sight, hearing, and smell) and brain function begin to diminish, but the extent to which this affects each person varies. Your patient may be a spry and alert 80-year-old or a frail and confused 60-year-old. Therefore, it is important not to stereotype older adults and expect them to be physically and/or mentally deficient. For example, the tendency may be to jump to the conclusion that someone who is hard of hearing is cognitively impaired. By the same token, many older adults often need special attention. The nurse needs to be aware of any physical limitations—any sensory condition (difficulty seeing or hearing), motor condition (difficulty walking or maintaining balance), or medical condition (back pain, cardiac or pulmonary deficits)—that could cause increased anxiety, stress, or physical discomfort for the patient during assessment of mental and emotional needs.

It is wise to identify any physical deficits at the onset of the assessment and make accommodations for them. If the patient is hard of hearing, speak a little more slowly in clear, louder tones (but not too loud), and seat the patient close to you without invading his or her personal space. Often times, a voice that is lower in pitch is easier for older adults to hear, although a higher-pitched voice may convey anxiety to some. Refer to Chapter 29 for more on assessing and communicating with the older adult.

BOX 8-1 The HEADSSS Psychosocial Interview Technique

H Home environment (e.g., relations with parents and siblings)

E Education and employment (e.g., school performance)

A Activities (e.g., sports participation, after-school activities, peer relations)

D Drug, alcohol, or tobacco use

S Sexuality (e.g., whether the patient is sexually active, practices safe sex, or uses contraception)

S Suicide risk or symptoms of depression or other mental disorder

S "Savagery" (e.g., violence or abuse in home environment or in neighborhood)

Language Barriers

It is becoming more and more apparent that psychiatric mental health nurses can best serve their patients if they have a thorough understanding of the complex cultural and social factors that influence health and illness. Awareness of individual cultural beliefs and health care practices can help nurses minimize stereotyped assumptions that can lead to ineffective care and interfere with the ability to evaluate care. There are many opportunities for misunderstandings when assessing a patient from a different cultural or social background from your own, particularly if the interview is conducted in English, and the patient speaks a different language or a different form of English (Fontes, 2008).

Often health care professionals require a translator to understand the patient's history and health care needs. There is a difference between an *interpreter* and a *translator*. An interpreter is more likely to unconsciously try to make sense of (interpret) what the patient is saying and therefore inserts his or her own understanding of the situation into the data base. A professional translator, on the other hand, tries to avoid interpreting. Fontes (2008) strongly advises against the use of untrained interpreters (e.g., family members, friends, neighbors).

For patients who do not speak English or have language difficulties, federal law mandates the use of a trained translator (Arnold & Boggs, 2007). In fact, Poole and Higgo state that the "use of a trained translator is essential wherever the patient's first language is not spoken English (even where the person has some English)" (2006, p. 135). A professionally trained translator is proficient in both English and the patient's spoken language, maintains confidentiality, and follows specific guidelines. Unfortunately, professional translators are not always readily available in many health care facilities.

Psychiatric Mental Health Nursing Assessment

The purpose of the psychiatric mental health nursing assessment is to:

- Establish rapport
- Obtain an understanding of the current problem or chief complaint
- Review physical status and obtain baseline vital signs
- Assess for risk factors affecting the safety of the patient or others
- Perform a mental status examination
- Assess psychosocial status
- Identify mutual goals for treatment
- Formulate a plan of care

Gathering Data

Review of Systems. The mind-body connection is significant in the understanding and treatment of psychiatric disorders. Many patients who are admitted for treatment of psychiatric conditions also are given a thorough physical examination by a primary care provider. Likewise, most nursing assessments include a baseline set of vital statistics, a historical and current review of body systems, and a documentation of allergic responses.

Poole and Higgo (2006) point out that several medical conditions and physical illnesses may mimic psychiatric illnesses (Box 8-2). Therefore, physical causes

---

BOX 8-2 Some Medical Conditions That May Mimic Psychiatric Illness

Depression

Neurological disorders:
- Cerebrovascular accident (stroke)
- Alzheimer's disease
- Brain tumor
- Huntington's disease
- Epilepsy (seizure disorder)
- Multiple sclerosis
- Parkinson's disease

Infections:
- Mononucleosis
- Encephalitis
- Hepatitis
- Tertiary syphilis
- Human immunodeficiency virus (HIV) infection

Endocrine disorders:
- Hypothyroidism and hyperthyroidism
- Cushing's syndrome
- Addison's disease
- Parathyroid disease

Gastrointestinal disorders:
- Liver cirrhosis
- Pancreatitis

Cardiovascular disorders:
- Hypoxia
- Congestive heart failure

Respiratory disorders:
- Sleep apnea

Nutritional disorders:
- Thiamine deficiency
- Protein deficiency
- B_{12} deficiency
- B_6 deficiency
- Folate deficiency

Collagen vascular diseases:
- Lupus erythematosus
- Rheumatoid arthritis

Cancer

Anxiety

Neurological disorders:
- Alzheimer's disease
- Brain tumor
- Stroke
- Huntington's disease

Infections:
- Encephalitis
- Meningitis

- Neurosyphilis
- Septicemia

Endocrine disorders:
- Hypothyroidism and hyperthyroidism
- Hypoparathyroidism
- Hypoglycemia
- Pheochromocytoma
- Carcinoid

Metabolic disorders:
- Low calcium
- Low potassium
- Acute intermittent porphyria
- Liver failure

Cardiovascular disorders:
- Angina
- Congestive heart failure
- Pulmonary embolus

Respiratory disorders:
- Pneumothorax
- Acute asthma
- Emphysema

Drug effects:
- Stimulants
- Sedatives (withdrawal)

Lead, mercury poisoning

Psychosis

Medical conditions:
- Temporal lobe epilepsy
- Migraine headaches
- Temporal arteritis
- Occipital tumors
- Narcolepsy
- Encephalitis
- Hypothyroidism
- Addison's disease
- HIV infection

Drug effects:
- Hallucinogens (e.g., LSD)
- Phencyclidine
- Alcohol withdrawal
- Stimulants
- Cocaine
- Corticosteroids

of symptoms must be ruled out. Conversely, psychiatric disorders can result in physical or somatic symptoms such as stomach aches, headaches, lethargy, insomnia, intense fatigue, and even pain. When depression is secondary to a known medical condition, it often goes unrecognized and thus untreated. Therefore, all patients who come into the health care system need to have both a medical and mental health evaluation to ensure a correct diagnosis and appropriate care.

Some people with certain physical conditions may be more prone to psychiatric disorders such as depression. It is believed, for example, that the disease process of multiple sclerosis or other autoimmune diseases may actually bring about depression. Other medical diseases typically associated with depression are coronary artery disease, diabetes, and stroke. Individuals need to be evaluated for any medical origins of their depression or anxiety.

When evidence suggests the presence of mental confusion or organic mental disease, a mental status examination should be performed.

Laboratory Data. Hypothyroidism may have the clinical appearance of depression, and hyperthyroidism may appear to be a manic phase of bipolar disorder; a simple blood test can usually differentiate between depression and thyroid problems. Abnormal liver enzyme levels can explain irritability, depression, and lethargy. People who have chronic renal disease often suffer from the same symptoms when their blood urea nitrogen and electrolyte levels are abnormal. Results of a toxicology screen for the presence of either prescription or illegal drugs also may provide useful information.

Mental Status Examination. Fundamental to the psychiatric mental health nursing assessment is a **mental status examination (MSE)**. In fact, an MSE is part of the assessment in all areas of medicine. The MSE in psychiatry is analogous to the physical examination in general medicine, and the purpose is to evaluate an individual's current cognitive processes. For acutely disturbed patients, it is not unusual for the mental health clinician to administer MSEs every day. Sommers-Flanagan and Sommers-Flanagan (2003) advise anyone seeking employment in the medical–mental health field to be competent in communicating with other professionals via MSE reports. Box 8-3 is an example of a basic MSE.

BOX 8-3 Mental Status Examination

Appearance
- Grooming and dress
- Level of hygiene
- Pupil dilation or constriction
- Facial expression
- Height, weight, nutritional status
- Presence of body piercing or tattoos, scars, etc.
- Relationship between appearance and age

Behavior
- Excessive or reduced body movements
- Peculiar body movements (e.g., scanning of the environment, odd or repetitive gestures, level of consciousness, balance and gait)
- Abnormal movements (e.g., tardive dyskinesia, tremors)
- Level of eye contact (keep cultural differences in mind)

Speech
- Rate: slow, rapid, normal
- Volume: loud, soft, normal
- Disturbances (e.g., articulation problems, slurring, stuttering, mumbling)
- Cluttering (e.g., rapid, disorganized, tongue-tied speech)

Mood
- Affect: flat, bland, animated, angry, withdrawn, appropriate to context
- Mood: sad, labile, euphoric

Disorders of the Form of Thought
- Thought process (e.g., disorganized, coherent, flight of ideas, neologisms, thought blocking, circumstantiality)
- Thought content (e.g., delusions, obsessions)

Perceptual Disturbances
- Hallucinations (e.g., auditory, visual)
- Illusions

Cognition
- Orientation: time, place, person
- Level of consciousness (e.g., alert, confused, clouded, stuporous, unconscious, comatose)
- Memory: remote, recent, immediate
- Fund of knowledge
- Attention: performance on serial sevens, digit span tests
- Abstraction: performance on tests involving similarities, proverbs
- Insight
- Judgment

Ideas of Harming Self or Others
- Suicidal or homicidal thoughts:
  - Presence of a plan
  - Means to carry out the plan
  - Opportunity to carry out the plan

The MSE, by and large, aids in collecting and organizing objective data. The nurse observes the patient's physical behavior, nonverbal communication, appearance, speech patterns, mood and affect, thought content, perceptions, cognitive ability, and insight and judgment.

Psychosocial Assessment. A psychosocial assessment provides additional information from which to develop a plan of care. It includes the following information about the patient:

- Central or chief complaint (in the patient's own words)
- History of violent, suicidal, or self-mutilating behaviors
- Alcohol and/or substance abuse
- Family psychiatric history
- Personal psychiatric treatment, including medications and complementary therapies
- Stressors and coping methods
- Quality of activities of daily living
- Personal background
- Social background, including support system
- Weaknesses, strengths, and goals for treatment
- Racial, ethnic, and cultural beliefs and practices
- Spiritual beliefs or religious practices

The patient's psychosocial history is most often the **subjective** part of the assessment. The focus of the history is the *patient's perceptions and recollections* of current lifestyle and life in general (family, friends, education, work experience, coping styles, and spiritual and cultural beliefs).

A psychosocial assessment elicits information about the systems in which a person operates. To conduct such an assessment, the nurse should have fundamental knowledge of growth and development, basic cultural and religious practices, pathophysiology, psychopathology, and pharmacology. Box 8-4 provides a basic psychosocial assessment tool.

Spiritual/Religious Assessment. Carson and Koenig (2004) stress the importance of a spiritual/religious assessment as integral to a holistic nursing assessment. The idea that spirituality or religious involvement are recognized as important influences on a person's health and behavior has long been recognized

---

BOX 8-4 Psychosocial Assessment

A. Previous hospitalizations
B. Educational background
C. Occupational background
  1. Employed? Where? What length of time?
  2. Special skills
D. Social patterns
  1. Describe family.
  2. Describe friends.
  3. With whom does the patient live?
  4. To whom does the patient go in time of crisis?
  5. Describe a typical day.
E. Sexual patterns
  1. Sexually active? Practices safe sex? Practices birth control?
  2. Sexual orientation
  3. Sexual difficulties
F. Interests and abilities
  1. What does the patient do in his or her spare time?
  2. What sport, hobby, or leisure activity is the patient good at?
  3. What gives the patient pleasure?
G. Substance use and abuse
  1. What medications does the patient take? How often? How much?
  2. What herbal or over-the-counter drugs does the patient take (caffeine, cough medicines, St. John's wort)? How often? How much?
  3. What psychotropic drugs does the patient take? How often? How much?

4. How many drinks of alcohol does the patient take per day? Per week?
5. What recreational drugs does the patient use (club drugs, marijuana, psychedelics, steroids)? How often? How much?
6. Does the patient overuse prescription drugs (benzodiazepines, pain medications)?
7. Does the patient identify the use of drugs as a problem?
H. Coping abilities
  1. What does the patient do when he or she gets upset?
  2. To whom can the patient talk?
  3. What usually helps to relieve stress?
  4. What did the patient try this time?
I. Spiritual assessment
  1. What importance does religion or spirituality have in the patient's life?
  2. Do the patient's religious or spiritual beliefs relate to the way the patient takes care of himself or herself or the illness? How?
  3. Does the patient's faith help the patient in stressful situations?
  4. Whom does the patient see when he or she is medically ill? Mentally upset?
  5. Are there special health care practices within the patient's culture that address his or her particular mental problem?

(Miller & Thoresen, 2003). Spirituality and religious beliefs have the potential to exert a positive influence on patients' views of themselves and how they interact and respond to others (Mackenzie et al., 2000).

A comprehensive analysis of empirical research published in more than 1200 studies and 400 reviews examined the relationships between religion and spirituality and many physical and mental conditions. The analysis found that there was a 60% to 80% correlation between better health and religion or spiritual beliefs. The studies covered a variety of physical conditions, such as heart disease, hypertension, immunological dysfunction, cancer, and pain. Psychiatric phenomena included depression, anxiety, and suicide, among others (Koenig et al., 2001).

Spirituality and religion are, however, quite different in their influences. **Spirituality** is more of an internal phenomenon. Spirituality is often understood as addressing universal human questions and needs (Anandarajab, 2008). Spirituality can be expressed as having three dimensions: (1) *cognitive* (beliefs, values, ideals, purpose, truth, wisdom), (2) *experiential* (love, compassion, connection forgiveness, altruism), and (3) a *behavioral* component (daily behavior, moral obligations, life choices, and medical choices) (Anandarajab, 2008). Spirituality is the part of us that seeks to understand life and may or may not be connected with the community or religious rituals. Spirituality can increase healthy behaviors, social support, and a sense of meaning, which are linked to decreased overall mental and physical illness (George et al., 2000).

In contrast, **religion** is an external system that includes beliefs, patterns of worship, and symbols and requirements of membership (Koenig, 2001; Miller & Thoresen, 2003). Although religion is often concerned with spirituality, religious groups are social entities and are often characterized by other nonspiritual goals as well (cultural, economic, political, social) (Miller & Thoresen, 2003). Religious involvement is associated with better physical health, better mental health, and longer survival (George et al., 2002). Religious affiliation is a choice to connect personal spiritual beliefs with a larger organized group or institution and typically involves specific rituals. Belonging to a religious community can provide support during difficult times, and prayer can be a source of hope, comfort, and support in healing.

Delgado (2007) notes that nurses and other health care providers may be uncomfortable with assessing for or discussing spiritual issues with patients, even though their proximity with patients and intimate patient needs gives them a unique opportunity to develop spiritual care theory and practices.

The following questions may be included in a spiritual or religious assessment:
- Who or what supplies you with strength and hope?
- Do you have a religious affiliation?
- Do you practice any spiritual activities (Yoga, Tai Chi, meditation)?
- Do you participate in any religious activities?
- What role does religion or spiritual practice play in your life?
- Does your faith help you in stressful situations?
- Do you pray or meditate?
- Has your illness affected your religious/spiritual practices?
- Would you like to have someone from your church/synagogue/temple or from our facility visit?

Cultural and Social Assessment. Because of the cultural diversity in most societies, there is a need for nursing assessments, diagnoses, and subsequent care to be planned around the unique cultural health care beliefs, values, and practices of each individual patient. Chapter 6 has a detailed discussion of the cultural implications for psychiatric mental health nursing and how to conduct a cultural and social assessment.

Some questions we can ask to help with a cultural and social assessment are:
- What is your primary language? Would you like a translator?
- How would you describe your cultural background?
- Who are you close to?
- Who do you seek in times of crisis?
- Who do you live with?
- Who do you seek when you are medically ill? Mentally upset or concerned?
- What do you do to get better when you have physical problems?
- What are the attitudes toward mental illness in your culture?
- How is your current problem viewed by your culture? Is it seen as a problem that can be fixed? A disease? A taboo? A fault or curse?
- Are there special foods that you eat?
- Are there special health care practices within your culture that address your particular mental or emotional health problem?
- Are there any special cultural beliefs about your illness that might help me give you better care?

After the cultural and social assessment, it is useful to summarize pertinent data with the patient. This summary provides patients with reassurance that they have been heard and gives them the opportunity to clarify any misinformation. The patient should be told what will happen next. For example, if the initial assessment takes place in the hospital, you should tell the patient who else he or she will be seeing. If the initial assessment was conducted by a psychiatric mental health nurse in a mental health clinic, the patient should be told when and how often he or she will meet with the nurse to work on the patient's problems. If you believe a referral is necessary, this should be discussed with the patient.

Validating the Assessment

To gain an even clearer understanding of your patient, it is helpful to look to outside sources. Emergency department records can be a valuable resource in understanding an individual's presenting behavior and problems. Police reports may be available in cases in which hostility and legal altercations occurred. Old medical records, most now accessible by computer, are a great help in validating information you already have or in adding new information to your database. If the patient was admitted to a psychiatric unit in the past, information about the patient's previous level of functioning and behavior gives you a baseline for making clinical judgments. Occasionally, consent forms may have to be signed by the patient or an appropriate relative to obtain access to records.

Using Rating Scales

A number of standardized rating scales are useful for psychiatric evaluation and monitoring. Rating scales are often administered by a clinician, but many are self-administered. Table 8-1 lists some of the common ones in use. Many of the clinical chapters in this book include a rating scale.

STANDARD 2: DIAGNOSIS

A nursing diagnosis is a clinical judgment about a patient's response, needs, actual and potential psychiatric disorders, mental health problems, and potential comorbid physical illnesses. A well-chosen and well-stated nursing diagnosis is the basis for selecting therapeutic outcomes and interventions (North American Nursing Diagnosis Association International [NANDA-I], 2009). Refer to inside back cover for a list of NANDA-I–approved nursing diagnoses.

A nursing diagnosis has three structural components:
1. Problem (unmet need)
2. Etiology (probable cause)
3. Supporting data (signs and symptoms)

The **problem**, or unmet need, describes the state of the patient at present. Problems that are within the nurse's domain to treat are termed *nursing diagnoses*. The nursing diagnostic title states what should change. For example: *Hopelessness*.

Etiology, or probable cause, is linked to the diagnostic title with the words *related to*. Stating the etiology or probable cause tells what needs to be addressed to effect the change and identifies causes the nurse can treat through nursing interventions. For example: *Hopelessness related to multiple losses*.

Supporting data, or signs and symptoms, state what the condition is like at present. It may be linked to the diagnosis and etiology with the words *as evidenced by*.

TABLE 8-1 Standardized Rating Scales*

Use	Scale
Depression	Beck Inventory
	Brief Patient Health Questionnaire (Brief PHQ)
	Geriatric Depression Scale (GDS)
	Hamilton Depression Scale
	Zung Self-Report Inventory
	Patient Health Questionnaire-9 (PHQ-9)
Anxiety	Brief Patient Health Questionnaire (Brief PHQ)
	Generalized Anxiety Disorder–7 (GAD-7)
	Modified Spielberger State Anxiety Scale
	Hamilton Anxiety Scale
Substance use disorders	Addiction Severity Index (ASI)
	Recovery Attitude and Treatment Evaluator (RAATE)
	Brief Drug Abuse Screen Test (B-DAST)
Obsessive-compulsive behavior	Yale-Brown Obsessive-Compulsive Scale (Y-BOCS)
Mania	Mania Rating Scale
Schizophrenia	Scale for Assessment of Negative Symptoms (SANS)
	Brief Psychiatric Rating Scale (BPRS)
Abnormal movements	Abnormal Involuntary Movement Scale (AIMS)
	Simpson Neurological Rating Scale
General psychiatric assessment	Brief Psychiatric Rating Scale (BPRS)
	Global Assessment of Functioning Scale (GAF)
Cognitive function	Mini-Mental State Examination (MMSE)
	St. Louis University Mental Status Examination (SLUMS)
	Cognitive Capacity Screening Examination (CCSE)
	Alzheimer's Disease Rating Scale (ADRS)
	Memory and Behavior Problem Checklist
	Functional Assessment Screening Tool (FAST)
	Global Deterioration Scale (GDS)
Family assessment	McMaster Family Assessment Device
Eating disorders	Eating Disorders Inventory (EDI)
	Body Attitude Test
	Diagnostic Survey for Eating Disorders

*These rating scales highlight important areas in psychiatric assessment. Because many of the answers are subjective, experienced clinicians use these tools as a guide when planning care and also draw on their knowledge of their patients.

Supporting data (defining characteristics) that validate the diagnosis include:

- The patient's statement (e.g., "It's no use; nothing will change.")
- Lack of involvement with family and friends
- Lack of motivation to care for self or environment

The complete nursing diagnosis might be: *Hopelessness related to multiple losses, as evidenced by lack of motivation to care for self.*

STANDARD 3: OUTCOMES IDENTIFICATION

Outcome criteria are the hoped-for outcomes that reflect the maximal level of patient health that can realistically be achieved through nursing interventions. Whereas nursing diagnoses identify nursing problems, outcomes reflect the desired change. The expected out-

comes provide direction for continuity of care (ANA et al., 2007). Outcomes should take into account the patient's culture, values, and ethical beliefs. Specifically, outcomes are stated in attainable and measurable terms and include a time estimate for attainment (ANA et al., 2007). Therefore, outcome criteria are patient-centered, geared to each individual, and documented as obtainable goals.

Moorhead and colleagues (2008) have compiled a standardized list of nursing outcomes in *Nursing Outcomes Classification (NOC)* (see Chapter 1). *NOC* includes a total of 385 standardized outcomes that provide a mechanism for communicating the effect of nursing interventions on the well-being of patients, families, and communities. Each outcome has an associated group of indicators used to determine patient status in relation to the outcome. Table 8-2 provides suggested *NOC* indicators for the

TABLE 8-2 *NOC* Indicators for Suicide Self-Restraint

Definition: Personal actions to refrain from gestures and attempts at killing self

Outcome target rating: Maintain at _____ Increase to _____

Suicide Self-Restraint Overall Rating	Never Demonstrated 1	Rarely Demonstrated 2	Sometimes Demonstrated 3	Often Demonstrated 4	Consistently Demonstrated 5	
Expresses feelings	1	2	3	4	5	NA
Expresses sense of hope	1	2	3	4	5	NA
Maintains connectedness in relationships	1	2	3	4	5	NA
Obtains assistance as needed	1	2	3	4	5	NA
Verbalizes suicidal ideas	1	2	3	4	5	NA
Controls impulses	1	2	3	4	5	NA
Refrains from gathering means for suicide	1	2	3	4	5	NA
Refrains from giving away possessions	1	2	3	4	5	NA
Refrains from inflicting serious injury	1	2	3	4	5	NA

Continued

TABLE 8-2 *NOC* Indicators for Suicide Self-Restraint—cont'd

Suicide Self-Restraint Overall Rating	Never Demonstrated 1	Rarely Demonstrated 2	Sometimes Demonstrated 3	Often Demonstrated 4	Consistently Demonstrated 5	
Refrains from using unprescribed mood-altering substances	1	2	3	4	5	NA
Discloses plan for suicide if present	1	2	3	4	5	NA
Upholds suicide contract	1	2	3	4	5	NA
Maintains self-control without supervision	1	2	3	4	5	NA
Refrains from attempting suicide	1	2	3	4	5	NA
Obtains treatment for depression	1	2	3	4	5	NA
Obtains treatment for substance abuse	1	2	3	4	5	NA
Reports adequate pain control for chronic pain	1	2	3	4	5	NA
Uses suicide prevention resources	1	2	3	4	5	NA
Uses social support group	1	2	3	4	5	NA
Uses available mental health care services	1	2	3	4	5	NA
Plans for future	1	2	3	4	5	NA

Modified from Moorhead, S., Johnson, M., Maas, M., & Swanson, E. (2008). *Nursing outcomes classification (NOC)* (4th ed.). St. Louis: Mosby.

outcome of *Suicide Self-Restraint*, along with the Likert scale that quantifies the achievement on each indicator from 1 (never demonstrated) to 5 (consistently demonstrated).

Although *NOC* is useful for communicating and standardizing language used in outcomes, it does not distinguish between short- and long-term outcomes. It is helpful to use long- and short-term outcomes, often stated as goals, when assessing the effective-

ness of nursing interventions. The use of long- and short-term outcomes or goals is particularly helpful for teaching and learning purposes. It is also valuable for providing guidelines for appropriate interventions. The use of goals guides nurses in building incremental steps toward meeting the desired outcome. All outcomes (goals) are written in positive terms, following the criteria set out by the Standards of Practice. Table 8-3 shows how specific outcome

TABLE 8-3 Examples of Long- and Short-Term Goals for a Suicidal Patient

Long-Term Goals or Outcomes	Short-Term Goals or Outcomes
1. Patient will remain free from injury throughout the hospital stay.	a. Patient will state he or she understands the rationale and procedure of the unit's protocol for suicide precautions shortly after admission. b. Patient will sign a "no-suicide" contract for the next 24 hours, renewable at the end of every 24-hour period (if approved for use by the mental health facility). c. Patient will seek out staff when feeling overwhelmed or self-destructive during hospitalization.
2. By discharge, patient will state he or she no longer wishes to die and has at least two people to contact if suicidal thoughts arise.	a,b. Patient will meet with social worker to find supportive resources in the community before discharge and work on trigger issues (e.g., housing, job). c. By discharge, patient will state the purpose of medication, time and dose, adverse effects, and who to call for questions or concerns. d. Patient will have the written name and telephone numbers of at least two people to turn to if feeling overwhelmed or self-destructive. e. Patient will have a follow-up appointment to meet with a mental health professional by discharge.

criteria might be stated for a suicidal individual with a nursing diagnosis of *Risk for suicide related to depression and suicide attempt*.

STANDARD 4: PLANNING

Inpatient and community-based facilities increasingly are using standardized care plans or clinical pathways for patients with specific diagnoses. Standardizing pathways or plans of care allows for inclusion of evidence-based practice and newly tested interventions as they become available. They are more time efficient, although less focused on the specific individual patient needs. Other health care facilities continue to devise individual plans of care. Whatever the care planning procedures in a specific institution, the nurse considers the following specific principles when planning care:

- *Safe*—Interventions must be safe for the patient, as well as for other patients, staff, and family.
- *Compatible and appropriate*—Interventions must be compatible with other therapies and with the patient's personal goals and cultural values, as well as with institutional rules.
- *Realistic and individualized*—Interventions should be (1) within the patient's capabilities, given the patient's age, physical strength, condition, and willingness to change; (2) based on the number of staff available; (3) reflective of the actual available community resources; and (4) within the student's or nurse's capabilities.
- *Evidence based*—Interventions should be based on scientific evidence and principles when available.

Using evidence-based interventions and treatments as they become available is the gold standard in health care (refer to Chapter 1). There are many definitions for evidence-based practice, but David Sackett's (an original founder of evidence-based medicine) definition remains among the most useful in today's practice. His definition clearly considers patient values and clinical experience together with the best research evidence (Sackett, 2000). **Evidence-based practice (EBP)** for nurses is a combination of clinical skill and the use of clinically relevant research in the delivery of effective patient-centered care. The combined use of the best available research, patient preferences, and sound clinical judgment and skills makes for an optimal patient-centered nurse-patient relationship (Sackett et al., 2000). Box 8-5 lists several online resources for evidence-based practice. Keep in mind that whatever interventions are planned, they must be acceptable and appropriate to the individual patient.

The *Nursing Interventions Classification (NIC)* (Bulechek et al., 2008) is a research-based, standardized listing of 542 interventions reflective of current clinical practice the nurse can use to plan care (see Chapter 1). Nurses in all settings can use *NIC* to support quality patient care and incorporate evidence-based nursing actions. Although many safe and appropriate interventions may not be included in *NIC*, it is a useful guide for standardized care. Individualizing interventions to meet a patient's special needs should always be part of the planning.

When choosing nursing interventions from *NIC* or other sources, the nurse uses not just those that fit the nursing diagnosis (e.g., *Risk for suicide*) but interventions that match the defining data. Although the outcome criteria *(NOC)* might be similar or the same (e.g.,

Suicide Self-Restraint), the safe and appropriate interventions may be totally different because of the defining data. For example, consider the nursing diagnosis *Risk for suicide related to feelings of despair as evidenced by two recent suicide attempts and repeated statements that "I want to die."* The planning of appropriate nursing interventions might include:

- Initiate suicide precautions (e.g., ongoing observations and monitoring of the patient, provision of a protective environment) for the person who is at serious risk for suicide.
- Search the newly hospitalized patient and personal belongings for weapons or potential weapons during the inpatient admission procedure, as appropriate.
- Use protective interventions (e.g., area restriction seclusion, physical restraints) if the patient lacks the restraint to refrain from harming self, as needed.
- Assign the hospitalized patient to a room located near the nursing station for ease in observations, as appropriate.

However, if the defining data are different, the appropriate interventions will be as well. For example: *Risk for suicide related to loss of spouse as evidenced by lack of self-care and statements evidencing loneliness.* The nurse might choose the following interventions for this patient's plan of care:

- Determine the presence and degree of suicidal risk.
- Facilitate support of the patient by family and friends.
- Consider strategies to decrease isolation and opportunity to act on harmful thoughts.

- Assist the patient in identifying a network of supportive personnel and resources within the community (e.g., support groups, clergy, care providers).
- Provide information about available community resources and outreach programs.

Chapter 24 addresses assessment of and interventions for suicidal patients in more depth.

STANDARD 5: IMPLEMENTATION

Psychiatric-Mental Health Nursing: Scope and Standards of Practice (ANA et al., 2007) identifies seven areas for intervention. Recent graduates and practitioners new to the psychiatric setting will participate in many of these activities with the guidance and support of more experienced health care professionals. The following four interventions are performed by both the psychiatric mental health registered nurse (RN-PMH) and the psychiatric mental health advanced practice registered nurse (APRN-PMH). (Refer to Chapter 1 for further discussion of these nursing roles.)

The basic implementation skills are accomplished through the nurse-patient relationship and therapeutic interventions. The nurse implements the plan using evidence-based practice whenever possible, uses community resources, and collaborates with nursing colleagues.

Basic Level Interventions

Standard 5A: Coordination of Care

The psychiatric mental health nurse coordinates the implementation of the plan and provides documentation.

Standard 5B: Health Teaching and Health Promotion

Psychiatric mental health nurses use a variety of health teaching methods adaptive to the patient's needs (e.g., age, culture, ability to learn, readiness, etc.), integrating current knowledge and research and seeking opportunities for feedback and effectiveness of care. **Health teaching** includes identifying the health education needs of the patient and teaching basic principles of physical and mental health, such as giving information about coping, interpersonal relationships, social skills, mental disorders, the treatments for such illnesses and their effects on daily living, relapse prevention, problem-solving skills, stress management, crisis intervention, and self-care activities. The last of these, **self-care activities**, assists the patient in assuming personal responsibility for activities of daily living (ADL) and focuses on improving the patient's mental and physical well-being.

Standard 5c: Milieu Therapy

Milieu therapy is an extremely important consideration in helping patients feel comfortable and safe. Milieu management includes orienting patients to their rights and responsibilities, selecting specific activities that meet patients' physical and mental health needs, and ensuring that patients are maintained in the least restrictive environment safety permits. It also includes informing patients about the need for limits and the conditions necessary to remove them in a culturally competent manner (see Chapter 6).

Standard 5d: Pharmacological, Biological, and Integrative Therapies

Nurses need to know the intended action, therapeutic dosage, adverse reactions, and safe blood levels of medications being administered and must monitor them when appropriate (e.g., blood levels for lithium). The nurse is expected to discuss and provide medication teaching tools to the patient and family regarding drug action, adverse side effects, dietary restrictions, and drug interactions and to provide time for questions. The nurse's assessment of the patient's response to psychobiological interventions is communicated to other members of the multidisciplinary mental health team. Interventions are also aimed at alleviating untoward effects of medication.

Advanced Practice Interventions

The following three interventions can be carried out by the APRN-PMH only.

Standard 5e: Prescriptive Authority and Treatment

The APRN-PMH is educated and clinically prepared to prescribe psychopharmacological agents for patients with mental health or psychiatric disorders in accordance with state and federal laws and regulations. Such prescriptions take into account individual variables such as culture, ethnicity, gender, religious beliefs, age, and physical health.

Standard 5f: Psychotherapy

The APRN-PMH is educationally and clinically prepared to conduct individual, couples, group, and family psychotherapy, using evidence-based psychotherapeutic frameworks and nurse-patient therapeutic relationships (ANA, 2007). Refer to Chapter 2 for an overview of various psychotherapies, Chapter 34 for a discussion of therapeutic groups, Chapter 35 for a discussion of family interventions, and Chapter 36 for a discussion of integrative therapies.

Standard 5g: Consultation

The APRN-PMH works with other clinicians to provide consultation, influence the identified plan, enhance the ability of other clinicians, provide services for patients, and effect change.

STANDARD 6: EVALUATION

Unfortunately, evaluation of patient outcomes is often the most neglected part of the nursing process. Evaluation of the individual's response to treatment should be systematic, ongoing, and criteria-based. Supporting data are included to clarify the evaluation. Ongoing assessment of data allows for revisions of nursing diagnoses, changes to more realistic outcomes, or identification of more appropriate interventions when outcomes are not met.

DOCUMENTATION

Documentation could be considered the seventh step in the nursing process. Keep in mind that medical records are legal documents and may be used in a court of law. (Chapter 7 has a detailed discussion of the various purposes and guidelines for use of medical records.) Besides the evaluation of stated outcomes, the medical record should include changes in patient condition, informed consents (for medications and treatments), reaction to medication, documentation of symptoms (verbatim when appropriate), concerns of the patient, and any untoward incidents in the health care setting. Documentation of patient progress is the responsibility of the entire mental health team.

Although communication among team members and coordination of services are the primary goals when choosing a system for documentation, practitioners in all settings must also consider professional standards, legal issues, requirements for reimbursement by insurers, and accreditation by regulatory agencies.

Information also must be in a format that is retrievable for quality assurance monitoring, utilization management, peer review, and research. Documentation—using the nursing process as a guide—is reflected in two of the formats commonly used in health care settings and described in Table 8-4. Electronic medical records are increasingly used in both inpatient and outpatient settings. Whatever format is used, documentation must be focused, organized, pertinent, and conform to certain legal and other generally accepted principles (Box 8-6).

TABLE 8-4 Narrative versus Problem-Oriented Charting

	Narrative Charting	Problem-Oriented Charting: SOAPIE
Characteristics	A descriptive statement of patient status written in chronological order throughout a shift. Used to support assessment findings from a flow sheet. In charting by exception, narrative notes are used to indicate significant symptoms, behaviors, or events that are exceptions to norms identified on an assessment flow sheet.	Developed in the 1960s for physicians to reduce inefficient documentation. Intended to be accompanied by a problem list. Originally SOAP, with IE added later. The emphasis is on problem identification, process, and outcome. **S:** Subjective data (patient statement) **O:** Objective data (nurse observations) **A:** Assessment (nurse interprets *S* and *O* and describes either a problem or a nursing diagnosis) **P:** Plan (proposed intervention) **I:** Interventions (nurse's response to problem) **E:** Evaluation (patient outcome)
Example	(Date/time/discipline) Patient was agitated in the morning and pacing in the hallway. Blinked eyes, muttered to self, and looked off to the side. Stated heard voices. Verbally hostile to another patient. Offered 2 mg haloperidol (Haldol) prn and sat with staff in quiet area for 20 minutes. Patient returned to community lounge and was able to sit and watch television.	(Date/time/discipline) **S:** "I'm so stupid. Get away, get away." "I hear the devil telling me bad things." **O:** Patient paced the hall, mumbling to self and looking off to the side. Shouted derogatory comments when approached by another patient. Watched walls and ceiling closely. **A:** Patient was having auditory hallucinations and increased agitation. **P:** Offered patient haloperidol prn. Redirected patient to less stimulating environment. **I:** Patient received 2 mg haloperidol PO prn. Sat with patient in quiet room for 20 minutes. **E:** Patient calmer. Returned to community lounge, sat and watched television.
Advantages	Uses a common form of expression (narrative writing) Can address any event or behavior Explains flow-sheet findings Provides multidisciplinary ease of use	Structured Provides consistent organization of data Facilitates retrieval of data for quality assurance and utilization management Contains all elements of the nursing process Minimizes inclusion of unnecessary data Provides multidisciplinary ease of use
Disadvantages	Unstructured May result in different organization of information from note to note Makes it difficult to retrieve quality assurance and utilization management data Frequently leads to omission of elements of the nursing process Commonly results in inclusion of unnecessary and subjective information	Requires time and effort to structure the information Limits entries to problems May result in loss of data about progress Not chronological Carries negative connotation

BOX 8-6 Legal Considerations for Documentation of Care

Do:

- Chart in a timely manner all pertinent and factual information.
- Be familiar with the nursing documentation policy in your facility, and make your charting conform to this standard. The policy generally states the method, frequency, and pertinent assessments, interventions, and outcomes to be recorded. If your agency's policies and procedures do not encourage or allow for quality documentation, bring the need for change to the administration's attention.
- Chart legibly in ink.
- Chart facts fully, descriptively, and accurately.
- Chart what you see, hear, feel, and smell.
- Chart pertinent observations: psychosocial observations, physical symptoms pertinent to the medical diagnosis, and behaviors pertinent to the nursing diagnosis.
- Chart follow-up care provided when a problem has been identified in earlier documentation. For example, if a patient has fallen and injured a leg, describe how the wound is healing.
- Chart fully the facts surrounding unusual occurrences and incidents.
- Chart *all* nursing interventions, treatments, and outcomes (including teaching efforts and patient responses) and safety and patient-protection interventions.
- Chart the patient's expressed subjective feelings.
- Chart each time you notify a physician, and record the reason for notification, the information that was communicated, the accurate time, the physician's instructions or orders, and the follow-up activity.
- Chart physicians' visits and treatments.
- Chart discharge medications and instructions given for use, as well as all discharge teaching performed, and note which family members were included in the process.

Don't:

- Do *not* chart opinions that are not supported by facts.
- Do *not* defame patients by calling them names or making derogatory statements about them (e.g., "an unlikable patient who is demanding unnecessary attention").
- Do *not* chart before an event occurs.
- Do *not* chart generalizations, suppositions, or pat phrases (e.g., "patient in good spirits").
- Do *not* obliterate, erase, alter, or destroy a record. If an error is made, draw one line through the error, write "mistaken entry," the date, and initial. Follow your agency's guidelines closely.
- Do *not* leave blank spaces for chronological notes. If you must chart out of sequence, chart "late entry." Identify the time and date of the entry and the time and date of the occurrence.
- If an incident report is filed, *do not note in the chart that one was filed.* This form is generally a privileged communication between the hospital and the hospital's attorney. Describing it in the chart may destroy the privileged nature of the communication.

KEY POINTS TO REMEMBER

- The nursing process is a six-step problem-solving approach to patient care.
- The *primary source* of assessment is the patient. *Secondary sources* of information include family members, neighbors, friends, police, and other members of the health team.
- A professional translator often is needed to prevent serious misunderstandings during assessment, treatment, and evaluation with non–English speaking patients.
- The assessment interview includes gathering objective data (mental or emotional status) and subjective data (psychosocial assessment).
- Medical examination, history, and systems review round out a complete assessment.
- Assessment tools and standardized rating scales may be used to evaluate and monitor a patient's progress.
- Determination of the nursing diagnosis (NANDA-I) defines the practice of nursing, improves communication between staff members, and assists in accountability of care.
- A nursing diagnosis consists of (1) an unmet need or problem, (2) an etiology or probable cause, and (3) supporting data.

- Outcomes are variable, measurable, and stated in terms that reflect a patient's actual state. *NOC* provides 385 standardized outcomes. Planning involves determining desired outcomes.
- Behavioral goals support outcomes. Goals are short, specific, and measurable; indicate the desired patient behavior(s); and include a set time for achievement.
- Planning nursing actions (using *NIC* or other sources) to achieve outcomes includes the use of specific principles. The plan should be (1) safe, (2) compatible with and appropriate for implementation with other therapies, (3) realistic and individualized, and (4) evidence based whenever possible. *NIC* provides nurses with 542 standardized nursing interventions applicable for use in all settings.
- Psychiatric mental health nursing practice includes four basic level interventions: coordination of care, health teaching and health promotion, milieu therapy, and pharmacological, biological, and integrative therapies.
- Advanced practice interventions are carried out by a nurse who is educated at the master's level or higher. Nurses certified for advanced practice psychiatric mental health nursing can prescribe certain medications, practice psychotherapy, and perform consulting work.

- The evaluation of care is a continual process of determining to what extent the outcome criteria have been achieved. The plan of care may be revised based on the evaluation.
- Documentation of patient progress through evaluation of the outcome criteria is crucial. The medical record is a legal document and should accurately reflect the patient's condition, medications, treatment, tests, responses, and any untoward incidents.

CRITICAL THINKING

1. Pedro Gonzales, a 37-year-old Hispanic man, arrived by ambulance from a supermarket where he had fallen. On his arrival to the emergency department (ED), his breath smelled "fruity." He appears confused and anxious, saying that "they put the evil eye on me, they want me to die, they are drying out my body…it's draining me dry…they are yelling, they are yelling…no, no I'm not bad…oh God, don't let them get me!" When his mother arrives in the ED, she tells the staff, through the use of a translator, that Pedro is a severe diabetic, has a diagnosis of paranoid schizophrenia, and this happens when he doesn't take his medications. In a group or in collaboration with a classmate, respond to the following:
   A. A number of nursing diagnoses are possible in this scenario. Given the above information, formulate at least two nursing diagnoses (problems), and include "related to" and "as evidenced by."
   B. For each of your nursing diagnoses, write out one long-term outcome (the problem, what should change, etc.). Include a time frame, desired change, and three criteria that will help you evaluate whether the outcome has been met, not met, or partially met.
   C. What specific needs might you take into account when planning nursing care for Mr. Gonzales?
   D. Using the SOAPIE format (see Table 8-4), formulate an initial nurse's note for Mr. Gonzales.

CHAPTER REVIEW

1. The nurse is assessing a 6-year-old patient. When assessing a child's perception of a difficult issue, which methods of assessment are appropriate? *Select all that apply.*
   1. Engage the child in a specific therapeutic game.
   2. Ask the child to draw a picture.
   3. Provide the child with an anatomically correct doll to act out a story.
   4. Allow the child to tell a story.

2. Which are the purposes of a thorough mental health nursing assessment? *Select all that apply.*
   1. Establish a rapport between the nurse and patient.
   2. Assess for risk factors affecting the safety of the patient or others.
   3. Allow the nurse the chance to provide counseling to the patient.
   4. Identify the nurse's goals for treatment.
   5. Formulate a plan of care.

3. The nurse is performing a spiritual assessment on a patient. Which patient statement would indicate to the nurse that there is an experiential concern in the patient's spiritual life?
   1. "I really believe that my spouse loves me."
   2. "My sister will never forgive me for what I did."
   3. "I try to find time every day to pray, even though it's not easy."
   4. "I am happy with my life choices, even if my mother is not."

4. The nurse is caring for a patient who states he has "given up on life." His wife left him, he was fired from his job, and he is four payments behind on his mortgage, meaning he will soon lose his house. Which nursing diagnosis is appropriate?
   1. Anxiety related to multiple losses
   2. Defensive coping related to multiple losses
   3. Ineffective denial related to multiple losses
   4. Hopelessness related to multiple losses

5. The nurse is documenting. Which statement is appropriate to include in the patient's chart?
   1. "Patient states, 'I am going to kill myself.'"
   2. "Patient is in good spirits today."
   3. "Patient has been nasty to the nursing staff this afternoon."
   4. "Patient is demanding and uncooperative."

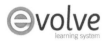

Visit the Evolve website for an **Audio Chapter Summary, Chapter Review Answers & Rationales, Critical Thinking Answer Guidelines,** and additional resources related to the content in this chapter: **http://evolve.elsevier.com/Varcarolis/foundations**

Companion CD Use the Companion CD to prepare for tests and the NCLEX® Examination with **Test-Taking Strategies** for psychiatric mental health nursing and hundreds of **Review Questions.**

References

American Nurses Association (ANA), American Psychiatric Nurses Association, & International Society of Psychiatric-Mental Health Nurses. (2007). *Psychiatric-mental health nursing: Scope and standards of practice*. Washington, DC: Nursesbooks.org.

Anandarajab, G. (2008). The 3 H and BMSEST models for spirituality in multicultural whole-person medicine. *Annals of Family Medicine*, 6(5).

Arnold, E. C., & Boggs, K. U. (2007). *Interpersonal relationships: Professional communication skills for nurses* (5th ed.). St. Louis: Saunders.

Bernzweig, J., Takayama, J. I., Phibbs, C., Lewis, C., & Pantell, R. H. (1997). Gender differences in physician-patient communication. *Archives of pediatric and Adolescent medicine*, 151(6), 586–591.

Bulechek, G. M., Butcher, H. K., & Dochterman, J. M. (2008). *Nursing interventions classification (NIC)* (5th ed.). St. Louis: Mosby.

Carson, V. B., & Koenig, H. G. (2004). *Spiritual caregiving as a ministry*. Philadelphia: Templeton.

Delgado, C. (2007). Meeting clients' spiritual needs. *Nursing Clinics of North America*, 42(2), 279–293.

Fontes, L. A. (2008). *Interviewing Across Cultures*. New York: The Guilford Press.

George, L. K., Ellison, C. G., & Larson, D. B. (2002). Explaining the relationships between religious involvement and health. *Psychological Inquiry*, 13(3), 190–200.

George, L. K., Larson, D. B., Koenig, H. G., & McCullough, M. E. (2000). Spirituality and health: What we know, what we need to know. *Journal of Social and Clinical Psychology*, 19(1), 102–116.

Koenig, H. G. (2001). *Handbook of religion and mental health*. New York: Oxford Press.

Koenig, H. G., McCullough, M., & Larson, D. B. (2001). *Handbook of religion and health*. New York: Oxford University Press.

Mackenzie, E., Rajagopal, D., Meibohm, M., & Lavizzo-Mourey, R. (2000). Spiritual support and psychological well-being: Older adults' perceptions of the religion and health connection. *Alternative Therapies in Health and Medicine*, 6(6), 37–45.

Miller, W. R., & Thoresen, C. E. (2003). Spirituality, religion, and health: An emerging research field. *American Psychological Association*, 58(1), 24–35.

Moorhead, S., Johnson, M., Maas, M. L., & Swanson, E. (2008). *Nursing outcomes classification (NOC)* (4th ed.). St. Louis: Mosby.

North American Nursing Diagnosis Association International (NANDA-I). (2009-2011). *NANDA-I nursing diagnoses: Definitions and classification 2009-2011*. Oxford, United Kingdom: Author.

Poole, R., & Higgo, R. (2006). *Psychiatric interviewing and assessment*. Liverpool, UK: Cambridge University Press.

Sackett, D. L., Straus, S. E., Richardson, W. S., Rosenberg, W., & Haynes, R. B. (2000). *Evidence-based medicine: How to practice and teach EBMB*. London: Churchill Livingstone.

Sommers-Flanagan, J., & Sommers-Flanagan, R. (2003). *Clinical interviewing* (3rd ed.). Hoboken, NJ: Wiley.

U.S. Department of Health and Human Services (USDHHS). (2003). *Summary of the HIPAA Privacy Act*. Washington, DC: Author.

Waseem, M., & Ryan, M. (2005). "Doctor" or "doctora": Do patients care? *Pediatric Emergency Care*, 21, 515–517.

CHAPTER 9

Therapeutic Relationships

Elizabeth M. Varcarolis

Key Terms and Concepts

clinical supervision, 158
contract, 167
countertransference, 160
empathy,170
genuineness, 169
orientation phase, 166
rapport, 166
social relationship, 157

termination phase, 168
therapeutic encounter, 159
therapeutic relationship, 158
therapeutic use of self, 157
transference, 159
values, 163
working phase, 167

Objectives

1. Compare and contrast the three phases of the nurse-patient relationship.
2. Compare and contrast a social relationship and a therapeutic relationship regarding purpose, focus, communications style, and goals.
3. Identify at least four patient behaviors a nurse may encounter in the clinical setting.
4. Explore qualities that foster a therapeutic nurse-patient relationship and qualities that contribute to a nontherapeutic nursing interactive process.
5. Define and discuss the roles of empathy, genuineness, and positive regard on the part of the nurse in a nurse-patient relationship.

6. Identify two attitudes and four actions that may reflect the nurse's positive regard for a patient.
7. Analyze what is meant by boundaries and the influence of transference and countertransference on boundary blurring.
8. Understand the use of attending behaviors (eye contact, body language, vocal qualities, and verbal tracking).
9. Discuss the influences of disparate values and cultural beliefs on the therapeutic relationship.

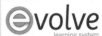 Visit the Evolve website for an **Audio Glossary & Flashcards, Concept Map Creator**, and additional resources related to the content in this chapter: **http://evolve.elsevier.com/Varcarolis/foundations**

Psychiatric mental health nursing is in many ways based on principles of *science*. A background in anatomy, physiology, and chemistry is the basis for providing safe and effective biological treatments. Knowledge of pharmacology—a medication's mechanism of action, indications for use, and adverse effects, based on evidence-based studies and trials—is vital to nursing practice. However, it is the caring relationship and the development of the interpersonal skills needed to enhance and maintain such a relationship that make up the *art* of psychiatric nursing. Quinlan (1996) states that "the development of that very human relationship allows a place for caring and healing to occur. This use of the essential humanness of the nurse as a person is the most critical part of the way nurses make themselves available to both patients and colleagues" (p. 7). Quinlan goes on to say that how this is achieved remains within the domain of the individual nurse.

CONCEPTS OF THE NURSE-PATIENT RELATIONSHIP

The nurse-patient relationship is the basis of all psychiatric mental health nursing treatment approaches, regardless of the specific goals. The very first connections between nurse and patient are to establish an understanding that the nurse is safe, confidential, reliable, consistent, and that the relationship will be conducted within appropriate and clear boundaries (LaRowe, 2004).

It is true that many psychiatric disorders, such as schizophrenia, bipolar disorder, and major depression, have strong biochemical and genetic components. However, many accompanying emotional problems like poor self-image, low self-esteem, and difficulties with adherence to a treatment regimen can be significantly improved through a therapeutic nurse-patient relationship (LaRowe, 2004). All too often, patients entering treatment have taxed or exhausted their familial and social resources and find themselves isolated and in need of emotional support.

The nurse-patient relationship is a creative process and unique to each nurse. Each of us has unique gifts that we can learn to use creatively to form positive bonds with others, historically referred to as the **therapeutic use of self**. Travelbee (1971) defined therapeutic use of self as "the ability to use one's personality consciously and in full awareness in an attempt to establish relatedness and to structure nursing interventions" (p. 19). It is important to note that the efficacy of this therapeutic use of self has been scientifically substantiated as an evidence-based intervention. A review of randomized clinical trials that studied patients with various disorders (e.g., mood, eating, personality) across a wide range of therapeutic modalities repeatedly found that the development of a therapeutic relationship (alliance) was an important and consistent predictor of a positive outcome in therapy (Butler Center for Research, 2006).

Therapeutic success is a result of the personal characteristics of the clinician and the patient, not necessarily the particular process employed (Korn, 2001). Furthermore, evidence suggests that psychotherapy (talk therapy) within a therapeutic relationship actually changes brain chemistry in much the same way as medication. Thus the adage that the best treatment for most psychiatric problems (less so with psychotic disorders) is a combination of medication and psychotherapy. Cognitive-behavioral therapy, in particular, has met with great success in the treatment of depression, phobias, obsessive-compulsive disorders, and others.

Establishing a therapeutic relationship with a patient takes time. Skills in this area gradually improve with guidance from those with more skill and experience.

Goals and Functions

The nurse-patient relationship is often loosely defined. However, a therapeutic nurse-patient relationship has specific goals and functions, including:

- Facilitating communication of distressing thoughts and feelings
- Assisting patients with problem solving to help facilitate activities of daily living
- Helping patients examine self-defeating behaviors and test alternatives
- Promoting self-care and independence

Social versus Therapeutic

A relationship is an interpersonal process that involves two or more people. Throughout life, we meet people in a variety of settings and share a variety of experiences. With some individuals, we develop long-term relationships; with others, the relationship lasts only a short time. Naturally, the kinds of relationships we enter vary from person to person and from situation to situation. Generally, relationships can be defined as *intimate*, *social*, or *therapeutic*. Intimate relationships occur between people who have an emotional commitment to each other. Within intimate relationships, mutual needs are met, and intimate desires and fantasies are shared. For our purposes in this chapter, we will limit our exploration to the aspects of social and therapeutic relationships.

Social Relationships

A **social relationship** can be defined as a relationship that is primarily initiated for the purpose of friendship, socialization, enjoyment, or accomplishment of a task. Mutual needs are met during social interaction (e.g., participants share ideas, feelings, and experiences). Communication skills may include giving advice and (sometimes) meeting basic dependency needs, such as lending money and helping with jobs. Often the content of the communication remains superficial. During social interactions, roles may shift. Within a social relationship, there is little emphasis on the evaluation of the interaction, as in the following example:

Patient: "Oh, gosh, I just hate to be alone. It's getting me down, and sometimes it hurts so much."

Nurse: "I know just how you feel. I don't like it either. What I do is get a friend and go to a movie or something. Do you have someone to hang out with?" (*In this response the nurse is minimizing the patient's feelings and giving advice prematurely.*)

Patient: "No, not really, but often I don't even feel like going out. I just sit at home feeling scared and lonely."

Nurse: "Most of us feel like that at one time or another. Maybe if you took a class or joined a group you could meet more people. I know of some great groups you could join. It's not good to be stuck in the house by yourself all of the time." *(Again, the nurse is not "hearing" the patient's distress and is minimizing her pain and isolation. The nurse goes on to give the patient unwanted and unhelpful advice, thus closing off the patient's feelings and experience.)*

Therapeutic Relationships

In a **therapeutic relationship**, the nurse maximizes his or her communication skills, understanding of human behaviors, and personal strengths to enhance the patient's growth. The focus of the relationship is on the patient's ideas, experiences, and feelings. Inherent in a therapeutic relationship is the nurse's focus on significant personal issues introduced by the patient during the clinical interview. The nurse and the patient identify areas that need exploration and periodically evaluate the degree of change in the patient.

Although the nurse may assume a variety of roles (e.g., teacher, counselor, socializing agent, liaison), the relationship is consistently focused on the patient's problem and needs. Nurses' needs must be met outside the relationship. When nurses begin to want the patient to "like them," "do as they suggest," "be nice to them," or "give them recognition," the needs of the patient cannot be adequately met, and the interaction could be detrimental (nontherapeutic) to the patient.

Working under **clinical supervision** is an excellent way to keep the focus and boundaries clear. Communication skills and knowledge of the stages and phenomena in a therapeutic relationship are crucial tools in the formation and maintenance of that relationship. Within the context of a therapeutic relationship, the following occur:

- The needs of the patient are identified and explored.
- Clear boundaries are established.
- Alternate problem-solving approaches are taken.
- New coping skills may be developed.
- Behavioral change is encouraged.

Just like staff nurses, nursing students may struggle with the boundaries between social and therapeutic relationships, because there is a fine line between the two. In fact, students often feel more comfortable "being a friend" because it is a more familiar role, especially with people close to their own age. However, when this occurs, the nurse or student needs to make it clear (to themselves and the patient) that the relationship is a therapeutic one. This does *not* mean that the nurse is not friendly toward the patient, and it does *not* mean that talking about everyday topics (television, weather, children's pictures) is forbidden. It *does* mean, however, that the nurse must follow the prior stated guidelines regarding a therapeutic relationship; essentially, the focus is on the patient, and the relationship is not designed to meet the nurse's needs. The patient's

problems and concerns are explored, potential solutions are discussed by both patient and nurse, and solutions are implemented by the patient, as in the following example:

Patient: "Oh, gosh, I just hate to be alone. It's getting me down, and sometimes it hurts so much."

Nurse: "Loneliness can be painful. What is going on now that you are feeling so alone?"

Patient: "Well, my mom died 2 years ago, and last month, my—oh, I am so scared." *(Patient takes a deep breath, looks down, and looks like she might cry.)*

Nurse: *(Sits in silence while the patient recovers.)* "Go on…"

Patient: "My boyfriend left for Iraq. I haven't heard from him, and they say he's missing. He was my best friend, and we were going to get married, and if he dies, I don't want to live."

Nurse: "Have you thought of harming yourself?"

Patient: "Well, if he dies, I will. I can't live without him."

Nurse: "Have you ever felt like this before?"

Patient: "Yes, when my mom died. I was depressed for about a year until I met my boyfriend."

Nurse: "It sounds like you're going through a very painful and scary time. Perhaps you and I can talk some more and come up with some ways for you to feel less anxious, scared, and overwhelmed. Would you be willing to work on this together?"

The ability of the nurse to engage in interpersonal interactions in a goal-directed manner to assist patients with their emotional or physical health needs is the foundation of the therapeutic nurse-patient relationship. Necessary behaviors of health care workers, including nurses, are:

- **Accountability**—Nurses assume responsibility for their conduct and the consequences of their actions.
- **Focus on patient needs**—The interest of the patient rather than the nurse, other health care workers, or the institution is given first consideration. The nurse's role is that of patient advocate.
- **Clinical competence**—The criteria on which the nurse bases his or her conduct are principles of knowledge and those that are appropriate to the specific situation. This involves awareness and incorporation of the latest knowledge made available from research (evidence-based practice).
- **Delaying judgment**—Ideally, nurses refrain from judging patients and avoid putting their own values and beliefs on others.
- **Supervision**—Supervision by a more experienced clinician or team is essential to developing one's competence in establishing therapeutic nurse-patient relationships.

Nurses interact with patients in a variety of settings: emergency departments, medical-surgical units, obstetric and pediatric units, clinics, community settings, schools, and patients' homes. Nurses who are sensitive to patients' needs and have effective assessment and communication skills can significantly help patients confront current problems and anticipate future choices.

Sometimes the type of relationship that occurs may be informal and not extensive, such as when the nurse and patient meet for only a few sessions. However, even though it is brief, the relationship may be substantial, useful, and important for the patient. This limited relationship is often referred to as a **therapeutic encounter**. When the nurse shows genuine concern for another's circumstances (has positive regard, empathy), even a short encounter can have a powerful effect.

At other times, the encounters may be longer and more formal, such as in inpatient settings, mental health units, crisis centers, and mental health facilities. This longer time span allows the therapeutic nurse-patient relationship to be more fully developed.

Relationship Boundaries and Roles

Establishing Boundaries

According to Su Fox (2008), boundaries can be thought of in terms of the following:
- **Physical boundaries**: general environment, office space, treatment room, conference room, corner of the day room, and other such places
- **The contract**: set time, confidentiality, agreement between nurse and patient as to roles, money, if involved with a licensed therapist
- **Personal space**: physical space, emotional space, space set by roles, and so forth

Blurring of Boundaries

A well-defined therapeutic nurse-patient relationship allows the establishment of clear boundaries that provide a safe space in which the patient can explore feelings and treatment issues (Peternelj-Taylor, 2002). Theoretically, the nurse's role in the therapeutic relationship can be stated rather simply as follows: The patient's needs are separated from the nurse's needs, and the patient's role is different from that of the nurse; therefore, the boundaries of the relationship are well defined. However, boundaries are constantly at risk of blurring, and a shift in the nurse-patient relationship may lead to nontherapeutic dynamics. Two common circumstances in which boundaries are blurred are (1) when the relationship is allowed to slip into a social context and (2) when the nurse's needs (for attention, affection, emotional support) are met at the expense of the patient's needs.

Boundaries are primarily necessary to protect the patient. The most egregious boundary violations are those of a sexual nature (Wheeler, 2008). This type of violation results in high levels of malpractice actions and the loss of professional licensure on the part of

the nurse. Other boundary issues are not as obvious. Table 9-1 illustrates some examples of patient and nurse behaviors that reflect blurred boundaries.

Blurring of Roles

Blurring of roles in the nurse-patient relationship is often a result of unrecognized transference or countertransference.

Transference. Transference is a phenomenon originally identified by Sigmund Freud when he used psychoanalysis to treat patients. **Transference** occurs when the patient unconsciously and inappropriately displaces (transfers) onto the nurse feelings and behaviors related to significant figures in the patient's past. The patient may even say, "You remind me of my (mother, sister, father, brother, etc.)."

TABLE 9-1 Patient and Nurse Behaviors That Reflect Blurred Boundaries

When the Nurse Is Overly Involved	When the Nurse Is Not Involved
More frequent requests by the patient for assistance, which causes increased dependency on the nurse	Patient's increased verbal or physical expression of isolation (depression)
Inability of the patient to perform tasks of which he or she is known to be capable prior to the nurse's help, which causes regression	Lack of mutually agreed-upon goals
Unwillingness on the part of the patient to maintain performance or progress in the nurse's absence	Lack of progress toward goals
Expressions of anger by other staff who do not agree with the nurse's interventions or perceptions of the patient	Nurse's avoidance of spending time with the patient
Nurse's keeping of secrets about the nurse-patient relationship	Failure of the nurse to follow through on agreed-upon interventions

Data from Pilette, P. C., Berck, C. B., & Achber, L. C. (1995). Therapeutic management of helping boundaries. *Journal of Psychosocial Nursing and Mental Health Services, 33*(1), 40-47.

Patient: "Oh, you are so high and mighty. Did anyone ever tell you that you are a cold, unfeeling machine, just like others I know?"

Nurse: "Tell me about one person who is cold and unfeeling toward you." (*In this example, the patient is experiencing the nurse in the same way she did with significant other[s] during her formative years. In this case, the patient's mother was very aloof, leaving her with feelings of isolation, worthlessness, and anger.*)

Although transference occurs in all relationships, it seems to be intensified in relationships of authority. This may occur because parental figures were the original figures of authority. Physicians, nurses, and social workers all are potential objects of transference. This transference may be positive or negative. If a patient is motivated to work with you, completes assignments between sessions, and shares feelings openly, it is likely the patient is experiencing positive transference (Wheeler, 2008).

Positive transference does not need to be addressed with the patient, whereas negative transference that threatens the nurse-patient relationship may need to be explored. Common forms of transference include the desire for affection or respect and the gratification of dependency needs. Other transferential feelings are hostility, jealousy, competitiveness, and love.

Sometimes patients experience positive or negative thoughts, feelings, and reactions that are realistic and appropriate and *not* a result of transference onto the health care worker. For example, if a nurse makes promises to the patient that are not kept; such as not showing up for a meeting, the patient may feel resentment and mistrust toward the nurse.

Countertransference. Countertransference occurs when the nurse unconsciously and inappropriately displaces onto the patient feelings and behaviors related to significant figures in the nurse's past. Frequently the patient's transference evokes countertransference in the nurse. For example, it is normal to feel angry when attacked persistently, annoyed when frustrated unreasonably, or flattered when idealized. A nurse might feel extremely important when depended on exclusively by a patient. If the nurse does not recognize his or her own omnipotent feelings as countertransference, encouragement of independent growth in the patient might be minimized at best.

Recognizing countertransference maximizes our ability to *empower* our patients. When we fail to recognize countertransference, the therapeutic relationship stalls, and essentially we *disempower* our patients by experiencing them not as individuals but rather as extensions of ourselves. Example:

Patient: "Yeah, well I decided not to go to that dumb group. 'Hi, I'm so-and-so, and I'm an alcoholic.' Who cares?" (*Patient sits slumped in a chair chewing gum, nonchalantly looking around.*)

Nurse: (*In a very impassioned tone*) "You always sabotage your chances. You need AA to get in control of your life. Last week you were going to go, and now you've disappointed everyone." (*Here the nurse is reminded of her mother, who was an alcoholic. The nurse had tried everything to get her mother into treatment and took it as a personal failure and deep disappointment that her mother never sought recovery. After the nurse sorts out her thoughts and feelings and realizes the frustration and feelings of disappointment and failure belonged with her mother and not the patient, the nurse starts out the next session with the following approach.*)

Nurse: "Look, I was thinking about last week, and I realize the decision to go to AA or find other help is solely up to you. It's true that I would like you to live a fuller and more satisfying life, but it's your decision. I'm wondering, however, what happened to change your mind about going to AA."

If the nurse feels either a strongly positive or a strongly negative reaction to a patient, the feeling most often signals countertransference. One common sign of countertransference is overidentification with the patient. In this situation, the nurse may have difficulty recognizing or objectively seeing patient problems that are similar to the nurse's own. For example, a nurse who is struggling with an alcoholic family member may feel disinterested, cold, or disgusted toward an alcoholic patient. Other indicators of countertransference are when the nurse gets involved in power struggles, competition, or arguments with the patient. Table 9-2 lists some common countertransference reactions.

Identifying and working through various transference and countertransference issues is crucial if we are to achieve professional and clinical growth and allow for positive change in the patient. Transference and countertransference, as well as numerous other issues, are best dealt with through the use of supervision by either the peer group or therapeutic team. Besides helping with boundary issues, supervision supplies practical and emotional support, education, and guidance regarding ethical issues. Regularly scheduled supervision sessions provide the nurse with the opportunity to increase self-awareness, clinical skills, and growth, as well as allow for continued growth of the patient. No matter how hard clinicians may try to examine their interactions objectively, professional support and help from an experienced supervisor is essential to good practice (Fox, 2008).

Self-Check on Boundaries

It is useful for all of us to take time out to be reflective and aware of our thoughts and actions with patients, as well as with colleagues, friends, and family. Figure 9-1 is a helpful boundary self-test you can use throughout your career, no matter what area of nursing you choose.

TABLE 9-2 Common Countertransference Reactions

As a nurse, you will sometimes experience countertransference feelings. Once you are aware of them, use them for self-analysis to understand those feelings that may inhibit productive nurse-patient communication.

Reaction to Patient	Behaviors Characteristic of the Reaction	Self-Analysis	Solution
Boredom (indifference)	Showing inattention Frequently asking the patient to repeat statements Making inappropriate responses	Is the content of what the patient presents uninteresting? Or is it the style of communication? Does the patient exhibit an offensive style of communication? Have you anything else on your mind that may be distracting you from the patient's needs? Is the patient discussing an issue that makes you anxious?	Redirect the patient if he or she provides more information than you need or goes "off track." Clarify information with the patient. Confront ineffective modes of communication.
Rescue	Reaching for unattainable goals Resisting peer feedback and supervisory recommendations Giving advice	What behavior stimulates your perceived need to rescue the patient? Has anyone evoked such feelings in you in the past? What are your fears or fantasies about failing to meet the patient's needs? Why do you want to rescue this patient?	Avoid secret alliances. Develop realistic goals. Do not alter meeting schedule. Let the patient guide interaction. Facilitate patient problem solving.
Overinvolvement	Coming to work early, leaving late Ignoring peer suggestions, resisting assistance Buying the patient clothes or other gifts Accepting the patient's gifts Behaving judgmentally at family interventions Keeping secrets Calling the patient when off duty	What particular patient characteristics are attractive? Does the patient remind you of someone? Who? Does your current behavior differ from your treatment of similar patients in the past? What are you getting out of this situation? What needs of yours are being met?	Establish firm treatment boundaries, goals, and nursing expectations. Avoid self-disclosure. Avoid calling the patient when off duty.
Overidentification	Having special agenda, keeping secrets Increasing self-disclosure Feeling omnipotent Experiencing physical attraction	With which of the patient's physical, emotional, cognitive, or situational characteristics do you identify? Recall similar circumstances in your own life. How did you deal with the issues now being created by the patient?	Allow the patient to direct issues. Encourage a problem-solving approach from the patient's perspective. Avoid self-disclosure.
Misuse of honesty	Withholding information Lying	Why are you protecting the patient? What are your fears about the patient learning the truth?	Be clear in your responses and aware of your hesitation; do not hedge. If you can provide information, tell the patient and give your rationale. Avoid keeping secrets. Reinforce the patient with regard to the interdisciplinary nature of treatment.

Continued

TABLE 9-2 Common Countertransference Reactions—cont'd

Reaction to Patient	Behaviors Characteristic of the Reaction	Self-Analysis	Solution
Anger	Withdrawing Speaking loudly Using profanity Asking to be taken off the case	What patient behaviors are offensive to you? What dynamic from your past may this patient be re-creating?	Determine the origin of the anger (nurse, patient, or both). Explore the roots of patient anger. Avoid contact with the patient if the anger is not understood.
Helplessness or hopelessness	Feeling sadness	Which patient behaviors evoke these feelings in you? Has anyone evoked similar feelings in the past? Who? What past expectations were placed on you (verbally and nonverbally) by this patient?	Maintain therapeutic involvement. Explore and focus on the patient's experience rather than on your own.

Data from Aromando, L. (1995). *Mental health and psychiatric nursing* (2nd ed.). Springhouse, PA: Springhouse.

NURSING BOUNDARY INDEX SELF-CHECK

Please rate yourself according to the frequency with which the following statements reflect your behavior, thoughts, or feelings within the past 2 years while providing patient care.*

1. Have you ever received any feedback about your behavior being overly intrusive with patients and their families?　Never _____　Rarely _____　Sometimes _____　Often _____

2. Do you ever have difficulty setting limits with patients?　Never _____　Rarely _____　Sometimes _____　Often _____

3. Do you ever arrive early or stay late to be with your patient for a longer period?　Never _____　Rarely _____　Sometimes _____　Often _____

4. Do you ever find yourself relating to patients or peers as you might to a family member?　Never _____　Rarely _____　Sometimes _____　Often _____

5. Have you ever acted on sexual feelings you have for a patient?　Never _____　Rarely _____　Sometimes _____　Often _____

6. Do you feel that you are the only one who understands the patient?　Never _____　Rarely _____　Sometimes _____　Often _____

7. Have you ever received feedback that you get "too involved" with patients or families?　Never _____　Rarely _____　Sometimes _____　Often _____

8. Do you derive conscious satisfaction from patients' praise, appreciation, or affection?　Never _____　Rarely _____　Sometimes _____　Often _____

9. Do you ever feel that other staff members are too critical of "your" patient?　Never _____　Rarely _____　Sometimes _____　Often _____

10. Do you ever feel that other staff members are jealous of your relationship with your patient?　Never _____　Rarely _____　Sometimes _____　Often _____

11. Have you ever tried to "match-make" a patient with one of your friends?　Never _____　Rarely _____　Sometimes _____　Often _____

12. Do you find it difficult to handle patients' unreasonable requests for assistance, verbal abuse, or sexual language?　Never _____　Rarely _____　Sometimes _____　Often _____

*Any item that is responded to with "Sometimes" or "Often" should alert the nurse to a possible area of vulnerability. If the item is responded to with "Rarely," the nurse should determine whether it is an isolated event or a possible pattern of behavior.

Figure 9-1 Nursing Boundary Index Self-Check. (From Pilette, P., Berck, C., & Achber, L. [1995]. Therapeutic management. *Journal of Psychosocial Nursing, 33*[1], 45.)

VALUES, BELIEFS, AND SELF-AWARENESS

Values are abstract standards and represent an ideal, either positive or negative. It is crucial that we have an understanding of our own values and attitudes so we may become aware of the beliefs or attitudes we hold that may interfere with establishing positive relationships with those under our care.

When working with patients, it is important for nurses to understand that our values and beliefs are not necessarily right and certainly are not right for everyone. It is helpful to realize that our values and beliefs (1) reflect our own culture/subculture, (2) are derived from a range of choices, and (3) are those we have *chosen* for ourselves from a variety of influences and role models. These chosen values (religious, cultural, societal) guide us in making decisions and taking actions that we hope will make our lives meaningful, rewarding, and fulfilled.

Interviewing others whose values, beliefs, cultures, or lifestyles are radically different from our own can be a challenge (Fontes, 2008). Several topics that cause controversy in society in general—including religion, gender roles, abortion, war, politics, money, drugs, alcohol, sex, and corporal punishment—also can cause conflict between nurses and patients (Fontes, 2008). Although we emphasize that the patient and nurse should identify outcomes together, what happens when the nurse's values, beliefs, and interpretive system are very different from those of a patient? Consider the following examples of possible conflicts:

- The patient wants an abortion, which is against the nurse's values.
- The nurse believes the patient who was raped should get an abortion, but the patient refuses.
- The patient engages in unsafe sex with multiple partners, which is against the nurse's values.
- The nurse cannot understand a patient who refuses medications on religious grounds.
- The patient puts material gain and objects far ahead of loyalty to friends and family, in direct contrast with the nurse's values.
- The nurse is deeply religious, whereas the patient is a nonbeliever who shuns organized religion.
- The patient's lifestyle includes taking illicit drugs, which is against the nurse's values.

How can nurses develop working relationships and help patients solve problems when patients' values, goals, and interpretive systems are so different from their own? Self-awareness requires that we understand what we value and those beliefs that guide our behavior. It is critical that as nurses we not only understand and accept our own values and beliefs but also are sensitive to and accepting of the unique and different values and beliefs of others. This is another area in which supervision by an experienced colleague can prove invaluable.

PEPLAU'S MODEL OF THE NURSE-PATIENT RELATIONSHIP

Hildegard Peplau introduced the concept of the nurse-patient relationship in 1952 in her groundbreaking book *Interpersonal Relations in Nursing*. This model of the nurse-patient relationship is well accepted in the United States and Canada and has become an important tool for all nursing practice. A **professional nurse-patient relationship** consists of a nurse who has skills and expertise and a patient who wants to alleviate suffering, find solutions to problems, explore different avenues to increased quality of life, and/or find an advocate (Fox, 2008).

Peplau (1952) proposed that the nurse-patient relationship "facilitates forward movement" for both the nurse and the patient (p. 12). This interactive nurse-patient process is designed to facilitate the patient's boundary management, independent problem solving, and decision making that promotes autonomy (Haber, 2000).

Peplau (1952, 1999) described the nurse-patient relationship as evolving through distinct interlocking and overlapping phases, generally recognized as follows:

1. Orientation phase
2. Working phase
3. Termination phase

An additional preorientation phase, during which the nurse prepares for the orientation phase, has also been identified. Most likely, you will not have time to develop all phases of the nurse-patient relationship in your brief psychiatric mental health nursing rotation. However, it is important to be aware of these phases in order to recognize and use them later. It is also important to remember that *any* contact that is caring, respectful, and demonstrative of concern for the situation of another person can have an enormous positive impact.

Preorientation Phase

Even before the first meeting, the nurse may have many thoughts and feelings related to the first clinical session. Beginning health care professionals usually have many concerns and experience anxiety on their first clinical day. These universal concerns include being afraid of people with psychiatric problems, saying "the wrong thing," and not knowing what to do in response to certain patient behaviors. Table 9-3 identifies common patient behaviors (e.g., crying, asking the nurse to keep a secret, threatening to commit suicide, giving a gift, wanting physical contact with the nurse) and gives examples of possible reactions by the nurse and suggested responses.

Talking with the instructor and participating in the supervised peer group discussion will promote confidence, feedback, and suggestions. Refer to Chapter 10 for a detailed discussion of communication strategies used in clinical practice.

TABLE 9-3 Common Patient Behaviors, Possible Nurse Reactions, and Suggested Nurse Responses

Possible Reactions	Useful Responses
IF THE PATIENT THREATENS SUICIDE	
The nurse may feel overwhelmed or responsible for "talking the patient out of it." The nurse may pick up some of the patient's feelings of hopelessness.	The nurse assesses whether the patient has a plan and the lethality of the plan. The nurse tells the patient that this is serious, that the nurse does not want harm to come to the patient, and that this information needs to be shared with other staff: "This is very serious, Mr. Lamb. I don't want any harm to come to you. I'll have to share this with the other staff." The nurse can then discuss with the patient the feelings and circumstances that led up to this decision. (Refer to Chapter 24 for strategies in suicide intervention.)
IF THE PATIENT ASKS THE NURSE TO KEEP A SECRET	
The nurse may feel conflict because the nurse wants the patient to share important information but is unsure about making such a promise.	The nurse *cannot* make such a promise. The information may be important to the health or safety of the patient or others: "I cannot make that promise. It might be important for me to share it with other staff." The patient then decides whether to share the information.
IF THE PATIENT ASKS THE NURSE A PERSONAL QUESTION	
The nurse may think that it is rude not to answer the patient's question. A new nurse might feel relieved to put off having to start the interview. The nurse may feel put on the spot and want to leave the situation. New nurses are often manipulated by a patient into changing roles. This keeps the focus off the patient and prevents the building of a relationship.	The nurse may or may not answer the patient's query. If the nurse decides to answer a natural question, he or she answers in a word or two, then refocuses back on the patient: *Patient:* Are you married? *Nurse:* Yes. Do you have a spouse? *Patient:* Do you have any children? *Nurse:* This time is for you . . . tell me about yourself. *Patient:* You can just tell me if you have any children. *Nurse:* This is your time to focus on your concerns. Tell me something about your family.
IF THE PATIENT MAKES SEXUAL ADVANCES	
The nurse feels uncomfortable but may feel conflicted about "rejecting" the patient or making him or her feel "unattractive" or "not good enough."	The nurse needs to set clear limits on expected behavior: "I'm not comfortable having you touch (kiss) me. This time is for you to focus on your problems and concerns." Frequently restating the nurse's role throughout the relationship can help maintain boundaries. If the patient doesn't stop, the nurse might say: "If you can't stop this behavior, I'll have to leave. I'll be back at [time] to spend time with you then." Leaving gives the patient time to gain control. The nurse returns at the stated time.
IF THE PATIENT CRIES	
The nurse may feel uncomfortable and experience increased anxiety or feel somehow responsible for making the person cry.	The nurse should stay with the patient and reinforce that it is all right to cry. Often it is at that time that feelings are closest to the surface and can be best identified: "You seem ready to cry." "You are still upset about your brother's death." "What are you thinking right now?" The nurse offers tissues when appropriate.

TABLE 9-3 Common Patient Behaviors, Possible Nurse Reactions, and Suggested Nurse Responses—cont'd

Possible Reactions	Useful Responses
IF THE PATIENT LEAVES BEFORE THE SESSION IS OVER	
The nurse may feel rejected, thinking it was something that he or she did. The nurse may experience increased anxiety or feel abandoned by the patient.	Some patients are not able to relate for long periods without experiencing an increase in anxiety. On the other hand, the patient may be testing the nurse: "I'll wait for you here for 15 minutes, until our time is up."
	During this time, the nurse does not engage in conversation with any other patient or even with the staff.
	When the time is up, the nurse approaches the patient, says the time is up, and restates the day and time the nurse will see the patient again.
IF THE PATIENT DOES NOT WANT TO TALK	
The nurse new to this situation may feel rejected or ineffectual.	At first, the nurse might say something to this effect: "It's all right. I would like to spend time with you. We don't have to talk."
	The nurse might spend short, frequent periods (e.g., 5 minutes) with the patient throughout the day: "Our 5 minutes is up. I'll be back at 10 AM and stay with you 5 more minutes."
	This gives the patient the opportunity to understand that the nurse means what he or she says and is back on time consistently. It also gives the patient time between visits to assess how he or she feels, what he or she thinks about the nurse, and perhaps to feel less threatened.
IF THE PATIENT GIVES THE NURSE A PRESENT	
The nurse may feel uncomfortable when offered a gift.	Possible guidelines:
The meaning needs to be examined. Is the gift (1) a way of getting better care, (2) a way to maintain self-esteem, (3) a way of making the nurse feel guilty, (4) a sincere expression of thanks, or (5) a cultural expectation?	If the gift is expensive, the only policy is to graciously refuse.
	If it is inexpensive, then (1) if it is given at the end of hospitalization when a relationship has developed, graciously accept; (2) if it is given at the beginning of the relationship, graciously refuse and explore the meaning behind the present: "Thank you, but it is our job to care for our patients. Are you concerned that some aspect of your care will be overlooked?"
	If the gift is money, it is always graciously refused.
IF ANOTHER PATIENT INTERRUPTS DURING TIME WITH YOUR CURRENT PATIENT	
The nurse may feel a conflict. The nurse does not want to appear rude. Sometimes the nurse tries to engage both patients in conversation.	The time the nurse had contracted with a selected patient is that patient's time. By keeping his or her part of the contract, the nurse demonstrates that the nurse means what he or she says and views the sessions as important: "I am with Mr. Rob for the next 20 minutes. At 10 AM, after our time is up, I can talk to you for 5 minutes."

Most experienced psychiatric mental health nursing faculty and staff monitor the unit atmosphere and have a sixth sense for behaviors that indicate escalating tension. They are trained in crisis interventions, and formal security is often available onsite to give the staff support. Your instructor will set the ground rules for safety during the first clinical day. For example, don't go into a patient's room alone, know if there are any patients not to engage, stay where other people are around in an open area, and know the signs and symptoms of escalating anxiety.

There are actions a nurse can take if a patient's anger begins to escalate, many of which are presented in Table 9-4. Chapter 25 offers a more detailed discussion of maintaining personal safety, recognizing potential agitation, and intervening with angry or aggressive patients. You should always trust your own instincts. If you feel uncomfortable for any reason, excuse yourself

TABLE 9-4 Guidelines for Maintaining Safety When a Patient's Anger Escalates

Nursing Intervention	Rationale
Pay attention to angry and aggressive behavior. Respond as early as possible.	Minimization of angry behaviors and ineffective limit setting are the most frequent factors contributing to the escalation of violence.
Assess for and provide for personal safety. Pay attention to the environment: Leave door open or use hallway. Choose a quiet place that is visible to staff. Have a quick exit available. The more angry the patient, the more space he/she will need to feel comfortable. Never turn your back on an angry patient. Leave immediately if there are signs behavior is escalating out of control or if you are uncomfortable. State, "I am leaving now, I will be back in 10 minutes," and seek out your clinical instructor or other staff member right away.	Exercising basic caution is essential to protecting yourself. Although the risk for violence may be minimal, it is easier to prevent a problem than to get out of a bad situation. These precautions are similar to using universal precautions (gloves, masks, gowns, etc.) on medical floors.
Appear calm and in control.	The perception that someone is in control can be comforting and calming to an individual whose anxiety is beginning to escalate.
Speak softly in a nonprovocative, nonjudgmental manner	When tone of voice is low and calm and the words are spoken slowly, anxiety levels in others may decrease.
Demonstrate genuineness and concern.	Even the most psychotic individual with schizophrenia may respond to nonprovocative interpersonal contact and expressions of concern and caring.
If patient is willing, both nurse and patient should sit at a 45-degree angle. Do not tower over or stare at the patient.	Sitting at a 45-degree angle puts you both on the same level but allows for frequent breaks in eye-contact. Towering over or staring can be interpreted as threatening or controlling by paranoid individuals.
When patient begins to talk, listen. Use clarification.	Allows patient to feel heard and understood, helps build rapport, and energy can be channeled productively.

for a moment, and discuss your feelings with your instructor or a staff member. In addition to getting reassurance and support, students can often provide valuable information about the patient's condition by sharing these perceptions.

Orientation Phase

The **orientation phase** can last for a few meetings or extend over a longer period. It is the first time the nurse and the patient meet and is the phase in which the nurse conducts the initial interview (see Chapter 10). When strangers meet, they interact according to their own backgrounds, standards, values, and experiences. The fact that each person has a unique frame of reference underlies the need for self-awareness on the part of the nurse. The initial interview includes the following aspects:

- An atmosphere is established in which rapport can grow.

- The nurse's role is clarified, and the responsibilities of both the patient and the nurse (parameters) are defined.
- The contract containing the time, place, date, and duration of the meetings is discussed.
- Confidentiality is discussed and assumed.
- The terms of termination are introduced (these are also discussed throughout the orientation phase and beyond).
- The nurse becomes aware of transference and countertransference issues.
- Patient problems are articulated, and mutually agreed-upon goals are established.

Establishing Rapport

A major emphasis during the first few encounters with the patient is on providing an atmosphere in which trust and understanding, or rapport, can grow. As in any relationship, **rapport** can be nurtured by demonstrating genuineness and empathy, developing positive regard, showing consistency, and offering assistance in problem solving and providing support.

Parameters of the Relationship

The patient needs to know about the nurse (who the nurse is and the nurse's background) and the purpose of the meetings. For example, a student might furnish the following information:

> **Student**: "Hello, Mrs. Rodriquez, I am Jim Thompson from the community college. I am in my psychiatric rotation and will be coming here for the next six Thursdays. I would like to spend time with you each Thursday if you are still here. I'm here to be a support person for you as you work on your treatment goals."

Formal or Informal Contract

A contract emphasizes the patient's participation and responsibility because it shows that the nurse does something *with* the patient rather than *for* the patient. The contract, either stated or written, contains the place, time, date, and duration of the meetings. During the orientation phase, the patient may begin to express thoughts and feelings, identify problems, and discuss realistic goals. Mutual agreement on those goals is also part of the contract.

> **Student**: "Mrs. Rodriquez, we will meet at 10 AM each Thursday in the consultation room at the clinic for 45 minutes from September 15 to October 27. We can use that time for further discussion of your feelings of loneliness and anger and explore some things you could do to make the situation better for yourself."

Confidentiality

The patient has a right to know (1) who else will be given the information shared with the nurse and (2) that the information may be shared with specific people, such as a clinical supervisor, the physician, the staff, or other students in conference. The patient also needs to know that the information will not be shared with relatives, friends, or others outside the treatment team, except in extreme situations. Extreme situations include (1) child or elder abuse, (2) threats of self-harm or harm to others, or (3) intention not to follow through with the treatment plan.

If information must be shared with others, this is usually done by the physician, according to legal guidelines (see Chapter 7). The nurse must be aware of the patient's right to confidentiality and must not violate that right. Safeguarding the privacy and confidentiality of patients is not only an ethical obligation but a legal responsibility as well (Erickson & Miller, 2005).

> **Student**: "Mrs. Rodriquez, I will be sharing some of what we discuss with my nursing instructor, and at times I may discuss certain concerns with my peers in conference or with the staff. However, I will *not* be sharing this information with your husband or any other members of your family or anyone outside the hospital without your permission."

Terms of Termination

Termination is that last phase in Peplau's model, but planning for termination actually begins in the orientation phase. It also may be mentioned when appropriate during the working phase if the nature of the relationship is time limited (e.g., six or nine sessions). The date of the termination phase should be clear from the beginning. In some situations, the nurse-patient contract may be renegotiated when the termination date has been reached. In other situations, when the therapeutic nurse-patient relationship is an open-ended one, the termination date is not known.

> **Student**: "Mrs. Rodriquez, as I mentioned earlier, our last meeting will be on October 27. We will have three more meetings after today."

Working Phase

The development of a strong working relationship can allow the patient to experience increased levels of anxiety and demonstrate dysfunctional behaviors in a safe setting while trying out new and more adaptive coping behaviors. In 1988, Moore and Hartman identified specific tasks of the working phase of the nurse-patient relationship that remain relevant in current practice:

- Maintain the relationship.
- Gather further data.
- Promote the patient's problem-solving skills, self-esteem, and use of language.
- Facilitate behavioral change.
- Overcome resistance behaviors.
- Evaluate problems and goals, and redefine them as necessary.
- Promote practice and expression of alternative adaptive behaviors.

During the working phase, the nurse and patient together identify and explore areas that are causing problems in the patient's life. Often, the patient's present ways of handling situations stem from earlier means of coping devised to survive in a chaotic and dysfunctional family environment. Although certain coping methods may have worked for the patient at an earlier age, they now interfere with the patient's interpersonal relationships and prevent attainment of current goals. The patient's dysfunctional behaviors and basic assumptions about the world are often defensive, and the patient is usually unable to change the dysfunctional behavior at will. Therefore, most of the problem behaviors or thoughts continue because of unconscious motivations and needs that are beyond the patient's awareness.

The nurse can work with the patient to identify unconscious motivations and assumptions that keep the patient from finding satisfaction and reaching potential. Describing, and often re-experiencing, old conflicts generally awakens high levels of anxiety. Patients may use various defenses against anxiety and displace their feelings onto the nurse. Therefore, during the working phase, intense emotions such as anxiety, anger, self-hate, hopelessness, and helplessness may surface. Defense mechanisms, such as acting out anger inappropriately, withdrawing, intellectualizing, manipulating, and denying are to be expected.

During the working phase, the patient may unconsciously transfer strong feelings that belong to significant others from the past into the present and onto the nurse (transference). The emotional responses and behaviors in the patient may also awaken strong countertransference feelings in the nurse. The nurse's awareness of personal feelings and reactions to the patient are vital for effective interaction with the patient.

Termination Phase

The **termination phase** is the final, integral phase of the nurse-patient relationship. Termination is discussed during the first interview and again during the working stage at appropriate times. Termination may occur when the patient is discharged or when the student's clinical rotation ends. Basically, the tasks of termination are:

- Summarizing the goals and objectives achieved in the relationship
- Discussing ways for the patient to incorporate into daily life any new coping strategies learned
- Reviewing situations that occurred during the nurse-patient relationship
- Exchanging memories, which can help validate the experience for both nurse and patient and facilitate closure of that relationship

Termination can stimulate strong feelings in both nurse and patient. Termination of the relationship signifies a loss for both, although the intensity and meaning of termination may be different for each. If a patient has unresolved feelings of abandonment, loneliness, being unwanted, or rejection, these feelings may be reawakened during the termination process. This process can be an opportunity for the patient to express these feelings, perhaps for the first time.

Important reasons for the student or nurse to address the termination phase are:

- Feelings are aroused in both the patient and the nurse with regard to the experience they have had; when these feelings are recognized and shared, patients learn that it is acceptable to feel sadness and loss when someone they care about leaves.

- Termination can be a learning experience; patients can learn that they are important to at least one person, and nurses learn continually from each clinical experience and patient encounter.
- By sharing the termination experience with the patient, the nurse demonstrates caring for the patient.
- This may be the first successful termination experience for the patient.

If a nurse has been working with a patient for a while, it is important for the nurse to bring into awareness any feelings and reactions the patient may be experiencing related to separations. If a patient denies that the termination is having an effect (assuming the nurse-patient relationship was strong), the nurse may say something like, "Goodbyes are difficult for people. Often they remind us of other goodbyes. Tell me about another separation in your past." If the patient appears to be displacing anger, either by withdrawing or by being overtly angry at the nurse, the nurse may use generalized statements such as, "People may experience anger when saying goodbye. Sometimes they are angry with the person who is leaving. Tell me how you feel about my leaving." Both new practitioners and students in the psychiatric setting need to give serious thought to their last clinical experience with their patient and work with their supervisor or instructor to facilitate communication during this time.

A common response of beginning practitioners and students is feeling guilty about terminating the relationship. These feelings may, in rare cases, be manifested by the student's giving the patient his or her telephone number, making plans to get together for coffee after the patient is discharged, continuing to see the patient afterward, or exchanging letters. Maintaining contact after discharge is not acceptable and is in opposition to the goals of a therapeutic relationship. Often this is in response to the student's need to (1) feel less guilty for "using the patient for learning needs," (2) maintain a feeling of being "important" to the patient, or (3) sustain the illusion that the student is the only one who "understands" the patient, among other student-centered rationales.

Indeed, part of the termination process may be to explore—after discussion with the patient's case manager—the patient's plans for the future: where the patient can go for help, which agencies to contact, and which people may best help the patient find appropriate and helpful resources.

WHAT HINDERS AND WHAT HELPS THE NURSE-PATIENT RELATIONSHIP

Not all nurse-patient relationships follow the classic phases outlined by Peplau. Some start in the orientation phase and move to a mutually frustrating phase and finally to mutual withdrawal (Figure 9-2).

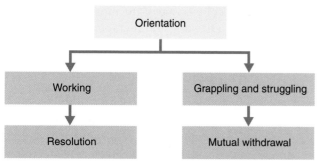

Figure 9-2 Phases of therapeutic and nontherapeutic relationships. (From Forchuk, C., Westwell, J., Martin, M., Bamber-Azzapardi, W., Kosterewa-Tolman, D., & Hux, M. [2000]. The developing nurse-client relationship: Nurses' perspectives. *Journal of the American Psychiatric Nurses Association, 6*[1], 3–10.)

Forchuk and associates (2000) conducted a qualitative study of the nurse-patient relationship. They examined the phases of both therapeutic and the nontherapeutic relationships. From this study, they identified certain behaviors that were beneficial to the progression of the nurse-patient relationship, as well as those that hampered the development of this relationship. The study emphasized the importance of consistent, regular, and private interactions with patients as essential to the development of a therapeutic relationship. Nurses in this study stressed the importance of consistency, pacing, and listening. Specifically, the study found evidence that the following factors enhanced the nurse-patient relationship, allowing it to progress in a mutually satisfying manner:

- **Consistency** includes ensuring that a nurse is always assigned to the same patient and that the patient has a regular routine for activities. Interactions are facilitated when they are frequent and regular in duration, format, and location. Consistency also refers to the nurse's being honest and consistent (congruent) in what is said to the patient.
- **Pacing** includes letting the patient set the pace and letting the pace be adjusted to fit the patient's moods. A slow approach helps reduce pressure, and at times it is necessary to step back and realize that developing a strong relationship may take a long time.
- **Listening** includes letting the patient talk when needed. The nurse becomes a sounding board for the patient's concerns and issues. **Listening is perhaps the most important skill for nurses to master**. Truly listening to another person (i.e., attending to what is behind the words) is a learned skill.
- **Initial impressions**, especially positive initial attitudes and preconceptions, are significant considerations in how the relationship will progress. Preconceived negative impressions and feelings toward the patient usually bode poorly for the

positive growth of the relationship. In contrast, the nurse's feeling that the patient is "interesting" or a "challenge" and a positive attitude about the relationship are usually favorable signs for the developing therapeutic relationship.

- **Promoting patient comfort** and **balancing control** usually reflect caring behaviors. *Control* refers to keeping a balance in the relationship: not too strict and not too lenient.
- **Patient factors** that seem to enhance the relationship include **trust** on the part of the patient and the patient's **active participation** in the nurse-patient relationship.

In relationships that did not progress to therapeutic levels, there seemed to be two major factors that hampered the development of positive relationships: inconsistency and unavailability (e.g., lack of contact, infrequent meetings, meetings in the hallway) on the part of the nurse, patient, or both. When nurse and patient are reluctant to spend time together, and meeting times become sporadic or superficial, the term *mutual avoidance* is used. This is clearly a lose-lose situation.

The nurse's personal feelings and lack of self-awareness are major elements that contribute to the lack of progression of positive relationships. Negative preconceived ideas and feelings (e.g., discomfort, dislike, fear, and avoidance) about the patient seem to be a constant in relationships that end in frustration and mutual withdrawal. Sometimes these feelings are known, and sometimes the nurse is only vaguely aware of them.

FACTORS THAT ENCOURAGE AND PROMOTE PATIENTS' GROWTH

Rogers and Truax (1967) identified three personal characteristics of the nurse that help promote change and growth in patients—factors still valued today as vital components for establishing a therapeutic relationship: (1) genuineness, (2) empathy, and (3) positive regard. These are some of the intangibles that are at the heart of the art of nursing.

Genuineness

Genuineness, or self-awareness of one's feelings as they arise within the relationship and the ability to communicate them when appropriate, is a key ingredient in building trust. When a person is genuine, one gets the sense that what is displayed on the outside of the person is congruent with the internal processes. Genuineness is conveyed by listening to and communicating with patients without distorting their messages and being clear and concrete in communications. Being genuine in a therapeutic relationship implies the ability to use therapeutic communication tools in an appropriately spontaneous manner, rather than rigidly or in a parrot-like fashion.

Empathy

Empathy is a complex multidimensional concept in which the helping person attempts to understand the world from the patient's perspective. It does not mean that the nurse condones or approves of the patient's actions but rather is nonjudgmental or uncritical of the patient's choices (Arkowitz et al., 2008). Essentially it means "temporarily living in the other's life, moving about in it delicately without making judgments" (Rogers, 1980, p. 142).

Therefore, empathy signifies a central focus and feeling with and in the patient's world. According to Mercer and Reynolds (2002), it involves:

- Accurately perceiving the patient's situation, perspective, and feelings
- Communicating one's understanding to the patient and checking with the patient for accuracy
- Acting on this understanding in a helpful (therapeutic) way toward the patient

Empathy versus Sympathy

There is much confusion regarding empathy versus sympathy. A simple way to distinguish them is that in empathy, we *understand* the feelings of others. In sympathy, we *feel* the feelings of others. When a helping person is feeling sympathy for another, objectivity is lost, and the ability to assist the patient in solving a personal problem ceases. Furthermore, sympathy is associated with feelings of pity and commiseration. Although these are considered nurturing human traits, they may not be particularly useful in a therapeutic relationship. When people express sympathy, they express agreement with another, which in some situations may discourage further exploration of a person's thoughts and feelings.

The following examples are given to clarify the distinction between empathy and sympathy. A friend tells you that her mother was just diagnosed with inoperable cancer. Your friend then begins to cry and pounds the table with her fist.

Sympathetic response: "I feel so sorry for you. I know exactly how you feel. My mother was hospitalized last year, and it was awful. I was so depressed. I still get upset just thinking about it." *(You go on to tell your friend about the incident.)*

Sometimes when nurses try to be sympathetic, they are apt to project their own feelings onto the patient's, which thus limits the patient's range of responses. A more useful response might be as follows:

Empathic response: "How upsetting this must be for you. Something similar happened to my mother last year, and I had so many mixed emotions. What thoughts and feelings are you having?" *(You continue to stay with your friend and listen to his or her thoughts and feelings.)*

Empathy is not a technique but rather an attitude that conveys respect, acceptance, and validation of the patient's strengths. In the practice of psychotherapy or counseling, empathy is one of the most important factors in building a trusting and therapeutic relationship (Wheeler, 2008).

Positive Regard

Positive regard implies respect. It is the ability to view another person as being worthy of caring about and as someone who has strengths and achievement potential. Positive regard is usually communicated indirectly by attitudes and actions rather than directly by words.

Attitudes

One attitude through which a nurse might convey positive regard, or respect, is willingness to work with the patient. That is, the nurse takes the patient and the relationship seriously. The experience is viewed not as "a job," "part of a course," or "time spent talking" but as an opportunity to work with patients to help them develop personal resources and actualize more of their potential in living.

Actions

Some actions that manifest an attitude of respect are attending, suspending value judgments, and helping patients develop their own resources.

Attending. Attending behavior is the foundation of interviewing. To succeed, nurses must pay attention to their patients in culturally and individually appropriate ways (Sommers-Flanagan & Sommers-Flanagan, 2003). *Attending* is a special kind of listening that refers to an intensity of presence, or being with the patient. At times, simply being with another person during a painful time can make a difference.

Posture, eye contact, and body language are nonverbal behaviors that reflect the degree of attending and are highly culturally influenced. Refer to Chapter 10 for a more detailed discussion of the cultural implications of the clinical interview.

Suspending Value Judgments. Although we will always have personal opinions, nurses are more effective when they guard against using their own value systems to judge patients' thoughts, feelings, or behaviors. For example, if a patient is taking drugs or is involved in risky sexual behavior, the nurse may recognize that these behaviors are hindering the patient from living a more satisfying life, posing a potential health threat, or preventing the patient from developing satisfying relationships. However, labeling these activities as bad or good is not useful. Rather, the nurse should focus on exploring the behavior and work toward identifying the thoughts and feelings that influence this behavior. Judgment on the part of the nurse will most likely interfere with further exploration.

The first steps in eliminating judgmental thinking and behaviors are to (1) recognize their presence, (2) identify how or where you learned these responses to the patient's behavior, and (3) construct alternative ways to view the patient's thinking and behavior. Denying judgmental thinking will only compound the problem.

Patient: "I guess you could consider me an addictive personality. I love to gamble when I have money and spend most of my time in the casino. It seems like I'm hooking up with a different woman every time I'm there, and it always ends in sex. This has been going on for at least 3 years."

A judgmental response would be:

Nurse A: "So your compulsive gambling and promiscuous sexual behaviors really haven't brought you much happiness, have they? You're running away from your problems and could end up with AIDS and broke."

A more helpful response would be:

Nurse B: "So your sexual and gambling activities are part of the picture also. You sound as if these activities are not making you happy."

In this example, Nurse B focuses on the patient's behaviors and the possible meaning they might have to the patient. Nurse B does not introduce personal value statements or prejudices regarding promiscuous behavior, as does Nurse A. Empathy and positive regard are essential qualities in a successful nurse-patient relationship.

Helping Patients Develop Resources. The nurse becomes aware of patients' strengths and encourages patients to work at their optimal level of functioning. It can be seen as one form of collaboration with the patient. The nurse does not act for patients unless absolutely necessary, and then only as a step toward helping them act on their own. It is important that patients remain as independent as possible to develop new resources for problem solving. The following are examples of helping the patient to develop independence:

Patient: "This medication makes my mouth so dry. Could you get me something to drink?"

Nurse: "There is juice in the refrigerator. I'll wait here for you until you get back."
or "I'll walk with you while you get some juice from the refrigerator."

Patient: "Could you ask the doctor to let me have a pass for the weekend?"

Nurse: "Your doctor will be on the unit this afternoon. I'll let her know that you want to speak with her."

Consistently encouraging patients to use their own resources helps minimize the patients' feelings of helplessness and dependency and validates their potential for change.

KEY POINTS TO REMEMBER

- The nurse-patient relationship is well defined, and the roles of the nurse and the patient must be clearly stated.
- It is important that the nurse be aware of the differences between a therapeutic relationship and a social or intimate relationship. In a therapeutic nurse-patient relationship, the focus is on the patient's needs, thoughts, feelings, and goals. The nurse is expected to meet personal needs outside this relationship in other professional, social, or intimate arenas.
- Although the boundaries and roles of the nurse-patient relationship generally are clearly defined, they can become blurred; this blurring can be insidious and may occur on an unconscious level. Usually, transference and countertransference phenomena are operating when boundaries are blurred.
- It is important to have a grasp of common countertransferential feelings and behaviors and of the nursing actions to counteract these phenomena.
- Supervision aids in promoting both the professional growth of the nurse and the nurse-patient relationship, allowing the patient's goals to be worked on and met.
- The phases of the nurse-patient relationship include orientation, working, and termination.
- Genuineness, empathy, and positive regard are personal strengths of the helping person; they foster growth and change in others.

CRITICAL THINKING

1. On your first clinical day, you are assigned to work with an older adult, Mrs. Schneider, who is depressed. Your first impression is, "Oh my, she looks like my nasty Aunt Helen. She even sits like her." You approach her with a vague feeling of uneasiness and say hello. Mrs. Schneider responds, "Who are you and how can you help me?"

   "My name is Alisha. I am a nursing student and I will be working with you today." She tells you that "a student" could never understand what she is going through. She then says, "If you really want to help me, you would get me a good job after I leave here."

   A. Identify transference and countertransference issues in this situation. What is your most important course of action?

   B. How could you best respond to Mrs. Schneider's question about who you are? What other information will you give her during this first clinical encounter? Be specific.

   C. What are some useful responses you could give her regarding her legitimate questions about ways you could be of help to her?

   D. Analyze Mrs. Schneider's request that you find her a job. Keeping in mind the aim of Peplau's interactive nurse-patient process, describe some useful ways you could respond to this request.

2. You are interviewing Tom Stone, a 17-year-old who was admitted to a psychiatric unit after a suicide attempt. How would you best respond to each of the following patient requests and behaviors?
   A. "I would feel so much better if you would sit closer to me and hold my hand."
   B. "I will tell you if I still feel like killing myself, but you have to promise not to tell anyone else. If you do, I just can't trust you, ever."
   C. "I don't want to talk to you. I have absolutely nothing to say."
   D. "I will be going home tomorrow, and you have been so helpful and good to me. I want you to have my watch to remember me by."
   E. Tom breaks down and starts sobbing.

CHAPTER REVIEW

1. Which of the following actions best represents the basis or foundation of all other psychiatric nursing care?
   1. The nurse assesses the patient at regular intervals.
   2. The nurse administers psychotropic medications.
   3. The nurse spends time sitting with a withdrawn patient.
   4. The nurse participates in team meetings with other professionals.

2. A male patient frequently inquires about the female student nurse's boyfriend, social activities, and school experiences. Which of the following initial responses by the student best addresses the issue raised by this behavior?
   1. The student requests assignment to a patient of the same gender as the student.
   2. She points out to the patient that he is making social inquiries and explores this behavior.
   3. She tells him that she cannot talk about her personal life and refocuses on his issues.
   4. She explains that if he persists in focusing on her she cannot work with him.

3. Mary, a patient in the psychiatric unit, had a very rejecting and abusive father and a difficult childhood, but from age 10 on was raised by a very warm and supportive grandmother who recently passed away. Mary frequently comments on how hard her nurse, Jane, works and on how other staff do not seem to care as much about their patients as Jane does. Jane finds herself agreeing with Mary and appreciating her insightfulness, recalling to herself that except for

her former head nurse, other staff do not seem to appreciate how hard she works and seem to take her for granted. Jane enjoys the time she spends with Mary and seeks out opportunities to interact with her. What phenomenon is occurring here, and which response by Jane would most benefit her and the patient?
   1. Mary is experiencing transference; Jane should help Mary to understand that she is emphasizing in Jane those qualities which were missing in her father.
   2. Jane is idealizing Mary, seeing in her strengths and abilities which Mary does not really possess; Jane should temporarily distance herself somewhat from Mary.
   3. Mary is overidentifying with Jane, seeing similarities that do not in reality exist; Jane should label and explore this phenomenon in her interactions with Mary.
   4. Jane is experiencing countertransference in response to Mary's meeting Jane's needs for greater appreciation; Jane should seek clinical supervision to explore these dynamics.

4. Which of the following statements would be appropriate during the orientation phase of the nurse-patient relationship? *Select all that apply.*
   1. "My name is Sarah, and I am a student nurse here to learn about mental health."
   2. "I will be here each Thursday from 8 AM until 12 noon if you would like to talk."
   3. "Tell me about what you think would best help you to cope with the loss of your wife."
   4. "Let's talk today about how our plan for improving your sleep has been working."
   5. "We will meet weekly for 1 hour, during which we will discuss how to meet your goals."
   6. "Being home alone while your wife was hospitalized must have been very difficult for you."

5. A student nurse exhibits the following behaviors or actions while interacting with her patient. Which of these are appropriate as part of a therapeutic relationship?
   1. Sitting attentively in silence with a withdrawn patient until the patient chooses to speak.
   2. Offering the patient advice on how he could cope more effectively with stress.
   3. Controlling the pace of the relationship by selecting topics for each interaction.
   4. Limiting the discussion of termination issues so as not to sadden the patient unduly.

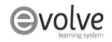

Visit the Evolve website for an **Audio Chapter Summary, Chapter Review Answers & Rationales, Critical Thinking Answer Guidelines,** and additional resources related to the content in this chapter: **http://evolve.elsevier.com/Varcarolis/foundations**

Companion CD Use the Companion CD to prepare for tests and the NCLEX® Examination with **Test-Taking Strategies** for psychiatric mental health nursing and hundreds of **Review Questions.**

References

Arkowitz, H., Westra, H. A., Miller, W. R., & Rollnick, R. (2008). *Motivational interviewing in the treatment of psychosocial problems*. New York: The Guilford Press.

Butler Center for Research. (2006). Therapeutic Alliance: Improving treatment outcome. *Research Update. Hazelden Foundation*. Retrieved July 15, 2008, from www.hazelden.org/web/public/bcrup 1006.pdf

Erickson, J. I., & Miller, S. (2005). Caring for patients while respecting their privacy: Renewing our commitment. *Online Journal of Issues in Nursing, 10*(2). Retrieved January 23, 2009 from http://www.nursingworld.org/MainMenuCategories/ANAMarketplace/ANA-Periodicals/OJIN/TableofContents/Volume102005/No2May05/tpc27_116017.aspx

Forchuk, C., Westwell, J., Martin, M., Bamber-Azzapardi, W., Kosterewa-Tolman, D., & Hux, M. (2000). The developing nurse-client relationship: Nurse's perspectives. *Journal of the American Psychiatric Nurses Association, 6*(1), 3–10.

Fontes, L. A. (2008). *Interviewing Clients Across Cultures*. New York: The Guilford Press.

Fox, S. (2008). *Relating to Clients*. Philadelphia: Jessica Kingsley Publishers.

Haber, J. (2000). Hildegard E. Peplau: The psychiatric nursing legacy of a legend. *Journal of the American Psychiatric Nurses Association, 6*(2), 56–62.

Korn, M. L. (2001). *Cultural aspects of the psychotherapeutic process*. Retrieved June 20, 2006, from http://doctor.medscape.com/viewarticle/418608

LaRowe, K. (2004). *The therapeutic relationship*. Retrieved February 3, 2005, from http://compassion-fatigue.com/Index.asp?PG=89

Mercer, S. W., & Reynolds, W. (2002). Empathy and quality of care. *British Journal of General Practice, 52*(Suppl.), S9–12.

Moore, J. C., & Hartman, C. R. (1988). Developing a therapeutic relationship. In C. K. Beck, R. P. Rawlins, & S. R. Williams (Eds.), *Mental health–psychiatric nursing*. St. Louis: Mosby.

Peplau, H. E. (1952). *Interpersonal relations in nursing: A conceptual frame of reference for psychodynamic nursing*. New York: Putnam.

Peplau, H. E. (1999). *Interpersonal relations in nursing: A conceptual frame of reference for psychodynamic nursing*. New York: Springer.

Peternelj-Taylor, C. (2002). Professional boundaries. A matter of therapeutic integrity. *Journal of Psychosocial Nursing and Mental Health Services, 40*(4), 22–29.

Quinlan, J. C. F. (1996). *Co-creating personal and professional knowledge through peer support and peer approval in nursing*. Submitted for degree of PhD of the University of Bath England, 1996. Retrieved July 17, 2006, from www.bath.ac.uk/carpp/jquinlan/titlepage.htm

Rogers, C. R. (1980). *A Way of Being*. Boston: Houghton Mifflin.

Rogers, C. R., & Truax, C. B. (1967). The therapeutic conditions antecedent to change: A theoretical view. In C. R. Rogers (Ed.), *The therapeutic relationship and its impact*. Madison: University of Wisconsin Press.

Sommers-Flanagan, J., & Sommers-Flanagan, R. (2003). *Clinical interviewing* (3rd ed.). Hoboken, NJ: Wiley.

Travelbee, J. (1971). *Interpersonal Aspects of Nursing* (2nd ed.). F.A. Davis Co.

Wheeler, K. (2008). *Psychotherapy for the advanced practice psychiatric nurse*. St. Louis: Mosby.

CHAPTER 10

Communication and the Clinical Interview

Elizabeth M. Varcarolis

Key Terms and Concepts

active listening, 179
closed-ended questions, 184
cultural filters, 187
double messages, 178
double-bind messages, 178
feedback, 175

nontherapeutic communication techniques, 184
nonverbal behaviors, 177
nonverbal communication, 177
open-ended questions, 181
therapeutic communication techniques, 179
verbal communication, 177

Objectives

1. Identify three personal and two environmental factors that can impede communication.
2. Discuss the differences between verbal and nonverbal communication, and identify five examples of nonverbal communication.
3. Identify two attending behaviors the nurse might focus on to increase communication skills.
4. Compare and contrast the range of verbal and nonverbal communication of different cultural groups in the areas of (a) communication style, (b) eye contact, and (c) touch. Give examples.
5. Relate problems that can arise when nurses are insensitive to cultural aspects of patients' communication styles.

6. Demonstrate the use of four techniques that can *enhance* communication, highlighting what makes them *effective*.
7. Demonstrate the use of four techniques that can *obstruct* communication, highlighting what makes them *ineffective*.
8. Identify and give rationales for suggested (a) setting, (b) seating, and (c) methods for beginning the nurse-patient interaction.
9. Explain to a classmate the importance of clinical supervision.

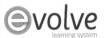 Visit the Evolve website for an **Audio Glossary & Flashcards, Concept Map Creator,** and additional resources related to the content in this chapter: **http://evolve.elsevier.com/Varcarolis/foundations**

Humans have a built-in need to relate to others, and our advanced ability to communicate with others gives substance and meaning to our lives. Our need to express ourselves to others is powerful; it is the foundation on which we form happy and productive relationships in our adult lives. By the same token, stress and negative feelings within a relationship are often the result of ineffective communication. All our actions, words, and facial expressions convey meaning to others. It has been said that we cannot *not* communicate. Even silence can convey acceptance, anger, or thoughtfulness.

In the provision of nursing care, communication takes on a new emphasis. Just as social relationships are different from therapeutic relationships, *basic communication* is different from professional, patient-centered, goal-directed, and scientifically based *therapeutic communication*.

The ability to form therapeutic relationships is fundamental and essential to effective nursing care, and therapeutic communication is crucial to the formation of a therapeutic relationship. Determining levels of pain in the postoperative patient, listening as parents express feelings of fear concerning their child's diagnosis, or understanding, without words, the needs of the intubated patient in the intensive care unit are essential skills in providing quality nursing care.

Ideally, therapeutic communication is a professional skill you learn and practice early in your nursing curriculum. But in psychiatric mental health nursing, communication skills take on a different and new emphasis. Psychiatric disorders cause not only physical symptoms (fatigue, loss of appetite, insomnia) but also emotional symptoms (sadness, anger, hopelessness, euphoria) that affect a patient's ability to relate to others.

It is often during the psychiatric rotation that students discover the utility of therapeutic communication and begin to rely on techniques they once considered artificial. For example, restating may seem like a funny thing to do. Using it in a practice session between students ("I felt sad when my dog ran away." "You felt sad when your dog ran away?") can derail communication and end the seriousness with laughter. Yet in the clinical setting, restating can become a powerful and profound tool:

Patient: "At the moment they told me my daughter would never be able to walk like her twin sister, I felt like I couldn't go on."

Student: *(after a short silence)* "You felt like you couldn't go on."

The technique, and the empathy it conveys, is appreciated in such a situation. Developing therapeutic communication skills takes time, and with continued practice, you will develop your own style and rhythm. Eventually, these techniques will become a part of the way you instinctively communicate with others in the clinical setting.

Beginning psychiatric practitioners are often concerned that they may say the wrong thing, especially when learning to apply therapeutic techniques. Will you say the wrong thing? Yes, you probably will, but that is how we all learn to find more useful and effective ways of helping individuals reach their goals. The challenge is to recover from your mistakes and use them for learning and growth (Sommers-Flanagan & Sommers-Flanagan, 2003).

One of the most common concerns students have is that they will say the one thing that will "push the patient over the edge," or maybe even be the cause for the patient to give up all hope. This is highly unlikely. Consider that symptoms of psychiatric disorders, such as irritability, agitation, negativity, disinterest in communication, or being hypertalkative, often frustrate and alienate friends and family. It is likely that the interactions the patient had been having were not always pleasant and supportive. Patients often see a well-meaning person who conveys genuine acceptance, respect, and concern for their well-being as a gift. Even if mistakes in communication are made or when the "wrong thing" is said, there is little chance that the comments will do actual harm.

THE COMMUNICATION PROCESS

Communication is an interactive process between two or more persons who send and receive messages to one another. The following is a simplified model of communication (Berlo, 1960):

1. One person has a need to communicate with another **(stimulus)** for information, comfort, or advice.
2. The person sending the message **(sender)** initiates interpersonal contact.
3. The message is the information sent or expressed to another. The clearest messages are those that are well organized and expressed in a manner familiar to the receiver.
4. The message can be sent through a **variety of media**, including auditory (hearing), visual (seeing), tactile (touch), smell, or any combination of these.
5. The person receiving the message **(receiver)** then interprets the message and responds to the sender by providing feedback. *Validating the accuracy of the sender's message is extremely important.* The nature of the feedback often indicates whether the meaning of the message sent has been correctly interpreted by the receiver. An accuracy check may be obtained by simply asking the sender, "Is this what you mean?" or "I notice you turn away when we talk about your going back to college. Is there a conflict there?"

Figure 10-1 shows this simple model of communication, along with some of the many factors that affect it.

Effective communication in therapeutic relationships depends on nurses' (1) knowing what they are trying to convey (the purpose of the message), (2) communicating what is really meant to the patient, and (3) comprehending the meaning of what the patient is intentionally or unintentionally conveying (Arnold & Boggs, 2007). Peplau (1952) identified two main principles that can guide the communication process during the nurse-patient interview, which is discussed in detail later in this chapter: (1) clarity, which ensures that the meaning of the message is accurately understood by both parties "as the result of joint and sustained effort of all parties concerned," and (2) continuity, which promotes connections among ideas "and the feelings, events, or themes conveyed in those ideas" (p. 290).

FACTORS THAT AFFECT COMMUNICATION

Personal Factors

Personal factors that can impede accurate transmission or interpretation of messages include emotional factors (e.g., mood, responses to stress, personal bias), social factors (e.g., previous experience, cultural differences, language differences), and cognitive factors (e.g., problem-solving ability, knowledge level, language use).

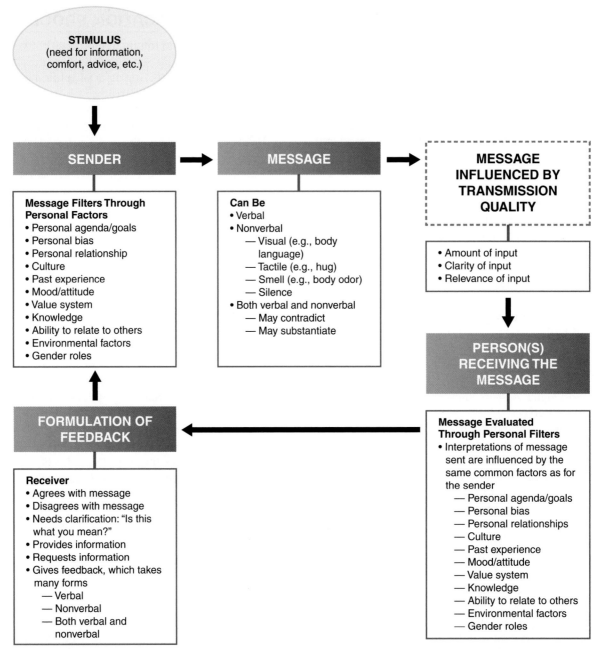

Figure 10-1 Operational definition of communication. (Data from Ellis, R., & McClintock, A. [1990]. *If you take my meaning.* London: Arnold.)

Environmental Factors

Environmental factors that may affect communication include physical factors (e.g., background noise, lack of privacy, uncomfortable accommodations) and societal determinants (e.g., sociopolitical, historical, and economic factors, the presence of others, expectations of others).

Relationship Factors

Relationship factors refer to the status of individuals in terms of social standing, power, relationship type, age, etc. Communication is influenced by this status.

Consider how you would describe your day in the clinical setting to your instructor, compared to how you would describe it to your friend. The fact that your instructor has more education than you and is in an evaluative role would likely influence how much you share and your choice of words.

Now think about the relationship between you and your patient. Your patient may be older or younger than you are, more or less educated, richer or poorer, successful at work or unemployed. These factors play into the dynamics of the communication, whether at a conscious or an unconscious level, and recognizing their influence is important. It may be difficult for you to work with a woman your mother's age, or you may feel impatient with a patient who is unemployed and an alcoholic.

It is sometimes difficult for students to grasp or remember that patients, regardless of their relationship factors, are in a position of vulnerability. The presence of a hospital identification band is a formal indication of a need for care, and as a caregiver, you are viewed in a role of authority. Part of the art of therapeutic communication is in finding a balance between your role as a professional and your role as a human being who has been socialized into complex patterns of interactions based, at least in part, on status.

Students sometimes fall back into time-tested and comfortable roles. One of the most common responses nursing students have is in treating the patient as a buddy. Imagine a male nursing student walking onto the unit, seeing his assigned patient and saying, "Hey, how's it going today?" while giving the patient a high-five. Or consider the female nursing student assigned to the 60-year-old woman who used to work as a registered nurse. This relationship has the potential to become unbalanced and nontherapeutic if the patient shifts the focus of concern onto the student.

VERBAL AND NONVERBAL COMMUNICATION

Verbal Communication

Verbal communication consists of all the words a person speaks. We live in a society of symbols, and our main social symbols are words. Talking is our most common activity. It is our public link with one another,

the primary instrument of instruction, a need, an art, and one of the most personal aspects of our private lives. When we speak, we:

- Communicate our beliefs and values
- Communicate perceptions and meanings
- Convey interest and understanding *or* insult and judgment
- Convey messages clearly *or* convey conflicting or implied messages
- Convey clear, honest feelings *or* disguised, distorted feelings

Words are culturally perceived; therefore, clarifying the intent of certain words is very important. Even if the nurse and patient have a similar cultural background, the mental image that each has for a given word may not be exactly the same. Although they believe they are talking about the same thing, the nurse and patient may actually be talking about two quite different things. Words are the symbols for emotions as well as mental images.

Nonverbal Communication

It is often said that "it's not what you say but how you say it." In other words, it is the **nonverbal behaviors** that may be sending the "real" message. The tone of voice, emphasis on certain words, and the manner in which a person paces speech are examples of **nonverbal communication**. Other common examples of nonverbal communication (often called *cues*) are physical appearance, facial expressions, body posture, amount of eye contact, eye cast (i.e., emotion expressed in the eyes), hand gestures, sighs, fidgeting, and yawning. Table 10-1 identifies examples of nonverbal behaviors.

TABLE 10-1 Nonverbal Behaviors

Behavior	Possible Nonverbal Cues	Example
Body behaviors	Posture, body movements, gestures, gait	The patient is slumped in a chair, puts her face in her hands, and occasionally taps her right foot.
Facial expressions	Frowns, smiles, grimaces, raised eyebrows, pursed lips, licking of lips, tongue movements	The patient grimaces when speaking to the nurse; when alone, he smiles and giggles to himself.
Eye cast	Angry, suspicious, and accusatory looks	The patient's eyes harden with suspicion.
Voice-related behaviors	Tone, pitch, level, intensity, inflection, stuttering, pauses, silences, fluency	The patient talks in a loud sing-song voice.
Observable autonomic physiological responses	Increase in respirations, diaphoresis, pupil dilation, blushing, paleness	When the patient mentions discharge, she becomes pale, her respirations increase, and her face becomes diaphoretic.
Personal appearance	Grooming, dress, hygiene	The patient is dressed in a wrinkled shirt, his pants are stained, his socks are dirty, and he is unshaven.
Physical characteristics	Height, weight, physique, complexion	The patient is grossly overweight, and his muscles appear flabby.

Nonverbal behaviors must be observed and interpreted in light of a person's culture, class, gender, age, sexual orientation, and spiritual norms. Cultural influences on communication are addressed later in this chapter.

Interaction of Verbal and Nonverbal Communication

Shawn Shea (1998), a nationally renowned psychiatrist and communication workshop leader, suggests that communication is roughly 10% verbal and 90% nonverbal. The high percentage he attributes to nonverbal behaviors may best describe our understanding of feelings and attitudes and not general communication. After all, it would be difficult to watch a foreign film and completely understand its meaning based solely on body language and vocal tones. However, nonverbal behaviors and cues influence communication to a surprising degree. Communication thus involves two radically different but interdependent kinds of symbols.

Spoken words represent our public selves and can be straightforward or used to distort, conceal, deny, or disguise true feelings. Nonverbal behaviors include a wide range of human activities, from body movements to facial expressions to physical reactions to messages from others. How a person listens and uses silence and sense of touch may also convey important information about the private self that is not available from conversation alone, especially in consideration of cultural norms.

Some elements of nonverbal communication, such as facial expressions, seem to be inborn and are similar across cultures. Matsumoto (2006) cited studies that found a high degree of agreement in spontaneous facial expressions or emotions across 10 different cultures. However, some cultural groups (e.g., Japanese) may control their facial expressions in public. Other types of nonverbal behaviors, such as how close people stand to each other when speaking, depend on cultural conventions. Some nonverbal communication is formalized and has specific meanings (e.g., the military salute, the Japanese bow).

Messages are not always simple; they can appear to be one thing when in fact they are another (Ellis et al., 2003). Often people have greater conscious awareness of their verbal messages than their nonverbal behaviors. The verbal message is sometimes referred to as the *content* of the message (what is said), and the nonverbal behavior is called the *process* of the message (nonverbal cues a person gives to substantiate or contradict the verbal message).

When the content is congruent with the process, the communication is more clearly understood and is considered healthy. For example, if a student says, "It's important that I get good grades in this class," that is

content. If the student has bought the books, takes good notes, and has a study buddy, that is *process.* Therefore, the content and process are congruent and straightforward, and there is a "healthy" message. If, however, the verbal message is not reinforced or is in fact contradicted by the nonverbal behavior, the message is confusing. For example, if the student does not have the books, skips several classes, and does not study, that is *process.* Here the student is sending two different messages.

Messages are sent to create meaning but also can be used defensively to hide what is actually going on, create confusion, and attack relatedness (Ellis et al., 2003). Conflicting messages are known as **double messages** or *mixed messages.* One way a nurse can respond to verbal and nonverbal incongruity is to reflect and validate the patient's feelings. For example, the nurse could say, "You say you are upset you did not pass this semester, but I notice you look more relaxed and less conflicted than you have all term. What do you see as some of the pros and cons of not passing the course this semester?"

Bateson and colleagues (1956) coined the term **double-bind messages**. A double-bind message is a mix of content (what is said) and process (what is conveyed nonverbally) that has both nurturing and hurtful aspects. The following vignette gives an example.

VIGNETTE

A 21-year-old female who lives at home with her chronically ill mother wants to go out for an evening with her friends. She is told by her frail but not helpless mother: "Oh, go ahead, have fun. I'll just sit here by myself, and I can always call 911 if I don't feel well; but you go ahead and have fun." The mother says this while looking sad, eyes downcast, slumped in her chair, and letting her cane drop to the floor. ▪

The recipient of this double-bind message is caught inside contradictory statements, so she cannot decide what is right. If she goes, the implication is that she is being selfish by leaving her sick mother alone. But if she stays, the mother could say, "I told you to go have fun." If she does go, the chances are she will not have much fun. The daughter is trapped in a no-win situation.

With experience, nurses become increasingly aware of patients' verbal and nonverbal communication. Nurses can compare patients' dialogue with their nonverbal behaviors to gain important clues about the real message. What individuals do may either express and reinforce or contradict what they say. So, as in the saying "actions speak louder than words," *actions* often reveal the true meaning of a person's intent, whether the intent is conscious or unconscious.

COMMUNICATION SKILLS FOR NURSES

Therapeutic Communication Techniques

Peplau emphasized the art of communication to highlight the importance of nursing interventions in facilitating achievement of quality patient care and quality of life (Haber, 2000). The nurse must establish and maintain a therapeutic relationship in which the patient will feel safe and hopeful that positive change is possible.

Once a therapeutic relationship is established, specific needs and problems can be identified, and the nurse can work with the patient on increasing problem-solving skills, learning new coping behaviors, and experiencing more appropriate and satisfying ways of relating to others. To do this, the nurse must have a sound knowledge of communication skills. Therefore, nurses must become more aware of their own interpersonal methods, eliminating obstructive, nontherapeutic communication techniques and developing additional responses that maximize nurse-patient interactions and increase the use of helpful therapeutic communication techniques. Useful tools for nurses when communicating with their patients are (1) the use of silence, (2) active listening, and (3) clarifying techniques.

Using Silence

Silence can sometimes intimidate both interviewers and patients (Sommers-Flanagan & Sommers-Flanagan, 2003). In the United States, there is an emphasis on action and a high level of verbal activity. Students and practicing nurses alike may find that when the flow of words stops, they become uncomfortable. They may rush to fill the void with "questions or chatter," thus cutting off potentially important thoughts and feelings the patient might be taking time to think about before articulating. Silence is not the absence of communication but a specific channel for transmitting and receiving messages; therefore, the practitioner needs to understand that silence is a significant means of influencing and being influenced by others.

Talking is a highly individualized practice. Some people find the telephone a nuisance, whereas others believe they cannot live without their cell phones on their persons at all times. In the initial interview, patients may be reluctant to speak because of the newness of the situation, the fact that the nurse is a stranger, or feelings of distrust, self-consciousness, embarrassment, or shyness. The nurse must recognize and respect individual differences in styles and tempos of responding. People who are quiet, those who have a language barrier or speech impediment, older adults, and those who lack confidence in their ability to express themselves may communicate a need for support and encouragement through their silence.

Although there is no universal rule concerning how much silence is too much, silence has been said to be worthwhile only as long as it is serving some function and not frightening the patient. Knowing when to speak during the interview largely depends on the nurse's perception about what is being conveyed through the silence. Icy silence may be an expression of anger and hostility; being ignored or given "the silent treatment" is recognized as an insult and is a particularly hurtful form of communication.

Silence may provide meaningful moments of reflection for both participants and gives an opportunity to contemplate thoughtfully what has been said and felt, weigh alternatives, formulate new ideas, and gain a new perspective on the matter under discussion. If the nurse waits to speak and allows the patient to break the silence, the patient may share thoughts and feelings that would otherwise have been withheld. Nurses who feel compelled to fill every void with words often do so because of their own anxiety, self-consciousness, and embarrassment. When this occurs, the nurse's need for comfort has taken priority over the needs of the patient.

It is crucial to recognize that some psychiatric disorders, such as major depression and schizophrenia, and medications may cause an overall slowing of thought processes. This slowing may be so severe, it may seem like an eternity before the patient responds. Patience and gentle prompting (e.g., "You were saying that you would like to get a pass this weekend to visit your niece.") can help patients gather their thoughts.

Silence is not always therapeutic. Prolonged and frequent silences by the nurse may hinder an interview that requires verbal articulation. Although a less talkative nurse may be comfortable with silence, this mode of communication may make the patient feel like a fountain of information to be drained dry. Moreover, without feedback, patients have no way of knowing whether or not what they said was understood. Additionally, children and adolescents in particular tend to feel uncomfortable with silence.

Active Listening

People want more than just a physical presence in human communication. Most people want the other person to be there for them psychologically, socially, and emotionally. Active listening in the nurse-patient relationship includes the following aspects:

- Observing the patient's nonverbal behaviors
- Understanding and reflecting on the patient's verbal message
- Understanding the patient in the context of the social setting of the patient's life

- Detecting "false notes" (e.g., inconsistencies or things the patient says that need more clarification)
- Providing feedback about himself or herself of which the patient might not be aware

Effective interviewers learn to become active listeners when the patient is talking, as well as when the patient becomes silent. During active listening, nurses carefully note verbal and nonverbal patient responses and monitor their own nonverbal responses. Using silence effectively and learning to listen actively—to both the patient and your own thoughts and reactions—are key ingredients in effective communication. Both skills take time to develop but can be learned; you will become more proficient with guidance and practice.

Some important principles of active listening (Mohl, 2003) include:

- The answer is always inside the patient.
- Objective truth is never as simple as it seems.
- Everything you hear is modified by the patient's filters.
- Everything you hear is modified by your own filters.
- It is okay to feel confused and uncertain.
- Listen to yourself too.

Active listening helps strengthen the patient's ability to solve problems. By giving the patient undivided attention, the nurse communicates that the patient is not alone. This kind of intervention enhances self-esteem and encourages the patient to direct energy toward finding ways to deal with problems. Serving as a sounding board, the nurse listens as the patient tests thoughts by voicing them aloud. This form of interpersonal interaction often enables the patient to clarify thinking, link ideas, and tentatively decide what should be done and how best to do it (Collins, 1983).

Listening with Empathy. Wheeler (2008) identifies empathy as the most important element in therapeutic communication. Research indicates that the connectedness that results from empathy actually improves brain function by increasing brain plasticity. Wheeler describes the empathetic process as the nurse entering and feeling the patient's world, the patient perceiving his or her own understanding of the world, and the patient experiencing acceptance and confirmation of himself or herself.

It is not enough for the nurse to feel empathy; an important part of this process is that empathy is communicated to the patient. One way to communicate empathy is through the following formula (Egan, 2005):
"You feel _____" *(name the emotion)* because _____ *(describe the experiences, thoughts, and behaviors).*
If we plug in a scenario, it would sound something like this, "You feel like a failure because you have let your father down by joining the Peace Corps rather than becoming a lawyer."

It is not always easy to be empathetic. A patient may describe brutal physical or sexual abuse they have experienced, the torment of watching a loved one die, hate and anger toward another person, or acts of violence or hurtful inconsideration they have committed. When people are self-pitying, critical, angry, sarcastic, or demeaning, the nurse's ability to listen with empathy may diminish. Chapter 9 offers a more detailed discussion of empathy.

Clarifying Techniques

Understanding depends on clear communication, which is aided by verifying the nurse's interpretation of the patient's messages. The nurse can request feedback on the accuracy of the message received from verbal and nonverbal cues. The use of clarifying techniques helps both participants identify major differences in their frame of reference, giving them the opportunity to correct misperceptions before they cause any serious misunderstandings. The patient who is asked to elaborate on or clarify vague or ambiguous messages needs to know that the purpose is to promote mutual understanding.

Paraphrasing. To clarify, the nurse might use paraphrasing, or restating in different (often fewer) words the basic content of a patient's message. Using simple, precise, and culturally relevant terms, the nurse may readily confirm interpretation of the patient's previous message before the interview proceeds. By prefacing statements with a phrase such as "I'm not sure I understand" or "In other words, you seem to be saying…," the nurse helps the patient form a clearer perception of what may be a bewildering mass of details. After paraphrasing, the nurse must validate the accuracy of the restatement and its helpfulness to the discussion. The patient may confirm or deny the perceptions through nonverbal cues or by direct response to a question such as "Was I correct in saying…?" As a result, the patient is made aware that the interviewer is actively involved in the search for understanding.

Restating. In restating, the nurse mirrors the patient's overt and covert messages, so the technique may be used to echo feeling as well as content. Restating differs from paraphrasing in that it involves repeating the same key words the patient has just spoken. If a patient remarks, "My life is empty…it has no meaning," additional information may be gained by restating: "Your life has no meaning?" The purpose of this technique is to explore more thoroughly subjects that may be significant. However, too frequent and indiscriminate use of restating might be interpreted by patients as inattention or disinterest.

It is easy to overuse this tool so that its application becomes mechanical. Parroting or mimicking what another has said may be perceived as poking fun at the person; therefore, the use of this nondirective approach can become a definite barrier to communication. To avoid overuse of restating, the nurse can combine restatements with direct questions that encourage descriptions: "What does your life lack?" "What kind of meaning is missing?" "Describe a day in your life that appears empty to you."

Reflecting. Reflection is a means of assisting people to better understand their own thoughts and feelings. Reflecting may take the form of a question or a simple statement that conveys the nurse's observations of the patient when sensitive issues are being discussed. The nurse might then describe briefly to the patient the apparent meaning of the emotional tone of the patient's verbal and nonverbal behavior. For example, to reflect a patient's feelings about his or her life, a good beginning might be, "You sound as if you have had many disappointments."

Sharing observations with a patient shows acceptance and that the patient has your full attention. When you reflect, you make the patient aware of inner feelings and encourage the patient to own them. For example, you may say to a patient, "You look sad." Perceiving your concern may allow the patient to spontaneously share feelings. The use of a question in response to the patient's question is another reflective technique (Arnold & Boggs, 2007). For example:

Patient: "Nurse, do you think I really need to be hospitalized?"

Nurse: "What do you think, Jane?"

Patient: "I don't know; that's why I'm asking you."

Nurse: "I'll be willing to share my impression with you at the end of this first session. However, you've probably thought about hospitalization and have some feelings about it. I wonder what they are."

Exploring. A technique that enables the nurse to examine important ideas, experiences, or relationships more fully is exploring. For example, if a patient tells you he does not get along well with his wife, you will want to further explore this area. Possible openers include:

> "*Tell me more* about your relationship with your wife."
> "*Describe* your relationship with your wife."
> "*Give me an example* of how you and your wife don't get along."
> Asking for an example can greatly clarify a vague or generic statement made by a patient.

Patient: "No one likes me."

Nurse: "Give me an example of one person who doesn't like you."

or

Patient: "Everything I do is wrong."

Nurse: "Give me an example of one thing you do that you think is wrong."

Table 10-2 lists more examples of therapeutic communication techniques.

Asking Questions and Eliciting Patient Responses

Open-Ended Questions. Many of the examples above and in Table 10-2 are open-ended. **Open-ended questions** and comments encourage lengthy responses and information about experiences, perceptions, or responses to a situation. For example:

- "What do you perceive as your biggest problem right now?"
- "Give me an example of some of the stresses you are under right now."
- "Tell me more about your relationship with your wife?"

Text continued on page 184

TABLE 10-2 Therapeutic Communication Techniques

Therapeutic Technique	Description	Example
Using silence	Gives the person time to collect thoughts or think through a point.	Encouraging a person to talk by waiting for the answers.
Accepting	Indicates that the person has been understood. An accepting statement does not necessarily indicate agreement but is nonjudgmental. (Nurse should not imply understanding when (s)he does not understand.)	"Yes." "Uh-huh." "I follow what you say."
Giving recognition	Indicates awareness of change and personal efforts. Does not imply good or bad, right or wrong.	"Good morning, Mr. James." "You've combed your hair today." "I see you've eaten your whole lunch."
Offering self	Offers presence, interest, and a desire to understand. Is not offered to get the person to talk or behave in a specific way.	"I would like to spend time with you." "I'll stay here and sit with you awhile."

Continued

TABLE 10-2 Therapeutic Communication Techniques—cont'd

Therapeutic Technique	Description	Example
Offering general leads	Allows the other person to take direction in the discussion. Indicates that the nurse is interested in what comes next.	"Go on." "And then?" "Tell me about it."
Giving broad openings	Clarifies that the lead is to be taken by the patient. However, the nurse discourages pleasantries and small talk.	"Where would you like to begin?" "What are you thinking about?" "What would you like to discuss?"
Placing the events in time or sequence	Puts events and actions in better perspective. Notes cause-and-effect relationships and identifies patterns of interpersonal difficulties.	"What happened before?" "When did this happen?"
Making observations	Calls attention to the person's behavior (e.g., trembling, nail biting, restless mannerisms). Encourages patient to notice the behavior and describe thoughts and feelings for mutual understanding. Helpful with mute and withdrawn people.	"You appear tense." "I notice you're biting your lips." "You appear nervous whenever John enters the room."
Encouraging description of perception	Increases the nurse's understanding of the patient's perceptions. Talking about feelings and difficulties can lessen the need to act them out inappropriately.	"What do these voices seem to be saying?" "What is happening now?" "Tell me when you feel anxious."
Encouraging comparison	Brings out recurring themes in experiences or interpersonal relationships. Helps the person clarify similarities and differences.	"Has this ever happened before?" "Is this how you felt when…?" "Was it something like…?"
Restating	Repeats the main idea expressed. Gives the patient an idea of what has been communicated. If the message has been misunderstood, the patient can clarify it.	*Patient:* "I can't sleep. I stay awake all night." *Nurse:* "You have difficulty sleeping?" *or* *Patient:* "I don't know…he always has some excuse for not coming over or keeping our appointments." *Nurse:* "You think he no longer wants to see you?"
Reflecting	Directs questions, feelings, and ideas back to the patient. Encourages the patient to accept his or her own ideas and feelings. Acknowledges the patient's right to have opinions and make decisions and encourages the patient to think of self as a capable person.	*Patient:* "What should I do about my husband's affair?" *Nurse:* "What do you think you should do?" *or* *Patient:* "My brother spends all of my money and then has the nerve to ask for more." *Nurse:* "You feel angry when this happens?"
Focusing	Concentrates attention on a single point. It is especially useful when the patient jumps from topic to topic. If a person is experiencing a severe or panic level of anxiety, the nurse should not persist until the anxiety lessens.	"This point you are making about leaving school seems worth looking at more closely." "You've mentioned many things. Let's go back to your thinking of 'ending it all.'"
Exploring	Examines certain ideas, experiences, or relationships more fully. If the patient chooses not to elaborate by answering no, the nurse does not probe or pry. In such a case, the nurse respects the patient's wishes.	"Tell me more about that." "Would you describe it more fully?" "Could you talk about how it was that you learned your mom was dying of cancer?"

TABLE 10-2 Therapeutic Communication Techniques—cont'd

Therapeutic Technique	Description	Example
Giving information	Makes facts the person needs available. Supplies knowledge from which decisions can be made or conclusions drawn. For example, the patient needs to know the role of the nurse; the purpose of the nurse-patient relationship; and the time, place, and duration of the meetings.	"My purpose for being here is..." "This medication is for..." "The test will determine..."
Seeking clarification	Helps patients clarify their own thoughts and maximize mutual understanding between nurse and patient.	"I am not sure I follow you." "What would you say is the main point of what you just said?" "Give an example of a time you thought everyone hated you."
Presenting reality	Indicates what is real. The nurse does not argue or try to convince the patient, just describes personal perceptions or facts in the situation.	"That was Dr. Todd, not a man from the Mafia." "That was the sound of a car backfiring." "Your mother is not here; I am a nurse."
Voicing doubt	Undermines the patient's beliefs by not reinforcing the exaggerated or false perceptions.	"Isn't that unusual?" "Really?" "That's hard to believe."
Seeking consensual validation	Clarifies that both the nurse and patient share mutual understanding of communications. Helps the patient become clearer about what he or she is thinking.	"Tell me whether my understanding agrees with yours."
Verbalizing the implied	Puts into concrete terms what the patient implies, making the patient's communication more explicit.	*Patient:* "I can't talk to you or anyone else. It's a waste of time." *Nurse:* "Do you feel that no one understands?"
Encouraging evaluation	Aids the patient in considering people and events from the perspective of the patient's own set of values.	"How do you feel about...?" "What did it mean to you when he said he couldn't stay?"
Attempting to translate into feelings	Responds to the feelings expressed, not just the content. Often termed *decoding*.	*Patient:* "I am dead inside." *Nurse:* "Are you saying that you feel lifeless? Does life seem meaningless to you?"
Suggesting collaboration	Emphasizes working with the patient, not doing things for the patient. Encourages the view that change is possible through collaboration.	"Perhaps you and I can discover what produces your anxiety." "Perhaps by working together, we can come up with some ideas that might improve your communications with your spouse."
Summarizing	Brings together important points of discussion to enhance understanding. Also allows the opportunity to clarify communications so that both nurse and patient leave the interview with the same ideas in mind.	"Have I got this straight?" "You said that..." "During the past hour, you and I have discussed..."
Encouraging formulation of a plan of action	Allows the patient to identify alternative actions for interpersonal situations the patient finds disturbing (e.g., when anger or anxiety is provoked).	"What could you do to let anger out harmlessly?" "The next time this comes up, what might you do to handle it?" "What are some other ways you can approach your boss?"

Adapted from Hays, J. S., & Larson, K. (1963). *Interacting with patients.* New York: Macmillan.

Since open-ended questions are not intrusive and do not put the patient on the defensive, they help the clinician illicit information, especially in the beginning of an interview or when a patient is guarded or resistant to answering questions. They are particularly useful when establishing rapport with a person.

Closed-Ended Questions. Nurses are usually urged to ask open-ended questions to elicit more than a "yes" or "no" response. However, closed-ended questions, when used sparingly, can give you specific and needed information. Closed-ended questions are most useful during an initial assessment or intake interview or to ascertain results, as in "Are the medications helping you?" "When did you start hearing voices?" "Did you

seek therapy after your first suicide attempt?" Care needs to be exercised with this technique. Frequent use of closed-ended questions during time spent with patients can close an interview down rapidly; this is especially true with guarded or resistant patients.

Nontherapeutic Communication Techniques

Although people may use "nontherapeutic" or ineffective communication techniques in their daily lives, they can cause problems for nurses because they tend to impede or shut down nurse-patient interaction. Table 10-3 describes nontherapeutic communication techniques and suggests more helpful responses.

TABLE 10-3 Nontherapeutic Communication Techniques			
Nontherapeutic Technique	**Description**	**Example**	**More Helpful Response**
Giving premature advice	Assumes the nurse knows best and the patient can't think for self. Inhibits problem solving and fosters dependency.	"Get out of this situation immediately."	**Encouraging problem solving**: "What are the pros and cons of your situation?" "What were some of the actions you thought you might take?" "What are some of the ways you have thought of to meet your goals?"
Minimizing feelings	Indicates that the nurse is unable to understand or empathize with the patient. Here the patient's feelings or experiences are being belittled, which can cause the patient to feel small or insignificant.	*Patient:* "I wish I were dead." *Nurse:* "Everyone gets down in the dumps." "I know what you mean." "You should feel happy you're getting better." "Things get worse before they get better."	**Empathizing and exploring**: "You must be feeling very upset. Are you thinking of hurting yourself?"
Falsely reassuring	Underrates a person's feelings and belittles a person's concerns. May cause the patient to stop sharing feelings if the patient thinks he or she will be ridiculed or not taken seriously.	"I wouldn't worry about that." "Everything will be all right." "You will do just fine, you'll see."	**Clarifying the patient's message:** "What specifically are you worried about?" "What do you think could go wrong?" "What are you concerned might happen?"
Making value judgments	Prevents problem solving. Can make the patient feel guilty, angry, misunderstood, not supported, or anxious to leave.	"How come you still smoke when your wife has lung cancer?"	**Making observations:** "I notice you are still smoking even though your wife has lung cancer. Is this a problem?"
Asking "why" questions	Implies criticism; often has the effect of making the patient feel defensive.	"Why did you stop taking your medication?"	**Asking open-ended questions; giving a broad opening:** "Tell me some of the reasons that led up to your not taking your medications."
Asking excessive questions	Results in the patient's not knowing which question to answer and possibly being confused about what is being asked.	*Nurse:* "How's your appetite? Are you losing weight? Are you eating enough?" *Patient:* "No."	**Clarifying:** "Tell me about your eating habits since you've been depressed."

TABLE 10-3 Nontherapeutic Communication Techniques—cont'd

Nontherapeutic Technique	Description	Example	More Helpful Response
Giving approval, agreeing	Implies the patient is doing the *right* thing—and that not doing it is wrong. May lead the patient to focus on pleasing the nurse or clinician; denies the patient the opportunity to change his or her mind or decision.	"I'm proud of you for applying for that job." "I agree with your decision."	**Making observations:** "I noticed that you applied for that job. What factors will lead up to your changing your mind?" **Asking open-ended questions; giving a broad opening:** "What led to that decision?"
Disapproving; disagreeing	Can make a person defensive.	"You really should have shown up for the medication group." "I disagree with that."	**Exploring:** "What was going through your mind when you decided not to come to your medication group?" "That's one point of view. How did you arrive at that conclusion?"
Changing the subject	May invalidate the patient's feelings and needs. Can leave the patient feeling alienated and isolated and increase feelings of hopelessness.	*Patient:* "I'd like to die." *Nurse:* "Did you go to Alcoholics Anonymous like we discussed?"	**Validating and exploring:** *Patient:* "I'd like to die." *Nurse:* "This sounds serious. Have you thought of harming yourself?"

Adapted from Hays, J. S., & Larson, K. (1963). *Interacting with patients.* New York: Macmillan.

Excessive Questioning

Excessive questioning—asking multiple questions (particularly closed-ended) consecutively or very rapidly—casts the nurse in the role of interrogator, who demands information without respect for the patient's willingness or readiness to respond. This approach conveys a lack of respect for and sensitivity to the patient's needs. Excessive questioning controls the range and nature of the responses, can easily result in a therapeutic stall, or may completely shut down an interview. It is a controlling tactic and may reflect the interviewer's lack of security in letting the patient tell his or her own story. It is better to ask more open-ended questions and follow the patient's lead. For example:

Excessive questioning: "Why did you leave your wife? Did you feel angry at her? What did she do to you? Are you going back to her?"

More therapeutic approach: "Tell me about the situation between you and your wife."

Giving Approval or Disapproval

"You look great in that dress." "I'm proud of the way you controlled your temper at lunch." "That's a great quilt you made." What could be bad about giving someone a pat on the back once in a while? Nothing, if it is done without conveying a positive or negative judgment. We often give our friends and family approval when they do something well. However, in a nurse-patient relationship, giving praise and approval becomes much more complex.

A patient may be feeling overwhelmed, experiencing low self-esteem, feeling unsure of where his or her life is going, and desperate for recognition, approval, and attention. Yet when people are feeling vulnerable, a value comment might be misinterpreted. For example:

Giving approval: "You did a great job in group telling John just what you thought about how rudely he treated you."

This message implies that the nurse was pleased by the manner in which the patient talked to John. The patient then sees such a response as a way to please the nurse by doing the right thing. To continue to please the nurse (and get approval), the patient may continue the behavior. The behavior might be useful for the patient, but when a behavior is being done to please another person, it is not coming from the individual's own volition or conviction. Also, when the other person the patient needs to please is not around, the motivation for the new behavior might not be there either. Thus the new response really is not a change in behavior as much as a ploy to win approval and acceptance from another.

Giving approval also cuts off further communication.

> **More therapeutic approach:** "I noticed that you spoke up to John in group yesterday about his rude behavior. How did it feel to be more assertive?"

This opens the way for finding out if the patient was scared, was comfortable, wants to work more on assertiveness, etc. It also suggests that this was a self-choice the patient made. The patient is given recognition for the change in behavior, and the topic is also opened for further discussion.

Giving disapproval implies that the nurse has the right to judge the patient's thoughts or feelings. Again, an observation should be made instead.

> **Giving disapproval:** "You really should not cheat, even if you think everyone else is doing it."
>
> **More therapeutic approach:** "Can you give me two examples of how cheating could negatively affect your goal of graduating?"

Giving Advice

Although we ask for and give advice all the time in daily life, giving advice to a patient is rarely helpful. Often when we ask for advice, our real motive is to discover whether we are thinking along the same lines as someone else or if they would agree with us. When a nurse gives advice to a patient, the nurse is interfering with the patient's ability to make personal decisions. When a nurse offers the patient solutions, the patient eventually begins to think the nurse does not view him or her as capable of making effective decisions. People often feel inadequate when they are given no choices over decisions in their lives. Giving advice to patients also can foster dependency ("I'll have to ask the nurse what to do about...") and undermine the patient's sense of competence and adequacy.

However, people do need information to make informed decisions. Often you can help a patient define a problem and identify what information might be needed to come to an informed decision. A useful approach would be to ask, "What do you see as some possible actions you can take?" It is much more constructive to encourage problem solving by the patient. At times you might suggest several alternatives a patient might consider (e.g., "Have you ever thought of telling your friend about the incident?"). The patient is then free to give you a yes or no answer and make a decision from among the suggestions.

Asking "Why" Questions

"Why did you come late?" "Why didn't you go to the funeral?" "Why didn't you study for the exam?" Very often, *why* questions imply criticism. We may ask our friends or family such questions, and in the context of a solid relationship, the *why* may be understood more as "What happened?" With people we do not know—especially those who may be anxious or overwhelmed—a *why* question from a person in authority (nurse, physician, teacher) can be experienced as intrusive and judgmental, which serves only to make the person defensive.

It is much more useful to ask *what* is happening rather than *why* it is happening. Questions that focus on who, what, where, and when often elicit important information that can facilitate problem solving and further the communication process. See Table 10-3 for additional ineffective communication techniques, as well as statements that would better facilitate interaction and patient comfort.

Cultural Considerations

The United States is becoming increasingly culturally diverse, and health care professionals need to be familiar with the verbal and nonverbal communication characteristics of a multicultural national population. The nurse's awareness of cultural meanings of certain verbal and nonverbal communications in initial face-to-face encounters with a patient can lead to the formation of a positive therapeutic relationship (Kavanaugh, 2003).

Unrecognized differences in cultural identities can result in assessment and interventions that are not optimally respectful of the patient and can be inadvertently biased or prejudiced. Health care workers need to have not only knowledge of various patients' cultures but also awareness of their own cultural identities. Especially important are nurses' attitudes and beliefs toward those from cultures other than their own, because these will affect their relationships with patients (Kavanaugh, 2003). Four areas that may prove problematic for the nurse interpreting specific verbal and nonverbal messages of the patient include:

1. Communication style
2. Use of eye contact
3. Perception of touch
4. Cultural filters

Communication Style

People may communicate in an intense and highly emotional manner. Some may consider it normal to use dramatic body language when describing emotional problems, and others may perceive such behavior as being out of control or reflective of some degree of pathology. For example, within the Hispanic community, intensely emotional styles of communication often are culturally appropriate and expected (Kavanaugh, 2003). French and Italian Americans typically show animated facial expressions and expressive hand gestures during communication, which can be misinterpreted by others.

In other cultures, a calm facade may mask severe distress. For example, in many Asian cultures, expression of positive or negative emotions is a private affair, and open expression of them is considered to be in bad taste and possibly a weakness. A quiet smile by an Asian American may express joy, an apology, stoicism, or even anger. German and British Americans also tend to value highly the concept of self-control and may show little facial emotion in the presence of great distress or emotional turmoil.

Eye Contact

Fontes (2008) warns that the presence or absence of eye contact should not be used to assess attentiveness, judge truthfulness, or make assumptions on the degree of engagement one has with a patient. Cultural norms dictate a person's comfort or lack of comfort with direct eye contact. Some cultures consider direct eye contact disrespectful and improper. For example, Hispanic individuals have traditionally been taught to avoid eye contact with authority figures such as nurses, physicians, and other health care professionals. Avoidance of direct eye contact is seen as a sign of respect to those in authority, but it could be misinterpreted as disinterest or even as a lack of respect.

In Japan, direct eye contact is considered to show lack of respect and to be a personal affront; preference is for shifting or downcast eyes or focus on the speaker's neck. With many Chinese, gazing around and looking to one side when listening to another is considered polite. In some Middle Eastern cultures, for a woman to make direct eye contact with a man may imply a sexual interest or even promiscuity. On the other hand, most Americans of European descent maintain eye contact during conversation; avoidance of eye contact by another person may be interpreted as being disinterested, not telling the truth, or avoiding the sharing of important information.

Touch

The therapeutic use of touch is a basic aspect of the nurse-patient relationship and is generally considered a gesture of warmth and friendship; however, the degree to which a patient is comfortable with the use of touch is often culturally determined. People from some cultures, Hispanic for example, are accustomed to frequent physical contact. Holding a patient's hand in response to a distressing situation or giving the patient a reassuring pat on the shoulder may be experienced as supportive and thus help facilitate openness (Kavanaugh, 2003). People from Italian and French backgrounds may also be accustomed to frequent touching during conversation, and in the Russian culture, touch is an important part of nonverbal communication used freely with intimate and close friends (Giger & Davidhizar, 2004).

However, personal touch within the context of an interview may perceived as an invasion of privacy or experienced as patronizing, intrusive, aggressive, or sexually inviting in other cultures. Among German, Swedish, and British Americans, touch practices are infrequent, although a handshake may be common at the beginning and end of an interaction. Chinese Americans may not like to be touched by strangers.

Even among people from similar cultures, the use of touch has different interpretations and rules regarding gender and class. Students are urged to find out if their facility has a "no touch" policy, particularly with adolescents and children who have experienced inappropriate touch and may not know how to interpret therapeutic touch from the health care worker.

Cultural Filters

It is important to recognize that it is impossible to listen to people in an unbiased way. In the process of socialization, we develop cultural filters through which we listen to ourselves, others, and the world around us (Egan, 2007). Cultural filters are a form of cultural bias or cultural prejudice that determine what we pay attention to and what we ignore. Egan stated that we need these cultural filters to provide structure for our lives and help us interpret and interact with the world. However, these cultural filters also unavoidably introduce various forms of bias into our communication, because they are bound to influence our personal, professional, familial, and sociological values and interpretations.

We all need a frame of reference to help us function in our world, but the trick is to understand that other people use many other frames of reference to help them function in their worlds. Acknowledging that everyone views the world differently and understanding that these various views impact each person's beliefs and behaviors can go a long way toward minimizing our personal distortions in listening. Building acceptance and understanding of cultural diversity is a skill that can be learned. Chapter 6 has a more in-depth discussion of cultural considerations in nursing.

Evaluation of Communication Skills

After you have had some introductory clinical experience, you may find the facilitative skills checklist in Figure 10-2 useful for evaluating your progress in developing interviewing skills. Note that some of the items might not be relevant for some of your patients (e.g., numbers 11 through 13 may not be possible when a patient is experiencing psychosis [disordered thought, delusions, and/or hallucinations]). Self-evaluation of clinical skills is a way to focus on therapeutic improvement. Role playing can help prepare you for clinical experience and practice effective and professional communication skills.

FACILITATIVE SKILLS CHECKLIST

Instructions: Periodically during your clinical experience, use this checklist to identify areas where growth is needed and progress has been made. Think of your clinical client experiences. Indicate the extent of your agreement with each of the following statements by marking the scale: *SA,* strongly agree; *A,* agree; *NS,* not sure; *D,* disagree; *SD,* strongly disagree.

1. I maintain good eye contact.	SA	A	NS	D	SD
2. Most of my verbal comments follow the lead of the other person.	SA	A	NS	D	SD
3. I encourage others to talk about feelings.	SA	A	NS	D	SD
4. I am able to ask open-ended questions.	SA	A	NS	D	SD
5. I can restate and clarify a person's ideas.	SA	A	NS	D	SD
6. I can summarize in a few words the basic ideas of a long statement made by a person.	SA	A	NS	D	SD
7. I can make statements that reflect the person's feelings.	SA	A	NS	D	SD
8. I can share my feelings relevant to the discussion when appropriate to do so.	SA	A	NS	D	SD
9. I am able to give feedback.	SA	A	NS	D	SD
10. At least 75% or more of my responses help enhance and facilitate communication.	SA	A	NS	D	SD
11. I can assist the person to list some alternatives available.	SA	A	NS	D	SD
12. I can assist the person to identify some goals that are specific and observable.	SA	A	NS	D	SD
13. I can assist the person to specify at least one next step that might be taken toward the goal.	SA	A	NS	D	SD

Figure 10-2 Facilitative Skills Checklist. (Adapted from Myrick, D., & Erney, T. [2000]. *Caring and sharing* [2nd ed., p. 168]. Copyright © 2000 by Educational Media Corporation, Minneapolis, Minnesota.)

THE CLINICAL INTERVIEW

Ideally, the content and direction of the clinical interview are decided and led by the patient. The nurse employs communication skills and active listening to better understand the patient's situation.

Preparing for the Interview

Pace

Helping a person with an emotional or medical problem is rarely a straightforward task, and the goal of assisting a patient to regain psychological or physiological stability can be difficult to achieve. Extremely important to any kind of counseling is permitting the patient to set the pace of the interview, no matter how slow or halting the progress may be (Arnold & Boggs, 2007).

Setting

Effective communication can take place almost anywhere. However, the quality of the interaction—whether in a clinic, a clinical unit, an office, or the patient's home—depends on the degree to which the nurse and patient feel safe; establishing a setting that enhances feelings of security is important to the therapeutic relationship. A health care setting, a conference room, or a quiet part of the unit that has relative privacy but is within view of others is ideal, but when the interview takes place in the patient's home, it offers the nurse a valuable opportunity to assess the patient in the context of everyday life.

Seating

In all settings, chairs should be arranged so conversation can take place in normal tones of voice and eye contact can be comfortably maintained or avoided. A nonthreatening physical environment for both nurse and patient would involve:

- Assuming the same height, either both sitting or both standing
- Avoiding a face-to-face stance when possible; a 90- to 120-degree angle or side-by-side position may be less intense, and patient and nurse can look away from each other without discomfort
- Providing safety and psychological comfort in terms of exiting the room—The patient should not be positioned between the nurse and the door, nor should the nurse be positioned in such a way that the patient feels trapped in the room.
- Avoiding a desk barrier between the nurse and the patient

Introductions

In the orientation phase, students tell the patient who they are, what the purpose of the meeting is, and how long and at what time they will be meeting with the patient. The issue of confidentiality is brought up during the initial interview. Remember that all health care professionals must respect the private, personal, and confidential nature of the patient's communication, except in the specific situations outlined earlier (e.g., harm to self or others, child abuse, elder abuse). What is discussed with staff and your clinical group in conference should not be discussed outside with others, no matter who they are (e.g., patient's relatives, news media, friends, etc.). The patient needs to know that whatever is discussed will stay confidential unless permission is given for it to be disclosed. Refer to Chapter 9 to review the nurse's responsibilities in the orientation phase.

Ask the patient how he or she would like to be addressed. This question conveys respect and gives the patient direct control over an important ego issue. (Some patients like to be called by their last names; others prefer being on a first-name basis with the nurse) (Arnold & Boggs, 2007).

Initiating the Interview

Once introductions have been made, you can turn the interview over to the patient by using one of a number of open-ended questions or statements:

- "Where should we start?"
- "Tell me a little about what has been going on with you."
- "What are some of the stresses you have been coping with recently?"
- "Tell me a little about what has been happening in the past couple of weeks."
- "Perhaps you can begin by letting me know what some of your concerns have been recently."
- "Tell me about your difficulties."

Communication can be facilitated by appropriately offering leads (e.g., "Go on"), making statements of acceptance (e.g., "Uh-huh"), or otherwise conveying interest.

Tactics to Avoid

Certain behaviors (Moscato, 1988) are counterproductive and should be avoided. For example:

Do Not:	Try To:
Argue with, minimize, or challenge the patient.	Keep focus on facts and the patient's perceptions.
Give false reassurance.	Make observations of the patient's behavior: "Change is always possible."
Interpret to the patient or speculate on the dynamics.	Listen attentively, use silence, and try to clarify the patient's problem.
Question or probe patients about sensitive areas they do not wish to discuss.	Pay attention to nonverbal communication. Strive to keep the patient's anxiety to a minimum.
Try to sell the patient on accepting treatment.	Encourage the patient to look at pros and cons.
Join in attacks patients launch on their mates, parents, friends, or associates.	Focus on facts and the patient's perceptions. Be aware of nonverbal communication.
Participate in criticism of another nurse or any other staff member.	Focus on facts and the patient's perceptions. Check out serious accusations with the other nurse or staff member. Have the patient meet with the nurse or staff member in question in the presence of senior staff member/clinician and clarify perceptions.

Helpful Guidelines

Meier and Davis (2001) offer some guidelines for conducting the initial interview:

- Speak briefly.
- When you do not know what to say, say nothing.
- When in doubt, focus on feelings.
- Avoid advice.
- Avoid relying on questions.
- Pay attention to nonverbal cues.
- Keep the focus on the patient.

Attending Behaviors: The Foundation of Interviewing

Engaging in attending behaviors and actively listening are two key principles of counseling on which almost everyone can agree (Sommers-Flanagan & Sommers-Flanagan, 2003). Positive attending behaviors serve to open up communication and encourage free expression, whereas negative attending behaviors are more likely to inhibit expression. All behaviors must be evaluated in terms of cultural patterns and past experiences of both the interviewer and the interviewee. There are no universals; however, there are guidelines students can follow.

Eye Contact

As previously discussed, cultural and individual variations influence a patient's comfort with eye contact. For some patients and interviewers, sustained eye contact is normal and comfortable. For others, it may be more comfortable and natural to make brief eye contact but look away or down much of the time. Sommers-Flanagan and Sommers-Flanagan (2003) state that in most situations, it is appropriate for nurses to maintain more eye contact when the patient speaks and less constant eye contact when the nurse speaks.

Body Language

Body language involves two elements: kinesics and proxemics. *Kinesics* is associated with physical characteristics, such as body movements and postures. Facial expressions, eye contact or lack thereof, the way someone holds the head, legs, and shoulders, and so on convey a multitude of messages. A person who slumps in a chair, rolls the eyes, and sits with arms crossed in front of the chest can be perceived as resistant and unreceptive to what another wants to communicate. On the other hand, a person who leans in slightly toward the speaker, maintains a relaxed and attentive posture, makes appropriate eye contact, makes hand gestures that are unobtrusive and smooth while minimizing the number of other movements, and matches their facial expressions to their feelings or to the patient's feelings can be perceived as open to and respectful of the communication.

Proxemics refers to the study of **personal space** and the significance of the physical distance between individuals. Proxemics takes into account that these distances may be different for different cultural groups. **Intimate distance** in the United States is 0 to 18 inches and is reserved for those we trust most and with whom we feel most safe. **Personal distance** (18 to 40 inches) is for personal communications such as those with friends or colleagues. **Social distance** (4 to 12 feet) applies to strangers or acquaintances, often in public places or formal social gatherings. **Public distance** (12 feet or more) relates to public space (e.g., public speaking). In public space, one may hail another, and the parties may move about while communicating.

Vocal Quality

Vocal quality, or paralinguistics, encompasses voice loudness, pitch, rate, and fluency. Sommers-Flanagan and Sommers-Flanagan (2003) say that "effective interviewers use vocal qualities to enhance rapport, communicate interest and empathy, and to emphasize special issues or conflicts" (p. 56). Paralinguistics provides a perfect example of "It's not *what* you say, but *how* you say it." Speaking in soft and gentle tones is apt to encourage a person to share thoughts and feelings, whereas speaking in a rapid, high-pitched tone may convey anxiety and create it in the patient. Consider, for example, how tonal quality can affect communication in a simple sentence like "I will see you tonight."

1. "*I* will see you tonight." (I will be the one who sees you tonight.)
2. "I *will* see you tonight." (No matter what happens, or whether you like it or not, I will see you tonight.)
3. "I will see *you* tonight." (Even though others are present, it is you I want to see.)
4. "I will see you *tonight*." (It is definite, tonight is the night we will meet.)

Verbal Tracking

Verbal tracking is just that: tracking what the patient is saying. Individuals cannot know if you are hearing or understanding what they are saying unless you provide them with cues. Verbal tracking is giving neutral feedback in the form of restating or summarizing what the patient has already said and does not include personal or professional opinions (Sommers-Flanagan & Sommers-Flanagan, 2003). For example:

> **Patient:** "I don't know what the fuss is about. I smoke marijuana to relax, and everyone makes a fuss."
>
> **Nurse:** "Do you see this as a problem for you?"
>
> **Patient:** "No, I don't. It doesn't affect my work...well, most of the time, anyway. I mean, of course, if I have to think things out and make important decisions, then obviously it can get in the way. But most of the time I'm cool."
>
> **Nurse:** "So when important decisions have to be made, then it interferes; otherwise, you don't see it affecting your functioning."
>
> **Patient:** "Yeah, well, most of the time I'm cool."

Meier and Davis (2001) state that verbal tracking involves pacing the interview with the patient by sticking closely with the patient's speech content (as well as speech volume and tone, as discussed earlier). It can be difficult to know which leads to follow if the patient introduces many topics at once. When this happens, the nurse can summarize what she has heard, respond to the feelings associated with so much to consider, and help the patient focus on and explore a specific topic. "With everything going on in your life recently, you must really feel overwhelmed. You're $2000 in debt and don't have a job, you've gained 30 pounds in 6 months, and your wife is frustrated with your drinking. Let's talk more about what is going on with your wife and her concerns about alcohol."

Clinical Supervision

Communication and interviewing techniques are acquired skills. You will learn to increase these abilities through practice and clinical supervision. In clinical supervision, the focus is on the nurse's behavior in the nurse-patient relationship; nurse and supervisor have opportunities to examine and analyze the nurse's feelings and reactions to the patient and the way they affect the relationship.

The importance of clinical supervision was stressed in Chapter 9. Farkas-Cameron (1995) writes that "the nurse who does not engage in the clinical supervisory process stagnates both theoretically and clinically, while depriving him- or herself of the opportunity to advance professionally" (p. 44). She observed that clinical supervision can be a therapeutic process for the nurse, during which feelings and concerns about the developing nurse-patient relationship are ventilated. The opportunity to examine interactions, obtain insights, and devise alternative strategies for dealing with various clinical issues enhances clinical growth and minimizes frustration and burnout. Clinical supervision is a necessary professional activity that fosters professional growth and helps minimize the development of nontherapeutic nurse-patient relationships.

Process Recordings

The best way to increase communication and interviewing skills is to review your clinical interactions exactly as they occur. This process offers the opportunity to identify themes and patterns in both your own and your patients' communications. As students, clinical review helps you learn to deal with the variety of situations that arise in the clinical interview.

Process recordings are written records of a segment of the nurse-patient session that reflect as closely as possible the verbal and nonverbal behaviors of both patient and nurse. Process recordings have some disadvantages because they rely on memory and are subject to distortions. However, they can be a useful tool for identifying communication patterns. Sometimes an observing clinician takes notes during the interview, but this practice also has disadvantages in that it may be distracting for both interviewer and patient. Some patients (especially those with a paranoid disorder) may resent or misunderstand the student's intent.

It is usually best to write notes verbatim (word for word) in a private area immediately after the interaction has taken place. You can carefully record your words and the patient's words, identify whether your responses are therapeutic or not, and recall your thinking and emotions at the time.

Table 10-4 gives an example of a process recording.

TABLE 10-4 Example of a Process Recording

Nurse	Patient	Communication Technique	Student's Thoughts and Feelings
"Good morning, Mr. Long."		**Therapeutic.** Giving recognition. Acknowledging a patient by name can enhance self-esteem and communicates that the patient is viewed as an individual by the nurse.	I was feeling nervous. He had attempted suicide, and I didn't know if I could help him. Initially I was feeling somewhat overwhelmed.
	"Who are you, and where the devil am I?" Gazes around with a confused look on his face—quickly sits on the edge of the bed.		
"I am Ms. Rodriguez. I am a student nurse from the college, and you are at Mt. Sinai Hospital. I would like to spend some time with you today."		**Therapeutic.** Giving information. Informing the patient of facts needed to make decisions or come to realistic conclusions. **Therapeutic.** Offering self. Making oneself available to the patient.	
	"What am I doing here? How did I get here?" (*Spoken in a loud, demanding voice.*)		I felt a bit intimidated when he raised his voice.
"You were brought in by your wife last night after swallowing a bottle of aspirin. You had to have your stomach pumped."		**Therapeutic.** Giving information. Giving needed facts so that the patient can orient himself and better evaluate his situation.	
	"Oh … yeah." Silence for 2 minutes. Shoulders slumped, Mr. Long stares at the floor and drops his head and eyes.		I was uncomfortable with the silence, but since I didn't have anything useful to say, I stayed with him in silence for the 2 minutes.

Continued

TABLE 10-4 Example of a Process Recording—cont'd

Nurse	Patient	Communication Technique	Student's Thoughts and Feelings
"You seem upset, Mr. Long. What are you thinking about?"		**Therapeutic.** Making observations. He looks sad. **Therapeutic.** Giving broad openings in an attempt to get at his feelings.	I began to feel sorry for him; he looked so sad and helpless.
	"Yeah, I just remembered... I wanted to kill myself." *(Said in a low tone almost to himself.)*		
"Oh, Mr. Long, you have so much to live for. You have such a loving family."		**Nontherapeutic.** Defending. **Nontherapeutic.** Introducing an unrelated topic.	I felt overwhelmed. I didn't know what to say—his talking about killing himself made me nervous. I could have said, "You must be very upset" *(verbalizing the implied)* or "Tell me more about this" *(exploring).*
	"What do you know about my life? You want to know about my family?...My wife is leaving me, that's what." *(Faces the nurse with an angry expression on his face and speaks in loud tones.)*		Again, I felt intimidated by his anger, but now I linked it with his wife's leaving him, so I didn't take it as personally as I did the first time.
"I didn't know. You must be terribly upset by her leaving."		**Therapeutic.** Reflective. Observing the angry tone and content of the patient's message and reflecting back the patient's feelings.	I really felt for him, and now I thought that encouraging him to talk more about this could be useful for him.

KEY POINTS TO REMEMBER

- Knowledge of communication and interviewing techniques is the foundation for development of any nurse-patient relationship. Goal-directed professional communication is referred to as *therapeutic communication.*
- Communication is a complex process. Berlo's communication model has five parts: stimulus, sender, message, medium, and receiver. Feedback is a vital component of the communication process for validating the accuracy of the sender's message.
- A number of factors can minimize, enhance, or otherwise influence the communication process: culture, language, knowledge level, noise, lack of privacy, presence of others, and expectations.
- There are verbal and nonverbal elements in communication; the nonverbal elements often play the larger role in conveying a person's message. Verbal communication consists of all words a person speaks. Nonverbal communication consists of the behaviors displayed by an individual, in addition to the actual content of speech.
- Communication has two levels: the content level (verbal speech) and the process level (nonverbal behavior). When content is congruent with process, the communication is said to be *healthy.* When the verbal message is not reinforced by the communicator's actions, the message is ambiguous; we call this a *double (or mixed) message.*
- Cultural background (as well as individual differences) has a great deal to do with what nonverbal behavior means to different individuals. The degree of eye contact and the use of touch are two nonverbal behaviors that can be misunderstood by individuals of different cultures.
- There are a number of therapeutic communication techniques nurses can use to enhance their nursing practices (see Table 10-2).

- There are also a number of nontherapeutic communication techniques that nurses can learn to avoid to enhance their effectiveness with people (see Table 10-3).
- Most nurses are most effective when they use nonthreatening and open-ended communication techniques.
- Effective communication is a skill that develops over time and is integral to the establishment and maintenance of a therapeutic relationship.
- The clinical interview is a key component of psychiatric mental health nursing, and the nurse must establish a safe setting and plan for appropriate seating, introductions, and initiation of the interview.
- Attending behaviors (e.g., eye contact, body language, vocal qualities, and verbal tracking) are key elements in effective communication.
- A meaningful therapeutic relationship is facilitated when values and cultural influences are considered. It is the nurse's responsibility to seek to understand the patient's perceptions.

CRITICAL THINKING

1. Keep a written log of a conversation you have with a patient. In your log, identify the therapeutic and nontherapeutic techniques you noticed yourself using. Then rewrite the nontherapeutic communications, and replace them with statements that would better facilitate discussion of thoughts and feelings. Share your log and discuss the changes you are working on with one classmate.

2. Role-play with a classmate at least five nonverbal communications, and have your partner identify the message he or she was receiving.

3. With the other students in your class watching, plan and role-play a nurse-patient conversation that lasts about three minutes. Use both therapeutic and nontherapeutic techniques. When you are finished have your other classmates try to identify the techniques that you used.

4. Demonstrate how the nurse would use touch and eye contact when working with patients from three different cultural groups.

CHAPTER REVIEW

1. You have been working closely with a patient for the past month. Today he tells you he is looking forward to meeting with his new psychiatrist but frowns and avoids eye contact while reporting this to you. Which of the following responses would most likely be therapeutic?
   1. "A new psychiatrist is a chance to start fresh; I'm sure it will go well for you."
   2. "You say you look forward to the meeting, but you appear anxious or unhappy."
   3. "I notice that you frowned and avoided eye contact just now; don't you feel well?"
   4. "I get the impression you don't really want to see your psychiatrist—can you tell me why?"

2. Which student behavior is consistent with therapeutic communication?
   1. Offering your opinion when asked in order to convey support.
   2. Summarizing the essence of the patient's comments in your own words.
   3. Interrupting periods of silence before they become awkward for the patient.
   4. Telling the patient he did well when you approve of his statements or actions.

3. Which statement about nonverbal behavior is accurate?
   1. A calm expression means that the patient is experiencing low levels of anxiety.
   2. Patients respond more consistently to therapeutic touch than to verbal interventions.
   3. The meaning of nonverbal behaviors varies with cultural and individual differences.
   4. Eye contact is a reliable measure of the patient's degree of attentiveness and engagement.

4. A nurse stops in to interview a patient on a medical unit and finds the patient lying supine in her bed with the head elevated at 10 degrees. Which initial response(s) would most enhance the chances of achieving a therapeutic interaction? *Select all that apply.*
   1. Apologize for the differential in height and proceed while standing to avoid delay.
   2. If permitted, raise the head of the bed and, with the patient's permission, sit on the bed.
   3. If permitted, raise the head of the bed to approximate the nurse's height while standing.
   4. Sit in whatever chair is available in the room to convey informality and increase comfort.
   5. Locate a chair or stool that would place the nurse at approximately the level of the patient.
   6. Remain standing and proceed so as not to create distraction by altering the arrangements.

5. A patient with schizophrenia approaches staff arriving for day shift and anxiously reports, "Last night demons came to my room and tried to rape me." Which response would be most therapeutic?
   1. "There are no such things as demons; what you saw were hallucinations."
   2. "It is not possible for anyone to enter your room at night; you are safe here."
   3. "You seem very upset; please tell me more about what you experienced last night."
   4. "That must have been very frightening, but we'll check on you at night and you'll be safe."

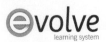

Visit the Evolve website for an **Audio Chapter Summary, Chapter Review Answers & Rationales, Critical Thinking Answer Guidelines,** and additional resources related to the content in this chapter: **http://evolve.elsevier.com/Varcarolis/foundations**

Companion CD Use the Companion CD to prepare for tests and the NCLEX® Examination with **Test-Taking Strategies** for psychiatric mental health nursing and hundreds of **Review Questions**.

References

Arnold, E. C., & Boggs, K. U. (2007). *Interpersonal relationships: Professional communication skills for nurses* (5th ed.). St. Louis: Saunders.

Bateson, G., Jackson, D., & Haley, J. (1956). Toward a theory of schizophrenia. *Behavioral Sciences, 1*(4), 251–264.

Berlo, D. K. (1960). *The process of communication.* San Francisco: Reinhart Press.

Collins, M. (1983). *Communication in health care: The human connection in the life cycle* (2nd ed.). St. Louis: Mosby.

Egan, G. (2007). *The skilled helper: A systematic approach to effective helping* (8th ed.). Pacific Grove, CA: Brooks/Cole.

Egan, G. (2005). *Essentials of skilled helping: Managing problems, developing opportunities.* Belmont, CA: Thomson Higher Education.

Ellis, R. B., Gates, B., & Kenworthy, N. (2003). *Interpersonal communicating in nursing* (2nd ed.). London: Churchill Livingstone.

Farkas-Cameron, M. M. (1995). Clinical supervision in psychiatric nursing. *Journal of Psychosocial Nursing and Mental Health Services, 33*(2), 40–47.

Fontes, L. A. (2008). *Interviewing clients across cultures: A practitioner's guide.* New York: Guilford.

Giger, J. N., & Davidhizar, R. E. (2004). *Transcultural nursing: Assessment and intervention* (4th ed.). St. Louis: Mosby.

Haber, J. (2000). Hildegard E. Peplau: The psychiatric nursing legacy of a legend. *Journal of the American Psychiatric Nursing Association, 6,* 510–562.

Kavanaugh, K. H. (2003). Transcultural perspectives in mental health nursing. In M. Andrews & J. Boyle (Eds.), *Transcultural concepts in nursing care.* Philadelphia: Lippincott Williams & Wilkins.

Matsumoto, D. (2006). Culture and nonverbal behavior. In V. L. Manusov, M. L. Patterson (Eds.), *The Sage handbook of nonverbal communication* (pp. 219–235). Newbury Park, CA: Sage.

Meier, S. T., & Davis, S. R. (2001). *The elements of counseling* (4th ed.). Pacific Grove, CA: Brooks/Cole.

Mohl, P. C. (2003). Psychiatry. In A. Tasman, J. Kay, J. A. Lieberman (Eds.), *Listening to the patient* (2nd ed.). West Sussex, England: Wiley.

Moscato, B. (1988). Psychiatric nursing. In H. S. Wilson, C. S. Kneisel (Eds.), *The one-to-one relationship* (3rd ed.). Menlo Park, CA: Addison-Wesley.

Peplau, H. E. (1952). *Interpersonal relations in nursing: A conceptual frame of reference for psychodynamic nursing.* New York: Putnam.

Shea, S. C. (1998). *Psychiatric interviewing: The art of understanding* (2nd ed.). Philadelphia: Saunders.

Sommers-Flanagan, J., & Sommers-Flanagan, R. (2003). *Clinical interviewing* (3rd ed.). Hoboken: Wiley.

Wheeler, K. (2008). *Psychotherapy for the advanced practice psychiatric nurse.* St. Louis: Mosby.

CHAPTER **11**

Understanding Responses to Stress

Margaret Jordan Halter and Elizabeth M. Varcarolis

Key Terms and Concepts

Benson's relaxation techniques, 204
biofeedback, 206
cognitive reframing, 206
coping styles, 201
distress, 197
eustress, 197
fight-or-flight response, 197
general adaptation syndrome (GAS), 197
guided imagery, 205

humor, 207
journaling, 207
meditation, 204
mindfulness, 206
physical stressors, 199
progressive muscle relaxation (PMR), 204
psychological stressors, 199
psychoneuroimmunology, 198
stressors, 196

Objectives

1. Recognize the short- and long-term physiological consequences of stress.
2. Compare and contrast Cannon's (fight-or-flight), Selye's (general adaptation syndrome), and psychoneuroimmunological models of stress.
3. Describe how responses to stress are mediated through perception, personality, social support, culture, and spirituality.
4. Assess stress level using the Recent Life Changes Questionnaire.
5. Identify and describe holistic approaches to stress management.
6. Teach a classmate or patient a behavioral technique to help lower stress and anxiety.
7. Explain how cognitive techniques can help increase a person's tolerance for stressful events.

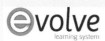 Visit the Evolve website for an **Audio Glossary & Flashcards, Concept Map Creator,** and additional resources related to the content in this chapter: **http://evolve.elsevier.com/Varcarolis/foundations**

Before turning our attention to the clinical disorders presented in the chapters that follow, we will explore the subject of stress. Stress and our responses to it are central to psychiatric disorders and the provision of mental health care. The interplay among stress, the development of psychiatric disorders, and the exacerbation (worsening) of psychiatric symptoms has been widely researched. The old adage "what doesn't kill you will make you stronger" does not hold true with the development of mental illness; early exposure to stressful events actually sensitizes people to stress in later life. In other words, we know that people who are exposed to high levels of stress as children—especially during stress-sensitive developmental periods—have a greater incidence of all mental illnesses as adults (Weber et al., 2008). However, we do not know if severe stress causes a vulnerability to mental illness or if vulnerability to mental illness influences the likelihood of adverse stress responses. It is most important to recognize that severe stress is unhealthy and can weaken biological resistance to psychiatric pathology in any individual; however, stress is especially harmful for those who have a genetic predisposition to these disorders.

While an understanding of the connection between stress and mental illness is essential in the psychiatric setting, it is also important when developing a plan of care for any patient, in any setting, with any diagnosis.

Imagine having an appendectomy and being served with an eviction notice on the same day. How well could you cope with either situation, let alone both simultaneously? The nurse's role is to intervene to reduce stress by promoting a healing environment, facilitating successful coping, and developing future coping strategies. In this chapter, we will explore how we are equipped to respond to stress, what can go wrong with the stress response, and how to care for our patients and even ourselves during times of stress.

RESPONSES TO AND EFFECTS OF STRESS

Early Stress Response Theories

The earliest research into the stress response (Figure 11-1) began as a result of observations that stressors brought about physical disorders or made existing conditions worse. Stressors are psychological or physical stimuli that are incompatible with current functioning

THE STRESS RESPONSE

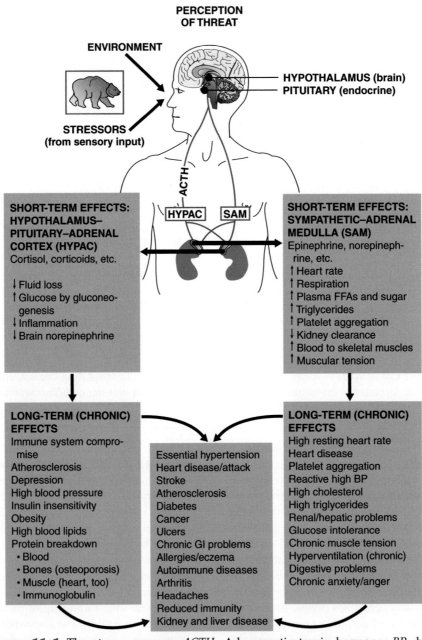

Figure 11-1 The stress response. *ACTH*, Adrenocorticotropic hormone; *BP*, blood pressure; *FFAs*, free fatty acids; *GI*, gastrointestinal. (From Brigham, D. D. [1994]. Imagery for getting well: Clinical applications of behavioral medicine. New York: W. W. Norton.)

and require adaptation. Walter Cannon (1871–1945) methodically investigated the sympathetic nervous system as a pathway of the response to stress, known more commonly as *fight* (aggression) *or flight* (withdrawal). The well-known **fight-or-flight response** is the body's way of preparing for a situation an individual perceives as a threat to survival. This response results in increased blood pressure, heart rate, and cardiac output.

While groundbreaking, Cannon's theory has been criticized for being simplistic, since not all animals or people respond by fighting or fleeing. In the face of danger, some animals become still (think of a deer) to avoid being noticed or to observe the environment in a state of heightened awareness. Also, Cannon's theory was developed primarily based on responses of animals and men. New research indicates that women may have unique physiological responses to stress. Physically, women have a lower hypothalamic-pituitary-adrenal axis and lower autonomic responses to stress at all ages, especially during pregnancy, and researchers hypothesize that estrogen exposure may reduce stress responses (Kajantie & Phillips, 2006). Men and women also have different neural responses to stress. While men experience altered prefrontal blood flow and increased salivary cortisol in response to stress, women experience increased limbic (emotional) activity and less significantly altered salivary cortisol (Wang et al., 2007).

Hans Selye (1907–1982) was another pioneer in stress research who introduced the concept of stress into both the scientific and popular literature. He expanded Cannon's theory of stress in 1956 in his formulation of the **general adaptation syndrome (GAS)**. The GAS occurs in three stages:

1. The *alarm* (or *acute stress*) stage is the initial, brief, and adaptive response (fight or flight) to the stressor. During the alarm stage, three principal *stress mediators* are involved:
   - The brain's cortex and hypothalamus signal the adrenal glands to release the catecholamine adrenalin. This increases sympathetic system activity (e.g., increased heart rate, respirations, and blood pressure) to enhance strength and speed. Pupils dilate for a broad view of the environment, and blood is shunted away from the digestive tract (resulting in dry mouth) and kidneys to more essential organs.
   - The hypothalamus also sends messages to the adrenal cortex. The adrenal cortex produces corticosteroids to help increase muscle endurance and stamina, whereas other nonessential functions (e.g., digestion) are decreased. Unfortunately, the corticosteroids also inhibit functions such as reproduction, growth, and immunity (Sadock & Sadock, 2008).

   - Endorphins are released that reduce sensitivity to pain and injury.

   The alarm stage is extremely intense, and no organism can sustain this level of reactivity and excitement for long. If the organism survives, the resistance stage follows.

2. The *resistance* stage could also be called the *adaptation stage*, because it is during this time sustained and optimal resistance to the stressor occurs. Usually stressors are successfully overcome; however, when they are not, the organism may experience the final exhaustion stage.

3. The *exhaustion* stage occurs when attempts to resist the stressor prove futile. At this point, resources are depleted, and the stress may become chronic, producing a wide array of psychological and physiological responses and even death.

The body responds the same physiologically regardless of whether the stress is real or only perceived as a threat and whether the threat is physical, psychological, or social. Additionally, the body cannot differentiate between the energy generated by positive and negative stimuli. Lazarus and colleagues (1980) described these reactions as *distress* and *eustress:*

- **Distress** is a negative, draining energy that results in anxiety, depression, confusion, helplessness, hopelessness, and fatigue. Distress may be caused by such stressors as a death in the family, financial overload, or school/work demands.
- **Eustress** is a positive, beneficial energy that motivates and results in feelings of happiness, hopefulness, and purposeful movement. Eustress may be the result of a much-needed vacation, being called in for an interview, the birth of a baby, or buying a new car. Eustress could lead to a depletion of physiological resources if sustained, but (fortunately/unfortunately) one does not typically become chronically happy and motivated.

Currently, Selye's GAS remains a popular theory, but it has been expanded and reinterpreted since the 1950s (McKewan, 2005). Some researchers question the notion of "nonspecific responses" and believe that different types of stressors bring about different patterns of responses. Furthermore, the GAS is most accurate in the description of how males respond when threatened. Females do not typically respond to stress by fighting or fleeing but rather by tending and befriending, a survival strategy that emphasizes the protection of young and a reliance on the social network for support.

Increased understanding of the exhaustion stage of the GAS has revealed that illness results from not only the depletion of reserves but also the stress mediators themselves. This is described in Immune Stress Responses on page 198. Table 11-1 describes some reactions to acute and prolonged (chronic) stress.

TABLE 11-1 Some Reactions to Acute and Prolonged (Chronic) Stress	
Acute Stress Can Cause	**Prolonged (Chronic) Stress Can Cause**
Uneasiness and concern	Anxiety and panic attacks
Sadness	Depression or melancholia
Loss of appetite	Anorexia or overeating
Suppression of the immune system	Lowered resistance to infections, leading to increase in opportunistic viral and bacterial infections
Increased metabolism and use of body fats	Insulin-resistant diabetes Hypertension
Infertility	Amenorrhea or loss of sex drive Impotence, anovulation
Increased energy mobilization and use	Increased fatigue and irritability Decreased memory and learning
Increased cardiovascular tone	Increased risk for cardiac events (e.g., heart attack, angina, and sudden heart-related death) Increased risk of blood clots and stroke
Increased cardiopulmonary tone	Increased respiratory problems

Neurotransmitter Stress Responses

Serotonin is a brain catecholamine that plays an important role in mood, sleep, sexuality, appetite, and metabolism. It is one of the main neurotransmitters implicated in depression, and many medications used to treat depression do so by increasing the availability of serotonin. During times of stress, serotonin synthesis becomes more active. This stress-activated turnover of serotonin is at least partially mediated by the corticosteroids, and researchers believe this activation may dysregulate (impair) serotonin receptor sights and the brain's ability to use serotonin (Sadock & Sadock, 2008). The influence of stressful life events on the development of depression is well documented, but researchers still do not understand fully the relationship. This neurotransmitter stress response research sheds some new light on the process.

Immune Stress Responses

Cannon and Selye focused on the physical and mental responses of the nervous and endocrine systems to acute and chronic stress. Later work revealed that there was also an interaction between the nervous system and the immune system that occurs during the alarm phase of the GAS. In one study, rats were given a mixture of saccharine along with a drug that reduces the immune system (Ader & Cohen, 1975). Afterward, when given *only* the saccharine, the rats continued to have decreased immune responses, which indicated that stress itself negatively impacts the body's ability to produce a protective structure.

Studies in **psychoneuroimmunology** continue to provide evidence that stress, through the hypothalamic-pituitary-adrenal and sympathetic-adrenal medullary axes, can induce changes in the immune system. This model helps explain what many researchers and clinicians have believed and witnessed for centuries: there are links among stress (biopsychosocial), the immune system, and disease—a clear mind-body connection that may alter health outcomes. Stress may result in malfunctions in the immune system that are implicated in autoimmune disorders, immunodeficiency, and hypersensitivities.

Stress influences the immune system in several complex ways. As discussed earlier, corticosteroids are released in response to stress and inhibit the immune system, which increases susceptibility to illness (Sadock & Sadock, 2008). Conversely, stress can enhance the immune system and prepare the body to respond to injury. Cytokines, which are proteins and glycoproteins used for communication between cells, are normally released by immune cells when a pathogen is detected; they serve to activate and recruit other immune cells. During times of stress, these cytokines are released, and immunity is profoundly activated. But the activation is limited, since the cytokines stimulate further release of corticosteroids, which inhibits the immune system.

The immune response and the resulting cytokine activity in the brain raise questions regarding their connection with psychological and cognitive states such as depression (Anisman & Merali, 2005). Some cancers are treated with a type of cytokine molecules known as *interleukins*. These chemotherapy drugs tend to cause or increase depression. Furthermore, elevated cytokines and immune activation are often seen during episodes of severe depression.

New research in this field is promising. Investigators are examining how psychosocial factors, such as optimism and social support, moderate the stress response. They are mapping the biological and cellular mechanisms by which stress affects the immune system and testing new theories (Borak, 2006).

MEDIATORS OF THE STRESS RESPONSE

Stressors

A variety of dissimilar situations (e.g., emotional arousal, fatigue, fear, loss, humiliation, loss of blood, extreme happiness, unexpected success) all are capable of producing stress and triggering the stress response (Selye, 1993). No individual factor can be singled out as the cause of the stress response; however, stressors can be divided into two categories: physical and psychological. **Physical stressors** include environmental conditions (e.g., trauma and excessive cold or heat), as well as physical conditions (e.g., infection, hemorrhage, hunger, and pain). **Psychological stressors** include such things as divorce, loss of a job, unmanageable debt, the death of a loved one, retirement, and fear of a terrorist attack, as well as changes we might consider positive, such as marriage, the arrival of a new baby, or unexpected success.

Perception

Researchers have looked at the degree to which various life events upset a specific individual and have found that the *perception* of a stressor determines the person's emotional and psychological reactions to it (Rahe, 1995). Responses to stress and anxiety are affected by factors such as age, gender, culture, life experience, and lifestyle, all of which may work to either lessen or increase the degree of emotional or physical influence and the sequelae of stress. For example, a man in his 40s who has a new baby, has just purchased a home, and is laid off with 6 months' severance pay may feel the stress of the job loss more intensely than a man in his 60s who is financially secure and is asked to take an early retirement.

Personality

As mentioned earlier, part of our response to stressors is based on our own individual perceptions, which are colored by a variety of factors, including genetic structure and vulnerability, childhood experiences, coping strategies, and personal outlook on life and the world. All these factors combine to form a unique personality with specific strengths and vulnerabilities.

Social Support

Social support is a mediating factor with significant implications for nurses and other health care professionals. Strong social support from significant others can enhance mental and physical health and act as a significant buffer against distress. A shared identity—whether with a family, social network, or colleagues—helps people overcome stressors more adaptively (Haslam & Reicher, 2006). Numerous studies have found a strong correlation between lower mortality rates and intact support systems (Koenig, McCullough, & Larson, 2001).

Self-Help Groups

The proliferation of self-help groups attests to the need for social supports, and the explosive growth of a great variety of support groups reflects their effectiveness for many people. Many of the support groups currently available are for people going through similar stressful life events: Alcoholics Anonymous (a prototype for 12-step programs), Gamblers Anonymous, Reach for Recovery (for cancer patients), and Parents Without Partners, to note but a few.

Low- and High-Quality Support

It is important to differentiate between social support relationships of low quality and those of high quality. Low-quality support relationships (e.g., living in an abusive home situation or with a controlling and demeaning person) often negatively affect a person's coping effectiveness in a crisis. On the other hand, high-quality relationships have been linked to less loneliness, more supportive behavior, and greater life satisfaction (Hobfall & Vaux, 1993). High-quality emotional support is a critical factor in enhancing a person's sense of control and rebuilding feelings of self-esteem and competency after a stressful event. Supportive, high-quality relationships are relatively free from conflict and negative interactions and are close, confiding, and reciprocal (Hobfall & Vaux, 1993).

Culture

Each culture not only emphasizes certain problems of living more than others but also interprets emotional problems differently from other cultures. For example, the specific characteristics of the dysphoria of depression vary cross-culturally (Kim, 2002; Neighbors, 2003). The Hopi of North America express depressive states through feelings of guilt, shame, and sinfulness. On the other hand, Puerto Ricans and other Hispanics describe irritability, rage, and "nervousness" as indicators of a depressive affect.

Although Western European and North American cultures subscribe to a psychophysiological view of stress and somatic distress, this is not the dominant view in other cultures. The overwhelming majority of Asians, Africans, and Central Americans "not only express subjective distress in somatic terms, but actually experience this distress somatically, such that psychological interpretations of suffering may not be much use cross-culturally" (Gonzalez, Griffith, & Ruiz, 1995). The following vignette illustrates this point.

VIGNETTE

A 62-year-old Puerto Rican woman was referred for evaluation of incapacitating abdominal pain after a medical diagnostic evaluation gave negative results. The pain began 9 months earlier, approximately 1 month after her substance-abusing son was jailed for killing his girlfriend, whom the patient loved "like a daughter." The patient expected that the psychiatrist would prescribe medication that would take her pain away, and she was initially distressed to learn that she was expected to talk about her life. Although not ruling out the use of medication, the therapist explained to the patient that her pain might be related to the wrenching emotional ordeal of the past year. The therapist made it a point to validate the patient's pain and took great care not to imply that the pain was "merely" the expression of unacknowledged emotion. In particular, the therapist told the patient that he understood her pain to be real and that he did not expect her pain to be gone overnight. This approach allowed the patient to engage in a course of brief psychotherapy, during which her conflicted feelings about her son were examined, although these feelings were never specifically identified as the cause of her pain. Eventually, the patient felt strong enough to make drastic changes in her role as enabler of her children, at which point she reported that her pain was much improved (Gonzalez et al., 1995, p. 60). ■

Spirituality and Religious Beliefs

Many spiritual and religious beliefs help people cope with stress, and these deserve closer scientific investigation. Studies have demonstrated that spiritual practices can enhance the immune system and sense of well-being (Koenig et al., 2001). Some scholars propose that spiritual well-being helps people deal with health issues, primarily because spiritual beliefs help people cope with issues of living. Thus people with spiritual beliefs have established coping mechanisms they employ in normal life and can use when faced with illness. People who include spiritual solutions to physical or mental distress often gain a sense of comfort and

support that can aid in healing and lowering stress. Even prayer, in and of itself, can elicit the relaxation response (discussed later in this chapter), which is known to reduce stress physically and emotionally and to reduce stress on the immune system.

Figure 11-2 operationally defines the process of stress and the positive or negative results of attempts to relieve stress, and Box 11-1 identifies several stress busters that can be incorporated into our lives with little effort.

NURSING MANAGEMENT OF STRESS RESPONSES

Measuring Stress

In 1967, Holmes and Rahe published the Social Readjustment Rating Scale. This life-change scale measures the level of positive or negative stressful life events over a 1-year period. The level, or life-change unit, of each event is assigned a score based on the degree of severity and/or disruption. This questionnaire has been rescaled twice, first in 1978 and again in 1997 when it was adapted as the Recent Life Changes Questionnaire.

According to Rahe, since the scale was developed in 1967, life has become more demanding and stressful (Jayson, 2008). For example, travel is perceived as much more stressful now compared to 30 years ago. In 2007, online interviews were conducted to collect data from 1306 participants and then compared to data collected in the original study by Holmes and Rahe

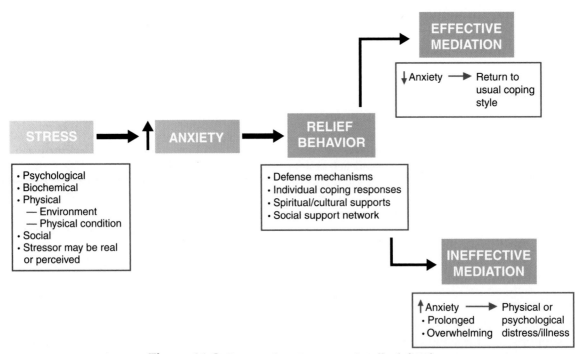

Figure 11-2 Stress and anxiety operationally defined.

BOX 11-1 Effective Stress Busters

Sleep
- Chronically stressed people are often fatigued, so go to sleep 30 to 60 minutes early each night for a few weeks.
- If you are still fatigued, try going to bed another 30 minutes earlier.
- Sleeping later in the morning is not helpful and can disrupt body rhythms.

Exercise (Aerobic)
- Exercise:
  - Can dissipate chronic and acute stress.
  - May decrease levels of anxiety, depression, and sensitivity to stress.
  - Can decrease muscle tension and increase endorphin levels.
- It is recommended you exercise for at least 30 minutes, three or more times a week.
- It is best to exercise at least 3 hours before bedtime.

Reduction or Cessation of Caffeine Intake
- Lowering or stopping caffeine intake can lead to more energy and fewer muscle aches and help you feel more relaxed.
- Slowly wean off coffee, tea, colas, and chocolate drinks.

Music (Classical or Soft Melodies of Choice)
- Listening to music increases your sense of relaxation.
- Increased healing effects may result.
- Therapeutically, music can:
  - Decrease agitation and confusion in older adults.
  - Increase quality of life in hospice settings.

Pets
- Pets can bring joy and reduce stress.
- They can be an important social support.
- Pets can alleviate medical problems aggravated by stress.

Massage
- Massage can slow the heart rate and relax the body.
- Alertness may actually increase.

TABLE 11-2 Perception of Life Stressors in 1967 and 2007

Life Change Event	1967	2007
Death of spouse	100	80
Death of family member	63	70
Divorce/separation	73/65	66
Job lay off or firing	47	62
Birth of child/pregnancy	40	60
Death of friend	50	50
Marriage	50	50
Retirement	45	49
Marital reconciliation	45	48
Change job field	36	47
Child leaves home	29	43

Data from First30Thirty Days. (2008). *Making changes today considered more difficult to handle than 30 years ago.* <http://www.first30days.com/pages/press_changereport.html> Accessed 23.4.09.

- Not all events are perceived to have the same degree of intensity or disruptiveness.
- Culture may dictate whether or not an event is stressful or how stressful it is.
- Different people may have different thresholds beyond which disruptions occur.
- The questionnaire equates change with stress.

Other stress scales that may be useful to nursing students have been developed. You might like to try the Perceived Stress Scale (Figure 11-3). Although there are no absolute scores, this scale measures how relatively uncontrollable, unpredictable, and overloaded you find your life. Try this scale in a clinical post-conference for comparison and discussion.

Assessing Coping Styles

People cope with life stressors in a variety of ways, and a number of factors can act as effective mediators to decrease stress in our lives. Rahe (1995) identified four discrete personal attributes (coping styles) people can develop to help manage stress:

1. Health-sustaining habits (e.g., medical compliance, proper diet, relaxation, pacing one's energy)
2. Life satisfactions (e.g., work, family, hobbies, humor, spiritual solace, arts, nature)
3. Social supports
4. Effective and healthy responses to stress

Examining these four coping categories can help nurses identify areas to target for improving their patients' responses to stress. Table 11-4 presents positive and negative responses to stress.

(First30Days, 2008). Although some life-change events were viewed as more stressful in 1967 (such as divorce and death of spouse), most events were viewed as more stressful in 2007 (Table 11-2).

Take a few minutes to assess your stress level for the past 6 to 12 months using the Recent Life Changes Questionnaire (Table 11-3). Keep in mind that when you administer the questionnaire, you must take into account the following:

TABLE 11-3 Recent Life Changes Questionnaire

Life-Changing Event	Life Change Unit*	Life-Changing Event	Life Change Unit*
HEALTH		Child leaving home:	
An injury or illness that:		To attend college	41
Kept you in bed a week or more or sent you to the hospital	74	Due to marriage	41
Was less serious than above	44	For other reasons	45
Major dental work	26	Change in arguments with spouse	50
Major change in eating habits	27	In-law problems	38
Major change in sleeping habits	26	Change in the marital status of your parents:	
Major change in your usual type and/or amount of recreation	28	Divorce	59
		Remarriage	50
WORK		Separation from spouse:	
Change to a new type of work	51	Due to work	53
Change in your work hours or conditions	35	Due to marital problems	76
Change in your responsibilities at work:		Divorce	96
More responsibilities	29	Birth of grandchild	43
Fewer responsibilities	21	Death of spouse	119
Promotion	31	Death of other family member:	
Demotion	42	Child	123
Transfer	32	Brother or sister	102
Troubles at work:		Parent	100
With your boss	29	**PERSONAL AND SOCIAL**	
With co-workers	35	Change in personal habits	26
With persons under your supervision	35	Beginning or ending of school or college	38
Other work troubles	28	Change of school or college	35
Major business adjustment	60	Change in political beliefs	24
Retirement	52	Change in religious beliefs	29
Loss of job:		Change in social activities	27
Laid off from work	68	Vacation	24
Fired from work	79	New close personal relationship	37
Correspondence course to help you in your work	18	Engagement to marry	45
		Girlfriend or boyfriend problems	39
HOME AND FAMILY		Sexual differences	44
Major change in living conditions	42	"Falling out" of a close personal relationship	47
Change in residence:		An accident	48
Move within the same town or city	25	Minor violation of the law	20
Move to a different town, city, or state	47	Being held in jail	75
Change in family get-togethers	25	Death of a close friend	70
Major change in health or behavior of family member	55	Major decision regarding your immediate future	51
Marriage	50	Major personal achievement	36
Pregnancy	67	**FINANCIAL**	
Miscarriage or abortion	65	Major change in finances:	
Gain of a new family member:		Increase in income	38
Birth of a child	66	Decrease in income	60
Adoption of a child	65	Investment and/or credit difficulties	56
A relative moving in with you	59	Loss or damage of personal property	43
Spouse beginning or ending work	46	Moderate purchase	20
		Major purchase	37
		Foreclosure on a mortgage or loan	58

*One-year totals ≥ 500 life change units are considered indications of high recent life stress.

From Miller, M. A., & Rahe, R. H. (1997). Life changes scaling for the 1990s. *Journal of Psychosomatic Research, 43* (3), 279–292.

Instructions: The questions in this scale ask you about your feelings and thoughts during the last month. In each case, please indicate with a check how often you felt or thought a certain way.

1. In the last month, how often have you been upset because of something that happened unexpectedly?

___0 never ___1 almost never ___2 sometimes ___3 fairly often ___4 very often

2. In the last month, how often have you felt that you were unable to control the important things in your life?

___0 never ___1 almost never ___2 sometimes ___3 fairly often ___4 very often

3. In the last month, how often have you felt nervous and "stressed"?

___0 never ___1 almost never ___2 sometimes ___3 fairly often ___4 very often

4. In the last month, how often have you felt confident about your ability to handle your personal problems?

___0 never ___1 almost never ___2 sometimes ___3 fairly often ___4 very often

5. In the last month, how often have you felt that things were going your way?

___0 never ___1 almost never ___2 sometimes ___3 fairly often ___4 very often

6. In the last month, how often have you found that you could not cope with all the things that you had to do?

___0 never ___1 almost never ___2 sometimes ___3 fairly often ___4 very often

7. In the last month, how often have you been able to control irritations in your life?

___0 never ___1 almost never ___2 sometimes ___3 fairly often ___4 very often

8. In the last month, how often have you felt that you were on top of things?

___0 never ___1 almost never ___2 sometimes ___3 fairly often ___4 very often

9. In the last month, how often have you been angered because of things that were outside of your control?

___0 never ___1 almost never ___2 sometimes ___3 fairly often ___4 very often

10. In the last month, how often have you felt difficulties were piling up so high that you could not overcome them?

___0 never ___1 almost never ___2 sometimes ___3 fairly often ___4 very often

Perceived stress scale scoring
Items 4, 5, 7, and 8 are the positively stated items. PSS-10 scores are obtained by reversing the scores on the positive items, e.g., 0=4, 1=3, 2=2, etc. and then adding all 10 items.

Figure 11-3 Perceived Stress Scale–10 Item (PSS-10). (Modified from the John D. and Catherine T. MacArthur Research Network on Socioeconomic Status and Health. <www.macses.ucsf.edu/Research/Psychosocial/notebook/PSS10.html>)

TABLE 11-4 Positive and Negative Responses to Stress

Positive Stress Responses	Negative Stress Responses
Problem solving—figuring out how to deal with the situation	Avoidance—choosing not to deal with the situation, letting negative feelings and situations fester and continue to become chronic
Using social support—calling in others who are caring and may be helpful	Self-blame—faulting oneself, which keeps the focus on minimizing one's self-esteem and prevents positive action toward resolution or working through of the feelings related to the event
Reframing—redefining the situation to see both positive and negative sides, as well as the way to use the situation to one's advantage	Wishful thinking—believing that things will resolve by themselves and that "everything will be fine" (a form of denial)

Adapted from Lazarus, R. S., & Folkman, S. (1984). *Stress, appraisal, and coping.* New York: Springer.

Managing Stress Through Relaxation Techniques

Poor management of stress has been correlated with an increased incidence of a number of physical and emotional conditions, such as heart disease, poor diabetes control, chronic pain, and significant emotional distress (Slater et al., 2003). Pychoneuroimmunology provides the foundation for several integrative therapies, also referred to as *mind-body therapies*. There is now considerable evidence that many mind-body therapies can be used as effective adjuncts to conventional medical treatment for a number of common clinical conditions (Astin et al., 2003). Chapter 36 offers a more detailed discussion of holistic, mind-body, and integrative therapies.

Nurses should be aware of a variety of stress and anxiety reduction techniques they can teach their patients. The following are some of the known benefits of stress reduction:

- Alters the course of certain medical conditions, such as high blood pressure, arrhythmias, arthritis, cancer, and peptic ulcers
- Decreases the need for medications such as insulin, analgesics, and antihypertensives
- Diminishes or eliminates the urge for unhealthy and destructive behaviors, such as smoking, addiction to drugs, insomnia, and overeating
- Increases cognitive functions such as learning and concentration and improves study habits
- Breaks up static patterns of thinking and allows fresh and creative ways of perceiving life events
- Increases the sense of well-being through endorphin release
- Reduces anxiety, increases comfort, and helps decrease sleep disturbances

Because no single stress-management technique is right for everyone, employing a mixture of techniques brings the best results. All are useful in a variety of situations for specific individuals. Essentially, there are stress-reducing techniques for every personality type, situation, and level of stress. Give them a try. Practicing relaxation techniques will help you not only help your patients reduce their stress levels but also manage your own physical responses to stressors. These techniques result in reduced heart and breathing rates, decreased blood pressure, improved oxygenation to major muscles, and reduced muscle tension. They also help manage subjective anxiety and improve appraisals of reality.

Relaxation Exercises

In 1938, Edmund Jacobson developed a rather simple procedure that elicits a relaxation response, which he coined **progressive muscle relaxation (PMR)** (Sadock & Sadock, 2008). This technique can be done without any external gauges or feedback and can be practiced almost anywhere. The premise behind PMR is that since anxiety results in tense muscles, one way to decrease anxiety is to nearly eliminate muscle contraction. This is accomplished by tensing groups of muscles (beginning with feet and ending with face) as tightly as possible for 8 seconds and suddenly releasing them. There is considerable research supporting the use of PMR as helpful for a number of medical conditions, such as "tension headaches" and psychiatric disorders, especially those with anxiety components (Conrad & Roth, 2006). Many good PMR scripts are available online.

Herbert Benson (1975, 1996) expanded on Jacobson's work by incorporating a state of mind that is conducive to relaxation. His techniques are influenced by Eastern practices and are achieved by adopting a calm and passive attitude and focusing on a pleasant mental image in a calm and peaceful environment. **Benson's relaxation techniques** allow the patient to switch from the sympathetic mode of the autonomic nervous system (fight-or-flight response) to a state of relaxation (the parasympathetic mode). Follow the steps in Box 11-2 to practice the relaxation response. Benson's relaxation techniques have been combined successfully with meditation and visual imagery to treat numerous disorders, such as diabetes, high blood pressure, migraine headaches, cancer, and peptic ulcers.

Meditation

Meditation follows the basic guidelines described for the relaxation response. It is a discipline for training the mind to develop greater calm and then using that calm to bring penetrative insight into one's experience. Meditation can be used to help people reach their deep inner resources for healing, calm the mind, and operate more efficiently in the world. It can help people develop strategies to cope with stress, make sensible adaptive choices under pressure, and feel more engaged in life (Miller, 2000).

BOX 11-2 Benson's Relaxation Technique

- Choose any word or brief phrase that reflects your belief system, such as *love, unity in faith and love, joy, shalom, one God, peace.*
- Sit in a comfortable position.
- Close your eyes.
- Deeply relax all your muscles, beginning at your feet and progressing up to your face. Keep them relaxed.
- Breathe through your nose. Become aware of your breathing. As you breathe out, say your word or phrase silently to yourself. For example, breathe IN... OUT (phrase), IN...OUT (phrase), and so forth. Breathe easily and naturally.
- Continue for 10 to 20 minutes. You may open your eyes and check the time but do not use an alarm. When you finish, sit quietly for several minutes, at first with your eyes closed and then with your eyes open. Do not stand up for a few minutes.
- Do not worry about whether you are successful in achieving a deep level of relaxation. Maintain a passive attitude, and permit relaxation to occur at its own pace. When distracting thoughts occur, try to ignore them by not dwelling on them, and return to repeating your word or phrase. With practice, the response should come with little effort. Practice the technique once or twice daily, but not within 2 hours after any meal, because the digestive process seems to interfere with the elicitation of the relaxation response.

From Benson, H. (1975). *The relaxation response.* New York: William Morrow & Company, Inc.

Meditation elicits a relaxation response by creating a hypometabolic state of quieting the sympathetic nervous system. Some people meditate using a visual object or a sound to help them focus. Others may find it useful to concentrate on their breathing while meditating. There are many meditation techniques, some with a spiritual base, such as Siddha meditation or prayer. Meditation is easy to practice anywhere. Some students find that meditating the morning of a test helps them focus and lessens anxiety. Keep in mind that meditation, like most other skills, must be practiced to produce the relaxation responses.

Guided Imagery

Guided imagery is a process whereby a person is led to envision images that are both calming and health enhancing and can be used in conjunction with Benson's relaxation technique. The content of the imagery exercises is shaped by the person helping with the imagery process. If a person has dysfunctional images, he or she can be helped to generate more effective and functional coping images to replace the depression- or anxiety-producing ones (Miller, 2000). For example, athletes have discovered that the use of images of positive coping and success can lead to improvement in performance (Aetna InteliHealth, 2008) (Box 11-3).

Imagery techniques are a useful tool in the management of many medical conditions and are an effective means of relieving pain for many people. Pain is reduced by inducing muscle relaxation and focusing the mind away from the pain. For some, imagery techniques are healing exercises in that they not only relieve the pain but also, in some cases, diminish the source of the pain (Koenig et al., 2001). Guided imagery is used by cancer patients to help reduce chronic high levels of cortisol, epinephrine, and catecholamines—which prevent the immune system from functioning effectively—and to produce β-endorphins—which increase pain thresholds and enhance lymphocyte proliferation (Koenig et al., 2001).

Often, audio recordings are made specifically for patients and their particular situations. However, many generic guided-imagery CDs and MP3s are available to patients and health care workers.

Breathing Exercises

Respiratory retraining, usually in the form of learning abdominal (diaphragmatic) breathing, has some definite merits in the modification of stress and anxiety reactions (Miller, 2000). One breathing exercise that has proved helpful for many patients with anxiety disorders has two parts (Box 11-4). The first part focuses on abdominal breathing, while the second part helps patients interrupt trains of thought, thereby quieting mental noise. With increasing skill, breathing becomes a tool for dampening the cognitive processes likely to induce stress and anxiety reactions.

Physical Exercise

Physical exercise can lead to protection from the harmful effects of stress on both physical and mental states. Regular physical activity was associated with lower incidence of all psychiatric disorders, except bipolar disorder, and comorbid conditions in subjects ages 14 to 24 in a study by Strohle and colleagues (2007). Researchers have been particularly interested in the influence exercise has over depression. Blumenthal and colleagues (2007) found that patients who had either 4 months of treatment with a selective serotonin reuptake inhibitor antidepressant or with aerobic exercise had similar relief of depression. Yoga, an ancient form of exercise, has been found to be helpful for depression when used

---

BOX 11-3 Script for Guided Imagery

- Imagine releasing all the tension in your body...letting it go.
- Now, with every breath you take, feel your body drifting down deeper and deeper into relaxation...floating down...deeper and deeper.
- Imagine a peaceful scene. You are sitting beside a clear, blue mountain stream. You are barefoot, and you feel the sun-warmed rock under your feet. You hear the sound of the stream tumbling over the rocks. The sound is hypnotic, and you relax more and more. You see the tall pine trees on the opposite shore bending in the gentle breeze. Breathe the clean, scented air, with each breath moving you deeper and deeper into relaxation. The sun warms your face.
- You are very comfortable. There is nothing to disturb you. You experience a feeling of well-being.
- You can return to this peaceful scene by taking time to relax. The positive feelings can grow stronger and stronger each time you choose to relax.
- You can return to your activities now, feeling relaxed and refreshed.

BOX 11-4 Deep Breathing Exercise

- Find a comfortable position.
- Relax your shoulders and chest; let your body relax.
- Shift to relaxed, abdominal breathing. Take a deep breath through your mouth, expanding the abdomen. Hold it for 3 seconds and then exhale slowly through the nose; exhale completely, telling yourself to relax.
- With every breath, turn attention to the muscular sensations that accompany the expansion of the belly.
- As you concentrate on your breathing, you will start to feel focused.
- Repeat this exercise for 2 to 5 minutes.

in conjunction with medication (Shapiro et al., 2007). Other popular forms of exercise that can decrease stress and improve well-being are walking, tai chi, dancing, cycling, aerobics, and water exercise.

Biofeedback

Through the use of sensitive instrumentation, biofeedback provides immediate and exact information regarding muscle activity, brain waves, skin temperature, heart rate, blood pressure, and other bodily functions. Indicators of the particular internal physiological process are detected and amplified by a sensitive recording device. An individual can achieve greater voluntary control over phenomena once considered to be exclusively involuntary if he or she knows instantaneously, through an auditory or visual signal, whether a somatic activity is increasing or decreasing.

Using biofeedback requires special training, and the technique is thought to be most effective for people with low to moderate hypnotic ability. For people with higher hypnotic ability, meditation, PMR, and other cognitive-behavioral therapy techniques produce the most rapid reduction in clinical symptoms.

With increasing recognition of the role of stress in a variety of medical illnesses, including diseases affected by immune dysfunction, biofeedback has emerged as an effective strategy for stress management. The necessity of using the complex instrumentation required to detect minute levels of muscle tension or certain patterns of electroencephalographic activity is uncertain, but it has been confirmed that teaching people to relax deeply and apply these skills in response to real-life stressors can be helpful in lowering stress levels.

Cognitive Reframing

Cognitive reframing has been found to be positively correlated with greater positive affect and higher self-esteem (Billingsley, Collins, & Miller, 2007). The goal of cognitive reframing is to change the individual's perceptions of stress by reassessing a situation and replacing irrational beliefs ("I can't pass this course.") with more positive self-statements ("If I choose to study for this course, I will increase my chances of success."). We can learn from most situations by asking ourselves:

- "What positive things came out of this situation or experience?"
- "What did I learn in this situation?"
- "What would I do in a different way?"

The desired result is to reframe a disturbing event or experience as less disturbing and to give the patient a sense of control over the situation. When the perception of the disturbing event is changed, there is less stimulation to the sympathetic nervous system, which in turn reduces the secretion of cortisol and catecholamines that destroy the balance of the immune system (Miller, 2000).

Cognitive distortions often include overgeneralizations ("He always…" or "I'll never…") and "should" statements ("I should have done better" or "He shouldn't have said that"). Table 11-5 shows some examples of cognitive reframing of anxiety-producing thoughts. Often, cognitive reframing is used along with progressive muscle relaxation and guided imagery to reduce stress.

Mindfulness

Mindfulness, a centuries-old form of meditation that has been dated back to Buddhist treatises, has received increased attention among health care professionals. It is based on the premise that we are not aware of ourselves moment-to-moment but operate on a sort of mental autopilot (Grossman et al., 2004). Mental activity often occurs unchecked; thoughts can become negative, untrue, unrealistic, and result in anxiety, depression, and lack of focus. Happiness or lack of happiness is not caused by outside forces but by our own perceptions and interpretations of reality.

TABLE 11-5 Cognitive Reframing of Irrational Thoughts

Irrational Thought	Positive Statements
"I'll never be happy until I am loved by someone I really care about."	"If I do not get love from one person, I can still get it from others and find happiness that way." "If someone I deeply care for rejects me, that will seem unfortunate, but I will hardly die." "If the only person I truly care for does not return my love, I can devote more time and energy to winning someone else's love and probably find someone better for me." "If no one I care for ever cares for me, I can still find enjoyment in friendships, in work, in books, and in other things."
"He should treat me better after all I do for him."	"I would like him to do certain things to show that he cares. If he chooses to continue to do things that hurt me after he understands what those things are, I am free to make choices about leaving or staying in this hurtful relationship."

Adapted from Ellis, A., & Harper, R. A. (1975). *A new guide to rational living.* North Hollywood, CA: Wilshire.

To become mindful, practitioners suggest observing and monitoring the content of our consciousness and recognize that thoughts are just thoughts. Negative interpretations ("Mowing the lawn is a hot, dirty, and exhausting job.") can become positive ("Mowing the lawn is fantastic exercise.") when mindfulness is practiced.

This moment-to-moment awareness also extends to the outer world. Being mindful includes being in the moment by paying attention to what is going on around you—what you are seeing, feeling, hearing. Imagine how much you miss during an ordinary walk to class if you spend it staring straight ahead as your mind wanders from one concern to the next. You miss the pattern of sunlight filtered through the leaves, the warmth of the sunshine on your skin, and the sounds of birds calling out to one another. By focusing on the here and now, rather than past and future, you are meditating and practicing mindfulness.

Mindfulness has been formalized as the Mindfulness Based Stress Reduction Program and is being used extensively throughout the United States. It is discussed in the bestselling book *Wherever You Go, There You Are* (2005) by Jon Kabat-Zinn. The goal of this program is to make mindfulness a continuous process. With practice, people can gradually learn to let go of destructive internal dialogue and reactiveness. Practicing mindfulness can be done at any time, and proponents suggest it becomes a way of life.

Journaling

Journaling is an extremely useful and surprisingly simple method of identifying stressors. It is a technique that can ease worry and obsession, help identify hopes and fears, increase energy levels and confidence, and facilitate the grieving process (Cullen, 2004). Keeping an informal diary of daily events and activities can reveal surprising information on sources of daily stress. Simply noting which activities put a strain on energy and time, which trigger anger or anxiety, and which precipitate a negative physical experience (e.g., headache, backache, fatigue) can be an important first step in stress reduction. Writing down thoughts and feelings is helpful not only in dealing with stress and stressful events but also in healing both physically and emotionally (Cullen, 2004). According to Cullen (2004), writing can strengthen the immune system, decrease reliance on pain medication, improve lung function in people with asthma, and reduce symptoms in people with rheumatoid arthritis.

Humor

The use of humor as a cognitive approach is a good example of how a stressful situation can be "turned upside down." The intensity attached to a stressful thought or situation can be dissipated when it is made to appear absurd or comical. Essentially, the bee loses its sting.

KEY POINTS TO REMEMBER

- Stress is a universal experience and an important concept when caring for any patient in any setting.
- The body responds similarly whether stressors are real or perceived and whether the stressor is negative or positive.
- Physiologically, the body reacts to anxiety and fear by arousal of the sympathetic nervous system. Specific symptoms include rapid heart rate, increased blood pressure, diaphoresis, peripheral vasoconstriction, restlessness, repetitive questioning, feelings of frustration, and difficulty concentrating.
- Cannon introduced the fight-or-flight model of stress, and Selye introduced the widely known general adaptation syndrome (GAS).
- The psychoneuroimmunology model describes the immune system's response to stress and effect on neural pathways in the brain.
- Prolonged stress can lead to chronic psychological and physiological responses when not mitigated at an early stage (see Table 11-1).
- There are basically two categories of stressors: physical (e.g., heat, hunger, cold, noise, trauma) and psychological (e.g., death of a loved one, loss of job, schoolwork, humiliation).
- Age, gender, culture, life experience, and lifestyle all are important in identifying the degree of stress a person is experiencing.
- Lowering the effects of chronic stress can alter the course of many physical conditions; decrease the need for some medications; diminish or eliminate the urge for unhealthy and destructive behaviors such as smoking, insomnia, and drug addiction; and increase a person's cognitive functioning.
- Perhaps the most important factor to assess is a person's support system. Studies have shown that high-quality social and intimate supports can go a long way toward minimizing the long-term effects of stress.
- Cultural differences exist in the extent to which people perceive an event as stressful and in the behaviors they consider appropriate to deal with a stressful event.
- Spiritual practices have been found to lead to an enhanced immune system and a sense of well-being.
- A variety of relaxation techniques are available to reduce the stress response and elicit the relaxation response, which results in improved physical and psychological functioning.

CRITICAL THINKING

1. Assess your level of stress using the Recent Life Changes Questionnaire found in Table 11-3, and evaluate your potential for illness in the coming year. Identify stress-reduction techniques you think would be useful to learn.

2. Teach a classmate the deep-breathing exercise identified in this chapter (see Box 11-4).

3. Assess a classmate's coping styles, and have the same classmate assess yours. Discuss the relevance of your findings.

4. Using Figure 11-1, explain to a classmate the short-term effects of stress on the sympathetic–adrenal medulla system, and identify three long-term effects if the stress is not relieved. How would you use this information to provide patient teaching? If your classmate were the patient, how would his or her response indicate that effective learning had taken place?

5. Using Figure 11-1, have a classmate explain to you the short-term effects of stress on the hypothalamus–pituitary–adrenal cortex and the eventual long-term effects if the stress becomes chronic. Summarize to your classmate your understanding of what was presented. Using your knowledge of the short-term effects of stress on the hypothalamus–pituitary–adrenal cortex and the long-term effects of stress, develop and present a patient education model related to stress for your clinical group.

6. In postconference discuss a patient you have cared for who had one of the stress-related effects identified in Figure 11-1. See if you can identify some stressors in the patient's life and possible ways to lower chronic stress levels.

CHAPTER REVIEW

1. The nurse is caring for a patient who is experiencing a crisis. Which symptoms would indicate that the patient is in the stage of alarm?
   1. Constricted pupils
   2. Dry mouth
   3. Decrease in heart rate
   4. Sudden drop in blood pressure

2. If it is determined that a patient will benefit from guided imagery, what teaching should the nurse provide?
   1. Focus on a visual object or sound.
   2. Become acutely aware of your breathing pattern.
   3. Envision an image of a place that is peaceful.
   4. Develop deep abdominal breathing.

3. A patient is going to undergo biofeedback. Which patient statement requires further teaching by the nurse?
   1. "This will measure my muscle activity, heart rate, and blood pressure."
   2. "It will help me recognize how my body responds to stress."
   3. "I will feel a small shock of electricity if I tell a lie."
   4. "The instruments will know if my skin temperature changes."

4. A patient has told the nurse that she knows she is going to lose her job, which scares her because she needs to work to pay her bills. Which nursing response reflects the positive stress response of *problem solving*?
   1. "What are your plans to find a new job?"
   2. "Can you call your parents to support you during this time?"
   3. "Is it possible that this job loss is an opportunity to find a better paying job?"
   4. "I'm sure everything will turn out just fine."

5. The nurse is caring for four patients. Which patient would be at highest risk for psychosocial compromise? The patient who has experienced:
   1. the death of a friend.
   2. a divorce.
   3. a recent job layoff.
   4. the death of a spouse.

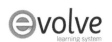 Visit the Evolve website for an **Audio Chapter Summary, Chapter Review Answers & Rationales, Critical Thinking Answer Guidelines,** and additional resources related to the content in this chapter: **http://evolve.elsevier.com/Varcarolis/foundations**

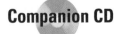 Use the Companion CD to prepare for tests and the NCLEX® Examination with **Test-Taking Strategies** for psychiatric mental health nursing and hundreds of **Review Questions**.

References

Ader, R., & Cohen, N. (1975). Behaviorally conditioned immunosuppression. *Psychosomatic Medicine, 37,* 333–340.

Aetna InteliHealth. (2008, April 30). *Guided imagery.* Retrieved August 19, 2008 from the Aetna InteliHealth website: http://www.intelihealth.com/IH/ihtIH/WSIHW000/8513/34968/358820.html?d=dmtContent

Anisman, H., & Merali, Z. (2005). Cytokines, stress, and depressive illness: Brain-immune interactions. *Annals of Medicine, 35*(1), 2–11.

Astin, J. A., Shapiro, S. L., Eisenberg, D. M., & Forys, K. L. (2003). Mind-body medicine: State of science, implications for practice. *Journal of the American Board of Family Practice, 16*(2), 131–147.

Benson, H. (1975). *The relaxation response* (2nd ed.). New York: William Morrow & Company, Inc.

Benson, H., & Stark, M. (1996). *Timeless healing.* New York: Scribner.

Billingsley, S. K., Collins, A. M., & Miller, M. (2007). Healthy student, healthy nurse: A stress management workshop. *Nurse Educator, 32*(2), 49–51.

Blumenthal, J. A., Babyak, M. A., Doraiswamy, P. M., Watkins, L., Hoffman, B. M., Barbour, K. A., et al. (2007). Exercise and pharmacotherapy in the treatment of major depressive disorder. *Psychosomatic Medicine, 69,* 587–596.

Borak, Y. (2006). The immune system and happiness. *Autoimmunity reviews, 5,* 523–537.

Conrad, A., & Roth, W. T. (2006). Muscle relaxation therapy for anxiety disorders: It works but how? *Journal of Anxiety Disorders, 21*(3), 243–264.

Cullen, D. (2004, February 10). *The power of the pen.* Retrieved February 3, 2005, from The Age website: http://www.theage.com.au/articles/2004/02/09/1076175101614.html?

Data from First30Thirty Days. (2008). *Making changes today considered more difficult to handle than 30 years ago.* <http://www.first30days.com/pages/press_changereport.html> Accessed 23.4.09.

Gonzalez, C. A., Griffith, E. E. H., & Ruiz, P. (1995). Cross-cultural issues in psychiatric treatment. In G. O. Gabbard (Ed.), *Treatment of psychiatric disorders* (2nd ed., Vol. I, pp. 55–74). Washington, DC: American Psychiatric Press.

Grossman, P., Niemann, L., Schmidt, S., & Walach, H. (2004). Mindfulness-based stress reduction and health benefits: A meta-analysis. *Journal of Psychosomatic Research, 57,* 35–43.

Haslam, S. A., & Reicher, S. (2006). Stressing the group: Social identity and the unfolding dynamics of responses to stress. *Journal of Applied Psychology, 91,* 1037–1052.

Hobfall, S. E., & Vaux, A. (1993). Social support: Social resources and social context. In L. Goldberger, S. Breznitz (Eds.), *Handbook of stress: Theoretical and clinical aspects* (2nd ed., pp. 685–705). New York: Free Press.

Holmes, T. H., & Rahe, R. H. (1967). The social readjustment rating scale. *Journal of Psychosomatic Research, 11,* 213.

Jayson, S. (2008, May 5). Survey: It's harder to readjust to life's changes these days. *USA Today.* Retrieved October 21, 2008 from http://www.usatoday.com/news/health/2008-05-05-life-changes_N.htm

Kabat-Zinn, J. (2005). *Wherever you go, there you are* (10th ed.). New York: Hyperion.

Kajantie, E., & Phillips, D. I. (2006). The effects of sex and hormonal status on the physiological response to acute psychosocial stress. *Psychoneuroendocrinology, 31,* 151–178.

Kim, M. (2002). Measuring depression in Korean Americans: Development of the Kim Depression Scale for Korean Americans. *Journal of Transcultural Nursing, 13*(2), 109–117.

Koenig, H. G., McCullough, M. E., & Larson, D. B. (2001). *Handbook of religion and health.* New York: Oxford University Press.

Lazarus, R. S., & DeLongis, A. (1983). Psychological stress and coping in aging. *American Psychologist, 38,* 245.

McKewan, B. S. (2005). Stressed or stressed out: What is the difference? *Journal of Psychiatry Neuroscience, 30*(5), 315–318.

Miller, W. R. (2000). *Integrating spirituality into treatment.* Washington, DC: American Psychological Association.

Neighbors, H. (2003, January 22). *The (mis)diagnosis of African Americans: Implementing DSM criteria in the hospital and community.* Retrieved April 4, 2004, from Psychiatry Grand Rounds, Department of Psychiatry, University of Michigan website: http://www.med.umich.edu/psych/mlk2003.htm

Rahe, R. H. (1995). Stress and psychiatry. In H. I. Kaplan, B. J. Sadock (Eds.), *Comprehensive textbook of psychiatry/VI* (6th ed., Vol. 2, pp. 1545–1559). Baltimore: Williams & Wilkins.

Sadock, V. A., & Sadock, B. J. (2008). *Kaplan and Sadock's concise textbook of clinical psychiatry* (3rd ed.).

Selye, H. (1974). *Stress without distress.* Philadelphia: Lippincott.

Selye, H. (1993). History of the stress concept. In L. Goldberger, S. Breznitz (Eds.), *Handbook of stress: Theoretical and clinical aspects* (2nd ed., pp. 7–17). New York: Free Press.

Shapiro, D., Cook, I. A., Davydov, D. M., Ottaviani, C., Leuchter, A. F., & Abrams, M. (2007). Yoga as a complementary treatment of depression: Effects of traits and moods on treatment outcome. *Evidenced Based Complementary and Alternative Medicine* [online]. Retrieved October 21, 2008 from http://ecam.oxfordjournals.org/cgi/content/abstract/nel114v1

Slater, M. A., Steptoe, A., Weickgenant, A., & Dimsdale, J. E. (2003). Psychiatry. In A. Tasman, J. Kay, J. A. Lieberman (Eds.), *Behavioral medicine* (2nd ed.). West Sussex, England: Wiley.

Strohle, A., Hofler, M., Pfister, H., Muller, A., Hoyer, J., Wittchen, H., et al. (2007). Physical activity and prevalence and incidence of mental disorders in adolescents and young adults. *Psychological Medicine, 37,* 1657–1666.

Wang, J., Korczykowski, M., Rao, H., Fan, Y., Pluta, J., Gur, R. C., et al. (2007). Gender difference in neural response to psychological stress. *Social Cognitive and Affective Neuroscience Advance Access, 2*(3), 227–239.

Weber, K., Rockstroh, B., Borgelt, J., Awiszus, B., Popov, T., Hoffmann, K., et al. (2008). Stress load during childhood affects psychopathology in psychiatric patients. *BioMedCentral Psychiatry, 8*(63). Retrieved August 19, 2008 from http://www.biomedcentral.com/1471–244X/8/63

Williamson, D., Dewey, A., & Steinberg, H. (2001). Mood change through physical exercise in nine- to ten-year-old children. *Perceptual and Motor Skills, 93*(1), 311–316.

Yang, E. V., & Glaser, R. (2002). Stress-associated immunomodulation and its implications for response to vaccination. *Expert Review of Vaccines, 1*(4), 453–459.

Unit 4

Psychobiological Disorders

A PATIENT SPEAKS

I am a 48-year-old woman, and I was born and raised in Maryland. I grew up with my parents and my older brother. I quit school in the twelfth grade when I had my first daughter. I have been married twice, and I am a widow. I have two daughters who are 30 and 26 years old. I have worked taking care of children and doing housekeeping. I first became aware of my obsessions and compulsions at the age of 12. I was cleaning my body all the time and always thinking of germs; it caused me a lot of stress. My hands used to get red, and touching things was awful for me. I went to a hospital to get help, but they did not know what it was; they just said that I was clean.

In my teens, I became depressed all the time. I went to the hospital again, but it did not seem to help. I know that my state of mind and OCD played a great part in my two marriages. I used to make my children clean up all the time, and I was always checking behind them. My husband did the same thing. They say, "Cleanliness is next to godliness." Drugs became a part of my life in my 30s and caused me great pain. I started to use cocaine after my husband died, and I used for 12 years.

Two years ago, I was hospitalized for depression, and I was homeless. The hospital referred me to a 28-day drug rehabilitation program. The drug program referred me to a women's recovery house shelter. I lived there for 6 months while I attended an outpatient mental health center. I got treatment for depression, hallucinations, OCD, and substance use. I had a therapist and psychiatrist in the clinic, along with dual-diagnosis group therapy. I also attended an intensive outpatient drug program right down the hall in the clinic. I worked on my OCD with my therapist, gradually touching on things that made me anxious. In the beginning, I could not stand to touch people or any of their belongings; I had to cover my hand to touch doorknobs. I learned to tolerate my anxiety about being around people.

After being drug-free for 6 months, I was eligible for an independent apartment in a group of apartments supervised by case managers. I love having my own apartment. I even got a part-time job as a receptionist at the YWCA. My life is good now that I am clean. My children are still in my life, and we get along better. I have great friends, and I am setting goals. I help my daughter take care of my mother, who has Alzheimer's disease. When I am nervous, the voices do come back, and I start to clean too much. But I take my medicine regularly, and I usually can calm myself with the help of my family. I still go to the clinic once a month.

CHAPTER 12

Anxiety and Anxiety Disorders

Margaret Jordan Halter, Elizabeth M. Varcarolis, and Nancy Christine Shoemaker

Key Terms and Concepts

Objectives

1. Compare and contrast the four levels of anxiety in relation to perceptual field, ability to learn, and physical and other defining characteristics.
2. Identify defense mechanisms and consider one adaptive and one maladaptive use of each.
3. Identify genetic, biological, psychological, and cultural factors that may contribute to anxiety disorders.
4. Describe clinical manifestations of each anxiety disorder.
5. Formulate four appropriate nursing diagnoses that can be used in treating a person with an anxiety disorder.
6. Name three defense mechanisms commonly found in patients with anxiety disorders.
7. Describe feelings that may be experienced by nurses caring for patients with anxiety disorders.
8. Propose realistic outcome criteria for a patient with (a) generalized anxiety disorder, (b) panic disorder, and (c) posttraumatic stress disorder.
9. Describe five basic nursing interventions used for patients with anxiety disorders.
10. Discuss three classes of medications appropriate for anxiety disorders.
11. Describe advanced practice and basic level interventions for anxiety disorders.

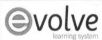 Visit the Evolve website for an **Audio Glossary & Flashcards, Concept Map Creator**, and additional resources related to the content in this chapter: **http://evolve.elsevier.com/Varcarolis/foundations**

For most people, anxiety is an everyday part of life. "I got really anxious when I couldn't find a parking space just before my final exam; I think I would have done better without that worry." For some people, however, anxiety-related symptoms become severely debilitating and interfere with normal functioning. "Today I got so worried I wouldn't find a parking space before the final exam, I stayed home." Or imagine being so incapacitated by anxiety, you live in dread of germs

to the point where hand washing has become the focal point of your day. Consider repeatedly feeling the immediate terror of emotionally reliving a horrific event in your life, such as hydroplaning on the expressway and finding yourself facing oncoming traffic in the opposite lanes. You would likely refuse to drive when it rains. In this chapter, we will examine the concept of anxiety, defenses against anxiety, and an overview of anxiety disorders and their treatment.

Anxiety

Anxiety is a universal human experience and is the most basic of emotions. It can be defined as a feeling of apprehension, uneasiness, uncertainty, or dread resulting from a real or perceived threat. **Fear** is a reaction to a specific danger, whereas anxiety is a vague sense of dread related to an unspecified or unknown danger. However, the body physiologically reacts in similar ways to both anxiety and fear. Another important distinction between anxiety and fear is that anxiety affects us at a deeper level. It invades the central core of the personality and erodes feelings of self-esteem and personal worth.

Dysfunctional behavior is often a defense against anxiety. When behavior is recognized as dysfunctional, nurses can initiate interventions to reduce anxiety. As anxiety decreases, dysfunctional behavior will frequently decrease, and vice versa.

Normal anxiety is a healthy reaction necessary for survival. It provides the energy needed to carry out the tasks involved in living and striving toward goals. Anxiety motivates people to make and survive change. It prompts constructive behaviors, such as studying for an examination, being on time for a job interview, preparing for a presentation, and working toward a promotion.

An understanding of the levels and defensive patterns used in response to anxiety is basic to psychiatric mental health nursing care. This understanding is essential for assessing and planning interventions to lower a patient's level of anxiety (as well as one's own) effectively. With practice, you will become skilled at identifying levels of anxiety, understanding the defenses used to alleviate anxiety, and evaluating the possible stressors that contribute to increased levels of anxiety.

LEVELS OF ANXIETY

As discussed in Chapter 2, Hildegard Peplau had a profound role in shaping the specialty of psychiatric mental health nursing. She identified anxiety as one of the most important concepts and developed an anxiety model that consists of four levels: mild, moderate, severe, and panic (Peplau, 1968). The boundaries between these levels are not distinct, and the behaviors and characteristics of individuals experiencing anxiety can and often do overlap. Identification of the specific level of anxiety is essential because interventions are based on the *degree* of the patient's anxiety.

Mild Anxiety

Mild anxiety, which occurs in the normal experience of everyday living, allows an individual to perceive reality in sharp focus. A person experiencing a mild level of anxiety sees, hears, and grasps more information, and problem solving becomes more effective. Physical symptoms may include slight discomfort, restlessness, irritability, or mild tension-relieving behaviors (e.g., nail biting, foot or finger tapping, fidgeting).

Moderate Anxiety

As anxiety increases, the perceptual field narrows, and some details are excluded from observation. The person experiencing **moderate anxiety** sees, hears, and grasps less information and may demonstrate **selective inattention**, in which only certain things in the environment are seen or heard unless they are pointed out. The ability to think clearly is hampered, but learning and problem solving can still take place, although not at an optimal level. Physical symptoms include tension, pounding heart, increased pulse and respiratory rate, perspiration, and mild somatic symptoms (gastric discomfort, headache, urinary urgency). Voice tremors and shaking may be noticed. Mild or moderate anxiety levels can be constructive, because anxiety may be a signal that something in the person's life needs attention or is dangerous (see the Case Study and Nursing Care Plan for Moderate Anxiety on the Evolve website).

Severe Anxiety

The perceptual field of a person experiencing severe anxiety is greatly reduced. A person with **severe anxiety** may focus on one particular detail or many scattered details and have difficulty noticing what is going on in the environment, even when it is pointed out by another. Learning and problem solving are not possible at this level, and the person may be dazed and confused. Behavior is automatic and aimed at reducing or relieving anxiety. Somatic symptoms (headache, nausea, dizziness, insomnia) often increase; trembling and a pounding heart are common, and the person may experience hyperventilation and a sense of impending doom or dread (see Case Study and Nursing Care Plan 12-1 on pages 239–241).

Panic

Panic is the most extreme level of anxiety and results in markedly disturbed behavior. Someone in a state of panic is unable to process what is going on in the environment and may lose touch with reality. The behavior that results may be manifested as pacing, running, shouting, screaming, or withdrawal. Hallucinations, or false sensory perceptions (e.g., seeing people or objects not really there), may be experienced. Physical behavior may become erratic, uncoordinated, and impulsive. Automatic behaviors are used to reduce and relieve anxiety, although such efforts may be ineffective. Acute panic may lead to exhaustion.

Review Table 12-1 which distinguishes among the levels of anxiety in regard to their (1) effects on perceptual field, (2) effects on ability to learn, and (3) physical and other defining characteristics.

TABLE 12-1 Levels of Anxiety

Mild	Moderate	Severe	Panic
PERCEPTUAL FIELD			
May have heightened perceptual field	Has narrow perceptual field; grasps less of what is going on	Has greatly reduced perceptual field	Unable to focus on the environment
Is alert and can see, hear, and grasp what is happening in the environment	Can attend to more *if pointed out by another* (selective inattention)	Focuses on details or one specific detail Attention scattered	Experiences the utmost state of terror and emotional paralysis; feels he or she "ceases to exist"
Can identify things that are disturbing and are producing anxiety		Completely absorbed with self	In panic, may have hallucinations or delusions that take the place of reality
		May not be able to attend to events in environment *even when pointed out by others*	
		In severe to panic levels of anxiety, the environment is blocked out. It is as if these events are not occurring.	
ABILITY TO LEARN			
Able to work effectively toward a goal and examine alternatives	Able to solve problems but not at optimal ability	Unable to see connections between events or details	May be mute or have extreme psychomotor agitation leading to exhaustion
	Benefits from guidance of others	Has distorted perceptions	Shows disorganized or irrational reasoning
Mild and moderate levels of anxiety can alert the person that something is wrong and can stimulate appropriate action.		**Severe and panic levels prevent problem solving and discovery of effective solutions. Unproductive relief behaviors are called into play, thus perpetuating a vicious cycle.**	
PHYSICAL OR OTHER CHARACTERISTICS			
Slight discomfort Attention-seeking behaviors Restlessness Irritability or impatience Mild tension-relieving behavior (foot or finger tapping, lip chewing, fidgeting)	Voice tremors Change in voice pitch Difficulty concentrating Shakiness Repetitive questioning Somatic complaints, (urinary frequency and urgency, headache, backache, insomnia) Increased respiration rate Increased pulse rate Increased muscle tension More extreme tension-relieving behavior (pacing, banging of hands on table)	Feelings of dread Ineffective functioning Confusion Purposeless activity Sense of impending doom More intense somatic complaints (dizziness, nausea, headache, sleeplessness) Hyperventilation Tachycardia Withdrawal Loud and rapid speech Threats and demands	Experience of terror Immobility or severe hyperactivity or flight Dilated pupils Unintelligible communication or inability to speak Severe shakiness Sleeplessness Severe withdrawal Hallucinations or delusions; likely out of touch with reality

DEFENSES AGAINST ANXIETY

Sigmund Freud and his daughter, Anna Freud, outlined most of the defense mechanisms we recognize today. Defense mechanisms are automatic coping styles that protect people from anxiety and maintain self-image by blocking feelings, conflicts, and memories. Although they operate all the time, defense mechanisms are not always apparent to the individual using them. Adaptive use of defense mechanisms helps people lower anxiety to achieve goals in acceptable ways. Maladaptive use of defense mechanisms occurs when

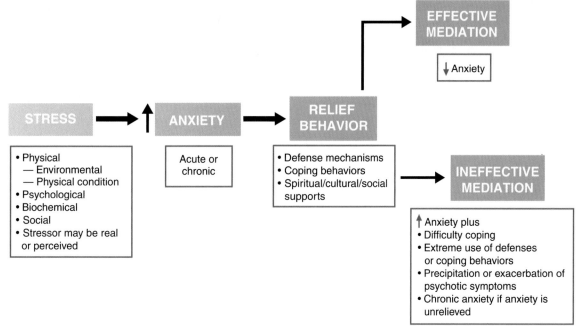

Figure 12-1 Anxiety operationally defined.

one or several are used in excess, particularly in the overuse of immature defenses. Figure 12-1 operationally defines anxiety and shows how defenses come into play.

With the exception of sublimation and altruism, which are always healthy coping mechanisms, all defense mechanisms can be used in both healthy and unhealthy ways. Most people use a variety of defense mechanisms but not always at the same level. Keep in mind that evaluating whether the use of defense mechanisms is adaptive or maladaptive is determined for the most part by their *frequency*, *intensity*, and *duration* of use. Table 12-2 describes defense mechanisms and their adaptive and maladaptive uses.

TABLE 12-2 Adaptive and Maladaptive Uses of Defense Mechanisms		
Defense Mechanism	**Adaptive Use**	**Maladaptive Use**
Compensation is used to make up for perceived deficiencies and cover up shortcomings related to these deficiencies to protect the conscious mind from recognizing them.	A shorter-than-average man becomes assertively verbal and excels in business.	An individual drinks alcohol when self-esteem is low to temporarily diffuse discomfort.
Conversion is the unconscious transformation of anxiety into a physical symptom with no organic cause. Often the symptom functions to gain attention or as an excuse.	A student is unable to take a final examination because of a terrible headache.	A man becomes blind after seeing his wife flirt with other men.
Denial involves escaping unpleasant, anxiety-causing thoughts, feelings, wishes, or needs by ignoring their existence.	A man reacts to news of the death of a loved one by saying, "No, I don't believe you. The doctor said he was fine."	A woman whose husband died 3 years earlier still keeps his clothes in the closet and talks about him in the present tense.
Displacement is the transference of emotions associated with a particular person, object, or situation to another nonthreatening person, object, or situation.	A patient criticizes a nurse after his family fails to visit.	A child who is unable to acknowledge fear of his father becomes fearful of animals.

Continued

TABLE 12-2 Adaptive and Maladaptive Uses of Defense Mechanisms—cont'd

Defense Mechanism	Adaptive Use	Maladaptive Use
Dissociation is a disruption in the usually integrated functions of consciousness, memory, identity, or perception of the environment. It may result in a separation between feeling and thought. This can also manifest itself in compartmentalizing uncomfortable or unpleasant aspects of oneself.	An art student is able to mentally separate herself from the noisy environment as she becomes absorbed in her work.	As the result of an abusive childhood and the need to separate from its realities, a woman finds herself perpetually in a world where she feels disconnected from reality.
Identification is attributing to oneself the characteristics of another person or group. This may be done consciously or unconsciously.	An 8-year-old girl dresses up like her teacher and puts together a pretend classroom for her friends.	A young boy thinks a neighborhood pimp with money and drugs is someone to look up to.
Intellectualization is a process in which events are analyzed based on remote, cold facts and without passion, rather than incorporating feeling and emotion into the processing.	Despite the fact that a man has lost his farm to a tornado, he analyzes his options and leads his child to safety.	A man responds to the death of his wife by focusing on the details of day care and operating the household, rather than processing the grief with his children.
Introjection is the process by which the outside world is incorporated or absorbed into a person's view of the self.	After his wife's death, a man has transient complaints of chest pains and difficulty breathing—the symptoms his wife had before she died.	A young child whose parents were overcritical and belittling grows up thinking that she is no good. She has taken on her parents' evaluation of her as part of her self-image.
Projection refers to the unconscious rejection of emotionally unacceptable features and attributing them to other people, objects, or situations. You can remember this defense through the childhood retort of "What you say is what you are."	A man who is unconsciously attracted to other women teases his wife about flirting.	A woman who has repressed an attraction toward other women refuses to socialize. She fears another woman will make homosexual advances toward her.
Rationalization consists of justifying illogical or unreasonable ideas, actions, or feelings by developing acceptable explanations that satisfy the teller as well as the listener.	An employee says, "I didn't get the raise because the boss doesn't like me."	A man who thinks his son was fathered by another man excuses his malicious treatment of the boy by saying, "He is lazy and disobedient," when that is not the case.
Reaction formation is when unacceptable feelings or behaviors are controlled and kept out of awareness by developing the opposite behavior or emotion.	A recovering alcoholic constantly preaches about the evils of drink.	A woman who has an unconscious hostility toward her daughter is overprotective and hovers over her to protect her from harm, interfering with her normal growth and development.
Regression is reverting to an earlier, more primitive and childlike pattern of behavior that may or may not have been previously exhibited.	A 4-year-old boy with a new baby brother starts sucking his thumb and wanting a bottle.	A man who loses a promotion starts complaining to others, hands in sloppy work, misses appointments, and comes in late for meetings.
Repression is a first-line psychological defense against anxiety. It is the temporary or long-term exclusion of unpleasant or unwanted experiences, emotions, or ideas from conscious awareness. This happens at an *unconscious* level.	A man forgets his wife's birthday after a marital fight.	A woman is unable to enjoy sex after having pushed out of awareness a traumatic sexual incident from childhood.

TABLE 12-2 Adaptive and Maladaptive Uses of Defense Mechanisms—cont'd

Defense Mechanism	Adaptive Use	Maladaptive Use
Splitting is the inability to integrate the positive and negative qualities of oneself or others into a cohesive image. Aspects of the self and of others tend to alternate between opposite poles; for example, either good, loving, worthy, and nurturing, or bad, hateful, destructive, rejecting, and worthless.	A toddler views her parents as superhuman and wants to be like them.	A 26-year-old woman has difficulty maintaining close relationships. Despite the fact that she can initially find many positive qualities about new acquaintances, eventually she becomes disillusioned when they turn out to be flawed.
Sublimation is an unconscious process of substituting mature, constructive, and socially acceptable activity for immature, destructive, and unacceptable impulses. Often these impulses are sexual or aggressive.	A woman who is angry with her boss writes a short story about a heroic woman.	The use of sublimation is always constructive.
Suppression is the *conscious* denial of a disturbing situation or feeling. For example, Jessica has been studying for the state board examination for a week solid. She says, "I won't worry about paying my rent until after my exam tomorrow."	A businessman who is preparing to make an important speech later in the day is told by his wife that morning that she wants a divorce. Although visibly upset, he puts the incident aside until after his speech, when he can give the matter his total concentration.	A woman who feels a lump in her breast shortly before leaving for a 3-week vacation puts the information in the back of her mind until after returning from her vacation.
Undoing is most commonly seen in children. It is when a person makes up for an act or communication.	After flirting with her male secretary, a woman brings her husband tickets to a concert he wants to see.	A man with rigid, moralistic beliefs and repressed sexuality is driven to wash his hands to gain composure when around attractive women.

Anxiety Disorders

Individuals with anxiety disorders use rigid, repetitive, and ineffective behaviors to try to control their anxiety. The common element of such disorders is that those affected experience a degree of anxiety so high that it interferes with personal, occupational, or social functioning. Recent studies also suggest that the presence of chronic anxiety disorders may increase the rate of cardiovascular system-related deaths. Anxiety disorders tend to be persistent and often disabling. Chapter 11 offers a more complete description of the debilitating effects of chronic stress and resultant anxiety.

CLINICAL PICTURE

The term *anxiety disorder* refers to a number of disorders, including:

- Panic disorders
- Phobias
- Obsessive-compulsive disorder
- Generalized anxiety disorder
- Posttraumatic stress disorder
- Acute stress disorder
- Substance-induced anxiety disorder
- Anxiety due to medical conditions
- Anxiety disorder not otherwise specified

Figure 12-2 presents the *Diagnostic and Statistical Manual of Mental Disorders,* 4th edition, text revision *(DSM-IV-TR)* criteria for various anxiety disorders.

Panic Disorders

Panic attacks are the key feature of **panic disorder (PD)**. The following vignette gives an example of a patient with signs and symptoms of a panic attack.

VIGNETTE

Sophia, a 30-year-old pharmacist, began to experience tension, irritability, and sleep disturbances after her mother's death from heart disease. On several occasions, Sophia has awakened gasping for breath. Her heart pounds and she feels a tight sensation like a band around her chest. Her pulse typically increases to more than 110 beats per minute, and she experiences dizziness. She fears that she is going to die.

On these occasions, Sophia telephones a friend to come over. The friend typically finds Sophia wringing her hands, moaning, and appearing totally disorganized. In each instance, the friend takes Sophia to the emergency department, where Sophia remains overnight for observation and tests. All diagnostic test results are normal. Because the physician finds no apparent organic basis for the episodes, she suggests they are likely panic attacks. ■

A **panic attack** is the sudden onset of extreme apprehension or fear, usually associated with feelings of impending doom. The feelings of terror present during a panic attack are so severe that normal function is suspended, the perceptual field is severely limited, and misinterpretation of reality may occur. Severe personality disorganization is evident. People experiencing panic attacks may believe they are losing their minds or having a heart attack. The attacks are often accompanied by highly uncomfortable physical symptoms such as palpitations, chest pain, breathing difficulties, nausea, and feelings of choking, chills, and hot flashes. Typically panic attacks come "out of the blue" (i.e., suddenly and not necessarily in response to stress), are extremely intense, last a matter of minutes, and then subside. Table 12-3 outlines a generic nursing care plan for PD.

Panic Disorder with Agoraphobia

Panic disorder with agoraphobia is a combination of panic-attack symptoms and agoraphobia. **Agoraphobia** is intense, excessive anxiety or fear about being in places or situations from which escape might be difficult or embarrassing or in which help might not be available if a panic attack occurred (APA, 2000). The feared places are avoided in an effort to control anxiety. Examples of situations that are commonly avoided by patients with agoraphobia are being alone outside; being alone at home; traveling in a car, bus, or airplane; being on

DSM-IV-TR CRITERIA FOR ANXIETY DISORDERS

ANXIETY DISORDERS

Panic Disorder	**Phobias**	**Obsessive-Compulsive Disorder (OCD)**	**Generalized Anxiety Disorder (GAD)**

1. Both A and B
  A. Recurrent episodes of panic attacks
  B. At least one of the attacks has been followed by 1 month (or more) of the following:
    1. Persistent concern about having additional attacks
    2. Worry about consequences ("going crazy," having a heart attack, losing control)
    3. Significant change in behavior
 	
2. A. Absence of agoraphobia = **Panic disorder without agoraphobia**
  B. Presence of agoraphobia = **Panic disorder with agoraphobia**
	1. Irrational fear of an object or situation that persists although the person may recognize it as unreasonable
	
	2. Types include:
	  • **Agoraphobia**: Fear of being alone in open or public places where escape might be difficult; may not leave home
	  • **Social phobia**: Fear of situations where one might be seen and embarrassed or criticized (e.g., speaking to authority figures, public speaking, or performing)
	  • **Specific phobia**: Fear of a single object, activity, or situation (e.g., snakes, closed spaces, flying)
	
	3. Anxiety is severe if the object, situation, or activity cannot be avoided.
		1. Either obsessions or compulsions
		  A. Preoccupation with persistent intrusive thoughts, impulses, or images (obsession)
		  or
		  B. Repetitive behaviors or mental acts that the person feels driven to perform in order to reduce distress or prevent a dreaded event or situation (compulsion)
		
		2. Person knows the obsessions/compulsions are excessive and unreasonable.
		
		3. The obsession/compulsion can cause increased distress and is time-consuming.
			1. A. Excessive anxiety or worry more days than not over 6 months
			  B. Inability to control the worrying
			
			2. Anxiety and worry associated with three or more of the following symptoms:
			  A. Restless, keyed-up
			  B. Easily fatigued
			  C. Difficulty concentrating, mind goes blank
			  D. Irritability
			  E. Muscle tension
			  F. Sleep disturbance
			
			3. Anxiety or worry or physical symptoms cause significant impairment in social, occupational, or other areas of important functioning.

Figure 12-2 Diagnostic criteria for various anxiety disorders. (Adapted from American Psychiatric Association. [2000]. *Diagnostic and statistical manual of mental disorders* [4th ed., text rev.]. Washington, DC: Author.)

TABLE 12-3 Generic Care Plan for Panic Disorder

Nursing diagnosis: *Anxiety* as evidenced by sudden onset of fear of impending doom or dying; increased pulse and respirations, shortness of breath, possible chest pain, dizziness, abdominal distress, panic attacks

Outcome criteria: Panic attacks will become less intense, and time between episodes will lengthen, so that patient can function comfortably at the usual level.

Short-Term Goal	Intervention	Rationale
1. Patient's anxiety will decrease to moderate by (date).	1a. If hyperventilation occurs, instruct patient to take slow, deep breaths. Breathing with the patient may be helpful.	1a. Focus is shifted away from distressing symptoms.
	1b. Keep expectations minimal and simple.	1b. Anxiety limits ability to attend to complex tasks.
2. Patient will gain mastery over panic episodes by (date).	2a. Help patient connect feelings before attack with onset of attack: • "What were you thinking about just before the attack?" • "Can you identify what you were feeling just before the attack?"	2a. Physiological symptoms of anxiety usually appear first as the result of a stressor. They are immediately followed by automatic thoughts, such as "I'm dying" or "I'm going crazy," which are distorted assessments.
	2b. Help patient recognize symptoms as resulting from anxiety, not from a catastrophic physical problem. *Examples:* • Explain physical symptoms of anxiety. • Discuss the fact that anxiety causes sensations similar to those of physical events, such as a heart attack.	2b. Factual information and alternative interpretations can help patient recognize distortions in thought.
	2c. Identify effective therapies for panic episodes.	2c. Cognitive-behavioral treatment is highly effective. Antianxiety medication is appropriate.
	2d. Teach patient abdominal breathing to be immediately used when anxiety is detected.	2d. Breathing exercises break the cycle of escalating symptoms of anxiety.
	2e. Teach patient to use positive self-talk, such as "I can control my anxiety."	2e. Cognitive restructuring is an effective way to replace negative self-talk.
	2f. Teach patient and family about any medication ordered for patient's panic attacks.	2f. Patient and family need to know what the medication can do, what the side effects and toxic effects are, and whom to call if untoward reactions occur.

a bridge; and riding in an elevator. Avoidance behaviors can be debilitating and life constricting. Consider the effect on a father whose agoraphobia renders him unable to leave home and prevents him from seeing his child's high school graduation; or the businesswoman whose avoidance of flying prevents her from attending distant business conferences. See Figure 12-2 for the *DSM-IV-TR* criteria for panic disorders.

VIGNETTE

Andrew is a 28-year-old man who suffers from panic attacks with agoraphobia. He once lived a very active life, often participating in thrill-seeking activities like bungee jumping and skydiving. Andrew's father, who had severe cardiovascular disease, died 2 years previously on his way to work. Since that time, Andrew has become increasingly fearful of the outdoors. He has gradually stopped leaving the family home, because he experiences panic attacks, fearing he will die if he leaves home. ■

Simple Agoraphobia

Agoraphobia without a history of PD (i.e., unaccompanied by panic attacks) occurs only rarely and early in the patient's history. Over time, agoraphobia with panic attacks usually develops (APA, 2000).

Phobias

A **phobia** is a persistent, irrational fear of a specific object, activity, or situation that leads to a desire for avoidance, or actual avoidance, of the object, activity, or situation (APA, 2000). **Specific phobias** are characterized by the

TABLE 12-4 Clinical Names for Common Phobias	
Clinical Name	**Feared Object or Situation**
Acrophobia	Heights
Agoraphobia	Open spaces
Astraphobia	Electrical storms
Claustrophobia	Closed spaces
Glossophobia	Talking
Hematophobia	Blood
Hydrophobia	Water
Monophobia	Being alone
Mysophobia	Germs or dirt
Nyctophobia	Darkness
Pyrophobia	Fire
Xenophobia	Strangers
Zoophobia	Animals

experience of high levels of anxiety or fear in response to specific objects or situations, such as dogs, spiders, heights, storms, water, blood, closed spaces, tunnels, and bridges (APA, 2000). Specific phobias are common and usually do not cause much difficulty, because people can contrive to avoid the feared object. Clinical names for common phobias are given in Table 12-4.

VIGNETTE
Daniel developed a morbid fear of elevators after being trapped in one for three hours during a power outage. As his fear and anxiety intensified, it became necessary for him to use only stairs or escalators. Daniel even became anxious if he had to enter closets or small storage rooms. He had developed claustrophobia, or a fear of closed spaces. ■

Social phobia, also called *social anxiety disorder (SAD)*, is characterized by severe anxiety or fear provoked by exposure to a social or a performance situation (e.g., fear of saying something that sounds foolish in public, not being able to answer questions in a classroom, eating in public, performing on stage). Fear of public speaking is the most common social phobia.

Characteristically, phobic individuals experience overwhelming and crippling anxiety when faced with the object or situation provoking the phobia. Phobic people go to great lengths to avoid the feared object or situation. A phobic person may not be able to think about or visualize the object or situation without becoming severely anxious. The life of a phobic person becomes more restricted as activities are given up so the phobic object can be avoided. All too frequently, complications ensue when people try to decrease anxiety through self-medication with alcohol or drugs. See Figure 12-2 for the *DSM-IV-TR* criteria for phobias.

VIGNETTE
William, a 22-year-old musical theater major, develops a fear of performing on stage. He suffers severe anxiety attacks whenever he is scheduled to appear in a student production. Recently he has become severely anxious when faced with giving classroom readings or singing solo in music class. He is thinking about changing his major. ■

Obsessive-Compulsive Disorder

Obsessions are defined as thoughts, impulses, or images that persist and recur, so that they cannot be dismissed from the mind. Obsessions often seem senseless to the individual who experiences them (egodystonic), and their presence causes severe anxiety.

Compulsions are ritualistic behaviors an individual feels driven to perform in an attempt to reduce anxiety. Performing the compulsive act temporarily reduces high levels of anxiety. Primary gain is achieved by compulsive rituals, but because the relief is only temporary, the compulsive act must be repeated again and again.

Although obsessions and compulsions can exist independently of each other, they most often occur together. Examples of common obsessions and compulsions are given in Table 12-5. Obsessive-compulsive behavior exists along a continuum. "Normal" individuals may experience mildly obsessive-compulsive behavior. For example, nearly everyone has had the experience of having a tune run persistently through the mind, despite attempts to push it away. Many people have had nagging doubts as to whether a door is locked or the stove is turned off. These doubts require the person to go back to check the door or stove. Minor compulsions, such as touching a lucky charm, knocking on wood, and making the sign of the cross upon hearing disturbing news, are not harmful to the individual. Mild compulsions about timeliness, orderliness, and reliability are valued traits in U.S. society.

At the pathological end of the continuum are obsessive-compulsive symptoms that typically involve issues of sexuality, violence, contamination, illness, or death. Pathological obsessions or compulsions cause marked distress to individuals, who often feel humiliation and shame regarding these behaviors. The rituals are time consuming and interfere with normal routines, social activities, and relationships with others. Severe OCD consumes so much of the individual's mental processes that the performance of cognitive tasks may be impaired. See Figure 12-2 for the *DSM-IV-TR* criteria for OCD and the Case Study and Nursing Care Plan for OCD on the Evolve website.

Generalized Anxiety Disorder

Generalized anxiety disorder (GAD) is characterized by excessive anxiety or worry about numerous things, lasting for 6 months or longer (APA, 2000).

TABLE 12-5 Common Obsessions and Compulsions

Type of Obsession	Example	Accompanying Compulsion
Doubt, need to check	"Did I turn off the stove?" repeatedly intrudes on the thinking of a woman who has recently gone from being a housewife to holding a secretarial position.	Checks to see if appliance is turned off, returning home several times each workday
Sexual imagery or ideation	A young woman has the recurrent thought "Pat his buttocks" when in the presence of a man.	Avoids the presence of men if possible; if with men, excuses self to wash hands every 10-15 minutes
Need for order	"Everything must be in its place" is the recurrent thought.	Arranges and rearranges items
Violence	A man repeatedly has the thought "I should kill her" when he sees a blonde woman.	Abruptly turns head away from women and squints eyes to try to avoid seeing blondes
Germs or dirt	A woman ruminates, "Everything is contaminated."	Avoids touching all objects; scrubs hands if forced to touch any object

The individual with GAD also displays many of the following symptoms:

- Restlessness
- Fatigue
- Poor concentration
- Irritability
- Tension
- Sleep disturbance

The individual's anxiety is out of proportion to the true impact of the event or situation about which the person is worried. Examples of worries typical in GAD are inadequacy in interpersonal relationships, job responsibilities, finances, health of family members, household chores, and lateness for appointments. Sleep disturbance is common because the individual worries about the day's events and real or imagined mistakes, reviews past problems, and anticipates future difficulties. Decision making is difficult, owing to poor concentration and dread of making a mistake. See Figure 12-2 for the *DSM-IV-TR* criteria for GAD, and refer to Table 12-6 for a generic care plan for GAD.

VIGNETTE

Angie is a 49-year-old legal secretary. She comes to the clinic complaining of feeling "so anxious I could jump out of my skin." She is shaky and diaphoretic; she has dilated pupils, an elevated pulse, and a quivering voice. She tells the nurse, "It was probably foolish to come here. Nobody understands me." Angie's only daughter is expecting her first child. Although the pregnancy is going well, Angie worries that something is wrong with the baby. "What if it's premature? What if it's deformed?"

Angie describes herself as tense and irritable. She has difficulty initiating sleep and cannot concentrate at her job. She worries about making mistakes at work, about being fired from her position, and about the financial problems that could result. She often says, "I just can't cope." Her daughter has begun calling several times a day to reassure her that all is well with the pregnancy and to try to decrease Angie's worry over other matters. The daughter has also begun shopping and housecleaning for Angie "to help her get some rest." ▪

Posttraumatic Stress Disorder

Posttraumatic stress disorder (PTSD) is characterized by persistent reexperiencing of a highly traumatic event that involved actual or threatened death or serious injury to self or others, to which the individual responded with intense fear, helplessness, or horror (APA, 2000). PTSD may occur after any traumatic event that is outside the range of usual experience. Examples are military combat; detention as a prisoner of war; natural disasters, such as floods, tornadoes, and earthquakes; human disasters, such as plane and train accidents; crime-related events, such as bombing, assault, mugging, rape, and being taken hostage; or diagnosis of a life-threatening illness. PTSD symptoms often begin within 3 months after the trauma, but a delay of months or years is not uncommon. Figure 12-3 presents the *DSM-IV-TR* criteria for PTSD.

The major features of PTSD are:

- Persistent reexperiencing of the trauma through recurrent intrusive recollections of the event, dreams about the event, and **flashbacks**—dissociative experiences during which the event is relived, and the person behaves as though he or she is experiencing the event at that time
- Persistent avoidance of stimuli associated with the trauma, causing the individual to avoid talking about the event or avoid activities, people, or places that arouse memories of the trauma

TABLE 12-6 Generic Care Plan for Generalized Anxiety Disorder

Nursing diagnosis: *Ineffective coping* related to persistent anxiety, fatigue, difficulty concentrating
Outcome criteria: Patient will maintain role performance.

Short-Term Goal	Intervention	Rationale
1. Patient will state that immediate distress is relieved by end of session.	1a. Stay with patient.	1a. Conveys acceptance and ability to give help.
	1b. Speak slowly and calmly.	1b. Conveys calm and promotes security.
	1c. Use short, simple sentences.	1c. Promotes comprehension.
	1d. Assure patient that you are in control and can assist him or her.	1d. Counters feeling of loss of control that accompanies severe anxiety.
	1e. Give brief directions.	1e. Reduces indecision. Conveys belief that patient can respond in a healthy manner.
	1f. Decrease excessive stimuli; provide quiet environment.	1f. Reduces need to focus on diverse stimuli. Promotes ability to concentrate.
	1g. After assessing level of anxiety, administer appropriate dose of anxiolytic agent if warranted.	1g. Reduces anxiety and allows patient to use coping skills.
	1h. Monitor and control own feelings.	1h. Anxiety is transmissible. Displays of negative emotion can cause patient anxiety.
2. Patient will be able to identify source of anxiety by (date).	2a. Encourage patient to discuss preceding events.	2a. Promotes future change through identification of stressors.
	2b. Link patient's behavior to feelings.	2b. Promotes self-awareness.
	2c. Teach cognitive therapy principles: • Anxiety is the result of a dysfunctional appraisal of a situation. • Anxiety is the result of automatic thinking.	2c. Provides a basis for behavioral change.
	2d. Ask questions that clarify and dispute illogical thinking: • "What evidence do you have?" • "Explain the logic in that." • "Are you basing that conclusion on fact or feeling?" • "What's the worst thing that could happen?"	2d. Helps promote accurate cognition.
	2e. Have patient give an alternative interpretation.	2e. Broadens perspective. Helps patient think in a new way about problem or symptom.
3. Patient will identify strengths and coping skills by (date).	3a. Provides awareness of self as individual with some ability to cope.	3a. Identify what has provided relief in the past.
	3b. Have patient write assessment of strengths.	3b. Increases self-acceptance.
	3c. Reframe situation in ways that are positive.	3c. Provides a new perspective and converts distorted thinking.

• Persistent numbing of general responsiveness, as evidenced by the individual's feeling detached or estranged from others, feeling empty inside, or feeling turned off to others
• Persistent symptoms of increased arousal, as evidenced by irritability, difficulty sleeping, difficulty concentrating, hypervigilance, or exaggerated startle response

Difficulty with interpersonal, social, or occupational relationships nearly always accompanies PTSD, and trust is a common issue of concern. Child and spousal abuse may be associated with hypervigilance and irritability, and chemical abuse may begin as an attempt to self-medicate to relieve anxiety (Case Study and Nursing Care Plan 12-2).

Acute Stress Disorder

Acute stress disorder occurs within 1 month after exposure to a highly traumatic event, such as those listed in the section on PTSD. To be diagnosed with acute stress disorder, the individual must display at least three dissociative symptoms either during or after the traumatic event, including a subjective sense of numbing, detachment, or absence of emotional responsiveness; a reduction in awareness of surroundings; derealization (a sense of unreality related to the environment); depersonalization (experience of a sense of unreality or self-estrangement); or dissociative amnesia (loss of memory) (APA, 2000). By definition, acute stress disorder resolves within 4 weeks. See Figure 12-3 for the *DSM-IV-TR* criteria for acute stress disorder.

VIGNETTE

Olivia, a 22-year-old college student, is sexually assaulted by a family friend. In the emergency department, she describes feeling detached from her body

DSM-IV-TR CRITERIA FOR ANXIETY DISORDERS: STRESS RELATED

ANXIETY DISORDERS: STRESS RELATED

Posttraumatic Stress Disorder

1. The person experienced, witnessed, or was confronted with an event that involved actual, threatened death to self or others, responding in fear, helplessness, or horror.

2. The event is persistently reexperienced by:
   (a) Recurrent and intrusive recollections of the event, including images, thoughts, or perceptions
   (b) Distressing dreams or images
   (c) Reliving the event through flashbacks, illusions, hallucinations

3. Persistent avoidance of stimuli associated with trauma:
   (a) Avoidance of thoughts, feelings, conversations
   (b) Avoidance of people, places, activities
   (c) Inability to recall aspects of trauma
   (d) Decreased interest in usual activities
   (e) Feelings of detachment, estrangement from others
   (f) Restriction in feelings (love, enthusiasm, joy)
   (g) Sense of shortened feelings

4. Persistent symptoms of increased arousal (two or more):
   (a) Difficulty falling/staying asleep
   (b) Irritability/outbursts of anger
   (c) Difficulty concentrating

5. **Duration more than 1 month:**
   • Acute: duration less than 3 months
   • Chronic: duration 3 months or more
   • Delayed: onset of symptoms is at least 6 months after stress

Acute Stress Disorder

1. The person experienced, witnessed, or was confronted with an event that involved actual, threatened death to self or others, responding in fear, helplessness, or horror.

2. Three or more of the following dissociative symptoms:
   (a) Sense of numbing, detachment, or absence of emotional response
   (b) Reduced awareness of surroundings (e.g., "in a daze")
   (c) Derealization
   (d) Depersonalization
   (e) Amnesia for an important aspect of the trauma

3. The event is persistently reexperienced by:
   (a) Distressing dreams or images
   (b) Reliving the event through flashbacks, illusions, hallucinations
   (c) Distress on exposure to reminders of the traumatic event

4. Marked avoidance of stimuli that arouse memory of trauma (thoughts, feelings, people, places, activities, conversations).

5. Marked symptoms of anxiety:
   (a) Difficulty falling/staying asleep
   (b) Irritability/outbursts of anger
   (c) Difficulty concentrating

6. Causes impairment in social, occupational, and other functioning, or impairs ability to complete some memory tasks.

7. **Not due to drug abuse/medications or medical condition.**

8. **Lasts from 2 days to 4 weeks and occurs within 4 weeks of the traumatic event.**

Figure 12-3 Diagnostic criteria for stress-related anxiety disorders. (Adapted from American Psychiatric Association. [2000]. *Diagnostic and statistical manual of mental disorders* [4th ed., text rev.]. Washington, DC: Author.)

and being unaware of her surroundings during the assault, "as though it took place in a vacuum." She displays virtually no affect (i.e., she does not cry or appear anxious, angry, or sad). Olivia finds it difficult to concentrate on the examiner's questions. Three days later, Olivia still feels as though her mind is detached from her body; she reports having difficulty sleeping, not being able to concentrate, and startling whenever anyone touches her. When she sees the nurse 4 weeks after the event, Olivia expresses feelings of anger and sadness over the assault, displays the ability to concentrate, and states that she no longer feels as though her mind and body are detached. She reports being able to sleep better and not being so jittery and easily startled. ■

Substance-Induced Anxiety Disorder

Substance-induced anxiety disorder is characterized by symptoms of anxiety, panic attacks, obsessions, and compulsions that develop with the use of a substance or within a month of stopping use of the substance (APA, 2000). For a diagnosis of substance-induced anxiety disorder, evidence of the use of a psychoactive substance (e.g., alcohol, cocaine, heroin, hallucinogens) must be obtained through the history, physical examination, or laboratory findings.

Anxiety Due to Medical Conditions

In **anxiety due to a medical condition**, the individual's symptoms of anxiety are a direct physiological result of a medical condition, such as hyperthyroidism, pulmonary embolism, or cardiac dysrhythmias (APA, 2000). To determine whether the anxiety symptoms are due to a medical condition, a careful and comprehensive assessment of multiple factors is necessary. Once again, evidence must be present in the history, physical examination, or laboratory findings for a diagnosis of anxiety due to a medical condition. Refer to Table 12-7 for a list of medical disorders that may contribute to anxiety symptoms.

Anxiety Disorder Not Otherwise Specified

Anxiety disorder not otherwise specified is a diagnosis used for disorders in which anxiety or phobic avoidance predominates but the symptoms do not meet full diagnostic criteria for a specific anxiety disorder.

EPIDEMIOLOGY

Anxiety disorders are the most common form of psychiatric disorders in the United States. They affect up to 40 million adults, or about 18% of the population aged 18 and older (Kessler, Chiu et al., 2005). Nearly three quarters of those with an anxiety disorder will have

TABLE 12-7 Common Medical Causes of Anxiety	
System	**Disorders**
Respiratory	Chronic obstructive pulmonary disease
	Pulmonary embolism
	Asthma
	Hypoxia
	Pulmonary edema
Cardiovascular	Angina pectoris
	Arrhythmias
	Congestive heart failure
	Hypertension
	Hypotension
	Mitral valve prolapse
Endocrine	Hyperthyroidism
	Hypoglycemia
	Pheochromocytoma
	Carcinoid syndrome
	Hypercortisolism
Neurological	Delirium
	Essential tremor
	Complex partial seizures
	Parkinson's disease
	Akathisia
	Otoneurological disorders
	Postconcussion syndrome
Metabolic	Hypercalcemia
	Hyperkalemia
	Hyponatremia
	Porphyria

their first episode by age 21.5 (Kessler, Berglund et al., 2005). People with anxiety disorders frequently seek health care services for relief of physical symptoms, at a cost of approximately $22 billion per year. Women are affected more frequently than men. Table 12-8 lists the 1-year prevalence rates (those who are affected within any given year) for specific anxiety disorders in the United States.

COMORBIDITY

Clinicians and researchers have clearly shown that anxiety disorders frequently co-occur with other psychiatric problems. Several studies suggest that other psychiatric disorders coexist about 90% of the time in people with generalized anxiety or panic disorder, 84% in those with agoraphobia, and about 70% in those with PTSD (Sadock & Sadock, 2008). Anxiety disorders are comorbid with major depression at a rate of 60%; in this type of comorbidity, anxiety symptoms tend to happen before depressive symptoms. In fact, treatments for both disorders are similar. This similarity leads to speculation that genetically, anxiety and depression may be two sides of the same coin and not distinct disorders (Kendler et al., 2007).

TABLE 12-8 One-Year Prevalence of Anxiety Disorders

Disorder	Prevalence in Adults (Any Given Year) (%)	Age of Onset	Gender Predilection
Panic disorder	2.7	Median age of onset 24 years	Two times more frequent in women
Generalized anxiety disorder	3.1	Median age of onset 31 years	Two times more frequent in women
Phobias (specific)	8.5	Median age of onset 7 years	Two times more frequent in women
Social anxiety disorder	6.8	Median age of onset 13 years	Equal prevalence in men and women
Obsessive-compulsive disorder	1.0	Median age of onset 19 years	Equal prevalence in men and women
Posttraumatic stress disorder	3.5	Median age of onset 19 years	Women more likely affected (rape is a major trigger)

Data from Kessler, R. C., Chiu, W. T., Demler, O, Walters, E. E. (2005). Prevalence, severity, and comorbidity of twelve-month *DSM-IV* disorders in the National Comorbidity Survey Replication (NCS-R). *Archives of General Psychiatry, 62*, 617–627; Kessler, R. C., Berglund, P. A., Demler O., Jin, R., Walters, E. E. (2005). Lifetime prevalence and age-of-onset distributions of *DSM-IV* disorders in the National Comorbidity Survey Replication (NCS-R). *Archives of General Psychiatry, 62*, 593–602; and Anxiety Disorders Association of America. (2008). *Statistics and facts about anxiety disorders.* <http://www.adaa.org/AboutADAA/PressRoom/Stats&Facts.asp> Accessed 22.10.08.

ETIOLOGY

There is no longer any doubt that biological factors predispose some individuals to pathological anxiety states (e.g., phobias, panic attacks). By the same token, traumatic life events, psychosocial factors, and sociocultural factors are also etiologically significant.

Biological Factors

Genetic

Numerous studies substantiate that anxiety disorders tend to cluster in families. Twin studies demonstrate the existence of a genetic component to both panic disorder and obsessive-compulsive disorder (OCD) (APA, 2000). First-degree biological relatives of those with OCD or phobias have a higher frequency of these disorders than exists in the general population. Nearly half of people with panic disorders have a relative who is also affected (Sadock & Sadock, 2008). Even for posttraumatic stress disorder and generalized anxiety disorder, there is evidence of inherited components (APA, 2000).

Neurobiological

Certain anatomic pathways (the limbic system) provide the transmission structure for the electrical impulses that occur when anxiety-related responses are sent or received. Neurons release chemicals (neurotransmitters) that convey these messages. The neurochemicals that regulate anxiety include epinephrine, norepinephrine, dopamine, serotonin, and gamma-aminobutyric acid (GABA).

There are various theories regarding the causes of anxiety disorders. One is the GABA benzodiazepine theory. Benzodiazepine receptors are linked to a receptor that inhibits the activity of the neurotransmitter GABA. The release of GABA slows neural transmission, which has a calming effect. Binding of benzodiazepine medications to benzodiazepine receptors facilitates the action of GABA (Sadock & Sadock, 2008). This theory proposes that abnormalities of the benzodiazepine receptors may lead to unregulated anxiety levels.

Studies suggest that the stress response of the hypothalamus-pituitary-adrenal system is abnormal in patients with PTSD. Repeated trauma or stress not only alters the release of neurotransmitters but also changes the anatomy of the brain. Neuroimaging has demonstrated that the size of the right hippocampus is significantly reduced in combat veterans who suffer from PTSD (Pavic et al., 2007).

Psychological Theories

Psychodynamic theories about the development of anxiety disorders center on the idea that unconscious childhood conflicts are the basis for symptom development. Sigmund Freud suggested that anxiety results from the threatened breakthrough of repressed ideas or emotions from the unconscious into consciousness. Freud also suggested that ego defense mechanisms are used by the individual to keep anxiety at manageable levels (see Chapter 2). The use of defense mechanisms results in behavior that is not wholly adaptive because of its rigidity and repetitive nature.

Harry Stack Sullivan (1953) believed that anxiety is linked to the emotional distress caused when early needs go unmet or disapproval is experienced (**interpersonal theory**). He also suggested that anxiety is "contagious," being transmitted to the infant from the mother or caregiver. Thus the anxiety experienced early in life becomes the prototype for anxiety experienced when unpleasant events occur later in life.

EVIDENCE-BASED PRACTICE

Teenage Pregnancy and the Trauma of Giving Birth

Anderson, C., & McGuiness, T. M. (2008). Do teenage mothers experience childbirth as traumatic? *Journal of Psychosocial Nursing and Mental Health Services, 46*(4), 21–24.

Problem

Despite the fact that hundreds of thousands of teenagers give birth every year in the United States, little is known about the psychological impact it has on these girls. Although giving birth can be a stressor at any age, teenagers often lack social support and resources for coping. Adverse psychological consequences can have a profoundly negative impact on both the mother's level of health and that of her infant.

Purpose of Study

The purpose of this study was to assess for posttraumatic stress (PTS) and postpartum depression (PPD) in teenage mothers.

Methods

For this pilot (initial) study, 28 teenage mothers were interviewed by telephone 9 months after childbirth. They were between the ages of 15 and 19 and included 13 Latina, 8 African Americans, and 6 Caucasians. The participants were asked to rate their perception of childbirth, respond to questions assessing for PTS, and respond to questions assessing for PPD.

Key Findings

- Most of the mothers rated their experience with childbirth at a midway point between *awful* and *great*.
- Fourteen of the participants were afraid of losing control during labor, and 13 believed that they would die in childbirth.
- Scores from a third of the participants indicated PTS as the result of childbirth experiences.
- Scores from more than half the participants indicated the presence of mild to severe depression.

Implications for Nursing Practice

Some teenage mothers are vulnerable to PTS and PPD because of lack of social support, low self-esteem, chaotic/harsh upbringing, and family conflict. Carefully assessing the patient's history for risk factors can be the first step in minimizing these vulnerabilities. Educational programs in which girls are provided with information related to the process of labor and delivery, pain management methods, and what to expect postpartum can reduce fear and possibly reduce psychiatric complications.

Psychiatric mental health nurses care for adolescent girls who have been abused or sexually assaulted, have eating disorders, and/or abuse alcohol and drugs. Understanding the additional stress childbirth may bring about should be considered when assessing and intervening with teenagers who have given birth. Collaboration between maternal-child health nurses and psychiatric mental health nurses could provide the ideal support for pregnant teenagers and teenagers who have given birth.

Behavioral theories suggest that anxiety is a learned response to specific environmental stimuli (classical conditioning). An example of classical conditioning is a boy who experiences anxiety when his abusive mother enters the room and then generalizes this anxiety as a response to all women (Sadock & Sadock, 2008). The social learning model suggests that anxiety is learned through the modeling of parents or peers. For example, a mother who is fearful of thunder and lightning and hides in closets during storms may transmit her anxiety to her children, who continue to adopt her behavior into adult life. Such individuals can unlearn this behavior by observing others who react normally to a storm by lighting candles and telling stories.

Cognitive theorists believe that anxiety disorders are caused by distortions in an individual's thoughts and perceptions. Because individuals with such distortions may believe that any mistake will have catastrophic results, they experience acute anxiety.

Cultural Considerations

Reliable data on the incidence of anxiety disorders are sparse, but sociocultural variation in symptoms of anxiety disorders has been noted. In some cultures, individuals express anxiety through somatic symptoms, whereas in other cultures, cognitive symptoms predominate. Panic attacks in Latin Americans and Northern Europeans often involve sensations of choking, smothering, numbness, or tingling, as well as fear of dying. In other cultural groups, panic attacks involve fear of magic or witchcraft. Social phobias in Japanese and Korean cultures may relate to beliefs that the individual's blushing, eye contact, or body odor is offensive to others (APA, 2000).

The *DSM-IV-TR* (APA, 2000) notes cultural aspects of each psychiatric disorder to alert the clinician to cultural contexts that must be considered before making a psychiatric diagnosis. The Considering Culture box discusses factors relevant to one anxiety disorder (ataque de nervios) primarily experienced by people from Hispanic cultures. Also review Chapter 6 for more discussion of cultural issues.

APPLICATION OF THE NURSING PROCESS

ASSESSMENT

General Assessment

People with anxiety disorders rarely need hospitalization unless they are suicidal or have compulsions that cause injury (cutting self, banging a body part). Most patients prone to anxiety disorders are encountered incidentally in a variety of community settings. A common example is someone taken to an emergency department to rule out a heart attack when in fact the individual is experiencing a panic attack. It is essential to determine whether the anxiety is *secondary* to another source (medical condition or substance) or the *primary* problem, as in an anxiety disorder.

As previously described, the main symptoms of anxiety disorders are panic attacks, excessive anxiety, severe reactions to stress or trauma, phobias, obsessions, and compulsions.

The Hamilton Rating Scale for Anxiety is a popular tool in measuring anxiety (Table 12-9). High scores may indicate GAD or PD, although it is important to note that high anxiety scores may also be a symptom of major depressive disorder. See how you rate on this tool. Keep in mind that although The Hamilton Rating Scale highlights important areas in the assessment of anxiety, it is intended for use by experienced clinicians as a guide for planning care and not as a method of self-diagnosis.

Self-Assessment

As a nurse working with an individual with an anxiety disorder, you may experience uncomfortable personal reactions. You may have feelings of frustration or anger while working with a patient with anxiety disorder; especially if it seems like that their symptoms are a matter of choice or under personal control. The rituals of the patient with OCD may hinder your ability to accomplish certain nursing tasks within the usual time. Communication with such patients can be difficult since patients with OCD often correct and clarify repeatedly, as though they cannot let go of any topic. Using therapeutic communication techniques (e.g., reflecting and paraphrasing [see Chapter 10]) may be ineffective; the patient may repeat the material, and angrily imply that you have not understood. Patience, the ability to provide clear structure, and empathy are assets when working with patients with anxiety disorders.

A person with a phobia may acknowledge that the fear is exaggerated and unrealistic, yet continues to practice avoidant behavior which may bewilder the nurse. Behavioral change is often accomplished slowly. The process of recovery is very different from that seen in a patient with an infection, who might be given antibiotics and demonstrates improvement in 24 hours. Nurses tend to become impatient with the patient experiencing anxiety and may feel angry when more rapid progress is not made. Negative feelings are easily transmitted to the patient, who then feels increasingly anxious.

The nurse who feels anger or frustration may withdraw from the patient emotionally and physically. As a result, the patient feels increasingly anxious and also

CONSIDERING CULTURE

Ataque de Nervios

It goes without saying that technology and the commonplace of travel have resulted in a "smaller" world. Psychiatric mental health nurses in the United States will be exposed to culture-bound syndromes with which they are unfamiliar. One example of a culture-bound syndrome is that of ataque de nervios, or in English, "attack of the nerves." This a disorder found primarily among Hispanic populations in response to stressful events, such as a death, acute family discord, or witnessing an accident. Symptoms are dramatic, and people afflicted by ataque de nervios exhibit sudden trembling, faintness, palpitations, out-of-control shouting, heat that moves from the chest to head, and seizure-like activities. After the episode, the affected individual often has little memory of it. This disorder is more common in socially disadvantaged females with less than a high school education.

What do these symptoms sound like to you? Although there is no category for this illness in the *DSM-IV-TR*, some clinicians and researchers believe that it is closely related to an anxiety disorder and could even be a form of panic attack. However, unlike people who have panic attacks, people with this disorder are responding to a precipitating event, and they do not typically experience fear or apprehension prior to the attack.

Hales, R. E., Yudofsky, S. C., & Gabbard, G. O. (2008). *The textbook of psychiatry* (5th ed.). Washington, DC: American Psychiatric Publishing; and Hinton, D. E., Chong, R., Pollack, M. H., Barlow, D. H., & McNally, R. J. (2008). Ataque de nervios: Relationship to anxiety sensitivity and dissociation predisposition. *Depression and Anxiety, 25,* 489–495.

TABLE 12-9 Hamilton Rating Scale for Anxiety

The symptom inventory provides scaled information that classifies anxiety behaviors and assists the clinician in targeting behaviors and achieving outcome measures. Provide a rating for each indicator based on the following scale: 0 = none; 1 = mild; 2 = moderate; 3 = disabling; 4 = severe, grossly disabling.

Item	Symptoms	Rating
1. Anxious mood	Worries, anticipation of the worst, fearful anticipation, irritability	_____
2. Tension	Feelings of tension, fatigability, startle response, moved to tears easily, trembling, feelings of restlessness, inability to relax	_____
3. Fear	Fearful of dark, strangers, being left alone, animals, traffic, crowds	_____
4. Insomnia	Difficulty in falling asleep, broken sleep, unsatisfying sleep and fatigue on waking, dreams, nightmares, night terrors	_____
5. Intellectual (cognitive) manifestations	Difficulty in concentration, poor memory	_____
6. Depressed mood swings	Loss of interest, lack of pleasure in hobbies, depression, early waking, diurnal	_____
7. Somatic (sensory) symptoms	Tinnitus, blurring of vision, hot and cold flushes, feelings of weakness, picking sensation	_____
8. Somatic (muscular) symptoms	Pains and aches, twitching, stiffness, myoclonic jerks, grinding of teeth, unsteady voice, increased muscular tone	_____
9. Cardiovascular symptoms	Tachycardia, palpitations, skipped beats, pain in chest, throbbing of vessels, fainting feelings	_____
10. Respiratory symptoms	Pressure of constriction in chest, choking feelings, sighing, dyspnea	_____
11. Gastrointestinal symptoms	Difficulty in swallowing, flatulence, abdominal pain, burning sensations, abdominal fullness, nausea, vomiting, borborygmi, looseness of bowels, loss of weight, constipation	_____
12. Genitourinary symptoms	Frequency of micturition, urgency of micturition, amenorrhea, menorrhagia, development of frigidity, premature ejaculation, loss of libido, impotence	_____
13. Autonomic symptoms	Dry mouth, flushing, pallor, tendency to sweat, giddiness, tension headache, raising of hair	_____
14. Behavior at interview	Fidgeting, restlessness or pacing, tremor of hands, furrowed brow, strained face, sighing or rapid respiration, facial pallor, swallowing, belching, brisk tendon jerks, dilated pupils, exophthalmos	_____

Scoring:
14-17 = mild anxiety
18-24 = moderate anxiety
25-30 = severe anxiety
Adapted from Hamilton, M. (1959). The assessment of anxiety states by rating. *British Journal of Medical Psychology, 32,* 50-55.

withdraws. Staging outcomes in small, attainable steps can help prevent you from feeling overwhelmed by the patient's slow progress and help the patient gain a sense of control.

At the very least, you are likely to experience increased tension and fatigue from mental strain when working with patients experiencing anxiety. Unlike the patient who needs a dressing changed several times a week, the patient with anxiety requires "emotional bandaging" much more often.

By having a clear understanding of the emotional pitfalls of working with patients who have anxiety disorders, a nurse is better prepared to minimize and avoid the guilt associated with strong negative feelings. By examining personal feelings, you can better understand their origin and respond objectively and constructively.

Assessment Guidelines Anxiety Disorders

1. Ensure that a sound physical and neurological examination is performed to help determine whether the anxiety is primary or secondary to another psychiatric disorder, medical condition, or substance use.
2. Determine current level of anxiety (mild, moderate, severe, or panic).
3. Assess for potential for self-harm and suicide; people suffering from high levels of intractable anxiety may become desperate and attempt suicide.
4. Perform a psychosocial assessment. Always ask the person, "What is going on in your life that may be contributing to your anxiety?" The patient may identify a problem that should be addressed by counseling (stressful marriage, recent loss, stressful job or school situation).
5. *Note:* Culture can affect how anxiety is manifested.

DIAGNOSIS

The North American Nursing Diagnosis Association International (NANDA-I) (2009) provides many nursing diagnoses that can be considered for patients experiencing anxiety and anxiety disorders. The "related-to" component will vary with the individual patient. Table 12-10 identifies potential nursing diagnoses for the patient experiencing anxiety. Signs and symptoms that might be found on assessment and support the diagnosis are included.

OUTCOMES IDENTIFICATION

The *Nursing Outcomes Classification (NOC)* identifies desired outcomes for patients with anxiety or anxiety-related disorders (Moorhead et al., 2008). Each outcome contains a definition and rating scale to

TABLE 12-10 Potential Diagnoses for Anxiety Disorders

Signs and Symptoms	Nursing Diagnoses
Concern that a panic attack will occur Exposure to phobic object or situation Presence of obsessive thoughts Recurrent memories of traumatic event Fear of panic attacks	*Anxiety (moderate, severe, panic)* *Fear*
High levels of anxiety that interfere with the ability to work, disrupt relationships, and change ability to interact with others Avoidance behaviors (phobia, agoraphobia) Hypervigilance after a traumatic event Inordinate time taken for obsession and compulsions	*Ineffective coping* *Deficient diversional activity* *Social isolation* *Ineffective role performance*
Difficulty with concentration Preoccupation with obsessive thoughts Disorganization associated with exposure to phobic object	*Disturbed thought processes**
Intrusive thoughts and memories of traumatic event	*Post-trauma syndrome*
Excessive use of reason and logic associated with overcautiousness and fear of making a mistake	*Decisional conflict*
Disruption in sleep related to intrusive thoughts, worrying, replaying of a traumatic event, hypervigilance, fear	*Insomnia* *Sleep deprivation* *Fatigue*
Feelings of hopelessness, inability to control one's life, low self-esteem related to inability to have some control in one's life	*Hopelessness* *Chronic low self-esteem* *Spiritual distress*
Inability to perform self-care related to rituals	*Self-care deficit*
Skin excoriation related to rituals of excessive washing or excessive picking at the skin	*Impaired skin integrity*
Inability to eat because of constant ritual performance Feeling of anxiety or excessive worrying that overrides appetite and need to eat	*Imbalanced nutrition: less than body requirements*
Excessive overeating to appease intense worrying or high anxiety levels	*Imbalanced nutrition: more than body requirements*

North American Nursing Diagnosis Association. (2009). *NANDA-I nursing diagnoses: Definitions and classification 2009–2011.* Oxford, United Kingdom: Author.
*Diagnosis retired from North American Nursing Diagnosis Association. (2007). *NANDA-I nursing diagnoses: Definitions and classification 2007–2008.* Philadelphia: Author.

measure the severity of the symptom or frequency of the desired response. This rating scale enables you to evaluate outcomes in the nursing care plan. Some of the *NOC*-recommended outcomes related to anxiety include *Anxiety Self-Control, Anxiety Level, Stress Level, Coping, Social Interaction Skills,* and *Symptom Control.* Refer to Table 12-11 for examples of intermediate and short-term indicators related to *NOC* outcomes.

PLANNING

Anxiety disorders are encountered in all health care settings. Nurses care for people with concurrent anxiety disorders in medical-surgical units, as well as in homes, day programs, and clinics. Usually patients with anxiety disorders do not require admission to inpatient psychiatric units, and planning for their care may involve selecting interventions that can be implemented in a community setting.

Whenever possible, the patient should be encouraged to participate actively in planning. By sharing decision making with the patient, you can increase the likelihood that positive outcomes will be attained. Shared planning is especially appropriate for someone with mild or moderate anxiety. When experiencing severe levels of anxiety, a patient may be unable to participate in planning, and the nurse may be required to take a more directive role.

IMPLEMENTATION

When working with patients with anxiety disorders, you must first determine what level of anxiety they are experiencing. A general framework for anxiety interventions can then be built on a solid foundation of understanding.

Mild to Moderate Levels of Anxiety

A person experiencing a mild to moderate level of anxiety is still able to solve problems; however, the ability to concentrate decreases as anxiety increases. A patient can be helped to focus and solve problems when you use specific nursing communication techniques, such as asking open-ended questions, giving broad openings, and exploring and seeking clarification. Closing off topics of communication and bringing up irrelevant topics can increase a person's anxiety, making the *nurse,* not the *patient,* feel better.

Reducing the patient's anxiety level and preventing escalation to more distressing levels can be aided by providing a calm presence, recognizing the anxious person's distress, and being willing to listen. Evaluation of effective past coping mechanisms is also useful. Often you can help the patient consider alternatives to problem situations and offer activities

TABLE 12-11 *NOC* Outcomes for Anxiety Disorders		
Nursing Outcome and Definition	**Intermediate Indicators**	**Short-Term Indicators**
Anxiety Self-Control: Personal actions to eliminate or reduce feelings of apprehension, tension, or uneasiness from an unidentifiable source	Controls anxiety response Maintains role performance	Monitors intensity of anxiety Uses relaxation techniques to decrease anxiety Decreases environmental stimuli when anxious Maintains adequate sleep
Coping: Personal actions to manage stressors that tax an individual's resources	Identifies multiple coping strategies Modifies lifestyle as needed	Reports decrease in physical symptoms of stress Identifies ineffective coping patterns Verbalizes need for assistance Seeks information concerning illness and treatment
Self-Esteem: Personal judgment of self-worth	Describes pride in self Describes success in social groups	Maintenance of eye contact Maintenance of grooming/hygiene Acceptance of self-limitations Acceptance of compliments from others
Knowledge: Disease Process: Extent of understanding conveyed about a specific disease process	Describes usual disease course	Description of signs and symptoms Description of cause or contributing factors Description of signs and symptoms of complications Description of precautions to prevent complications

Data from Moorhead, S., Johnson, M., Maas, M., & Swanson, E. (2008). *Nursing outcomes classification (NOC)* (4th ed.). St. Louis, MO: Mosby.

TABLE 12-12 Interventions for Mild to Moderate Levels of Anxiety

Nursing diagnosis: *Anxiety (moderate)* related to situational event or psychological stress, as evidenced by increase in vital signs, moderate discomfort, narrowing of perceptual field, and selective inattention

Intervention	Rationale
Help the patient identify anxiety. "Are you comfortable right now?"	It is important to validate observations with the patient, name the anxiety, and start to work with the patient to lower anxiety.
Anticipate anxiety-provoking situations.	Escalation of anxiety to a more disorganizing level is prevented.
Use nonverbal language to demonstrate interest (e.g., lean forward, maintain eye contact, nod your head).	Verbal and nonverbal messages should be consistent. The presence of an interested person provides a stabilizing focus.
Encourage the patient to talk about his or her feelings and concerns.	When concerns are stated aloud, problems can be discussed and feelings of isolation decreased.
Avoid closing off avenues of communication that are important for the patient. Focus on the patient's concerns.	When staff anxiety increases, changing the topic or offering advice is common but leaves the person isolated.
Ask questions to clarify what is being said. "I'm not sure what you mean. Give me an example."	Increased anxiety results in scattering of thoughts. Clarifying helps the patient identify thoughts and feelings.
Help the patient identify thoughts or feelings before the onset of anxiety. "What were you thinking right before you started to feel anxious?"	The patient is assisted in identifying thoughts and feelings, and problem solving is facilitated.
Encourage problem solving with the patient.*	Encouraging patients to explore alternatives increases sense of control and decreases anxiety.
Assist in developing alternative solutions to a problem through role play or modeling behaviors.	The patient is encouraged to try out alternative behaviors and solutions.
Explore behaviors that have worked to relieve anxiety in the past.	The patient is encouraged to mobilize successful coping mechanisms and strengths.
Provide outlets for working off excess energy (e.g., walking, playing ping-pong, dancing, exercising).	Physical activity can provide relief of built-up tension, increase muscle tone, and increase endorphin levels.

*Patients experiencing mild to moderate anxiety levels can problem solve.

that may temporarily relieve feelings of inner tension. Table 12-12 identifies interventions useful in assisting people experiencing mild to moderate levels of anxiety.

Severe to Panic Levels of Anxiety

A person experiencing a severe to panic level of anxiety is unable to solve problems and may have a poor grasp of what is happening in the environment. Unproductive relief behaviors may take over, and the person may not be in control of his or her actions. Extreme regression and running about aimlessly are behavioral manifestations of a person's intense psychic pain.

Appropriate nursing interventions are to provide for the safety of the patient and others, and to meet physical needs (e.g., fluids, rest) to prevent exhaus-

tion. Anxiety reduction measures may take the form of removing the person to a quiet environment with minimal stimulation and providing gross motor activities to drain some of the tension. The use of medications may have to be considered, but both medications and restraints should be used only after other more personal and less restrictive interventions have failed to decrease anxiety to safer levels. Although a patient's communication may be scattered and disjointed, feeling understood can decrease the overwhelming sense of isolation and reduce anxiety.

Because individuals experiencing severe to panic levels of anxiety are unable to solve problems, the techniques suggested for communicating with persons with mild to moderate levels of anxiety may not be effective at more severe levels. Patients experiencing severe to panic anxiety levels are out of control, so they need to know they are safe from their own impulses. Firm, short, and simple statements are useful. Reinforcing commonalities in the environment and pointing out reality when there are distortions can also be useful interventions for severely anxious persons. Table 12-13 suggests some basic nursing interventions for patients with severe to panic levels of anxiety.

Anxiety management and reduction are primary concerns when working with patients who have anxiety disorders, but they may have a variety of other needs. When developing a plan of care, the psychiatric mental health nurse can utilize the *Psychiatric-Mental Health Nursing: Scope and Standards of Practice* (American Nurses Association [ANA] et al., 2007). The *Nursing Interventions Classification (NIC)* offers pertinent interventions in the behavioral and safety domains (Bulechek, Butcher, & Dochterman, 2008). Refer to Box 12-1 for potential nursing interventions for patients experiencing anxiety.

Guidelines for basic nursing interventions are:

1. Identify community resources that can offer the patient specialized treatment proven to be highly effective for people with a variety of anxiety disorders.
2. Identify community support groups for people with specific anxiety disorders and their families.
3. Use counseling, milieu therapy, promotion of self-care activities, and psychobiological and health teaching interventions as appropriate.

TABLE 12-13 Interventions for Severe to Panic Levels of Anxiety

Nursing diagnosis: *Anxiety (severe, panic)* related to severe threat (biochemical, environmental, psychosocial), as evidenced by verbal or physical acting out, extreme immobility, sense of impending doom, inability to differentiate reality (possible hallucinations or delusions), and inability to problem solve

Intervention	Rationale
Maintain a calm manner.	Anxiety is communicated interpersonally. The quiet calm of the nurse can serve to calm the patient. The presence of anxiety can escalate anxiety in the patient.
Always remain with the person experiencing an acute severe to panic level of anxiety.	Alone with immense anxiety, a person feels abandoned. A caring face may be the patient's only contact with reality when confusion becomes overwhelming.
Minimize environmental stimuli. Move to a quieter setting and stay with the patient.	Helps minimize further escalation of patient's anxiety.
Use clear and simple statements and repetition.	A person experiencing a severe to panic level of anxiety has difficulty concentrating and processing information.
Use a low-pitched voice; speak slowly.	A high-pitched voice can convey anxiety. Low pitch can decrease anxiety.
Reinforce reality if distortions occur (e.g., seeing objects that are not there or hearing voices when no one is present).	Anxiety can be reduced by focusing on and validating what is going on in the environment.
Listen for themes in communication.	In severe to panic levels of anxiety, verbal communication themes may be the only indication of the patient's thoughts or feelings.
Attend to physical and safety needs when necessary (e.g., need for warmth, fluids, elimination, pain relief, family contact).	High levels of anxiety may obscure the patient's awareness of physical needs.
Because safety is an overall goal, physical limits may need to be set. Speak in a firm, authoritative voice: "You may not hit anyone here. If you can't control yourself, we will help you."	A person who is out of control is often terrorized. Staff must offer the patient and others protection from destructive and self-destructive impulses.
Provide opportunities for exercise (e.g., walk with nurse, punching bag, ping-pong game).	Physical activity helps channel and dissipate tension and may temporarily lower anxiety.
When a person is constantly moving or pacing, offer high-calorie fluids.	Dehydration and exhaustion must be prevented.
Assess need for medication or seclusion after other interventions have been tried and not been successful.	Exhaustion and physical harm to self and others must be prevented.

BOX 12-1 *NIC* **Interventions for Anxiety Disorders**

Coping Enhancement

Definition: Assisting a patient to adapt to perceived stressors, changes, or threats that interfere with meeting life demands and roles

Activities*:
- Provide an atmosphere of acceptance.
- Encourage verbalization of feelings, perceptions, and fears.
- Acknowledge the patient's spiritual/cultural background.
- Discourage decision making when the patient is under severe stress.

Hope Inspiration

Definition: Enhancing the belief in one's capacity to initiate and sustain actions

Activities*:
- Assist the patient to identify areas of hope in life.
- Demonstrate hope by recognizing the patient's intrinsic worth and viewing the patient's illness as only one facet of the individual.
- Avoid masking the truth.
- Help the patient expand spiritual self.

Self-Esteem Enhancement

Definition: Assisting a patient to increase his or her personal judgment of self-worth

Activities:*
- Make positive statements about the patient.
- Monitor frequency of self-negating verbalizations.
- Explore previous achievements.
- Explore reasons for self-criticism or guilt.

Relaxation Therapy

Definition: Use of techniques to encourage and elicit relaxation for the purpose of decreasing undesirable signs and symptoms such as pain, muscle tension, or anxiety

Activities:*
- Demonstrate and practice the relaxation technique with the patient.
- Provide written information about preparing and engaging in relaxation techniques.
- Anticipate the need for the use of relaxation.
- Evaluate and document the response to relaxation therapy.

---

*Partial list.

Data from Bulechek, G. M., Butcher, H. K., & Dochterman, J. M. (2008). *Nursing interventions classification (NIC)* (5th ed.). St. Louis: Mosby.

Counseling

Basic level psychiatric mental health nurses use counseling to reduce anxiety, enhance coping and communication skills, and intervene in crises. When patients request or prefer to use integrative therapies, the nurse performs assessment and teaching as appropriate.

Milieu Therapy

As mentioned earlier, most patients who demonstrate anxiety disorders can be treated successfully as outpatients. Hospital admission is necessary only if severe anxiety or symptoms interfere with the individual's health or if the individual is suicidal. When hospitalization is necessary, the following features of the therapeutic milieu can be especially helpful to the patient:

- Structuring the daily routine to offer physical safety and predictability, thus reducing anxiety over the unknown
- Providing daily activities to promote sharing and cooperation
- Providing therapeutic interactions, including one-on-one nursing care and behavior contracts
- Including the patient in decisions about his or her own care

Promotion of Self-Care Activities

Patients with anxiety disorders are usually able to meet their own basic physical needs. Self-care activities that are most likely to be affected are discussed in the following sections.

Nutrition and Fluid Intake

Patients who engage in ritualistic behaviors may be too involved with their rituals to take time to eat and drink. Some phobic patients may be so afraid of germs, they cannot eat. In general, nutritious diets with snacks should be provided. Adequate intake should be firmly encouraged, but a power struggle should be avoided. Weighing patients frequently (e.g., three times a week) is useful in assessing nutrition.

Personal Hygiene and Grooming

Some patients, especially those with OCD and phobias, may be excessively neat and engage in time-consuming rituals associated with bathing and dressing. Hygiene, dressing, and grooming may take several hours. Maintenance of skin integrity may become a problem when the rituals involve excessive washing and skin becomes excoriated and infected.

Some patients are indecisive about bathing or about what clothing should be worn. For the latter, limiting choices to two outfits is helpful. In the event of severe indecisiveness, simply presenting the patient with the clothing to be worn may be necessary. You may also need to remain with the patient to give simple directions: "Put on your shirt. Now put on your slacks." Matter-of-fact support is effective in assisting patients to independently perform as much of a task as possible. Encourage patients to express thoughts and feelings about self-care. This communication can provide a basis for later health teaching or for ongoing dialogue about the patient's abilities.

Elimination

Patients with OCD may be so involved with the performance of rituals that they may suppress the urge to void and defecate. Constipation and urinary tract infections may result. Interventions may include creating a regular schedule for taking the patient to the bathroom.

Sleep

Patients experiencing anxiety frequently have difficulty sleeping. Patients may perform rituals to the exclusion of resting and sleeping, and physical exhaustion may occur. Patients with GAD, PTSD, and acute stress disorder often experience sleep disturbance from nightmares. Teaching them how to discover ways to promote sleep (e.g., warm bath, warm milk, relaxing music) and monitoring sleep through a sleep record

are useful interventions. Chapter 20 offers an in-depth discussion of sleep disturbances.

Pharmacological Interventions

Several classes of medications have been found to be effective in the treatment of anxiety disorders. Table 12-14 identifies medications approved by the U.S. Food and Drug Administration (FDA) for the treatment of anxiety, as well as medications that do not have specific approval but are commonly used "off-label" for anxiety disorders. Review Chapter 3 for more detailed explanation of the actions of psychotropic medications.

Antidepressants

Selective serotonin reuptake inhibitors (SSRIs) are the first-line treatment for acute stress disorders and PTSD (Sadock & Sadock, 2008). They are preferable to the tricyclic antidepressants (TCAs) because they have a more rapid onset of action and fewer problematic side effects.

TABLE 12-14 Drug Treatment of Patients with Anxiety Disorders

Generic (Trade)	FDA-Approved Uses	Off-Label Uses
ANTIDEPRESSANTS		
Selective Serotonin Reuptake Inhibitors		
Citalopram (Celexa)		Panic disorder Social anxiety disorder Obsessive-compulsive disorder Generalized anxiety disorder Posttraumatic stress disorder
Escitalopram (Lexapro)	Generalized anxiety disorder	Panic disorder Social anxiety disorder Obsessive-compulsive disorder Posttraumatic stress disorder
Fluoxetine (Prozac)	Panic disorder Obsessive-compulsive disorder	Social anxiety disorder Generalized anxiety disorder Posttraumatic stress disorder
Fluvoxamine (Luvox)	Obsessive-compulsive disorder Social anxiety disorder	Panic disorder Generalized anxiety disorder Posttraumatic stress disorder
Paroxetine (Paxil)	Panic disorder Social anxiety disorder Obsessive-compulsive disorder Generalized anxiety disorder Posttraumatic stress disorder	
Sertraline (Zoloft)	Panic disorder Social anxiety disorder Obsessive-compulsive disorder Posttraumatic stress disorder	Generalized anxiety disorder

TABLE 12-14 Drug Treatment of Patients with Anxiety Disorders—cont'd

Generic (Trade)	FDA-Approved Uses	Off-Label Uses
Selective Serotonin Norepinephrine Reuptake Inhibitors		
Duloxetine (Cymbalta)	Panic disorder Generalized anxiety disorder	Obsessive-compulsive disorder Posttraumatic stress disorder
Venlafaxine (Effexor)	Generalized anxiety disorder Social anxiety disorder Panic disorder	Obsessive-compulsive disorder Posttraumatic stress disorder
Tricyclics		
Amitriptyline (Elavil)		Panic disorder Generalized anxiety disorder Posttraumatic stress disorder
Clomipramine (Anafranil)	Obsessive-compulsive disorder	Panic disorder Generalized anxiety disorder Posttraumatic stress disorder
Desipramine (Norpramin)		Panic disorder Generalized anxiety disorder Posttraumatic stress disorder
Doxepin (Adapin, Sinequan)		Panic disorder Generalized anxiety disorder Posttraumatic stress disorder
Imipramine (Tofranil)		Panic disorder Generalized anxiety disorder Posttraumatic stress disorder
Nortriptyline (Aventyl, Pamelor)		Panic disorder Generalized anxiety disorder Posttraumatic stress disorder
Monoamine Oxidase Inhibitors		
Phenelzine (Nardil)		Panic disorder Social anxiety disorder Generalized anxiety disorder Posttraumatic stress disorder
Tranylcypromine (Parnate)		Panic disorder Social anxiety disorder Generalized anxiety disorder Posttraumatic stress disorder
ANTIANXIETY AGENTS		
Benzodiazepines		
Alprazolam (Xanax)	Panic disorder Generalized anxiety disorder	Social anxiety disorder
Chlordiazepoxide (Librium)		Panic disorder Social anxiety disorder Generalized anxiety disorder
Clonazepam (Klonopin)	Panic disorder	Generalized anxiety disorder Social anxiety disorder
Diazepam (Valium)	Generalized anxiety disorder	Panic disorder Social anxiety disorder
Lorazepam (Ativan)		Panic disorder Social anxiety disorder Generalized anxiety disorder

Continued

TABLE 12-14 Drug Treatment of Patients with Anxiety Disorders—cont'd

Generic (Trade)	FDA-Approved Uses	Off-Label Uses
Oxazepam (Serax)		Panic disorder Social anxiety disorder Generalized anxiety disorder
Nonbenzodiazepines Buspirone (BuSpar)	Generalized anxiety disorder	Social anxiety disorder Obsessive-compulsive disorder
OTHER CLASSES		
Antihistamines Hydroxyzine hydrochloride (Atarax)		Generalized anxiety disorder
Hydroxyzine pamoate (Vistaril)		Generalized anxiety disorder
β-Blockers Atenolol (Tenormin)		Social anxiety disorder
Propranolol (Inderal)		Social anxiety disorder
Anticonvulsants Carbamazepine (Tegretol)		Posttraumatic stress disorder Panic disorder
Gabapentin (Neurontin)		Panic disorder Social anxiety disorder Generalized anxiety disorder Posttraumatic stress disorder
Valproic acid (Depakote)		Panic disorder Social anxiety disorder Generalized anxiety disorder Posttraumatic stress disorder

Data from Clip & Save: Drug Chart. (2008). *Journal of Psychosocial and Mental Health Services, 46,* 5; Stahl, S. M. (2006). *Essential psychopharmacology: The prescriber's guide* (Revised and updated ed.). New York: Cambridge; and Pollack, M. H., Kinrys, G., Delong, H., Vasconcelos, D., & Simon, N. (2008). The pharmacotherapy of anxiety disorders. In T. A. Stern, J. F. Rosenbaum, M. Fava, J. Biederman, & S. L. Rauch (Eds.). *Massachusetts General Hospital comprehensive clinical psychiatry: Expert consult.* Philadelphia: Mosby.

Duloxetine (Cymbalta) and Venlafaxine (Effexor) are serotonin-norepinephrine reuptake inhibitors (SNRIs) that are also useful for treatment of some anxiety disorders.

Monoamine oxidase inhibitors (MAOIs) are reserved for treatment-resistant conditions because of the risk of life-threatening hypertensive crisis if the patient does not follow dietary restrictions (patients cannot eat foods containing tyramine and must be given specific dietary instructions). The risk of hypertensive crisis also makes the use of MAOIs contraindicated in patients with comorbid substance abuse.

Antidepressants have the secondary benefit of treating comorbid depressive disorders. Some of the SSRIs exert more of an "activating" effect than others and may increase anxiety. Sertraline (Zoloft) and paroxetine (Paxil) seem to have a more calming effect than the other SSRIs.

Antianxiety Drugs

Antianxiety drugs (also called *anxiolytics*) are often used to treat the somatic and psychological symptoms of anxiety disorders (Pollock et al., 2008). When moderate or severe anxiety is reduced, patients are better able to participate in treatment of their underlying problems. Benzodiazepines are most commonly used because they have a quick onset of action. However, due to the potential for dependence these medications ideally should be used for short periods only until other medications or treatments reduce symptoms. An important nursing intervention is to monitor for side effects of the benzodiazepines, including sedation, ataxia, and decreased cognitive function. Benzodiazepines are not recommended for patients with a known substance abuse problem and should not be given to women during pregnancy or breast feeding. Box 12-2 gives other important information for patient teaching.

BOX 12-2   Patient and Family Teaching: Antianxiety Medications

1. Caution the patient:
   - Not to increase dose or frequency of ingestion without prior approval of therapist.
   - That these medications reduce the ability to handle mechanical equipment (e.g., cars, saws, and machinery).
   - Not to drink alcoholic beverages or take other antianxiety drugs, because depressant effects of both would be potentiated.
   - To avoid drinking beverages containing caffeine, because they decrease the desired effects of the drug.
2. Recommend that the patient taking benzodiazepines avoid becoming pregnant, because these drugs increase the risk of congenital anomalies.
3. Advise the patient not to breast-feed, because these drugs are excreted in the milk and would have adverse effects on the infant.
4. Teach a patient who is taking monoamine oxidase inhibitors about the details of a tyramine-restricted diet (see Chapter 3).
5. Teach the patient that:
   - Cessation of benzodiazepine use after 3 to 4 months of daily use may cause withdrawal symptoms such as insomnia, irritability, nervousness, dry mouth, tremors, convulsions, and confusion.
   - Medications should be taken with or shortly after meals or snacks to reduce gastrointestinal discomfort.
   - Drug interactions can occur: Antacids may delay absorption; cimetidine interferes with metabolism of benzodiazepines, causing increased sedation; central nervous system depressants, such as alcohol and barbiturates, cause increased sedation; serum phenytoin concentration may build up because of decreased metabolism.

Buspirone (BuSpar) is an alternative antianxiety medication that does not cause dependence, but 2 to 4 weeks are required for it to reach full effects. The drug may be used for long-term treatment and should be taken regularly.

Other Classes of Medications

Other classes of medications sometimes used to treat anxiety disorders include β-blockers, antihistamines, and anticonvulsants. These agents are often added if the first course of treatment is ineffective. β-Blockers block the nerves that stimulate the heart to beat faster and have been used to treat SAD. Anticonvulsants have shown some benefit in the management of GAD, PD, PTSD, and SAD (Sadock & Sadock, 2008). Antihistamines are a safe, nonaddictive alternative to benzodiazepines to lower anxiety levels, and again

are helpful in treating patients with substance use problems.

Another therapeutic strategy may come in a most unusual form. D-cycloserine is an antibiotic used to treat tuberculosis that has also been demonstrated to enhance learning. D-cycloserine binds with N-methyl-D-aspartate (NMDA) receptors in the area of the brain that mediates fears and phobic responses, the amygdale and may help patients *unlearn* fear responses more quickly (Stahl, 2008). Administration of this drug while undergoing cognitive behavioral therapy actually promotes fear extinction, not just fear conditioning, in phobic individuals. It has also been useful when combined with extinction-based exposure therapy in the treatment of obsessive-compulsive disorder and social anxiety disorder (Kushner et al., 2007; Hoffman et al., 2006).

Integrative Therapy

Chapter 36 identifies a number of complementary practices or integrative therapies that people use to cope with stress in their lives. Herbal and complementary therapy is very popular, and an estimated $34 billion is spent in the United States annually for these products (Alsawaf & Aminah, 2007). However, herbs and dietary supplements are not subject to the same rigorous testing as prescription medications. Also, herbs and dietary supplements are not required to be uniform, and there is no guarantee bioequivalence of the active compound among preparations.

Problems that can occur with the use of psychotropic herbs include toxic side effects and herb-drug interactions. Nurses and other health care providers do well to improve their knowledge of these products so that discussions with their patients provide informed and reliable information. The Integrative Therapy box discusses kava kava, an herb often used for its sedative and antianxiety effects.

Health Teaching

Health teaching is a significant nursing intervention for patients with anxiety disorders. Patients may conceal symptoms for years before seeking treatment and often come to the attention of health care providers during a co-occurring problem. People with PD and GAD seem more motivated than those with other anxiety disorders to get treatment; most seek help during the first year of symptoms (Wang et al., 2005). Only 7% of people with PTSD seek help during the first year of symptoms; in fact, on average they wait 12 years before getting help for their symptoms.

Teaching about the specific disorder and available effective treatments is a major step to improving the quality of life for those with anxiety disorders. Whether in a community or hospital setting, nurses can

INTEGRATIVE THERAPY

Kava Kava

Kava kava is prepared from a South Pacific plant *(Piper methysticum)* and is used as an herbal sedative with anti-anxiety effects. Prior to seeking psychiatric treatment, patients with anxiety disorders may try kava kava in the belief that herbs are safer than medications, but it may have a darker side. Kava kava is known to dramatically inhibit a liver enzyme (P450) necessary for the metabolism of many medications. This inhibition could result in liver failure, especially when taken along with alcohol or other medications such as central nervous system depressants (antianxiety agents fall into this category).

This potentially dangerous interaction highlights the need for the nurse to ask about all medications the patient is taking—both prescribed and over-the-counter—before administering medications to those with anxiety disorders. Several countries have actually taken kava kava off of the market, but some researchers believe that the benefits of this drug may outweigh the risks, compared to other medications used to treat anxiety. The bottom line is that kava kava is considered to be beneficial for short-term use in mild to moderate anxiety. But as with any drug, it should be used carefully.

Saeed, S. A., Bloch, R. M., & Antonacci, D. J. (2007). Herbal and dietary supplements for treatment of anxiety disorders. *Complementary and Alternative Medicine, 76,* 549–556.

teach patients about signs and symptoms of anxiety disorders, presumed causes or risk factors (especially substance abuse), medications, the use of relaxation techniques, and the benefits of psychotherapy.

Advanced Practice Interventions

Advanced practice nurses use several cognitive and behavioral treatment approaches, including relaxation training, modeling, systematic desensitization, flooding, response prevention, and thought stopping.

Cognitive Therapy

Cognitive therapy is based on the belief that patients make errors in thinking that lead to mistaken negative beliefs about self and others. For example, "I have to be perfect or my boyfriend will not love me." Through a process called **cognitive restructuring**, the therapist helps the patient (1) identify automatic negative beliefs that cause anxiety, (2) explore the basis for these thoughts, (3) reevaluate the situation realistically, and (4) replace negative self-talk with supportive ideas.

Behavioral Therapy

There are currently several forms of **behavioral therapy**, which involve teaching and physical practice of activities to decrease anxious or avoidant behavior:

- **Relaxation training**—Relaxation exercises for breathing or muscle groups are taught. The relaxation response is the opposite of the stress response and results in a reduced heart rate and breathing and relaxed muscles. Refer to Chapter 11 for a description of different approaches to relaxation training.
- **Modeling**—The therapist or significant other acts as a role model to demonstrate appropriate behavior in a feared situation, and then the patient imitates it. For example, the role model rides in an elevator with a claustrophobic patient.
- **Systemic desensitization**—The patient is gradually introduced to a feared object or experience through a series of steps, from the least frightening to the most frightening (graduated exposure). The patient is taught to use a relaxation technique at each step when anxiety becomes overwhelming. For example, a patient with agoraphobia would start with opening the door to the house to go out on the steps and advance to attending a movie in a theater. The therapist may start with imagined situations in the office before moving on to in vivo (live) exposures.
- **Flooding**—Unlike systemic desensitization, this method exposes the patient to a large amount of an undesirable stimulus in an effort to extinguish the anxiety response. The patient learns through prolonged exposure that survival is possible and that anxiety diminishes spontaneously. For example, an obsessive patient who usually touches objects with a paper towel may be forced to touch objects with a bare hand for 1 hour. By the end of that period, the anxiety level is lower.
- **Response prevention**—This method is used for compulsive behavior. The therapist does not allow the patient to perform the compulsive ritual (e.g., hand washing), and the patient learns that anxiety does subside even when the ritual is not completed. After trying this in the office, the patient learns to set time limits at home to gradually lengthen the time between rituals until the urge fades away.
- **Thought stopping**—In this technique a negative thought or obsession is interrupted. The patient may be instructed to say "Stop!" out loud when the idea comes to mind or to snap a rubber band worn on the wrist. This distraction briefly blocks the automatic undesirable thought and cues the patient to select an alternative, more positive idea. (After learning the exercise, the patient gives the command silently.)

Cognitive-Behavioral Therapy

Cognitive-behavioral therapy combines cognitive therapy with specific behavioral therapies to reduce the anxiety response. Cognitive-behavioral therapy includes cognitive restructuring, psychoeducation, breathing restraining and muscle relaxation, teaching of self-monitoring for panic and other symptoms, and in vivo (real life) exposure to feared objects or situations.

EVALUATION

Identified outcomes serve as the basis for evaluation. Each *NOC* outcome has a built-in rating scale that helps the nurse measure improvement. In general, evaluation of outcomes for patients with anxiety disorders deals with questions such as the following:

- Is the patient experiencing a reduced level of anxiety?
- Does the patient recognize symptoms as anxiety related?
- Does the patient continue to display obsessions, compulsions, phobias, worrying, or other symptoms of anxiety disorders? If still present, are they more or less frequent? More or less intense?

- Is the patient able to use newly learned behaviors to manage anxiety?
- Can the patient adequately perform self-care activities?
- Can the patient maintain satisfying interpersonal relations?
- Can the patient assume usual roles?

KEY POINTS TO REMEMBER

- Anxiety has an unknown or unrecognized source, whereas fear is a reaction to a specific threat.
- Peplau operationally defined four levels of anxiety (mild, moderate, severe, and panic). The patient's perceptual field, ability to learn, and physical and other characteristics are different at each level (see Table 12-1).
- Defenses against anxiety can be adaptive or maladaptive and in a hierarchy from healthy to intermediate to immature. Table 12-2 provides adaptive and maladaptive examples of many of the more common defense mechanisms.

Case Study and Nursing Care Plan 12-1   Severe Level of Anxiety

The following case study describes a man experiencing a severe level of acute anxiety. See if you can match his signs and symptoms with those in Table 12-1.

Matt Michaels, a 63-year-old man, comes into the emergency department (ED) with his wife Anne, who has taken an overdose of sleeping pills and antidepressant medications. Ten years earlier, Anne's mother died, and since that time Anne has suffered several episodes of severe depression with suicide attempts. She has needed hospitalization during these episodes. Anne Michaels had been released from the hospital 2 weeks earlier after treatment for depression and threatened suicide.

Matt has a long-established routine of giving his wife her antidepressant medications in the morning and her sleeping medication at night and keeping the bottles hidden when he is not at home. Today he had forgotten to hide the medications before he went to work. His wife had

taken the remaining pills from both bottles with large quantities of alcohol. When Matt returned home for lunch, Anne was comatose. In the ED, Anne suffers cardiac arrest and is taken to the intensive care unit (ICU).

Matt appears very jittery. He moves about the room aimlessly. He drops his hat, a medication card, and his keys. His hands are trembling, and he looks around the room, bewildered. He appears unable to focus on any one thing. He says over and over, in a loud, high-pitched voice, "Why didn't I hide the bottles?" He is wringing his hands and begins stomping his feet, saying, "It's all my fault. Everything is falling apart."

Other people in the waiting room appear distracted and alarmed by his behavior. Matt seems to be oblivious to his surroundings.

ASSESSMENT

Gabriel Brown, the psychiatric nurse clinician working in the ED, comes into the waiting room and assesses Matt's behavior as indicative of a severe anxiety level. After talking with Matt briefly, Gabriel believes nursing intervention is indicated. Gabriel bases his conclusion on the following assessment of the patient:

Objective Data

Unable to focus on anything
Engaging in purposeless activity (walking around aimlessly)
Oblivious to his surroundings
Showing unproductive relief behavior (stomping, wringing hands, dropping things)

Subjective Data

"Everything is falling apart."
"Why didn't I hide the bottles?"
"It's all my fault."

Continued

DIAGNOSIS

Gabriel formulates the following nursing diagnosis:

Anxiety (severe) related to the patient's perception of responsibility for his wife's coma and possible death, as evidenced by inability to focus, confusion, and the feeling that "everything is falling apart"

OUTCOMES IDENTIFICATION

Patient will demonstrate effective coping strategies.

PLANNING

Gabriel thinks that if he can lower Matt's anxiety to a moderate level, he can work with Matt to get a clear picture of his situation and place the events in a more realistic perspective. He also thinks Matt needs to talk to someone and share some of his pain and confusion to help sort out his feelings. Gabriel identifies two short-term goals:

1. Patient's anxiety will decrease from severe to moderate by 4 PM
2. Patient will verbalize his feelings and a need for assistance by 4 PM

IMPLEMENTATION

Gabriel takes Matt to a quiet room in the back of the ED. He introduces himself to Matt and comments that he notices that Matt is upset. He says, "I will stay with you." At first, Matt finds it difficult to sit down and continues pacing around the room. Gabriel sits quietly and calmly while listening to Matt's self-recriminations. He attends carefully to what Matt is saying—and what he is not saying—to identify themes.

After a while, Matt becomes calmer and is able to sit next to Gabriel. Gabriel offers him orange juice, which he accepts and holds tightly.

Gabriel speaks calmly, using simple, clear statements. He uses communication tools that are helpful to Matt in sorting out his feelings and naming them.

Dialogue	Therapeutic Tool/Comment
Matt: Yes…yes…I forgot to hide the bottles. She usually tells me when she feels bad. Why didn't she tell me?	
Nurse: You think that if she had told you she wanted to kill herself you would have hidden the pills?	Gabriel asks for clarification on Matt's thinking.
Matt: Yes, if I had only known, this wouldn't have happened.	
Nurse: It sounds as if you believe you should have known what your wife was thinking without her telling you.	Here Gabriel clarifies Matt's expectations that he should be able to read his wife's mind.
Matt: Well…yes…when you put it that way…I just don't know what I'll do if she dies.	

When Gabriel thinks that Matt has discussed his feelings of guilt sufficiently, he asks Matt to clarify his thinking about his wife's behavior. Matt is able to place his feelings of guilt in a more realistic perspective. Next, Gabriel brings up another issue—the question of whether Matt's wife will live or die.

Dialogue	Therapeutic Tool/Comment
Nurse: You said that if your wife dies, you don't know what you will do.	Gabriel reflects Matt's feelings back to him.
Matt: Oh, God (he begins to cry); I can't live without her…she's all I have in the world.	
Silence	
Nurse: She means a great deal to you.	Gabriel reflects Matt's feelings back to him.
Matt: Everything. Since her mother died, we are each other's only family.	
Nurse: What would it mean to you if your wife died?	Gabriel asks Matt to evaluate his feelings about his wife.

Dialogue	Therapeutic Tool/Comment
Matt: I couldn't live by myself, alone. I couldn't stand it. (Starts to cry again.)	
Nurse: It sounds as if being alone is very frightening to you.	Gabriel restates in clear terms Matt's experience and feelings.
Matt: Yes…I don't know how I'd manage by myself.	
Nurse: A change like that could take time to adjust to.	Gabriel validates that if Matt's wife died, it would be very painful. At the same time, he implies hope that Matt could work through the death in time.
Matt: Yes…it would be very hard.	

Again Gabriel gives Matt a chance to sort out his feelings and fears. Gabriel helps him focus on the reality that his wife may die and encourages him to express fears related to her possible death. After a while, Gabriel offers to go up to the ICU with Matt to see how his wife is doing. When they arrive at the ICU, although Anne is still comatose, her condition has stabilized, and she is breathing on her own.

After his arrival at the ICU, Matt starts to worry about whether he remembered to lock the door at home. Gabriel suggests that he call neighbors and ask them to check the door. At this time, Matt is able to focus on everyday things. Gabriel makes arrangements to see Matt the next day when he comes in to visit his wife.

The next day, Anne has regained consciousness. She is discharged 1 week later. At the time of discharge, Matt and Anne Michaels are considering family therapy with the psychiatric nurse clinician once a week in the outpatient department.

EVALUATION

The first short-term goal is to lower anxiety from severe to moderate. Gabriel can see that Matt has become more visibly calm: his trembling, wringing of hands, and stomping of feet have ceased, and he is able to focus on his thoughts and feelings with Gabriel's help.

The second short-term goal established for Matt is that he will verbalize his feelings and his need for assistance. Matt is able to identify and discuss with Gabriel his feelings of guilt and fear of being left alone in the world if his wife should die. Both these feelings are overwhelming him. He is also able to state that he needs assistance in coping with these feelings in order to make tentative plans for the future.

Case Study and Nursing Care Plan **12-2** Posttraumatic Stress Disorder

Mr. Blake, 46, is brought to the emergency department by his very distraught wife after she finds him writing a suicide note and planning to shoot himself in the woods with a hand gun. Mr. Blake is subdued, shows minimal affect, and his breath has the distinct odor of alcohol. When asked about suicidal thoughts, he states that he is worthless and that his wife and family would be better off if he were dead. He refuses to contract for safety. The decision is made to hospitalize him to protect him from danger to himself.

Mr. Blake's wife gives further history. Her husband is a construction contractor who served in the United States National Guard during the Iraq War. He lost half his squad from a roadside bombing, narrowly escaping with his life. He walks with a permanent limp due to the attack. Upon

returning home he showed no signs of anxiety and refused offers of crisis treatment, stating, "I was in a war, I can handle stress." But 6 months later, Mrs. Blake noticed that her husband had trouble sleeping, his mood was irritable or withdrawn, he avoided news reports on television, and he started drinking daily. He complained of nightmares but would not talk to her about his fears. He only agreed to go to the primary care provider, a nurse practitioner, to request sleeping medication.

Mr. Blake was admitted to the psychiatric unit and his care assigned to Ms. Dawson, a registered nurse. She observes that Mr. Blake is quiet and passive as he is oriented to the unit, but that he looks around vigilantly and is easily startled by sounds on the unit.

Continued

ASSESSMENT

Self-Assessment

Ms. Dawson is a registered nurse with an associate degree and 3 years of experience on this unit. Initially she feels sympathy for Mr. Blake, and he reminds her of her Uncle James, who served in Vietnam. She is concerned because his suicide plan was lethal and he is guarded in his speech, not revealing his thoughts or feelings. She realizes that as she implements suicide precautions, she must demonstrate an attitude of hope and acceptance to encourage him to develop trust. Also, she must stay neutral and not convey any pity or sympathy.

Objective Data

Sleep difficulty, nightmares
Hypervigilance
Alcohol use
Irritability
Withdrawn mood
Constricted/reduced range of affect
Feels estranged from wife and children
Avoidance of news coverage with potential for emergency
  reports
Refusal of treatment and safety contract
Plan for suicide

Subjective Data

"I don't deserve to live; I should have died with the
  others."
"You can't stop me."

DIAGNOSIS

Risk for suicide related to anger and hopelessness due to severe trauma, as evidenced by suicidal plan and verbalization
  of intent
Lethal plan with saved prescription medication and alcohol
Refusal to contract for safety
Emotional withdrawal from wife

OUTCOMES IDENTIFICATION

Patient will consistently refrain from attempting suicide.

PLANNING

The initial plan is to maintain safety for Mr. Blake while encouraging him to express feelings and recognize that his situation is not hopeless.

IMPLEMENTATION

Mr. Blake's plan of care is personalized as follows:

Short-Term Goal	Intervention	Rationale	Evaluation
1. Patient will speak to staff whenever experiencing self-destructive thoughts.	1a. Administer medications with mouth checks.	1a. Addresses risk of hiding medications	GOAL MET After 8 hours, patient contracts for safety every shift and starts to discuss feelings of self-harm.
	1b. Provide ongoing surveillance of patient and environment.	1b. Provides one-to-one monitoring for safety.	
	1c. Contract for "no self-harm" for specified periods.	1c. Encourages increased self-control.	

Short-Term Goal	Intervention	Rationale	Evaluation
	1d. Use direct, nonjudgmental approach in discussing suicide.	1d. Shows acceptance of patient's situation with respect.	
	1e. Provide illness teaching regarding PTSD.	1e. Offers reality of treatment.	
2. Patient will express feelings by the third day of hospitalization.	2a. Interact with patient at regular intervals to convey caring and openness and to provide an opportunity to talk.	2a. Encourages development of trust.	GOAL MET By second day, patient occasionally answers questions about feelings and admits to anger and grief.
	2b. Use silence and listening to encourage expression of feelings.	2b. Shows positive expectation that patient will respond.	
	2c. Be open to expressions of loneliness and powerlessness.	2c. Allows patient to voice these uncomfortable feelings.	
	2d. Share observations or thoughts about patient's behavior or response.	2d. Directs attention to here-and-now treatment situation.	
3. Patient will express will to live by discharge from unit.	3a. Listen to expressions of grief.	3a. Supports patient, communicates that such feelings are natural.	GOAL MET By third day, patient becomes tearful and states that he does not want to hurt his wife and daughter.
	3b. Encourage patient to identify own strengths and abilities.	3b. Affirms patient's worth and potential to survive.	
	3c. Explore with patient previous methods of dealing with life problems.	3c. Reinforces patient's past coping skills and ability to problem solve now.	
	3d. Assist in identifying available support systems.	3d. Addresses fact that anxiety has narrowed patient's perspective, distorting reality about loved ones.	
	3e. Refer to spiritual advisor of individual's choice.	3e. Allows opportunity to explore spiritual values and self-worth.	

EVALUATION

See individual outcomes and evaluation within the care plan.

- Anxiety disorders are the most common psychiatric disorders in the United States and frequently co-occur with depression or substance abuse.
- Research has identified genetic and biological factors in the etiology of anxiety disorders.
- Psychological theories and cultural influences are also pertinent to the understanding of anxiety disorders.
- Patients with anxiety disorders suffer from panic attacks, irrational fears, excessive worrying, uncontrollable rituals, or severe reactions to stress.
- People with anxiety disorders are often too embarrassed or ashamed to seek psychiatric help. Instead, they may go to primary care providers with multiple somatic complaints.
- Psychiatric treatment is effective for anxiety disorders.
- Basic level nursing interventions include counseling, milieu therapy, promotion of self-care activities, psychobiological intervention, and health teaching.
- Advanced practice nursing interventions include behavioral and cognitive-behavioral therapies.

CRITICAL THINKING

1. Ethan is a senior in college and is taking his final examinations for an engineering course. The professor catches him copying from the examination of his willing partner, Jessica, and takes his exam away. Ethan's heart immediately begins to pound, his pulse and respiration rates increase, and he has to wipe perspiration from his hands and face several times. He feels as if he has to vomit and has a throbbing in his head.

   When talking with the professor after the examination, he initially has difficulty focusing; when he starts to speak, his voice trembles. Ethan says that Jessica convinced him that cheating was done all the time—in fact, it was her idea. Ethan goes on to say that this "silly little exam" doesn't mean anything anyway, that he already passed the important courses. He tells the professor, "I thought you were the greatest, and now I see that you're a fool." The professor remains calm and explains that regardless of Ethan's thoughts on this matter, Ethan was caught cheating, he will have to take responsibility for his actions, and the choice to cheat was his. The professor will have Ethan go before the disciplinary board, which is the well-known procedure when one is caught cheating. When Ethan realizes that this incident could affect his graduating on time, he begins to yell at the professor and call him offensive names. Another professor walking past the classroom witnesses this encounter.
   A. Identify the level of anxiety Ethan was experiencing once he was caught cheating, and describe the signs and symptoms that helped you determine this level.
   B. Identify and define five defense mechanisms Ethan used to lessen his anxiety.
   C. Given the circumstances once Ethan was caught, how could he have reacted using healthier coping defenses in a manner that would have reflected more self-responsibility?

2. Ms. Smith, a patient with OCD, washes her hands until they are cracked and bleeding. Your nursing goal is to promote healing of her hands. What interventions will you plan?

3. This is Mr. Olivetti's third emergency department visit in a week. He is experiencing severe anxiety accompanied by many physical symptoms. He clings to you, desperately crying, "Help me! Help me! Don't let me die!" Diagnostic tests have ruled out a physical disorder. The patient outcome has been identified as "Patient anxiety level will be reduced to moderate/mild within one hour."
   A. What interventions should you use? Be comprehensive in your approach.
   B. Mr. Olivetti is given an appointment at the anxiety disorders clinic. How will you explain the importance of keeping the clinic appointment? Are there any factors you would have to consider while providing patient education?

4. Mrs. Valenti is a patient with GAD. She has a history of substance abuse and is now a recovering alcoholic. During a clinic visit, she tells you she plans to ask the psychiatrist to prescribe diazepam (Valium) to use when she feels anxious. She asks whether you think this is a good idea. How would you respond? What action could you take?

CHAPTER REVIEW

1. Since learning that he will have a trial pass to a new group home tomorrow, Bill's usual behavior has changed. He has started to pace rapidly, has become very distracted, and is breathing rapidly. He has trouble focusing on anything other than the group home issue and complains that he suddenly feels very nauseated. Which initial nursing response is most appropriate for Bill's level of anxiety?
   1. "You seem anxious. Would you like to talk about how you are feeling?"
   2. "If you do not calm down, I will have to give you prn medicine to calm you."
   3. "Bill, slow down. Listen to me. You are safe. Take a nice, deep breath.."
   4. "We can delay the visit to the group home if that would help you calm down."

2. A patient, who seems to be angry when his family again fails to visit as promised, tells the nurse that he is fine and that the visit wasn't important to him anyway. When the nurse suggests that perhaps he might be disappointed or even a little angry that the family has again let him down, the patient responds that it is his family that is angry, not him, or else they would have visited. What defense mechanism(s) is this patient using to deal with his feelings? *Select all that apply.*
   1. Rationalization
   2. Introjection
   3. Projection
   4. Regression
   5. Denial
   6. Dissociation

3. John, a construction worker, is on duty when a wall under construction suddenly falls, crushing a number of co-workers. Shaken initially, he seems to be coping well with the tragedy but later begins to experience tremors, nightmares, and periods during which he feels numb or detached from his environment. He finds himself frequently thinking about the tragedy and feeling guilty that he was spared while many others died. Which statement about this situation is most accurate?
   1. John is experiencing posttraumatic stress disorder (PTSD) and requires therapy.
   2. John has acute stress disorder and should be treated with antianxiety medications.
   3. John is experiencing anxiety and grief and should be monitored for PTSD symptoms.
   4. John is experiencing mild anxiety and a normal grief reaction; no intervention is needed.

4. A variety of medications are used in the treatment of severe anxiety disorders. Which class of medication used to treat anxiety is potentially addictive?

1. Benzodiazepines
2. Selective serotonin reuptake inhibitors (SSRIs)
3. Beta-blockers
4. Antihistamines
5. Buspirone

5. An older adult in the outpatient internal medicine clinic complains of feeling a sense of dread and fearfulness without apparent cause. It has been growing steadily worse and is to the point where it is interfering with the patient's sleep and volunteer work. After a brief interview and cursory physical exam, the APRN diagnoses the patient with generalized anxiety disorder and suggests a referral to the mental health clinic. Which response(s) by the clinic nurse would be appropriate? *Select all that apply.*

1. Complete a neurological history and neurological examination.
2. Examine the patient's extremities for edema, and listen to her lungs.
3. Observe the patient's respirations, and obtain a pulse oximetry reading.
4. Review the patient's current medications, and observe the patient's gait.
5. Suggest that a battery of blood tests, including a CBC, be ordered and reviewed.
6. Ask the APRN to review the nurse's findings before ordering the referral.

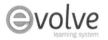

Visit the Evolve website for an **Audio Chapter Summary, Chapter Review Answers & Rationales, Critical Thinking Answer Guidelines,** and additional resources related to the content in this chapter: **http://evolve.elsevier.com/Varcarolis/foundations**

Companion CD   Use the Companion CD to prepare for tests and the NCLEX® Examination with **Test-Taking Strategies** for psychiatric mental health nursing and hundreds of **Review Questions**.

References

Alsawaf, M. A., & Aminah, J. (2007). Shopping for nutrition-based complementary and alternative medicine on the internet. *Journal of Cancer Education, 22*(3), 174–176.

American Nurses Association, American Psychiatric Nurses Association, & International Society of Psychiatric-Mental Health Nurses. (2007). *Psychiatric-mental health nursing: Scope and standards of practice.* Silver Spring, MD: NurseBooks.org.

Bulechek, G. M., Butcher, H. K., & Dochterman, J. M. (Eds.). (2008). *Nursing Interventions Classification (NIC)* (5th ed.). St. Louis: Mosby.

Hofmann, S. G., Meuret, A. E., Smits, J. A. J., Simon, N. M., Pollack, M. H., Eisenmenger, K., et al. (2006). Augmentation of exposure therapy with d-cycloserine for social anxiety disorder. *Archives of General Psychiatry, 63,* 298–304.

Kendler, K. S., Gardner, C. O., Gatz, M., & Pedersen, N. L. (2007). The sources of co-morbidity between major depression and generalized anxiety disorder in a Swedish national twin sample. *Psychological Medicine, 37,* 453–462.

Kessler, R. C., Chiu, W. T., Demler, O., & Walters, E. E. (2005). Prevalence, severity, and comorbidity of twelve-month *DSM-IV* disorders in the National Comorbidity Survey Replication (NCS-R). *Archives of General Psychiatry, 62,* 617–627.

Kessler, R. C., Berglund, P. A., Demler, O., Jin, R., & Walters, E. E. (2005). Lifetime prevalence and age-of-onset distributions of *DSM-IV* disorders in the National Comorbidity Survey Replication (NCS-R). *Archives of General Psychiatry, 62*(6), 593–602.

Kushner, M. G., Kim, S. W., Donahue, C., Thuras, P., Adson, D., Kotlyar, J., et al. (2007). D-cycloserine augmented exposure therapy for obsessive-compulsive disorder. *Biological Psychiatry, 62,* 835–838.

Moorhead, S., Johnson, M., Maas, M., & Swanson, E. (Eds.). (2008). *Nursing Outcomes Classification (NOC)* (4th ed.). St. Louis: Mosby.

North American Nursing Diagnosis Association International. (2009). *NANDA-I nursing diagnoses: Definitions and classification 2009–2011.* Oxford, United Kingdom: Author.

Pavic, R., Gregurek, M., Rados, B., Brkljacic, L., Brajkovic, I., Simetin-Pavic, G., et al. (2007). Smaller right hippocampus in war veterans with posttraumatic stress disorder. *Psychiatry Research: Neuroimaging, 154*(2), 191–198.

Peplau, H. E. (1968). A working definition of anxiety. In S. F. Burd & M. A. Marshall (Eds.), *Some clinical approaches to psychiatric nursing.* New York: Macmillan.

Pollock, M. H., Kinrys, G., Delong, H., Vasconcelos, D., & Simon, N. (2008). The pharmacotherapy of anxiety disorders. In T. A. Stern, J. F. Rosenbaum, M. Fava, J. Biederman, & S. L. Rauch (Eds.) *Massachusetts General Hospital comprehensive clinical psychiatry: Expert consult* (pp. 565–575). Philadelphia: Mosby.

Sadock, B. J., & Sadock, V. A. (2008). *Kaplan and Sadock's concise textbook of clinical psychiatry* (3rd ed.). Philadelphia: Lippincott.

Stahl, S. M. (2008). *Stahl's essential psychopharmacology* (3rd ed.). Cambridge: Cambridge University Press.

Sullivan, H. S. (1953). *The interpersonal theory of psychiatry.* New York: W. W. Norton.

Wang, P. S., Berglund, P., Olfson, M., Pincus, H. A., Wells, K. B., & Kessler, R. C. (2005). Failure and delay in initial treatment contact after first onset of mental disorders in the national comorbidity survey replication. *Archives of General Psychiatry, 62,* 603–613.

CHAPTER 13

Depressive Disorders

Mallie Kozy and Elizabeth M. Varcarolis

Key Terms and Concepts

Objectives

1. Compare and contrast major depressive disorder and dysthymic disorder.
2. Discuss the links between the stress model of depression and the biological model of depression.
3. Assess behaviors in a patient with depression in regard to each of the following areas: (a) affect, (b) thought processes, (c) feelings, (d) physical behavior, and (e) communication.
4. Formulate five nursing diagnoses for a patient with depression, and include outcome criteria.
5. Name unrealistic expectations a nurse may have while working with a patient with depression, and compare them to your own personal thoughts.
6. Role-play six principles of communication useful in working with patients with depression.
7. Evaluate the advantages of the selective serotonin reuptake inhibitors (SSRIs) over the tricyclic antidepressants (TCAs).

8. Explain the unique attributes of two of the atypical antidepressants for use in specific circumstances.
9. Write a medication teaching plan for a patient taking a tricyclic antidepressant, including (a) adverse effects, (b) toxic reactions, and (c) other drugs that can trigger an adverse reaction.
10. Write a medication teaching plan for a patient taking a monoamine oxidase inhibitor, including foods and drugs that are contraindicated.
11. Write a nursing care plan incorporating the recovery model of mental health.
12. Describe the types of depression for which electroconvulsive therapy (ECT) is most helpful.

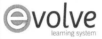 Visit the Evolve website for an **Audio Glossary & Flashcards, Concept Map Creator**, and additional resources related to the content in this chapter: **http://evolve.elsevier.com/Varcarolis/foundations**

No textbook chapter can adequately convey the personal pain and suffering experienced by the individual with depression, not to mention the pain, helplessness, and frustration felt by the affected individual's friends and loved ones. However, it is essential for nursing students to gain a fundamental

understanding of this group of disorders. People of all ethnicities, cultures, ages, socioeconomic groups, education levels, and geographic areas are susceptible to depressive episodes, but some individuals are more susceptible than others. Virtually all nurses will come into contact with patients with depression or whose primary condition is complicated by depression. This chapter includes basic information and therapeutic tools that will facilitate the care of patients with depression.

CLINICAL PICTURE

Figure 13-1 presents diagnostic criteria for major depressive disorder and dysthymic disorder, the two depressive disorders defined by the *Diagnostic and Statistical Manual of Mental Disorders*, fourth edition, text revision *(DSM-IV-TR)* (American Psychiatric Association [APA], 2000a). Several subtypes of major depressive disorder, as well as other proposed depressive types currently being researched to determine whether they should be considered disorders, are described in detail in this chapter.

Major Depressive Disorder

Patients with a **major depressive disorder (MDD)** experience substantial pain and suffering, as well as

DSM-IV-TR CRITERIA FOR DEPRESSIVE DISORDERS

DEPRESSIVE DISORDERS

Major Depressive Disorder

1. Represents a change in previous functions.

2. Symptoms cause clinically significant distress or impair social, occupational, or other important areas of functioning.

3. **Five or more** of the following occur nearly every day for most waking hours over the same 2-week period:
   - Depressed mood most of day, nearly every day
   - Anhedonia
   - Significant weight loss or gain (more than 5% of body weight in 1 month)
   - Insomnia or hypersomnia
   - Increased or decreased motor activity
   - Anergia (fatigue or loss of energy)
   - Feelings of worthlessness or inappropriate guilt (may be delusional)
   - Decreased concentration or indecisiveness
   - Recurrent thoughts of death or suicidal ideation (with or without plan)

Specifiers Describing Most Recent Episode

1. Chronic

2. Atypical features

3. Catatonic features

4. Melancholic features

5. Postpartum onset

Dysthymic Disorder

1. Occurs over a 2-year period (1 year for children and adolescents), depressed mood.

2. Symptoms cause clinically significant distress in social, occupational, and other important areas of functioning.

3. **Two or more** of the following are present:
   - Decreased or increased appetite
   - Insomnia or hypersomnia
   - Low energy or chronic fatigue
   - Decreased self-esteem
   - Poor concentration or difficulty making decisions
   - Feelings of hopelessness or despair

Specify If

1. Early onset (before 21 years of age)

2. Late onset (21 years of age or older)

3. Atypical features

Figure 13-1 Diagnostic criteria for major depressive disorder and dysthymic disorder. (Adapted from American Psychiatric Association. [2000]. *DSM-IV-TR*. Washington, DC: Author.)

psychological, social, and occupational disability. A patient with MDD presents with a history of one or more major depressive episodes and no history of manic or hypomanic episodes. In MDD, the symptoms interfere with the person's social or occupational functioning and in some cases may include psychotic features. Delusional or psychotic major depression is a severe form of mood disorder characterized by delusions or hallucinations. For example, patients might have delusional thoughts that interfere with their nutritional status (e.g., "God put snakes in my stomach and told me not to eat").

The emotional, cognitive, physical, and behavioral symptoms experienced during a major depressive episode represent a change in the person's usual functioning. The course of MDD is variable. At least 60% of people can expect to have a second episode, individuals who have experienced two episodes of major depression have a 70% chance of experiencing a third, and those who have had three episodes have a 90% chance of future episodes (APA, 2000a).

Subtypes

The diagnosis for MDD may include one of the following specifiers to describe the most recent episode of depression:

- **Psychotic features.** Indicates the presence of disorganized thinking, delusions (e.g., delusions of guilt or being punished for sins, somatic delusions of horrible disease or body rotting, delusions of poverty or going bankrupt), or hallucinations (usually auditory, voices berating person for sins).
- **Melancholic features.** This outdated term indicates a severe form of endogenous depression (not attributable to environmental stressors) characterized by severe apathy, weight loss, profound guilt, symptoms that are worse in the morning, early morning awakening, and often suicidal ideation.
- **Atypical features.** Refers to people who have dominant vegetative symptoms (overeating and oversleeping). Onset is younger, psychomotor activities are slow, and anxiety is often an accompanying problem, which may cause misdiagnosis.
- **Catatonic features.** Marked by nonresponsiveness, extreme psychomotor retardation (may seem paralyzed), withdrawal, and negativity.
- **Postpartum onset.** Indicates onset within 4 weeks after childbirth. It is common for psychotic features to accompany this depression. *Severe ruminations or delusional thoughts about the infant signify increased risk of harm to the infant.*
- **Seasonal features (seasonal affective disorder, [SAD]).** Indicates that episodes mostly begin in fall or winter and remit in spring. These patients have reduced cerebral metabolic activity. SAD is characterized by anergia, hypersomnia, overeating, weight gain, and a craving for carbohydrates; it responds to light therapy.

CONSIDERING CULTURE

Postpartum Depression in Immigrant Women

Women who deliver a baby in a country different from the one in which they were born may be at higher risk for postpartum depression (PPD). Various studies have shown that among immigrant populations, postpartum depression rates are around 37% compared to 7% among nonimmigrants (Zelkowitz et al., 2008). Research shows that risk factors for PPD are the same for immigrants as nonimmigrants, specifically prenatal depression, anxiety, somatic symptoms, and marital relationship. So why is there a higher rate in immigrant women?

One reason is lack of support. Immigrant women report support networks as strong and as large as nonimmigrant women; however, a larger portion of the social network is located in a different country. This can put a strain on a marital relationship because immigrant women may expect and need more support from their spouses. Husbands may not be prepared to take on the kind of supportive role required by their wives.

It may be hard to detect PPD in immigrant women because of language barriers and because PPD may manifest itself in somatic complaints. Zelkowitz and colleagues found that immigrant women with PPD had more somatic complaints than women who did not have depression.

Immigrant women have special needs because of language barriers, geographically distant support networks, increased somatic symptoms, and paternal role strain (Ozeki, 2008). Nurses can design interventions geared toward increasing support and alleviating physical complaints of female immigrants who have recently delivered.

Zelkowitz, P., Saucier, J. F., Wang, T., Katofsky, L., Valenzuela, M., & Westreich, R. (2008). Stability and change in depressive symptoms from pregnancy to two months postpartum in childbearing immigrant women. *Archives of Women's Mental Health, 11,* 1–11. Ozeki, N. (2008). Transcultural stress factors of Japanese mothers living in the United Kingdom. *Journal of Transcultural Nursing, 19,* 47–54.

Proposed Subtypes

The following subtypes of MDD represent areas of dysfunction proposed by clinicians and researchers and are currently being researched for inclusion as diagnoses in the fifth edition of the *Diagnostic and Statistical Manual of Mental Disorders (DSM-V)*:

- **Premenstrual dysphoric disorder.** Characterized by more severe symptoms than premenstrual syndrome. Symptoms begin toward last week of luteal phase, are absent in the week following menses, and include depressed mood, anxiety, affective lability, or persistent and marked anger or irritability. Other symptoms include anergia, overeating, difficulty concentrating, and feeling out of control or overwhelmed, among others.
- **Mixed anxiety-depression.** Prevalence of 5% has been estimated. Characterized by significant functional disability. Criteria include at least 1 month of persistent dysphoric mood with possible hypervigilance, difficulty concentrating, fatigue, low self-esteem, and irritability, among others—all of which cause significant distress or impairment in functioning.
- **Recurrent brief depression.** Meets criteria for MDD, but episodes last 1 day to 1 week. Depressive episode must recur at least once per month over 12 months or more. *Carries a high risk for suicide.*
- **Minor depression.** Characterized by sustained depressed mood without the full depressive syndrome. Pessimistic attitude and self-pity are required for the diagnosis. May be chronic and may be complicated by a superimposed major depressive episode.

Dysthymic Disorder

Dysthymic disorder (DD) is characterized by a chronic depressive syndrome that is usually present for most of the day, more days than not, for at least 2 years (APA, 2000b). The depressive mood disturbance, because of its chronic nature, cannot be distinguished from the person's usual pattern of functioning ("I've always been this way.") (APA, 2000b). Although people with dysthymia suffer from social and occupational distress, it is not usually severe enough to warrant hospitalization unless the person becomes suicidal. The age of onset is usually from early childhood and teenage years to early adulthood. Patients with DD are at risk for developing major depressive episodes and other psychiatric disorders.

Differentiating MDD from DD can be difficult because the disorders have similar symptoms. The main differences are in the duration and severity of the symptoms (APA, 2000b).

EPIDEMIOLOGY

Depression is the leading cause of disability in the United States. The lifetime prevalence of a major depressive episode—or the total number of people in the United States who will experience the disorder within their lifetime—is 8.6% (Center for Mental Health Services [CMHS], 2006). Studies find that MDD is twice as common in women (11.2%) as in men (6.0%), although one may question the validity of these statistics, considering that men commit suicide at a far higher rate than women. The CMHS has determined that MDD and DD tend to have higher prevalence rates in lower-income groups; DD (chronic mild depression) occurs in about 3.4% of people during their lifetimes. About 40% of people with DD also meet the criteria for MDD or bipolar disorder (BD) in any given year.

Children and Adolescents

Children as young as 3 years of age have been diagnosed with depression. MDD is said to occur in as many as 18% of preadolescents, which is perhaps a low estimate because depression in this age group is often underdiagnosed. Children and adolescents between 9 and 17 years of age have a 6% prevalence of depression, and 4.9% have MDD (National Institute of Mental Health [NIMH], 2007a). Girls 15 years and older are twice as likely to experience a major depressive episode as boys. The dominant symptom of depression in children and adolescents tends to be irritability (Joska & Stein, 2008).

Older Adults

Although depression in older adults is common, it is *not* a normal result of aging. It is estimated that of the 35 million people over age 65, 2 million (almost 6%) suffer from severe depression, and another 5 million (around 14%) suffer from less severe forms of depression (NIMH, 2007b). Many older adults suffer from *subsyndromal depression* in which they experience many, but not all, the symptoms of a major depressive episode. These individuals have an increased risk of developing major depression (NIMH, 2007b), and a disproportionate number of older adults with depression are likely to die by suicide. Unfortunately, the symptoms of depression often go unrecognized in this population, although older adults generally make frequent medical visits. Thus older individuals suffering from depression are at risk for being untreated.

COMORBIDITY

A depressive syndrome frequently accompanies other psychiatric disorders, such as anxiety disorders, schizophrenia, substance abuse, eating disorders, and schizoaffective disorder. People with anxiety disorders (e.g., panic disorder, generalized anxiety disorder, obsessive-compulsive disorder) commonly present with depression, as do people with personality disorders (particularly borderline personality disorder), adjustment disorder, and brief depressive reactions.

Mixed anxiety-depression is perhaps one of the most common psychiatric presentations. Symptoms of anxiety occur in an average of 70% of cases of major depression.

The presence of comorbid anxiety disorder and depression has a negative impact on the disease course. Comorbidity has been shown to result in a higher rate of suicide, greater severity of depression, greater impairment in social and occupational functioning, and poorer response to treatment (Simon & Rosenbaum, 2003). This is especially true in older adults with depression who have concurrent symptoms of anxiety or an anxiety disorder (Lenze, 2003).

The incidence of major depression greatly increases with the occurrence of a medical disorder, and people with chronic medical problems are at a higher risk for depression than those in the general population. Depression is often secondary to a medical condition and may also be secondary to use of substances such as alcohol, cocaine, marijuana, heroin, and even anxiolytics and other prescription medications (Table 13-1). Depression can also be a sequela, or consequence, of bereavement and grief. Chapter 32 has an in-depth discussion of end-of-life issues and bereavement.

ETIOLOGY

Although many theories attempt to explain the cause of depression, many psychological, biological, and cultural variables make identification of any one cause difficult; furthermore, it is unlikely there is a single cause for depression. The high variability in symptoms, response to treatment, and course of the illness supports the supposition that depression may result from a complex interaction of causes. For example, genetic predisposition to the illness combined with childhood stress may lead to significant changes in the central nervous system (CNS) that result in depression. However, there seem to be several common risk factors for depression, listed in Box 13-1 (Sadock & Sadock, 2008).

Biological Factors

Genetic

Twin studies consistently show that genetic factors play a role in the development of depressive disorders. Various studies reveal that the average concordance rate for mood disorders among monozygotic twins (twins sharing the same genetic material) is about 37%. That is, if one twin is affected, the second has a 37% chance of being affected as well (Joska &

TABLE 13-1	Depression Secondary to Medical Conditions and Substances/Medications
MEDICAL CONDITIONS	
Neurological	Epilepsies, Parkinson's disease, multiple sclerosis, Alzheimer's disease
Infectious or inflammatory	Neurosyphilis, AIDs
Cardiac disorders	Ischemic heart disease, cardiac failure, cardiomyopathies
Endocrine	Hypothyroidism, diabetes mellitus, vitamin deficiencies, parathyroid disorders
Inflammatory disorders	Collagen-vascular diseases, irritable bowel syndrome, chronic liver disorders
Neoplastic disorders	Central nervous system tumors, paraneoplastic syndromes
SUBSTANCES/MEDICATIONS	
Central nervous system depressants	Alcohol, barbiturates, benzodiazepines, clonidine
Central nervous system medications	Amantadine, bromocriptine, levodopa, phenothiazines, phenytoin
Psychostimulants	Amphetamines
Systemic medications	Corticosteroids, digoxin, diltiazem, enalapril, ethionamide, isotretinoin, mefloquine, methyldopa, metoclopramide, quinolones, reserpine, statins, thiazides, vincristine

Data from Joska, J. A., & Stein, D. J. (2008). Mood disorders. In R. E. Hales, S. C. Yudofsky, & G. O. Gabbard (Eds.), *Textbook of psychiatry* (5th ed.) (p. 464). Washington, DC: American Psychiatric Publishing.

Stein, 2008). Increased heritability of mood disorders is associated with an earlier age of onset, greater rate of comorbidity, and increased risk of recurrent illness. For depression to develop, however, a genetic predisposition must also be affected by environmental factors (Sadock & Sadock, 2008).

Biochemical

The brain is a highly complex organ that contains billions of neurons. There is much evidence to support the concept that many CNS neurotransmitter abnormalities may cause clinical depression. These neurotransmitter abnormalities may be the result of genetic or environmental factors or even of other medical conditions, such as cerebral infarction, hypothyroidism, acquired immunodeficiency syndrome (AIDS), or drug use.

BOX 13-1 Primary Risk Factors for Depression

- Female gender
- Being unmarried
- Low socioeconomic class
- Early childhood trauma
- The presence of a negative life event, especially loss and humiliation
- Family history of depression, especially in first-degree relatives
- High levels of neuroticism (predisposition to respond to stress poorly)
- Postpartum period
- Medical illness
- Absence of social support
- Alcohol or substance abuse

From Joska, J. A., & Stein, D. J. (2008). Mood disorders. In R. E. Hales, S. C. Yudofsky, & G. O. Gabbard (Eds.), *Textbook of psychiatry* (5th ed.) (pp. 457–504). Washington, DC: American Psychiatric Publishing.

Specific neurotransmitters in the brain are believed to be related to altered mood states. Two of the main neurotransmitters involved are **serotonin** (5-hydroxytryptamine [5-HT]) and **norepinephrine**. Serotonin is an important regulator of sleep, appetite, and libido; therefore, serotonin-circuit dysfunction can result in sleep disturbances, decreased appetite, low sex drive, poor impulse control, and irritability (Joska & Stein, 2008). Norepinephrine modulates attention and behavior. It is stimulated by stressful situations, which may result in overuse and a deficiency of norepinephrine. A deficiency, an imbalance as compared to other neurotransmitters, or an impaired ability to use available norepinephrine can result in apathy, reduced responsiveness, and slowed psychomotor activity.

At present, research suggests that depression results from the dysregulation of a number of neurotransmitter systems in addition to serotonin and norepinephrine. The dopamine, acetylcholine, and GABA systems are also believed to be involved in the pathophysiology of a major depressive episode (Sadock & Sadock, 2008).

Stressful life events, especially losses, seem to be a significant factor in the development of depression. Norepinephrine, serotonin, and acetylcholine play a role in stress regulation. When these neurotransmitters become overtaxed through stressful events, neurotransmitter depletion may occur.

At this time, no single mechanism of depressant action has been found. The relationships among the serotonin, norepinephrine, dopamine, acetylcholine, and GABA systems are complex and need further assessment and study. However, treatment with medication that helps regulate these neurotransmitters has proved empirically successful in the treatment of many patients. Figure 13-2 shows a positron emission tomographic (PET) scan of the brain of a woman with depression before and after taking medication. Refer to Figure 3-7 for PET scans comparing brain activity in an individual with depression and an individual without depression.

Alterations in Hormonal Regulation

Although neuroendocrine findings are as yet inconclusive, the neuroendocrine characteristic most widely studied in relation to depression has been hyperactivity of the hypothalamic-pituitary-adrenal cortical axis. People with major depression have increased urine

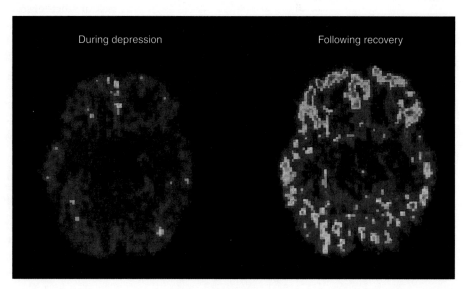

Figure 13-2 Positron emission tomographic (PET) scans of a 45-year-old woman with recurrent depression. The scan on the left was taken when the patient was on no medication and very depressed. The scan on the right was taken several months later when the patient was well, after she had been treated with medication for her depression. Note that her entire brain, particularly the left prefrontal cortex, is more active when she is well. (Courtesy Mark George, MD, Biological Psychiatry Branch, National Institute of Mental Health.)

cortisol levels and elevated corticotrophin-releasing hormone (Joska & Stein, 2008). Dexamethasone, an exogenous steroid that suppresses cortisol, is used in the dexamethasone suppression test for depression. Results of this test are abnormal in about 50% of people with depression, which indicates hyperactivity of the hypothalamic-pituitary-adrenal cortical axis. However, the findings may also be abnormal in people with obsessive-compulsive disorder (OCD) and other medical conditions. Significantly, patients with MDD with psychotic features are among those with the highest rates of nonsuppression of cortisol on the dexamethasone suppression test.

Diathesis-Stress Model

The diathesis-stress model of depression takes into account the interplay of biology and life events in the development of depressive disorders. It is believed that psychosocial stressors and interpersonal events trigger neurophysical and neurochemical changes in the brain. Early life trauma may result in long-term hyperactivity of the CNS corticotropin-releasing factor (CRF) and norepinephrine systems, with a consequent neurotoxic effect on the hippocampus, which leads to overall neuronal loss. These changes could cause sensitization of the CRF circuits to even mild stress in adulthood, leading to an exaggerated stress response (Gillespie & Nemeroff, 2005).

According to the stress-diathesis model, depression results from a dynamic interplay of biology and environment. Some people may be born with a predisposition toward depression which is triggered by experiencing a stressful life event. The experience of depression further alters the neurological connections in the brain, increasing the predisposition toward depression. The result is a vicious cycle of recurrent depressive disorder. Early, effective treatment is needed to break the cycle.

Psychological Factors

Cognitive Theory

In cognitive theory, the underlying assumption is that a person's thoughts will result in emotions. If a person looks at a life in a positive way, the person will experience positive emotions, but negative interpretation of life events can result in sorrow, anger, and hopelessness. Cognitive theorists believe that people may acquire a psychological predisposition to depression due to early life experiences. These experiences contribute to negative, illogical, and irrational thought processes that may remain dormant until they are activated during times of stress (Beck & Rush, 1995). Beck found that persons with depression disorders process

information in negative ways, even in the midst of positive factors. He believed that automatic, negative, repetitive, unintended, and not-readily-controllable thoughts perpetuate depression. Three thoughts constitute **Beck's cognitive triad:**

1. A negative, self-deprecating view of self
2. A pessimistic view of the world
3. The belief that negative reinforcement (or no validation for the self) will continue in the future

Coming to realize that one has an ability to interpret life events in positive ways helps a person recognize that he or she has an element of control over emotions and therefore depression.

Learned Helplessness

An older but still plausible theory of depression is that of learned helplessness. Seligman (1973) stated that although anxiety is the initial response to a stressful situation, it is replaced by depression if the person feels no control over the outcome of a situation. A person who believes that an undesired event is his or her fault and that nothing can be done to change it is prone to depression. The theory of learned helplessness has been used to explain the development of depression in certain social groups, such as older adults, people living in impoverished areas, and women.

APPLICATION OF THE NURSING PROCESS

ASSESSMENT

Undiagnosed and untreated depression is often associated with more severe presentation of symptoms, greater risk of suicide, somatic problems, and severe anxiety or anxiety disorders. A study by Bijl and associates (2004) concluded that individuals with depression who manifested psychological symptoms were recognized as having depression 90% of the time, in contrast to those who showed somatic symptoms (e.g., chronic pain, insomnia), who were recognized as having depression 50% of the time, and those who had a medical disorder, in whom depression was identified 20% of the time.

General Assessment

Assessment Tools

Numerous standardized depression screening tools that help assess the type of depression are available, including the Beck Depression Inventory, the Hamilton Depression Scale, the Zung Depression

Scale, and the Geriatric Depression Scale. The Patient Health Questionnaire-9 (PHQ-9), a short inventory that highlights predominant symptoms seen in depression, is presented here because of its ease of use (Figure 13-3).

The website www.depression-screening.org, sponsored by the National Mental Health Association (NMHA), enables people to take an online confidential screening test for depression and find reliable information on the illness.

PATIENT HEALTH QUESTIONNAIRE-9 (PHQ-9)

Over the <u>last 2 weeks</u>, how often have you been bothered by any of the following problems?	Not at all	Several days	More than half the days	Nearly every day
1. Little interest or pleasure in doing things	0	1	2	3
2. Feeling down, depressed, or hopeless	0	1	2	3
3. Trouble falling or staying asleep, or sleeping too much	0	1	2	3
4. Feeling tired or having little energy	0	1	2	3
5. Poor appetite or overeating	0	1	2	3
6. Feeling bad about yourself — or that you are a failure or have let yourself or your family down	0	1	2	3
7. Trouble concentrating on things, such as reading the newspaper or watching television	0	1	2	3
8. Moving or speaking so slowly that other people could have noticed? Or the opposite — being so fidgety or restless that you have been moving around a lot more than usual	0	1	2	3
9. Thoughts that you would be better off dead or of hurting yourself in some way	0	1	2	3

<u> 0 </u> + _____ + _____ + _____

= Total score: _____

If you checked off <u>any</u> problems, how <u>difficult</u> have these problems made it for you to do your work, take care of things at home, or get along with other people?

Not difficult at all	Somewhat difficult	Very difficult	Extremely difficult
☐	☐	☐	☐

I confirm this information is accurate.	Patient's/Subject's initials:	Date:

A

PHQ-9 SCORING CARD FOR SEVERITY DETERMINATION

for healthcare professional use only

Scoring—add up all checked boxes on PHQ-9

Total Score	Depression Severity
0-4	None
5-9	Mild
10-14	Moderate
15-19	Moderately severe
20-27	Severe

B

Figure 13-3 **A,** Patient Health Questionnaire-9 (PHQ-9). **B,** Scoring the PHQ-9. (© 2005 Pfizer, Inc. Developed by Drs. Robert L. Spitzer, Janet B. Williams, Kurt Kroenke, and colleagues.)

Assessment of Suicide Potential

The patient should always be evaluated for suicidal or homicidal ideation. About 15% of people with clinical depression commit suicide (Brendel et al., 2008). Initial suicide assessment might include the following statements or questions:

- You have said you are depressed. Tell me what that is like for you.
- When you feel depressed, what thoughts go through your mind?
- Have you gone so far as to think about taking your own life?
  - Do you have a plan?
  - Do you have the means to carry out your plan?
  - Is there anything that would prevent you from carrying out your plan?

Refer to Chapter 24 for a detailed discussion of suicide, critical risk factors, warning signs, and strategies for suicide prevention. Also see Case Study and Nursing Care Plan 13-1 on pages 274–276.

Key Assessment Findings

A depressed mood and anhedonia are the key symptoms in depression. Almost 97% of people with depression have anergia (lack of energy or passivity). Anxiety, a common symptom in depression, is seen in about 60% to 90% of patients with depression.

When people experience a depressive episode, their thinking is slow, and their memory and concentration are usually negatively affected. They also dwell on and exaggerate their perceived faults and failures and are unable to focus on their strengths and successes. A person with major depression may experience delusions of being punished for doing bad deeds or being a terrible person. Feelings of worthlessness, guilt, anger, and helplessness are common.

Psychomotor agitation may be evidenced by constant pacing and wringing of hands. The slowed movements of psychomotor retardation, however, are more common. Somatic complaints (headaches, malaise, backaches) are also common. Vegetative signs of depression (change in bowel movements and eating habits, sleep disturbances, and disinterest in sex) are usually present. In primary care, people with MDD experience chronic pain at a rate of 66% and disabling pain at a rate of 41%, compared to 43% and 10% respectively of patients who do not have depression (Arnow et al., 2006).

Areas to Assess

Affect

Affect is the outward representation of a person's internal state of being and is an objective finding based on the nurse's assessment. A person who has depression sees the world through gray-colored glasses. Posture is poor, and the patient may look older than the stated age. Facial expressions convey sadness and dejection, and the patient may have frequent bouts of weeping. Conversely, the patient may say that he or she is unable to cry. Feelings of hopelessness and despair are readily reflected in the person's affect. For example, the patient may not make eye contact, may speak in a monotone, may show little or no facial expression (flat affect), and may make only yes or no responses. Frequent sighing is common.

Thought Processes

During a depressive episode, the person's ability to solve problems and think clearly is negatively affected. Judgment is poor, and indecisiveness is common. The individual may claim that the mind is slowing down. Memory and concentration are poor. Evidence of delusional thinking may be seen in a person with major depression. Common statements of delusional thinking are "I have committed unpardonable sins," "God wants me dead," and "I am wicked and should die."

Mood

Mood is the patient's subjective experience of sustained emotions or feelings. Feelings frequently reported by people with depression include anxiety, worthlessness, guilt, helplessness, hopelessness, and anger. Feelings of worthlessness range from feeling inadequate to having an unrealistically negative evaluation of self-worth. These feelings reflect the low self-esteem that is a painful partner to depression. Statements such as "I am no good, I'll never amount to anything" are common.

Feelings

Guilt is a common accompaniment to depression. A person may ruminate over present or past failings. Extreme guilt can assume psychotic proportions (e.g., "I have committed terrible sins, and God is punishing me for my evil ways").

Helplessness is evidenced by the inability to carry out the simplest tasks (e.g., grooming, doing housework, working, caring for children), because they seem too difficult to accomplish. With feelings of helplessness come feelings of hopelessness, which are particularly correlated with suicidality (Beck et al., 2006). Even though most depressive episodes are time limited, people experiencing them believe things will never change. This feeling of utter hopelessness can lead people to view suicide as a way out of constant mental pain. Hopelessness, one of the core characteristics of depression and risk factors for suicide, is a combined cognitive and emotional state that includes the following attributes:

- Negative expectations for the future
- Loss of control over future outcomes
- Passive acceptance of the futility of planning to achieve goals
- Emotional negativism, as expressed in despair, despondency, or depression

Anger and **irritability** are natural outcomes of profound feelings of helplessness. Anger in depression is often expressed inappropriately through destruction of property, hurtful verbal attacks, or physical aggression toward others. However, anger may be directed toward the self in the form of suicidal or subsuicidal behaviors (e.g., alcohol abuse, substance abuse, overeating, smoking, etc.). These behaviors often result in feelings of low self-esteem and worthlessness.

Physical Behavior

Lethargy and fatigue may result in psychomotor retardation, in which movements are extremely slow, facial expressions are decreased, and gaze is fixed. The continuum of **psychomotor retardation** may range from slowed and difficult movements to complete inactivity and incontinence. **Psychomotor agitation**, in which patients constantly pace, bite their nails, smoke, tap their fingers, or engage in some other tension-relieving activity, may also be observed. At these times, patients commonly feel fidgety and unable to relax.

Grooming, dress, and personal hygiene are markedly neglected. People who usually take pride in their appearance and dress may be poorly groomed and allow themselves to look shabby and unkempt.

Vegetative signs of depression are universal. *Vegetative signs* refer to alterations in those activities necessary to support physical life and growth (eating, sleeping, elimination, sex). For example, **changes in eating patterns** are common. About 60% to 70% of people with depression report having anorexia; overeating occurs more often in DD.

Change in sleep patterns is a cardinal sign of depression. Often, people experience **insomnia**, wake frequently, and have a total reduction in sleep, especially deep-stage sleep (Sadock & Sadock, 2008). One of the hallmark symptoms of depression is waking at 3 or 4 AM and then staying awake or sleeping for only short periods. The light sleep of a person with depression tends to prolong the agony of depression over a 24-hour period. For some, sleep is increased (**hypersomnia**) and provides an escape from painful feelings. In any event, sleep is rarely restful or refreshing.

Changes in bowel habits are common. Constipation is seen most frequently in patients with psychomotor retardation. Diarrhea occurs less frequently, often in conjunction with psychomotor agitation.

Interest in sex declines (loss of libido) during depression. Some men experience impotence, and a declining interest in sex often occurs among both men and women, which can further complicate marital and social relationships.

Communication

A person with depression may speak and comprehend very slowly. The lack of an immediate response by the patient to a remark does not necessarily mean the patient has not heard or chooses not to reply; the patient may need more time to comprehend what was said and then compose a reply. In extreme depression, however, a person may become mute.

Religious Beliefs and Spirituality

The role of religious beliefs and spirituality in depression is just beginning to be understood. Arehart-Treichel (2006) found that among people with depression, there was a concern with spiritual questions, such as "What is the meaning of life?" The author concluded that people with depression and anxiety, like people with other serious illnesses, are concerned with the greater meaning of their experience and look beyond themselves for answers. Doolitte and Farrell (2004) found that certain aspects of faith and religious beliefs, such as belief in a higher power, belief in prayer, and the ability to find meaning in suffering were associated with lower rates of depression. Nurses must assess patients' spiritual health by asking how their depression has affected their faith. Encouraging a connection with religious or spiritual practices that have brought them comfort in the past may be therapeutic.

Age Considerations

Assessment of Children and Adolescents

Depression often is overlooked in children and adolescents because mood changes in children are frequently seen as behavioral problems and in adolescents as a part of normal development. Although children with depression may display irritability and disruptive behavior, sadness and hopelessness are often the core issues (Grayson, 2004). Although it is normal for teens to experience a degree of mood lability, adolescents with depression will have a sustained change in mood, thinking, and motivation; they may become sexually promiscuous or engage in alcohol or substance abuse. Both age groups may withdraw from friends and become preoccupied with death.

Assessment of Older Adults

It can be easy to overlook depression in older adults, because they are more likely to complain of aches and pains than acknowledge feelings of sadness or grief. Depression may exist alongside other illnesses or occur as the result of vascular changes in the brain (NIMH, 2007b). Patients and health care professionals may falsely believe that depression is a normal part of aging, but

EVIDENCE-BASED PRACTICE

Depression, Spirituality, and Symptom Burden

Gusick, G. (2008). The contribution of depression and spirituality to symptom burden in chronic heart failure. *Archives of Psychiatric Nursing, 22,* 53–55.

Problem
Heart failure (HF) adds greatly to disease burden in the United States. While the role of psychological factors and symptom burden in chronic illness has been explored, the role of spirituality is less well understood.

Purpose of Study
The purpose of the study was to see if spirituality had any relationship to depression and symptom burden in patients with HF.

Methods
Adults with HF attending an outpatient clinic were recruited to participate in this exploratory correlational study. The 102 participants completed questionnaires to measure depression, spiritual beliefs, and symptom burden.

Key Findings
- There was a positive correlation between depression scores and the frequency and intensity of HF symptoms.

- There was not a significant relationship between spirituality and symptom burden; however, the interaction between depression and spirituality accounted for a greater variance in symptom burden than depression alone. In other words, if a person had a higher depression score, spiritual beliefs appeared to have an influence on symptom burden.

Implications for Nursing Practice
When symptoms of heart failure worsen, it is usually assumed that the underlying pathology is physical, but this study underscores the fact that heart failure patients need to be screened and treated for depression. Nurses can assess for symptoms of depression in patients with HF, thus contributing to appropriate reduction in symptom burden.

---

the nurse must assess older adults to see if the level of functioning represents a change from normal patterns.

Self-Assessment

Patients with depression often reject the advice, encouragement, and understanding of the nurse and others, and they often do not appear to respond to nursing interventions and seem resistant to change. When this occurs, you may experience feelings of frustration, hopelessness, and annoyance. These problematic responses can be altered by the following:
- Recognizing any unrealistic expectations for yourself or the patient
- Identifying feelings that originate with the patient
- Understanding the roles biology and genetics play in the precipitation and maintenance of a depressed mood

Unrealistic Expectations of Self

Nursing students and others new to caring for individuals with depression may have unrealistic expectations of themselves and their patients, and problems result when these expectations are not met. Unmet expectations usually result in a nurse's feeling anxious, hurt, angry, helpless, or incompetent. Unrealistic expectations

of self and others may be held even by experienced health care workers, and this phenomenon contributes to staff burnout. Many of your nursing expectations may not be conscious, but when these expectations are made conscious and are worked through with peers and more experienced clinicians (supervisors), more realistic expectations can be formed and attainable outcomes identified. Realistic expectations of self and the patient can decrease feelings of helplessness and increase a nurse's self-esteem and therapeutic potential.

Feeling What the Patient Is Feeling

It is not uncommon for nurses and other health professionals to experience intense anxiety, frustration, annoyance, hopelessness, and helplessness while caring for individuals with depression; nurses empathetically sense what the patient is feeling. The novice nurse may interpret these emotions as personal reactions toward the patient with whom he or she is working. However, these feelings can be important diagnostic clues to the patient's experience. You can discuss feelings of annoyance, hopelessness, and helplessness with peers and supervisors to separate personal feelings from those originating with the patient. If personal feelings are not recognized, named, and examined, withdrawal by the nurse is likely to occur.

VIGNETTE

Juanita is working with David, a patient with depression, who is living at a homeless shelter after losing his job and being evicted from his apartment. David expresses a lot of hopelessness about his future and believes he will never get another job or be able to live on his own. During clinical conference, Juanita states that she is feeling threatened and frustrated because David rejects her suggestions and her attempts to help. She confesses that she thinks David is not trying to feel better or improve his situation. Juanita spends time reviewing the illness of depression, common behaviors, and patient needs. She also reviews the recovery model of mental illness. In subsequent visits, she refocuses on David and stops giving him suggestions. After 4 weeks, David has worked out a plan to live with relatives while he undergoes vocational training. He thanks Juanita for listening and not making him "feel like a failure." ∎

People instinctively avoid situations and persons that arouse feelings of frustration, annoyance, or intimidation. If the nurse also has unresolved feelings of anger and depression, the complexity of the situation is compounded. There is no substitute for competent and supportive supervision to facilitate growth, both professionally and personally. Supervision by a more experienced clinician and sharing with peers help minimize feelings of confusion, frustration, and isolation and can increase your therapeutic potential and self-esteem while you care for individuals with depression.

Assessment Guidelines Depression

1. Always evaluate the patient's risk of harm to self or others. Overt hostility is highly correlated with suicide (see Chapter 24).
2. Depression is a mood disorder that can be secondary to a host of medical or other psychiatric disorders, as well as medications. A thorough medical and neurological examination helps determine if the depression is primary or secondary to another disorder. Essentially, evaluate whether:
   - The patient is psychotic.
   - The patient has taken drugs or alcohol.
   - Medical conditions are present.
   - The patient has a history of a comorbid psychiatric syndrome (eating disorder, borderline or anxiety disorder).
3. Assess the patient's past history of depression, and determine what happened and what worked and did not work.
4. Assess support systems, family, significant others, and the need for information and referrals.

DIAGNOSIS

Depression is a complex disorder, and individuals with depression have a variety of needs; therefore, nursing diagnoses are many. However, a high priority for the nurse is determining the risk of suicide, and the nursing diagnosis of *Risk for suicide* is always considered. Refer to Chapter 24 for assessment guidelines and interventions for suicidal individuals. Other key targets for nursing interventions are represented by the diagnoses of *Hopelessness, Ineffective coping, Social isolation, Spiritual distress,* and *Self-care deficit (bathing, dressing, feeding, toileting).* Table 13-2 identifies signs and symptoms commonly experienced in depression and offers potential nursing diagnoses.

OUTCOMES IDENTIFICATION
The Recovery Model

The 2003 report from the President's New Freedom Commission on Mental Illness articulated that national health priorities should focus on recovery from mental illness rather than treatment of it. The **recovery model** emphasizes that healing is possible and attainable for individuals with mental illnesses, including depression. Recovery is attained through partnership with health care providers who focus on the patient's strengths. Treatment goals are mutually developed based on the patient's personal needs and values, and interventions are evidenced-based (New York State Office of Mental Health, 2004).

Remember that MDD can be a recurrent and chronic illness. Care should be directed not only at resolution of the acute phase but also at long-term management. The nurse and the patient identify realistic outcome criteria and formulate concrete, measurable short-term and intermediate indicators. Each patient is different, and indicators should be selected according to individual needs.

Table 13-3 presents some outcome criteria from the *Nursing Outcomes Classification (NOC)* (Moorhead et al., 2008). Indicators for the outcomes of the vegetative or physical signs of depression (e.g., *reports adequate sleep*) are formulated to show, for example, evidence of weight gain, return to normal bowel activity, sleep duration of 6 to 8 hours per night, or return of sexual desire.

PLANNING

The planning of care for patients with depression is geared toward the patient's phase of depression, particular symptoms, and personal goals. At all times during the care of a person with depression, nurses and members of the health care team must be

TABLE 13-2 Potential Nursing Diagnoses for Depression

Signs and Symptoms	Potential Nursing Diagnoses
Previous suicidal attempts, putting affairs in order, giving away prized possessions, suicidal ideation (has plan, ability to carry it out), overt or covert statements regarding killing self, feelings of worthlessness, hopelessness, helplessness	*Risk for suicide* *Risk for self-mutilation*
Lack of judgment, memory difficulty, poor concentration, inaccurate interpretation of environment, negative ruminations, cognitive distortions	*Disturbed thought processes**
Difficulty with simple tasks, inability to function at previous level, poor problem solving, poor cognitive functioning, verbalizations of inability to cope	*Ineffective coping* *Interrupted family processes* *Risk for impaired attachment* *Ineffective role performance*
Difficulty making decisions, poor concentration, inability to take action	*Decisional conflict*
Feelings of helplessness, hopelessness, powerlessness	*Hopelessness* *Powerlessness*
Questioning of meaning of life and own existence, inability to participate in usual religious practices, conflict over spiritual beliefs, anger toward spiritual deity or religious representatives	*Spiritual distress* *Impaired religiosity* *Risk for impaired religiosity*
Feelings of worthlessness, poor self-image, negative sense of self, self-negating verbalizations, feeling of being a failure, expressions of shame or guilt, hypersensitivity to slights or criticism	*Chronic low self-esteem* *Situational low self-esteem*
Withdrawal, noncommunicativeness, speech that is only in monosyllables, avoidance of contact with others	*Impaired social interaction* *Social isolation* *Risk for loneliness*
Vegetative signs of depression: changes in sleeping, eating, grooming and hygiene, elimination, sexual patterns	*Self-care deficit (bathing, dressing, feeding, toileting)* *Imbalanced nutrition: less than body requirements* *Disturbed sleep pattern* *Constipation* *Sexual dysfunction*

Data from North American Nursing Diagnosis Association International (NANDA-I). (2009). *NANDA-I nursing diagnoses: Definitions and classification 2009-2011.* Oxford, United Kingdom: Author.
*Diagnosis retired from North American Nursing Diagnosis Association. (2007). *NANDA-I nursing diagnoses: Definitions and classification 2007–2008.* Philadelphia: Author.

TABLE 13-3 *NOC* Outcomes Related to Depression

Nursing Outcome and Definition	Intermediate Indicators	Short-Term Indicators
Depression Self-Control: Personal actions to minimize melancholy and maintain interest in life events	Reports improved mood Adheres to therapy schedule Takes medication as prescribed Follows treatment plan	Monitors intensity of depression Identifies precursors of depression Plans strategies to reduce effects of precursors Reports changes in symptoms to health care provider

Data from Moorhead, S., Johnson, M., Maas, M., Swanson, E. (2008). *Nursing outcomes classification (NOC)* (4th ed.). St. Louis, MO: Mosby.

cognizant of the potential for suicide; assessment of risk for self-harm (or harm to others) is ongoing. A combination of therapy (cognitive, behavioral, and interpersonal) and psychopharmacology is an effective approach to the treatment of depression across all age groups.

Be aware that the vegetative signs of depression (changes in eating, sleeping, sexual satisfaction, etc.), as well as changes in concentration, activity level, social interaction, care for personal appearance, and so on, often need targeting. The planning of care for a patient with depression is based on the individual's symptoms and goals and attempts to encompass a variety of areas in the person's life. Safety is always the highest priority.

IMPLEMENTATION

There are three phases in treatment and recovery from major depression:

1. The **acute phase** (6 to 12 weeks) is directed at reduction of depressive symptoms and restoration of psychosocial and work function. Hospitalization may be required.
2. The **continuation phase** (4 to 9 months) is directed at prevention of relapse through pharmacotherapy, education, and depression-specific psychotherapy.
3. The **maintenance phase** (1 year or more) of treatment is directed at prevention of further episodes of depression.

It is important to keep in mind that both the continuation and maintenance phases are geared toward maintaining the patient as a functional and contributing member of the community after recovery from the acute phase.

Counseling and Communication Techniques

Nurses often have great difficulty communicating with patients without talking. However, some patients with depression are so withdrawn that they are unwilling or unable to speak, and just sitting with them in silence may seem like a waste of time or be uncomfortable. As your anxiety increases, you may start daydreaming, feel bored, remember something that "must be done now," and so on. It is important to be aware that this time can be meaningful, especially if you have a genuine interest in learning about the patient with depression.

It is difficult to say when a withdrawn patient will be able to respond. However, certain techniques are known to be useful in guiding effective nursing interventions. Some communication techniques to use with a severely withdrawn patient are listed in Table 13-4. Counseling guidelines for use with patients with depression are offered in Table 13-5.

Health Teaching and Health Promotion

One basic premise of the recovery model of mental illness is that each individual controls his or her treatment based on individual goals. Within this model, health teaching is paramount because it allows patients to make informed choices. Health teaching is also an avenue for providing hope to the patient and should include:

- Depression is an illness that is beyond a person's voluntary control.
- Although it is beyond voluntary control, depression can be managed through medication and lifestyle.

TABLE 13-4 Guidelines for Communication with Severely Withdrawn Persons

Intervention	Rationale
When a patient is mute, use the technique of *making observations:* "There are many new pictures on the wall." "You are wearing your new shoes."	When a patient is not ready to talk, direct questions can raise the patient's anxiety level and frustrate the nurse. Pointing to commonalities in the environment draws the patient into and reinforces reality.
Use simple, concrete words.	Slowed thinking and difficulty concentrating impair comprehension.
Allow time for the patient to respond.	Slowed thinking necessitates time to formulate a response.
Listen for covert messages and ask about suicide plans.	People often experience relief and decrease in feelings of isolation when they share thoughts of suicide.
Avoid platitudes such as "Things will look up." "Everyone gets down once in a while."	Platitudes tend to minimize the patient's feelings and can increase feelings of guilt and worthlessness, because the patient cannot "look up" or "snap out of it."

TABLE 13-5 Guidelines for Counseling People with Depression

Intervention	Rationale
Help the patient question underlying assumptions and beliefs and consider alternate explanations to problems.	Reconstructing a healthier and more hopeful attitude about the future can alter depressed mood.
Work with the patient to identify cognitive distortions that encourage negative self-appraisal. For example: a. Overgeneralizations b. Self-blame c. Mind reading d. Discounting of positive attributes	Cognitive distortions reinforce a negative, inaccurate perception of self and world. a. The patient takes one fact or event and makes a general rule out of it ("He always…"; "I never…"). b. The patient consistently blames self for everything perceived as negative. c. The patient assumes others don't like him or her, without any real evidence that assumptions are correct. d. The patient focuses on the negative
Encourage activities that can raise self-esteem. Identify need for (a) problem-solving skills, (b) coping skills, and (c) assertiveness skills.	Many people with depression, especially women, are not taught a range of problem solving and coping skills. Increasing social, family, and job skills can change negative self-assessment.
Encourage exercise, such as running and/or weight lifting.	Exercise can improve self-concept and potentially shift neurochemical balance.
Encourage formation of supportive relationships, such as through support groups, therapy, and peer support.	Such relationships reduce social isolation and enable the patient to work on personal goals and relationship needs.
Provide information referrals, when needed, for religious or spiritual information (e.g., readings, programs, tapes, community resources).	Spiritual and existential issues may be heightened during depressive episodes; many people find strength and comfort in spirituality or religion.

- Illness management depends in large part on understanding personal signs and symptoms of relapse.
- Illness management depends on understanding the role of medication and possible medication side effects.
- Long-term management is best assured if the patient undergoes psychotherapy along with taking medication.
- Identifying and coping with the stress of interpersonal relationships—whether they are familial, social, or occupational—is key to illness management.

Including the family in discharge planning is also important and helps the patient in the following ways:

- Increases the family's understanding and acceptance of the family member with depression during the aftercare period
- Increases the patient's use of aftercare facilities in the community
- Contributes to higher overall adjustment in the patient after discharge

Promotion of Self-Care Activities

In addition to feelings of hopelessness, despair, and physical discomfort, signs of physical neglect may be apparent. Nursing measures for improving physical well-being and promoting adequate self-care are initiated. Some effective interventions targeting physical needs are listed in Table 13-6. Nurses in the community can work with family members to encourage a family member with depression to perform and maintain his or her self-care activities.

Milieu Management

When a person has acute and severe depression, admission to an inpatient setting may be indicated. The patient with depression needs protection from suicidal acts and a supervised environment for regulating treatments. Often, being removed from a stressful interpersonal situation increases therapeutic value. Hospitals have protocols regarding the care and protection of the suicidal patient (see Chapter 24).

TABLE 13-6 Interventions Targeting the Vegetative Signs of Depression

Intervention	Rationale
NUTRITION—ANOREXIA	
Offer small, high-calorie and high-protein snacks frequently throughout the day and evening.	Low weight and poor nutrition render the patient susceptible to illness. Small, frequent snacks are more easily tolerated than large plates of food when the patient is anorexic.
Offer high-protein and high-calorie fluids frequently throughout the day and evening.	These fluids prevent dehydration and can minimize constipation.
When possible, encourage family or friends to remain with the patient during meals.	This strategy reinforces the idea that someone cares, can raise the patient's self-esteem, and can serve as an incentive to eat.
Ask the patient which foods or drinks he or she likes. Offer choices. Involve the dietitian.	The patient is more likely to eat the foods provided.
Weigh the patient weekly and observe the patient's eating patterns.	Monitoring the patient's status gives the information needed for revision of the intervention.
SLEEP—INSOMNIA	
Provide periods of rest after activities.	Fatigue can intensify feelings of depression.
Encourage the patient to get up and dress and to stay out of bed during the day.	Minimizing sleep during the day increases the likelihood of sleep at night.
Encourage the use of relaxation measures in the evening (e.g., tepid bath, warm milk).	These measures induce relaxation and sleep.
Reduce environmental and physical stimulants in the evening—provide decaffeinated coffee, soft lights, soft music, and quiet activities.	Decreasing caffeine and epinephrine levels increases the possibility of sleep.
SELF-CARE DEFICITS	
Encourage the use of toothbrush, washcloth, soap, makeup, shaving equipment, and so forth.	Being clean and well groomed can temporarily increase self-esteem.
When appropriate, give step-by-step reminders such as "Wash the right side of your face, now the left."	Slowed thinking and difficulty concentrating make organizing simple tasks difficult.
ELIMINATION—CONSTIPATION	
Monitor intake and output, especially bowel movements.	Many patients with depression are constipated. If the condition is not checked, fecal impaction can occur.
Offer foods high in fiber, and provide periods of exercise.	Roughage and exercise stimulate peristalsis and help evacuation of fecal material.
Encourage the intake of fluids.	Fluids help prevent constipation.
Evaluate the need for laxatives and enemas.	These measures prevent fecal impaction.

Pharmacological Interventions

Because mood disorders are caused by problems with neurotransmitters, it follows that medications that alter brain chemistry are an important component in the treatment of them. Antidepressant therapy benefits about 80% of people with major depression (Mental Health America, 2008). It should be noted, however, the combination of specific psychotherapies (e.g., CBT, IPT, behavioral) and antidepressant therapy is superior to either psychotherapy or psychopharmacological treatment alone (Reynolds et al., 2006).

Antidepressant Drugs

Antidepressant drugs can positively alter poor self-concept, degree of withdrawal, vegetative signs of depression, and activity level. Target symptoms include:

- Sleep disturbance
- Appetite disturbance (decreased or increased)
- Fatigue
- Decreased sex drive
- Psychomotor retardation or agitation
- Diurnal variations in mood (often worse in the morning)
- Impaired concentration or forgetfulness

- **Anhedonia** (loss of ability to experience joy or pleasure in living)

A drawback of antidepressant drugs is that improvement in mood may take 1 to 3 weeks or longer. If a patient is acutely suicidal, electroconvulsive therapy (discussed in detail later in this chapter) can be a reliable and effective alternative.

The goal of antidepressant therapy is the complete remission of symptoms (Stahl, 2008). Often, the first antidepressant prescribed is not the one that will ultimately bring about remission; aggressive treatment helps in finding the proper treatment. An adequate trial for the treatment of depression is 3 months. Individuals experiencing their first depressive episode are maintained on antidepressants for 6 to 9 months after symptoms of depression remit. Some people may have multiple episodes of depression or may have a chronic form (similar to the chronicity of diabetes) and benefit from indefinite antidepressant therapy.

Antidepressants may precipitate a psychotic episode in a person with schizophrenia or a manic episode in a patient with bipolar disorder. Patients with bipolar disorder often receive a mood stabilizing drug along with an antidepressant.

Choosing an Antidepressant. All antidepressants work to increase the availability of one or more of the neurotransmitters, serotonin, norepinephrine, and dopamine. All antidepressants work equally well; however, a variety of antidepressants or a combination of antidepressants may need to be tried before the most effective regimen is found for an individual patient. Each of the antidepressants has different adverse effects, costs, safety issues, and maintenance considerations. Selection of the appropriate antidepressant is based on the following considerations (Suehs et al., 2008):

- Side-effect profile (e.g., sexual dysfunction, weight gain)
- Ease of administration
- History of past response
- Safety and medical considerations

Table 13-7 provides an overview of antidepressants used in the United States.

Selective Serotonin Reuptake Inhibitors. The **selective serotonin reuptake inhibitors (SSRIs)** are recommended as first-line therapy for most types of depression. Essentially, the SSRIs selectively block the neuronal uptake of serotonin (e.g., 5-HT, 5-HT$_1$ receptors), which increases the availability of serotonin in the synaptic cleft. Refer to Chapter 3 for a more detailed discussion of how the SSRIs work.

SSRI antidepressant drugs have a relatively low side-effect profile compared with the older antidepressants (tricyclics—discussed later in this chapter); they do not create dry mouth, blurred vision, or urinary retention, making it easier for patients to take these medications as prescribed. Adherence to the medication regimen is a crucial step toward recovery or remission of symptoms. The SSRIs are effective in depression with anxiety features and depression with psychomotor agitation.

Because the SSRIs cause relatively few adverse effects and have low cardiotoxicity, they are less dangerous than older antidepressants when taken in overdose. The SSRIs, selective serotonin-norepinephrine reuptake inhibitors (SNRIs), and atypical antidepressants have a low lethality risk in suicide attempts, whereas the tricyclic antidepressants have a very high potential for lethality with overdose.

Indications. The SSRIs have a broad base of clinical use. In addition to their use in treating depressive disorders, the SSRIs have been prescribed with success to treat some of the anxiety disorders—in particular, obsessive-compulsive disorder and panic disorder (see Chapter 12). Fluoxetine has been found to be effective in treating some women who suffer from late-luteal-phase dysphoric disorder and bulimia nervosa.

Common adverse reactions. Agents that selectively enhance synaptic serotonin within the CNS may induce agitation, anxiety, sleep disturbance, tremor, sexual dysfunction (primarily anorgasmia), or tension headache. The effect of the SSRIs on sexual performance may be the most significant undesirable outcome reported by patients. Autonomic reactions (e.g., dry mouth, sweating, weight change, mild nausea, and loose bowel movements) may also be experienced with the SSRIs.

Potential toxic effects. One rare and life-threatening event associated with SSRIs is **serotonin syndrome**. This syndrome is thought to be related to overactivation of the central serotonin receptors, caused by either too high a dose or interaction with other drugs. Symptoms include abdominal pain, diarrhea, sweating, fever, tachycardia, elevated blood pressure, altered mental state (delirium), myoclonus (muscle spasms), increased motor activity, irritability, hostility, and mood change. Severe manifestations can induce hyperpyrexia (excessively high fever), cardiovascular shock, or death. The risk of this syndrome seems to be greatest when an SSRI is administered in combination with a second serotonin-enhancing agent, such as a monoamine oxidase inhibitor (MAOI). A patient should discontinue all SSRIs for 2 to 5 weeks before starting an MAOI. Box 13-2 lists the signs and symptoms of serotonin syndrome and gives emergency treatment guidelines. Box 13-3 is a useful tool for patient and family teaching about the SSRIs.

Tricyclic Antidepressants. The **tricyclic antidepressants (TCAs)** inhibit the reuptake of norepinephrine and serotonin by the presynaptic neurons in the CNS, increasing the amount of time norepinephrine

TABLE 13-7 Drug Treatment of Patients with Major Depression

Generic (Trade)	Action	Notes	Side Effects	Warnings
SELECTIVE SEROTONIN REUPTAKE INHIBITORS (SSRIs)				
Citalopram (Celexa) Escitalopram (Lexapro) Fluoxetine (Prozac) Fluvoxamine (Luvox) Paroxetine (Paxil) Sertraline (Zoloft)	Blocks the reuptake of serotonin	First line of treatment for major depression Some SSRIs activate and others sedate; choice depends on patient symptoms Risk of lethal overdose minimized with SSRIs	Agitation, insomnia, headache, nausea and vomiting, sexual dysfunction, and hyponatremia	Discontinuation syndrome— dizziness, insomnia, nervousness, irritability, nausea, and agitation—may occur with abrupt withdrawal (depending on half-life). Taper slowly. Contraindicated in people taking MAOIs
SEROTONIN NOREPINEPHRINE REUPTAKE INHIBITORS (SNRIs)				
Venlafaxine (Effexor) Duloxetine (Cymbalta)	Blocks the reuptake of serotonin and norepinephrine	Effexor is a popular next-step strategy after trying SSRIs Cymbalta has the advantage of decreasing neuropathic pain	Hypertension (venlafaxine), nausea, insomnia, dry mouth, sweating, agitation, headache, sexual dysfunction	Monitor blood pressure with Effexor, especially at higher doses and with a history of hypertension Discontinuation syndrome (see SSRIs above) Contraindicated in people taking MAOIs
NOREPINEPHRINE REUPTAKE INHIBITORS (NRIs)				
Reboxetine (Vestra)	Blocks the reuptake of norepinephrine and enhances its transmission	Antidepressant effects similar to SSRIs and TCAs Useful with severe depression and impaired social functioning	Insomnia, sweating, dizziness, dry mouth, constipation, urinary hesitancy, tachycardia, decreased libido	Contraindicated in people taking MAOIs
SEROTONIN RECEPTOR ANTAGONISTS/AGONISTS				
Nefazodone (formerly sold as Serzone)	Selective blockage of serotonin$_2$ receptors and α_1-adrenergic receptors	Lower risk of long-term weight gain than SSRIs or TCAs Lower risk of sexual side effects than SSRIs	Sedation, hepatotoxicity, dizziness, hypotension, paresthesias	Life-threatening liver failure is possible but rare Priapism of penis and clitoris is a rare but serious side effect Contraindicated in people taking MAOIs
NOREPINEPHRINE DOPAMINE REUPTAKE INHIBITOR (NDRI)				
Bupropion (Wellbutrin)	Blocks the reuptake of norepinephrine and dopamine	Stimulant action may reduce appetite May increase sexual desire Used as an aid to quit smoking	Agitation, insomnia, headache, nausea and vomiting, seizures (0.4%)	Contraindicated in people taking MAOIs High doses increase seizure risk, especially in people who are predisposed to them

Continued

TABLE 13-7 Drug Treatment of Patients with Major Depression—cont'd

Generic (Trade)	Action	Notes	Side Effects	Warnings
SEROTONIN NOREPINEPHRINE DISINHIBITORS (SNDIs)				
Mirtazapine (Remeron)	Blocks α_1- adrenergic receptors that normally inhibit norepinephrine and serotonin	Antidepressant effects equal SSRIs and may occur faster	Weight gain, sedation, dizziness, headache; sexual dysfunction is rare	Drug-induced somnolence exaggerated by alcohol, benzodiazepines, and other CNS depressants Contraindicated in people taking MAOIs
TRICYCLIC ANTIDEPRESSANTS (TCAs)				
Amitriptyline (Elavil) Clomipramine (Anafranil) Desipramine (Norpramin) Doxepin (Adapin, Sinequan) Imipramine (Tofranil) Nortriptyline (Aventyl, Pamelor) Protriptyline (Vivactil)	Inhibits the reuptake of serotonin and norepinephrine. Antagonizes adrenergic, histaminergic, and muscarinic receptors	Therapeutic effects similar to SSRIs, but side effects are more prominent May work better in melancholic depression TCAs can worsen many cardiac and medical conditions	Dry mouth, constipation, urinary retention, blurred vision, orthostatic hypotension, cardiac toxicity, sedation	Lethal in overdose Use cautiously in older adults and those with cardiac disorders, elevated intraocular pressure, urinary retention, hyperthyroidism, seizure disorders, and liver or kidney dysfunction. Contraindicated in people taking MAOIs
MONOAMINE OXIDASE INHIBITORS (MAOIs)				
Phenelzine (Nardil) Selegiline Transdermal System Patch (EMSAM) Tranylcypromine (Parnate)	Inhibits the enzyme monoamine oxidase, which normally breaks down neurotransmitters, including serotonin and norepinephrine	Efficacy similar to other antidepressants, but dietary restrictions and potential drug interactions make this drug less desirable	Insomnia, nausea, agitation, and confusion Potential for hypertensive crises or serotonin syndrome with concurrent use of other antidepressants	Contraindicated in people taking other antidepressants Tyramine-rich food could bring about a hypertensive crisis Many other drug interactions

Data from Martinez, M., Marangell, L. B., & Martinez, J. M. (2008). Psychopharmacology. In R. E. Hales, S. C. Yudofsky, & G. O. Gabbard (Eds.), *Textbook of Psychiatry*. Arlington, VA: American Psychiatric Publishing; Lehne, R. A. (2010). *Pharmacology for nursing care* (7th ed.). St. Louis: Saunders.

BOX 13-2 Serotonin Syndrome: Symptoms and Interventions

Symptoms
- Hyperactivity or restlessness
- Tachycardia → cardiovascular shock
- Fever → hyperpyrexia
- Elevated blood pressure
- Altered mental states (delirium)
- Irrationality, mood swings, hostility
- Seizures → status epilepticus
- Myoclonus, incoordination, tonic rigidity
- Abdominal pain, diarrhea, bloating
- Apnea → death

Interventions
- Remove offending agent(s)
- Initiate symptomatic treatment:
  - Serotonin-receptor blockade with cyproheptadine, methysergide, propranolol
  - Cooling blankets, chlorpromazine for hyperthermia
  - Dantrolene, diazepam for muscle rigidity or rigors
  - Anticonvulsants
  - Artificial ventilation
  - Paralysis

BOX 13-3 Patient and Family Teaching: Selective Serotonin Reuptake Inhibitors (SSRIs)

- May cause sexual dysfunction or lack of sex drive. Inform nurse or primary care provider if this occurs.
- May cause insomnia, anxiety, and nervousness. Inform nurse or primary care provider if this occurs.
- May interact with other medications. Tell primary care provider about other medications patient is taking (digoxin, warfarin). SSRIs should not be taken within 14 days of the last dose of a monoamine oxidase inhibitor.
- No over-the-counter drug should be taken without first notifying primary care provider.
- Common side effects include fatigue, nausea, diarrhea, dry mouth, dizziness, tremor, and sexual dysfunction or lack of sex drive.
- Because of the potential for drowsiness and dizziness, patient should not drive or operate machinery until these side effects are ruled out.
- Alcohol should be avoided.
- Liver and renal function tests should be performed and blood counts checked periodically.
- Medication should not be discontinued abruptly. If side effects become bothersome, patient should ask primary care provider about changing to a different drug. Abrupt cessation can lead to serotonin withdrawal.
- Any of the following symptoms should be reported to the primary care provider immediately:
  - Increase in depression or suicidal thoughts
  - Rash or hives
  - Rapid heartbeat
  - Sore throat
  - Difficulty urinating
  - Fever, malaise
  - Anorexia and weight loss
  - Unusual bleeding
  - Initiation of hyperactive behavior
  - Severe headache

---

and serotonin are available to the postsynaptic receptors. This increase in norepinephrine and serotonin in the brain is believed to be responsible for mood elevations.

Indications. The sedative effects of the TCAs are attributed to the blockade of histamine receptors (Lehne, 2010). Patients must take therapeutic doses of TCAs for 10 to 14 days or longer before they begin to work; full effects may not be seen for 4 to 8 weeks. An effect on some symptoms of depression, such as insomnia and anorexia, may be noted earlier. Choosing a TCA for a patient is based on what has worked for the patient or a family member in the past and the drug's adverse effects.

A stimulating TCA, such as desipramine (Norpramin) or protriptyline (Vivactil) may be best for a patient who is lethargic and fatigued. If a more sedating effect is needed for agitation or restlessness, drugs such as amitriptyline (Elavil) and doxepin (Sinequan) may be more appropriate choices. Regardless of which TCA is given, the initial dose should always be low and increased gradually.

Common adverse reactions. The chemical structure of the TCAs closely resembles that of antipsychotic medications, and the **anticholinergic** actions are similar (e.g., dry mouth, blurred vision, tachycardia, constipation, urinary retention, and esophageal reflux). These side effects are more common and more severe in patients taking antidepressants. They usually are not serious and are often transitory, but **urinary retention** and **severe constipation** warrant immediate medical attention. Weight gain is also a common complaint among people taking TCAs.

The α-adrenergic blockade of the TCAs can produce postural-orthostatic hypotension and tachycardia. Postural hypotension can lead to dizziness and increase the risk of falls.

Administering the total daily dose of TCA at night is beneficial for two reasons. First, most TCAs have sedative effects and thereby aid sleep. Second, the minor side effects occur while the individual is sleeping, which increases compliance with drug therapy.

Potential toxic effects. The most serious effects of the TCAs are cardiovascular: dysrhythmias, tachycardia, myocardial infarction, and heart block have been reported. Because the cardiac side effects are so serious, TCA use is considered a risk in older adults and patients with cardiac disease. Patients should have a thorough cardiac workup before beginning TCA therapy.

Adverse drug interactions. Use of an MAOI along with a TCA is contraindicated. A few of the more common medications usually *not* given while TCAs are being used are listed in Box 13-4. A patient who is taking any of these medications along with a TCA should have medical clearance, because some of the reactions can be fatal.

Contraindications. People who have recently had a myocardial infarction (or other cardiovascular problems), those with narrow-angle glaucoma or a history of seizures, and women who are pregnant should not be treated with TCAs, except with extreme caution and careful monitoring.

Patient and family teaching. Areas for the nurse to discuss when teaching patients and their families about TCA therapy are presented in Box 13-5.

Monoamine Oxidase Inhibitors. The enzyme monoamine oxidase is responsible for inactivating, or breaking down, certain monoamine neurotransmitters in the brain, such as norepinephrine, serotonin, dopamine, and tyramine. When a person ingests an MAOI, these amines do not get inactivated, and there is an increase of neurotransmitters available for synaptic release in the brain. The increase in norepinephrine, serotonin, and dopamine is the desired effect, because it results in mood elevation. The increase in tyramine, on the other hand, poses a problem. When the level of tyramine increases, and it is not inactivated by monoamine oxidase, high blood pressure, hypertensive crisis, and eventually cerebrovascular accident can occur. Therefore, people taking these drugs must reduce or eliminate their intake of foods and drugs that contain high amounts of tyramine (Table 13-8 and Box 13-6).

Because people with depression are often lethargic, confused, and apathetic, adherence to strict dietary limitations may not be realistic. That is why MAOIs, although highly effective, are not often given as a first-line treatment.

Indications. MAOIs are particularly effective for people with atypical depression (characterized by mood reactivity, oversleeping, and overeating), as well as panic disorder, social phobia, generalized anxiety disorder, obsessive-compulsive disorder, posttraumatic stress disorder, and bulimia. The MAOIs commonly used in the United States at present are phenelzine (Nardil) and tranylcypromine sulfate (Parnate). Selegiline (Emsam), a newer MAOI delivered transdermally in a patch, does not seem to affect tyramine sensitivity.

Common adverse reactions. Some common and troublesome long-term side effects of the MAOIs are orthostatic hypotension, weight gain, edema, change in cardiac rate and rhythm, constipation, urinary hesitancy, sexual dysfunction, vertigo, overactivity, muscle twitching, hypomanic and manic behavior, insomnia, weakness, and fatigue.

BOX 13-4 Drugs to Be Used with Caution with Tricyclic Antidepressants (TCAs)

- Monoamine oxidase inhibitors
- Phenothiazines
- Barbiturates
- Disulfiram (Antabuse)
- Oral contraceptives (or other estrogen preparations)
- Anticoagulants
- Some antihypertensives (clonidine, guanethidine, reserpine)
- Benzodiazepines
- Alcohol
- Nicotine

BOX 13-5 Patient and Family Teaching: Tricyclic Antidepressants (TCAs)

- The patient and family should be told that mood elevation may take from 7 to 28 days. Up to 6 to 8 weeks may be required for the full effect to be reached and for major depressive symptoms to subside.
- The family should reinforce this frequently to the family member with depression, who may have trouble remembering and respond to ongoing reassurance.
- The patient should be reassured that drowsiness, dizziness, and hypotension usually subside after the first few weeks.
- When the patient starts taking TCAs, the patient should be cautioned to be careful working around machines, driving cars, and crossing streets because of possible altered reflexes, drowsiness, or dizziness.
- Alcohol can block the effects of antidepressants. The patient should be told to refrain from drinking.
- If possible, the patient should take the full dose at bedtime to reduce the experience of side effects during the day.
- If the patient forgets the bedtime dose (or the once-a-day dose), the patient should take the dose within 3 hours; otherwise the patient should wait until the usual medication time the next day. The patient should *not* double the dose.
- Suddenly stopping TCAs can cause nausea, altered heartbeat, nightmares, and cold sweats in 2 to 4 days. The patient should call the primary care provider or take one dose of TCA until the primary care provider can be contacted.

TABLE 13-8 Foods That Can Interact with Monoamine Oxidase Inhibitors (MAOIs)

	FOODS THAT CONTAIN TYRAMINE	
Category	Unsafe Foods (High Tyramine Content)	Safe Foods (Little or No Tyramine)
Vegetables	Avocados, especially if overripe; fermented bean curd; fermented soybean; soybean paste	Most vegetables
Fruits	Figs, especially if overripe; bananas, in large amounts	Most fruits
Meats	Meats that are fermented, smoked, or otherwise aged; spoiled meats; liver, unless very fresh	Meats that are known to be fresh (exercise caution in restaurants; meats may not be fresh)
Sausages	Fermented varieties; bologna, pepperoni, salami, others	Nonfermented varieties
Fish	Dried or cured fish; fish that is fermented, smoked, or otherwise aged; spoiled fish	Fish that is known to be fresh; vacuum-packed fish, if eaten promptly or refrigerated only briefly after opening
Milk, milk products	Practically all cheeses	Milk, yogurt, cottage cheese, cream cheese
Foods with yeast	Yeast extract (e.g., Marmite, Bovril)	Baked goods that contain yeast
Beer, wine	Some imported beers, Chianti wines	Major domestic brands of beer; most wines
Other foods	Protein dietary supplements; soups (may contain protein extract); shrimp paste; soy sauce	
	FOODS THAT CONTAIN OTHER VASOPRESSORS	
Food	Comments	
Chocolate	Contains phenylethylamine, a pressor agent; large amounts can cause a reaction.	
Fava beans	Contain dopamine, a pressor agent; reactions are most likely with overripe beans.	
Ginseng	Headache, tremulousness, and mania-like reactions have occurred.	
Caffeinated beverages	Caffeine is a weak pressor agent; large amounts may cause a reaction.	

From Lehne, R. A. (2010). *Pharmacology for nursing* (7th ed.) (p. 351). Philadelphia: Saunders.

BOX 13-6 Drugs That Can Interact with Monoamine Oxidase Inhibitors (MAOIs)

- Over-the-counter medications for colds, allergies, or congestion (any product containing ephedrine, phenylephrine hydrochloride, or phenylpropanolamine)
- Tricyclic antidepressants (imipramine, amitriptyline)
- Narcotics
- Antihypertensives (methyldopa, guanethidine, reserpine)
- Amine precursors (levodopa, l-tryptophan)
- Sedatives (alcohol, barbiturates, benzodiazepines)
- General anesthetics
- Stimulants (amphetamines, cocaine)

Potential toxic effects. The most serious reaction to the MAOIs is an increase in blood pressure, with the possible development of intracranial hemorrhage, hyperpyrexia, convulsions, coma, and death. Therefore, routine monitoring of blood pressure, especially during the first 6 weeks of treatment, is necessary.

Because many drugs, foods, and beverages can cause an increase in blood pressure in patients taking MAOIs, hypertensive crisis is a constant concern. The beginning of a hypertensive crisis usually occurs within a few hours of ingestion of the contraindicated substance. The crisis may begin with headaches, stiff or sore neck, palpitations, increase or decrease in heart rate (often associated with chest pain), nausea, vomiting, or increase in temperature (pyrexia). When a hypertensive crisis is suspected, immediate medical attention is crucial. Antihypertensive medications such as the calcium channel blocker, nifedipine, or an alpha-adrenergic blocker such as phentolamine may be given (Martinez et al., 2008). Pyrexia is treated with hypothermic blankets or ice packs.

Table 13-9 identifies common side effects and toxic effects of the MAOIs, and Box 13-7 can be used as an MAOI teaching guide for patients and their families.

TABLE 13-9 Adverse Reactions to and Toxic Effects of Monoamine Oxidase Inhibitors (MAOIs)

Adverse Reactions	Comments
Hypotension Sedation, weakness, fatigue Insomnia Changes in cardiac rhythm Muscle cramps Anorgasmia or sexual impotence Urinary hesitancy or constipation Weight gain	Hypotension is a normal side effect of MAOIs. Orthostatic blood pressures should be taken–first lying down, then sitting or standing after 1-2 minutes. This may be a dangerous side effect, especially in older adults who may fall and sustain injuries as the result of dizziness from the blood pressure drop.

Toxic Effects	Comments
Hypertensive crisis: • Severe headache • Tachycardia, palpitations • Hypertension • Nausea and vomiting	Patient should go to local emergency department immediately—blood pressure should be checked. One of the following may be given to lower blood pressure: • 5 mg intravenous phentolamine (Regitine) *or* • Sublingual nifedipine to promote vasodilation Patients may be prescribed a 10 mg nifedipine capsule to carry in case of emergency

Data from Lehne, R. A. (2010). *Pharmacology for nursing* (7th ed.). Philadelphia: Saunders; Fava, M., & Papakostas, G. I. (2008). Antidepressants in T. A. Stern, J. F. Rosenbaum, M. Fava, J. Biederman, & S. L. Rauch (Eds.). Comprehensive clinical psychiatry (pp. 595–619). Philadelphia: Mosby.

BOX 13-7 Patient and Family Teaching: Monoamine Oxidase Inhibitors (MAOIs)

- Tell the patient and family to avoid certain foods and all medications (especially cold remedies) unless prescribed by and discussed with the patient's primary care provider (see Table 13-8 and Box 13-6 for specific food and drug restrictions).
- Give the patient a wallet card describing the MAOI regimen.
- Instruct the patient to avoid Chinese restaurants (sherry, brewer's yeast, and other contraindicated products may be used).
- Tell the patient to go to the emergency department immediately if he or she has a severe headache.
- Ideally, blood pressure should be monitored during the first 6 weeks of treatment (for both hypotensive and hypertensive effects).
- After the MAOI is stopped, instruct the patient that dietary and drug restrictions should be maintained for 14 days.

Contraindications. The use of MAOIs may be contraindicated with each of the following:
- Cerebrovascular disease
- Hypertension and congestive heart failure
- Liver disease
- Consumption of foods containing tyramine, tryptophan, and dopamine (see Table 13-8)
- Use of certain medications (see Box 13-6)
- Recurrent or severe headaches
- Surgery in the previous 10 to 14 days
- Age younger than 16 years

Use of Antidepressants by Pregnant Women. Within the last few years, there have been increasing concerns about the safety of antidepressants taken during pregnancy. Early studies demonstrated an association between TCAs and congenital malformations of the heart and limbs, and MAOI use has been associated with severe hypertension and stroke (Mayo Foundation, 2007). The use of SSRIs has been associated with breathing problems and withdrawal symptoms in infants (Tracy, 2006). One study indicated that women who took either SSRIs or TCAs had an increased risk of preterm birth (Agency for Healthcare Research and Quality, 2008). Another study demonstrated a higher risk for spontaneous abortion with use of antidepressants (Hemels et al., 2005).

Although these problems have been documented, the overall risk remains small (Mayo Foundation, 2007), and untreated depression presents its own problems. Pregnant women with depression have a higher risk of preterm birth, low-birth-weight infants, substance abuse, and nicotine use (Doskoch, 2001). The decision to take antidepressants while pregnant is one that must be made by carefully weighing the risks and benefits involved.

Use of Antidepressants by Children and Adolescents. In 2005, the U.S. Food and Drug

Administration (FDA) (2004) issued a black-box warning for all antidepressants, alerting the public to the increased risk of suicidal thinking or attempts in children or adolescents taking antidepressants. Following the black-box warning, the number of prescriptions written for SSRIs for children and young adults decreased, but suicides in those age groups actually increased (Dudley et al., 2008). Dudley and colleagues concluded that the risk for suicide is greater in children and adolescents with depression who do not take antidepressants. To minimize the risk of suicide in people taking antidepressants, close monitoring by health care professionals and patient/caregiver education are essential. Chapter 24 has a more detailed discussion of suicide risk factors and warning signs.

Use of Antidepressants by Older Adults. Polypharmacy and the normal process of aging contribute to concerns about prescribing antidepressants for older adults. SSRIs are a first-line treatment for older adults, but they have the potential for aggravated side effects. Starting doses are recommended to be half the lowest adult dose, with dose adjustments occurring no more frequently than every 7 days. TCAs and MAOIs have side-effect profiles that are more dangerous for older adults, specifically cardiotoxicity with TCAs and hypotension with both classes. Any medication with a side effect of hypotension or sedation in older adults increases the risk of falls. Older adults should be cautioned against abrupt discontinuation of antidepressants because of the possibility of discontinuation syndrome, which causes anxiety, dysphoria, flulike symptoms, dizziness, excessive sweating, and insomnia (Akpafflong et al., 2008).

Electroconvulsive Therapy

Despite being a highly effective somatic (physical) treatment for psychiatric disorders, electroconvulsive therapy (ECT) has a bad reputation. This may be due to media portrayals of patients being restrained on a gurney while having a full-blown seizure induced. Given the current sophistication of anesthetic and paralytic agents, ECT is actually not dramatic at all. Another possible reason for ECT's stigmatized status is that how it works remains a mystery (Stahl, 2008), although researchers have speculated as to its mechanism of action. It is likely that the seizure that is induced results in mobilization and activity of neurotransmitters.

Indications

ECT is used most commonly for depression. While as many as 50% of people taking antidepressants fail to achieve full remission, clinical trials of ECT report a rate of 70% to 90% remission (Welch, 2008). Suicidal thoughts respond to ECT in 80% of cases. Psychotic

illnesses are the second most common indication for ECT. For drug-resistant patients, a combination of ECT and antipsychotic medication has resulted in sustained improvement about 80% of the time.

While medication is generally the first line of treatment, according to Sadock and Sadock (2008), ECT may be a primary treatment in the following cases:

- When a patient is suicidal or homicidal, and there is a need for a rapid, definitive response
- If previous medication trials have failed
- When there is marked agitation, marked vegetative symptoms, or catatonia
- For major depression with psychotic features

ECT is useful in treating patients with major depression, especially when psychotic symptoms are present. Patients who have depression with marked psychomotor retardation and stupor also respond well. ECT is also indicated for manic patients whose conditions are resistant to treatment with lithium and antipsychotic drugs and for rapid cyclers. A **rapid cycler** is a patient with bipolar disorder who has many episodes of mood swings close together (four or more in 1 year). People with schizophrenia (especially catatonic), those with schizoaffective syndromes, psychotic patients who are pregnant, and patients with Parkinson's disease can also benefit from ECT.

ECT is not necessarily effective, however, in patients with DD, atypical depression, personality disorders, drug dependence, or depression secondary to situational or social difficulties.

The usual course of ECT for a patient with depression is 2 or 3 treatments per week to a total of 6 to 12 treatments. Although no absolute contraindications to ECT exist, several conditions pose risks and require careful workup and management. Since the heart can be stressed at the onset of the seizure and for up to 10 minutes after, careful assessment and management in hypertension, congestive heart failure, cardiac arrhythmias, and other cardiac conditions is warranted (Welch, 2008). ECT also stresses the brain as a result of increased cerebral oxygen, blood flow, and intracranial pressure. Conditions such as brain tumors and subdural hematomas may increase the risk of using ECT. Providers of care and patients need to weigh the risk of continued disability or potential suicide from depression against ECT treatment risks.

Initiating Electroconvulsive Therapy

The procedure is explained to the patient, and informed consent is obtained if the patient is being treated voluntarily. For a patient treated involuntarily, permission may be obtained from the next of kin, although in some states treatment must be court ordered. The patient is usually given a general anesthetic to induce sleep (e.g., a short-acting barbiturate such as methohexital sodium [Brevital]) and a muscle-paralyzing agent (e.g., succinylcholine) to prevent muscle distress and even fractures. These medications have revolutionized the comfort and safety of ECT. An electroencephalogram (EEG) monitors brain waves, and an electrocardiogram (ECG) monitors cardiac responses. Brief seizures (30 to 60+ seconds) are deliberately induced by an electric current (as brief as 1 second) transmitted through electrodes attached to one or both sides of the head.

Potential Adverse Reactions

Patients wake about 15 minutes after the procedure. After awakening from ECT, the patient may be confused and disoriented. The nurse and family may need to orient the patient frequently during the course of treatment. Many patients state that they have memory deficits for the first few weeks after the course of treatment, but memory usually, although not always, recovers. ECT is not a permanent cure for depression, and maintenance treatment with TCAs or lithium decreases the relapse rate. Maintenance ECT (once a week to once a month) may also help to decrease relapse rates for patients with recurrent depression.

Transcranial Magnetic Stimulation

Transcranial magnetic stimulation (TMS) is a noninvasive treatment modality that uses MRI-strength magnetic pulses to stimulate focal areas of the cerebral cortex. Mitchell and Loo (2006) analyzed 25 studies involving the use of TMS for patients with depression and concluded that benefits were statistically significant and treatment was safe. Ongoing research is needed to determine optimum treatment guidelines (frequency, intensity, and duration) and who would benefit most from this type of procedure.

Indications

In 2008, the United States Food and Drug Administration (FDA) approved the use of TMS for patients who have been unresponsive to other methods of treatment for depression. A large-scale, multisite, randomized controlled trial reported that TMS is an effective stand-alone (without antidepressants) treatment (O'Reardon et al., 2007). Studies have been conducted and are underway to research the safety and efficacy of TMS in the treatment of schizophrenia, anxiety disorders, and pain (George et al., 2008).

Initiating Transcranial Magnetic Stimulation

Outpatient treatment with TMS takes about 30 minutes and is typically ordered for 5 days a week for 4 to 6 weeks. Patients are awake and alert during the procedure. An electromagnet is placed on the patient's scalp, and short magnetic pulses pass into the prefrontal

EVIDENCE-BASED PRACTICE

Electroconvulsive Therapy (ECT) and Older Adults

Amazon, J., McNeely, E., Lehr, S., & Marquardt, M. G. (2008). The decision-making process of older adults who elect to receive ECT. *Journal of Psychosocial Nursing, 46* (5), 45–52.

Problem

Electroconvulsive therapy (ECT) remains an effective treatment option for people experiencing late-life depression; however, the decision making process of older adults opting for ECT remains largely misunderstood. Nurses must have a better understanding of this process in order to assist older adults as they make decisions about whether or not to have ECT.

Purpose of Study

The purpose of the study was to explore the decision-making process of older adults electing to receive ECT.

Methods

Seven older adults between the ages of 60 and 90 who had received ECT participated in this exploratory phenomenological study. Each participant engaged in a 1-hour, in-depth interview in which they were asked to describe the process of deciding to receive ECT. The participants' responses were analyzed for common themes.

Key Findings

- Four key themes that emerged were:
  - Trust in family, their physician, and God
  - Support from family, friends, and significant others
  - Past experience with positive results from ECT, either for themselves or a friend or acquaintance
  - A sense of desperation for the need to get well
- The overriding substantive theme involved the negative impact of the stigma of both mental illness and ECT. Participants feared what other people would think if knowledge of their ECT was made known.

Implications for Nursing Practice

In addition to providing education and information to older adults considering whether or not to receive ECT, psychiatric mental health nurses must also work to break through the stigma and discrimination these patients face.

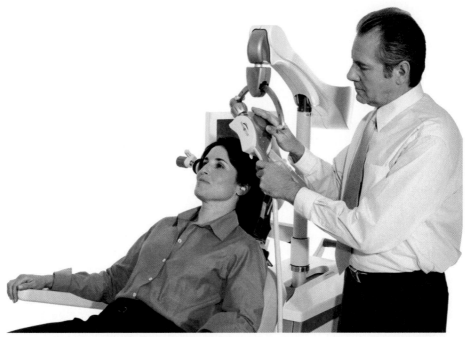

Figure 13-4 Transcranial magnetic stimulation. (Photo courtesy of Neuronetics.)

cortex of the brain (Figure 13-4). These pulses are similar to those used by MRI scanners but are more focused. The pulses cause electrical charges to flow and induce neurons to fire or become active. During TMS, patients feel a slight tapping or knocking in the head, contraction of the scalp, and tightening of the jaws.

Potential Adverse Reactions

After the procedure, patients may experience a headache and lightheadedness. No neurological deficits or memory problems have been noted. Seizures are a rare complication of TMS; one research study that analyzed 10,000 treatment sessions reported no occurrence of seizures (Janicak et al., 2008). Most of the common side effects of TMS are mild and include scalp tingling and discomfort at the administration site.

Vagus Nerve Stimulation

The use of **vagus nerve stimulation (VNS)** originated as a treatment for epilepsy. Clinicians noted that while VNS decreased seizures, it also appeared to improve mood in a population that normally experiences increased rates of depression (Dougherty & Rauch, 2008). The theory behind VNS relates to the action of the vagus nerve, the longest cranial nerve, which extends from the brainstem to organs in the neck, chest, and abdomen. Researchers believe that electrical stimulation of the vagus nerve results in boosting the level of neurotransmitters, thereby improving mood and also improving the action of antidepressants (Stahl, 2008).

Indications

Nearly a decade after VNS was approved for use in Europe, the FDA granted approval for VNS use in the United States for treatment-resistant depression. The efficacy of VNS in treating depression is still being established. Other potential applications of VNS include anxiety, obesity, and pain (George et al., 2008).

Initiating Vagus Nerve Stimulation

The surgery to implant VNS is typically outpatient. A pacemaker-like device is implanted surgically into the left chest wall (Stahl, 2008). The device is connected to a thin, flexible wire that is threaded up and wrapped around the vagus nerve on the left side of the neck. After surgery, an infrared magnetic wand is held against the chest while a personal computer or personal digital assistant (PDA) is used to program the frequency of pulses. Pulses are usually delivered for 30 seconds, every 5 minutes, for 24 hours a day. Antidepressant action typically occurs in several weeks.

Potential Adverse Reactions

The implantation of VNS (Figure 13-5) is a surgical procedure, carrying with it the risks inherent in any surgical procedure (e.g., pain, infection, sensitivity to anesthesia). Side effects of active VNS therapy are due to the proximity of the lead on the vagus nerve, which is close to the laryngeal and pharyngeal branches of the left vagus nerve (Dougherty & Rauch, 2008). Voice alteration occurs in nearly 60% of patients. Other side effects include neck pain, cough, paresthesia, and dyspnea, which tend to decrease with time. The device can

INTEGRATIVE THERAPY

Pilkington, Rampes, and Richardson (2006) highlight an array of complementary, alternative, and integrative approaches in the treatment of depression, including the use of dietary supplements, acupuncture, aromatherapy, meditation, light therapy, homeopathy, and yoga. Herbal products and supplements for depression have become a multimillion-dollar industry; however, the long-term effects of these products have just begun to be studied. Pilkington and colleagues warn that because many of these methods are not well supported by research, they should be used with caution. The approaches briefly discussed here are light therapy, use of St. John's Wort, and exercise.

Light Therapy

Light therapy has been researched for nearly 20 years and is accepted as a first-line treatment for seasonal affective disorder (SAD). People with SAD often live in regions in which there are marked seasonal differences in the amount of daylight, which is thought to disrupt melatonin production, circadian rhythms, or the ability to process dopamine and norepinephrine. Whatever the cause, the effect is a seasonal depression. Light therapy may also be useful as an adjunct in treating chronic MDD or DD with seasonal exacerbations (APA, 2000b).

Light therapy is thought to be effective because of the influence of light on melatonin. Melatonin is secreted by the pineal gland and is necessary for maintaining and shifting biological rhythms. Exposure to light suppresses the nocturnal secretion of melatonin, which seems to have a therapeutic effect on people with SAD (Harvard Medical School, 2008). Ideal treatment consists of 30 to 45 minutes of exposure daily to a 10,000-lux light source. Morning exposure is best; however, success has been reported when exposure occurs at other times of the day or in divided doses. Anecdotal reports suggest that increasing the available light by adding additional light sources may also help to elevate mood. For those affected by SAD, light therapy has been found to be as effective in reducing depressive symptoms as medications. Negative side effects include headache, eyestrain, and (rarely) hypomania. Concerns about eye damage from light exposure have not been validated (Harvard Medical School, 2008).

St. John's Wort

St. John's Wort *(Hypericum perforatum)* is a flower that can be processed into tea or tablets. It is thought to increase the amount of serotonin, norepinephrine, and dopamine in the brain, resulting in antidepressant effects. Studies of St. John's Wort used in the treatment of depression offer mixed results. It has generally been found to be as effective as antidepressants in the treatment of mild to moderate depression (Randlov et al., 2006), but usefulness in severe depression has not been established (Hypericum Depression Trial Study Group, 2002). Because St. John's Wort is not regulated by the FDA, concentrations of the active ingredients may vary from preparation to preparation, which may account for some variation in research results. St. John's Wort has the potential for adverse reactions when taken with other medications, and safety has not been established for use during pregnancy or in children.

Exercise

Substantial evidence suggests that exercise can enhance mood and counteract symptoms of depression (Harris et al., 2006). Cripps (2008) reports that the effects of exercise on symptoms of depression are biological, social, and psychological. Research shows that exercise increases available serotonin, typically low in depression. It has also been demonstrated to dampen the activity of the hypothalamic-pituitary-adrenocorticoid (HPA) axis, which is believed to be overly active in depression. People with depression who exercise regularly report feeling an elevated mood, greater happiness, and being more socially involved. Additional benefits of exercise are that it is more easily accessed, less expensive, and results in fewer side effects than antidepressants.

American Psychiatric Association. (2000b). *Practice guidelines for the treatment of psychiatric disorders: Compendium 2000.* Washington, DC: Author.

Cripps, F. (2008). Exercise your mind: Physical activity as a therapeutic technique for depression. *International Journal of Therapy and Rehabilitation, 15,* 460–464.

Harris, A. H., Cronkite, R., & Moos, R. (2006). Physical activity, exercise coping, and depression in a 10-year cohort study of depressed patients. *Journal of Affective Disorders, 93*(1-3), 79–85.

Harvard Medical School. (2008, January). A SAD story: Light therapy and antidepressants help people who get depressed during the winter. *Harvard Health Letter.* Retrieved October 29, 2008, from http://www.health.harvard.edu/fhg/updates/Seasonal-affective-disorder.shtml

Hypericum Depression Study Trial Group. (2002). Effect of *Hypericum perforatum* (St. John's Wort) in major depressive disorder. *Journal of the American Medical Association, 287,* 1807–1814.

Pilkington, K., Rampes, H., & Richardson, J. (2006). Complementary medicine for depression. *Expert Review of Neurotherapeutics, 6,* 1741–1751.

Randlov, C., Mehlsen, J., Thomsen, C. F., Hedman, C., Von Fircks, H., & Winther, K. (2006). The efficacy of St. John's Wort in patients with minor depressive symptoms or dysthymia—a double-blind placebo-controlled study. *Phytomedicine, 13*(4), 215–221.

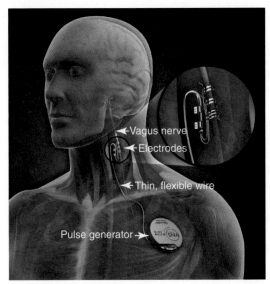

Figure 13-5 Vagus nerve stimulation. (Image courtesy of Cyberonics, Inc.)

be turned off at any time by placing a special magnet over the implant. This may be especially helpful when engaging in public speaking or heavy exercise.

Advanced Practice Interventions

The advanced practice nurse is qualified to provide psychotherapy, social skills training, and group therapy (American Psychiatric Nurses Association et al., 2007). In some states, nurses who have met appropriate educational standards may be certified to prescribe medication to treat depression.

Psychotherapy

Cognitive behavioral therapy (CBT), interpersonal therapy (IPT), time-limited focused psychotherapy, and behavioral therapy all are especially effective in the treatment of depression. However, only CBT and IPT demonstrate superiority in the maintenance phase. CBT helps people change their negative thought patterns and behaviors, whereas IPT focuses on working through personal relationships that may contribute to depression (NIMH, 2007c).

Group Therapy

Group therapy is a widespread modality for the treatment of depression; it increases the number of people who can receive treatment at a decreased cost per individual. Another advantage is that groups offer patients an opportunity to socialize and share common feelings and concerns, which decreases feelings of isolation, hopelessness, helplessness, and alienation.

Future of Treatment

There is a great need for earlier detection, earlier intervention, prevention of progression, achievement of remission, and integration of neuroscience and behavioral science in the treatment of depression (Greden, 2004). Goals include:

- Improved screening for high-risk ages and groups, including:
  - Individuals in late adolescence and early adulthood
  - Women in reproductive years
  - Adults and older adults with medical problems (e.g., pain)
  - People with a family history of depression
- Increased education, particularly about the linkage between physical symptoms and depression
- Psychopharmacological treatment augmented with cognitive-behavioral therapies
- Inclusion of more supplementary strategies, such as:
  - Promotion of sleep hygiene
  - Increase in exercise
  - Better overall health care

EVALUATION

Short-term indicators and outcome criteria are frequently evaluated during the course of treatment for depression. For example, if the patient with depression came into the unit with suicidal thoughts, the nurse evaluates whether suicidal thoughts are still present, the person is able to state alternatives to suicidal impulses in the future, the patient is able to explore thoughts and feelings that precede suicidal impulses, and so forth. Outcomes relating to thought processes, self-esteem, and social interactions are frequently formulated, because these areas are often problematic in people with depression.

Physical needs warrant nursing or medical attention. If a patient has lost weight because of anorexia, is the appetite returning? If the patient was constipated, are the bowels now functioning normally? If the patient was suffering from insomnia, is sleep improving to 6 to 8 hours of sleep per night? If indicators have not been met, an analysis of the data, nursing diagnoses, goals, and planned nursing interventions is made. The care plan is reassessed and reformulated as necessary.

Case Study and Nursing Care Plan 13-1   Depression

Ms. Glessner is a 35-year-old executive secretary. She has been divorced for 3 years and has two sons, 11 and 13 years of age. She is brought into the emergency department (ED) by her neighbor. She has some slashes on her wrists and is bleeding. The neighbor states that both of Ms. Glessner's sons are visiting their father for the summer. Ms. Glessner has become more and more despondent since terminating a 2-year relationship with a married man 4 weeks previously. According to the neighbor, for 3 years after her divorce, Ms. Glessner talked constantly about not being pretty or good enough and doubted that anyone could really love her. The neighbor states that Ms. Glessner has been withdrawn for at least 3 years. After the relationship with her boyfriend ended, she became even more withdrawn and sullen. Ms. Glessner is about 20 lb overweight, and her neighbor states that Ms. Glessner often stays awake late into the night, drinking by herself and watching television. She sleeps through most of the day on the weekends.

After receiving treatment in the ED, Ms. Glessner is seen by a psychiatrist. The initial diagnosis is dysthymic disorder with suicidal ideation. A decision is made to hospitalize her briefly for suicide observation and evaluation for appropriate treatment.

The nurse, Ms. Ward, admits Ms. Glessner to the unit from the ED.

Nurse: Hello, Ms. Glessner, I'm Marcia Ward. I'll be your primary nurse.

Ms. Glessner: Yeah…I don't need a nurse, a doctor, or anyone else. I just want to get away from this pain.

Nurse: You want to get away from your pain?

Ms. Glessner: I just said that, didn't I? Oh, what's the use? No one understands.

Nurse: I would like to understand, Ms. Glessner.

Ms. Glessner: Look at me. I'm fat…ugly…and no good to anyone. No one wants me.

Nurse: Who doesn't want you?

Ms. Glessner: My husband didn't want me…and now Jerry left me to go back to his wife.

Nurse: You think because Jerry went back to his wife that no one else could care for you?

Ms. Glessner: Well…he doesn't anyway.

Nurse: Because he doesn't care, you believe that no one else cares about you?

Ms. Glessner: Yes…

Nurse: Who do you care about?

Ms. Glessner: No one…except my sons…. I do love my sons, even though I don't often show it.

Nurse: Tell me more about your sons.

Ms. Ward continues to speak with Ms. Glessner. Ms. Glessner talks about her sons with some affect and apparent affection; however, she continues to state that she does not think of herself as worthwhile.

ASSESSMENT

Self-Assessment

Ms. Ward is aware that when patients have depression, they can be negative, think life is hopeless, and be hostile toward those who want to help. When Ms. Ward was new to the unit, she withdrew from patients with depression and sought out patients who appeared more hopeful and appreciative of her efforts. The unit coordinator was very supportive of Ms. Ward when she was first on the unit. Ms. Ward, along with other staff, was sent to in-service education sessions on working with patients with depression and was encouraged to speak up in staff meetings about the feelings many of these patients evoked in her. As a primary nurse, she was assigned a variety of patients. She found that as time went on, with the support of her peers and the opportunity to speak up at staff meetings, she was able to take what patients said less personally and not feel so responsible when patients did not respond as fast as she would like.

After 2 years, she had had the experience of seeing many patients who seemed hopeless and despondent on admission respond well to nursing and medical interventions and go on to lead full and satisfying lives. This also made it easier for Ms. Ward to understand that even though the patient with depression may think life is hopeless and may believe there is nothing in life to live for, change is always possible.

Objective Data

Slashed her wrists
Recently broke off with boyfriend
Has thought poorly of herself for 3 years, since divorce
Has two sons she cares about
Is 20 lb overweight
Stays awake late at night, drinking by herself
Has been withdrawn since divorce

Subjective Data

"No one could ever love me."
"I'm not good enough."
"I just want to get rid of this pain."
"I'm fat and ugly…no good to anyone."
"I do love my sons, although I don't always show it."

DIAGNOSIS

The nurse evaluates Ms. Glessner's strengths and weaknesses and decides to concentrate on two initial nursing diagnoses that seem to have the highest priority.

1. *Risk for suicide* related to separation from 2-year relationship, as evidenced by actual suicide attempt
   - Slashed her wrists
   - Recently broke off with boyfriend
   - Drinks at night by herself
   - Withdrawn for 3 years since divorce
2. *Situational low self-esteem* related to divorce and recent termination of love relationship, as evidenced by derogatory statements about self
   - "I'm not good enough."
   - "No one could ever love me."
   - "I'm fat and ugly…no good to anyone."
   - "I do love my sons, although I don't always show it."

OUTCOMES IDENTIFICATION

Patient refrains from attempting suicide.

PLANNING

Because Ms. Glessner is discharged after 48 hours, the issue of disturbance in self-esteem continues to be addressed in her therapy after discharge. Ms. Ward later reviews the goals for her work with Ms. Glessner in the community.

IMPLEMENTATION

Ms. Glessner's plan of care is personalized as follows:

Short-Term Goal	Intervention	Rationale	Evaluation
1. Patient expresses at least one reason to live, and this is apparent by the second day of hospitalization.	1a. Observe patient every 15 minutes while she is suicidal. 1b. Remove all dangerous objects from patient.	1a, b. Patient safety is ensured. Impulsive self-harmful behavior is minimized.	GOAL MET By the end of the second day, Ms. Glessner states she really did not want to die, she just couldn't stand the loneliness in her life. She states that she loves her sons and would never want to hurt them.
	1c. Obtain a "no self-harm" contract with patient for a specific period of time, to be renegotiated.	1c. May help patient gain a sense of control and a feeling of responsibility.	
	1d. Spend regularly scheduled periods of time with patient throughout the day.	1d. This interaction reinforces that patient is worthwhile and builds up experience to begin to relate better to nurse on one-to-one basis.	
	1e. Assist patient in evaluating both positive and negative aspects of her life.	1e. A person with depression is often unable to acknowledge any positive aspects of life unless they are pointed out by others.	
	1f. Encourage appropriate expression of angry feelings.	1f. Providing for expression of pent-up hostility in a safe environment can reinforce more adaptive methods of releasing tension and may minimize need to act out self-directed anger.	
	1g. Accept patient's negativism	1g. Acceptance enhances feelings of self-worth.	

Continued

Short-Term Goal	Intervention	Rationale	Evaluation
2. Patient will identify two outside supports she can call upon if she feels suicidal in the future.	2a. Explore usual coping behaviors.	2a. Behaviors that need reinforcing and new coping skills that need to be introduced can be identified.	GOAL MET By discharge, Ms. Glessner states that she is definitely going to try cognitive-behavioral therapy. She also discusses joining a women's support group that meets once a week in a neighboring town.
	2b. Assist patient in identifying members of her support system.	2b. Strengths and weaknesses in support available can be evaluated.	
	2c. Suggest a number of community-based support groups she might wish to discuss or visit (e.g., hotlines, support groups, women's groups).	2c. Patient needs to be aware of community supports to use them.	
	2d. Assist patient in identifying realistic alternatives she is willing to use.	2d. Unless patient is in agreement with any plan, she will be unable or unwilling to follow through in a crisis.	

EVALUATION

During the course of her work with Ms. Ward, Ms. Glessner decides to go to some meetings of Parents Without Partners. She states that she is looking forward to getting back to work and feels much more hopeful about her life. She has also lost 3 lb while attending Weight Watchers. She states, "I need to get back into the world." Although Ms. Glessner still has negative thoughts about herself, she admits to feeling more hopeful and better about herself, and she has learned important tools to deal with her negative thoughts.

KEY POINTS TO REMEMBER

- Depression is the most common psychiatric disorder.
- There are a number of subtypes of depression and depressive clinical phenomena. The two primary depressive disorders are major depressive disorder (MDD) and dysthymic disorder (DD).
- The symptoms of major depression are usually severe enough to interfere with a person's social or occupational functioning. A person with MDD may or may not have psychotic symptoms, and the symptoms usually exhibited during an episode of major depression are different from the characteristics of the normal premorbid personality.
- The symptoms of DD are often chronic (lasting at least 2 years) and are considered mild to moderate. Usually a person's social or occupational functioning is not greatly impaired. The symptoms in a DD are often congruent with the person's usual pattern of functioning.
- Many theories exist about the cause of depression. The most accepted is psychophysiological theory; however, cognitive theory, learned helplessness theory, and the diathesis-stress theory help explain triggers to depression and maintenance of depressive thoughts and feelings.
- Nursing assessment includes the evaluation of affect, thought processes (especially suicidal thoughts), mood, feelings, physical behavior, communication, and religious beliefs and spirituality. The nurse also must be aware of the symptoms that may mask depression.
- Nursing diagnoses can be numerous. Individuals with depression are always evaluated for risk for suicide. Some other common nursing diagnoses are Disturbed thought processes, Chronic low self-esteem, Imbalanced nutrition, Constipation, Disturbed sleep pattern, Ineffective coping, and Disabled family coping.
- Working with people who have depression can evoke intense feelings of hopelessness and frustration in health care workers. Nurses must clarify expectations of themselves and their patients and sort personal feelings from those communicated by the patient via empathy. Peer supervision and individual supervision by an experienced nurse clinician, psychiatric social worker, or psychologist are useful in increasing therapeutic potential.

- Interventions with patients who have depression involve several approaches. Basic-level interventions include using specific principles of communication, planning activities of daily living, administering or participating in psychopharmacological therapy, maintaining a therapeutic environment, and teaching patients about the biochemical aspects of depression.
- Advanced practice interventions may include several short-term psychotherapies that are effective in the treatment of depression, including IPT, CBT, skills training (assertiveness and social skills), and some forms of group therapy.
- Depression is often overlooked in children, adolescents, and older adults because symptoms of depression are often mistaken for signs of normal development.
- Planning and interventions for patients with depression are based on the recovery model, which involves a therapeutic alliance with health care professionals in order to achieve outcomes based on individual patient needs and values.
- Evaluation is ongoing throughout the nursing process, and patients' outcomes are compared with the stated outcome criteria and short-term and intermediate indicators. The care plan is revised when indicators are not being met.

CRITICAL THINKING

1. You are spending time with Mr. Plotsky, who is undergoing a workup for depression. He hardly makes eye contact, slouches in his seat, and wears a blank but sad expression. Mr. Plotsky has had numerous bouts of major depression in the past and says to you, "This will be my last depression. I will never go through this again."
   A. Since safety is the first concern, what are the appropriate questions to ask Mr. Plotsky at this time?
   B. In terms of behaviors, thought processes, activities of daily living, and ability to function at work and home, give examples of the kinds of signs and symptoms you might find when assessing a patient with depression.
   C. Mr. Plotsky tells you that he has been on every medication there is, but none have worked. He asks you about the herb St. John's wort. What should you tell him about its effectiveness for severe depression, interactions with other antidepressants, and regulatory status?
   D. What might be some somatic options for a person who is resistant to antidepressant medications?
   E. Mr. Plotsky asks what causes depression. In simple terms, how might you respond to his query?
   F. Mr. Plotsky tells you that he has never tried therapy because he thinks it is for weaklings. What information could you give him about various therapeutic modalities that have proven effective for other patients with depression?

2. You are working with Ms. Folk, a 28-year-old with MDD on long-term antidepressant therapy. She asks you about the possibility of pregnancy while taking her SSRIs.
   A. What are some of the things Ms. Folk might want to consider about taking antidepressants if she plans to get pregnant?
   B. If she decides to stop taking her antidepressants, what are some things she might do to help manage her depression?

CHAPTER REVIEW

1. The nurse is caring for a patient who exhibits disorganized thinking and delusions. The patient repeatedly states, "I hear voices of aliens trying to contact me." The nurse should recognize this presentation as which type of major depressive disorder (MDD)?
   1. Catatonic
   2. Atypical
   3. Melancholic
   4. Psychotic

2. Which patient statement indicates learned helplessness?
   1. "I am a horrible person."
   2. "Everyone in the world is just out to get me."
   3. "It's all my fault that my husband left me for another woman."
   4. "I hate myself."

3. The nurse is planning care for a patient with depression who will be discharged to home soon. What aspect of teaching should be the priority on the nurse's discharge plan of care?
   1. Pharmacological teaching
   2. Safety risk
   3. Awareness of symptoms increasing depression
   4. The need for interpersonal contact

4. The nurse is reviewing orders given for a patient with depression. Which order should the nurse question?
   1. A low starting dose of a tricyclic antidepressant
   2. An SSRI given initially with an MAOI
   3. Electroconvulsive therapy to treat suicidal thoughts
   4. Elavil to address the patient's agitation

5. A female patient tells the nurse that he would like to begin taking St. John's wort for depression. What teaching should the nurse provide?
   1. "St. John's wort should be taken several hours after your other antidepressant."
   2. "St. John's wort has generally been shown to be effective in treating depression."
   3. "This supplement is safe to take if you are pregnant."
   4. "St. John's wort is regulated by the FDA, so you can be assured of its safety."

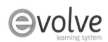

Visit the Evolve website for an **Audio Chapter Summary, Chapter Review Answers & Rationales, Critical Thinking Answer Guidelines**, and additional resources related to the content in this chapter: **http://evolve.elsevier.com/Varcarolis/foundations**

Companion CD Use the Companion CD to prepare for tests and the NCLEX® Examination with **Test-Taking Strategies** for psychiatric mental health nursing and hundreds of **Review Questions**.

References

Akpafflong, M. J., Wilson-Lawson, M., & Kunik, M.E. (2008). Antidepressant-associated side effects in older adult depressed patients. *Geriatrics, 63*(4), 18–23.

American Psychiatric Association. (2000a). *Diagnostic and statistical manual of mental disorders* (4th ed., text rev.) *(DSM-IV-TR)*. Washington, DC: Author.

American Psychiatric Association. (2000b). *Practice guidelines for the treatment of psychiatric disorders: Compendium 2000*. Washington, DC: Author.

Arehart-Treichel, J. (2006). Spirituality tied to higher depression, anxiety rates. *Psychiatric News, 41*(21), 26–28.

Arnow, B. A., Hunkeler, E. M., Blasey, C. M., Lee, J., Constantino, M. J., Fireman, B., Kraemer, H. C., Dea, R., et al. (2006). Comorbid depression, chronic pain, and disability in primary care. *Psychosomatic Medicine, 68*, 262–268.

Beck, A. T., Brown, G., Berchick, R. J., Stewart, B. L., & Steer, R. A. (2006). Relationship between hopelessness and ultimate suicide: A replication with psychiatric outpatients. *Focus, 4*, 291–296.

Beck, A. T., & Rush, A. J. (1995). Cognitive therapy. In H. I. Kaplan & B. J. Sadock (Eds.), *Comprehensive textbook of psychiatry/VI* (6th ed., Vol. 2) (pp. 1847–1856). Baltimore: Williams & Wilkins.

Bijl, D., van Marwijk, H. W., de Haan, M., van Tilburg, W., & Beekman, A. J. (2004). Effectiveness of disease management programmes for recognition, diagnosis and treatment of depression in primary care. *European Journal of General Practice, 10*, 6–12.

Brendel, R. W., Lagomasino, I. T., Perlis, R. H., & Stern, T. A. (2008). The suicidal patient. In T. A. Stern, J. F. Rosenbaum, M. Fava, J. Biederman, & S. L. Rauch (Eds.). *Comprehensive Clinical Psychiatry* (pp. 733–745). St. Louis: Mosby.

Bulechek, G. M., Butcher, H. K., Dochterman, J. M. (2008). *Nursing interventions classification (NIC)* (5th ed.). St. Louis: Mosby.

Doolitte, B., & Farrell, M. (2004). The association between spirituality and depression in an urban clinic. *Primary Care Companion Journal of Clinical Psychiatry, 6*, 114–118.

Doskoch, P. (2001). Which is more toxic to a fetus—antidepressants or maternal depression? *Neuropsychiatry Reviews, 2*(5), 1.

Dougherty, D. D., & Rauch, S. L. (2008). Neurotherapeutics. In T. A. Stern, J. F. Rosenbaum, M. Fava, J. Biederman, & S. L. Rauch (Eds.), *Comprehensive Clinical Psychiatry* (pp. 645–650). St. Louis: Mosby.

Dudley, M., Hadzi-Pavlovic, D., Andrews, D., & Perich, T. (2008). New-generation antidepressants, suicide and depressed adolescents: How should clinicians respond to changing evidence? *The Australian and New Zealand Journal of Psychiatry, 42*, 456–466.

George, M. S., Nahas, Z. H., Borckardt, J. J., Anderson, B., & Foust, M. J. (2008). Nonpharmacological somatic treatments. In R. E. Hales, S. C. Yudofsky, & G. O. Gabbard (Eds.), *Textbook of psychiatry* (5th ed., pp. 1133–1153). Washington, DC: American Psychiatric Publishing.

C. F., & Nemeroff, C. B. (2007). Corticotropin-releasing factor and the psychobiology of early-life stress. *Current directions in psychological science, 16*(2), 85–89.

Grayson, C. E. (2004). Can children really suffer from depression? *Depression in Children*. Retrieved July 2, 2008 from http://www.medicinenet.com/depression_in_children/article.htm#suffer

Greden, J. F. (2004, May 1–6). *Best practices for achieving remission in depression with physical symptoms: Current and future trends*. Paper presented in Symposium 10E conducted at the American Psychiatric Association Annual Meeting, New York.

Gusick, G. (2008). The contribution of depression and spirituality to symptom burden in chronic heart failure. *Archives of Psychiatric Nursing, 22*(1), 53–55.

Hemels, M.E.H., Einarson, A., Koren, G., Lanctot, C.L., & Einarson, T.R. (2005). Antidepressant use during pregnancy and the rates of spontaneous abortions: A meta-analysis *The Annals of Pharmacotherapy, 39*, 803–809.

Janicak, P. G., O'Reardon, J. P., Sampson, S. M., Husain, M. M., Lisanby, S. H., Rado, J. T., Heart, K. L., & Demitrack, M. A. (2008). Transcranial magnetic stimulation in the treatment of major depressive disorder: A comprehensive summary of safety experience from acute exposure, extended exposure, and during reintroduction treatment. *Journal of Clinical Psychiatry, 69*(2), 222–232.

Joska, J.A., & Stein, D.J. (2008). Mood disorders. In R. E. Hales, S. C. Yudofsky, & G. O. Gabbard (Eds.), *Textbook of psychiatry* (5th ed., pp. 457–504). Washington, DC: American Psychiatric Publishing.

Lehne, R. A. (2010). *Pharmacology for nursing care* (7th ed.). St. Louis: Saunders.

Lenze, E. J. (2003). Comorbidity of depression and anxiety in the elderly. *Current Psychiatric Reports, 5*, 62–67.

Martinez, M., Marangell, L. B., & Martinez, J. M. (2008). Psychopharmacology. In R. E. Hales, S. C. Yudofsky, & G. O. Gabbard (Eds.), *Textbook of psychiatry* (5th ed., p. 1073). Arlington, VA: American Psychiatric Publishing.

Mayo Foundation for Medical Education and Research. (2007). *Antidepressants: Are they safe during pregnancy?* Retrieved June 26, 2008, from http://www.mayoclinic.com/health/antidepressants/DN00007

Mental Health America. (2008, Jan. 24). *Factsheet: Depression: What you need to know*. Retrieved June 26, 2008, from http://www.mentalhealthamerica.net/go/information/get-info/depression/depression-what-you-need-to-know/depression-what-you-need-to-know

Moorhead, S., Johnson, M., Maas, M. L., & Swanson, E. (2008). *Nursing outcomes classification (NOC)* (4th ed.). St. Louis: Mosby.

National Institute of Mental Health. (2007a). *Depression in children and adolescents: A fact sheet for primary care providers* (NIH Publication No. 004744). Washington, DC: Author. Retrieved October 31, 2008, from http://www.mental-health-matters.com/articles/article.php?artID = 320

National Institute of Mental Health. (2007b). *Older adults: Depression and suicide facts* (NIH publication No. 03–4593). Bethesda, MD: National Institutes of Health. Retrieved October 31, 2008, from http://www.nimh.nih.gov/health/publications/older-adults-depression-and-suicide-facts.shtml

National Institute of Mental Health. (2007c). *Depression research at the National Institute of Mental Health (NIH Publication No. 004501)*. Bethesda, MD: National Institutes of Health.

North American Nursing Diagnosis Association International (NANDA-I). (2009). *NANDA-I nursing diagnoses: Definitions and classification 2009–2011*. Oxford, United Kingdom: Author.

Ozeki, N. (2008). Transcultural stress factors of Japanese mothers living in the United Kingdom. *Journal of Transcultural Nursing, 19*, 47–54.

O'Reardon, J. P., Solvason, H. B., Janicak, P. G., Sampson, S., Isenberg, Z. N., McDonald, W. M., Avery, D., Fitzgerald, P. B., et al. (2007). Efficacy and safety of transcranial magnetic stimulation in the acute treatment of major depression: A multisite randomized controlled trial. *Biological Psychiatry, 62*(11), 1208–1216.

Reynolds, C. F. III, Dew, M. A., Pollock, B. G., Mulsant, B. H., Frank, E., Miller, M. D., et al. (2006). Maintenance treatment of major depression in old age. *New England Journal of Medicine, 354*, 1130–1138.

Sadock, B. J., & Sadock, V. A. (2008). *Concise textbook of clinical psychiatry* (3rd ed.). Philadelphia: Lippincott, Williams, and Wilkins.

Seligman, M. E. (1973). Fall into hopelessness. *Psychology Today, 7*, 43.

Simon, N. M., & Rosenbaum, J. F. (2003, March 27). *Anxiety and depression comorbidity: Implications and intervention.* Retrieved January 16, 2005, from Medscape website: http://www.medscape.com/viewarticle/451325.

Stahl, S. M. (2008). *Stahl's essential pharmacology.* New York: Cambridge.

Suehs, B. T., Argo, T. R., Bendele, S. D., Crismon, M. L., Trivedi, M. H., & Kurian, B. (2008). *Texas Medication Algorithm Project procedural manual: Major depressive disorder algorithms.* The Texas Department of State Health Services. Retrieved March 4, 2009 from http://www.dshs.state.tx.us/mhprograms/pdf/TIMA_MDD_Manual_080608.pdf

Tracy, T. (2006). *Is it safe to take antidepressants during pregnancy?* Retrieved June 26, 2008, from http://www1.umn.edu/umnnews/Columns/Health_Talk_and_You/Is_it_safe_to_take_antidepressants_during_pregnanc.html#

U.S. Food and Drug Administration, Center for Drug Evaluation and Research. (2004). *Worsening depression and suicidality in patients being treated with antidepressant medications.* Retrieved January 16, 2005, from http://www.fda.gov/cder/drug/antidepressants/Antidepressants PHA.htm

Welch, C. A. (2008). Electroconvulsive therapy. In T. A. Stern, J. F. Rosenbaum, M. Fava, J. Biederman, & S. L. Rauch (Eds.), *Comprehensive Clinical Psychiatry* (pp. 635–644). St. Louis: Mosby.

Zelkowitz, P., Saucier, J.F., Wang, T., Katofsky, L., Valenzuela, M., & Westreich, R. (2008). Stability and change in depressive symptoms from pregnancy to two months postpartum in childbearing immigrant women. *Archives of Women's Mental Health, 11*, 1–11.

CHAPTER **14**

Bipolar Disorders

Margaret Jordan Halter and Elizabeth M. Varcarolis

Key Terms and Concepts

acute phase, 288
anticonvulsant drugs, 294
bipolar I disorder, 281
bipolar II disorder, 281
clang associations, 287
continuation phase, 288
cyclothymia, 281
flight of ideas, 286

grandiosity, 287
hypomania, 281
lithium carbonate, 292
maintenance phase, 288
mania, 281
mood stabilizers, 299
rapid cycling, 281
seclusion protocol, 297

Objectives

1. Assess a patient experiencing mania for (a) mood, (b) behavior, and (c) thought processes, and be alert to possible dysfunction.
2. Formulate three nursing diagnoses appropriate for a patient with mania, and include supporting data.
3. Explain the rationales behind five methods of communication that may be used with a patient experiencing mania.
4. Teach a classmate at least four expected side effects of lithium therapy.
5. Distinguish between signs of early and severe lithium toxicity.
6. Write a medication care plan specifying five areas of patient teaching regarding lithium carbonate.

7. Compare and contrast basic clinical conditions that may respond better to anticonvulsant therapy with those that may respond better to lithium therapy.
8. Evaluate specific indications for the use of seclusion for a patient experiencing mania.
9. Defend the use of electroconvulsive therapy for a patient in specific situations.
10. Review at least three of the items presented in the patient and family teaching plan (see Box 14-2) with a patient with bipolar disorder.
11. Distinguish the focus of treatment for a person in the acute manic phase from the focus of treatment for a person in the continuation or maintenance phase.

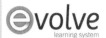 Visit the Evolve website for an **Audio Glossary & Flashcards, Concept Map Creator,** and additional resources related to the content in this chapter: **http://evolve.elsevier.com/Varcarolis/foundations**

Once commonly known as *manic-depression*, bipolar disorder is a chronic, recurrent illness that must be carefully managed throughout a person's life. Bipolar disorder frequently goes unrecognized, and people suffer for an average of 6 years before receiving a proper diagnosis and treatment (Wang et al., 2005). Bipolar disorder is marked by shifts in mood, energy, and ability to function. The course of the illness is variable, and symptoms range from severe mania—an exaggerated euphoria or irritability—to severe depression (Figure 14-1). Periods of normal functioning may alternate with periods of illness (highs, lows, or a combination of both). However, many individuals continue to experience chronic interpersonal or occupational difficulties even during remission. The mortality rate for bipolar disorder is severe; 25% to 60% of individuals with bipolar disorder will make a suicide attempt at least once in their lifetime, and nearly 20% of all deaths among this population are from suicide (Tondo & Baldessarini et al., 2006).

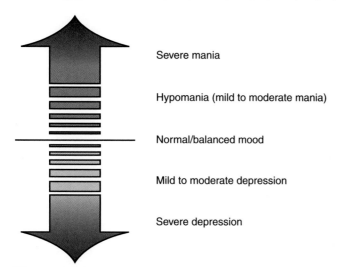

Severe mania

Hypomania (mild to moderate mania)

Normal/balanced mood

Mild to moderate depression

Severe depression

Figure 14-1 Spectrum of symptoms in bipolar disorders. (Redrawn from *Bipolar disorder*. http://www.nimh.nih.gov/health/publications/bipolar-disorder/nimhbipolar.pdf. [p. 5] Accessed 18.7.08.)

CLINICAL PICTURE

The three types of bipolar disorder currently identified include the following (listed from most to least severe):

- **Bipolar I disorder**: At least one episode of mania alternates with major depression. Psychosis may accompany the manic episode.
- **Bipolar II disorder**: Hypomanic episode(s) alternate with major depression. Psychosis is not present in bipolar II. The hypomania of bipolar II disorder tends to be euphoric and often increases functioning (Benazzi, 2007), and the depression tends to put people at particular risk for suicide.
- **Cyclothymia**: Hypomanic episodes alternate with minor depressive episodes (at least 2 years in duration). Individuals with cyclothymia tend to have irritable hypomanic episodes.

The specifier **rapid cycling** (four or more mood episodes in a 12-month period) is used to indicate more severe symptoms, such as poorer global functioning, high recurrence risk, and resistance to conventional somatic treatments. It is estimated to be present in 12% to 24% of patients who go to specialized clinics for mood disorders (Bauer et al., 2008). The *Diagnostic and Statistical Manual of Mental Disorders*, fourth edition, text revision *(DSM-IV-TR)* (American Psychiatric Association [APA], 2000) distinguishes between **mania** and **hypomania** for diagnostic purposes, as shown in Figure 14-2.

EPIDEMIOLOGY

The lifetime prevalence, or the percentage of the population that has ever experienced bipolar disorder in the United States, has been estimated at 3.9%. The lifetime risk, or the percentage of the population that will have a bipolar disorder by age 75, is 5.1% (Kessler et al., 2005).

The median age of onset for bipolar I is 18 years; for bipolar II, the median age of onset is 20 years (Merikangas et al., 2007). Bipolar I tends to begin with a depressive episode—in women 75% of the time, in men 67% of the time (Sadock & Sadock, 2008). The episodes tend to increase in number and severity during the course of the illness.

Bipolar I disorder seems to be somewhat more common among males, but bipolar II disorder (characterized by the milder form of mania—hypomania—and increased depression) is more common among females (Baldassano et al., 2005). Women with bipolar disorders are more likely to abuse alcohol, commit suicide, and develop thyroid disease; men with bipolar disorder are more likely to have legal problems and commit acts of violence.

According to Vieta and Suppes (2008), bipolar II disorder is underdiagnosed and often mistaken for major depression or personality disorders, when it actually may be the most common form of bipolar disorder. Clinicians may downplay bipolar II and consider it to simply be the milder version of bipolar disorders. However, it is a source of significant morbidity and mortality, particularly due to the occurrence of severe depression. According to Benazzi (2007), one out of two people with depression may have bipolar II.

Cyclothymia usually begins in adolescence or early adulthood. There is a 15% to 50% risk that an individual with cyclothymia will subsequently develop bipolar I or bipolar II disorder.

COMORBIDITY

One large-scale study with 9282 participants revealed that more than half of people with bipolar disorder have another Axis I psychiatric disorder (Merikangas et al., 2007). Within a lifetime, the most commonly co-occurring disorders for all bipolar disorders were panic attacks (62%), alcohol abuse (39%), social phobia (38%), oppositional defiant disorder (37%), specific phobia (35%), and seasonal affective disorder (35%). Substance use disorders were much higher in bipolar I than in bipolar II disorders. Treatment for substance abuse and bipolar disorder should proceed concurrently whenever possible (APA, 2000).

The incidence of borderline personality disorder occurring along with bipolar disorder is high. Patients who have borderline personality disorder have a 19.4% higher rate of bipolar disorder than do people with other personality disorders (Gunderson et al., 2006).

With advances in a global scientific database, trends are emerging that were previously unknown. One such trend is the relationship between psychiatric illnesses and physically-based illnesses. In a study of nearly 37,000 people, several physical disorders were found to be associated with bipolar I (McIntyre et al., 2006). The rates of the following disorders were significantly higher: chronic fatigue syndrome, asthma,

DSM-IV-TR CRITERIA FOR BIPOLAR DISORDER

1. A distinct period of abnormality and persistently elevated, expansive, or irritable mood for at least:
   * 4 days for hypomania
   * 1 week for mania

2. During the period of mood disturbance, **three or more** of the following symptoms have persisted (four if the mood is only irritable) and have been present to a significant degree:
   * Inflated self-esteem or grandiosity
   * Decreased need for sleep (e.g., the person feels rested after only 3 hours of sleep)
   * More talkative than usual or pressure to keep talking
   * Flight of ideas or subjective experience that thoughts are racing
   * Distractibility (i.e., the person's attention is too easily drawn to unimportant or irrelevant external stimuli)
   * Increase in goal-directed activity (either socially, at work or school, or sexually) or psychomotor agitation
   * Excessive involvement in pleasurable activities that have a high potential for painful consequences (e.g., the person engages in unrestrained buying sprees, sexual indiscretions, or foolish business investments)

Hypomania

1. The episode is associated with an unequivocal change in functioning that is uncharacteristic of the person when not symptomatic.

2. The disturbance in mood and the change in functioning are observed by others.

3. Absence of marked impairment in social or occupational functioning.

4. Hospitalization is not indicated.

5. Symptoms are not due to direct physiological effects of substance (e.g., drug abuse, medication, or other medical conditions).

Mania

1. Severe enough to cause marked impairment in occupational activities, usual social activities, or relationships.

   or

2. Necessitate hospitalization to prevent harm to self or others, or there are psychotic features.

3. Symptoms are not due to direct physiological effects of substance (drug abuse, medication) or general medical condition (e.g., hyperthyroidism).

Figure 14-2 Diagnostic criteria for bipolar disorder. (Adapted from American Psychiatric Association. *Diagnostic and statistical manual of mental disorders* [4th ed., text rev.]. Washington, DC: Author.)

migraine, chemical sensitivity, hypertension, bronchitis, and gastric ulcers. The presence of these diseases further complicates the lives of people with bipolar I by impairing their ability to work, increasing their dependence on others, and increasing their need for health care.

ETIOLOGY

Bipolar disorders are thought to be distinctly different from one another; for example, bipolar I disorder, bipolar II disorder, and cyclothymia have different characteristics. Other variants of bipolar disease, including a number of other diseases whose end-result is bipolar symptomatology, are currently being evaluated (Baum et al., 2008; Wellcome Trust Case Council Consortium, 2007; Sklar et al., 2008).

Episodes of depression in bipolar disorders are different from unipolar depression (i.e., depression without episodes of mania—see Chapter 13). Depressive episodes in bipolar disorder affect younger people, produce more episodes of illness, and require more frequent hospitalization. They are also characterized by higher rates of divorce and marital conflict.

Theories of the development of bipolar disorders focus on biological, psychological, and environmental factors. Most likely, multiple independent variables contribute to the occurrence of bipolar disorder. For this reason, a biopsychosocial approach will likely be the most successful approach to treatment.

Biological Factors

Genetic

The bipolar disorders have a strong heritability (i.e., the influence of genetic factors is much greater than the influence of external factors). Bipolar disorders are 80% to greater than 90% heritable, whereas Parkinson's disease, for example, is only 13% to 30% heritable (Burmeister et al., 2008). The rate of bipolar disorders may be as much as 5 to 10 times higher for people who have a relative with bipolar disorder than the rates found in the general population.

It is likely that bipolar disorder is a polygenic disease, which means that a number of genes contribute to its expression. In a landmark study at the National Institute of Mental Health (NIMH), researchers found a connection between bipolar disorder and a genome that encodes an enzyme called *diacylglycerol kinase eta* (DGKH). Lithium is the first-line therapy for bipolar disorder, and DGKH is a crucial part of a lithium-sensitive pathway (Baum et al., 2008). Other research has focused on abnormal circadian genes that may result in a superfast biological clock, which manifests itself in extreme insomnia (McClung, 2007).

The scientific community has been increasingly drawn to the concept of bipolar disorders and schizophrenia having similar genetic origins and pathology (Owen et al., 2007). Both disorders exhibit irregularities on chromosomes 13 and 15. It may be that the genotype has more to do with the specific expression of psychoses (altered thought, delusions, and hallucinations) than are reflected in traditional classification systems. Current psychiatric diagnostic systems will undoubtedly be modified as advances are made in molecular genetics, which will revolutionize our understanding and treatment of many psychotic disorders.

Neurobiological

Neurotransmitters (norepinephrine, dopamine, and serotonin) have been studied since the 1960s as causal factors in mania and depression. One simple explanation is that too few of these chemical messengers will result in depression, and an oversupply will cause mania. However, proportions of neurotransmitters in relation to one another may be more important. Receptor site insensitivity could also be at the root of the problem—even if there is enough of a certain neurotransmitter, it is not going where it needs to go.

Additional research has found that the interrelationships in the neurotransmitter system are complex, and more elaborate theories have been developed since the amine hypotheses were originally proposed. Mood disorders are most likely a result of interactions among various chemicals, including neurotransmitters and hormones.

Brain pathways implicated in the pathophysiology of bipolar disorder are located in subregions of the prefrontal cortex (PFC) and medial temporal lobe (MTL). Dysregulation in the neurocircuits surrounding these areas have been viewed through functional imaging (e.g., positron emission tomography [PET] scans, magnetic resonance imaging [MRI]) (Pollock & Kuo, 2004). Neuroimaging studies reveal structural and functional brain changes in people with bipolar disorder. Some structural changes seem to cause the disorder, and some seem to be *caused by* the disorder. For example, prefrontal cortical changes are evident in the early stages of the illness, whereas lateral ventricle abnormalities develop with repeated episodes of mania and/or depression (Strakowski et al., 2005). Functional imaging also reveals differences in the anterior limbic regions of the brain, which are associated with emotion, motivation, memory, and fear—the areas most deeply affected by bipolar disorder.

Neuroendocrine

The hypothalamic-pituitary-thyroid-adrenal (HPTA) axis has been closely scrutinized in people with mood disorders. Hypothyroidism is known to be associated with depressed moods, and hypothyroidism is seen in some patients experiencing rapid cycling. High-dose thyroid hormone administration has been suggested as a method to improve outcomes in treatment-resistant bipolar disorder (Gitlin, 2007).

Psychological Factors

Although there is increasing evidence for genetic and biological vulnerabilities in the etiology of the mood disorders, psychological factors may play a role in precipitating manic episodes for many individuals. In the absence of severe stressful events, it is possible that a person with a genetic predisposition and a neurochemical imbalance may never experience symptoms of bipolar disorder. However, once the disease has been triggered by an event that is perceived as stressful—loss of a relationship, financial difficulties, failing an exam, being accepted to a highly desirable graduate school—it no longer requires environmental stress to continue.

Environmental Factors

Bipolar disorder is a worldwide problem that generally affects all races and ethnic groups equally, but some evidence suggests that bipolar disorders may be more prevalent in upper socioeconomic classes. The exact reason for this is unclear; however, people with bipolar disorders appear to achieve higher levels of education and higher occupational status than individuals with unipolar depression. The educational levels of individuals with unipolar depressive disorders, on the other hand, appear to be no different from those of individuals with no symptoms of depression within the same socioeconomic class. Also, the proportion of patients with bipolar disorders among creative writers, artists, highly educated men and women, and professional people is higher than in the general population.

APPLICATION OF THE NURSING PROCESS

ASSESSMENT

Individuals with bipolar disorder are often misdiagnosed or underdiagnosed. Early diagnosis and proper treatment can help people avoid:

- Suicide attempts
- Alcohol or substance abuse
- Marital or work problems
- Development of medical comorbidity

Figure 14-3 presents the Mood Disorder Questionnaire (MDQ). This is *not* a definitive diagnostic test; however, it is a helpful initial screening device.

General Assessment

The characteristics of mania discussed in the following sections are (1) mood, (2) behavior, (3) thought processes and speech patterns, and (4) cognitive function.

Mood

The euphoric mood associated with mania is unstable. During euphoria, the patient may state that he or she is experiencing an intense feeling of well-being, is "cheerful in a beautiful world," or is becoming "one with God." The overly joyous mood may seem out of proportion to what is going on, and cheerfulness may be inappropriate for the circumstances. This mood may change quickly to irritation and anger when the person is thwarted. The irritability and belligerence may be short-lived, or it may become the prominent feature of the manic phase of bipolar disorder.

People experiencing a manic state may laugh, joke, and talk in a continuous stream, with uninhibited familiarity. They often demonstrate boundless enthusiasm, treat others with confidential friendliness, and incorporate everyone into their plans and activities. They know no strangers, and energy and self-confidence seem boundless.

Elaborate schemes to get rich and famous and acquire unlimited power may be frantically pursued, despite objections and realistic constraints. Excessive phone calls and e-mails are made, often to famous and influential people all over the world. People in the manic phase are busy during all hours of the day and night, furthering their grandiose plans. To the person experiencing mania, no aspirations are too high, and no distances are too far. No boundaries exist to curtail them.

In the manic state, a person often gives away money, prized possessions, and expensive gifts. The person experiencing a manic episode may throw lavish parties, frequent expensive nightclubs and restaurants, and spend money freely on friends and strangers alike. This excessive spending, use of credit cards, and high living continue even in the face of bankruptcy. Intervention is often needed to prevent financial ruin.

As the clinical course progresses from hypomania to mania, sociability and euphoria are replaced by a stage of hostility, irritability, and paranoia. The following is a patient's description of the painful transition from hypomania to mania (Jamison, 1995):

> At first when I'm high, it's tremendous...ideas are fast...like shooting stars you follow until brighter ones appear...all shyness disappears, the right words and gestures are suddenly there...uninteresting people, things become intensely interesting. Sensuality is pervasive; the desire to seduce and be seduced is irresistible. Your marrow is infused with unbelievable feelings of ease, power, well-being, omnipotence, euphoria... you can do anything...but somewhere this changes....
>
> The fast ideas become too fast and there are far too many...overwhelming confusion replaces clarity... you stop keeping up with it—memory goes. Infectious humor ceases to amuse—your friends become frightened...everything now is against the grain...you are irritable, angry, frightened, uncontrollable, and trapped in the blackest caves of the mind—caves you never knew were there. It will never end. Madness carves its own reality.

Behavior

When people experience hypomania, they have voracious appetites for social engagement, spending, and activity, even indiscriminate sex. Constant activity and a reduced need for sleep prevent proper rest. Although short periods of sleep are possible, some patients may not sleep for several days in a row. **This nonstop physical activity and the lack of sleep and food can lead to physical exhaustion and even death if not treated; it therefore constitutes an emergency.**

When in full-blown mania, a person constantly goes from one activity, place, or project to another. Many projects may be started, but few if any are completed. Inactivity is impossible, even for the shortest period of time. Hyperactivity may range from mild, constant motion to frenetic, wild activity. Flowery and lengthy letters are written, and excessive phone calls are made. Individuals become involved in pleasurable activities that can have painful consequences. For example, spending large sums of money on frivolous items, giving money

MOOD DISORDER QUESTIONNAIRE

Instructions: Please answer each question as best you can.

	Yes	No
1. **Has there ever been a period of time when you were not your usual self and....**		
you felt so good or so hyper that other people thought you were not your normal self or you were so hyper that you got into trouble?	O	O
you were so irritable that you shouted at people or started fights or arguments?	O	O
you felt much more self-confident than usual?	O	O
you got much less sleep than usual and found you didn't really miss it?	O	O
you were much more talkative or spoke much faster than usual?	O	O
thoughts raced through your head or you couldn't slow down your mind?	O	O
you were so easily distracted by things around you that you had trouble concentrating or staying on track?	O	O
you had much more energy than usual?	O	O
you were much more active or did many more things than usual?	O	O
you were much more social or outgoing than usual; for example, you telephoned friends in the middle of the night?	O	O
you were much more interested in sex than usual?	O	O
you did things that were unusual for you or that other people might have thought were excessive, foolish, or risky?	O	O
spending money got you or your family into trouble?	O	O
2. **If you answered "Yes" to more than one of the above, have several of these ever happened during the same period of time?**	O	O

3. **How much of a problem did any of these cause you — like being unable to work; having family, money, or legal troubles; or getting into arguments or fights? Please select one response only.**

    O No problem   O Minor problem   O Moderate problem   O Serious problem

	Yes	No
4. **Have any of your blood relatives (children, siblings, parents, grandparents, aunts, uncles) had manic-depressive illness or bipolar disorder?**	O	O
5. **Has a health care professional ever told you that you have manic-depressive illness or bipolar disorder?**	O	O

Criteria for Results: Answering "Yes" to 7 or more of the events in question 1, answering "Yes" to question 2, and answering "Moderate problem" or "Serious problem" to question 3 is considered a positive screen result for bipolar disorder.

Figure 14-3 The Mood Disorder Questionnaire (MDQ). (From Hirschfeld, R., Williams, J., Spitzer, R., Calabrese, J., Flynn, L., Keck, P., Lewis, L. et al. [2000]. Development and validation of a screening instrument for bipolar spectrum disorder: The Mood Disorder Questionnaire, *American Journal of Psychiatry, 157*[11], 1873–1875. © 2004 Eli Lilly and Company.)

away indiscriminately, or making foolish business investments can leave an individual or family penniless. Sexual indiscretion can dissolve relationships and marriages and lead to sexually transmitted diseases. Religious preoccupation is a common symptom of mania.

Individuals experiencing mania may be manipulative, profane, fault finding, and adept at exploiting others' vulnerabilities. They constantly push limits. These behaviors often alienate family, friends, employers, health care providers, and others.

EVIDENCE-BASED PRACTICE

Sleep Disruption in the Manic Phase of Bipolar Disorder

Roybal, K., Theobold, D., Graham, A., DiNieri, J., Russo, S., Krishnan, V. et al. (2007). Mania-like behavior induced by disruption of *CLOCK*. *Proceedings of the National Academy of Sciences, USA, 104*, 6406-6411.

Problem

One of the most dramatic symptoms of bipolar disorder in the manic phase is sleep disruption. If you have ever stayed awake all night and tried to function the next day, you may have a partial appreciation for the thought impairment, decreased judgment, and emotional dysregulation experienced by people who have been awake for 3 nights. Researchers believe that a faulty circadian rhythm, the natural 24- to 25-hour sleep/wake cycle monitored by a body clock in the hypothalamus, may be to blame. This connection is strengthened by our knowledge that normal sleep/wake cycles are essential to mood stabilization and that sleep disruptions can trigger mania.

Purpose of Study

The purpose of this study was to examine the role of a specific gene in the disruption of circadian rhythms. This gene is the central transcriptional activator of molecular rhythms, or *Clock* gene.

Methods

Researchers mutated the *Clock* gene in mice that served in the study. Next, they implanted electrodes in the medial forebrain bundle of their brains, the area which allowed mice to give themselves pleasurable sensations. They then measured the degree of current, or reward, that the mice gave themselves.

Key Findings

- *Clock* mutant mice are similar to bipolar patients in a manic state in their increased preference for stimuli that is rewarding, including brain stimulation and cocaine.

- The experimental mice displayed other behaviors associated with mania, including less depressive behavior and decreased anxiety.
- Lithium treatment reverses manic-like behavior in *Clock* mutant mice.
- Once *Clock* mutant mice had their Functional CLOCK restored, their abnormal behavior ceased.

Implications for Nursing

The study of molecular genetics holds great promise for how people are diagnosed and treated. At a personal level, understanding the mechanics of mania may lessen professional stigma (negative attitudes of health care workers) and even our own attitudes toward people experiencing mania. When you are dealing with someone who is hypertalkative, hypersexual, and constantly making requests, it is fairly easy to become irritated and even resentful. An increased understanding of the physiology behind the disorder can go a long way.

At a hands-on level, the importance of promoting an adaptive sleep/wake cycle in people with mood disorders, particularly people with mania, is highlighted by this study. Teaching aimed at understanding the importance of not "burning the midnight oil" (staying awake all night) is important for everyone but imperative for people with bipolar disorder. Furthermore, recognizing disturbed sleep patterns may aid people to recognize symptoms of impending mania.

Modes of dress often reflect the person's grandiose yet tenuous grasp of reality. Dress may be described as outlandish, bizarre, colorful, and noticeably inappropriate. Makeup may be garish and overdone. People with mania are highly distractible. Concentration is poor, and individuals with mania go from one activity to another without completing anything. Judgment is poor. Impulsive marriages and divorces can take place.

People often emerge from a manic state startled and confused by the shambles of their lives. The following description conveys one patient's experience (Jamison, 1995):

Now there are only others' recollections of your behavior—your bizarre, frenetic, aimless behavior—at least

mania has the grace to dim memories of itself...now it's over, but is it?...Incredible feelings to sort through... Who is being too polite? Who knows what? What did I do? Why? And most hauntingly, will it, when will it, happen again? Medication to take, to resist, to resent, to forget...but always to take. Credit cards revoked... explanations at work...bad checks and apologies overdue...memory flashes of vague men (what did I do?)...friendships gone, a marriage ruined.

Thought Processes and Speech Patterns

Flight of ideas is a nearly continuous flow of accelerated speech with abrupt changes from topic to topic that are usually based on understandable associations or plays on words. At times, the attentive listener can keep up with the flow of words, even though direction changes from moment to moment. Speech is rapid, verbose, and circumstantial (including minute and unnecessary details). When the condition is severe, speech may be disorganized and incoherent. The incessant talking often includes joking, puns, and teasing:

> How are you doing, kid, no kidding around, I'm going home…home sweet home…home is where the heart is, the heart of the matter is I want out and that ain't hay…hey, Doc…get me out of this place.

The content of speech is often sexually explicit and ranges from grossly inappropriate to vulgar. Themes in the communication of the individual with mania may revolve around extraordinary sexual prowess, brilliant business ability, or unparalleled artistic talents (e.g., writing, painting, and dancing). The person may actually have only average ability in these areas.

Speech is not only profuse but also loud, bellowing, or even screaming. One can hear the force and energy behind the rapid words. As mania escalates, flight of ideas may give way to clang associations. **Clang associations** are the stringing together of words because of their rhyming sounds, without regard to their meaning:

> Cinema I and II, last row. Row, row, row your boat. Don't be a cutthroat. Cut your throat. Get your goat. Go out and vote. And so I wrote.

Grandiosity (inflated self-regard) is apparent in both the ideas expressed and the person's behavior. People with mania may exaggerate their achievements or importance, state that they know famous people, or believe they have great powers. The boast of exceptional powers and status can take delusional proportions during mania. Grandiose persecutory delusions are common. For example, people may think that God is speaking to them or that the FBI is out to stop them from saving the world. Sensory perceptions may become altered as the mania escalates, and hallucinations may occur. However, no evidence of delusions or hallucinations is present during hypomania.

Cognitive Function

The onset of bipolar disorder is often preceded by comparatively high cognitive function. However, there is growing evidence that about one third of patients with bipolar disorder display significant and persistent cognitive problems and difficulties in psychosocial areas. Cognitive deficits in bipolar disorder are milder but similar to those in patients with schizophrenia (Schretlen et al., 2007). Cognitive impairments exist in both bipolar I and bipolar II, but are more pronounced in bipolar I (Torrent et al., 2006).

The potential cognitive dysfunction among many people with bipolar disorder has specific clinical implications (Robinson et al., 2006):

- Cognitive function greatly affects overall function.
- Cognitive deficits correlate with a greater number of manic episodes, history of psychosis, chronicity of illness, and poor functional outcome.
- Early diagnosis and treatment are crucial to prevent illness progression, cognitive deficits, and poor outcome.
- Medication selection should consider not only the efficacy of the drug in reducing mood symptoms but also the cognitive impact of the drug on the patient.

Self-Assessment

The patient experiencing mania (who is often out of control and resists being controlled) can elicit numerous intense emotions in a nurse. The patient may use humor, manipulation, power struggles, or demanding behavior to prevent or minimize the staff's ability to set limits on and control dangerous behavior. People with mania have the ability to staff split, or divide the staff into either the good guys or the bad guys. "The nurse on the day shift is always late with my medication and never talks with me. You are the only one who seems to care." This divisive tactic may pit one staff member or group against another, undermining a unified front and consistent plan of care. Frequent staff meetings to deal with the behaviors of the patient and the nurses' responses to these behaviors can help minimize staff splitting and feelings of anger and isolation. Limit-setting (e.g., lights out after 11 PM) is the main theme in treating a person in mania. **Consistency among staff is imperative if the limit setting is to be carried out effectively.**

The patient can become aggressively demanding, which often triggers frustration, worry, and exasperation in health care professionals. The behavior of a patient experiencing mania is often aimed at decreasing the effectiveness of staff control, which could be accomplished by getting involved in power plays. For example, the patient might taunt the staff by pointing out faults or oversights and drawing negative attention to one or more staff members. Usually, this is done in a loud and disruptive manner, which provokes staff to become defensive and thereby escalates the environmental tension and the patient's degree of mania.

If you are working with a patient experiencing mania, you may find yourself feeling helplessness, confusion, or even anger. Understanding, acknowledging, and sharing these responses and countertransference reactions will enhance your professional ability to care for the patient and perhaps promote your personal development as well. Collaborating with the multidisciplinary team, accessing supervision with your nursing faculty member, and sharing your experience with peers in post-conference may be helpful, perhaps essential.

Assessment Guidelines Bipolar Disorder

1. Assess whether the patient is a danger to self and others:
   - Patient experiencing manias can exhaust themselves to the point of death.
   - Patients may not eat or sleep, often for days at a time.
   - Poor impulse control may result in harm to others or self.
   - Uncontrolled spending may occur.
2. Assess the need for protection from uninhibited behaviors. External control may be needed to protect the patient from such things as bankruptcy, because patients experiencing mania may give away all of their money or possessions.
3. Assess the need for hospitalization to safeguard and stabilize the patient.
4. Assess medical status. A thorough medical examination helps to determine whether mania is primary (a mood disorder—bipolar disorder or cyclothymia) or secondary to another condition.
   - Mania may be secondary to a general medical condition.
   - Mania may be substance-induced (caused by use or abuse of a drug or substance or by toxin exposure).
5. Assess for any coexisting medical condition or other situation that warrants special intervention (e.g., substance abuse, anxiety disorder, legal or financial crises).
6. Assess the patient's and family's understanding of bipolar disorder, knowledge of medications, and knowledge of support groups and organizations that provide information on bipolar disorder.

DIAGNOSIS

Nursing diagnoses vary among patients experiencing mania. A primary consideration for a patient in acute mania is the prevention of exhaustion and death from cardiac collapse. Because of the patient's poor judgment, excessive and constant motor activity, probable dehydration, and difficulty evaluating reality, *Risk for injury* is a likely and appropriate diagnosis. Table 14-1 lists potential nursing diagnoses for bipolar disorders.

OUTCOMES IDENTIFICATION

Outcome criteria will be based on which of the three phases of the illness the patient is experiencing. The *Nursing Outcomes Classification (NOC)* (Moorhead et al., 2008) provides useful outcomes for each phase.

Acute Phase

The overall outcome of the acute phase is injury prevention. Outcomes in the acute phase reflect both physiological and psychiatric issues. For example, the patient will:
- Be well hydrated.
- Maintain stable cardiac status.
- Maintain/obtain tissue integrity.
- Get sufficient sleep and rest.
- Demonstrate thought self-control.
- Make no attempt at self-harm.

Relevant *NOC* outcomes for this phase include *Hydration, Cardiac Pump Effectiveness, Tissue Integrity: Skin and Mucous Membranes, Sleep, Distorted Thought Self-Control,* and *Suicide Self-Restraint.*

Continuation Phase

The continuation phase lasts for 4 to 9 months. Although the overall outcome of this phase is relapse prevention, many other outcomes must be accomplished to achieve relapse prevention. These outcomes include:
- Psychoeducational classes for patient and family related to:
  - Knowledge of disease process
  - Knowledge of medication
  - Consequences of substance addictions for predicting future relapse
  - Knowledge of early signs and symptoms of relapse
- Support groups or therapy (cognitive-behavioral, interpersonal)
- Communication and problem-solving skills training

Relevant *NOC* outcomes for this phase include *Compliance Behavior, Knowledge: Disease Process, Social Support,* and *Substance Addiction Consequences.*

Maintenance Phase

The overall outcomes for the maintenance phase continue to focus on prevention of relapse and limitation of the severity and duration of future episodes. Relevant *NOC* outcomes include *Knowledge: Disease Process, Compliance Behavior,* and *Family Support During Treatment.* Additional outcomes include:
- Participation in learning interpersonal strategies related to work, interpersonal, and family problems
- Participation in psychotherapy, group, or other ongoing supportive therapy modality

PLANNING

Planning care for an individual with bipolar disorder usually is geared toward the particular phase of mania the patient is in (acute, continuation, or maintenance),

TABLE 14-1 Potential Nursing Diagnoses For Bipolar Disorders

Signs and Symptoms	Nursing Diagnoses
Excessive and constant motor activity Poor judgment Lack of rest and sleep Poor nutritional intake (excessive or relentless mix of above behaviors can lead to cardiac collapse)	*Risk for injury*
Loud, profane, hostile, combative, aggressive, demanding behaviors	*Risk for other-directed violence* *Risk for self-directed violence* *Risk for suicide*
Intrusive and taunting behaviors Inability to control behavior Rage reaction	*Ineffective coping*
Manipulative, angry, or hostile verbal and physical behaviors Impulsive speech and actions Property destruction or lashing out at others in a rage reaction	*Defensive coping* *Ineffective coping*
Racing thoughts, grandiosity, poor judgment	*Disturbed thought processes** *Ineffective coping*
Giving away of valuables, neglect of family, impulsive major life changes (divorce, career changes)	*Interrupted family processes* *Caregiver role strain*
Continuous pressured speech, jumping from topic to topic *(flights of ideas)*	*Impaired verbal communication*
Constant motor activity, going from one person or event to another Annoyance or taunting of others, loud and crass speech Provocative behaviors	*Impaired social interaction*
Failure to eat, groom, bathe, dress self because patient is too distracted, agitated, and disorganized	*Imbalanced nutrition: less than body requirements* *Deficient fluid volume* *Self-care deficit (bathing, dressing, feeding, toileting)*
Inability to sleep because patient is too frantic and hyperactive (sleep deprivation can lead to exhaustion and death)	*Disturbed sleep pattern*

Data from North American Nursing Diagnosis Association International (NANDA-I). (2009). *NANDA-I nursing diagnoses: Definitions and classification 2009-2011.* Oxford, United Kingdom, Author.

*Diagnosis retired from North American Nursing Diagnosis Association. (2007). *NANDA-I nursing diagnoses: Definitions and classification 2007–2008.* Philadelphia: Author.

as well as any other co-occurring issues identified in the assessment (e.g., risk of suicide, risk of violence to person or property, family crisis, legal crises, substance abuse, risk-taking behaviors).

Acute Phase

During the acute phase, planning focuses on medically stabilizing the patient while maintaining safety, and the hospital is usually the safest environment for accomplishing this (see Case Study and Nursing Care Plan 14-1 on pages 300–302). Nursing care is geared toward managing medications, decreasing physical activity, increasing food and fluid intake, ensuring at least 4 to 6 hours of sleep per night, alleviating any bowel or bladder problems, and intervening to see that self-care

needs are met. Some patients may require seclusion or even electroconvulsive therapy (ECT).

Continuation Phase

During the continuation phase, planning focuses on maintaining adherence to the medication regimen and prevention of relapse. Interventions are planned in accordance with the assessment data regarding the patient's interpersonal and stress-reduction skills, cognitive functioning, employment status, substance-related problems, and social support systems. During this time, psychoeducational teaching is necessary for the patient and family. The need for referrals to community programs, groups, and support for any co-occurring disorders or problems (e.g., substance abuse, family problems, legal issues, and financial crises) is evaluated.

Evaluation of the need for communication skills training and problem-solving skills training is also an important consideration. People with bipolar disorders often have interpersonal and emotional problems that affect their work, family, and social lives. Residual problems resulting from reckless, violent, withdrawn, or bizarre behavior that may have occurred during a manic episode often leave lives shattered and family and friends hurt and distant. For some patients, cognitive-behavioral therapy (in addition to medication management) is useful to address these issues, although the focus of psychotherapeutic treatment will vary over time for each individual.

Maintenance Phase

During the maintenance phase, planning focuses on preventing relapse and limiting the severity and duration of future episodes. Patients with bipolar disorders require medications over long periods of time or even an entire lifetime. Psychotherapy, support groups, psychoeducational groups, and periodic evaluations help patients maintain their family, social, and occupational lives.

IMPLEMENTATION

Patients with bipolar disorders are often ambivalent about treatment. Only 39% of people experiencing symptoms of bipolar disorder seek treatment within the first year, and the median delay of treatment is 6 years (Wang et al., 2005). Patients may minimize the destructive consequences of their behaviors or deny the seriousness of the disease, and some are reluctant to give up the increased energy, euphoria, and heightened sense of self-esteem of hypomania (Hirschfeld et al., 2000).

Unfortunately, nonadherence to the regimen of mood-stabilizing medication is a major cause of relapse, so establishing a therapeutic alliance with the individual with bipolar disorder is crucial.

Acute Phase

Depressive Episodes

Depressive episodes of bipolar disorder have the same symptoms and risks as major depression (see Chapter 13), although they are often more intense. Hospitalization may be required if suicidal ideation, psychosis, or catatonia is present. Lithium and lamotrigine (Lamictal) are the first line of treatment for a person with bipolar disorder experiencing an acute depressive episode (APA, 2008). Treatment with antidepressants is not recommended (particularly for bipolar I disorder), since the patient's central nervous system (CNS) may

become overactive, which results in hypomania or mania. Patients who experience depression while taking maintenance levels of medications may benefit from increased doses of the original drugs. When depressive episodes have psychotic features, an atypical antipsychotic may be added to the medication regimen.

Manic Episodes

Hospitalization provides safety for a patient experiencing acute mania (bipolar I disorder), imposes external controls on destructive behaviors, and provides for medication stabilization. There are unique approaches to communicating with and maintaining the safety of the patient during the hospitalization period (Table 14-2). Staff members continuously set limits in a firm, nonthreatening, and neutral manner to prevent further escalation of mania and provide safe boundaries for the patient and others.

Continuation Phase

The continuation phase is crucial for patients and their families. The outcome for this phase is prevention of relapse, and community resources are chosen based on the needs of the patient, the appropriateness of the referral, and the availability of resources. Frequently a case manager evaluates appropriate follow-up care for patients and their families.

Medication adherence during this phase is perhaps the most important treatment outcome. This follow-up is frequently handled in a mental health center. However, adherence to the medication regimen is also addressed in day hospitals and psychiatric home-care visits. Some patients may attend day hospitals if they are not too excitable and are able to tolerate a certain level of stimuli. In addition to medication management, day hospitals offer structure, decrease social isolation, and help patients channel their time and energy. If a patient is homebound, psychiatric home care is the appropriate modality for follow-up care.

Maintenance Phase

The goal of the maintenance phase is to prevent recurrence of an episode of bipolar disorder. The community resources cited earlier are helpful, and patients and their families often greatly benefit from mutual support and self-help groups that will be discussed later in this chapter.

Pharmacological Interventions

Individuals with bipolar disorder often require multiple medications. For severe manic episodes, lithium or valproate (Depakote) and an atypical antipsychotic such as olanzapine (Zyprexa) or risperidone (Risperdal) are recommended. Individuals experiencing less severe symptoms may be given

TABLE 14-2 Interventions for the Patient Experiencing Acute Mania

Intervention	Rationale
COMMUNICATION	
Use firm and calm approach: "John, come with me. Eat this sandwich."	Structure and control are provided for patient who is out of control. Feelings of security can result: "Someone is in control."
Use short and concise explanations or statements.	Short attention span limits comprehension to small bits of information.
Remain neutral; avoid power struggles and value judgments.	Patient can use inconsistencies and value judgments as justification for arguing and escalating mania.
Be consistent in approach and expectations.	Consistent limits and expectations minimize potential for patient's manipulation of staff.
Have frequent staff meetings to plan consistent approaches and set agreed-on limits.	Consistency of all staff is needed to maintain controls and minimize manipulation by patient.
With other staff, decide on limits, tell patient in simple, concrete terms with consequences. Example: "John, do not yell at or hit Peter. If you cannot control yourself, we will help you." Or "The seclusion room will help you feel less out of control and prevent harm to yourself and others."	Clear expectations help patient experience outside controls, as well as understand reasons for medication, seclusion, or restraints (if he or she is not able to control behaviors).
Hear and act on legitimate complaints.	Underlying feelings of helplessness are reduced, and acting-out behaviors are minimized.
Firmly redirect energy into more appropriate and constructive channels.	Distractibility is the nurse's most effective tool with the patient experiencing mania.
STRUCTURE IN A SAFE MILIEU	
Maintain low level of stimuli in patient's environment (e.g., away from bright lights, loud noises, and people).	Escalation of anxiety can be decreased.
Provide structured solitary activities with nurse or aide.	Structure provides security and focus.
Provide frequent high-calorie fluids.	Serious dehydration is prevented.
Provide frequent rest periods.	Exhaustion is prevented.
Redirect violent behavior.	Physical exercise can decrease tension and provide focus.
When warranted in acute mania, use phenothiazines and seclusion to minimize physical harm.	Exhaustion and death can result from dehydration, lack of sleep, and constant physical activity.
Observe for signs of lithium toxicity.	There is a small margin of safety between therapeutic and toxic doses.
Protect patient from giving away money and possessions. Hold valuables in hospital safe until rational judgment returns.	Patient's "generosity" is a manic defense that is consistent with irrational, grandiose thinking.
PHYSIOLOGICAL SAFETY: SELF-CARE NEEDS	
Nutrition Monitor intake, output, and vital signs.	Adequate fluid and caloric intake are ensured; development of dehydration and cardiac collapse is minimized.
Offer frequent, high-calorie, protein drinks and finger foods (e.g., sandwiches, fruit, milkshakes).	Constant fluid and calorie replacement are needed. Patient may be too active to sit at meals. Finger foods allow "eating on the run."
Frequently remind patient to eat. "Tom, finish your milkshake." "Sally, eat this banana."	The patient experiencing mania is unaware of bodily needs and is easily distracted. Needs supervision to eat.

Continued

TABLE 14-2 Interventions for the Patient Acute Mania—cont'd	
Intervention	**Rationale**
Sleep	
Encourage frequent rest periods during the day.	Lack of sleep can lead to exhaustion and death.
Keep patient in areas of low stimulation.	Relaxation is promoted, and manic behavior is minimized.
At night, provide warm baths, soothing music, and medication when indicated. Avoid giving patient caffeine.	Relaxation, rest, and sleep are promoted.
Hygiene	
Supervise choice of clothes; minimize flamboyant and bizarre dress (e.g., garish stripes or plaids and loud, unmatching colors).	The potential is decreased for ridicule, which lowers self-esteem and increases the need for manic defense. The patient is helped to maintain dignity.
Give simple step-by-step reminders for hygiene and dress. "Here is your razor. Shave the left side...now the right side. Here is your toothbrush. Put the toothpaste on the brush."	Distractibility and poor concentration are countered through simple, concrete instructions.
Elimination	
Monitor bowel habits; offer fluids and foods that are high in fiber. Evaluate need for laxative. Encourage patient to go to the bathroom.	Fecal impaction resulting from dehydration and decreased peristalsis is prevented.

only one of these. There may be times when a benzodiazepine antianxiety agent can help reduce agitation or anxiety. Antidepressants that may have been prescribed previously are often tapered and possibly discontinued to reduce mania or hypomania (APA, 2008).

Lithium Carbonate

The chemical name for **lithium carbonate** is $LiCO_3$, although you may see it abbreviated as Li+. Lithium is effective in the treatment of bipolar I acute and recurrent manic and depressive episodes. Lithium inhibits about 80% of acute manic and hypomanic episodes within 10 to 21 days (Sadock & Sadock, 2008). Lithium is less effective in people with mixed mania (elation and depression), those with rapid cycling, and those with atypical features.

Indications. Lithium is particularly effective in reducing:
- Elation, grandiosity, and expansiveness
- Flight of ideas
- Irritability and manipulation
- Anxiety

To a lesser extent, lithium controls:
- Insomnia
- Psychomotor agitation
- Threatening or assaultive behavior
- Distractibility
- Hypersexuality
- Paranoia

Lithium must reach therapeutic levels in the patient's blood to be effective. This usually takes 7 to 14 days, or longer for some patients. An antipsychotic or benzodiazepine can be used to prevent exhaustion, coronary collapse, and death until lithium reaches therapeutic levels. Antipsychotics act promptly to slow speech, inhibit aggression, and decrease psychomotor activity. As lithium becomes effective in reducing manic behavior, the antipsychotic drugs are usually discontinued. Although lithium is an effective intervention for treating the acute manic phase of a bipolar disorder, it is not a cure. Many patients receive lithium for maintenance indefinitely and experience manic and depressive episodes if the drug is discontinued.

Actress Patty Duke describes her response to lithium after years of alternating depression, elation, and bad choices (Moore, 2008):

"Lithium saved my life. After just a few weeks on the drug, death-based thoughts were no longer the first I had when I got up and last when I went to bed. The nightmare that had spanned 30 years was over. I'm not a Stepford wife; I still feel the exultation and sadness that any person feels. I'm just not required to feel them 10 times as long or as intensively as I used to. "

Therapeutic and Toxic Levels. Trade names for lithium carbonate include Lithane, Eskalith, and Lithonate. During the active phase, 300 mg to 600 mg is given 2 or 3 times a day by mouth to reach a clear therapeutic result or a lithium level of 0.8 to 1.4 mEq/L. The maintenance blood levels should range between 0.4 and 1.3 mEq/L. To avoid serious toxicity, lithium levels should not exceed 1.5 mEq/L (Lehne, 2010). At serum levels above 1.5 mEq/L, early signs of toxicity can occur; at 1.5 to 2.0 mEq/L, advanced signs of toxicity may be seen; and at 2.0 to 2.5 mEq/L or above, severe lithium toxicity and death can occur, and emergency measures should be taken immediately. Gastric lavage and treatment with urea, mannitol, and aminophylline can hasten lithium excretion. Hemodialysis may also be necessary in extreme cases.

A small increment exists between the therapeutic and toxic levels of lithium. Lithium levels should be measured at least 5 days after beginning lithium therapy and after any dosage change, until the therapeutic level has been reached (Perlis & Ostacher, 2008). After therapeutic levels have been reached, blood levels are determined every month. After 6 months to a year of stability, measurement of blood levels every 3 months may suffice. Blood should be drawn in the morning, 8 to 12 hours after the last dose of lithium is taken. Table 14-3 details expected side effects of lithium, signs of lithium toxicity, and interventions for both.

For older adult patients, the principle of **start low and go slow** still applies. Levels are often monitored every 3 or 4 days. As mentioned earlier, toxic effects are usually associated with lithium levels of 2.0 mEq/L or higher, although they can occur at much lower levels (even within a therapeutic range).

Maintenance Therapy. Some clinicians suggest that patients with bipolar disorder need to be given lithium for 9 to 12 months, and some patients may need life-long lithium maintenance to prevent further relapses. Many patients respond well to lower dosages during maintenance or prophylactic lithium therapy.

Lithium is unquestionably effective in preventing both manic and depressive episodes in patients with bipolar disorder. However, complete suppression occurs in only 50% of patients or fewer, even with adherence to the maintenance therapy regimen. Therefore, the patient and family should be given careful instructions about (1) the purpose and requirements of lithium therapy, (2) its adverse effects, (3) its toxic

TABLE 14-3 Lithium Side Effects and Signs of Lithium Toxicity		
Level	**Signs**	**Interventions**
EXPECTED SIDE EFFECTS		
<0.4-1.0 mEq/L (therapeutic level)	Fine hand tremor, polyuria, and mild thirst Mild nausea and general discomfort Weight gain	Symptoms may persist throughout therapy. Symptoms often subside during treatment. Weight gain may be helped with diet, exercise, and nutritional management.
EARLY SIGNS OF TOXICITY		
<1.5 mEq/L	Nausea, vomiting, diarrhea, thirst, polyuria, lethargy, slurred speech, muscle weakness, and fine hand tremor	Medication should be withheld, blood lithium levels measured, and dosage reevaluated. Dehydration, if present, should be addressed.
ADVANCED SIGNS OF TOXICITY		
1.5-2.0 mEq/L	Coarse hand tremor, persistent gastrointestinal upset, mental confusion, muscle hyperirritability, electroencephalographic changes, incoordination, sedation	Interventions outlined above or below should be used, depending on severity of circumstances.
SEVERE TOXICITY		
2.0-2.5 mEq/L	Ataxia, confusion, large output of dilute urine, serious electroencephalographic changes, blurred vision, clonic movements, seizures, stupor, severe hypotension, coma; death is usually secondary to pulmonary complications.	Hospitalization is indicated. The drug is stopped, and excretion is hastened. If patient is alert, an emetic is administered.
>2.5 mEq/L	Convulsions, oliguria, and death can occur.	In addition to the interventions above, hemodialysis may be used in severe cases.

Data from Lehne, R. A. (2010). *Pharmacology for nursing care* (7th ed., p. 357). Philadelphia: Saunders; and Sadock, B.J., & Sadock, V.A. (2008). *Concise textbook of clinical psychiatry* (3rd ed.). Philadelphia: Lippincott, Williams & Wilkins.

effects and complications, and (4) situations in which the physician should be contacted. The patient and family should also be advised that suddenly stopping lithium can lead to relapse and recurrence of mania. Health care providers must stress to patients and their families the importance of discontinuing maintenance therapy gradually. Box 14-1 outlines patient and family teaching regarding lithium therapy.

Patients need to know that **two major long-term risks of lithium therapy are hypothyroidism and impairment of the kidney's ability to concentrate urine.** Therefore, a person receiving lithium therapy must have periodic follow-ups to assess thyroid and renal function.

Contraindications. Before lithium is administered, a medical evaluation is performed to assess the patient's ability to tolerate the drug. In particular, baseline physical and laboratory examinations should include assessment of renal function; determination of thyroid status, including levels of thyroxine and thyroid-stimulating hormone; and evaluation for dementia or neurological disorders, which presage a poor response to lithium. Other clinical and laboratory assessments, including an electrocardiogram, are performed as needed, depending on the individual's physical condition.

Lithium therapy is generally contraindicated in patients with cardiovascular disease, brain damage, renal disease, thyroid disease, or myasthenia gravis. Whenever possible, lithium is not given to women who

are pregnant, because it may harm the fetus. The fear of becoming pregnant and the wish to become pregnant are both major concerns for many women taking lithium. Lithium use is also contraindicated in mothers who are breast-feeding and in children younger than 12 years of age.

Anticonvulsant Drugs

In the 1980s, researchers hypothesized that mood instability could be viewed much the same as epilepsy and that a chain reaction of sensitivity, or *kindling*, was responsible for the worsening of bipolar symptoms over time (Ostacher & Tilley, 2008). This hypothesis led to the use of carbamazepine and valproate as a treatment for mania and the incorporation of anticonvulsant therapy. Subsequent research did not support the kindling theory, however. It is likely that symptom improvement for bipolar disorder is based on a different mechanism of action than seizure prevention.

Three anticonvulsant drugs have demonstrated efficacy and been approved for the treatment of mood disorders: valproate (Depakote), carbamazepine (Tegretol), and lamotrigine (Lamictal) (APA, 2008). Anticonvulsant drugs are thought to be:
- Superior for continuously cycling patients
- More effective when there is no family history of bipolar disease
- Effective at dampening affective swings in schizoaffective patients

---

BOX 14-1 Patient and Family Teaching: Lithium Therapy

The patient and the patient's family should receive the following teaching, be encouraged to ask questions, and be given the material in written form as well.
1. Lithium treats your current emotional problem and also helps prevent relapse. Therefore, it is important to continue taking the drug after the current episode is over.
2. Because therapeutic and toxic dosage ranges are so close, it is important to monitor lithium blood levels very closely—more frequently at first, then once every several months after that.
3. Lithium is not addictive.
4. It is important to eat a normal diet with normal salt and fluid intake (1500-3000 mL/day or six 12-oz glasses of fluid). Lithium decreases sodium reabsorption in the kidneys, which could lead to a deficiency of sodium. A low sodium intake leads to a relative increase in lithium retention, which could produce toxicity.
5. You should stop taking lithium if you have excessive diarrhea, vomiting, or sweating. All of these symptoms can lead to dehydration. Dehydration can raise lithium levels in the blood to toxic levels. **Inform your physician if you have any of these problems.**
6. Do not take diuretics (water pills) while you are taking lithium.
7. Lithium is irritating to the lining of your stomach. Take lithium with meals.
8. It is important to have your kidneys and thyroid checked periodically, especially if you are taking lithium over a long period. Talk to your doctor about this follow-up.
9. Do not take any over-the-counter medicines without checking first with your doctor.
10. If you find that you are gaining a lot of weight, you may need to talk this over with your doctor or nutritionist.
11. Many self-help groups are available to provide support for people with bipolar disorder and their families. The local self-help group is (give name and telephone number).
12. You can find out more information by calling (give name and telephone number).
13. Keep a list of side effects and toxic effects handy, along with the name and number of a contact person (see Table 14-3).
14. If lithium is to be discontinued, your dosage will be tapered gradually to minimize the risk of relapse.

- Effective at diminishing impulsive and aggressive behavior in some nonpsychotic patients
- Helpful in cases of alcohol and benzodiazepine withdrawal
- Beneficial in controlling mania (within 2 weeks) and depression (within 3 weeks or longer)

Valproate. Valproate (available as divalproex sodium [Depakote] and valproic acid [Depakene]) is useful in treating lithium nonresponders who are in acute mania, experience rapid cycles, are in dysphoric mania, or have not responded to carbamazepine. Valproate is also helpful in preventing future manic episodes. It is important to monitor liver function and platelet count periodically, although serious complications are rare.

Carbamazepine. Some patients with treatment-resistant bipolar disorder improve after taking carbamazepine (Tegretol) and lithium, or carbamazepine and an antipsychotic. Carbamazepine seems to work better in patients with rapid cycling and in severely paranoid, angry, patients experiencing manias than in euphoric, overactive, overfriendly patients experiencing manias. It is also thought to be more effective in dysphoric patients experiencing manias.

As with valproate, liver function and platelet count should be monitored periodically. Blood levels of carbamazepine should be monitored at least weekly for the first 8 weeks of treatment, because the drug can increase levels of liver enzymes that can speed its own metabolism. In some instances, this can cause bone-marrow suppression and liver inflammation.

Lamotrigine. Lamotrigine (Lamictal) is a first-line treatment for bipolar depression and is approved for acute and maintenance therapy. Lamotrigine is generally well tolerated, but there is one serious but rare dermatological reaction: a potentially life-threatening rash. Patients should be instructed to seek immediate medical attention if a rash appears, although most are likely benign (Preston et al., 2005).

Antianxiety Drugs

Clonazepam and Lorazepam. Clonazepam (Klonopin) and lorazepam (Ativan) are antianxiety (anxiolytic) drugs useful in the treatment of acute mania in some patients who are resistant to other treatments. These drugs are also effective in managing the psychomotor agitation seen in mania. They should be avoided, however, in patients with a history of substance abuse.

Atypical Antipsychotics

In addition to showing sedative properties during the early phase of treatment (help with insomnia, anxiety, agitation), the atypical antipsychotics seem to have mood-stabilizing properties. Most evidence supports the use of olanzapine (Zyprexa) or risperidone (Risperdal). For example, an initial study showed that olanzapine is better tolerated and prevents mania relapse more effectively than lithium (Tohen, 2003).

Table 14-4 provides an overview of drugs used to treat bipolar disorder. It identifies drugs with U.S. Food and Drug Administration (FDA) approval for bipolar disorder and also drugs that are commonly prescribed "off label" even though they are not specifically approved. Additionally, American Psychiatric Association (2008) pharmacological recommendations for management of bipolar depression, mania, and maintenance are described.

TABLE 14-4 Drug Treatment of Patients with Bipolar Disorder

Generic (Trade)	FDA-Approved Uses	Off-Label Uses	American Psychiatric Association (APA) Recommendations
Lithium (Eskalith, Lithobid)	Acute mania Maintenance	Depression	A first line for bipolar depression Recommended for acute mania A first line of maintenance treatment of bipolar disorder
ANTICONVULSANTS			
Valproic Acid (Depakene, Depakote, Depacon)	Acute mania	Depression Maintenance	Recommended for acute mania A first line of maintenance treatment of bipolar disorder
Carbamazepine (Tegretol)	Acute mania	Depression Maintenance	Recommended for maintenance treatment of bipolar disorder
Lamotrigine (Lamictal)	Maintenance	Depression (can worsen mania)	A first line for bipolar depression Recommended for maintenance treatment of bipolar disorder
Oxcarbazepine (Trileptal)		Acute mania Maintenance	Recommended for maintenance treatment of bipolar disorder

Continued

TABLE 14-4 Drug Treatment of Patients with Bipolar Disorder—cont'd

Generic (Trade)	FDA Approval	Off-Label	American Psychiatric Association (APA) Recommendations
ATYPICAL ANTIPSYCHOTICS			
Aripiprazole (Abilify)	Mania Maintenance	Depression	
Olanzapine (Zyprexa)	Mania Maintenance	Depression	Recommended for acute mania
Quetiapine fumarate (Seroquel)	Depression Mania Maintenance		
Risperidone (Risperdal)	Mania	Depression Maintenance	First line treatment for severe mania
Ziprasidone (Geodon)	Mania	Depression Maintenance	
ANTIANXIETY AGENTS			
Clonazepam (Klonopin) Lorazepam (Ativan)		Mania	May be helpful in mania Recommended for agitation or severe symptoms

Data from Hales, R. E., Yudofsky, S. C., & Gabbard, G. O. (2008). *Textbook of psychiatry* (5th ed.). Washington, DC: American Psychiatric Publishing. (2009). *Practice guideline for the treatment of patients with bipolar disorder* (2nd ed.). Retrieved March 17, 2009 from http://www.psychiatryonline.com/popup.aspx?aID=50099&print=yes

CONSIDERING CULTURE

Racial Influence on the Types of Medications Prescribed for Bipolar Disorder

Imagine that Jason, a 28-year-old, Caucasian male, arrives at a community mental health center complaining of an inability to sleep. His speech is rapid, he paces, and he talks about the inability of the mayor to cleanse the sewers of chlorine gas. He jumps from topic to topic but seems to always return to his family being Russian rulers in exile. After some amount of deliberation, the nurse practitioner tentatively diagnoses him as having bipolar disorder, manic phase, and prescribes a mood stabilizer, lithium, and an antipsychotic, Zyprexa.

Shortly after that, George, a 32-year-old, African American male, arrives at the center. He is irritated that his wife threw him out for running up their credit card debt, being involved with another woman, and keeping her awake at night with loud music and incessant talking. George says that he is superhuman and no longer needs to eat or sleep. During the assessment, he wrings his hands, jumps up from his chair, and looks nervously around the room as if he is afraid or is hearing something. After further assessment, the nurse practitioner diagnoses him with a psychotic disorder (with a need to rule out schizophrenia) and prescribes Zyprexa.

What's the big difference between the two patients? It is probably not their symptoms but quite likely their races. Research demonstrates that African Americans are less likely to receive lithium treatment for bipolar disorder and are far more likely to be prescribed antipsychotics (Kilbourne & Pincus, 2006). Implications of this study and many others are that bipolar disorder is not being treated uniformly among different races and that people are suffering needlessly when cost-effective pharmacotherapy is available (lithium is less expensive than either atypical antipsychotic agents or mood stabilizers).

Shi and colleagues (2007) suggest that African Americans are also more likely to be prescribed long-acting injectable antipsychotics, a form of medicating that is typically reserved for non-adherent patients. The reason for this is unclear, but it may point to communication difficulties or barriers between prescriber and patient or racial stereotypes and misperceptions.

Kilbourne, A. M., & Pincus, H. A. (2006). Brief reports: Patterns of psychotropic medication use by race among veterans with bipolar disorder. *Psychiatric Services, 57* (1), 123-126.
Shi, L., Ascher-Svanum, H., Zhu, B., Faries, D., Montgomery, W., & Marder, S. (2007). Characteristics and use patterns of patients taking first-generation depot antipsychotics or oral antipsychotics for schizophrenia. *Psychiatric Services, 58,* 482-488.

Electroconvulsive Therapy

Electroconvulsive therapy (ECT) is used to subdue severe manic behavior, especially in patients with treatment-resistant mania and patients with rapid cycling (i.e., those who experience four or more episodes of illness a year). Depressive episodes—particularly those with severe, catatonic, or treatment-resistant depression—are an indication for this treatment and may be helpful for mania during pregnancy (APA, 2008). ECT is effective for patients with bipolar disorder who have rapid cycling, for those with paranoid-destructive features (who often respond poorly to lithium therapy), and in acutely suicidal patients. Chapter 13 offers a more detailed discussion of ECT.

Milieu Management

Control of hyperactive behavior during the acute phase almost always includes immediate treatment with an antipsychotic drug. However, when a patient is dangerously out of control, use of the seclusion room or restraints may also be indicated. The seclusion room provides comfort and relief to many patients who can no longer control their own behavior. Seclusion serves the following purposes:

- Reduces overwhelming environmental stimuli

- Protects a patient from injuring self, others, or staff
- Prevents destruction of personal property or property of others

Seclusion is warranted when documented data collected by the nursing and medical staff reflect the following points:

- Substantial risk of harm to others or self is clear.
- The patient is unable to control his or her actions.
- Problematic behavior has been sustained (continues or escalates despite other measures).
- Other measures have failed (e.g., setting limits beginning with verbal de-escalation or using chemical restraints).

The use of seclusion or restraints is associated with complex therapeutic, ethical, and legal issues. Most state laws prohibit the use of unnecessary physical restraint or isolation. Barring an emergency, the use of seclusion and restraints warrants the patient's consent. Therefore, most hospitals have well-defined protocols for treatment with seclusion. **Seclusion protocol** includes a proper reporting procedure through the chain of command when a patient is to be secluded. For example, the use of seclusion and restraint is permitted only on the written order of a physician, which must be reviewed and rewritten every 24 hours. The order must include the type of restraint to be used. Only in an emergency may the charge nurse place a

INTEGRATIVE THERAPY

Omega-3 Fatty Acids as a Treatment for Bipolar Disorder

A few generations ago, youngsters actively resisted a nightly dose of cod liver oil that mothers swore by as a method to prevent constipation. While the foul-tasting, rancid-smelling liquid undoubtedly helped win that particular battle, it may have had other benefits as well. Cod liver oil is rich in omega-3 fatty acids, which have drawn increasing attention as being important in mood regulation. Fish oil is the target of this attention. It contains two omega-3 fatty acids, eicosapentaenoic acid (EPA) and docosahexaenoic acid (DHA), which are important in CNS functioning. EPA seems to be particularly important to behavior and mood.

The interest in these particular fatty acids developed as research began to suggest that people who live in areas with low seafood consumption (especially coldwater seafood) exhibited higher rates of depression and bipolar disorder. This led researchers to explore the influence of omega-3 fatty acids as protective for bipolar disorder (Parker et al., 2006). Alternative treatments are especially attractive for the depressive phase of the disorder, since drugs that are normally used to treat depression can catapult a person into a dangerous manic episode.

The jury is still out on the absolute benefits of either eating more fish or taking fish oil supplements (delivered in pleasant-tasting gel capsules). In a review of published trials, one group of researchers was unable to come up with clear support for increasing dietary intake of omega-3 fatty acids (Appleton et al., 2006). But Kidd (2007) conducted another large-scale analysis of current research and concluded just the opposite: that multiple studies support the benefits of fish oil for the mood swings of bipolar disorder. Given the array of health benefits some researchers have identified, adding this dietary recommendation to patients with bipolar disorder may be helpful.

Appleton, K. M., Hayward, R. C., Gunnell, D., Peters, T. J., Rogers, P. J., Kessler, D., et al. (2006). Effects of n-3 long-chain polyunsaturated fatty acids on depressed mood: Systematic review of published trials. *American Journal of Clinical Nutrition*, 84, 1308–1316.

Kidd, P. M. (2007). Omega-3 DHA and EPA for cognition, behavior, and mood: Clinical findings and structural-functional synergies with cell membrane phospholipids. *Alternative Medicine Review*, 12(3), 207–227.

Parker, G., Gibson, N. A., Brotchie, H., Heruc, G., Rees, A., & Hadzi-Pavlovic, D. (2006). Omega-3 fatty acids and mood disorders. *The American Journal of Psychiatry*, 163, 969–978.

patient in seclusion or restraint; under these circumstances, a written physician's order must be obtained within a specified period of time (15 to 30 minutes).

Seclusion protocols also identify specific nursing responsibilities, such as how often the patient's behavior is to be observed and documented (e.g., every 15 minutes), how often the patient is to be offered food and fluids (e.g., every 30 to 60 minutes), and how often the patient is to be toileted (e.g., every 1 to 2 hours). Because phenothiazines are often administered to patients in seclusion, vital signs should be measured frequently (e.g., every 1 to 2 hours).

Careful and precise documentation is a legal necessity. The nurse documents the following:

- The behavior leading up to the seclusion or restraint
- The actions taken to provide the least restrictive alternative
- The time the patient was placed in seclusion
- Every 15 minutes, the patient's behavior, needs, nursing care, and vital signs
- The time and type of medications given and their effects on the patient

When a patient requires seclusion to prevent self-harm or violence toward others, it is ideal to have one nurse on each shift work with the patient on a continuous basis. Communication with a patient in seclusion is concrete and direct but also empathetic and limited to brief instructions. Patients need reassurance that seclusion is only a temporary measure and that they will be returned to the unit when their behavior is more controlled and they demonstrate the ability to safely be around others.

Frequent staff meetings regarding personal feelings are necessary to prevent using seclusion as a form of punishment or leaving a patient in seclusion for long periods of time without proper supervision. **Restraints and seclusion are never to be used as punishment or for the convenience of the staff.** Refer to Chapter 7 for a more detailed discussion of the legal implications of seclusion and restraints and Chapter 25 for further discussion and guidelines.

Support Groups

Patients with bipolar disorder, as well as their friends and families, benefit from forming mutual support groups, such as those sponsored by the Depression and Bipolar Support Alliance (DBSA), the National Alliance for the Mentally Ill (NAMI), the National Mental Health Association, and the Manic-Depressive Association.

Health Teaching and Health Promotion

Patients and families need information about bipolar illness, with particular emphasis on its chronic and highly recurrent nature. In addition, patients and families need to be taught the warning signs and symptoms of impending episodes. For example, changes in

---

BOX 14-2 Patient and Family Teaching: Bipolar Disorder

1. Patients with bipolar disorder and their families need to know:
   - The chronic and episodic nature of bipolar disorder
   - The fact that bipolar disorder is long term and that maintenance treatment therefore will require that one or more mood-stabilizing agents be taken for a long time
   - The expected side effects and toxic effects of the prescribed medication, as well as whom to call and where to go in case of a toxic reaction
   - The signs and symptoms of relapse that may "come out of the blue"
   - The role of family members and others in preventing a full relapse
   - The phone numbers of emergency contact people, which should be kept in an easily accessed place
2. The use of alcohol, drugs of abuse, even small amounts of caffeine, and over-the-counter medications can produce a relapse.
3. Good sleep hygiene is critical to stability. Frequently, the early symptom of a manic episode is lack of sleep. In

some cases, mania may be averted by the use of sleep medications (e.g., temazepam [Restoril]).
4. Psychosocial strategies are important for dealing with work, interpersonal, and family problems; for lowering stress; for enhancing a sense of personal control; and for increasing community functioning.
5. Group and individual psychotherapy are invaluable for gaining insight and skills in relapse prevention, providing social support, increasing coping skills in interpersonal relations, improving adherence to the medication regimen, reducing functional morbidity, and decreasing rehospitalizations.

Health care workers need to remember the following:

- Minimization and denial are common defenses that require gradual introduction of facts.
- Anger and abusive remarks, although aimed at the health care provider, are symptoms of the disease and are not personal.

Adapted from Zerbe, K. J. (1999). *Women's mental health in primary care.* Philadelphia: Saunders; and Milkowitz, D. J. (2003). Bipolar disorder. In D. H. Barlow (Ed.), *Clinical handbook of psychological disorders* (pp. 523-560). New York: Guilford Press.

sleep patterns are especially important because they usually precede, accompany, or precipitate mania. Even a single night of unexplainable sleep loss can be taken as an early warning of impending mania. Health teaching stresses the importance of establishing regularity in sleep patterns, meals, exercise, and other activities. Box 14-2 lists health-teaching guidelines for patients with bipolar disorder and their families.

Mood stabilizers may cause weight gain and other metabolic disturbances such as altered metabolism of lipids and glucose (Fagiolini et al., 2008). These alterations increase the risk for diabetes, high blood pressure, dyslipidemia, cardiac problems, or all of these in combination (metabolic syndrome). Not only do these disturbances impair quality of life and lifespan, they are also a major reason for nonadherence. Teaching aimed at weight reduction and management is essential to keeping patients physically healthy and emotionally stable.

Recovery concepts are particularly important for patients with bipolar disorder, who often have issues with adherence to treatment. The best method of addressing this problem is to follow a collaborative-care model in which responsibilities for treatment adherence are shared (Sajatovic et al., 2005). In this model, patients are responsible for making it to appointments and openly communicating information, and the health care provider is responsible for keeping current on treatment methods and listening carefully as the patient shares perceptions. Through this sharing, treatment adherence becomes a self-managed responsibility.

Advanced Practice Interventions

When a patient with bipolar disorder is not experiencing acute mania, advanced practice registered nurses (APRNs) may utilize psychotherapy to help the patient cope more adaptively to stresses in the environment and decrease the risk of relapse. Specific approaches to psychotherapy include cognitive-behavioral therapy, family therapy, and interpersonal therapy. APRNs who hold prescriptive authority may also prescribe any of the medications used to treat bipolar disorders.

Psychotherapy

Pharmacotherapy and psychiatric management are essential in the treatment of acute manic attacks and during the continuation and maintenance phases of bipolar disorder. Individuals with bipolar disorder must deal with the psychosocial consequences of their past episodes and their vulnerability to experiencing future episodes. They also have to face the burden of long-term treatments that may involve unpleasant side effects. Many patients have strained interpersonal relationships, marriage and family problems, academic and occupational problems, and legal or other social difficulties. Psychotherapy can help them work through these difficulties, decrease some of the psychic

distress, and increase self-esteem. Psychotherapeutic treatments can also help patients improve their functioning between episodes and attempt to decrease the frequency of future episodes.

Cognitive-behavioral therapy (CBT) is typically used as an adjunct to pharmacotherapy and involves identifying maladaptive cognitions and behaviors that may be barriers to a person's recovery and ongoing mood stability. It is also used for bipolar disorder in children (Barclay, 2003). CBT focuses on adherence to the medication regimen, early detection and intervention for manic or depressive episodes, stress and lifestyle management, and the treatment of depression and comorbid conditions (Lam et al., 2003; Otto et al., 2003). Patients treated with cognitive therapy are more likely to take their medications as prescribed than are patients who do not participate in therapy, and psychotherapy results in greater adherence to the lithium regimen (Lam et al., 2003).

A formalized psychotherapy called *interpersonal and social rhythm therapy* has been tested in combination with pharmacotherapy in randomized clinical trials as treatment for patients during the maintenance phase of bipolar illness. This therapy addresses the variables that relate to recurrence of symptoms, especially nonadherence with medication, stress management, and maintenance of social supports (Frank, 2007).

Often the patients receiving medication and therapy place more value on psychotherapy than do clinicians. A patient describes her feelings about drug therapy and psychotherapy as follows (Jamison, 1995):

> I cannot imagine leading a normal life without lithium. From startings and stoppings of it, I now know it is an essential part of my sanity. Lithium prevents my seductive but disastrous highs, diminishes my depressions, clears out the weaving of my disordered thinking, slows me, gentles me out, keeps me in my relationships, in my career, out of a hospital, and in psychotherapy. It keeps me alive, too. But psychotherapy heals, it makes some sense of the confusion, it reins in the terrifying thoughts and feelings, it brings back hope and the possibility of learning from it all. Pills cannot, do not, ease one back into reality. They bring you back headlong, careening, and faster than can be endured at times. Psychotherapy is a sanctuary, it is a battleground, and it is where I have come to believe that someday I may be able to contend with all of this. No pill can help me deal with the problem of not wanting to take pills, but no amount of therapy alone can prevent my manias and depressions. I need both.

EVALUATION

Outcome criteria often dictate the frequency of evaluation of short-term and intermediate indicators. Are the patient's vital signs stable? Is he or she well hydrated? Is the patient able to control personal behavior or respond to external controls? Is the patient able to sleep for 4 or 5 hours a night or take frequent, short rest periods during the day? Does the family have a clear understanding of the patient's disease and need for medication? Do the patient and family know which community agencies may help them?

If outcomes or related indicators are not achieved satisfactorily, the preventing factors are analyzed. Were the data incorrect or insufficient? Were nursing diagnoses inappropriate or outcomes unrealistic? Was intervention poorly planned? After the outcomes and care plan are reassessed, the plan is revised, if indicated. Longer-term outcomes include adherence to the medication regimen; resumption of functioning in the community; achievement of stability in family, work, and social relationships and in mood; and improved coping skills for reducing stress.

Case Study and Nursing Care Plan 14-1   Mania

Ms. Horowitz is brought to the emergency department after being found on the highway shortly after her car broke down. She is dressed in a long red dress, a blue and orange scarf, many long chains, and a yellow and green turban. The police report that when they came to her aid, she told them she was "driving to fame and fortune." She appeared overly cheerful and was constantly talking, laughing, and making jokes. At the same time, she paced up and down beside the car, sometimes tweaking the cheek of one of the policemen. She was coy and flirtatious with the police officers, saying at one point, "Boys in blue are fun to do."

When she reached into the car and started drinking from an open bottle of bourbon, the police decided that her behavior and general condition might result in harm to herself or others. When they explained to Ms. Horowitz that they wanted to take her to the hospital for a general checkup, her jovial mood turned to anger and rage, yet 2

minutes after getting into the police car, she was singing "Carry Me Back to Old Virginny."

On admission to the emergency department, Ms. Horowitz is seen by a psychiatrist, and her sister is called. The sister states that Ms. Horowitz stopped taking her lithium about 5 weeks ago and is becoming more and more agitated and out of control. She reports that Ms. Horowitz has not eaten in 2 days, has stayed up all night calling friends and strangers all over the country, and finally fled the house when the sister called an ambulance to take her to the hospital. The psychiatrist contacts Ms. Horowitz's physician, and her previous history and medical management are discussed. It is decided that she should be hospitalized during the acute manic phase and restarted on lithium therapy. It is hoped that medications and a controlled environment will prevent further escalation of the manic state and prevent possible exhaustion and cardiac collapse.

ASSESSMENT

Self-Assessment

Mr. Atkins has worked as a nurse on the psychiatric unit for 2 years. He has learned to deal with many of the challenging behaviors associated with the manic defense. For example, he no longer takes most of the verbal insults personally, even when the remarks are cutting and hit close to home. He is also better able to recognize and set limits on some of the tactics used by the patient experiencing mania to split the staff. The staff on this unit work closely with each other, making the atmosphere positive and supportive; therefore, communication is good among staff. Frequent and effective communication is needed to prevent staff splitting, maximize external controls, and maintain consistency in nursing care.

The only aspects of Ms. Horowitz's behavior Mr. Atkins thinks he may have difficulty with are the sexual advances and loud sexual comments she makes toward him. He knows that this could make him anxious, and his concern is that his anxiety might be picked up by the patient. When he discusses this with the unit coordinator, they decide that two nurses should provide care for Ms. Horowitz. A female nurse will spend time with her in her room, and Mr Atkins will spend time with her in quiet areas on the unit. It is decided that neither Mr. Atkins nor any male staff member will be alone with Ms. Horowitz in her room at any time. Mr. Atkins will ask for relief if Ms. Horowitz's sexual remarks and acting-out behaviors make him anxious.

Objective Data

Little if anything to eat for days
Little if any sleep for days
History of mania
History of lithium maintenance
Constant physical activity: unable to sit
Very loud and distracting to others
Anger when wishes are curtailed
Flight of ideas
Dress loud and inappropriate

Remarks suggestive of sexual themes: calls nurse "lover"
Behavior that some patients find amusing
Remarks that suggest grandiose thinking
Poor judgment

Subjective Data

"Driving myself to fame and fortune."
"I'm untouchable...I'll get the FBI to set me free."
"Let me be...set me free, lover."

DIAGNOSIS

1. *Risk for injury* related to dehydration and faulty judgment, as evidenced by inability to meet own physiological needs and set limits on own behavior
   - Has not slept for days
   - Has not consumed food or fluids for days
   - Engages in constant physical activity, unable to sit
2. *Defensive coping* related to biochemical changes, as evidenced by change in usual communication patterns
   - Very loud and distracting to others
   - Remarks suggest sexual themes
   - Behavior some patients find amusing
   - Remarks suggesting grandiose thinking
   - Flight of ideas
   - Loud, hostile, and sexual remarks to other patients

OUTCOMES IDENTIFICATION

Physical status will remain stable during manic phase.

PLANNING

The nurse plans interventions that will help de-escalate Ms. Horowitz's activity to minimize potential physical injury (dehydration, cardiac instability) through the use of medication and provision of a nonstimulating environment.

IMPLEMENTATION

Mr. Atkins makes the following nursing care plan.

Short-Term Goal	Intervention	Rationale	Evaluation
1. Patient will be well hydrated, as evidenced by good skin turgor and normal urinary output and specific gravity, within 24 hours.	1a. Give haloperidol (Haldol) intramuscularly immediately and as ordered.	1a. Continuous physical activity and lack of fluids can eventually lead to cardiac collapse and death.	GOAL MET After 3 hours, patient takes small amounts of fluid (2-4 oz per hour).
	1b. Check vital signs frequently (every 1-2 hours).	1b. Cardiac status is monitored.	After 5 hours, patient starts taking 8 oz per hour with a lot of reminding and encouragement.
	1c. Place patient in private or quiet room (whenever possible).	1c. Environmental stimuli are reduced—escalation of mania and distractibility is minimized.	After 24 hours, urine specific gravity is within normal limits.
	1d. Stay with patient and divert patient away from stimulating situations.	1d. Nurse's presence provides support. Ability to interact with others is temporarily impaired.	
	1e. Offer high-calorie, high-protein drink (8 oz) every hour in quiet area.	1e. Proper hydration is mandatory for maintenance of cardiac status.	
	1f. Frequently remind patient to drink: "Take two more sips."	1f. Patient's concentration is poor; she is easily distracted.	
	1g. Offer finger food frequently in quiet area.	1g. Patient is unable to sit; snacks she can eat while pacing are more likely to be consumed.	
	1h. Maintain record of intake and output.	1h. Such a record allows staff to make accurate nutritional assessment for patient's safety.	
	1i. Weigh patient daily.	1i. Monitoring of nutritional status is necessary.	

Continued

Short-Term Goal	Intervention	Rationale	Evaluation
2. Patient will sleep or rest 3 hours during the first night in the hospital with aid of medication and nursing interventions.	2a. Continue to direct patient to areas of minimal activity. 2b. When possible, try to direct energy into productive and calming activities (e.g., pacing to slow, soft music; slow exercise; drawing alone; or writing in quiet area). 2c. Encourage short rest periods throughout the day (e.g., 3-5 minutes every hour) when possible. 2d. Patient should drink decaffeinated drinks only— decaffeinated coffee, tea, or colas. 2e. Provide nursing measures at bedtime that promote sleep—warm milk, soft music.	2a. Lower levels of stimulation can decrease excitability. 2b. Directing patient to paced, nonstimulating activities can help minimize excitability. 2c. Patient may be unaware of feelings of fatigue. Can collapse from exhaustion if hyperactivity continues without periods of rest. 2d. Caffeine is a central nervous system stimulant that inhibits needed rest or sleep. 2e. Such measures promote nonstimulating and relaxing mood.	Patient is awake most of the first night. Sleeps for 2 hours from 4 to 6 AM. Patient is able to rest on the second day for short periods and engage in quiet activities for short periods (5-10 minutes).
3. Patient's blood pressure (BP) and pulse (P) will be within normal limits within 24 hours with the aid of medication and nursing interventions.	3a. Continue to monitor BP and P frequently throughout the day (every 30 minutes). 3b. Keep staff informed by verbal and written reports of baseline vital signs and patient progress.	3a. Physical condition is presently a great strain on patient's heart. 3b. Alerting all staff regarding patient's status can increase medical intervention if a change in status occurs.	GOAL MET Baseline measures on unit are not obtained because of hyperactive behavior. Information from family physician states that baseline BP is 130/90 mm Hg and baseline P is 88 beats per minute. BP at end of 24 hours is 130/70 mm Hg; P is 80 beats per minute.

EVALUATION

After 2 days, the medical staff think that Ms. Horowitz's physical status is stable. Her vital signs are within normal limits, she is consuming sufficient fluids, and her urinary output is normal. Although her hyperactivity persists, it does so to a lesser degree; she is able to get periods of rest during the day and is sleeping 3 to 4 hours during the night.

Ms. Horowitz's hyperactivity continues to be a challenge to the nurses; however, she is able to participate in some activities that require gross motor movement. These activities are useful in channeling some of her aggressive energy. Shortly after her arrival on the unit, Ms. Horowitz starts a fight with another patient, but seclusion is avoided because she is able to refrain from further violent episodes as a result of medication and nursing interventions. She can be directed toward solitary activities, which channel some of her energies, at least for short periods.

As the effect of the drugs progresses, Ms. Horowitz's activity level decreases, and by discharge, she is able to discuss issues of concern with the nurse and make some useful decisions about her future. She is to come for follow-up at the community center and agrees to join a family psychoeducational group for patients with bipolar disorder and their families, which she will attend with her sister.

KEY POINTS TO REMEMBER

- Biological factors appear to play a role in the etiology of the bipolar disorders. Strong genetic correlates have been revealed, especially through twin studies. In addition, little doubt exists that neurotransmitter (norepinephrine, dopamine, serotonin) excess and imbalance are also related to bipolar mood swings, which supports the existence of neurobiological influences. Neuroendocrine and neuroanatomical findings provide strong evidence for biological influences.

- Early detection of bipolar disorder can help diminish comorbid substance abuse, suicide, and decline in social and personal relationships and may help promote more positive outcomes. Unfortunately, bipolar disorder often goes unrecognized.

- The nurse assesses the patient's level of mood (hypomania, acute mania), behavior, and thought processes, and is alert to cognitive dysfunction.

- Analyzing the objective and subjective data helps the nurse formulate appropriate nursing diagnoses. Some of the nursing diagnoses appropriate for patients with mania are *Risk for violence, Defensive coping, Ineffective coping, Disturbed thought processes*, and *Situational low self-esteem*.

- During the acute phase of mania, physical needs often take priority and demand nursing interventions. Therefore, *Deficient fluid volume* and *Imbalanced nutrition or elimination*, as well as *disturbed sleep pattern*, are usually addressed in the nursing plan.

- The diagnosis *Interrupted family processes* is vital. Support groups, psychoeducation, and guidance for the family can greatly affect the patient's adherence to the medication regimen.

- Planning involves identifying the specific needs of the patient and family during the three phases of mania (acute, continuation, and maintenance). Can the patient benefit from communication-skills training, improvement in coping skills, legal or financial counseling, or further psychoeducation? What community resources does the patient need at this time?

- Patients experiencing mania can be demanding and manipulative. Examples of manipulative behavior include pitting members of the staff against one another, loudly and persistently pointing to faults and shortcomings in staff, constantly demanding attention and favors from the staff, and provoking both patients and staff with profane and lewd remarks. The patient experiencing mania constantly interrupts activities and distracts groups with continuous physical motion and incessant joking and talking. The nurse sets limits in a firm, neutral manner and tailors communication techniques and interventions to maintain the patient's safety.

- Health care workers, family, and friends often feel angry and frustrated by the patient's disruptive behaviors. When these feelings are not examined and shared with others, the therapeutic potential of the staff is reduced, and feelings of confusion and helplessness remain.

- Antimanic medications are available. Lithium has a narrow therapeutic index, which necessitates thorough patient and family teaching and regular follow-up. Anticonvulsant drugs such as carbamazepine and valproic acid are useful, especially in treating people with disease refractory to lithium therapy. Anticonvulsant drugs are also useful in treating patients who need rapid de-escalation and do not respond to other treatment approaches.

- Antipsychotic agents may be used for their sedating and mood-stabilizing properties, especially during initial treatment.

- For some patients, ECT may be the most appropriate medical treatment.

- Patient and family teaching takes many forms and is most important in encouraging adherence to the medication regimen and reducing the risk of relapse.

- Evaluation includes examining the effectiveness of the nursing interventions, changing the outcomes as needed, and reassessing the nursing diagnoses. Evaluation is an ongoing process and is part of each of the other steps in the nursing process.

CRITICAL THINKING

1. Donald has been diagnosed with bipolar disorder and has been taking lithium for 4 months. During a clinic visit, he tells you that he does not think he will be taking his lithium anymore because he feels fine and misses his old "intensity." He says he is able to function well at his job and at home with his family and that his wife agrees that he "has this thing licked."
   A. What are Donald's needs in terms of teaching?
   B. What are the needs of his family?

2. Write a teaching plan for Donald, or use an already constructed plan that includes the following teaching topics with sound rationales:
   A. Use of alcohol, drugs, caffeine, over-the-counter medications
   B. Need for sleep, hygiene
   C. Types of community resources available
   D. Signs and symptoms of relapse

CHAPTER REVIEW

1. Which behavior exhibited by a patient with mania should the nurse choose to address first?
   1. Indiscriminate sexual relations
   2. Excessive spending of money
   3. Declaration of "being at one with the world"
   4. Demonstration of flight of ideas

2. The nurse is caring for a patient experiencing mania. Which is the most appropriate nursing intervention?
   1. Provide consistency among staff members when working with the patient.
   2. Negotiate limits so the patient has a voice in the plan of care.

3. Allow only certain staff members to interact with the patient.

4. Attempt to control the patient's emotions.

3. The nurse is planning care for a patient experiencing the acute phase of mania. Which is the priority intervention?

1. Prevent injury.

2. Maintain stable cardiac status.

3. Get the patient to demonstrate thought self-control.

4. Ensure that the patient gets sufficient sleep and rest.

4. What critical information should the nurse provide about the use of lithium?

1. "You will still have hypersexual tendencies, so be certain to use protection when engaging in intercourse."

2. "Lithium will help you to only feel the euphoria of mania but not the anxiety."

3. "It will take 1 to 2 weeks and maybe longer for this medication to start working fully."

4. "This medication is a cure for bipolar disorder."

5. The nurse has provided education for a patient in the continuation phase after discharge from the hospital. What indicates that the plan of care has been successful? *Select all that apply.*

1. Patient identifies three signs and symptoms of relapse.

2. Patient states, "My wife doesn't mind if I still drink a little."

3. Patient describes the purpose of each medication he has been prescribed.

4. Patient states, "I no longer have a disease."

5. Patient identifies two ways to problem-solve a specific situation.

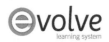

Visit the Evolve website for an **Audio Chapter Summary, Chapter Review Answers & Rationales, Critical Thinking Answer Guidelines,** and additional resources related to the content in this chapter: **http://evolve.elsevier.com/Varcarolis/foundations**

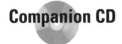

Companion CD   Use the Companion CD to prepare for tests and the NCLEX® Examination with **Test-Taking Strategies** for psychiatric mental health nursing and hundreds of **Review Questions**.

References

American Psychiatric Association. (2000). *Diagnostic and statistical manual of mental disorders (DSM-IV-TR)* (4th ed. text rev.). Washington, DC: Author.

American Psychiatric Association. (2008). *Practice guidelines for the treatment of patients with bipolar disorder* (2nd ed.). Retrieved July 18, 2008 from www.psychiatryonline.com/popup.aspx?aID=50099&print=yes

Baldassano, C. F., Marangell, L. B., Gyulai, L., Nassir Ghaemi, S., Joffe, H., Kim, D. R., et al. (2005). Gender differences in bipolar disorder: Retrospective data from the first 500 STEP-BD participants. *Bipolar Disorder, 5,* 465–470.

Barclay, L. (2003, October 20). *Cognitive behavioral therapy useful for bipolar disorder in children* [Abstract C6]. Paper presented at the 50th Annual Meeting of the American Academy of Child and Adolescent Psychiatry, Miami, FL.

Bauer, M., Beaulieu, S., Dunner, D. L., Lafer, B., & Kupka, R. (2008). Rapid cycling bipolar disorder—diagnostic concepts. *Bipolar Disorders, 10*(2), 153–162.

Baum, A. E., Akula, N., Cabanero, M., Cardona, I., Corona, W., Klemens, B., et al. (2008). A genome-wide association study implicates diacylglycerol kinase eta (DGKH) and several other genes in the etiology of bipolar disorder. *Molecular Psychiatry, 13,* 197–207.

Benazzi, F. (2007). Bipolar II disorder: Epidemiology, diagnosis, and management. *CNS Drugs, 21,* 727–740.

Burmeister, M., McInnis, M. G., & Zollner, S. (2008). Psychiatric genetics: Progress amid controversy. *Nature Reviews Genetics, 9,* 527–540.

Fagiolini, A., Chengappa, K. N., Soreca, I., & Chang, J. (2008). Bipolar disorder and the metabolic syndrome: Causal factors, psychiatric outcomes and economic burden. *CNS Drugs, 22,* 655–669.

Frank, E. (2007). Interpersonal and social rhythm therapy: A means of improving depression and preventing relapse in bipolar disorder. *Journal of Clinical Psychology, 63,* 463–473.

Gitlin, M. (2007). Treatment resistant bipolar disorder. *Focus, 5,* 49–63.

Gunderson, J. G., Weinberg, I., Daversa, M. T., Kueppenbender, K. D., Zanarini, M. C., Shea, M. T., et al. (2006). Descriptive and longitudinal observations on the relationship of borderline personality disorder and bipolar disorder. *American Journal of Psychiatry, 163,* 1173–1178.

Hirschfeld, R. M. A., Bowden, C., Gitlin, M., Keck, P., Suppes, T., Thase, M., et al. (2000). Practice guidelines for the treatment of patients with bipolar disorder. In American Psychiatric Association, *Practice guidelines for the treatment of psychiatric disorders: Compendium 2000.* Washington, DC: Author.

Jamison, K. R. (1995). *An unquiet mind.* New York: Knopf.

Kessler, R. C., Berglund, P. A., Demler, O., Jin, R., & Walters, E. E. (2005). Lifetime prevalence and age-of-onset distributions of *DSM-IV* disorders in the National Comorbidity Survey Replication (NCS-R). *Archives of General Psychiatry, 62,* 593–602.

Kilbourne, A. M., & Pincus, H. A. (2006). Patterns of psychotropic medication use by race among veterans with bipolar disorder. *Psychiatric Services, 57*(1), 123–126.

Lam, D. H., Watkins, E. R., Hayward, P., Bright, J., Wright, K., Kerr, N., et al. (2003). A randomized controlled study of cognitive therapy for relapse prevention for bipolar affective disorder: Outcome of the first year. *Archives of General Psychiatry, 60,* 145–152.

Lehne, R. A. (2010). *Pharmacology for nursing care* (7th ed.). Philadelphia: Saunders.

McClung, C. A. (2007). Circadian genes, rhythms, and the biology of mood disorders. *Pharmacology and Therapeutics, 114,* 222–232.

McIntyre, R. S., Konarski, J. Z., Soczynska, J. K., Wilkins, K., Panjwani, G., Bouffard, B., et al. (2006). Medical comorbidity in bipolar disorder: Implications for functional outcomes and health service utilization. *Psychiatric Services, 57,* 1140–1144.

Merikangas, K. R., Akiskal, H. S., Angst, J., Greenberg, P. E., Hirschfeld, R. M., Petukhova, M., et al. (2007). Lifetime and 12-month prevalence of bipolar spectrum disorder in the National Comorbidity Survey Replication. *Archives of General Psychiatry, 64,* 543–552.

Moore, M. (2008, November 2). Patty Duke puts celebrity face on bipolar disorder. *Missoulian.* Retrieved November 2, 2008 from http://missoulian.com/articles/2008/10/11/news/local/news05.txt

Moorhead, S., Johnson, M., Maas, M., & Swanson, E. (Eds.). (2008). *Nursing outcomes classification (NOC)* (3rd ed.). St. Louis: Mosby.

North American Nursing Diagnosis Association International (NANDA-I). (2009). *NANDA-I nursing diagnoses: Definitions and classification. 2009–2011.* Oxford, United Kingdom: Author.

Ostacher, M. J., & Tilley, C. A. (2008). Anticonvulsants. In T. A. Stern, J. F. Rosenbaum, M. Fava, J. Biederman, & S. L. Rauch (Eds.), *Comprehensive Clinical Psychiatry* (pp. 661–666). Philadelphia: Mosby Elsevier.

Otto, M. W., Reilly-Harrington, N., & Sachs, G. S. (2003). Psychoeducational and cognitive-behavioral strategies in the management of bipolar disorder [Abstract]. *Journal of Affective Disorders, 73,* 171–181.

Owen, M. J., Craddock, N., & Jablensky, A. (2007). The genetic deconstruction of psychosis. *Schizophrenia Bulletin, 33,* 905–911.

Perlis, R. H., & Ostacher, M. J. (2008). Anticonvulsants. In T. A. Stern, J. F. Rosenbaum, M. Fava, J. Biederman, & S. L. Rauch (Eds.), *Comprehensive Clinical Psychiatry* (pp. 651–659). Philadelphia: Mosby Elsevier.

Pollock, R., & Kuo, I. (2004, February 9–13). *Neuroimaging in bipolar disorder.* Paper presented at the 5th Invitational Congress of Biological Psychiatry, Sydney, Australia.

Preston, J. D., O'Neal, J. H., & Talaga, M. C. (2005). *Handbook of clinical psychopharmacology for therapists* (4th ed.). Oakland, CA: New Harbinger.

Robinson, L. J., Thompson, J. M., Gallagher, P., Goswami, U., Young, A., Ferrier, I., et al. (2006). A meta-analysis of cognitive deficits in euthymic patients with bipolar disorder. *Journal of Effective Disorders, 93,* 105–115.

Sadock, B. J., & Sadock, V. A. (2008). *Concise textbook of clinical psychiatry* (3rd ed.). Philadelphia: Lippincott Williams & Wilkins.

Sajatovic, M., Davies, M., Bauer, M., McBride, L., Hays, R., Safavi, R., et al. (2005). Attitudes regarding the collaborative practice model and treatment adherence among individuals with bipolar disorder. *Comprehensive Psychiatry, 46,* 272–277.

Schretlen, D. J., Cascella, N. G., Meyer, S. M., Kingery, L. R., Testa, M., & Munro, C. A. (2007). Neuropsychological functioning in bipolar disorder and schizophrenia. *Biological Psychiatry, 62*(2), 179–186.

Sklar, P., Smoller, J. W., Fan, J., Ferreira, M. A. R., Perlis, R. H., Chambert, K., et al. (2008). Whole-genome association study of bipolar disorder. *Molecular Psychiatry, 13,* 558–569.

Strakowski, S. M., DelBello, M. P., & Adler, C. M. (2005). The functional neuroanatomy of bipolar disorder: A review of neuroimaging findings. *Molecular Psychiatry, 10,* 105–116.

Tohen, M. (2003, June 18). *Olanzapine more effective for preventing mania relapse.* Paper presented at the 5th Invitational Congress of Bipolar Disorders, Pittsburgh, PA.

Tondo, L., & Baldessarini, R. J. (2005). Suicidal risk in bipolar disorder. *Clinical Neuropsychiatry, 2,* 55–65.

Torrent, C., Sanchez-Moreno, J., Comes, M., Goikolea, J. M., Salamero, M., & Vieta, E. (2006). Cognitive impairment in bipolar II disorder. *The British Journal of Psychiatry, 189,* 254–259.

Vieta, E., & Suppes, T. (2008). Bipolar II disorder: Arguments for and against a distinct diagnostic entity. *Bipolar Disorders, 10*(1), 163–178.

Wang, P. S., Berglund, P., Olfson, M., Pincus, H. A., Wells, K. B., & Kessler, R. C. (2005). Failure and delay in initial treatment contact after first onset of mental disorders in the National Comorbidity Survey Replication. *Archives of General Psychiatry, 62,* 603–613.

Wellcome Trust Case Control Consortium. (2007). Genome-wide association study of 14, 000 cases of seven common diseases and 3, 000 shared controls. *Nature, 447,* 661–678.

CHAPTER 15

Schizophrenia

Edward A. Herzog and Elizabeth M. Varcarolis

Key Terms and Concepts

acute dystonia, 328
affect, 307
affective symptoms, 312
akathisia, 328
ambivalence, 307
anosognosia, 318
associative looseness, 307
atypical antipsychotics, 326
autism, 307
clang association, 315
cognitive symptoms, 312
command hallucinations, 316
concrete thinking, 313
conventional antipsychotics, 326
delusions, 313
depersonalization, 315
derealization, 315
echolalia, 317

echopraxia, 317
extrapyramidal side effects (EPSs), 327
hallucinations, 315
ideas of reference, 333
illusions, 315
metabolic syndrome, 327
negative symptoms, 312
neologisms, 315
neuroleptic malignant syndrome (NMS), 331
paranoia, 331
positive symptoms, 312
pseudoparkinsonism, 328
reality testing, 315
recovery model, 320
stereotyped behaviors, 317
tardive dyskinesia (TD or TDK), 328
word salad, 315

Objectives

1. Describe the progression of symptoms, focus of care, and intervention needs for the prepsychotic through maintenance phases of schizophrenia.
2. Discuss at least three of the neurobiological-anatomical-genetic findings that indicate that schizophrenia is a brain disorder.
3. Differentiate among the positive and negative symptoms of schizophrenia in terms of psychopharmacological treatment and effect on quality of life.
4. Discuss how to deal with common reactions the nurse may experience while working with a patient with schizophrenia.
5. Develop teaching plans for patients taking conventional antipsychotic drugs (e.g., haloperidol [Haldol])

and atypical antipsychotic drugs (e.g., risperidone [Risperdal]).
6. Compare and contrast the conventional antipsychotic medications with atypical antipsychotics.
7. Create a nursing care plan that incorporates evidence-based interventions for key areas of dysfunction in schizophrenia, including hallucinations, delusions, paranoia, cognitive disorganization, anosognosia, and impaired self-care.
8. Role-play intervening with a patient who is hallucinating, delusional, and exhibiting disorganized thinking.

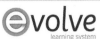

Visit the Evolve website for an **Audio Glossary & Flashcards, Concept Map Creator**, and additional resources related to the content in this chapter: **http://evolve.elsevier.com/Varcarolis/foundations**

Schizophrenia is a potentially devastating brain disorder that affects a person's thinking, language, emotions, social behavior, and ability to perceive reality accurately. It affects one in every 100 people (over 3 million people in the United States) and is among the most disruptive and disabling of mental disorders. Unfortunately, people with this disorder are often misunderstood and stigmatized by not only the general population but even the medical community. Negative attitudes toward patients can interfere with recovery and impair their quality of life (Crowe et al., 2006).

For example, many believe that people with schizophrenia are likely to be violent, but the rate of violence for schizophrenia overall is no greater than that of the general public. Schizophrenia is a psychotic disorder, meaning that delusions, hallucinations, and disorganized thinking, speech and/or behavior are prominent elements of the disorder (American Psychiatric Association [APA], 2000).

CLINICAL PICTURE

Adding to observations made by Emil Kraepelin (1856-1926), Eugen Bleuler (1857-1939) coined the term *schizophrenia*. He first proposed that schizophrenia was not one illness but a heterogeneous group of illnesses with different characteristics and clinical courses. Bleuler's fundamental signs of schizophrenia are referred to as the *four A's*:

1. **Affect**: The outward manifestation of a person's feelings and emotions. Schizophrenia may cause flat, blunted, inappropriate, or bizarre affect.
2. **Associative looseness**: Disorganized thinking, manifested as jumbled and illogical speech and impaired reasoning, is displayed (also known as *looseness of association*).
3. **Autism**: Thinking is not bound to reality but reflects the private perceptual world of the individual. Delusions, hallucinations, and neologisms are examples of autistic thinking.
4. **Ambivalence**: Simultaneously holding two opposing emotions, attitudes, ideas, or wishes toward the same person, situation, or object. Ambivalence occurs in all relationships but becomes pathological and paralyzing when a person continuously vacillates between opposing positions.

VIGNETTE

Sam, a 25-year-old man soon to be discharged from the hospital, constantly tells the social worker he wants his own apartment. When Sam is told that an apartment has been found for him, he asks, "But who will take care of me?" Sam is acting out his ambivalence between his desire to be independent and his desire to be taken care of. ∎

DSM-IV-TR Criteria for Schizophrenia

A. Characteristic Symptoms
Two or more of the following during a 1-month period (or less if successfully treated)
  1. Delusions
  2. Hallucinations
  3. Disorganized speech (e.g., associative looseness)
  4. Grossly disorganized or catatonic behavior
  5. Negative symptoms (e.g., affective flattening, avolition, alogia)
If delusions bizarre or auditory hallucinations and
  a. voices keep a running commentary about person's thoughts/behaviors **or**
  b. two or more voices converse with each other
Then only one criterion is needed.

B. Social/Occupational Dysfunction
If one or more major areas of the person's life are markedly below premorbid functioning (work, interpersonal relationships, or self-care) **or**
If childhood or adolescence failure to achieve expected level of interpersonal, academic, or occupational achievement
Then meets criteria of **B**.

C. Duration
Continuous signs persist for at least 6 months with at least 1 month that meets criteria of **A** (active phase) and may include prodromal or residual symptoms.

D. 1. All other mental diseases (e.g., schizoaffective/mood disorder) have been ruled out.
  2. **All other medical conditions** (substance use/medications or general medical conditions) have been ruled out.
  3. **If history of pervasive developmental disorders**, then prominent hallucinations or delusions for 1 month are needed to make the diagnosis of schizophrenia.

Figure 15-1 Diagnostic criteria for schizophrenia. (Adapted from American Psychiatric Association. [2000]. *Diagnostic and statistical manual of mental disorders* [4th ed., text rev.] [DSM-IV-TR]. Washington, DC: Author.)

Clinicians in the United States use the criteria of the *Diagnostic and Statistical Manual of Mental Disorders*, fourth edition, text revision *(DSM-IV-TR)* for the diagnosis of schizophrenia (APA, 2000). Figure 15-1 presents the *DSM-IV-TR* criteria for schizophrenia.

Other psychotic disorders (e.g., schizophreniform and schizoaffective disorders) are described in Box 15-1.

EPIDEMIOLOGY

The lifetime prevalence of schizophrenia is 1% worldwide with no differences related to race, social status, or culture. It is more common in males (1.4:1) and among persons growing up in urban areas (Tandon et al., 2008). Schizophrenia usually develops during the late teens and early twenties, although onset before the age of 10 has been reported (Masi et al., 2006). Childhood

---

BOX 15-1 Psychotic Disorders Other Than Schizophrenia

Schizophreniform Disorder

The features of schizophreniform disorder are similar to schizophrenia except:
- The total duration of the illness is at least 1 month but less than 6 months.
- Impaired social or occupational functioning may not be apparent (although it may appear later).

This disorder may or may not develop into schizophrenia; persons who do not develop schizophrenia have a good prognosis. This diagnosis may be given when a person appears to have schizophrenia but has not yet been symptomatic for the 6 months required by *DSM-IV-TR* criteria.

Brief Psychotic Disorder

This disorder involves a sudden onset of psychosis (delusions, hallucinations, disorganized speech) or grossly disorganized or catatonic behavior lasting at least 1 day but less than 1 month. It is often precipitated by extreme stressors and is followed by a return to premorbid functioning.

Schizoaffective Disorder

Schizoaffective disorder is characterized by a major depressive, manic, or mixed mood episode presenting concurrently with symptoms of schizophrenia. The symptoms are not due to any substance use or to a medical condition.

Delusional Disorder

Delusional disorder involves nonbizarre delusions (e.g., situations that could occur in real life, such as being followed, deceived by a spouse, or having a disease) of at least 1 month's duration. One's ability to function is not markedly impaired, nor is behavior otherwise odd or psychotic. Common themes include delusions of control, reference, persecution, grandeur, somatic, erotomania, or jealousy. A related disorder, Capgras Syndrome, involves a delusion about a significant other (e.g., family member or pet) being replaced by an imposter; this disorder may be due to psychiatric or organic brain disease (Denes, 2007).

Shared Psychotic Disorder (Folie à Deux)

Folie à deux ("madness between two") is a condition in which one individual comes to share the delusional beliefs of another with whom there is a close, sustained relationship. Impairment is usually much less than that of the person who has the psychotic disorder. For example, a man living with a wife and daughter who both had schizophrenia came to share their belief that standing too close to the stove while cooking caused their obesity.

Induced or Secondary Psychosis

Psychosis may be induced by substances (drugs of abuse, alcohol, medications, or toxins) (Mauri et al., 2006) or caused by a medical condition (delirium, neurological or metabolic conditions, hepatic or renal diseases, and many others). Medical conditions and substance abuse must always be ruled out before a diagnosis of schizophrenia or other psychotic disorder can be made.

---

schizophrenia, although rare, does exist, occurring in 1 out of 40,000 children. Early onset (18 to 25 years) occurs more often in males and is associated with poor functioning before onset, more structural brain abnormality, and increased levels of apathy (APA, 2000). Individuals with a later onset (25 to 35 years) are more likely to be female, have less structural brain abnormality, and have better outcomes (APA, 2000).

COMORBIDITY

Substance abuse disorders occur in nearly 50% of persons with schizophrenia (Green et al., 2008). When substance abuse occurs in people with schizophrenia, it is associated with treatment nonadherence, relapse, incarceration, homelessness, violence, suicide, and a poorer prognosis (Mauri et al., 2006). **Nicotine depen-**

dence rates in schizophrenia range from 70% to 90% and contribute to an increased incidence of cardiovascular and respiratory disorders (Green et al., 2006).

Anxiety, depression, and suicide co-occur frequently in schizophrenia. Anxiety may be a response to symptoms (e.g., hallucinations) or circumstances (e.g, isolation, overstimulation) and may worsen schizophrenia symptoms and prognosis (Mauri et al., 2008). Almost half of all persons with schizophrenia attempt suicide at some point in their lives, and approximately 10% succeed (Hayashi et al., 2005). Both depression and suicide attempts can occur at any point in the illness (Osborn et al., 2008).

Physical health illnesses are more common among people with schizophrenia than in the general population. The risk of premature death is 1.6 to 2.8 times greater than that in the general population; on average, patients with schizophrenia die 28 years prematurely due to disorders such as hypertension (22%), obesity (24%), cardiovascular disease (21%), diabetes (12%), chronic obstructive pulmonary disease (COPD) (10%), and trauma (6%) (Miller et al., 2007).

People with psychotic disorders may be at greater risk due to apathy, poor health habits, medications (see the discussion of metabolic syndrome later in this chapter), or failure to recognize signs of illness. Owing to poverty, stigma, or stereotyping (e.g., emergency department personnel assuming that because a patient has a psychotic disorder, his chest pain is imaginary), they may not receive adequate health care.

Polydipsia can lead to fatal water intoxication (indicated by hyponatremia, confusion, worsening psychotic symptoms, and ultimately coma). It is characterized by a seemingly insatiable thirst that results in a dangerous intake of water. It occurs in 7% of inpatients with schizophrenia (Gonzalez & Perez, 2007). Factors that contribute to excess water intake include taking antipsychotic medication (causes dry mouth), compulsive behavior, and neuroendocrine abnormalities (Bralet et al., 2007).

ETIOLOGY

Schizophrenia typically manifests early in adulthood. It becomes chronic or recurrent in at least 80% of those who develop it; on average, everyone has about a 0.7% chance of developing schizophrenia (Tandon et al., 2008).

Schizophrenia is a complicated disorder. In fact, what we call "schizophrenia" actually may be a group of disorders with common but varying features and multiple, overlapping etiologies. What is known is that brain chemistry, structure, and activity are different in a person with schizophrenia than in a person who does not have the disorder.

The scientific consensus is that schizophrenia occurs when multiple inherited gene abnormalities combine with nongenetic factors (e.g., viral infections, birth injuries, prenatal malnutrition), altering the structures of the brain, affecting the brain's neurotransmitter systems, and/or injuring the brain directly (Tandon et al., 2008). This is called the *diathesis-stress model of schizophrenia* (Walker & Tessner, 2008).

Biological Factors

Genetic

Schizophrenia and schizophrenia-like symptoms, such as eccentric thinking, occur at an increased rate in relatives of individuals with schizophrenia. According to Smoller and colleagues (2008):

- Compared to the usual 1% risk in the population, having a first-degree relative with schizophrenia increases the risk to 10%.

- There is variability of expression of schizophrenia, depending upon environmental factors; schizoaffective disorder and cluster-A personality disorders are more common in relatives of people with schizophrenia.
- Concordance rates in twins (how often one twin will have the disorder when the other one has it) is about 50% for identical twins and about 15% for fraternal twins.

Evidence suggests that multiple genes on different chromosomes interact with each other in complex ways to create vulnerability for schizophrenia. Genes potentially linked to schizophrenia continue to be identified, suggesting a high degree of complexity (Tandon et al., 2008).

Neurobiological

Dopamine Theory. The dopamine theory of schizophrenia is derived from the study of the action of the first antipsychotic drugs, collectively known as *conventional* (or *first-generation*) *antipsychotics* (e.g., haloperidol and chlorpromazine). These drugs block the activity of dopamine-2 (D_2) receptors in the brain, limiting the activity of dopamine and reducing some of the symptoms of schizophrenia. Amphetamines, cocaine, methylphenidate (Ritalin), and levodopa increase the activity of dopamine in the brain and in biologically susceptible persons may precipitate schizophrenia's onset. If schizophrenia is already present, they may exacerbate its symptoms. However, because the dopamine-blocking agents do not alleviate all the symptoms of schizophrenia, the dopamine hypothesis is no longer considered conclusive.

Other Neurochemical Hypotheses. A newer class of drugs, collectively known as *atypical* (or *second-generation*) *antipsychotics*, block serotonin as well as dopamine, which suggests that serotonin may play a role in schizophrenia as well. If we can better understand how atypical agents modulate the expression and targeting of 5-hydroxytryptamine 2A (5-HT2A) and its receptors, we may better understand schizophrenia.

Researchers have long been aware that phencyclidine piperidine (PCP) induces a state closely resembling schizophrenia. This observation led to interest in the *N*-methyl-D-aspartate (NMDA) receptor complex and the possible role of **glutamate** in the pathophysiology of schizophrenia. Glutamate is a crucial neurotransmitter during periods of neuromaturation; abnormal maturation of the central nervous system (CNS) is considered to be a central factor contributing to schizophrenia (Goff, 2005).

Brain Structure Abnormalities

Disruptions in communication pathways in the brain are thought to be severe in schizophrenia. Therefore, it is conceivable that structural abnormalities cause disruption of the brain's functioning. Using brain imaging techniques—computed tomography (CT), magnetic resonance imaging (MRI), and positron emission tomography (PET)—researchers (Broome et al., 2005) have provided substantial evidence that some people with schizophrenia have structural brain abnormalities, including:

- Enlargement of the lateral cerebral ventricles, third ventricle dilation, and/or ventricular asymmetry
- Reduced cortical, frontal lobe, hippocampal and/or cerebellar volumes
- Increased size of the sulci (fissures) on the surface of the brain

In addition, MRI and CT scans demonstrate lower brain volume and more cerebrospinal fluid in people with schizophrenia. PET scans also show a lowered rate of blood flow and glucose metabolism in the frontal lobes, which govern planning, abstract thinking, social adjustment, and decision making, all of which are affected in schizophrenia. (Figure 3-5 in Chapter 3 shows a PET scan demonstrating reduced brain activity in the frontal lobe of a patient with schizophrenia.) Such structural changes may worsen as the disorder continues. Postmortem studies on individuals with schizophrenia reveal a reduced volume of gray matter in the brain, especially in the temporal and frontal lobes; those with the most tissue loss had the worst symptoms (e.g., hallucinations, delusions, bizarre thoughts, and depression).

Psychological and Environmental Factors

A number of stressors, particularly those occurring during vulnerable periods of neurological development, are believed to combine with genetic vulnerabilities to produce schizophrenia. Reducing such stressors is believed to have the potential to reduce the severity of the disorder or even prevent it (Compton, 2004).

CONSIDERING CULTURE

The Stigma of Schizophrenia

Mrs. Chou, a 25-year-old woman, left China for the United States 6 months ago to join her husband. In China, she lived with her parents and had learned English. She was shy and looked to her parents and later to her husband for guidance and support. Shortly after arrival in the United States, her mother developed pneumonia and died. Mrs. Chou later told her husband that if she had stayed in China, her mother would not have become ill, and that evil would now come to their 1-year-old child because Mrs. Chou had not taken proper care of her mother.

Mrs. Chou became increasingly lethargic, staring into space and mumbling to herself. When Mr. Chou asked who she was talking to, she answered, "My mother."

Mr. Chou realized that something was terribly wrong with his wife, yet he was reluctant to ask either relatives or professionals for assistance, since mental illness is strongly stigmatized in the Chinese culture. In fact, mental illness may be believed to be a punishment for personal failings.

Mrs. Chou was finally admitted to a psychiatric unit when Mr. Chou noticed she had quit eating and taking care of herself and was certainly unable to care for their child. During her admission assessment, she sat motionless and mute. Mr. Nolan, her primary nurse, noticed that after he checked her pulse, her arm remained in midair until he lowered it for her. Mrs. Chou was unkempt and pale, and her skin turgor was poor.

Mr. Nolan also spoke with Mr. Chou, who was visibly distressed by his wife's condition. He discovered that Mr. Chou blamed himself for his wife's illness, because his relocation to the United States prevented her from caring for her ailing mother. He agreed with his wife that their mutual failings placed their child at risk of retribution. He conceded that coming to the hospital had been very difficult, owing to embarrassment both about his wife's mental illness and his own belief that he should not burden others with the care of himself and his wife. Mr. Nolan helped Mr. Chou recognize that in U.S. culture, family members shared caregiving burdens, professional help was more available, and stigmatization was less intense.

Gradually, Mr. Chou's distress lessened as he came to appreciate that he would not have to carry the level of burden he had anticipated. As Mrs. Chou's psychosis abated, both she and Mr. Chou came to ascribe more culpability for the illness to fate, reducing their burden of self-blame. They agreed to meet with a Chinese-American healer who helped them integrate the beliefs and resources of their original and adopted cultures, further reducing their guilt and distress.

Wong, D. F. K., Tsui, H. K. P., Pearson, V., Chen, E. Y. H., & Chui, S. N. (2004). Family burdens, Chinese health beliefs, and the mental health of Chinese caregivers in Hong Kong. *Transcultural Psychiatry, 4*, 497–513.

Prenatal Stressors

A history of pregnancy or birth complications is associated with an increased risk for schizophrenia. Prenatal risk factors include viral infection, poor nutrition, hypoxia, and exposure to toxins. Psychological trauma to the mother during pregnancy (e.g., the death of a relative) can also contribute to the development of schizophrenia (Khashan et al., 2008). Other risk factors include a father older than 35 at the child's conception and being born during late winter or early spring (Tandon et al., 2008).

Psychological Stressors

Although there is no evidence that stress alone causes schizophrenia, stress increases cortisol levels, impeding hypothalamic development and causing other changes that may precipitate the illness in vulnerable individuals. Schizophrenia often manifests at times of developmental and family stress, such as beginning college or moving away from one's family. Social, psychological, and physical stressors may play a significant role in both the severity and course of the disorder and the person's quality of life. Other factors increasing the risk of schizophrenia include cannabis use and exposure to psychological trauma or social defeat (Tandon et al., 2008).

Environmental Stressors

Environmental factors are also believed to contribute to the development of schizophrenia in vulnerable persons. These include exposure to social adversity (e.g., living in chronic poverty or high-crime environments) and migration to or growing up in a foreign culture (Tandon et al., 2008; Broome et al., 2005).

Course of the Disorder

The onset of symptoms or forewarning (prodromal) symptoms may appear a month to a year before the first psychotic break or full-blown manifestations of the illness; such symptoms represent a clear deterioration in previous functioning. The course thereafter typically includes recurrent exacerbations separated by periods of reduced or dormant symptoms. Occasionally a person will have a single episode of schizophrenia without recurrences or have several episodes and none thereafter. For most patients, however, schizophrenia is a chronic or recurring disorder which, like diabetes or heart disease, is managed but rarely cured.

Frequently the history of a person with schizophrenia reveals that prior to the illness, the person was socially awkward, lonely, perhaps depressed, and expressed himself or herself in vague, odd, or unrealistic ways. In this prodromal phase, complaints about anxiety, phobias, obsessions, dissociative features, and compulsions may be noted. As anxiety mounts, indications of a thought disorder become evident. Concentration, memory, and completion of school- or job-related work deteriorate.

Intrusive thoughts, "mind wandering," and the need to devote more time to maintaining one's thoughts are reported.

The person may feel that something "strange" or "wrong" is happening. Events are misinterpreted, and mystical or symbolic meanings may be given to ordinary events. For example, the patient may think that certain colors have special powers or that a song on the radio is a message from God. Discerning others' emotions becomes more difficult, and other people's actions or words may be mistaken for signs of hostility or evidence of harmful intent (Chung et al., 2008).

Sexuality is frequently altered in psychotic disorders. Preoccupation with homosexual themes may occur, particularly in people with paranoid schizophrenia. Doubts regarding sexual identity, exaggerated sexual needs, altered sexual performance, and fears of intimacy are prominent in schizophrenia. The person may engage in public masturbatory behavior.

Prognostic Considerations

For the majority of patients, most symptoms can be at least somewhat controlled through medications and psychosocial interventions. With support and effective treatments, many people with schizophrenia experience a good quality of life and success within their families, occupations, and other roles. Associates may not even realize the person has schizophrenia.

However, in most cases, schizophrenia does not respond fully to available treatments, leaving residual symptoms and causing varying degrees of disability. Some cases require repeated or lengthy inpatient care or institutionalization. An abrupt onset of symptoms is usually a favorable prognostic sign, and those with good premorbid social, sexual, and occupational functioning have a greater chance for a good remission or a complete recovery. A slow, insidious onset over 2 to 3 years is more ominous, and the younger one is at the onset of schizophrenia, the more discouraging the prognosis. A childhood history of withdrawn, reclusive, eccentric, and tense behavior is also an unfavorable diagnostic sign, as is a preponderance of negative symptoms (Möller, 2007).

Phases of Schizophrenia

Schizophrenia usually progresses through predictable phases, although the presenting symptoms during a given phase and the length of the phase can vary widely. The phases of schizophrenia are as follows (Chung et al., 2008; APA, 2004):

- **Phase I—Acute:** Onset or exacerbation of florid, disruptive symptoms (e.g., hallucinations, delusions, apathy, withdrawal) with resultant loss of functional abilities; increased care or hospitalization may be required.

- **Phase II—Stabilization:** Symptoms are diminishing, and there is movement toward one's previous level of functioning (baseline); day hospitalization or care in a residential crisis center or a supervised group home may be needed.
- **Phase III—Maintenance:** The patient is at or nearing baseline (or premorbid) functioning; symptoms are absent or diminished; level of functioning allows the patient to live in the community. Ideally, recovery with few or no residual symptoms has occurred. Most persons in this phase live in their own residences.

Some clinicians also designate an earlier **Prodromal (or Prepsychotic) Phase** in which subtle symptoms or deficits associated with schizophrenia are present; such symptoms may or may not herald the onset of schizophrenia.

APPLICATION OF THE NURSING PROCESS

ASSESSMENT

Nursing assessment of patients who have or may have a psychotic disorder focuses largely on symptoms, coping, functioning, and safety. Assessment involves interviewing the patient and observing behavior and other outward manifestations of the disorder. It also should include mental status and spiritual, cultural, biological, psychological, social, and environmental elements. Sound therapeutic communication skills, an understanding of the disorder and the ways patients may be experiencing their world, and establishing trustworthiness and a therapeutic nurse-patient relationship all strengthen the assessment.

During the Prepsychotic Phase

Experts believe that detection and treatment of symptoms that may warn of schizophrenia's onset lessens the risk of developing the disorder or the severity of the disorder if it does develop. A delay in diagnosis and treatment allows the psychotic process to become more entrenched; it can also result in relational, work, housing, and school problems (Riecher-Rössler et al., 2006).

Therefore, early assessment plays a key role in improving the prognosis for persons with schizophrenia (Chung et al., 2008). This form of primary prevention involves monitoring those at high risk (e.g., children of parents with schizophrenia) for symptoms such as abnormal social development and cognitive dysfunction. Intervening to reduce stressors (i.e., reduce or avoid exposure to triggers), enhancing social and coping skills (i.e., build resiliency), and prophylactic antipsychotic medication administration may also be of benefit (Bechdolf et al., 2006).

Similarly, in patients who have already developed the disorder, minimizing the onset and duration of relapses is believed to improve the prognosis. Research suggests that with each relapse of psychosis, there is an increase in residual dysfunction and deterioration. Recognition of the early warning signs of relapse—such as reduced sleep and concentration—followed by close monitoring and intensification of treatment is essential (van Meijel et al., 2004). For this reason, adherence to antipsychotics can be more important than the risk of side effects, because most side effects are reversible, whereas the consequences of relapse may not be.

General Assessment

Not all people with schizophrenia (or even people with the same subtype of the disorder) have the same symptoms, and some of the symptoms of schizophrenia are also found in other disorders. Figure 15-2 describes the four main symptom groups of schizophrenia:

1. **Positive symptoms:** the presence of something that is not normally present (e.g., hallucinations, delusions, bizarre behavior, paranoia)
2. **Negative symptoms:** the absence of something that should be present but is not (e.g., apathy, lack of motivation, anhedonia, and poor thought processes)
3. **Cognitive symptoms:** abnormalities in how a person thinks
4. **Affective symptoms:** symptoms involving emotions and their expression

The positive symptoms usually appear early in the illness, and their dramatic nature captures our attention and often precipitates hospitalization. They are also the symptoms most lay people associate with insanity, making schizophrenia the disorder most associated with being "crazy." However, positive psychotic symptoms are perhaps less important prognostically and usually respond to antipsychotic medication. The negative symptoms, however, tend to be persistent and crippling because they render the person inert and unmotivated. Box 15-2 gives a more detailed listing of the positive and negative symptoms of schizophrenia.

Positive Symptoms

Positive symptoms—such as hallucinations, delusions, bizarre behavior, and paranoia—are associated with:
- Acute onset
- Normal premorbid functioning
- Normal social functioning during remissions
- Normal CT findings
- Normal neuropsychological test results
- Favorable response to antipsychotic medication

The positive symptoms presented here are categorized as alterations in thinking, speech, perception, and behavior.

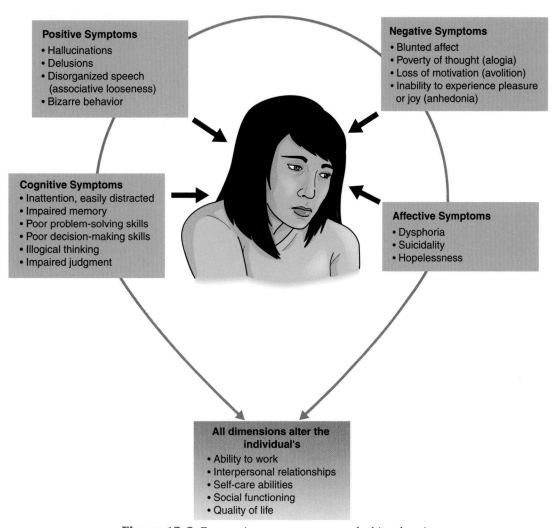

Positive Symptoms
• Hallucinations
• Delusions
• Disorganized speech
  (associative looseness)
• Bizarre behavior

Negative Symptoms
• Blunted affect
• Poverty of thought (alogia)
• Loss of motivation (avolition)
• Inability to experience pleasure
  or joy (anhedonia)

Cognitive Symptoms
• Inattention, easily distracted
• Impaired memory
• Poor problem-solving skills
• Poor decision-making skills
• Illogical thinking
• Impaired judgment

Affective Symptoms
• Dysphoria
• Suicidality
• Hopelessness

**All dimensions alter the
individual's**
• Ability to work
• Interpersonal relationships
• Self-care abilities
• Social functioning
• Quality of life

Figure 15-2 Four main symptom groups of schizophrenia.

Alterations in Thinking. All people experience occasional and momentary errors in thinking (e.g., "Why are all these lights turning red when I'm already late? Someone must be trying to slow me down!"), but most can catch and correct the error by using intact **reality testing**. People with impaired reality testing, however, maintain the error, which contributes to delusions. **Delusions** are false fixed beliefs that cannot be corrected by reasoning. A person experiencing delusions is convinced that what he or she believes to be real *is* real. Student nurses sometimes try unsuccessfully to argue a patient out of delusions by offering evidence of reality; this may irritate the patient and slow the development of a therapeutic relationship. Table 15-1 provides definitions and examples of frequent types of delusions.

About 75% of people with schizophrenia experience delusions at some time. The most common delusions are persecutory, grandiose, or those involving religious or hypochondriacal ideas. A delusion may be a response to anxiety or reflect areas of concern for a person; for example, someone with poor self-esteem may believe he is Beethoven or an emissary of God, allowing him to feel more powerful or important. Looking for and addressing such underlying themes or needs can be a key nursing intervention. At times, delusions hold a kernel of truth. One patient repeatedly told the staff that the Mafia was out to kill him. Later, staff learned that he had been selling drugs, had not paid his contacts, and gang members *were* trying to find him to hurt or even kill him.

Concrete thinking refers to an impaired ability to think abstractly. For example, the nurse might ask what brought the patient to the hospital, and the patient might answer, concretely, "a cab" (rather than explaining that he had attempted suicide). Concreteness is often assessed through the patient's interpretation of proverbs; a concrete interpretation of "The grass is always greener on the other side of the fence" would be "That side gets more sun, so it's greener there." Concreteness reduces one's ability to understand and address abstract concepts such as love or the passage of time.

BOX 15-2 Positive and Negative Symptoms of Schizophrenia

Positive Symptoms
Hallucinations
- Auditory
  - Voices commenting
  - Voices conversing
- Tactile
- Olfactory
- Gustatory
- Visual

Delusions
- Persecutory
- Jealousy
- Grandiose
- Religious
- Somatic
- Reference
- Being controlled
- Thought broadcasting, insertion, withdrawal

Bizarre Behavior
- Inappropriate clothing, appearance, and social/sexual behavior
- Aggressive, agitated behavior
- Repetitive, stereotyped behavior

Positive Formal Thought Disorder and Speech Patterns
- Disorganization
- Associative looseness
- Flight of ideas (FOI)
- Rapid or pressured speech
- Tangentiality
- Blocking
- Incoherence
- Illogicality
- Circumstantiality
- Distractibility
- Clang associations

- Concreteness
- Memory impairment

Inappropriate Affect
- Incongruent affect for situation
- Bizarre affect

Negative Symptoms
Affective Flattening
- Blunted or flattened affect
- Paucity of expressive gestures
- Lack of vocal inflections

Alogia
- Poverty of speech
- Poverty of content of speech

Avolition, Apathy
- Decreased spontaneous movement and behavior
- Inattention to grooming and hygiene
- Reduced task completion at work, home, or school
- Physical anergia

Anhedonia, Asociality
- Poor eye contact
- Few recreational interests or activities
- Reduced sexual interest or activity
- Impaired intimacy and closeness
- Reduced mirthfulness, joy
- Few relationships with friends or peers

Attention Deficits
- Social inattentiveness
- Impaired task completion

Other
- Reduced ability to "read" others' emotions or intent

Alterations in Speech. Associations are the threads that tie one thought logically to another. In associative looseness, these threads are interrupted or illogically connected; thinking becomes haphazard, illogical, and difficult to follow:

> **Nurse:** Are you going to the picnic today?
> **Patient:** I'm not an elephant hunter, no tiger teeth for me.

At times, the nurse may be able to decipher or decode the patient's messages and begin to understand the patient's feelings and needs. Any exchange in which a person feels understood is useful. Therefore, the nurse might respond to the patient in this way:

> **Nurse:** Are you saying that you're afraid to go out with the others today?
> **Patient:** Yeah…no tiger getting me today.

Sometimes it is not possible to understand what the patient may mean, because the patient's speech is too fragmented. For example:

> **Patient:** I sang out for my mother…for this to hell I went. These little hills hop aboard, share the Christmas mice spread…the devil will be washed away.

If the nurse does not understand what the patient is saying, it is important to let the patient know this. Clear messages and honesty are an important part of working effectively in psychiatric mental health

TABLE 15-1 Summary of Delusions*

Delusion	Definition	Example
Control	Believing that another person, group of people, or external force controls thoughts, feelings, impulses, or behavior	Brian always wears a hat so that aliens don't insert thoughts into his brain.
Ideas of Reference	Giving personal significance to trivial events; perceiving events as relating to you when they are not	When Maria saw staff talking together, she believed they were plotting against her.
Persecution	Believing that one is being singled out for harm by others; this belief often takes the form of a plot by people in power	Peter believed that the Secret Service was planning to kill him by poisoning his food. Therefore, he would only eat food he bought from machines.
Grandeur	Believing that one is a very powerful or important person	Sam believed he was a famous playwright and tennis pro.
Somatic Delusions	Believing that the body is changing in an unusual way (e.g., rotting inside)	David told the doctor that his heart had stopped and his insides were rotting away.
Erotomanic	Believing that another person desires you romantically	Although he barely knew her, Mary insisted that Mr. Johnson would marry her if only his current wife would stop interfering.
Jealousy	Believing that one's mate is unfaithful	Harry wrongly accused his girlfriend of going out with other men. His proof was that she came home from work late twice that week, even though the girlfriend's boss explained that everyone had worked late.

*A false belief held and maintained as true regardless of evidence to the contrary. This does not include sharing unusual beliefs maintained by one's culture or subculture.

nursing. An honest response lets the patient know that the nurse does not understand, would like to understand, and can be trusted to be honest.

Neologisms are made-up words (or idiosyncratic uses of existing words) that have meaning for the patient but a different or nonexistent meaning to others. ("I was going to tell him the *mannerologies* of his hospitality won't do.") This eccentric use of words represents disorganized thinking and interferes with communication.

Echolalia is the pathological repeating of another's words and is often seen in catatonia.

Nurse: Mary, come get your medication.

Mary: Come get your medication.

Echopraxia is the mimicking of *movements* of another. It is also seen in catatonia.

Clang association is the choice of words based on their sound rather than their meaning, often rhyming and sometimes having a similar beginning sound ("On the track...have a Big Mac;" "Click, clack, clutch, close"). Clanging may also be seen in neurological disorders.

Word salad is a jumble of words that is meaningless to the listener—and perhaps to the speaker as well—because of an extreme level of disorganization.

Alterations in Perception. Alterations in perception involve errors in how one perceives reality. The most common form of altered perception in psychosis is hallucination, but depersonalization and derealization are sometimes experienced as well.

Depersonalization is a nonspecific feeling that a person has lost his or her identity and that the self is different or unreal. People may feel that body parts do not belong to them or may suddenly sense that their body has drastically changed. For example, a patient may see her fingers as snakes or her arms as rotting wood.

Derealization is a false perception that the environment has changed. For example, everything seems bigger or smaller, or familiar surroundings have become somehow strange and unfamiliar. Both depersonalization and derealization can be interpreted as **loss of ego boundaries** (sometimes called *loose ego boundaries*).

Hallucinations involve perceiving a sensory experience for which no external stimulus exists (e.g., hearing a voice when no one is speaking). Hallucinations differ from **illusions** in that illusions are misperceptions or misinterpretations of a real experience; for example, a man sees his coat on a coat rack and believes it is a bear about to attack. He does see something real but misinterprets what it is.

Causes of hallucinations include psychiatric disorders, drug abuse, medications, organic disorders, hyperthermia, toxicity (e.g., digitalis), and other conditions. Types of hallucination include:

- **Auditory**—hearing voices or sounds
- **Visual**—seeing persons or things
- **Olfactory**—smelling odors
- **Gustatory**—experiencing tastes
- **Tactile**—feeling bodily sensations

Table 15-2 provides definitions and examples of these types of hallucinations.

Auditory hallucinations are experienced by up to 15% of persons without psychotic disorders and 60% of people with schizophrenia at some time during their lives (Hubl et al., 2004). Voices typically seem to come from outside the person's head, and auditory processing areas of the brain are activated during auditory hallucinations just as they are when a genuine external sound is heard (Hubl et al., 2004). This abnormal activation may cause hallucinations, but another leading theory is that "voices" are a misperception of one's internally-generated conversation (Hoffman & Varanko, 2006).

John Nash, the world-renowned mathematician portrayed in the film *A Beautiful Mind* (2001), describes the voices he heard during the acute phase of his illness:

> I thought of the voices as…something a little different from aliens. I thought of them more like angels…It's really my subconscious talking, it was really that…I know that now.

Voices may be of persons familiar or unknown, single or multiple. They may be perceived as supportive and pleasant or derogatory and frightening. Voices commenting on the person's behavior or conversing with the person are most common. A person who hears voices when no one is present often struggles to understand the experience, sometimes developing related delusions to explain the voices (e.g., the patient may believe the voices are from God, the devil, or deceased relatives). Persons with chronic hallucinations may attempt to cope by drowning them out with loud music or competing with them by talking loudly (Farhall et al., 2007).

Command hallucinations are "voices" that direct the person to take an action. All hallucinations must be assessed and monitored carefully, because the voices may command the person to hurt self or others. For example, voices might command a patient to "jump out the window" or "take a knife and kill my child." Command hallucinations are often terrifying and may herald a psychiatric emergency. In all cases, it is essential to assess what the patient hears, the patient's ability to recognize the hallucination as real or not real, and the patient's ability to resist any commands. Patients may falsely deny hallucinations, requiring behavioral assessment to support (validate) or refute the patient's report. Outward indications of possible hallucinations include turning or tilting the head as if to listen to someone, suddenly stopping current activity as if interrupted, and moving the lips silently.

Visual hallucinations occur less frequently in schizophrenia and are more likely to occur in organic disorders such as acute alcohol withdrawal or dementia. Olfactory, tactile, or gustatory hallucinations are unusual; when present, other physical sources should be investigated (Sadock & Sadock, 2008).

Boundary impairment is an impaired ability to sense where one's body ends and others' bodies begin. For example, a patient might drink another's beverage, believing that because it is in his vicinity, it is his.

Alterations in Behavior. Alterations in behavior include bizarre and agitated behaviors involving such things as stilted, rigid demeanor or eccentric dress,

TABLE 15-2 Summary of Hallucinations

Hallucination	Definition	Example
Auditory	Hearing voices or sounds that do not exist in the environment but are misperceptions of inner thoughts or feelings	John hit the ambulance attendant when a voice told him the attendant was taking him to a concentration camp.
Visual	Seeing a person, object, animal, colors, or visual patterns that do not exist in the environment	Charles became very frightened and screamed, "There are rats coming at me!"
Olfactory	Smelling odors that do not exist	Theresa "smells" her insides rotting.
Gustatory	Tasting sensations that do not exist	Sam will not eat his food because he "tastes" the poison they are putting in it.
Tactile	Feeling strange sensations on the skin where no external objects stimulate such feelings; common in delirium tremens	Jack "feels" electrical impulses tingling as they control his mind, and he covers his walls in tinfoil to block them out.

grooming, and rituals. Other behavioral changes seen in schizophrenia include:

- **Catatonia:** a pronounced increase or decrease in the rate and amount of movement; the most common form is stuporous behavior in which the person moves little or not at all.
- **Motor retardation:** a pronounced slowing of movement.
- **Motor agitation:** excited behavior such as running or pacing rapidly, often in response to internal or external stimuli; it can pose a risk to others and to the patient, who is at risk for exhaustion, collapse, and even death.
- **Stereotyped behaviors:** repeated motor behaviors that do not presently serve a logical purpose.
- **Automatic obedience:** the performance by a catatonic patient of all simple commands in a robot-like fashion.
- **Waxy flexibility:** the extended maintenance of posture, usually seen in catatonia. For example, the nurse raises the patient's arm, and the patient continues to hold this position in a statue-like manner.
- **Negativism:** akin to resistance but may not be intentional. In *active negativism*, the patient does the opposite of what he or she is told to do; *passive negativism* is a failure to do what is requested.
- **Impaired impulse control:** a reduced ability to resist one's impulses. Examples include socially inappropriate behaviors such as grabbing another's cigarette, throwing food on the floor, pushing staff, and changing TV channels while others are watching.

Negative Symptoms

Negative symptoms develop slowly and are those that most interfere with a person's adjustment and ability to cope. Negative symptoms impede one's ability to:

- Initiate and maintain conversations and relationships
- Obtain and maintain a job
- Make decisions and follow through on plans
- Maintain adequate hygiene and grooming

Negative symptoms contribute to poor social functioning and social withdrawal. During the acute phase, they are difficult to assess because positive symptoms (such as delusions and hallucinations) dominate. Selected negative symptoms are outlined in Table 15-3.

Affect is the observable behavior that indicates a person's emotional state. In schizophrenia, affect may not always coincide with inner emotions. Affect in schizophrenia can usually be categorized in one of four ways:

- **Flat**—immobile or blank facial expression
- **Blunted**—reduced or minimal emotional response
- **Inappropriate**—emotional response incongruent with the tone or circumstances of the situation (e.g., a man laughs when told that his father has died)
- **Bizarre**—odd, illogical, emotional state that is grossly inappropriate or unfounded; especially prominent in disorganized schizophrenia and includes grimacing and giggling

Cognitive Symptoms

Cognitive symptoms represent the third symptom dimension and are evident in most people with schizophrenia. They involve difficulty with attention, memory, information processing, cognitive flexibility, and executive functions (e.g., decision

TABLE 15-3 Negative Symptoms of Schizophrenia	
Negative Symptom	**Description**
Affective blunting	A reduction in the expression, range, and intensity of affect (In *flat affect*, no facial expression is present.)
Anergia	Lack of energy; passivity, lack of persistence at work or school
Anhedonia	Inability to experience pleasure in activities that usually produce it; result of profound emotional barrenness
Avolition	Reduced motivation; inability to initiate tasks such as social contacts, grooming, and other activities of daily living (ADLs)
Poverty of content of speech	While adequate in amount, speech conveys little information because of vagueness or superficiality
Poverty of speech	Reduced amount of speech—responses range from brief to one-word answers
Thought blocking	A sudden interruption in the thought process, usually due to internal stimuli *Example:* A patient abruptly stops talking in the middle of a sentence and remains silent. **Nurse:** What just happened now? **Patient:** I forgot what I was saying. Something took my thoughts away.

making, judgment, planning, and problem solving) (Braw et al., 2008). These impairments can leave the patient unable to manage personal health care, hold a job, initiate or maintain a support system, or live alone.

Affective Symptoms

Affective symptoms, the fourth dimension, are common and increase patients' suffering. Assessment for depression is crucial because it:

- May herald an impending relapse
- Increases substance abuse
- Increases suicide risk
- Further impairs functioning

Self-Assessment

Working with individuals with schizophrenia produces strong emotional reactions in most health care workers. The patient's intensely anxious, lonely, dependent, and distrustful presentation evokes similarly intense, uncomfortable, and frightening emotions in others. The chronicity, repeated exacerbations, and slow response to treatment many patients experience can lead to feelings of helplessness and powerlessness in staff. Patient behavior (especially violent behavior) can produce strong emotional responses (called *countertransference*) such as fear or anger (see Chapter 9).

Without support and the opportunity and willingness to explore these feelings with more experienced staff, the nurse may adopt nontherapeutic behaviors—denial, withdrawal, patient avoidance, and anger most commonly. These behaviors thwart the patient's progress and undermine the nurse's self-esteem. Comments such as "These patients are hopeless," and "All you can do is babysit these people" are indications of unrecognized or unresolved countertransference that, if left uncorrected, interfere with both treatment and work satisfaction. Examining whether one's expectations of patients are realistic and seeking new ways of helping patients can help staff overcome feelings of helplessness and reduce countertransference.

Patients may experience fear, stigma, or shame related to their mental illness, leading them to conceal some aspects of their experience. Negativism and alogia (reduced verbalization) can also limit patient responses. Many patients with schizophrenia experience anosognosia, an inability to realize they are ill that is caused by the illness itself. The resulting lack of insight can make assessment (and treatment) challenging, delaying completion of a full assessment and requiring additional skills on the part of the nurse. Selected techniques that may help you overcome these challenges can be found in Table 15-4.

Assessment Guidelines Schizophrenia and Other Psychotic Disorders

1. Determine if the patient has had a medical workup. Are there any indications of medical problems that might mimic psychosis (e.g., digitalis or anticholinergic toxicity, brain trauma, drug intoxication, delirium, fever)?
2. Assess whether the patient abuses or is dependent on alcohol or drugs.
3. Assess for risk to self or others.
4. Assess for command hallucinations (e.g., voices telling the person to harm self or another). If present, ask the patient:
   - Do you recognize the voices?
   - Do you believe the voices are real?
   - Do you plan to follow the command? (A positive response to any of these questions suggests an increased risk that the patient will act on the commands.)
5. Assess the patient's belief system. Is it fragmented or poorly organized? Is it systematized? Are the beliefs delusional? If yes, then:
   - Does the patient feel that he or loved ones are being threatened or in danger?
   - Does the patient feel the need to act against a person or organization to protect or avenge himself or loved ones? (A positive response to either of these questions suggests an increased risk of danger to others.)
6. Assess for suicide risk (see Chapters 9 and 24).
7. Assess for ability to ensure self safety, addressing:
   - Adequacy of food and fluid intake
   - Hygiene and self-care
   - Handling of potentially hazardous activities, such as smoking and cooking
   - Ability to transport self safely
   - Impulse control and judgment
   - Appropriate dress for weather conditions
8. Assess for co-occurring disorders:
   - Depression
   - Anxiety
   - Substance abuse or dependency
   - Medical disorders (especially brain trauma, toxicity, delirium, cardiovascular disease, obesity, and diabetes)
9. Assess medications the patient has been prescribed, whether and how the patient is taking the medications, and what factors (e.g., costs, mistrust of staff, side effects) are affecting adherence.
10. Assess for the presence and severity of positive and negative symptoms. Complete a mental status examination, noting which

Assessment Guidelines Schizophrenia and
Other Psychotic Disorders—cont'd

symptoms are present, how they affect functioning, and how the patient is managing them.

11. Assess the patient's insight, knowledge of the illness, relationships and support systems, other coping resources, and strengths.

12. Assess the family's knowledge of and response to the patient's illness and its symptoms. Are family members overprotective? Hostile? Anxious? Are they familiar with family support groups and respite resources?

DIAGNOSIS

People with schizophrenia have multiple disturbing and disabling symptoms that require a multifaceted approach to care and treatment of both the patient and the family. Table 15-5 lists potential nursing diagnoses for a person with schizophrenia.

OUTCOMES IDENTIFICATION

Desired outcomes vary with the phase of the illness. *Nursing Outcomes Classification (NOC)* (Moorhead et al., 2008) is a useful guide. Ideally, outcomes

TABLE 15-4 Interventions for Overcoming Obstacles to Assessment

Intervention	Rationale	Example
Use empathic comments and observations to prompt the patient to provide information.	Empathy conveys understanding and builds trust and rapport.	**Nurse:** "It must be difficult to find yourself in a psych hospital." **Patient:** "Yes...I'm frightened."
Minimize questioning, especially closed-ended questioning. Seek data conversationally using prompts and open-ended questions.	Extended questioning can increase suspiciousness, and closed questions elicit minimal information. Both become wearying and off-putting.	"Could you please tell me more about...?" "Tell me what life has been like for you lately."
Directly but supportively seek the needed information, explaining the reasons for the assessment.	Being direct but supportive conveys genuineness, builds rapport, and helps reduce anxiety.	"I know we have not known each other very long, but you seem very sad, and sometimes sad people think about hurting themselves. So it is important for me to find out if you are safe. Have you ever thought about hurting yourself?"
Judiciously use indirect, supportive (therapeutic) confrontation.	Blunt contradiction or premature confrontation increases resistance.	"I realize admitting to voices might be difficult to do, but although you say you do not hear voices, I notice you talking as if to others when no one is there."
Seek other data to support (validate) the patient's report (obtain further history from third parties, past medical records, and other treatment providers when possible), preferably with the patient's permission.	Patients may be unable or unwilling to provide information fully and reliably. Validating their reports assures the validity of the assessment.	"Your brother reports he works at a factory. Is that your understanding?"
Prioritize the data you seek, and avoid seeking nonessential data.	Patients may have limited tolerance for the assessment interview and answer only a limited amount of inquiries. Seeking nonessential information does not benefit the patient or assessment.	**Patient:** "I hate school! I wish they'd all die!" **Nurse:** (less-therapeutic) "Which school do you go to?" **Nurse:** (more-therapeutic) "Things would be better if they were dead..." (Paraphrasing prompts patient elaboration and confirmation/refutation of the comment.)

TABLE 15-5 Potential Nursing Diagnoses for Schizophrenia

Symptom	Nursing Diagnoses
POSITIVE SYMPTOMS	
Hears voices that others do not (auditory hallucinations)	Disturbed sensory perception: auditory
Hears voices telling him or her to hurt self or others (command hallucinations)	Risk for self-directed violence Risk for other-directed violence
Delusions	Disturbed thought processes*
Shows loose association of ideas (associative looseness) Conversation is derailed by unnecessary and tedious details (circumstantiality)	Disturbed thought processes* Impaired verbal communication
NEGATIVE SYMPTOMS	
Uncommunicative, withdrawn Expresses feelings of rejection or aloneness (lies in bed all day, positions back to door)	Social isolation Impaired social interaction Risk for loneliness
Talks about self as "bad" or "no good" Feels guilty because of "bad thoughts"; extremely sensitive to real or perceived slights	Chronic low self-esteem Risk for self-directed violence
Shows lack of energy (anergia) Shows lack of motivation (avolition), unable to initiate tasks (social contact, grooming, and other aspects of daily living)	Ineffective coping Self-care deficit (bathing, dressing, feeding, toileting) Constipation
OTHER	
Families and significant others become confused or overwhelmed, lack knowledge about disorder or treatment, feel powerless in coping with patient	Compromised family coping Caregiver role strain Deficient knowledge
Stops taking medication (because of anosognosia, side effects, drugs costs, mistrust of staff), stops going to therapy, is not supported in treatment by significant others	Nonadherence

Data from North American Nursing Diagnosis Association International (NANDA-I) (2009). *NANDA-I nursing diagnoses: Definitions and classification 2009–2011*. Oxford, United Kingdom: Author.
*Diagnosis retired from North American Nursing Diagnosis Association. (2007). *NANDA-I nursing diagnoses: Definitions and classification 2007–2008*. Philadelphia: Author.

should focus on enhancing strengths and minimizing the effects of the patient's deficits and symptoms. Outcomes should be consistent with the recovery model (see Chapter 30), which stresses hope, living a full and productive life, and eventual recovery rather than focusing on controlling symptoms and adapting to disability.

Phase I—Acute

For the acute phase, the overall goal is **patient safety and medical stabilization**. Therefore, if the patient is at risk for violence to self or others, initial outcome criteria address safety issues (e.g., *patient refrains from self injury*). Another outcome is *patient consistently labels hallucinations as "not real—a symptom of an illness."* Table 15-6 gives selected short-term and interme-

diate indicators for the outcome *Distorted Thought Self-Control*.

Phase II—Stabilization

Outcome criteria during phase II focus on helping the patient adhere to treatment, become stabilized on medications, and control or cope with symptoms. The outcomes target the negative symptoms and may include ability to succeed in social, vocational, or self-care activities.

Phase III—Maintenance

Outcome criteria for phase III focus on maintaining achievement, preventing relapse, and achieving independence and a satisfactory quality of life.

TABLE 15-6 *NOC* Outcomes Realted to Distorted Thought Self-Control		
Nursing Outcome and Definition	**Intermediate Indicators**	**Short-Term Indicators**
Distorted Thought Self-Control: Self-restraint of disruptions in perception, thought processes, and thought content	Maintains affect consistent with mood Interacts appropriately Perceives environment and the ideas of others accurately Exhibits logical thought flow patterns Exhibits reality-based thinking Exhibits appropriate thought content	Recognizes that hallucinations or delusions are occurring Refrains from attending to and responding to hallucinations or delusions Describes content of hallucinations or delusions Reports decrease in hallucinations or delusions Asks for validation of reality

Data from Moorhead, S., Johnson, H., Maas, M., & Swanson, E. (2008). *Nursing outcomes classification (NOC)* (4th ed.). St. Louis: Mosby.

PLANNING

The planning of appropriate interventions is guided by the phase of the illness and the strengths and needs of the patient. It is influenced by cultural considerations, available resources, and patient preferences.

Phase I—Acute

Hospitalization is indicated if the patient is considered a danger to self or others, refuses to eat or drink, or is too disorganized or otherwise impaired to function safely in the community without supervision. The planning process focuses on the best strategies to ensure patient safety and provide symptom stabilization.

In discharge planning, the patient and multidisciplinary treatment team identify aftercare needs for follow-up and support. Discharge planning considers not only external factors, such as the patient's living arrangements, economic resources, social supports, and family relationships, but also internal factors, such as resilience and repertoire of coping skills. Because relapse can be devastating to the patient's circumstances (resulting in loss of employment, housing, and relationships) and worsen the long-term prognosis, vigorous efforts are made to connect the patient and family with (not simply refer them to) community resources that provide therapeutic programming and social, financial, and other needed support.

Phase II—Stabilization/Phase III—Maintenance

Planning during the stabilization and maintenance phases focuses on providing patient and family education and skills training (psychosocial education).

Relapse prevention skills are vital. Planning identifies interpersonal, coping, health care, and vocational needs and addresses how and where these needs can best be met within the community.

IMPLEMENTATION

Interventions are geared toward the phase of schizophrenia the patient is experiencing. For example, during the acute phase, the clinical focus is on crisis intervention, medication for symptom stabilization, and safety. Interventions are often hospital based; however, many patients in the acute stage increasingly are being treated in the community.

Phase I—Acute

Settings

A number of factors that affect the choice of treatment setting include the following (APA, 2004):
- Level of care/restrictiveness needed to protect the person from harm to self or others
- Patient's needs for external structure and support
- Patient's ability to cooperate with treatment
- Need for a particular treatment available only in particular settings
- Need for treatment of a concurrent medical condition
- Availability of supportive others who can provide critical information and treatment history to staff and permit stabilization in less restrictive settings

The use of less restrictive and more cost-effective alternatives to hospitalization that work for many patients include:
- **Partial hospitalization:** Patients sleep at home and attend treatment sessions (similar to what

they would receive if admitted) during the day or evening.

- **Residential crisis centers:** Patients who are unable to remain in the community but do not require full inpatient services can be admitted (usually for 1 to 14 days) to receive increased supervision, guidance, and medication stabilization.
- **Halfway houses:** Patients live in the community with a group of other patients, sharing expenses and responsibilities. Staff are present in the house 24 hours a day, 7 days a week to provide supervision and therapeutic activities.
- **Day treatment programs:** Patients reside in the community and attend structured programming during the day.

These programs may include group and individual therapy, supervised activities, and specialized skill training. It is vital that staff be aware of these and other community resources and make this information available to discharged patients and their families, ideally by directly connecting them with these resources. Patients and family members should be given telephone numbers and addresses of local support groups that are affiliated with the National Alliance on Mental Illness (NAMI) (www.nami.org).

Other community resources include community mental health centers (usually providing medication services, day treatment, access to 24-hour emergency services, psychotherapy, psychoeducation, and case management), home health services, supported employment programs (wherein patients receive services from job training to on-site coaches who help them learn to succeed in the work environment, often via the Bureau of Vocational Rehabilitation [BVR]), peer-led services (e.g., drop-in centers, sometimes called "clubhouses," that offer social contact, constructive activities, and sometimes employment opportunities), family educational/skills groups (e.g., NAMI's "Family-to-Family" program), and respite care for caregivers.

Interventions

Acute phase interventions include:
- Psychiatric, medical, and neurological evaluation
- Psychopharmacological treatment
- Support, psychoeducation, and guidance
- Supervision and limit setting in the milieu

The length of hospitalization or other intensive treatment programs during the acute phase is often short (days). As soon as the acute symptoms are adequately stabilized, the patient is discharged to the community, where appropriate treatment can be continued during the stabilization and maintenance phases.

Phase II—Stabilization/Phase III—Maintenance

Effective long-term care of an individual with schizophrenia relies on a three-pronged approach: medication administration/adherence, nursing intervention, and community support. **Family psychoeducation, a key role of the nurse, is an essential intervention**. All interventions and strategies are geared to the patient's strengths, culture, personal preferences, and needs.

Milieu Management

Effective hospital care provides (1) protection from stressful or disruptive environments and (2) structure; patients in the acute phase of schizophrenia show greater improvement in a structured milieu than on an open unit that allows more freedom. Hospital alternatives (e.g., crisis centers) also provide a structured milieu. A therapeutic milieu is consciously designed to maximize safety, opportunities for learning skills, therapeutic activities, and access to resources. The milieu also provides guidance, supportive peer contact, and opportunities for practicing conflict resolution, stress reduction techniques, and dealing with symptoms.

Activities and Groups

Participation in activities and groups appropriate to the patient's level of functioning may decrease withdrawal, enhance motivation, modify unacceptable behaviors, develop friendships, and increase social competence. Activities such as drawing, reading poetry, and listening to music are used to focus conversation and promote the recognition and expression of feelings. Self-esteem is enhanced as patients experience successful task completion. Recreational activities such as picnics and outings to stores and restaurants are not simply diversions; they teach constructive leisure skills, increase social comfort, facilitate growth in social concern and interactional skills, and enhance the ability to develop boundaries and set limits on self and others. After discharge, group therapy can provide necessary structure within the patient's community milieu.

Safety

A small percentage of patients with schizophrenia, especially during the acute phase, may exhibit a risk for physical violence, typically in response to hallucinations, delusions, paranoia, impaired judgment or impulse control, or self-referentiality (believing neutral, everyday occurrences carry special personal meaning). When the potential for violence exists, measures to protect the patient and others become the priority. Interventions include increasing staff supervision, reducing stimulation (e.g., noise, crowds), addressing paranoia and other contributing symptoms, providing constructive diversion and outlets for physical energy, teaching and practicing coping skills, implementing cognitive-behavioral approaches (to correct unrealistic expectations or selectively extinguish aggression), de-escalating tension verbally, and when necessary, using seclusion or chemical (medication) or physical restraints. Refer to Chapter 25 for a more detailed discussion of caring for the aggressive patient, seclusion, and restraints.

Counseling and Communication Techniques

Therapeutic communication techniques for patients with schizophrenia aim to lower the patient's anxiety, build trust, encourage clear communication by the patient, decrease defensiveness, encourage interaction, enhance self-esteem, and reinforce skills such as reality testing and assertiveness. It is important to remember that patients with schizophrenia may have memory impairment and require repetition. They may also have limited tolerance for interaction, owing to the stimulation it creates. Therefore, shorter (<30 minutes) but more frequent interactions may be more therapeutic. Interventions for paranoia and other selected presentations are discussed later in this chapter.

Hallucinations

When a patient is having a hallucination, the nursing focus is on understanding the patient's experiences and responses. Suicidal or homicidal themes or commands necessitate appropriate safety measures. For example, "voices" that tell a patient a particular individual plans to harm him may lead him to act aggressively against that person; one-to-one supervision of the patient or transfer of the potential victim to another unit is often essential.

Hallucinations are real to the person who is experiencing them and may be distracting during nurse-patient interactions. Call the patient by name, speak simply but in a louder voice than usual, approach the patient in a nonthreatening and nonjudgmental manner, maintain eye contact, and redirect the patient's focus to the conversation as needed (Farhall et al., 2007). Box 15-3 lists other techniques for communicating with patients experiencing hallucinations.

Delusions

Delusions may be the patient's attempts to understand confusion and distorted experiences. They reflect the misperception of one's circumstances, which go uncorrected in schizophrenia due to impaired reality testing. When as a nurse, you attempt to see the world through the eyes of the patient, it is easier to understand the patient's delusional experience. For example:

BOX 15-3 Guidelines for Communication with Patients Experiencing Hallucinations

- Ask the patient directly about the hallucinations. Example: "Are you hearing voices?" followed by "What are you hearing?"
- Watch the patient for cues that he or she is hallucinating, such as eyes darting to one side, muttering, appearing distracted, or watching a vacant area of the room.
- Avoid reacting to hallucinations as if they are real. Do not argue back to the voices.
- Do not negate the patient's experience, but offer your own perceptions. Example: "I don't see the devil standing over you, but I understand how upsetting that must be for you."
- Focus on reality-based, "here-and-now" diversions such as conversations or simple projects. Tell the patient, "The voice you hear is part of your illness; it cannot hurt you. Try to listen to me and the others you can see around you."
- Be alert to signs of anxiety in the patient, which may indicate that hallucinations are increasing.

Data from Farhall, J., Greenwood, K. M., & Jackson, H. J. (2007). Coping with hallucinated voices in schizophrenia: A review of self-initiated strategies and therapeutic interventions. *Clinical Psychology Review, 27,* 476–493.

Patient: You people are all alike...all in on the FBI plot to destroy me.

Nurse: I don't want to hurt you, Tom. Thinking that people are out to destroy you must be very frightening.

In this example, the nurse acknowledges the patient's experience, conveys empathy about the patient's fearfulness, avoids focusing on the content of the delusion (FBI and plot to destroy), but labels the patient's feelings so they can be explored as tolerated. Note that talking about the feelings is helpful, but extended focus on delusional material is not.

It is *never* useful to debate or attempt to dissuade the patient regarding the delusion. Doing so can intensify the patient's retention of irrational beliefs and cause the patient to view you as rejecting or oppositional. However, it *is* helpful to clarify misinterpretations of the environment and gently suggest, as tolerated, a more reality-based perspective. For example:

Patient: I see the doctor is here; he is out to destroy me.

Nurse: It is true the doctor wants to see you, but he wants to talk to you about your treatment. Would you feel more comfortable talking to him in the day room?

Focusing on specific reality-based activities and events in the environment helps to minimize the focus

BOX 15-4 Guidelines for Communication with Patients Experiencing Delusions

- To build trust, be open, honest, and reliable.
- Respond to suspicions in a matter-of-fact, empathic, supportive, and calm manner.
- Ask the patient to describe the delusions. Example: "Tell me more about someone trying to hurt you."
- Avoid debating the delusional content, but interject doubt where appropriate. Example: "It seems like it would be hard for that petite girl to hurt you."
- Focus on the feelings that underlie or flow from the delusions. Example: "You seem to wish you could be more powerful," or "It must feel frightening to think others want to hurt you."
- Once it is understood and addressed, do not dwell further on the delusion. Instead, focus on more reality-based topics. If the patient obsesses about delusions, set firm limits on the amount of time you will talk about them, and explain your reason.
- Observe for events that trigger delusions. If possible, help the patient find ways to reduce or manage them.
- Validate if part of the delusion is real. Example: "Yes, there was a man at the nurse's station, but I did not hear him talk about you."

Data from Farhall, J., Greenwood, K. M., & Jackson, H. J. (2007). Coping with hallucinated voices in schizophrenia: A review of self-initiated strategies and therapeutic interventions. *Clinical Psychology Review, 27*, 476–493.

BOX 15-5 Patient and Family Teaching: Coping with Auditory Hallucinations or Delusions

Distraction
- Listening to music
- Reading (aloud may help more)
- Counting backwards from 100
- Watching television

Interaction
- Looking at others—do they seem to be hearing/fearing what you are? If not, ignore the voices/thoughts.
- Talking with another person

Activity
- Walking
- Cleaning the house
- Having a relaxing bath
- Playing the guitar or singing
- Going to the gym (or anyplace you enjoy being, where others will be present)

Talking to Yourself
- Telling the voices or thoughts to go away
- Telling yourself that the voices and thoughts are a symptom and not real
- Telling yourself that no matter what you hear, voices can be safely ignored

Social Action
- Talking to a trusted friend or member of the family
- Calling a help line or going to a drop-in center
- Visiting a favorite place or a comfortable public place

Physical Action
- Taking extra medication when ordered (call your prescriber)
- Going for a walk or doing other exercise
- Using breathing exercises and other relaxation methods

Data from Farhall, J., Greenwood, K. M., & Jackson, H. J. (2007). Coping with hallucinated voices in schizophrenia: A review of self-initiated strategies and therapeutic interventions. *Clinical Psychology Review, 27*, 476-493; and Jenner, J. A., Neinhuis, F. J., van de Willige, G., & Wiersma, D. (2006). "Hitting" voices of schizophrenia patients may lastingly reduce persistent auditory hallucinations and their burden: 18-month outcome of a randomized controlled trial. *Canadian Journal of Psychiatry, 51*(3), 169–177.

on delusional thoughts. The more time the patient spends engaged in activities or with people, the more opportunities there are to receive feedback about and become comfortable with reality.

Work with the patient to find out which coping strategies succeed and how the patient can make the best use of them. Box 15-4 lists techniques for communicating with patients experiencing delusions, and Box 15-5 presents patient and family teaching topics for coping with hallucinations and delusions.

Associative Looseness

Associative looseness often mirrors the patient's autistic thoughts and reflects poorly organized thinking. An increase in associative looseness often indicates that the patient is feeling increased anxiety or overwhelmed by internal and external stimuli. The patient's ramblings may also produce confusion and frustration in the nurse. The following guidelines are useful for intervention with a patient whose speech is confused and disorganized:

- Do *not* pretend you understand the patient's words or meaning when you don't; tell the patient you are having difficulty understanding.
- Place the difficulty in understanding on yourself, *not* on the patient. Example: "I'm having trouble following what you are saying," *not* "You're not making any sense."
- Look for recurring topics and *themes* in the patient's communications, and *tie these to events*

and timelines. Example: "You've mentioned trouble with your brother several times, usually after your family has visited. Tell me about your brother and your visits with him."

- Summarize or paraphrase the patient's communications to role-model more effective ways of making his point and to give the patient a chance to correct anything you may have misunderstood.
- Reduce stimuli in the vicinity, and speak concisely, clearly, and concretely.
- Tell the patient what you *do* understand, and reinforce clear communication and accurate expression of needs, feelings, and thoughts.

Health Teaching and Health Promotion

Education is an essential strategy and includes teaching the patient and family about the illness, including possible causes, medications and medication side effects, coping strategies, what to expect, and prevention of relapse. Understanding these things helps the patient and family to recognize the impact of stress, enhances their understanding of the importance of treatment to a good outcome, encourages involvement in (and support of) therapeutic activities, and identifies resources for consultation and ongoing support in dealing with the illness.

Including family members in any strategies aimed at reducing psychotic symptoms reduces family anxiety and distress and enables the family to reinforce staff's efforts. The family plays an important role in the stability of the patient. The patient who returns to a warm, concerned, and supportive environment is less likely to experience relapse. An environment in which people are critical or their involvement in the patient's life is intrusive is associated with relapse and poorer outcomes.

Lack of understanding of the disease and its symptoms can lead others to misinterpret the patient's apathy and lack of drive as laziness, fostering a hostile response by family members, caregivers, or community. Thus public education about the symptoms of schizophrenia can reduce tensions in families, as well as communities. The most effective education occurs over time and is available when the family is most receptive (Weisman et al., 2006). Box 15-6 offers guidelines for patient and family teaching about schizophrenia.

BOX 15-6 Patient and Family Teaching: Schizophrenia

1. Learn all you can about the illness.
   - Attend psychoeducational and support groups.
   - Join the National Alliance on Mental Illness (NAMI).
   - Contact the National Institute of Mental Health (NIMH).
2. Develop a relapse prevention plan.
   - Know the early warning signs of relapse (e.g., avoiding others, trouble sleeping, troubling thoughts).
   - Know whom to call, what to do, and where to go when early signs of relapse appear. Make a list and keep it with you.
   - Relapse is part of the illness, not a sign of failure.
3. Take advantage of all psychoeducational tools.
   - Participate in family, group, and individual therapy.
   - Learn new ways to act and coping skills to help handle family, work, and social stress. Get information from your nurse, case manager, doctor, NAMI, community mental health groups, or a hospital.
   - Have a plan, on paper, of what to do to cope with stressful times.
   - Everyone needs a place to address their fears and losses and to learn new ways of coping.
4. Adhere to treatment.
   - People who adhere to treatment that works for them do the best in coping with the disorder.

- Engaging in struggles over adherence does not help, but tying adherence to the patient's own goals does. ("Staying in treatment will help you keep your job and avoid trouble with the police.")
- Share concerns about troubling side effects or concerns (e.g., sexual problems, weight gain, "feeling funny") with your nurse, case manager, doctor, or social worker; most side effects can be helped.
- Keeping side effects a secret or stopping medication can prevent you from having the life you want.
5. Avoid alcohol and/or drugs; they can act on the brain and cause a relapse.
6. Keep in touch with supportive people.
7. Keep healthy—stay in balance.
   - Taking care of one's diet, health, and hygiene helps prevent medical illnesses.
   - Maintain a regular sleep pattern.
   - Keep active (hobbies, friends, groups, sports, job, special interests).
   - Nurture yourself, and practice stress-reduction activities daily.

Data from *Beyond symptom control: Moving towards positive patient outcomes*. Paper presented at the American Psychiatric Association 55th Institute on Psychiatric Services, 10/29-11/2/2003, Boston, MA. <www.medscape.com/viewprogram/2835_pnt> Accessed 21.01.05.
Further information can be found in the Substance Abuse and Mental Health Services Administration (SAMHSA) pamphlet *Developing A Recovery And Wellness Lifestyle: A Self-Help Guide*, available at http://mentalhealth.samhsa.gov/publications/allpubs/SMA-3718 or via the Wellness Recovery Action Plan (WRAP) website (M. A. Copeland and staff): www.mentalhealthrecovery.com

INTEGRATIVE THERAPY
Yoga as an Adjunctive Treatment for Schizophrenia

Social and occupational functioning is a problem for people with schizophrenia. Studies indicate that yoga, in conjunction with conventional medical treatment, may improve symptoms of schizophrenia, social and occupational functioning, and quality of life. Yoga is based on an ancient Indian spiritual practice that has been reported to improve the connection between the mind, body, and spirit.

In a randomized controlled study by Duraiswamy and colleagues (2007), 61 patients with a diagnosis of schizophrenia participated in a study that compared the efficacy of physical exercise (stretching and aerobic) and yoga. Participants were supervised as they performed one or the other and also practiced independently for 1 hour each day. After 4 months, both groups experienced symptom reduction, but subjects who had practiced yoga had greater improvement in both negative symptoms of schizophrenia and psychological quality of life.

Machleidt and Ziegenbein (2008) found that yoga together with traditional medical treatment improved not only quality of life but also occupational and social functioning. Another randomized controlled study (Koss-Chioino, 2008) focused on 45 people with schizophrenia who were assigned to either a physical exercise group (brisk walking and jogging) or a traditional yoga group for 1 hour 5 times a week. Both groups functioned better in terms of symptoms of schizophrenia and social and occupational functioning, but people in the yoga group did better for overall quality of life measures.

Yoga is a promising adjunctive treatment for schizophrenia that provides participants with an essential experience of grounding, especially in distinguishing themselves from the outside world. It may be the centering quality of the breathing work, in particular, that improves the interrelationship of mind, body, and spirit.

Duraiswamy, G., Thirhalli, J., Nagendra, H. R., & Gandahar, B. N. (2007). Yoga therapy as an add-on treatment in the management of patients with schizophrenia—a randomized controlled trial. *Acta Psychiatrica Scandinavica, 3,* 226–32.
Koss-Chioino, J. D. (2008). Complementary and alternative treatments in mental health care. Journal of Nervous and Mental Disease, 196, 468–474.
Machleidt, W., & Ziegenbein, M. (2008). Complementary and alternative treatments. Acta Psychiatrica Scandinavica, 117, 397–398.

Pharmacological Interventions

Drugs used to treat psychotic disorders, **antipsychotics**, first became available in the 1950s. Before that time, the available medications provided only sedation, not treatment of the disorder itself. Until the 1960s, patients who had even one episode of schizophrenia usually spent months or years in state or private hospitals. Psychotic episodes resulted in great emotional and financial burdens to families and patients. The advent of antipsychotic drugs at last provided symptom control and allowed patients to be managed in the community.

Two groups of antipsychotic drugs exist: **conventional antipsychotics** (traditional dopamine antagonists [D_2 dopamine receptor antagonists]), also known as *typical* or *first-generation antipsychotics*, and **atypical antipsychotics** (serotonin-dopamine antagonists [$5\text{-}HT_{2A}$ receptor antagonists]), also known as *second-generation antipsychotics*. Newer "third-generation" drugs (aripiprazole [now available] and bifeprunox [pending]) give hope for enhanced effectiveness and side-effect reduction (Wadenberg, 2007). Other drugs, such as anticonvulsants and antiparkinsonian drugs, are used to augment antipsychotics for patients who do not respond fully. For example, D-serine—an amino acid that enhances NMDA activity—has been shown to increase the effectiveness of selected antipsychotics (Heresco-Levy et al., 2005).

All antipsychotics are effective for most exacerbations of schizophrenia and for reduction or mitigation of relapse. The conventional antipsychotics affect primarily the positive symptoms of schizophrenia (e.g., hallucinations, delusions, disordered thinking, etc.). The atypical antipsychotics can improve negative symptoms (e.g., asociality, blunted affect, lack of motivation) as well.

Antipsychotic agents usually take effect 2 to 6 weeks after the regimen is started. Only about 10% of patients with schizophrenia fail to respond to antipsychotic drug therapy; such patients should not continue to take medication that holds only risks and no benefit for them.

Atypical Antipsychotics

Atypical antipsychotics first emerged in the early 1990s with clozapine (Clozaril). Unfortunately, clozapine produces agranulocytosis in 0.8% to 1% of those who take it and also increases the risk for seizures. Clozapine produced dramatic improvement in some patients whose disorder had been resistant to the earlier antipsychotics. Due to the risk for agranulocytosis, however, patients taking clozapine must have weekly white blood cell counts for the first 6 months, then frequent monitoring thereafter, to obtain the medication. As a result, clozapine use is declining.

Atypicals are often chosen as first-line antipsychotics because they treat both the positive and negative symptoms of schizophrenia. Furthermore, they produce minimal to no extrapyramidal side effects (EPSs) or tardive dyskinesia. Side effects tend to be significantly less and result in greater adherence to treatment.

Atypical antipsychotics include risperidone (Risperdal), olanzapine (Zyprexa), quetiapine (Seroquel), ziprasidone (Geodon), and aripiprazole (Abilify), which technically is a third-generation drug. These atypicals are free of the potential hematological side effects of clozapine and are all first-line agents because of their lower side-effect profile.

One significant disadvantage of the atypicals, with the exception of ziprasidone and aripiprazole, is that they have a tendency to cause significant weight gain. Metabolic syndrome—which includes weight gain,

dyslipidemia, and altered glucose metabolism—is a significant concern in most atypicals and increases the risk of diabetes, hypertension, and atherosclerotic heart disease (Tschoner et al., 2007). An additional disadvantage of atypicals is that they are more expensive than conventional antipsychotics. Table 15-7 lists the classification, route, and side-effect profile of the anti-psychotic drugs.

Conventional Antipsychotics

Conventional antipsychotics are antagonists at the D_2 dopamine receptor site in both the limbic and motor centers. This blockage of D_2 dopamine receptor sites in the motor areas causes extrapyramidal side effects (EPSs), which include akathisia, acute dystonias, pseudoparkinsonism, and tardive dyskinesia. Other adverse reactions include anticholinergic effects, orthostasis, photosensitivity, and lowered seizure threshold.

TABLE 15-7 Antipsychotic Drugs: Classification, Route, and Side-Effect Profile

Generic (Brand)	Route	EPSs	Sedation	OH	ACh	Weight Gain	Diabetes
ATYPICAL ANTIPSYCHOTICS–TREAT POSITIVE AND NEGATIVE SYMPTOMS							
Aripiprazole (Abilify)	PO	Very low	Low	Low	None	Low	Low
Clozapine (Clozaril)	PO	Very low	High	Moderate	High	High	High
Olanzapine (Zyprexa)	PO, IM	Very low	High	Moderate	High	High	High
Paliperidone (Invega)	PO	Moderate	Low	Low	None	Moderate	*
Quetiapine (Seroquel)	PO	Very low	Moderate	Moderate	None	Moderate	Moderate
Risperidone (Risperdal)	PO, IM	Very low	Low	Low	None	Moderate	Moderate
Ziprasidone (Geodon)	PO, IM	Moderate	Moderate	Moderate	None	Low	Low
CONVENTIONAL ANTIPSYCHOTICS–TREAT POSITIVE SYMPTOMS							
Low Potency							
Chlorpromazine (Thorazine)	PO, IM, IV, R	Moderate	High	High	Moderate	Moderate	—
Thioridazine (Mellaril)	PO	Low	High	High	High	Moderate	—
Medium Potency							
Loxapine (Loxitane)	PO	Moderate	Moderate	Low	Low	Low	—
Molindone (Moban)	PO	Moderate	Moderate	Low	Low	Low	—
Perphenazine (Trilafon)	PO	Moderate	Moderate	Low	Low	—	—
High Potency							
Trifluoperazine (generic only)	PO, IM	High	Low	Low	Low	—	—
Thiothixene (Navane)	PO	High	Low	Moderate	Low	Moderate	—
Fluphenazine (Prolixin)	PO, IM	High	Low	Low	Low	—	—
Haloperidol (Haldol)	PO, IM	High	Low	Low	Low	Moderate	—
Pimozide (Orap)	PO	High	Moderate	Low	Moderate	—	—

*Data unavailable.

ACh, Anticholinergic side effects; *EPSs,* extrapyramidal side effects; *OH,* orthostatic hypotension.

Data from Martinez, M., Marangell, L. B., & Martinez, J. M. (2008). Psychopharmacology. In R. E. Hales, S. C. Yudofsky, & G. O. Gabbard (Eds.), *Textbook of psychiatry.* Arlington, VA: American Psychiatric Publishing; and Lehne, R. A. (2010). *Pharmacology for nursing care* (7th ed.). St. Louis: Saunders.

Specific drugs are often chosen for their side-effect profiles. For example, chlorpromazine (Thorazine) is the most sedating agent and has fewer EPSs than do other antipsychotic agents, but it causes significant hypotension. Haloperidol (Haldol) is less sedating and induces less hypotension but has a high incidence of EPSs. As a result, haloperidol has value for treating hallucinations because of its effectiveness in controlling positive symptoms with minimal hypotension and sedation. Patients may prefer less sedating drugs, but those who are agitated or excitable may do better with a more sedating medication.

Conventional antipsychotics are becoming less common in the treatment of schizophrenia because of their minimal impact on negative symptoms and their side effects. However, conventional antipsychotics are effective against positive symptoms, are much less expensive than atypicals, and come in a depot (long-acting injectable) form, which is given once or twice a month. (*Note:* Risperidone, an atypical antipsychotic, also is available in a depot form [Risperdal Consta].) For patients who respond to them and can tolerate their side effects, conventional antipsychotics remain an appropriate choice (Swartz et al., 2007), especially when metabolic syndrome or cost are concerns.

The conventional antipsychotics are often divided into low-potency and high-potency drugs on the basis of their anticholinergic (ACh) side effects, EPSs, and sedative profiles:

Low potency = high sedation + high ACh + low EPSs
High potency = low sedation + low ACh + high EPSs

Conventional antipsychotics are used cautiously in people with seizure disorders; they can lower the seizure threshold. Three of the more common EPSs are **acute dystonia** (acute sustained contraction of muscles, usually of the head and neck), **akathisia** (psychomotor restlessness evident as pacing or fidgeting, sometimes pronounced and very distressing to patients), and **pseudoparkinsonism** (a medication-induced, temporary constellation of symptoms associated with Parkinson's disease: tremor, reduced accessory movements, impaired gait, and stiffening of muscles). Most patients develop tolerance to them after a few months.

EPSs can usually be minimized by lowering dosages and/or adding antiparkinsonian drugs, especially cent-rally acting anticholinergic drugs such as trihexyphenidyl and benztropine mesylate (Cogentin). Diphenhydramine hydrochloride (Benadryl) and amantadine hydrochloride (Symmetrel) are also useful. Lorazepam, a benzodiazepine, may be helpful in reducing akathisia. Table 15-8 identifies some of the drugs most commonly used to treat EPSs.

Unfortunately, antiparkinsonian drugs can cause significant anticholinergic side effects and worsen

TABLE 15-8 Antiparkinsonian and Anticholinergic Agents for Treatment of Extrapyramidal Side Effects

Note: All anticholinergic agents (ACAs) can contribute to risk of anticholinergic toxicity. Practice caution when using multiple ACA agents.

Generic (Trade) Name	Chemical Type
Trihexyphenidyl*	ACA
Benztropine mesylate (Cogentin)*	ACA
Biperiden (Akineton)*	ACA
Diphenhydramine hydrochloride (Benadryl)	Antihistamine (used for its anticholinergic properties)

*Antiparkinsonian agent.
ACA, Anticholinergic agent (after 1 to 6 months of long-term maintenance antipsychotic therapy, most ACAs can be withdrawn).
Data from Tirgobov, E., Wilson, B. A., Shannon, M. T., & Stang, C. L. (2005). *Psychiatric drug guide.* Upper Saddle River, NJ: Pearson/Prentice Hall.

the anticholinergic side effects of conventional antipsychotics and other anticholinergic medications. These side effects include urinary retention, dilated pupils, constipation, reduced visual accommodation [blurred vision], dry mucous membranes, reduced peristalsis, and cognitive impairment. *Anticholinergic (Ach) toxicity*, a potentially life-threatening side effect usually seen in older adults or those on multiple antipsychotic drugs, produces hyperthermia, hot/dry/red skin, paralytic ileus, agitation, delirium, fluctuating vital signs, tachycardia, marked mydriasis, confusion, mental status changes, worsening of psychotic symptoms, and coma (Kemmerer, 2007).

Other troubling side effects of conventional antipsychotics include weight gain, sexual dysfunction, endocrine disturbances (e.g., galactorrhea), drooling, and tardive dyskinesia, discussed in the following section. Weight gain, frequently a problem for women, can be more than 100 pounds; therefore, changing the antipsychotic may be necessary. Impotence and sexual dysfunction are occasionally reported (but frequently experienced) by men and may also necessitate a medication change.

Table 15-9 identifies common side effects of the conventional antipsychotic medications, their usual times of onset, and related nursing and medical interventions.

Tardive dyskinesia (TD or TDK) is a persistent EPS that usually appears after prolonged treatment and persists even after the medication has been discontinued. TDK consists of involuntary tonic muscular contractions that typically involve the tongue, fingers, toes, neck, trunk, or pelvis. This potentially serious EPS is most frequently seen in women and older patients and affects up to 50% of individuals receiving long-term, high-dose therapy. TDK varies from mild

TABLE 15-9 Side Effects of Conventional Antipsychotics and Related Nursing Interventions

Side Effect	Nursing Interventions
Dry mouth	Provide frequent sips of water, ice chips, and sugarless candy or gum. If severe, provide Xero-Lube—a saliva substitute.
Urinary retention and hesitancy	Check voiding. Try warm towel on abdomen, and consider catheterization if no result.
Constipation	Usually short term. May use stool softener. Ensure adequate fluid intake. Increase fiber intake. Use dietary laxatives (e.g., prune juice).
Blurred vision	Usually abates in 1 to 2 weeks. May require use of reading or magnifying glasses. If intolerable, consider consult regarding change in medication.
Photosensitivity	Encourage patient to wear sunglasses, sunscreen, sun-blocking clothing. Limit exposure to sunlight.
Dry eyes	Use artificial tears.
Inhibition of ejaculation or impotence in men	Consult prescriber—patient may need alternative medication.
Anticholinergic toxicity: dry mucous membranes; reduced or absent peristalsis; mydriasis; nonreactive pupils; hot, dry, red skin; hyperpyrexia without diaphoresis; tachycardia; agitation; unstable vital signs; worsening of psychotic symptoms; delirium; urinary retention; seizure; repetitive motor movements	***Potentially life-threatening medical emergency*** Consult prescriber immediately. Hold all medications. Implement emergency cooling measures as ordered (cooling blanket, alcohol, or ice bath). Implement urinary catheterization prn. Administer benzodiazepines or other prn sedation as ordered. Physostigmine may be ordered.
Pseudoparkinsonism: masklike facies, stiff and stooped posture, shuffling gait, drooling, tremor, "pill-rolling" phenomenon *Onset: 5 hours-30 days*	Administer prn antiparkinsonian agent (e.g., trihexyphenidyl or benztropine) If intolerable, consult prescriber regarding medication change. Provide towel or handkerchief to wipe excess saliva.
Acute dystonic reactions: acute contractions of tongue, face, neck, and back (usually tongue and jaw first) Opisthotonos: tetanic heightening of entire body, head and belly up Oculogyric crisis: eyes locked upward Laryngeal dystonia: could threaten airway (rare) *Onset: 1-5 days*	Administer antiparkinsonian agent as above. Also consider diphenhydramine hydrochloride (Benadryl) 25-50 mg IM/IV. Relief usually occurs in 5-15 minutes. Prevent further dystonias with antiparkinsonian agent (see Table 15-8). Experience can be frightening, and patient may fear choking. Accompany to quiet area to provide comfort and support. Assist patient to understand the event and avert distortion or mistrust of medications. Monitor airway.
Akathisia: motor inner-driven restlessness (e.g., tapping foot incessantly, rocking forward and backward in chair, shifting weight from side to side) *Onset: 2 hours-60 days*	Consult prescriber regarding possible medication change. Give antiparkinsonian agent. Tolerance to akathisia does not develop, but akathisia disappears when neuroleptic is discontinued. Propranolol (Inderal), lorazepam (Ativan), or diazepam (Valium) may be used. In severe cases, may cause great distress and contribute to suicidality.

Continued

TABLE 15-9 Side Effects of Conventional Antipsychotics and Related Nursing Interventions—cont'd

Side Effect	Nursing Interventions

Tardive dyskinesia (TD):
Face: protruding and rolling tongue, blowing, smacking, licking, spastic facial distortion, smacking movements
Limbs:
  Choreic: rapid, purposeless, and irregular movements
  Athetoid: slow, complex, and serpentine movements
Trunk: neck and shoulder movements, dramatic hip jerks and rocking, twisting pelvic thrusts
Onset: Months-years
	No known treatment.
	Discontinuing the drug rarely relieves symptoms.
	Possibly 20% of patients taking these drugs for >2 years may develop TD.
	Nurses and doctors should encourage patients to be screened for TD at least every 3 months.
	Onset may merit reconsideration of meds.
	Changes in appearance may contribute to stigmatizing response.
	Teach patient actions to conceal involuntary movements (purposeful muscle contraction overrides involuntary tardive movements).

Hypotension and postural hypotension	Check blood pressure before giving agent. A systolic pressure of 80 mm Hg when standing is indication not to give the current dose. Advise patient to arise slowly to prevent dizziness and hold onto railings/furniture while arising to reduce falls. Effect usually subsides when drug is stabilized in 1 to 2 weeks. Elastic bandages may prevent pooling. If condition is dangerous, consult prescriber regarding medication change, volume expanders, or pressure agents.
Tachycardia	Always evaluate patients with existing cardiac problems before antipsychotic drugs are administered. Haloperidol (Haldol) is usually the preferred drug because of its low ACh effects.
Agranulocytosis: symptoms include sore throat, fever, malaise, and mouth sores. It is a rare occurrence, but a possibility the nurse should be aware of. Any flulike symptoms should be carefully evaluated. *Onset:* During the first 12 weeks of therapy, occurs suddenly	***A potentially dangerous blood dyscrasia*** Blood work usually done every week for 6 months, then every 2 months. Physician may order blood work to determine presence of leukopenia or agranulocytosis. If test results are positive, the drug is discontinued, and reverse isolation may be initiated. Mortality is high if the drug is not ceased and if treatment is not initiated. Teach patient to observe for signs of infection.
Cholestatic jaundice: rare, reversible, and usually benign if caught in time; prodromal symptoms are fever, malaise, nausea, and abdominal pain; jaundice appears 1 week later	Consult prescriber regarding possible medication change. Bed rest and high-protein, high-carbohydrate diet if ordered. Liver function tests should be performed every 6 months.
Neuroleptic malignant syndrome (NMS): rare, potentially fatal *Severe extrapyramidal:* severe muscle rigidity, oculogyric crisis, dysphasia, flexor-extensor posturing, cogwheeling *Hyperpyrexia:* elevated temperature (over 103° F or 39° C) *Autonomic dysfunction:* hypertension, tachycardia, diaphoresis, incontinence *Delirium, stupor, coma* *Onset:* Variable, progresses rapidly over 2-3 days *Risk Factors:* Concomitant use of psychotropics, older age, female, presence of a mood disorder, and rapid dose titration (increase)	***Acute, life-threatening medical emergency*** Stop neuroleptic. Transfer STAT to medical unit. Bromocriptine (Parlodel) can relieve muscle rigidity and reduce fever. Dantrolene (Dantrium) may reduce muscle spasms. Cool body to reduce fever (cooling blankets, alcohol, cool water, or ice bath as ordered). Maintain hydration with oral and IV fluids; correct electrolyte imbalance. Arrhythmias should be treated. Small doses of heparin may decrease possibility of pulmonary emboli. Early detection increases patient's chance of survival.

Data from Kemmerer, D. A. (2007). Anticholinergic syndrome. *Journal of Emergency Nursing, 33*(1), 76–78.

to moderate and can be disfiguring or incapacitating; a common presentation is a guppy-like mouth movement sometimes accompanied by tongue protrusion. Its appearance can contribute to the stigmatization of mentally ill persons.

Early symptoms of tardive dyskinesia are fasciculations of the tongue (described as looking like a bag of worms) or constant smacking of the lips. These can progress into uncontrollable biting, chewing, or sucking motions; an open mouth; and lateral movements of the jaw. No reliable treatment exists for tardive dyskinesia. The National Institute of Mental Health (NIMH) developed the Abnormal Involuntary Movement Scale (AIMS), a brief test for the detection of tardive dyskinesia and other involuntary movements (Figure 15-3). It examines facial, oral, extremity, and trunk movement. Regular administration of the AIMS exam to detect TDK as early as possible is a key nursing role.

Potentially Dangerous Responses to Antipsychotics

Nurses need to know about some rare—but serious and potentially fatal—effects of antipsychotic drugs, including neuroleptic malignant syndrome, agranulocytosis, and liver impairment.

Neuroleptic malignant syndrome (NMS) occurs in about 0.2% to 1% of patients who have taken conventional antipsychotics; it can occur with atypicals as well. Acute reduction in brain dopamine activity plays a role in its development. NMS is a life-threatening medical emergency and is fatal in about 10% of cases. It usually occurs early in therapy but has been reported in people after 20 years of treatment.

NMS is characterized by reduced consciousness, increased muscle tone (muscular rigidity), and autonomic dysfunction—including hyperpyrexia, labile hypertension, tachycardia, tachypnea, diaphoresis, and drooling. Treatment consists of early detection, discontinuation of the antipsychotic, management of fluid balance, temperature reduction, and monitoring for complications. Mild cases of neuroleptic malignant syndrome are treated with bromocriptine (Parlodel). More severe cases are treated with intravenous dantrolene (Dantrium) and even with electroconvulsive therapy (ECT) in some cases (Haddad & Dursun, 2007).

Agranulocytosis is a serious side effect and can be fatal. **Liver impairment** may also occur. Nurses need to be aware of the prodromal signs and symptoms of these side effects and teach them to their patients and patients' families (see Table 15-9).

Adjuncts to Antipsychotic Drug Therapy

Antidepressants are recommended along with antipsychotic agents for the treatment of depression, which is common in schizophrenia. Refer to Chapter 13 for a more detailed discussion of depression and antidepressant drugs.

Antimanic (mood stabilizing) **agents** have been helpful in enhancing the effectiveness of antipsychotics. Valproate is used during acute exacerbations of psychosis to hasten response to antipsychotics (Freudenriech et al., 2008). Lamotrigine may be given along with clozapine to improve therapeutic affects.

Augmentation with **benzodiazepines** (e.g., clonazepam) can reduce anxiety and agitation and contribute to improvement in positive and negative symptoms (Tirgobov, 2005).

When to Change an Antipsychotic Regimen

The following circumstances suggest a need to adjust or change the antipsychotic agent or add supplemental medications (e.g., lithium, carbamazepine, valproate):

- Inadequate improvement in target symptoms despite an adequate trial of the drug
- Persistence of dangerous or intolerable side effects

Specific Interventions for Paranoid, Catatonic, and Disorganized Schizophrenia

The *DSM-IV-TR* criteria for the subtypes of schizophrenia are presented in Figure 15-4 on page 334. The following sections discuss the paranoid, catatonic (excited and withdrawn phases), and disorganized subtypes and identifies pertinent communication guidelines, self-care needs, and milieu needs.

Paranoia

Any intense and strongly defended irrational suspicion can be regarded as paranoia. Paranoia is evident, at least intermittently, in many people without psychotic disorders but is verified as irrational and discarded by the **reality-testing** process. This process fails in patients experiencing paranoia concomitant with psychotic disorders. For them, paranoid ideas cannot be corrected by experiences or modified by facts or reality. **Projection** is the most common defense mechanism used in paranoia; when individuals with paranoia feel angry (or self-critical), they project the feeling onto others and believe others are angry with (or harshly critical toward) them—as if to say, "I'm not angry, you are!"

Paranoid schizophrenia usually has a later age of onset (late 20s to 30s), develops rapidly in individuals with good premorbid functioning, tends to be intermittent during the first 5 years of the illness, and in some cases is associated with a good outcome or complete recovery. People with a paranoid disorder are usually frightened and may behave defensively (e.g., a delusion that another person is planning to kill the patient

ABNORMAL INVOLUNTARY MOVEMENT SCALE (AIMS)

Public Health Service
Alcohol, Drug Abuse, and Mental Health Administration
National Institute of Mental Health

Name: _____
Date: _____
Prescribing Practitioner: _____

Code: 0 = None
1 = Minimal, may be extreme normal
2 = Mild
3 = Moderate
4 = Severe

Instructions: Complete Examination Procedure before making ratings.

Movement ratings: Rate highest severity observed. Rate movements that occur upon activation one *less* than those observed spontaneously. Circle movement as well as code number that applies.		Rater Date	Rater Date	Rater Date	Rater Date
Facial and Oral Movements	**1. Muscles of facial expression** (e.g., movements of forehead, eyebrows, periorbital area, cheeks, including frowning, blinking, smiling, grimacing)	0 1 2 3 4	0 1 2 3 4	0 1 2 3 4	0 1 2 3 4
	2. Lips and perioral area (e.g., puckering, pouting, smacking)	0 1 2 3 4	0 1 2 3 4	0 1 2 3 4	0 1 2 3 4
	3. Jaw (e.g., biting, clenching, chewing, mouth opening, lateral movement)	0 1 2 3 4	0 1 2 3 4	0 1 2 3 4	0 1 2 3 4
	4. Tongue: Rate only increases in movement both in and out of mouth — *not* inability to sustain movement. Darting in and out of mouth.	0 1 2 3 4	0 1 2 3 4	0 1 2 3 4	0 1 2 3 4
Extremity Movements	**5. Upper (arms, wrists, hands, fingers):** Include choreic movements (i.e., rapid, objectively purposeless, irregular, spontaneous) and athetoid movements (i.e., slow, irregular, complex, serpentine) *Do not include tremor* (i.e., repetitive, regular, rhythmic).	0 1 2 3 4	0 1 2 3 4	0 1 2 3 4	0 1 2 3 4
	6. Lower (legs, knees, ankles, toes) (e.g., lateral knee movement, foot tapping, heel dropping, foot squirming, inversion and eversion of foot)	0 1 2 3 4	0 1 2 3 4	0 1 2 3 4	0 1 2 3 4
Trunk Movements	**7. Neck, shoulder, hips** (e.g., rocking, twisting, squirming, pelvic gyrations)	0 1 2 3 4	0 1 2 3 4	0 1 2 3 4	0 1 2 3 4
Global Judgments	**8. Severity of abnormal movements overall**	0 1 2 3 4	0 1 2 3 4	0 1 2 3 4	0 1 2 3 4
	9. Incapacitation due to abnormal movements	0 1 2 3 4	0 1 2 3 4	0 1 2 3 4	0 1 2 3 4
	10. Patient's awareness of abnormal movements: Rate only patient's report. No awareness 0 Aware, no distress 1 Aware, mild distress 2 Aware, moderate distress 3 Aware, severe distress 4	0 1 2 3 4	0 1 2 3 4	0 1 2 3 4	0 1 2 3 4
Dental Status	**11. Current problems with teeth and/or dentures**	No Yes	No Yes	No Yes	No Yes
	12. Are dentures usually worn?	No Yes	No Yes	No Yes	No Yes
	13. Edentia	No Yes	No Yes	No Yes	No Yes
	14. Do movements disappear in sleep?	No Yes	No Yes	No Yes	No Yes

Figure 15-3 Abnormal Involuntary Movement Scale (AIMS).

Continued

AIMS Examination Procedure
Either before or after completing the Examination Procedure, observe the patient unobtrusively, at rest (e.g., in waiting room).

The chair to be used in this examination should be a hard, firm one without arms.

1. Ask patient to remove shoes and socks.
2. Ask patient whether there is anything in his or her mouth (e.g., gum, candy) and, if there is, to remove it.
3. Ask patient about the *current* condition of his or her teeth. Ask patient if he or she wears dentures. Do teeth or dentures bother the patient *now?*
4. Ask patient whether he or she notices any movements in mouth, face, hands, or feet. If yes, ask to describe and to what extent they *currently* bother patient or interfere with his or her activities.
5. Have patient sit in chair with hands on knees, legs slightly apart, and feet flat on floor. Look at entire body movements while in this position.
6. Ask patient to sit with hands hanging unsupported: if male, between legs; if female and wearing a dress, hanging over knees. Observe hands and other body areas.
7. Ask patient to open mouth. Observe tongue at rest within mouth. Do this twice.
8. Ask patient to protrude tongue. Observe abnormalities of tongue movement. Do this twice.
9. Ask patient to tap thumb, with each finger, as rapidly as possible for 10 to 15 seconds, separately with right hand, then with left hand. Observe each facial and leg movement.
10. Flex and extend patient's left and right arms (one at a time). Note any rigidity.
11. Ask patient to stand up. Observe in profile. Observe all body areas again, hips included.
12. Ask patient to extend both arms outstretched in front with palms down. Observe trunk, legs, and mouth.
13. Have patient walk a few paces, turn, and walk back to chair. Observe hands and gait. Do this twice.

Figure 15-3—cont'd

can result in the patient attacking or killing that person first). The paranoia is often a defense against painful feelings of loneliness, despair, helplessness, and fear of abandonment. Useful nursing strategies are outlined in the following sections.

Communication Guidelines. Because persons with paranoia have difficulty trusting those around them, they are usually guarded, tense, and reserved. To ensure interpersonal distance, they may adopt a superior, aloof, hostile, or sarcastic attitude, disparaging and dwelling on the shortcomings of others to maintain their self-esteem. Although they may shun interpersonal contact, functional impairment other than paranoia may be minimal. Patients frequently misinterpret the intent or actions of others, perceiving oversights as personal rejection. They also may personalize unrelated events (**ideas of reference**, or **referentiality**). For example, a patient might see a nurse talking to the psychiatrist and believe they are talking about him.

During care, a patient suffering from paranoia may make offensive yet accurate criticisms of staff and of unit policies. It is important that responses focus on reducing the patient's anxiety and fear and not be defensive reactions or rejections of the patient. Staff conferences and clinical supervision help maintain objectivity and a therapeutic perspective about the patient's motivation and behavior, increasing professional effectiveness.

Self-Care Needs. People with paranoid schizophrenia usually have stronger ego resources than do individuals with other schizophrenic disorders; this is particularly evident in occupational functioning and capacity for independent living. Grooming, dress, and self-care may not be problems and may in fact be meticulous. Nutrition, however, may be affected by a delusion that the food is poisoned. Providing foods in commercially sealed packaging—for example, peanut butter and crackers or nutritional drinks in cartons—can improve nutrition. If patients worry that others will harm them when they are asleep, they may be fearful of going to sleep—a problem that impairs restorative rest and warrants nursing intervention.

Milieu Needs. A person with paranoia may become physically aggressive in response to their paranoid hallucinations or delusions. The patient projects hostile drives onto others and then acts on these drives. Homosexual urges are projected onto others as well, and fear of sexual advances from others may stimulate aggression. An environment that provides a sense of security and safety minimizes anxiety and environmental distortions. Activities that distract the patient from ruminating on paranoid themes also decrease anxiety.

Case Study and Nursing Care Plan 15-1 on pages 338–340 discusses a patient with paranoid schizophrenia.

Catatonia: Withdrawn Phase

The essential feature of catatonia is abnormal levels of motor behavior, either extreme motor agitation or extreme motor retardation. Other associated behaviors include posturing, waxy flexibility, stereotyped behavior, muteness, extreme negativism or automatic obedience, echolalia, and echopraxia (discussed earlier in

DSM-IV-TR CRITERIA FOR SCHIZOPHRENIA SUBTYPES

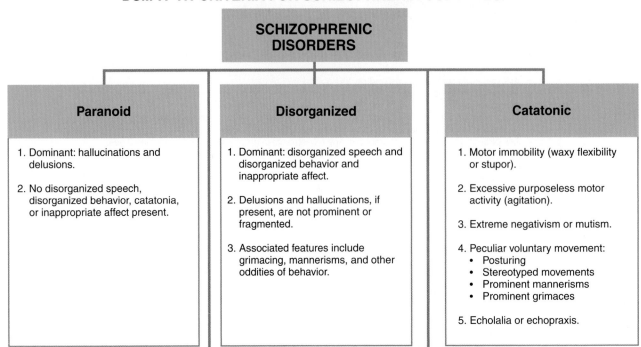

Figure 15-4 Diagnostic criteria for schizophrenia subtypes. (Adapted from American Psychiatric Association. [2000]. *Diagnostic and statistical manual of mental disorders* [4th ed., text rev.] [*DSM-IV-TR*]. Washington, DC: Author.)

this chapter). The onset of catatonia is usually abrupt, and the prognosis favorable. With pharmacotherapy and improved individual management, severe catatonic symptoms are rarely seen today. Useful nursing strategies for intervening in catatonia are discussed in the following sections.

Communication Guidelines. Patients with catatonia can be so withdrawn they appear stuporous or comatose. They can be mute and may remain so for

hours, days, or even weeks or months if untreated. Although such patients may not appear to pay attention to events going on around them, they are acutely aware of the environment and may accurately remember events at a later date. Developing skill and confidence in working with withdrawn patients takes practice. The patient's inability or refusal to cooperate or participate in activities challenges staff to work to remain objective and avert frustration and anger.

Self-Care Needs. In extreme withdrawal, a patient may need to be hand- or tube-fed to maintain adequate nutritional status. Aspiration is a risk. Normal control over bladder and bowel functions may be interrupted, so the assessment and management of urinary or bowel retention or incontinence is essential. When physical movements are minimal or absent, range-of-motion exercises can reduce muscular atrophy, calcium depletion, and contractures. Dressing and grooming usually require direct assistance.

Milieu Needs. The catatonic person's appearance may range from decreased spontaneous movement to complete stupor. Waxy flexibility is often seen; for example, if the patient raises his arms over his head, he may maintain that position for hours or longer. Caution is advised, because even after holding a single posture for long periods, the patient may suddenly and without provocation show brief outbursts of gross motor activity in response to inner hallucinations, delusions, and change in neurotransmitter levels.

Catatonia: Excited Phase

Communication Guidelines. During the excited stage of catatonia, the person is in a state of greatly increased motor activity. They may talk or shout continually and incoherently, requiring the nurse's communication to be clear, direct, and loud (enough to focus the patient's attention on the nurse) and to reflect concern for the safety of the patient and others.

Self-Care Needs. A person who is constantly and intensely hyperactive can become completely exhausted and even die if medical attention is not available. Patients with concurrent medical conditions (e.g., congestive heart failure) are most at risk. Intramuscular administration of a sedating antipsychotic is often required to reduce psychomotor agitation to a safer level. During heightened physical activity, the patient requires stimulation reduction and additional fluids, calories, and rest. It is not unusual for the agitated patient to be destructive or aggressive to others in response to hallucinations or delusions or inner distress. Many of the concerns and interventions are the same as those for mania.

Disorganized Schizophrenia

Disorganized schizophrenia represents the most regressed and socially impaired of all the subtypes. A person with disorganized schizophrenia may have marked associative looseness, grossly inappropriate affect, bizarre mannerisms, and incoherence of speech and may display extreme social withdrawal. Delusions and hallucinations are fragmentary and poorly organized. Behavior may be considered odd, and a giggling or grimacing response to internal stimuli is common.

Disorganized schizophrenia has an earlier age of onset (early to middle teens), often develops insidiously, is associated with poor premorbid functioning and a significant family history of psychiatric disorders, and carries a poor prognosis. Often these patients reside in state hospitals and can live safely in the community only in a structured, well-supervised setting. Families of patients living at home need significant community support, respite care, and access to day hospital services. Unfortunately, a good portion of these patients become homeless. See the Case Study and Nursing Care Plan for Disorganized Thinking on the Evolve website.

Communication Guidelines. People with disorganized schizophrenia experience persistent and severe perceptual and communication problems. Communication should be concise, clear, and concrete. Tasks should be broken into discrete tasks that are taken one at a time. Repeated refocusing may be needed to keep the patient on topic or to allow task completion. This repetition can be frustrating to the nurse and others, requiring special effort to identify and correct countertransference and nontherapeutic responses.

Self-Care Needs. In patients with disorganized schizophrenia, grooming is neglected; hair is often dirty and matted, and clothes are unclean and often inappropriate for the weather (presenting a risk to self). Cognition, memory, and executive function are grossly impaired, and the patient is frequently too disorganized to carry out simple activities of daily living (ADLs). Areas of nursing focus include encouraging optimal levels of functioning, preventing further regression, and offering alternatives for inappropriate behaviors whenever possible. Significant direct assistance for ADLs is needed.

Milieu Needs. Patients with disorganized schizophrenia need assistance to conform their behavior to social expectations. Nurses should provide for the patient's privacy needs. Peer education about the disorder may reduce peer frustration and acting out.

VIGNETTE

Martin Taylor, a 36-year-old man, is accompanied to the mental health center by his mother. Ms. Lamb, Martin's nurse, obtains background information from his mother. According to her, he had been in a state hospital for treatment of schizophrenia for 3 months and after his discharge was doing well at home until recently. His only employment history was 5 months as a janitor after high school graduation. His mother states that as a teenager Martin was an excellent athlete and received average grades. At age 17, he had his first psychotic break when he took various street drugs. His behavior became markedly bizarre (e.g., eating cat food and swallowing a rubber-soled heel, which precipitated an emergency laparotomy).

Ms. Lamb meets with Martin. He is unshaven and disheveled. He is wearing a headband that holds Popsicle sticks and paper scraps. He chain smokes, paces, and frequently changes position. He reports that he is Alice from Alice in the Underground and that people from space hurt him with needles. His speech is marked by associative looseness and occasional blocking, and he often stops in the middle of a phrase and giggles to himself.

He starts to giggle, and Ms. Lamb asks what he is thinking about. He states, "You interrupted me." He then begins to shake his head while repeating in a sing-song voice, "Shake them tigers...shake them tigers...." He denies suicidal or homicidal ideation. Ms. Lamb notes that Martin has great difficulty accurately perceiving what is going on around him. He exhibits regressed social behaviors (e.g., eating with his hands and picking his nose in public). He has no apparent insight into his problems, telling Ms. Lamb that his biggest problem is the people in space. ■

Undifferentiated Schizophrenia

In the undifferentiated type of schizophrenia, active signs of the disorder (positive and/or negative symptoms) are present, but the individual does not meet the criteria for any of the other subtypes. As with disorganized schizophrenia, undifferentiated schizophrenia begins early (early to middle teens) and has an insidious onset. However, the premorbid state is less predictable, and the disability remains fairly stable and persistent over time.

Residual Schizophrenia

In the residual type of schizophrenia, active-phase symptoms are no longer present, but evidence of two or more residual symptoms persists. Residual symptoms typically include:
- Reduced initiative, interests, or energy
- Social withdrawal
- Impaired role function (as employee, student, homemaker)
- Speech deficits (e.g., circumstantiality, vague speech, and poverty of speech or content of speech)
- Odd beliefs, magical thinking, and unusual perceptual experiences

Nursing care for undifferentiated and residual schizophrenia is similar to that for withdrawn,

paranoid, and disorganized schizophrenia, as dictated by the patient's behavior.

Advanced Practice Interventions

Services that may, in most locations, be provided by Advanced Practice Registered Nurses (APRNs) include psychotherapy, cognitive-behavioral therapy (CBT), group therapy, medication administration, social skills training, cognitive remediation, and family therapy. Family therapy is one of the most important interventions the APRN can implement for the patient with schizophrenia.

Family Therapy

Family therapy is a service usually delivered by APRNs or other independently licensed personnel. Families of persons with schizophrenia often endure considerable hardships while coping with the psychotic and residual symptoms of the illness, particularly if they are direct caregivers. The patient and family may become isolated from other relatives, communities, and support systems. In fact, until the 1970s (and sometimes even today) families were often blamed for causing schizophrenia in the affected family member. NAMI and the National Alliance for Research in Schizophrenia and Depression (NARSD) are actively involved in countering this image and in making families full partners in the treatment process.

Family education and family therapy improve the quality of life for the patient with schizophrenia and reduce the relapse rate for many patients. The following example shows how a family came to distinguish between "Martha's problem" and "the problem caused by schizophrenia."

It was a good idea, us all meeting in our own home to discuss my sister's illness. We were all able to say how it felt, and for the first time I realized that I knew very little about what she was suffering or how much—the word *schizophrenia* meant nothing to me before. I used to think she was just being lazy until she told me what it was really like (Gamble & Brennan, 2000, p. 192).

Programs that provide support, education, coping skills training, and social network development are extremely effective. This **psycho-educational** approach brings educational and behavioral approaches into family treatment and does not blame families but rather recognizes them as secondary victims of a biological illness. In family therapy sessions, fears, faulty communication patterns, and distortions are identified, problem-solving skills are taught, healthier alternatives to conflict are explored, and guilt and anxiety can be lessened.

EVIDENCE-BASED PRACTICE

Cognitive Interventions for Auditory Hallucinations

England, M. (2007). Efficacy of cognitive nursing intervention for voice hearing. *Perspectives in Psychiatric Care, 43*(2), 69–76.

Problem
Medications alone do not always fully relieve hallucinations. Research has suggested that cognitive interventions can reduce distress stemming from residual hallucinations.

Purpose of Study
This study sought to determine whether structured cognitive nursing interventions would produce significant improvement in a population of patients who hear voices.

Methods
A sample of patients was divided into a usual-care control group and an experimental structured-cognitive-interventions group. Symptom reports, treatment adherence, and other parameters were measured pre- and post-intervention. A clinical nurse specialist provided 12, 90-minute, individual cognitive sessions focusing on patients' thoughts about their hallucinations and alternate ways of thinking about their hallucinations that would be more reality-based and less distressing.

Key Findings
The cognitive-intervention group demonstrated significant improvement in self-esteem and subject distress related to symptoms. This outcome is consistent with research showing that hearing voices is tied to poor self-esteem and the nature of one's relationship with the voices.

Implications for Nursing Practice
Existing cognitive interventions, when added to traditional psychopharmacology, can significantly enhance symptom management. Although within the scope of practice for nurses, such interventions are not consistently used at present, training nurses in their use and providing other support to increase their use has the potential to contribute to a higher quality of life for persons with residual hallucinations.

EVALUATION

Evaluation is especially important in planning care for people who have psychotic disorders. Outcome expectations that are unrealistic discourage patient and staff alike. It is critical for staff to remember that change is a process that occurs over time. For a person with schizophrenia, progress may occur erratically, and gains may be difficult to discern in the short term.

It is important to reassess chronically ill patients regularly so that new data can be considered and treatment adjusted when needed. Questions to be asked include:

- Is the patient not progressing because a more important need is not being met?
- Is the staff making the best use of the patient's strengths and interests to promote treatment and achieve desired outcomes?
- Are other possible interventions being overlooked?
- Are new or better interventions available?

- How is the patient responding to existing or recently changed medications or other treatments?
- Is the patient becoming discouraged, anxious, or depressed?
- Is the patient treatment adherent? Are side effects controlled or troubling?
- Is functioning improving or regressing?
- What is the patient's quality of life, and is it improving?
- Is the family involved, supportive, and knowledgeable regarding the patient's disorder and treatment?

Active staff involvement and interest in the patient's progress communicates concern and caring, helps the patient to maximize progress, promotes treatment adherence, and reduces staff feelings of helplessness and burnout. Input from the patient can offer valuable information about why a certain desired outcome has not occurred.

Case Study and Nursing Care Plan 15-1   **Paranoid Schizophrenia**

Tom, a 32-year-old man, is an inpatient at a Veterans Administration hospital. He has been separated from his wife and 4 children for 3 years. His records state that he has been in and out of hospitals for 13 years. Tom is a former Marine who first "heard voices" at the age of 19 while he was serving in the Gulf War. He subsequently received a medical discharge.

The hospitalization was precipitated by an exacerbation of auditory hallucinations. "I thought people were following me. I hear voices, usually a woman's voice, and she's tormenting me. People say that it happens because I don't take my medications. The medications make me tired, and I can't have sex." Tom also uses marijuana, which he knows increases his paranoia. "It makes me feel good, and not much else does." Tom finished 11 years of school but did not graduate. He says he has no close friends. He spent 5 years in prison for manslaughter and was abusing alcohol and drugs when the crime occurred. Drug abuse has also been a contributing factor to Tom's psychiatric hospitalizations.

Ms. Lally is Tom's nurse. Tom is dressed in pajamas and bathrobe, his hygiene is good, and he is well nourished. He reports that he does not sleep much because "the voices get worse at night." Ms. Lally notes in Tom's medical record that he has had two episodes of suicidal ideation, during which the voices were telling him to jump "off rooftops"

and "in front of trains." During the first interview, Tom rarely makes eye contact and speaks in a low monotone. At times, he glances about the room as if distracted, mumbles to himself, and appears upset.

Nurse: Tom, my name is Ms. Lally. I will be your nurse in the hospital. If it is okay with you, we will meet every day for 30 minutes at 10 AM. We can talk about areas of concern to you.

Tom: Well…don't believe what they say about me. I want to start…. Are you married?

Nurse: This time is for you to talk about your concerns.

Tom: Oh…(looks furtively around the room, then lowers his eyes) I think someone is trying to kill me….

Nurse: You seem to be focusing on something other than our conversation.

Tom: The voices tell me things…I can't say….

Nurse: I don't hear any voices except yours and mine. I will stay with you. Tell me what is happening, and I will try to help you.

Tom: The voices tell me bad things.

Ms. Lally stays with Tom and encourages him to communicate with her. As Tom focuses more on the conversation, his anxiety appears to lessen. His thoughts become more connected, he is able to concentrate more, and he mumbles to himself less.

ASSESSMENT

Self-Assessment

On the first day of admission, Tom assaults another male patient, stating that the patient accused him of being a homosexual and touched him on the buttocks. After assessing the incident, the staff agrees that Tom's provocation came more from his own projections (Tom's sexual attraction to the other patient) than from anything the other patient did or said.

Tom's difficulty with impulse control frightens Ms. Lally. She has concerns regarding Tom's ability to curb his impulses and the possibility of Tom's striking out at her, especially when Tom is hallucinating and highly delusional. Ms. Lally mentions her concerns to the nursing coordinator, who suggests that Ms. Lally meet with Tom in the day room until he demonstrates more control and less suspicion of others. After 5 days, Tom is less excitable, and the sessions are moved to a room set aside for patient interviews. Ms. Lally also speaks with a senior staff nurse regarding her fears. By talking to the senior nurse and understanding more clearly her own fear, Ms. Lally is able to manage her fear and identify interventions to help Tom regain a better sense of control.

Objective Data

Speaks in low monotone

Makes poor eye contact

Weight appropriate for height

Clean, bathed, clothes match

Impaired reality testing

Has a history of drug abuse (cocaine and marijuana) which
appears to contribute to relapses

Has no close friends, separated from wife and children

Was first hospitalized at age 19 and has not worked since
that time

Has had suicidal impulses twice, both associated with
command hallucinations

Was imprisoned for 5 years for violence (manslaughter)
and assaulted a peer in the hospital

Thoughts scattered when anxious

Subjective Data

"I hear voices"

"Someone is trying to kill me, I think."

"I don't take my medications. They make me tired, and
I can't have sex."

"The voices get worse at night, and I can't sleep."

"(Drugs) make me feel good…not much else does."

Voices have told him to "jump off rooftops" and "in front
of trains."

DIAGNOSIS

1. *Disturbed thought processes* related to alteration in neurological function, as evidenced by persecutory hallucinations and paranoia:
   - Voices have told him to "jump off rooftops" and "in front of trains."
   - "Someone is trying to kill me, I think."
   - Abuses cocaine and marijuana (although these increase paranoia) because "They make me feel good."
2. *Nonadherence* to medication regimen related to side effects of therapy, as evidenced by verbalization of noncompliance and persistence of symptoms:
   - Failure to take prescribed medications because "They make me tired, and I can't have sex."
   - Chronic history of relapse of symptoms

OUTCOMES IDENTIFICATION

1. Tom consistently refrains from acting upon his "voices" and suspicions.
2. Tom consistently adheres to treatment regimen.

PLANNING

The nurse plans intervention that will (1) help Tom deal with his disturbing thoughts and (2) minimize drug abuse and adverse effects of medication to increase adherence and decrease the potential for relapse and violence.

IMPLEMENTATION

Nursing diagnosis: *Disturbed thought processes* related to schizophrenia as evidenced by patient stating, "Voices are scaring me."
Outcome: Tom consistently refrains from acting upon his "voices" and suspicions when they occur.

Short-Term Goal	Intervention	Rationale	Evaluation
1. By the end of the first week, Tom will recognize the presence of hallucinations and identify one or more contributing factors, as evidenced by telling his nurse when they occur and what preceded them.	1a. Meet with Tom each day for 30 minutes to establish trust and rapport. 1b. Explore those times when voices are most threatening and disturbing, noting the circumstances that precede them. 1c. Provide noncompetitive activities that focus on the here and now.	1a. Short, consistent meetings help decrease anxiety and establish trust. 1b. Identifies events that increase anxiety and trigger "voices"; by learning to manage triggers, hallucinations can be reduced. 1c. Increased time spent in reality-based activities decreases focus on hallucinations.	GOAL MET By the end of the first week, Tom tells the nurse when he is experiencing hallucinations.
2. By the end of the first week, Tom will recognize hallucinations as "not real" and ascribe them to his illness.	2a. Explore content of hallucinations with Tom. 2b. Educate Tom about the nature of hallucinations and ways to determine if "voices" are real.	2a. Identifies suicidal or aggressive themes or command hallucinations. 2b. Improves Tom's reality testing and helps him begin to attribute his experiences to schizophrenia.	GOAL MET Tom identifies that the voices tell him he is a loser and he needs to be careful "because someone is after me." He identifies that the voices are worse at nighttime. He notes that others do not seem to hear what he hears and also states that smoking marijuana and taking cocaine produce very threatening voices.
3. By discharge, Tom will consistently report a decrease in hallucinations.	3. Explore with Tom possible actions that can minimize anxiety and/or reduce hallucinations, such as whistling or reading aloud.	3. Offers alternatives while anxiety level is relatively low.	GOAL MET Tom states that he is hearing voices less, and they are less threatening to him. Tom identifies that if he whistles or sings, he stays calm and can control the voices.

Nursing diagnosis: Nonadherence
Outcome: Tom consistently adheres to medication regimen.

Continued

Short-Term Goal	Intervention	Rationale	Evaluation
1. By the end of week 1, Tom will discuss his concerns about medication with staff.	1a. Evaluate medication response and side-effect issues.	1a. Identify drugs and dosages that have increased therapeutic value and decreased side effects.	GOAL MET Tom identifies the reasons for stopping his medication. He agrees to try olanzapine because he trusts staff's assurances that the side effects will be reduced. Tom states that he sleeps better at night but is still tired during the day.
	1b. Initiate medication change to olanzapine (Zyprexa). A large dose is taken at bedtime to increase sleep, and a small dose is taken during the day to decrease fatigue.	1b. Olanzapine causes no known sexual difficulties.	
	1c. Educate Tom regarding side effects—how long they last and what actions can be taken.	1c. Can give increased sense of control over symptoms.	
2. By the end of week 2, Tom will describe two ways to reduce or cope with side effects and two ways the medications help him meet his goals (e.g., avoiding jail and reducing fear).	2a. Connect Tom with the local NAMI support group.	2a. Provides peer support and a chance to hear from others (further along in recovery) how medications can be helpful and side effects can be managed. NAMI group can also offer suggestions for dealing with his loneliness and other problems.	GOAL MET Week 1: Tom attends meeting. Week 2: He speaks in the group about "not feeling good." Several group members say they understand and try to help him figure out why he is not feeling good. Peers say how taking medication has helped them feel better.

Evaluation

By discharge, Tom expresses hope that the medicines will help him feel better and avoid problems like jail. He has a better understanding of his medications and what to do for side effects. He knows that marijuana and cocaine increase his symptoms and explains that when he gets lonely, he now has ideas of things other than drugs he can do to "feel good." Tom continues with the support group and outpatient counseling, stating that it's because Ms. Lally really cared about him; this made him want to get better and led him to trust what staff told him. He reports sleeping much better and says that he has more energy during the day.

KEY POINTS TO REMEMBER

- Schizophrenia is a biological disorder of the brain. It is not one disorder but a group of disorders with overlapping symptoms and treatments.
- The primary differences among subtypes involve the spectrum of symptoms that dominate, their severity, the impairment in affect and cognition, and the impact on social and other areas of functioning.
- Psychotic symptoms are often more pronounced and obvious than are symptoms found in other disorders, making schizophrenia more likely to be apparent to others and increasing the risk of stigmatization.
- Neurochemical (catecholamines and serotonin), genetic, and neuroanatomical findings help explain the symptoms of schizophrenia. However, no one theory accounts fully for the complexities of schizophrenia.
- When the nurse works with patients with schizophrenia, four categories of symptoms may be evident. The positive and negative symptoms of schizophrenia are two of the major categories of symptoms. Symptoms vary considerably among patients and fluctuate over time.
- The *positive symptoms* of schizophrenia (e.g., hallucinations, delusions, associative looseness) are more pronounced and respond best to antipsychotic drug therapy.
- The *negative symptoms* of schizophrenia (e.g., social withdrawal and dysfunction, lack of motivation, reduced affect) respond less well to antipsychotic therapy and tend to be more debilitating.

- The degree of cognitive impairment warrants careful assessment and active intervention to increase the patient's ability to adapt, function, and maximize the ultimate quality of life.
- Comorbid depression must be identified and treated to reduce the potential for suicide, substance abuse, nonadherence, and relapse.
- Some applicable nursing diagnoses include *Disturbed sensory perception, Disturbed thought processes, Impaired communication, Ineffective coping, Risk for self-directed or other-directed violence, and Impaired family coping.*
- Outcomes are chosen based on the type and phase of schizophrenia and the patient's individual needs, strengths, and level of functioning. Short-term and intermediate indicators are also developed to better track the incremental progress typical of schizophrenia.
- Interventions for people with schizophrenia include trust-building, therapeutic communication techniques, support, assistance with self-care, promotion of independence, stress management, promotion of socialization, psycho-education to promote understanding and adaptation, milieu management, cognitive-behavioral interventions, cognitive enhancement/remediation techniques, and medication administration.
- Because antipsychotic medications are essential in the care of patients with schizophrenia, the nurse must understand the properties, adverse and toxic effects, and dosages of conventional and atypical antipsychotics and other medications used to treat schizophrenia. The nurse helps the patient and family understand and appreciate the importance of medication to recovery.
- Schizophrenia can produce countertransference responses in staff; clinical supervision and self-assessment help the nurse remain objective and therapeutic.

CRITICAL THINKING

1. Jamie, a 24-year-old woman, is hospitalized after an abrupt onset of psychosis and is diagnosed with paranoid schizophrenia. Jamie is recently divorced and works as a legal secretary. Her work had become erratic, and her suspiciousness was attracting negative responses. Jamie is being discharged in two days to her mother's care until she is able to resume her job. Jamie's mother is overwhelmed and asks the nurse how she is going to cope: "I can hardly say anything to Jamie without her getting upset. She is still mad at me because I called 911 and had her admitted. She says there is nothing wrong with her, and I'm worried she'll stop her medication once she is home. What am I going to do?"
   A. Explain Jamie's behavior and symptoms to a classmate as you would for Jamie's mother.
   B. How would you respond to the mother's immediate concerns?

C. What are some of the priority concerns the nurse should address before discharge?
D. Identify interventions that are based on the concepts of the recovery model.
E. What are some community resources that can help support this family? Describe how each could be helpful to this family.
F. What do you think of the prognosis for Jamie? Support your position with data regarding Jamie's diagnosis and the treatment you have planned.

CHAPTER REVIEW

1. A patient is found in a closet with an empty 2-liter bottle of cola taken from the staff refrigerator. The bottle was full but now is empty. Recently, staff have noticed an increase in this patient's response to auditory hallucinations and the recent addition of confusion to his symptoms. For the past several days, the patient has been seen drinking from the hallway water cooler and taking items from his peers' dinner trays. Which response is most appropriate?
   1. Place the patient on every-15-minute checks to identify any further deterioration.
   2. Restrict his access to fluids, and evaluate for water intoxication via daily weights.
   3. Attempt to distract the patient from excess fluid intake and other bizarre behavior.
   4. Request an increase in antipsychotic medication, owing to the worsening of his psychosis.

2. Jim is sometimes seen moving his lips silently or murmuring to himself when he does not realize others are watching. Sometimes when he is conversing with others, he suddenly stops, appears distracted for a moment, and then resumes. Based on these observations, Jim most likely is experiencing which symptom(s)? *Select all that apply.*
   1. Illusions
   2. Paranoia
   3. Delusional thinking
   4. Auditory hallucinations
   5. Impaired reality testing
   6. Stereotyped behaviors

3. Mary, a patient diagnosed with schizophrenia, is encouraged to attend groups but stays in her room instead. Staff and peers encourage her participation, but her hygiene remains poor. She does not seem to care that others wish that she would behave differently. Which is the most likely explanation for Mary's failure to respond to others' efforts to help her behave in a more adaptive fashion? *Select all that apply.*
   1. She is avolitional.
   2. She is displaying anergia.
   3. She is displaying negativism.
   4. She is exhibiting paranoid delusions.

5. She is being resistant or oppositional.
6. She is experiencing social withdrawal.
7. She is apathetic due to her schizophrenia.

4. You are attempting to interview Mr. Jones, a newly admitted involuntary patient with schizophrenia. Mr. Jones seems evasive and uncomfortable and gives one-word responses that are minimally informative. Which response would be most useful for facilitating the interview?
    1. "Why did you come to the hospital today?"
    2. "It must be difficult to be admitted to a hospital against your will."
    3. "If you could cooperate for just a few minutes, we could get this done."
    4. "Did your schizophrenia get worse because you stopped taking your medication?"

5. A week later, Mr. Jones has begun to take the conventional antipsychotic haloperidol. You approach him with his bedtime dose and notice that he is sitting very stiffly and immobile. When you approach, you notice that he is diaphoretic, and when you ask if he is okay he seems unable to turn towards you or to respond verbally. You also notice that his eyes are aimed sharply upward and he seems frightened. How should the nurse respond? *Select all that apply.*
    1. Begin to wipe him with a washcloth wet with cold water or alcohol.
    2. Hold his medication, stat page his doctor, and check his temperature.
    3. Administer a medication such as benztropine IM to correct his dystonic reaction.
    4. Reassure him that although there is no treatment for his tardive dyskinesia, it will pass.
    5. Explain that he has anticholinergic toxicity, hold his meds, and give IM physostigmine.
    6. Hold his medication tonight, and consult his doctor after completing medication rounds.

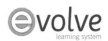 Visit the Evolve website for an **Audio Chapter Summary, Chapter Review Answers & Rationales, Critical Thinking Answer Guidelines**, and additional resources related to the content in this chapter: **http://evolve.elsevier.com/Varcarolis/foundations**

Companion CD Use the Companion CD to prepare for tests and the NCLEX® Examination with **Test-Taking Strategies** for psychiatric mental health nursing and hundreds of **Review Questions**.

References

American Psychiatric Association. (2000). *Diagnostic and statistical manual of mental disorders* (4th ed., text rev.) *(DSM-IV-TR)*. Washington, DC: Author.

American Psychiatric Association. (2004). *Practice guidelines for the treatment of patients with schizophrenia* (2nd ed.). Washington, DC: Author.

Bechdolf, A., Phillips, L. J., Francey, S. M., Leicester, S., Morrison, A. P., Veith, V. et al. (2006). Recent approaches to psychological interventions for people at risk of psychosis. *European Archive of Psychiatry and Clinical Neuroscience, 256,* 159–173.

Bralet, M., Ton, T., & Falissard, B. (2007). Schizophrenic patients with polydipsia and water intoxication more often have a form of schizophrenia first described by Kraepelin. *Psychiatry Research, 152,* 267–271.

Braw, Y., Bloch, Y., Mendelovich, S., Ratzoni, G., Gal., G., Harari, H. et al. (2008). Cognition in young schizophrenia outpatients: Comparison of first episode with multiepisode patients. *Schizophrenia Bulletin, 34,* 544–554.

Broome, M. R., Woolley, J. B., Tabraham, P., Johns, L. C., Bramon, E., Murray, G.K. et al. (2005). What causes the onset of psychosis? *Schizophrenia Research, 79,* 23–34.

Chung, Y. S., Kang, D., Shin, N. Y., Yu, S. Y., & Kwon, J. S. (2008). Deficit of theory of mind in individuals at ultra-high risk for schizophrenia. *Schizophrenia Research, 99,* 111–118.

Compton, M. T. (2004). Considering schizophrenia from a prevention perspective. *American Journal of Preventive Medicine, 26*(2), 178–185.

Crowe, T. P., Deane, F. P., Oades, L. G., Caputi, P., & Morland, K. G. (2006). Effectiveness of a collaborative recovery training program in Australia in promoting positive views about recovery. *Psychiatric Services, 57,* 1497–1500.

Denes, G. (2007). Capgras delusion. *Neurological Sciences, 28*(4), 163–164.

Farhall, J., Greenwood, K. M., & Jackson, H. J. (2007). Coping with hallucinated voices: A review of self-initiated strategies and therapeutic interventions. *Clinical Psychology Review, 27,* 476–493.

Freudenreich, O., Weiss, A. P., & Goff, D. C. (2008). Psychosis and schizophrenia. In T. A. Stern, J. F. Rosenbaum, M. Fava, J. Biederman, & S. L. Rauch (Eds.), *Massachusetts General Hospital comprehensive clinical psychiatry* (pp. 371–389). St. Louis: Mosby.

Gamble, C., & Brennan, G. (2000). Working with families and informed careers. In C. Gamble & G. Brennan (Eds.), *Working with serious mental illness: A manual for clinical practice.* London: Baillière Tindall.

Goff, D. C. (2005). Pharmacologic implications of neurobiological models of schizophrenia. *Harvard Review of Psychiatry, 13,* 352–359.

Gonzalez, I., & Perez, N. (2007). High risk of polydipsia and water intoxication in schizophrenia patients. *Schizophrenia Research, 99*(1-3), 377–378.

Green, A. I., Noordsy, D. L., Brunette, M. F., & O'Keefe, C. O. (2008). Substance abuse and schizophrenia: Pharmacotherapeutic intervention. *Journal of Substance Abuse Treatment, 34*(1), 61–71.

Haddad, P. M., & Dursun, S. M. (2007). Neurological complications of psychiatric drugs: Clinical features and management. *Human Psychopharmacology, 23*(1), 15–26.

Hayashi, T., Ishida, Y., Miyashita, T., Kiyokawa, H., Kimora, A., & Kondo, T. (2005). Fatal water intoxication in a schizophrenia patient—an autopsy case. *Journal of Clinical Forensic Medicine, 12*(3), 157–159.

Heresco-Levy, U., Javitt, D. C., Ebstein, R., Vass, A., Lichtenberg, T., Bar, G. et al. (2005). D-serine efficacy as add-on pharmacotherapy to risperidone and olanzapine for treatment-refractory schizophrenia. *Biological Psychiatry, 57*, 577–585.

Hoffman, R. E. & Varanko, M. (2006). Seeing voices: Fused visual/auditory verbal hallucinations reported by three persons with schizophrenia-spectrum disorder. *Acta Psychiatrica Scandinavica, 114*, 290–293.

Hubl, D., Koenig, T., Strik, W., Federspiel, A., Kreis, R., Boesch, C. et al. (2004). Pathways that make voices: White matter changes in auditory hallucinations. *Archives of General Psychiatry, 61*, 658–668.

Khashan, A. S., Abel, K. M, McNamee, R., Pedersen, M. G., Webb, R. T., Baker, P. N., et al. (2008). Higher risk of offspring schizophrenia following antenatal maternal exposure to severe adverse life events. *Archives of General Psychiatry, 65*(2), 146–152.

Masi, G., Mucci, M., & Pari, C. (2006). Children with schizophrenia: Clinical picture and pharmacological treatment. *CNS Drugs, 20*, 841–866.

Mauri, M. C., Volonteri, L. S., De Gaspari, I. F., Colasanti, A., Brambilla, M. A., & Cerruti, L. (2006). Substance abuse in first-episode schizophrenic patients: A retrospective study. *Clinical Practice and Epidemiology in Mental Health* [online], 2(4). Retrieved November 1, 2008 from http://www.pubmedcentral.nih.gov/articlerender.fcgi?artid=1435752

Mauri, M. C., Moliterno, D., Rossattini, M., & Colasanti, A. (2008). Depression in schizophrenia: Comparison of first- and second-generation antipsychotic drugs. *Schizophrenia Research, 99*(1-3), 7–12.

Miller, B. J., Paschall, C. B., & Svendsen, D. P. (2007). *Mortality and medical co-morbidity in patients with serious mental illness.* Poster presentation at the 8th Annual All-Ohio Institute on Community Psychiatry, 3/16/2007, Beachwood, OH.

Möller, H. J. (2007). Clinical evaluation of negative symptoms in schizophrenia. *European Psychiatry, 22*, 380–386.

Moorhead, S., Johnson, M., Maas, M. L., & Swanson, E. (2008). *Nursing outcomes classification (NOC)* (4th ed.). St. Louis: Mosby.

Nash, J. *John Nash quotes.* Retrieved November 2, 2008, from http://thinkexist.com/quotes/john_nash/

North American Nursing Diagnosis Association International (NANDA-I) (2009). *NANDA-I nursing diagnoses: Definitions and classification 2009-2011.* Oxford, United Kingdom: Author.

Osborn, D., Levy, G., Nazareth, I., & King, M. (2008). Suicide and severe mental illnesses. *Schizophrenia Research, 99*(1-3), 134–138.

Riecher-Rössler, A., Gschwandtner, U., Borgwardt, S., Aston, J., Pflüger, M., Rössler, W. (2006). Early detection and treatment of schizophrenia: How early? *Acta Psychiatrica Scandinavica, 113*(suppl 429), 73–80.

Sadock, B. J., & Sadock, V. A. (2008). *Concise textbook of clinical psychiatry* (3rd ed.). Philadelphia: Lippincott Williams & Wilkins.

Smoller, J. W., Finn, C. T., & Gardner-Schuster, E. E. (2008). Genetics and psychiatry. In T. A Stern, J. F. Rosenbaum, M. Fava, J. Biederman, & S. L. Rauch (Eds.), *Massachusetts General Hospital comprehensive clinical psychiatry* (pp. 853–883). St. Louis: Mosby.

Swartz, M. S., Perkins, D. O., Stroup, T. S., Davis, S. M., Capuano, G., Rosenheck, R. A. et al. (2007). Effects of antipsychotic medications on psychosocial functioning in patients with chronic schizophrenia: Findings from the NIMH CATIE study. *American Journal of Psychiatry, 164*, 428–436.

Tandon, R., Keshavan, M. S., & Nasrallah, H. A. (2008). Schizophrenia, "just the facts": What we know in 2008, (part 2) epidemiology and etiology. *Schizophrenia Research, 102*(1-3), 1–18.

Tschoner, A., Engl, J., Laimer, M., Kaser, S., Rettenbacher, M., Fleischhacker, W., et al. (2007). Metabolic side effects of antipsychotic medication. *International Journal of Clinical Practice, 61*, 1356–1370.

van Meijel, B., van der Gaag, M., Sylvain, R. K., & Grypdonck, M. (2004). Recognition of early warning signs in patients with schizophrenia: A review of the literature. *International Journal of Mental Health Nursing, 13*, 107–116.

Wadenberg, M. G. (2007). Bifeprunox: A novel antipsychotic agent with partial agonist properties at dopamine D_2 and serotonin $5-HT_{1A}$ receptors. *Future Neurology, 2*(2), 153–165.

Walker, E., & Tessner, K. (2008). Schizophrenia. *Perspectives on Psychological Science, 3*(1), 30–37.

Weisman, A., Duarte, E., Koneru, V., & Wasserman, S. (2006). The development of culturally informed, family-focused treatment for schizophrenia. *Family Process, 45*(2), 171–186.

CHAPTER 16

Eating Disorders

Carissa R. Enright and Kathleen Ibrahim

Key Terms and Concepts

anorexia nervosa, 344
binge eating disorder, 345
bulimia nervosa, 344

cognitive distortions, 352
ideal body weight, 351

Objectives

1. Discuss four theories of eating disorders.
2. Compare and contrast the signs and symptoms (clinical picture) of anorexia nervosa and bulimia nervosa.
3. Identify three life-threatening conditions, stated in terms of nursing diagnoses, for a patient with an eating disorder.
4. Identify three realistic outcome criteria for (a) a patient with anorexia nervosa and (b) a patient with bulimia nervosa.

5. Describe therapeutic interventions appropriate for anorexia nervosa and bulimia nervosa in the acute phase and long-term phase of treatment.
6. Explain the basic premise of cognitive-behavioral therapy in the treatment of eating disorders.
7. Differentiate between the long-term prognoses of anorexia nervosa, bulimia nervosa, and binge eating disorder.

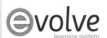 Visit the Evolve website for an **Audio Glossary & Flashcards, Concept Map Creator**, and additional resources related to the content in this chapter: **http://evolve.elsevier.com/Varcarolis/foundations**

Of all the psychiatric disorders, eating disorders may be the most perplexing. The eating and sharing of food is usually pleasurable and culturally important. It is difficult for many of us to understand how people could starve themselves or induce vomiting and seem to have little regard for how it affects them physically and socially. Cases of anorexia nervosa are documented in ancient writings; however, bulimia and binge eating necessitates an abundance of food and may be a more recent disorder of eating. Many theories of the etiology of these disorders have been postulated, but to date, the reasons behind the behavior are still a mystery that drives research.

CLINICAL PICTURE

The main types of eating disorders are anorexia nervosa, bulimia nervosa, and eating disorder not otherwise specified (NOS). A fourth disorder, binge eating disorder, is mentioned in the *Diagnostic and Statistical Manual of Mental Disorders*, fourth edition, text revision *(DSM-IV-TR)*, as a diagnosis requiring additional research (American Psychiatric Association [APA], 2000). Individuals with anorexia nervosa refuse to maintain a minimally normal weight for height and express intense fear of gaining weight. The term *anorexia* is a misnomer, because loss of appetite is rare. Some people with anorexia nervosa restrict their intake of food; others engage in binge eating and purging. Individuals with bulimia nervosa engage in repeated episodes of binge eating followed by inappropriate compensatory behaviors, such as self-induced vomiting; misuse of laxatives, diuretics, or other medications; fasting; or excessive exercise. Eating disorder NOS is a category that includes disorders of eating that do not meet the criteria for either anorexia nervosa or bulimia nervosa. All of these disorders are characterized by a significant disturbance in the perception of body shape and weight (APA, 2000). Individuals with binge eating disorder engage in repeated episodes of binge eating, after which they experience significant distress. These individuals do not regularly use compensatory behaviors, such as self-induced vomiting, misuse of laxatives and other medications, fasting, and excessive exercise that are seen in patients with bulimia nervosa.

Figure 16-1 identifies the diagnostic criteria for anorexia nervosa, bulimia nervosa, and eating disorders not otherwise specified.

EPIDEMIOLOGY

For women, the lifetime incidence of anorexia nervosa, bulimia nervosa, and binge eating disorder are 0.9%, 1.5%, and 3.5%, respectively; and the lifetime incidence for men is 0.3%, 0.5%, and 2% (Hudson et al., 2007). It is extremely difficult to determine the specific number of people afflicted with eating disorders, since fewer than half seek health care for their illness. Many people with disordered eating patterns do not meet full *DSM-IV-TR* criteria and are not included in these

statistics. In the United States, rates of eating disorders in Hispanic, Caucasian, and Native American women are similar, whereas African American women have a lower rate (APA, 2006).

Most eating disorders begin in the early teens to mid-20s, although they commonly occur following puberty, with bulimia occurring in later adolescence. Anorexia nervosa may start early (between ages 7 and 12), but bulimia nervosa is rarely seen in children younger than 12 years.

The rate of eating disorders among middle-aged women seems to have increased with the baby boomer generation (those born in the mid-1900s) (APA, 2006). Women are particularly at risk in industrialized nations, where there is an abundance of food and physical attractiveness is linked with being thin. Although anorexia is found in all cultures, bulimia and binge eating disorder are more common in countries most influenced by Western culture (Keel & Klump, 2003). There is some concern that adolescents who go on "extreme diets" that either restrict calories or involve avoiding certain food groups are at risk for developing an eating disorder, but it does not appear that caloric restriction

EVIDENCE-BASED PRACTICE

Prevention of Eating Disorders

Meyer, T. A., Gast, J. (2008) The effects of peer influence on disordered eating behavior. *The Journal of School Nursing, 24* (1): 36–42.

Problem
With a rise in eating-disorder cases in the United States, early education has emerged as a prevention program starting in the preteen years.

Purpose of Study
Although peer pressure is well known to influence the behavior of children ages 9 to 13, little is known about this influence on disordered eating behaviors which may progress to an eating disorder as these children grow older. This study is designed to examine how peer influence on both males and females affects eating behavior.

Methods
A randomized cross-sectional design was used. Two hundred students in seven homeroom classes at a middle school were randomly chosen from grades six through eight. Eighty-three subjects were male, mean age 12.61, and 117 subjects were female, mean age 12.59. Three paper-and-pencil instruments were used: a survey to collect demographics, the Eating Disorder Inventory (EDI), and the Inventory of Peer Influence on Eating Concerns (I-PIEC).

The EDI is a measurement tool that assesses a number of psychological and behavioral traits commonly found in individuals who have anorexia nervosa or bulimia nervosa. The I-PIEC is used to measure peer influence on children's eating and body concerns that consisted of three constructs: messages, interactions, and likability.

Key Findings
- Likability was the most significant predictor of disordered eating symptoms followed by the message subscale.
- Both males and females were influenced by peers, with males more sensitive to messages and girls more sensitive to likability.
- Both males and females had similar rates of disordered eating at ages younger than the normal teen years when eating disorders are usually diagnosed.

Implications for Nursing Practice
School nurses are often responsible for promoting health through education. At present, few programs designed to prevent disordered eating in young men and women include guidance in how to handle the urge to engage in unhealthy eating patterns to remain compatible among their peers.

DSM-IV-TR CRITERIA FOR EATING DISORDERS

EATING DISORDERS

Anorexia Nervosa

A. Refusal to maintain body weight at or above a minimally normal weight for age and height (e.g., weight loss leading to maintenance of body weight less than 85% of that expected) or failure to make expected weight gain during period of growth, leading to body weight less than 85% of that expected.

B. Intense fear of gaining weight or becoming fat, even though underweight.

C. Disturbance in the way in which one's body weight or shape is experienced, undue influence of body weight or shape on self-evaluation, or denial of the seriousness of the current low body weight.

D. In females, postmenarcheal amenorrhea (i.e., the absence of at least three consecutive menstrual cycles). (A woman is considered to have amenorrhea if her periods occur only after hormone [e.g., estrogen] administration.)

Specify type:

Binge eating/purging type: During the episode of anorexia nervosa, the person engages in recurrent episodes of binge eating or purging behaviors.

Restricting type: During the episode of anorexia nervosa, the person does *not* engage in recurrent episodes of binge eating or purging behaviors.

Bulimia Nervosa

A. Recurrent episodes of binge eating. An episode of binge eating is characterized by both of the following:

(1) Eating in a discrete period (e.g., within any 2-hour period) an amount of food that is definitely larger than most people would eat during a similar period and under similar circumstances.
(2) A sense of lack of control over eating during the episode (e.g., a feeling that one cannot stop eating or control what or how much one is eating).

B. Recurrent inappropriate compensatory behavior to prevent weight gain such as self-induced vomiting; misuse of laxatives, diuretics, enemas, or other medications; fasting; or excessive exercise.

C. The binge eating and inappropriate compensatory behavior both occur on average at least twice a week for 3 months.

D. Self-evaluation is unduly influenced by body shape and weight.

E. The disturbance does not occur exclusively during episodes of anorexia nervosa.

Specify type:

Purging type: During the current episode of bulimia nervosa, the person has regularly engaged in self-induced vomiting or the misuse of laxatives, diuretics, or enemas.

Nonpurging type: During the current episode of bulimia nervosa, the person has used other inappropriate compensatory behaviors such as fasting or excessive exercise but has not regularly engaged in self-induced vomiting or the misuse of laxatives, diuretics, or enemas.

Eating Disorder Not Otherwise Specified (NOS)

The eating disorder not otherwise specified category is for disorders of eating that do not meet the criteria for any specific eating disorder. Examples include:

1. For females, all the criteria for anorexia nervosa are met except that the individual has regular menses.

2. All the criteria for anorexia nervosa are met except that despite significant weight loss, the individual's current weight is in the normal range.

3. All the criteria for bulimia nervosa are met except that the binge eating and inappropriate compensatory mechanisms occur at a frequency of less than twice a week for a duration of less than 3 months.

4. The regular use of inappropriate compensatory behavior by an individual of normal body weight after eating small amounts of food (i.e., self-induced vomiting after the consumption of two cookies).

5. Repeatedly chewing and spitting out, but not swallowing, large amounts of food.

6. Binge eating disorder: recurrent episodes of binge eating in the absence of the regular use of inappropriate compensatory behaviors characteristic of bulimia nervosa.

Figure 16-1 Diagnostic criteria for eating disorders. (Adapted from American Psychiatric Association. [2000]. *Diagnostic and statistical manual of mental disorders* [4th ed., text rev.] *[DSM-IV-TR]*. Washington, DC: Author.)

as a method to reduce body weight in individuals who are overweight is in itself responsible for this risk (Williamson et al., 2008).

Although patients with eating disorders are at risk of medical complications that may result in death, the major cause of death among those affected by eating disorders is suicide. Patients diagnosed with anorexia nervosa or bulimia nervosa may have a suicide rate that is 6.7 times greater than the norm for their age group (Pompili et al., 2006).

COMORBIDITY

Depression and anxiety are common comorbid conditions in people with all types of eating disorders. The estimated lifetime prevalence of mood disorders in anorexia nervosa ranges from 31% to 89% and in bulimia nervosa ranges from 24% to 90%. The fact that depressive symptoms accompany any type of starvation makes it difficult to determine an exact prevalence (Godart et al., 2007).

The incidence of obsessive-compulsive disorder (OCD) has been reported to be as high as 25% in patients with anorexia nervosa. The OCD symptoms center on food preoccupation and may be manifested in collecting cookbooks, preparing elaborate meals for others, and hoarding food. Anxiety disorders, particularly social phobia, are also common. In addition, substance abuse has been found in as many as 23% to 40% of patients with bulimia nervosa and ranged from 12% to 18% among patients with anorexia nervosa (APA, 2006).

People with eating disorders who also have depression, substance abuse, and/or poor impulse control are at greater risk for relapse. There is some evidence that the younger the person is when anorexic symptoms begin, the better the chance for positive outcomes (Berkman et al., 2007).

Personality disorders may occur in 42% to 75% of people with eating disorders. There is a high rate of avoidant personality disorders in all the eating disorders. This avoidance fits the clinical picture of being overly concerned with acceptance and approval and fear of criticism or rejection. Patients with anorexia nervosa are more likely to have a Cluster C personality disorder (avoidant, dependent, obsessive-compulsive, or passive aggressive) (Berkman et al., 2007). Obsessive-compulsive and dependent personality disorders are also common in patients with bulimia. Borderline personality disorder is common in patients with binge eating disorder.

Sexual abuse has been reported in 20% to 50% of patients with eating disorders. It appears that such early trauma may predispose individuals to binge-and-purge eating behavior. In general, bulimia is more common in girls than in boys. However, among those who have been sexually or physically abused, nearly twice as many boys present with binge-and-purge symptoms as do girls (APA, 2006).

ETIOLOGY

The eating disorders—anorexia nervosa, bulimia nervosa, and eating disorder NOS, which includes binge eating disorder—are actually entities or syndromes and are not considered to be specific diseases. It is not known if they share a common cause and pathology; therefore, it is more appropriate to conceptualize them as syndromes on the basis of the cluster of symptoms they present (Halmi, 2008). A number of theories attempt to explain eating disorders.

Biological Factors

Genetic

There is a strong genetic link for eating disorders. In fact, data from community-based twin studies have suggested that the heritability is greater than 50% (Keel & Klump, 2003). A genetic vulnerability may lead to poor affect and impulse control or to an underlying neurotransmitter dysfunction, but no single causative gene has been discovered to date. However, there is evidence that certain gene abnormalities may predispose a person to have symptoms of eating disorders and even confer a risk for developing full-blown eating disorders (Frieling et al., 2006).

Neurobiological

Research demonstrates that altered brain serotonin function contributes to dysregulation of appetite, mood, and impulse control in the eating disorders. These patients consistently exhibit personality traits of perfectionism, obsessive-compulsiveness, and dysphoric mood, all of which are modulated through serotonin pathways in the brain. Because these traits appear to begin in childhood—before the onset of actual eating-disorder symptoms—and persist into recovery, they are believed to contribute to a vulnerability to disordered eating (Kaye, 2007).

Tryptophan, an amino acid essential to serotonin synthesis, is only available through diet. A normal diet boosts serotonin in the brain and regulates mood. Temporary drops in dietary tryptophan may actually relieve symptoms of anxiety and dysphoria and provide a reward for caloric restriction. However, continued malnutrition will result in a physiological dysphoria. This cycle of temporary relief, followed by more dysphoria, sets up a positive feedback loop that reinforces the disordered eating behavior (Kaye, 2007). This dietary need for tryptophan may account for the fact that antidepressants that boost serotonin do not improve mood symptoms until after an underweight patient has been restored to 90% of optimal weight.

Newer brain imaging capabilities allow for more research into etiological factors of anorexia nervosa and bulimia nervosa. Overall, there is a consistent finding that patients with eating disorders who are acutely ill and those who have recovered show differences in frontal, cingulated, temporal, and/or parietal regions of the brain in comparison to controls. More studies will be necessary before conclusions can be made about the significance of these differences (Kaye, 2007).

Psychological Factors

Because anorexia nervosa was observed primarily in girls approaching puberty, early psychoanalytic theories linked the symptoms to an unconscious aversion to sexuality. By maintaining a childlike body, the patient avoids the anxiety associated with developing into a mature sexual being. Throughout the 1900s, many authors examined the family dynamics of these patients and concluded that a failure to separate from parents and a rebellion against the maternal bond explained the disordered eating behaviors. Further work by Bruch in the 1970s explored the symptoms as a defense against an overwhelming feeling of ineffectiveness and powerlessness. Even with further insight into the intrapsychic origin of the behavior, the process of psychoanalysis—with the goal of making unconscious processes conscious—failed to effect a cure for these syndromes (Caparrotta & Ghaffari, 2006).

Currently, cognitive-behavioral theorists suggest that eating disorders are based on learned behavior that has positive reinforcement. For example, a mildly overweight 14-year-old has the flu and loses a little weight. She returns to school, and her friends say, "Wow, you look great." Now she purposefully strives to lose weight. When people say, "Wow, you look really skinny," she hears, "Wow, you look great." Her behavior is powerfully reinforced by these comments despite the fact that her health is at risk.

Family theorists maintain that eating disorders are a problem of the whole family, and often the symptoms in the child serve to take the attention away from a distressed marriage. Families with a child who has anorexia are often described as enmeshed and perfectionistic; the child feels smothered by protectiveness and at the same time abandoned.

Environmental Factors

The Western cultural ideal that equates feminine beauty to tall, thin models has received much attention in the media as an etiology for the eating disorders. Studies have shown that culture influences the development of self-concept and satisfaction with body size. The rate of obesity in the United States is at an alarming level: 35% of adult women are obese, and 16% of 2- to 19-year-old girls are obese (Centers for Disease Control and Prevention [CDC], 2006).

Record numbers of men and women are on diets to reduce body weight, but no study has been able to explain why only an estimated 0.3% to 3% of the population develops an eating disorder. Although a causal link between cultural norms of thinness and the eating disorders has not been proved, all patients with eating disorders have low self-esteem that is negatively impacted by their inability to conform to an impossible cultural standard of beauty (Stein & Corte, 2003).

CONSIDERING CULTURE

The Concept of Weight

Although cultural beliefs about physical beauty do not *cause* eating disorders, they influence self-esteem and set the standard of beauty for men and women. If this cultural ideal is unhealthy, it can pose health risks if not addressed.

For centuries, body weight indicated the availability of food. Only persons with wealth had the luxury of fat, and therefore the ideal was to achieve a large body. With the recent media focus on the effect of the Western fashion industry and unnaturally thin models, it is of interest that other cultures still have the more traditional standards that equate obesity with beauty.

The Saharawi of Morocco are a nomadic people who see those who are thin as ill. Young women, as they reach marriageable age, seek to rapidly increase their weight. To accomplish this, they eat large amounts of traditional foods, restrict their activity, and even take drugs such as corticosteroids to increase appetite and promote weight gain. Of the 249 women interviewed in this study, 225 were unsatisfied with their current weight. The group had a mean BMI of 29.6, with a range from 17.3 to 41.4. Only eight women wished to lose weight; the rest sought to become heavier. The authors suggest that a change in the cultural norm for beauty will be necessary to prevent the known health risks of obesity in that population.

Culturally competent care planning is made very difficult when the cultural ideal is unhealthy. In seeking to change behavior, the cultural norm must be acknowledged as important to the individual. The nurse's role is to provide adequate education about the risks and health consequences of the norm and help individuals find a solution that respects their culture but promotes health.

Rguibi, M., & Belahsen, R. (2006). Fattening practices among Moroccan Saharawi women. *Eastern Mediterranean Health Journal, 12*, 619–624.

Anorexia Nervosa

APPLICATION OF THE NURSING PROCESS

ASSESSMENT

Anorexia nervosa and bulimia nervosa are two separate syndromes that present two clinical pictures on assessment. Box 16-1 lists several thoughts and behaviors associated with anorexia nervosa, and Table 16-1 identifies clinical signs and symptoms of anorexia nervosa found on assessment, together with their causes.

Eating disorders are serious and in extreme cases can lead to death. Box 16-2 identifies a number of medical complications that can occur in individuals with anorexia nervosa and the laboratory findings that may result. Because the eating behaviors in these conditions are so extreme, hospitalization may become necessary (often via the emergency department). Box 16-3 identifies physical and psychiatric criteria for hospitalization of an individual with an eating disorder.

Fundamental to the care of individuals with eating disorders is establishing and maintaining a therapeutic alliance. This will take both time and diplomacy on the part of the nurse. In treating patients who have been sexually abused or who have otherwise been victims of boundary violations, it is critical that the nurse and other health care workers maintain and respect clear boundaries (APA, 2006).

General Assessment

Individuals with the binge-purge type of anorexia nervosa may present with severe electrolyte imbalance (as a result of purging) and enter the health care

TABLE 16-1 Possible Signs and Symptoms of Anorexia Nervosa	
Clinical Presentation	**Cause**
Low weight	Caloric restriction, excessive exercising
Amenorrhea	Low weight
Yellow skin	Hypercarotenemia
Lanugo	Starvation
Cold extremities	Starvation
Peripheral edema	Hypoalbuminemia and refeeding
Muscle weakening	Starvation, electrolyte imbalance
Constipation	Starvation
Abnormal laboratory values (low triiodothyronine, thyroxine levels)	Starvation
Abnormal computed tomographic scans, electroencephalographic changes	Starvation
Cardiovascular abnormalities (hypotension, bradycardia, heart failure)	Starvation, dehydration Electrolyte imbalance
Impaired renal function	Dehydration
Hypokalemia (low potassium)	Starvation
Anemic pancytopenia	Starvation
Decreased bone density	Estrogen deficiency, low calcium intake

system through admission to an intensive care unit. The patient with anorexia will be severely underweight and may have growth of fine, downy hair (lanugo) on the face and back. The patient will also have mottled, cool skin on the extremities and low blood pressure, pulse, and temperature readings, consistent with a malnourished, dehydrated state (see Table 16-1).

As with any comprehensive psychiatric nursing assessment, a complete evaluation of biopsychosocial function is mandatory. The areas to be covered include the patient's:
- Perception of the problem
- Eating habits
- History of dieting
- Methods used to achieve weight control (restricting, purging, exercising)
- Value attached to a specific shape and weight
- Interpersonal and social functioning
- Mental status and physiological parameters

BOX 16-1 Thoughts and Behaviors Associated with Anorexia Nervosa

- Terror of gaining weight
- Preoccupation with thoughts of food
- View of self as fat even when emaciated
- Peculiar handling of food:
  - Cutting food into small bits
  - Pushing pieces of food around plate
- Possible development of rigorous exercise regimen
- Possible self-induced vomiting, use of laxatives and diuretics
- Cognition so disturbed that individual judges self-worth by his or her weight

INTEGRATIVE THERAPY

Ma Huang

In an attempt to lose weight and fight hunger, many patients with eating disorders turn to weight-loss products that contain herbs. *Ma huang*, the Chinese name for the *Ephedra sinica* plant, is a stimulant banned from the United States by the FDA because of the risk of stroke and sudden death, but it may still be contained in natural products sold over the Internet. In a small study of patients with eating disorders, 42% of patients who actually experienced adverse side effects on ephedra products decided to continue taking the herb.

Steffen, K. J., Roerig, J. L., Mitchell, J. E., Crosby, R. D. (2006). A survey of herbal and alternative medication use among participants with eating-disorder symptoms. *International Journal of Eating Disorders, 39*, 741–746.

BOX 16-2 Medical Complications of Anorexia Nervosa

- Bradycardia
- Orthostatic changes in pulse or blood pressure
- Cardiac arrhythmias
- Prolonged QT interval and ST-T wave abnormalities
- Peripheral neuropathy
- Acrocyanosis
- Symptomatic hypotension
- Leukopenia
- Lymphocytosis
- Carotenemia (elevated carotene levels in blood), which produces skin with yellow pallor
- Hypokalemic alkalosis (with self-induced vomiting or use of laxatives and diuretics)
- Elevated serum bicarbonate levels, hypochloremia, and hypokalemia
- Electrolyte imbalances, which lead to fatigue, weakness, and lethargy
- Osteoporosis, indicated by decrease in bone density
- Fatty degeneration of liver, indicated by elevation of serum enzyme levels
- Elevated cholesterol levels
- Amenorrhea
- Abnormal thyroid functioning
- Hematuria
- Proteinuria

Data from Halmi, K. A. (2008). Eating disorders: Anorexia nervosa, bulimia nervosa, and obesity. In R. E. Hales, S. C. Yudofsky, G. O. Gabbard (Eds.), *Textbook of psychiatry* (5th ed., pp. 762, 769–770). Washington, DC: American Psychiatric Publishing.

BOX 16-3 Criteria for Hospital Admission of Patients with Eating Disorders

Physical Criteria
- Weight loss over 30% over 6 months
- Rapid decline in weight
- Inability to gain weight with outpatient treatment
- Severe hypothermia due to loss of subcutaneous tissue or dehydration (temperature lower than 36° C or 96.8° F)
- Heart rate less than 40 beats per minute
- Systolic blood pressure less than 70 mm Hg
- Hypokalemia (less than 3 mEq/L) or other electrolyte disturbances not corrected by oral supplementation
- Electrocardiographic changes (especially arrhythmias)

Psychiatric Criteria
- Suicidal or severely out-of-control, self-mutilating behaviors
- Out-of-control use of laxatives, emetics, diuretics, or street drugs
- Failure to comply with treatment contract
- Severe depression
- Psychosis
- Family crisis or dysfunction

Self-Assessment

When caring for the patient with anorexia, you may find it difficult to appreciate the compelling force of the illness, incorrectly believing that weight restriction, bingeing, and purging are self-imposed. If we see such self-destructive behaviors as choices, it is only natural to blame the patient for any consequent health problems. The common personality traits of these patients—perfectionism, obsessive thoughts and actions relating to food, intense feelings of shame, people pleasing, and the need to have complete control over their therapy—pose additional challenges.

In your efforts to motivate such patients and take advantage of their decision to seek help and be healthier, take care not to allow encouragement to cross the line into authoritarianism and assumption of a parental role. A patient's terror at gaining weight and her or his resistance to clinical interventions may engender significant frustration in the nurse struggling to build a therapeutic relationship and be empathetic. Guard against any tendency to be coercive in your approach, and be aware that one of the primary goals of treatment—weight gain—is the very thing the patient fears. When patients appear to be resistant to change, it is helpful to acknowledge the constant struggle that so characterizes the treatment.

Assessment Guidelines Anorexia Nervosa

Determine whether:

1. The patient has a medical or psychiatric condition that warrants hospitalization (see Box 16-3).
2. A thorough physical examination with appropriate blood work has been done.
3. Other medical conditions have been ruled out.
4. The patient is amenable to receiving or compliant with appropriate therapeutic modalities.
5. The family and patient need further teaching or information regarding the patient's treatment plan (e.g., psychopharmacological interventions, behavioral therapy, cognitive therapy, family therapy, individual psychotherapy).
6. The patient and family desire to participate in a support group.
7. The patient and family have been provided referral to a support group.

DIAGNOSIS

Imbalanced nutrition: less than body requirements is usually the most appropriate initial nursing diagnosis for individuals with anorexia (North American Nursing Diagnosis Association International, 2009). *Imbalanced nutrition: less than body requirements* generates further nursing diagnoses—for example, *Decreased cardiac output*, *Risk for injury* (electrolyte imbalance), and *Risk for imbalanced fluid volume* (which would have first priority when problems are addressed). Other nursing diagnoses include *Anxiety*, *Chronic low self-esteem*, *Disturbed body image*, *Deficient knowledge*, *Ineffective coping*, *Powerlessness*, and *Hopelessness*.

OUTCOMES IDENTIFICATION

To evaluate the effectiveness of treatment, outcome criteria are established to measure treatment results. Relevant categories of the *Nursing Outcomes Classification (NOC)* (Moorhead et al., 2008) include *Weight Gain Behavior*, *Weight Maintenance Behavior*, *Anxiety Self-control*, *Nutritional Status: Nutrient Intake*, and *Self-esteem*. Refer to Table 16-2 for examples of short-term NOC indicators for the patient with anorexia nervosa.

PLANNING

Planning is affected by the acuity of the patient's situation. When a patient with anorexia is experiencing extreme electrolyte imbalance or weighs below 75% of ideal body weight, the plan is to provide immediate medical stabilization, most likely in an inpatient unit (APA, 2006). If a specialized eating-disorder unit is not available, hospitalization on a cardiac or medical unit is usually brief, providing only limited weight restoration and addressing only the acute complications (e.g., electrolyte imbalance and dysrhythmias) and acute psychiatric symptoms (e.g., significant depression).

TABLE 16-2 *NOC* Outcomes Related to Anorexia Nervosa

Nursing Outcome and Definition	Short-Term Indicators
Nutritional Status: Nutrient Intake: Nutrient intake to meet metabolic needs	Caloric intake Protein intake Fat intake Carbohydrate intake
Weight Gain Behavior: Personal actions to gain weight following voluntary or involuntary significant weight loss	Sets achievable weight gain goals Selects a healthy target weight Commits to a healthy eating plan Monitors exercise for caloric requirements
Anxiety Self-Control: Personal action to eliminate or reduce feelings of apprehension, tension, or uneasiness from an unidentifiable source.	Monitors intensity of anxiety Plans coping strategies for stressful situations Uses effective coping strategies
Self-Esteem: Personal judgment of self-worth	Verbalization of self-acceptance Description of self Acceptance of compliments from others Feelings about self-worth

Data from Moorhead, S., Johnson, M., Maas, M. L., & Swanson, E. (Eds.). (2008). *Nursing outcome classification (NOC)* (4th ed.) St. Louis: Mosby.

With the initiation of therapeutic nutrition, malnourished patients may need treatment on a medical unit, owing to **refeeding syndrome**, a potentially catastrophic treatment complication involving a metabolic alteration in serum electrolytes, vitamin deficiencies, and sodium retention (Lauts, 2005).

Once a patient is medically stable, the plan addresses the issues underlying the eating disorder. These psychological issues are usually addressed on an outpatient basis. The plan of care will include individual, group, and family therapy, as well as psychopharmacological therapy during different phases of the illness. The nature of the treatment is determined by the intensity of the symptoms—which may vary over time—and the experienced disruption in the patient's life.

Discharge planning is a critical component in treatment. Often, family members benefit from counseling. The discharge planning process must address living arrangements, school, work, the feasibility of independent financial status, applications for state and/or federal program assistance (if needed), and follow-up outpatient treatment.

IMPLEMENTATION

Acute Care

Typically a patient with an eating disorder is admitted to the inpatient psychiatric facility in a crisis state. The initial focus depends on the results of a comprehensive assessment. Any acute psychiatric symptoms, such as suicidal ideation, are addressed immediately. The nurse is challenged to establish trust and monitor the eating pattern.

Psychosocial Interventions

After intervention for any acute symptoms, the patient with anorexia begins a weight restoration program that allows for incremental weight gain. Based on the patient's height, a treatment goal is set at 90% of ideal body weight, the weight at which most women are able to menstruate.

As patients begin to refeed, they ideally begin to participate in milieu therapy, in which the cognitive distortions that perpetuate the illness are consistently confronted by all members of the interdisciplinary team. Box 16-4 identifies some common types of cognitive distortions characteristic of people with

---

BOX 16-4 Cognitive Distortions

Overgeneralization

A single event affects unrelated situations.
- "He didn't ask me out. It must be because I'm fat."
- "I was happy when I wore a size 6. I must get back to that weight."

All-or-Nothing Thinking

Reasoning is absolute and extreme, in mutually exclusive terms of black or white, good or bad.
- "If I have one popsicle, I must eat five."
- "If I allow myself to gain weight, I'll blow up like a balloon."

Catastrophizing

The consequences of an event are magnified.
- "If I gain weight, my weekend will be ruined."
- "When people say I look better, I know they think I'm fat."

Personalization

Events are overinterpreted as having personal significance.
- "I know everybody is watching me eat."
- "I think people won't like me unless I'm thin."

Emotional reasoning

Subjective emotions determine reality.
- "I know I'm fat, because I feel fat."
- "When I'm thin, I feel powerful."

Adapted from Bowers, W. A. (2001). Basic principles for applying cognitive-behavioral therapy to anorexia nervosa. *Psychiatric Clinics of North America, 24,* 293–303.

---

eating disorders. Focus should be on the eating behavior and underlying feelings of anxiety, dysphoria, low self-esteem, and lack of control. When possible, the distortions in body image are avoided, because attempts to change this perception are often misinterpreted, as shown in the following vignette.

VIGNETTE

Alicia, a 17-year-old cheerleader, did not come to treatment for weight loss until she fainted at a football game. She insisted that she only needed to "get more energy, not get fat." When the nurse pointed out that Alicia's ribs were clearly visible and that her backbone looked like a skeleton, Alicia grinned and said, "Thank you." ▪

Pharmacological Interventions

There are no drugs approved by the U.S. Food and Drug Administration (FDA) for the treatment of anorexia nervosa, and research does not support the use of pharmacological agents to treat the core symptoms (Becker et al., 2008). However, the selective serotonin reuptake inhibitor (SSRI) fluoxetine (Prozac) has proven useful in reducing obsessive-compulsive behavior *after* the patient has reached a maintenance weight. Conventional antipsychotics such as chlorpromazine (Thorazine) may be helpful for delusional or overactive patients (Halmi, 2008). Atypical antipsychotic agents such as olanzapine (Zyprexa) are helpful in improving mood and decreasing obsessional behaviors and resistance to weight gain (Attia & Walsh, 2007).

Health Teaching and Health Promotion

Self-care activities are an important part of the treatment plan. These activities include learning more constructive coping skills, improving social skills, and developing problem-solving and decision-making skills. The skills become the focus of both therapy sessions and supervised food-shopping trips. As the patient approaches the goal weight, she or he is encouraged to expand the repertoire to include eating out in a restaurant, preparing a meal, and eating forbidden foods. The following vignette illustrates the need for supportive education.

VIGNETTE

A nursing assessment of a small group of three young women and one young man in a nutrition group finds that all the participants are very knowledgeable about the caloric value of common foods; as a group, they all avoid any "fatty" foods. The topic of fat-soluble vitamins and the consequences of vitamin deficiencies on the body was new information to all of the participants, and one of the young women started to cry, saying, "I had no idea I was doing that to my body." This show of emotion promoted a supportive interaction among the other group members as they shared their own stories of symptoms they could now identify as vitamin deficits. ▪

Milieu Management

Patients admitted to an inpatient unit designed to treat eating disorders participate in a combination of therapeutic modalities provided by a multidisciplinary team. These modalities are designed to normalize eating patterns and begin to address the medical, family, and social issues raised by the illness.

The milieu of an eating-disorder unit is purposefully organized to assist the patient in establishing more adaptive behavioral patterns, including normalization of eating. The highly structured milieu includes precise meal times, adherence to the selected menu, observation during and after meals, and regularly scheduled weighing.

Close monitoring of patients includes monitoring all trips to the bathroom after eating to prevent self-induced vomiting. Patients may also need monitoring on bathroom trips after seeing visitors and after any hospital pass to ensure they have not had access to and ingested any laxatives or diuretics. Often, patient privileges are linked to weight gain and treatment-plan adherence. The following vignette demonstrates monitoring the bathroom as a therapeutic intervention.

VIGNETTE

A 20-year-old woman who primarily restricts her eating but resorts to purging when forced to eat by her family became visibly distressed after eating all of her therapeutic meal. Although her treatment plan was to join other patients in group therapy, the patient requested permission to go to the bathroom alone because she had "embarrassing gas" she did not want overheard. The nurse negotiated to stand away from the bathroom door if the patient agreed not to flush the toilet until the nurse was able to inspect the contents. However, the patient flushed the toilet before inspection. Even if this patient had not used this bathroom break to purge, the breaking of the contract with the nurse was discussed in treatment team as an indication that this patient was not able to adhere to her prescribed treatment without additional structure. The treatment team established a new expectation that until the patient had gained 2 pounds, she was to wait 30 minutes after every meal before she was allowed supervised bathroom breaks. ▪

VIGNETTE

In an outpatient eating-disorder treatment facility, Nicole made friends with another patient, Stacy. Later Nicole told the nurse, "I found out that Stacy was so sick she needed a feeding tube and was in the hospital for 2 weeks. I'm sicker than Stacy is. I needed to stay in the hospital for 3 weeks! ▪

Advanced Practice Interventions

Anorexia nervosa is a chronic illness that waxes and wanes. The 1-year relapse rate approaches 50% and long-term studies show that up to 20% of patients continue to meet full criteria for anorexia nervosa after several years (Attia & Walsh, 2007). Recovery is evaluated as a stage in the process rather than a fixed event. Factors that influence the stage of recovery include percentage of ideal body weight that has been achieved, the extent to which self-worth is defined by shape and weight, and the amount of disruption existing in the patient's personal life.

The patient will require long-term treatment that might include periodic brief hospital stays, outpatient psychotherapy, and pharmacological interventions. The combination of individual, group, couples, and family therapy (especially for the younger patient) provides the patient with the greatest chance for a successful outcome.

Psychotherapy

The advanced practice nurse provides individual, group, or family therapy in a variety of settings. The goals of treatment are weight restoration with normalization of eating habits and initiation of the treatment of psychological, interpersonal, and social issues that personally affect each individual patient.

Outpatient partial hospitalization programs designed to treat eating disorders are structured to achieve outcomes comparable to those of inpatient eating-disorder units. The advanced practice nurse, along with other therapists, might contract with patients with anorexia regarding the terms of treatment. For example, outpatient treatment can continue only if the patient maintains a contracted weight. If weight falls below the goal, other treatment arrangements must be made until the patient returns to the goal weight. This highly structured approach to treating patients whose weight is below 75% of ideal body weight is necessary, even for therapists who approach treatment from a more emotional or cognitive model of therapy. Assisting the patient with a daily meal plan, reviewing a journal of meals and dietary intake maintained by the patient, and providing for weekly weighing (ideally two to three times a week) are essential if the patient is to reach a medically stable weight.

Families frequently report feeling powerless in the face of behavior that is mystifying. For instance, patients are often unable to experience compliments as supportive and therefore are unable to internalize the support. They often seek attention from others but feel shamed when they receive it. Patients express that they want their families to care for and about them but are unable to recognize expressions of care. When others do respond with love and support, patients do not perceive this as positive. The following vignette demonstrates this phenomenon.

VIGNETTE

In a multifamily group on an inpatient unit, Mrs. Demi (who last saw her daughter before she had gained 40 lbs) is asked by the group leader how she regards her daughter, Lila. Mrs. Demi replies, "She looks healthy." Her daughter responds with an angry, sullen look. She ultimately verbalizes that she interprets comments about her "healthy" appearance as "You look fat." The group leader points out that it is interesting that Lila equates "healthy" with "fat." In the multifamily group, there is a commonly expressed view that the illness "is not about weight" but that thinness confers a feeling of being special and that being at a normal weight (i.e., healthy) means this special status is lost. ■

Often family members and significant others seek ways to communicate clearly with the patient with anorexia but find that they are frequently misunderstood and that overtures of concern are misinterpreted. Consequently, families experience the tension of saying or doing the wrong thing and then feeling responsible if a setback occurs. Advanced practice psychiatric mental health nurses have an important role in assisting families and significant others to develop strategies for improved communication and search for ways to be comfortably supportive to the patient.

EVALUATION

The process of evaluation is built into the outcomes specified by *NOC*. Evaluation is ongoing, and short-term indicators are revised as necessary to achieve the treatment outcomes established. The indicators provide a daily guide for evaluating success and must be continually reevaluated for their appropriateness. Case Study and Nursing Care Plan 16-1 on pages 359–362 presents a patient with anorexia nervosa.

Bulimia Nervosa

Bulimia first entered the *DSM* as a diagnosis in the third edition in 1980 but without purging or inappropriate compensatory behaviors as criteria. The diagnosis became bulimia nervosa with the addition of the preceding criteria in 1987. In the current *DSM-IV-TR* (APA, 2000), it is further subcategorized as purging or nonpurging type (see Figure 16-1).

APPLICATION OF THE NURSING PROCESS

ASSESSMENT

General Assessment

Initially, patients with bulimia nervosa do not appear to be physically or emotionally ill. They are often at or slightly above or below ideal body weight. However, as the assessment continues and the nurse makes further observations, the physical and emotional problems of the patient become apparent. On inspection, the patient demonstrates enlargement of the parotid glands, with dental erosion and caries if the patient has been inducing vomiting. Box 16-5 identifies a number of medical complications that can occur and the laboratory findings that may result in individuals with bulimia nervosa. The disclosed history may reveal great difficulties with both impulsivity and compulsivity. Family relationships are frequently chaotic and reflect a lack of nurturing. Patients' lives reflect instability and troublesome interpersonal relationships as well. It is not uncommon for patients to have a history of impulsive stealing of items such as food, clothing, or jewelry (Halmi, 2008).

VIGNETTE

During the initial assessment, the nurse wonders if Brittany is actually in need of hospitalization on the eating-disorders unit. The nurse is struck by how well the patient appears, seeming healthy, well dressed, and articulate. As Brittany continues to relate her history, she tells of restricting her intake all day until early evening, when she buys her food and begins to binge as she is shopping. She arrives home and immediately induces vomiting. For the remainder of the evening and into the early morning hours, she "zones out" while watching television and binge eating. Periodically she goes to the bathroom to vomit. She does this about 15 times during the evening. The nurse admitting Brittany to the unit reminds her of the goals of the hospitalization, including interrupting the binge-purge cycle and normalizing eating. The nurse further explains to Brittany that she has the support of the eating-disorder treatment team and the milieu of the unit to assist her toward recovery. ■

Box 16-6 lists several thoughts and behaviors associated with bulimia nervosa, and Table 16-3 identifies possible signs and symptoms found on assessment and their causes.

BOX 16-5 Medical Complications of Bulimia Nervosa

- Sinus bradycardia
- Orthostatic changes in pulse or blood pressure
- Cardiac arrhythmias
- Cardiac arrest from electrolyte disturbances or Ipecac intoxication
- Cardiac murmur; mitral valve prolapse
- Electrolyte imbalances
- Elevated serum bicarbonate levels (although can be low, which indicates a metabolic acidosis)
- Hypochloremia
- Hypokalemia
- Dehydration, which results in volume depletion, leading to stimulation of aldosterone production, which in turn stimulates further potassium excretion from kidneys; thus there can be both an indirect renal loss of potassium and a direct loss through self-induced vomiting
- Severe attrition and erosion of teeth, producing irritating sensitivity and exposing the pulp of the teeth
- Loss of dental arch
- Diminished chewing ability
- Parotid gland enlargement associated with elevated serum amylase levels
- Esophageal tears caused by self-induced vomiting
- Severe abdominal pain indicative of gastric dilation
- Russell's sign (callus on knuckles from self-induced vomiting)

Data from Halmi, K. A. (2008). Eating disorders: Anorexia nervosa, bulimia nervosa, and obesity. In R. E. Hales, S. C. Yudofsky, & G. O. Gabbard (Eds.), *Textbook of psychiatry* (5th ed., pp. 762, 769–770). Washington, DC: American Psychiatric Publishing.

BOX 16-6 Thoughts and Behaviors Associated with Bulimia Nervosa

- Binge eating behaviors
- Often self-induced vomiting (or laxative or diuretic use) after bingeing
- History of anorexia nervosa in one fourth to one third of individuals
- Depressive signs and symptoms
- Problems with:
  - Interpersonal relationships
  - Self-concept
  - Impulsive behaviors
- Increased levels of anxiety and compulsivity
- Possible chemical dependency
- Possible impulsive stealing

TABLE 16-3 Possible Signs and Symptoms of Bulimia Nervosa

Clinical Presentation	Cause
Normal to slightly low weight	Excessive caloric intake with purging, excessive exercising
Dental caries, tooth erosion	Vomiting (HCl reflux over enamel)
Parotid swelling	Increased serum amylase levels
Gastric dilation, rupture	Binge eating
Calluses, scars on hand (Russell's sign)	Self-induced vomiting
Peripheral edema	Rebound fluid, especially if diuretic used
Muscle weakening	Electrolyte imbalance
Abnormal laboratory values (electrolyte imbalance, hypokalemia, hyponatremia)	Purging: vomiting, laxative and/or diuretic use
Cardiovascular abnormalities (cardiomyopathy, electrocardiographic changes)	Electrolyte imbalance—**can lead to death**
Cardiac failure (cardiomyopathy)	Ipecac intoxication

Self-Assessment

In working with someone with bulimia, be aware that the patient is sensitive to the perceptions of others regarding this illness and may feel significant shame and totally out of control. In building a therapeutic alliance, try to empathize with the patient's feelings of low self-esteem, unworthiness, and dysphoria. If you believe the patient is not being honest (e.g., active bingeing or purging goes unreported) or is being manipulative, acknowledge such obstacles and the frustration they provoke, and construct alternative ways to view the patient's thinking and behavior. An accepting, nonjudgmental approach, along with a comprehensive understanding of the subjective experience of the patient with bulimia, will help to build trust.

Assessment Guidelines Bulimia Nervosa

1. Medical stabilization is the first priority. Problems resulting from purging are disruptions in electrolyte and fluid balance and cardiac function. Therefore, a thorough medical examination is vital.

Continued

2. Medical evaluation usually includes a thorough physical examination, as well as pertinent laboratory testing, including:
   - Electrolyte levels
   - Glucose level
   - Thyroid function tests
   - Complete blood count
   - ECG
3. Psychiatric evaluation is advised because treatment of psychiatric comorbidity is important to outcome.

DIAGNOSIS

The assessment of the patient with bulimia nervosa yields nursing diagnoses that result from the disordered eating and weight-control behaviors. Problems resulting from purging are a first priority because electrolyte and fluid balance and cardiac function are affected. Common nursing diagnoses include *Decreased cardiac output, Powerlessness, Chronic low self-esteem, Anxiety,* and *Ineffective coping* (substance abuse, impulsive responses to problems).

OUTCOMES IDENTIFICATION

Relevant *NOC* outcomes include *Vital Signs, Electrolyte and Acid/Base Balance, Weight Maintenance Behavior, Self-esteem, Hope,* and *Coping.* Table 16-4 lists selected short-term indicators for patients with bulimia nervosa.

PLANNING

The criteria for inpatient admission of a patient with bulimia nervosa are included in the criteria for inpatient admission of a patient with an eating disorder presented in Box 16-3. Like the patient with anorexia nervosa, the patient with bulimia may be treated for life-threatening complications such as gastric rupture (rare), electrolyte imbalance, and cardiac dysrhythmias in an acute care unit of a hospital. If the patient is admitted to a general inpatient psychiatric unit because of acute suicidal risk, only the acute psychiatric manifestations are addressed short term. Planning will also include appropriate referrals for continuing outpatient treatment.

VIGNETTE

Iris weighs 85% of her ideal body weight. She has a history of diuretic abuse, and she becomes very edematous when she stops their use and enters treatment. The nurse informs Iris that the edema is related to the use of diuretics and thus is transient, and that it will resolve after Iris begins to eat normally and discontinues the diuretics. Iris cannot tolerate the weight gain and the accompanying edema that occurs when she stops taking diuretics. She restarts the diuretics, perpetuating the cycle of fluid retention and the risk of kidney damage. The nurse empathizes with Iris's inability to tolerate the feelings of anxiety and dread she experiences because of her markedly swollen extremities. ■

IMPLEMENTATION

Acute Care

A patient who is medically compromised as a result of bulimia nervosa is referred to an inpatient eating-disorder unit for comprehensive treatment of the illness. The cognitive-behavioral model of treatment is highly effective and frequently serves as the cornerstone of the therapeutic approach. Inpatient units designed to treat eating disorders are especially structured to interrupt the cycle of binge eating and purging and to normalize eating habits. Therapy is begun to examine the underlying conflicts and distorted perceptions of shape and

TABLE 16-4 *NOC* Outcomes Related to Bulimia Nervosa	
Nursing Outcome and Definition	**Short-Term Indicators**
Vital Signs: Extent to which temperature, pulse, respiration, and blood pressure are within normal range	Body temperature Apical heart rate Apical heart rhythm Respiratory rate Systolic blood pressure
Impulse Self-Control: Self-restraint of compulsive or impulsive behaviors	Identifies harmful impulsive behaviors Identifies feelings that lead to impulsive actions Identifies consequences of impulsive actions Controls impulses
Weight Maintenance Behavior: Personal actions to maintain optimum body weight	Maintains recommended eating pattern Retains ingested foods Maintains fluid balance Plans for situations that affect food and fluid intake Expresses realistic body image
Hope: Optimism that is personally satisfying and life-supporting	Expresses faith Expresses will to live Expresses optimism Sets goals

Data from Moorhead, S., Johnson, M., Maas, M. L., & Swanson, E. (Eds.). (2008). *Nursing outcome classification (NOC)* (4th ed.) St. Louis: Mosby

weight that sustain the illness. Evaluation for treatment of comorbid disorders, such as major depression and substance abuse, is also undertaken. In most cases of substance dependence, the treatment of the eating disorder must occur after the substance dependence is treated.

Milieu Management

The highly structured milieu of an inpatient eating-disorder unit has as its primary goals the interruption of the binge-purge cycle and the prevention of disordered eating behaviors. Observation during and after meals (to prevent purging), normalization of eating patterns, and maintenance of appropriate exercise are integral elements of such a unit. The multidisciplinary team uses a comprehensive treatment approach to address the emotional and behavioral problems that arise when the patient is no longer binge eating or purging. Like the interruption of other obsessive-compulsive behaviors, preventing the binge-purge pattern allows underlying anxiety to come to the surface and be examined.

Pharmacological Interventions

Antidepressant medication together with cognitive-behavioral psychotherapy has been shown to bring about improvement in bulimic symptoms. Limited research suggests that the SSRIs and tricyclic antidepressants helped reduce binge eating and vomiting over short terms. Fluoxetine (Prozac) treatment may help prevent relapse. Bupropion (Wellbutrin) may be effective, but due to an increased risk for seizures, it is contraindicated in patients who purge (Williams & Goodie, 2007).

Counseling

Compared with the patient with anorexia, the patient with bulimia nervosa often more readily establishes a therapeutic alliance with the nurse, because the eating-disordered behaviors are seen as a problem. The therapeutic alliance allows the nurse, along with other members of the multidisciplinary team, to provide counseling that gives useful feedback regarding the patient's distorted beliefs.

Health Teaching and Health Promotion

Health teaching focuses on not only the eating disorder but also meal planning, use of relaxation techniques, maintenance of a healthy diet and exercise, coping skills, the physical and emotional effects of bingeing and purging, and the impact of cognitive distortions. This preparation lays the foundation for the second phase of treatment, in which there are carefully planned challenges to the patient's newly developed skills. For instance, the patient is expected to have an unsupervised meal at home and share the feelings this event provoked with others in a group therapy setting.

Once a patient reaches therapeutic goals, it is recommended that patients seek long-term care to solidify those goals and address the attitudes, perceptions, and psychodynamic issues that maintain the eating disorder and attend the illness.

Advanced Practice Interventions

Psychotherapy

Cognitive-behavioral therapy is the most effective treatment for bulimia nervosa. Restructuring faulty perceptions and helping individuals develop accepting attitudes toward themselves and their bodies is a primary focus of therapy. When patients do not indulge in bulimic behaviors, issues of self-worth and interpersonal functioning become more prominent.

VIGNETTE

Becky, a 23-year-old patient with a 6-year history of bulimia nervosa, struggles with issues of self-esteem. She expresses much guilt about "letting her father down" in the past by drinking alcohol excessively and binge eating and purging. She is determined that this time she is not going to fail at treatment. After her initial success in stopping the disordered behaviors, she says defiantly, "I'm doing this for *me*." Becky usually experiences her behavior as either pleasing or disappointing to others, but she begins to realize that her feeling of self-worth is very much dependent on how others see her and that she needs to develop a better sense of herself. ∎

Box 16-7 presents relevant *Nursing Interventions Classification (NIC)* interventions for the management of eating disorders (Bulechek et al., 2008).

EVALUATION

Evaluation of treatment effectiveness is ongoing and built into the *NOC* categories. Outcomes are revised as necessary to reach the desired outcomes. Case Study and Nursing Care Plan 16-2 on pages 363–364 presents a patient with bulimia nervosa.

Binge Eating Disorder

Binge eating disorder as a variant of compulsive overeating is described here. In the *DSM-IV-TR* appendix, research criteria are listed for further study of binge

BOX 16-7 *NIC* Interventions for Eating Disorders Management

Definition: Prevention and treatment of severe diet restriction and overexercising or bingeing and purging of food and fluids.

Activities:

- Collaborate with other members of health care team to develop treatment plan; involve patient and/or significant others as appropriate.
- Confer with team and patient to set a target weight if patient is not within a recommended weight range for age and body frame.
- Establish the amount of daily weight gain that is desired.
- Confer with dietitian to determine daily caloric intake necessary to attain and/or maintain target weight.
- Teach and reinforce concepts of good nutrition with patient (and significant others as appropriate).
- Encourage patient to discuss food preferences with dietitian.
- Develop a supportive relationship with patient.
- Monitor physiological parameters (vital signs, electrolyte levels) as needed.
- Weigh on a routine basis (e.g., at same time of day and after voiding).
- Monitor intake and output of fluids, as appropriate.
- Monitor daily caloric intake.
- Encourage patient self-monitoring of daily food intake and weight gain/maintenance as appropriate.
- Establish expectations for appropriate eating behaviors, intake of food/fluid, and amount of physical activity.
- Use behavioral contracting with patient to elicit desired weight gain or maintenance behaviors.
- Restrict food availability to scheduled, pre-served meals and snacks.
- Observe patient during and after meals/snacks to ensure that adequate intake is achieved and maintained.
- Accompany patient to bathroom during designated observation times following meals/snacks.
- Limit time spent in bathroom during periods when not under direct supervision.
- Monitor patient for behaviors related to eating, weight loss, and weight gain.
- Use behavior modification techniques to promote behaviors that contribute to weight gain and limit weight-loss behaviors, as appropriate.
- Provide reinforcement for weight gain and behaviors that promote weight gain.
- Provide remedial consequences in response to weight loss, weight-loss behaviors, or lack of weight gain.
- Provide support (e.g., relaxation therapy, desensitization exercises, opportunities to talk about feelings) as patient integrates new eating behaviors, changing body image, and lifestyle changes.
- Encourage patient use of daily logs to record feelings and circumstances surrounding urge to purge, vomit, or overexercise.
- Limit physical activity as needed to promote weight gain.
- Provide a supervised exercise program when appropriate.
- Allow opportunity to make limited choices about eating and exercise as weight gain progresses in desirable manner.
- Assist patient (and significant others, as appropriate) to examine and resolve personal issues that may contribute to the eating disorder.
- Assist patient to develop a self-esteem that is compatible with a healthy body weight.
- Confer with the health care team on a routine basis about patient's progress.
- Initiate maintenance phase of treatment when patient has achieved target weight and has consistently shown desired eating behaviors for designated period of time.
- Monitor patient weight on routine basis.
- Determine acceptable range of weight variation in relation to target range.
- Place responsibility for choices about eating and physical activity with patient, as appropriate.
- Provide support and guidance as needed.
- Assist patient to evaluate the appropriateness/consequences of choices about eating and physical activity.
- Reinstitute weight-gain protocol if patient is unable to remain within target weight range.
- Institute a treatment program and follow-up care (medical, counseling) for home management.

From Bulechek, G. M., Butcher, H. K., & Dochterman, J. M. (2008). *Nursing interventions classification (NIC)* (5th ed., pp. 278–279). St. Louis: Mosby.

DSM-IV-TR CRITERIA FOR BINGE EATING DISORDER

Binge Eating Disorder (Compulsive Overeating)

A. Recurrent episodes of binge eating. An episode of binge eating is characterized by both of the following:
   1. Eating, in a discrete period (e.g., within any 2-hour period), an amount of food that is definitely larger than most people would eat in a similar period under similar circumstances.
   2. A sense of lack of control over eating during the episode (e.g., a feeling that one cannot stop eating or control what or how much one is eating).

B. The binge eating episodes are associated with three or more of the following:
   1. Eating much more rapidly than normal
   2. Eating until feeling uncomfortably full
   3. Eating large amounts of food when not feeling physically hungry
   4. Eating alone because of being embarrassed by how much one is eating
   5. Feeling disgusted with oneself, depressed, or very guilty after overeating

C. Marked distress regarding binge eating is present.

D. The binge eating occurs, on average, at least 2 days a week for 6 months.

   Note: The method of determining frequency differs from that used for bulimia nervosa; future research should address whether the preferred method of setting a frequency threshold is counting the number of days on which binges occur or counting the number of episodes of binge eating.

E. The binge eating is not associated with the regular use of inappropriate compensatory behaviors (e.g., purging, fasting, excessive exercise) and does not occur exclusively during the course of anorexia nervosa or bulimia nervosa.

Figure 16-2 Diagnostic criteria for binge eating disorder. (Adapted from American Psychiatric Association. [2000]. *Diagnostic and statistical manual of mental disorders* [4th ed., text rev.] [DSM-IV-TR]. Washington, DC: Author.)

eating disorder (Figure 16-2). Because the individual engages in no compensatory behaviors (purging, exercise) in an attempt to control weight in this disorder, it is currently diagnosed as *eating disorder NOS.*

Overeating is frequently noted as a symptom of an affective disorder (e.g., atypical depression). Higher rates of affective and personality disorders are found among binge eaters. Binge eaters report a history of major depression significantly more often than non–binge eaters, with lifetime rates of 46% to 58% (APA, 2006).

There is little research into binge eating disorder, and all studies to date have followed participants for less than 6 years and therefore cannot be used to make long-term predictions of efficacy. Also, results are variable due to a strong placebo effect; even subjects on placebo treatments showed improvement.

Because of their efficacy with bulimia, the use of SSRIs at or near the high end of the dosage range have been studied to treat binge eating disorder and seem to help in the short term; however, patients regained significant weight after discontinuance of medication. Other medications that are under investigation include the tricyclic antidepressants, antiepileptic agents, and appetite suppressants (Williams & Goodie, 2007).

Cognitive-behavioral therapy, behavior therapy, dialectical behavior therapy, and interpersonal therapy have all been associated with binge frequency reduction rates of 67% or more and significant abstinence rates during active treatment (APA, 2006). Many advanced practice nurses are qualified to provide these therapies. Case Study and Nursing Care Plan 16-3 on pages 364–366 presents a patient with binge eating disorder.

Case Study and Nursing Care Plan 16-1   Anorexia Nervosa

Cynthia is a 20-year-old woman who is brought to the inpatient eating-disorder unit of a psychiatric research hospital by two older brothers, who support her on either side. She is profoundly weak, holding her head up with her hands.

ASSESSMENT

Self-Assessment

Mindy Jacobs, RN, is assigned to care for Cynthia. Although Mindy is a young nurse, she has spent the last 3 years working on the eating-disorders unit. When she began working on the unit, she had difficulty with overidentifying with patients. During college, Mindy struggled with bulimia, but with treatment she has done well. She seeks guidance from her nursing supervisor and the multidisciplinary team. This support allows her to maintain appropriate boundaries while creating a therapeutic alliance with patients.

Continued

Objective Data	**Subjective Data**
Height: 62 inches (5 feet 2 inches)	Denies being underweight: "I need treatment because I get fatigued so easily."
Weight: 58 lb—50% of ideal body weight	"I check my legs every night. I'm so afraid of getting fat. I hate it if my legs touch each other."
Blood pressure: 74/50 mm Hg	"I don't like to start anything until I know I can do it perfectly the first time. I wouldn't want anyone to see me make a mistake."
Pulse: 54 beats per minute	Depressed mood
Anemic—hemoglobin: 9 g/dL	
Cachectic appearance, pale, with fine lanugo	
Sad facial expression	
Bruising on inside of each knee from sleeping on her side with knees touching	

DIAGNOSIS

1. *Imbalanced nutrition: less than body requirements* related to restriction of caloric intake secondary to extreme fear of weight gain
2. *Chronic low self-esteem* related to perception that others are always judging her

OUTCOMES IDENTIFICATION

Patient will reach 75% of ideal weight (92 lb) by discharge.

PLANNING

The initial plan is to address Cynthia's unstable physiological state.

IMPLEMENTATION

Cynthia's care plan is personalized as follows:

Short-Term Goal	Intervention	Rationale	Evaluation
1. Patient will gain a minimum of 2 lb and a maximum of 3 lb weekly through inpatient stay.	1a. Acknowledge the emotional and physical difficulty patient is experiencing. Use patient's extreme fatigue to engage cooperation in the treatment plan.	1a. A first priority is to establish a therapeutic alliance.	**WEEK 1:** Patient increases caloric intake with liquid supplement only. Patient unable to eat solid food. Patient does not gain weight. Patient remains hypotensive, bradycardic, anemic (hemoglobin [HGB] = 9 g/dL).
	1b. Weigh patient daily for the first week, then three times a week. Patient should be weighed in bra and panties only. There should be no oral intake, including a drink of water, before the early morning weigh-in.	1b. These measures ensure that weight is accurate.	**WEEK 2:** Patient gains 2 lb drinking liquid supplement—minimal solid food. Patient remains hypotensive, bradycardic (HGB = 10 g/dL).
	1c. Do not negotiate weight with patient or reweigh. Patient may choose not to look at the scale or request that she not be told the weight.	1c. Patient may try to control and sabotage treatment.	**WEEK 3:** Patient gains I lb drinking liquid supplement. Patient selects meal plan but is unable to eat most of solid food. Patient's blood pressure (BP) = 84/60 mm Hg; pulse = 68 beats per minute, regular; HGB = 11 g/dL.
	1d. Measure vital signs tid until stable, then daily. Repeat ECG and laboratory tests until stable.	1d. As patient begins to increase in weight, cardiovascular status improves to within normal range, and monitoring is less frequent.	

Short-Term Goal	Intervention	Rationale	Evaluation
	1e. Provide a pleasant, calm atmosphere at mealtimes. Patient should be told the specific times and duration (usually a half hour) of meals.	1e. Mealtimes become episodes of high anxiety, and knowledge of regulations decreases tension in the milieu, particularly when patient has given up so much control by entering treatment.	**WEEKS 4-6:** Patient gains an average of 2.5 lb/wk. Patient samples more of solid food selected from meal plan. Patient's BP = 90/60 mm Hg; pulse = 68 beats per minute, regular; HGB = 11.5 g/dL.
	1f. Administer liquid supplement as ordered.	1f. Patient may be unable to eat solid food at first.	**WEEK 7:** Patient weighs 71 lb (almost 60% of ideal body weight); calories are mostly from liquid supplement.
	1g. Observe patient during meals to prevent hiding or throwing away of food and for at least 1 hour after meals and snacks to prevent purging.	1g, 1h. The compelling force of the illness is such that these behaviors are difficult to stop. A power struggle between staff and patient may emerge, in which patient appears to comply but defies the rules (appearing to eat but throwing away food).	Patient selects balanced meals, eating more varied solid food: turkey, carrots, lettuce, fruit. Patient's HGB = 12.5 g/dL; normal range of BP and pulse are maintained.
	1h. Encourage patient to try to eat some solid food. Preparation of patient's meals should be guided by likes and dislikes list, because patient is unable to make own selections to complete menu.		Patient continues to increase participation in social aspects of eating.
	1i. Be empathetic with patient's struggle to give up control of her eating and her weight as she is expected to make minimum weight gain on a regular basis. Permit patient to verbalize feelings at these times.	1i. Patient is expected to gain at least 0.5 lb on a specific schedule, usually three times a week (Monday, Wednesday, Friday).	**WEEKS 8-12:** Patient gains an average of 2.5 lb/wk and weighs 82 lb (approx. 68% of ideal body weight). Patient is eating more varied solid food, but most caloric intake is still from liquid supplement.
	1j. Monitor patient's weight gain. A weight gain of 2 to 3 lb/wk is medically acceptable.	1j. Weight gain of more than 5 lb in 1 week may result in pulmonary edema.	Patient maintains normal vital signs and HGB levels. Patient maintains social interaction during mealtimes and snacks.
	1k. Provide teaching regarding healthy eating as the basis of a healthy lifestyle.	1k. Healthy aspects of eating (e.g., increased energy, rather than gaining weight) are reinforced.	**WEEKS 13-16:** Patient has reached medically stable weight at the end of 16th week—92 lb (75% of ideal body weight). Patient continues to eat more solid food with relatively less liquid supplement. Patient is not able to participate in planned exercise program until patient reaches 85% of ideal body weight.
	1l. Use a cognitive-behavioral approach to address patient's expressed fears regarding weight gain. Identify and examine dysfunctional thoughts; identify and examine values and beliefs that sustain these thoughts.	1l. Confronting irrational thoughts and beliefs is crucial to changing eating behaviors.	

Continued

Short-Term Goal	Intervention	Rationale	Evaluation
	1m. As patient approaches her target weight, there should be encouragement to make her own choices for menu selection.	1m. Patient can assume more control of her meals, which is empowering for the patient with anorexia.	
	1n. Emphasize social nature of eating. Encourage conversation that does not have the theme of food during mealtimes.	1n. Eating as a social activity, shared with others and with participation in conversation, serves as both a distraction from obsessional preoccupations and a pleasurable event.	
	1o. Focus on the patient's strengths, including her good work in normalizing her weight and eating habits.	1o. Patient who is beginning to normalize weight and eating behaviors has achieved a major accomplishment, of which she should be proud. Noneating activities are explored as a source of gratification.	
	1p. Provide for a planned exercise program when patient reaches target weight.	1p. Patient experiences a strong drive to exercise; this measure accommodates this drive by planning a reasonable amount.	
	1q. Encourage patient to apply all the knowledge, skills, and gains made from the various individual, family, and group therapy sessions.	1q. Patient has been receiving intensive therapy and education, which have provided tools and techniques that are useful in maintaining healthy behaviors.	

EVALUATION

By the end of the 16th week, Cynthia has achieved a stable weight of 92 lb. This weight is approaching congruency with Cynthia's height, frame, and age. Her vital signs and hemoglobin levels are consistently demonstrated as normal. She is participating in therapy and consistently communicating satisfaction with her body appearance.

Case Study and Nursing Care Plan 16-2   Bulimia Nervosa

Sally is a 30-year-old college graduate who reports that she is an aspiring actress. She is being admitted to a partial hos-pitalization program designed for patients with eating disor-ders. Sally has bulimia nervosa.

ASSESSMENT

Self-Assessment

Matthew, a seasoned nurse in the area of eating disorders, is assigned to care for Sally. Matthew enjoys working with patients with bulimia because he believes he can help patients move toward health. When he first encounters Sally, he experiences an immediate negative response that surprises him. He speaks to his supervisor about these feelings and raises the question of whether or not he is the appropriate nurse to care for Sally. As he and the supervisor discuss his feelings, Matthew is able to recognize that Sally reminds him of a girlfriend he had many years earlier. The relationship ended badly. Matthew experiences an emotional release with this realization and believes that he will be able to separate his earlier negative experience from his work with Sally.

Objective Data

Height: 65 inches (5 feet 5 inches)
Weight: 127 lb—95% of ideal body weight
Blood pressure: 120/80 mm Hg sitting; 90/60 mm Hg standing
Pulse: 70 beats/min sitting; 96 beats/min standing
Potassium level of 2.7 mmol/L (normal range, 3.3 to 5.5 mmol/L)

ECG: abnormal—consistent with hypokalemia
Erosion of enamel, enlarged parotid glands, consistent with a history of binge eating/purging.

Subjective Data

"I can't stand to be fat."
"I'm ashamed that I can't control my bingeing and vomiting—I know it's not good."

DIAGNOSIS

1. *Risk for injury* related to low potassium and other physical changes secondary to binge eating and purging
2. *Powerlessness* related to inability to control bingeing and vomiting cycles

OUTCOMES IDENTIFICATION

Sally will demonstrate ability to regulate eating patterns, resulting in consistently normal electrolyte balance.

PLANNING

Sally is admitted to a partial hospitalization program designed for patients with eating disorders. She attends the program 3 or 4 days a week and participates in individual and group therapy. She will continue to work as a "temp" for a publishing house.

IMPLEMENTATION

Sally's care plan is personalized as follows:

Short-Term Goal	Intervention	Rationale	Evaluation
1. Patient will identify signs and symptoms of low potassium (K⁺) level, and K⁺ level will remain within normal limits throughout hospitalization.	1a. Educate patient regarding the ill effects of self-induced vomiting, low K⁺ level, dental erosion.	1a. Health teaching is crucial to treatment. The patient needs to be reminded of the benefits of normalization of eating behavior.	**WEEK 1:** Patient begins to select balanced meals. Patient demonstrates knowledge of untoward effects of vomiting and K⁺ deficiency. Patient begins to demonstrate understanding of repetitive nature of binge-purge cycle.
	1b. Educate patient about binge-purge cycle and its self-perpetuating nature.	1b, 1c. The compulsive nature of the binge-purge cycle is maintained by the sequence of intake restriction, hunger, bingeing, purging accompanied by feelings of guilt, and then repetition of the cycle over and over.	
	1c. Teach patient that fasting sets one up to binge eat.		

Continued

Short-Term Goal	Intervention	Rationale	Evaluation
	1d. Explore ideas about trigger foods.	1d. Patient needs to understand beliefs about trigger foods to challenge irrational thoughts.	**WEEK 2:** Patient begins to challenge irrational thoughts and beliefs. Patient continues to plan nutritionally balanced meals, including dinner at home. Patient begins to sample "forbidden foods" and discuss thoughts and attitudes about same.
	1e. Challenge irrational thoughts and beliefs about "forbidden" foods.	1e. Challenge forces patient to examine own thinking and beliefs.	**WEEK 3:** Patient discusses triggers to binge and resultant behavior. Patient continues to challenge irrational thoughts and beliefs in individual and group sessions. Patient plans meals, including "forbidden foods".
	1f. Teach patient to plan and eat regularly scheduled, balanced meals.	1f. This teaching helps to ensure success in maintaining abstinence from binge-purge activity.	**WEEK 4:** Patient reports no binge-purge behaviors at day program or outside. Patient demonstrates understanding of repetitive nature of binge-purge cycle. Patient continues to challenge irrational thoughts and beliefs.

EVALUATION

At the end of 4 weeks, Sally reports no binge-purge cycles, and her potassium level remains consistently within normal limits. She is beginning to plan meals and challenge irrational thoughts and beliefs.

Case Study and Nursing Care Plan 16-3   Binge Eating (Eating Disorder Not Otherwise Specified)

Angela is a 25-year-old schoolteacher who gives a history of overeating since the age of 10 years. She seeks treatment at *a community mental health center because she has recently felt more depressed.*

ASSESSMENT

Self-Assessment

The nurse assigned to Angela is Bernice. Bernice is new to the community mental health center, and her experience as a psychiatric nurse is primarily with the seriously mentally ill. She has never worked with a patient with an eating disorder. During Bernice's initial contact with Angela, she feels revulsion with regard to Angela's weight. Bernice speaks to her nurse supervisor about this feeling because she is unable to identify where this feeling comes from and is not sure she can control it. The supervisor recognizes that Bernice's feelings will interfere with creating a therapeutic alliance with Angela and decides to reassign Bernice and provide her with additional support and education regarding the care of the patient with an eating disorder.

Objective Data	Subjective Data
Height: 61 inches (5 feet 1 inch)	"I'll eat anything in sight."
Weight: 200 lb—180% of ideal weight	"I wish I wouldn't wake up in the morning."
Uncontrollable eating pattern	"I once showed promise, and look at me now."
Sad facial expression	"I don't take laxatives or diuretics, and I don't vomit."
Minimal success with participation in Weight Watchers and Overeating Anonymous programs	"I am not suicidal."

DIAGNOSIS

Imbalanced nutrition: more than body requirements related to compulsive overeating, including episodes of bingeing

OUTCOMES IDENTIFICATION

Patient will normalize eating pattern and achieve a specific target weight according to a predetermined plan.

IMPLEMENTATION

Angela's care plan is personalized as follows:

Short-Term Goal	Intervention	Rationale	Evaluation
1. Patient will demonstrate at least two coping strategies that result in adhering to a structured meal schedule.	1a. Clinical nurse specialist can use many techniques of cognitive-behavioral therapy in addressing the issues of overweight and disordered eating. Patient should begin a journal.	1a. Cognitive-behavioral techniques can be useful in addressing automatic behaviors. Recording what, when, and where one eats begins to identify patterns that can be modified.	**WEEK 1:** Patient selects a meal plan with structured times and places; begins journal and maintains it consistently. Patient begins to relate feelings about eating. **WEEK 2:** Patient is able to adhere to structured meal schedule approximately 25% of the time. Patient expresses the struggle and feelings of tension around implementing structured meal schedule; some modifications are made to allow the patient to be more successful. Patient shares contents of journal, which she consistently maintains.
	1b. Teach the patient to structure and plan ahead for times and places where she will have her meals and snacks for the day.	1b. Organization and structure can allow for a different choice.	
	1c. Teach patient not to abstain from eating for longer periods of time than planned to avoid rebound binge eating.	1c, 1d. Extended periods of abstinence, restrictive dietary intake, or very-low-calorie diet can result in rebound overeating.	Patient reports weight is unchanged; patient was unable to change pattern of exercise. **WEEK 3:** Patient is adhering to schedule 50% of the time. Patient shares journal entries and relates thoughts and feelings concerning eating. Patient reports 0.5-lb weight loss. Patient is beginning to walk for a half hour as part of her daily routine.
	1d. Review the nutritional content of dietary intake to ensure consumption of a balanced diet.		
	1e. Review journal with patient to identify areas for improvement in adhering to the treatment plan.	1e. The journal is an important tool in modifying eating behaviors.	**WEEK 4:** Patient continues to adhere to structured schedule approximately 75% of the time.

Continued

Short-Term Goal	Intervention	Rationale	Evaluation
	1f. Explore with patient the thoughts and feelings she is experiencing about this new regimen.	1f, 1g. Nurse must be empathetic and supportive of patient's experience, which is one of struggle accompanied by feelings of tension.	Patient walks regularly, experiencing a better sense of well-being. Patient thinks she is up to the challenge of continuing the plan to normalize her eating pattern and increase her energy expenditure. Patient's weight is 196 lb (− 4 lb); she acknowledges that progress has and will continue to be slow.
	1g. Identify thoughts, beliefs, and underlying assumptions that reinforce disordered eating patterns.		
	1h. Establish a once-a-week schedule of weighing.	1h. From day to day, there may be minimal or no weight reduction, which can lead to discouragement.	

EVALUATION

At the end of 4 weeks, Angela's weight is 196 lb. She adheres to a structured meal plan 75% of the time and has increased her exercise by incorporating daily walks into her routine.

KEY POINTS TO REMEMBER

- A number of theoretical models help explain the origins of eating disorders.
- Neurobiological theories identify an association among eating disorders, depression, and neuroendocrine abnormalities.
- Psychological theories explore issues of control in anorexia and affective instability and poor impulse control in bulimia.
- Genetic theories postulate the existence of vulnerabilities that may predispose people toward eating disorders.
- Sociocultural models look at our present societal ideal of being thin.
- Men with eating disorders share many of the characteristics of women with eating disorders.
- The suicide rate of patients suffering with eating disorders is much higher than predicted rates in similar age groups.
- Anorexia nervosa is a potentially life-threatening eating disorder that includes severe underweight; low blood pressure, pulse, and temperature; dehydration; and low serum potassium level and dysrhythmias.
- Anorexia may be treated in an inpatient treatment setting in which milieu therapy, psychotherapy (cognitive), development of self-care skills, and psychobiological interventions can be implemented.
- Long-term treatment is provided on an outpatient basis and aims to help patients maintain healthy weight. It includes treatment modalities such as individual therapy, family therapy, group therapy, psychopharmacology, and nutrition counseling.
- Patients with bulimia nervosa are typically within the normal weight range, but some may be slightly below or above ideal body weight.
- Assessment of the bulimic patient may show enlargement of the parotid glands and dental erosion and caries if the patient has induced vomiting.
- Acute care may be necessary when life-threatening complications such as gastric rupture (rare), electrolyte imbalance, and cardiac dysrhythmias are present.
- The goal of interventions is to interrupt the binge-purge cycle.
- Psychotherapy and self-care skill training are included in the treatment plan.
- Long-term treatment focuses on therapy aimed at addressing any coexisting depression, substance abuse, and/or personality disorders that are causing the patient distress and interfering with the quality of life. Self-worth and interpersonal functioning eventually become issues that are useful for the patient to target.
- Eating disorders NOS include a variety of patterns, among them binge eating disorder.
- People with binge eating disorder report a history of major depression significantly more often than people who do not binge eat.
- Effective treatment for obese patients with binge eating disorder integrates modification of the disordered eating, improvement of depressive symptoms, and achievement of an appropriate weight for the individual.

CRITICAL THINKING

1. Logan, a 19-year-old male model, has experienced a rapid decrease in weight over the last four months after his agent told him he would have to lose some weight or lose a coveted account. Logan is 6 feet 2 inches tall and weighs 132 lb, down from his usual 176 lb. He is brought to the emergency department with a pulse of 40 beats per minute and severe arrhythmias. His laboratory workup reveals severe hypokalemia. He has become extremely depressed, saying, "I'm too fat.... I don't want anything to eat.... If I gain weight, my life will be ruined. There is nothing to live for if I can't model." Logan's parents are startled and confused, and his best friend is worried and feels powerless to help Logan. "I tell Logan he needs to eat or he will die.... I tell him he is a skeleton, but he refuses to listen to me. I don't know what to do."
   A. Which physical and psychiatric criteria suggest that Logan should be immediately hospitalized?
   B. What are some of the questions you would eventually ask Logan when evaluating his biopsychosocial functioning?
   C. What are your feelings toward someone with anorexia? Can you make a distinction between your thoughts and feelings toward women with anorexia and toward men with anorexia?
   D. What are some things you could do for Logan's parents and friend in terms of offering them information, support, and referrals? Identify specific referrals.
   E. Explain the kinds of interventions or restrictions that may be used while Logan is hospitalized (e.g., weighing, observation after eating or visits, exercise, therapy, self-care).
   F. How would you describe partial hospitalization programs or psychiatric home care programs when asked if Logan will have to be hospitalized for an extended period?
   G. What are some of Logan's cognitive distortions that would be a target for therapy?
   H. Identify at least five criteria that, if met, would indicate that Logan was improving.

2. You and Heather have been close friends since nursing school and are now working on the same surgical unit. Heather told you that in the past she has made several suicide attempts. Today you accidentally come upon her bingeing off unit, and she looks embarrassed and uncomfortable when she sees you. Several times you notice that she spends time in the bathroom, and you hear sounds of retching. In response to your concern, she admits that she has been binge-purging for several years but that now she is getting out of control and feels profoundly depressed.
   A. Although Heather doesn't show any physical signs of bulimia nervosa, what would you look for when assessing an individual with bulimia?
   B. What kinds of emergencies could result from bingeing and purging?
   C. What would be the most useful type of psychotherapy for Heather initially, and what issues would need to be addressed?
   D. What kinds of new skills does a person with bulimia need to learn to lessen the compulsion to binge and purge?
   E. What would be some signs that Heather is recovering?

CHAPTER REVIEW

1. Which female patient should the nurse recognize as having the highest risk to have or develop bulimia nervosa? The one who:
   1. grew up in an underserved area.
   2. lives in a society influenced by Eastern cultural beliefs.
   3. is 20 years old.
   4. is African-American.

2. The nurse is caring for a 16-year-old female patient with anorexia nervosa. What should the initial nursing intervention be upon the patient's admission to the unit?
   1. Build a therapeutic relationship.
   2. Increase the patient's caloric consumption.
   3. Involve the patient in group therapy to build a support group.
   4. Self-assess to decrease tendencies towards authoritarianism.

3. The nurse is caring for a patient with bulimia. Which nursing intervention is appropriate?
   1. Monitoring patient on bathroom trips after eating.
   2. Allow patient extensive private time with family members.
   3. Provide meals whenever the patient requests them.
   4. Encourage patient to select foods that she likes.

4. The nurse is admitting a patient who weighs 100 pounds, is 66 inches tall, and is below ideal body weight. The patient's blood pressure is 130/80 mm Hg, pulse is 72 beats per minute, potassium is 2.5 mmol/L, and ECG is abnormal. Her teeth enamel is eroded, her hands are visibly shaking, and her parotid gland is enlarged. The patient states, "I am really worked up about coming to this unit." What is the priority nursing diagnosis?
   1. *Powerlessness*
   2. *Risk for injury*
   3. *Imbalanced nutrition: Less than body requirements*
   4. *Anxiety*

5. The nurse is planning care for a patient with an eating disorder. What outcomes are appropriate? *Select all that apply.*
   1. The patient will experience a decrease in depression.
   2. The patient will identify four methods to control anxiety.
   3. The patient will collect different kinds of cookbooks.
   4. The patient will identify two people to contact if suicidal thoughts occur.

Ⓔvolve
learning system

Visit the Evolve website for an **Audio Chapter Summary, Chapter Review Answers & Rationales, Critical Thinking Answer Guidelines,** and additional resources related to the content of this chapter: **http://evolve.elsevier.com/Varcarolis/foundations**

Companion CD

Use the Companion CD to prepare for tests and the NCLEX® Examination with **Test-Taking Strategies** for psychiatric mental health nursing and hundreds of **Review Questions**.

References

American Psychiatric Association. (2000). *Diagnostic and statistical manual of mental disorders (DSM-IV-TR)* (4th ed., text rev.). Washington, DC: Author.

American Psychiatric Association. (2006). *Practice guideline for the treatment of patients with eating disorders* (3rd ed.). Washington, DC: Author.

Attia, E., & Walsh, B. T. (2007). Anorexia nervosa. *The American Journal of Psychiatry, 164*(12), 1805–1810.

Becker, A. E., Mickley, D. W., Derenne, J. L., & Klibanski, M. (2008). Eating disorders: Evaluation and management. In T. A. Stern, J. F. Rosenbaum, M. Fava, J. Biederman, & S. L. Rauch (Eds.), *Massachusetts General Hospital comprehensive clinical psychiatry* (pp. 499–518). St. Louis: Mosby.

Berkman, N. D., Lohr, K. N., & Bulik, C. M. (2007). Outcomes of eating disorders: A systematic review of the literature. *International Journal of Eating Disorders, 40,* 293–309.

Bulechek, G. M., Butcher, H. K., & Dochterman, J. M. (Eds.). (2008). *Nursing interventions classification (NIC)* (5th ed.). St. Louis: Mosby.

Caparrotta, L., & Ghaffari, K. (2006). A historical overview of the psychodynamic contributions to the understanding of eating disorders. *Psychoanalytic Psychotherapy, 20*(3), 175–196.

Casazza, K., & Ciccazzo, M. (2007). The method of delivery of nutrition and physical activity information may play a role in eliciting behavior changes in adolescents. *Eating Behaviors, 8,* 73–82.

Cassin, S. E., & von Ranson, K. M. (2005). Personality and eating disorders: A decade in review. *Clinical Psychology Review, 25,* 895–916.

Centers for Disease Control and Prevention. (2006). *Overweight and obesity.* Retrieved March 18, 2009 from http://www.cdc.gov/NCCDPHP/DNPA/obesity/

Frieling, H., Romer, K. D., Wilhelm, J., Hillemacher, T., Kornhuber, J., deZwaan, M., et al. (2006). Association of catecholamine-*O*-methyltransferase and 5-HTTLPR genotype with eating disorder–related behavior and attitudes in females with eating disorders. *Psychiatric Genetics, 16*(5), 205–208.

Godart, N. T., Perdereau, F., Rein, Z., Berthoz, S. Wallier, J., Jeammet, P., et al. (2007). Comorbidity studies of eating disorders and mood disorders. Critical review of the literature. *Journal of Affective Disorders, 97*(1–3), 37–49.

Halmi, K. A. (2008). Eating disorders: Anorexia nervosa, bulimia nervosa, and obesity. In R. E. Hales, S. C. Yudofsky, & G. O. Gabbard (Eds.), *Textbook of psychiatry* (pp. 971–998). Washington, DC: American Psychiatric Publishing.

Hudson, J. I., Hiripi, E., Pope, H. G. Jr., & Kessler, R. C. (2007). The prevalence and correlates of eating disorders in the National Comorbidity Survey Replication. *Biological Psychiatry, 61,* 348–358.

Kaye, W. (2007). Neurobiology of anorexia and bulimia nervosa. *Physiology & Behavior, 94,* 112–135.

Keel, P. K., & Klump, K. L. (2003). Are eating disorders culture-bound syndromes? Implications for conceptualizing their etiology. *Psychological Bulletin, 129,* 747–769.

Lauts, N. M. (2005). Management of the patient with refeeding syndrome. *Journal of Infusion Nursing, 28*(5), 337–342.

Moorhead, S., Johnson, M., Maas, M. L., & Swanson, E. (Eds.). (2008). *Nursing outcomes classification (NOC)* (4th ed.). St. Louis: Mosby.

North American Nursing Diagnosis Association International (NANDA-I). (2009). *NANDA-I nursing diagnoses: Definitions and classification 2009–2011.* Oxford, United Kingdom: Author.

Pompili, M., Girardi, P., Tatarelli, G., Ruberto, A., & Tatarelli, R. (2006). Suicide and attempted suicide in eating disorders, obesity and weight-image concern. *Eating Behaviors, 7,* 384–394.

Stein, K. F., & Corte, C. (2003). Reconceptualizing causative factors and intervention strategies in the eating disorders: A shift from body image to self-concept impairments. *Archives of Psychiatric Nursing, 17*(2), 57–66.

Williams, P. M., & Goodie, J. (2007). Identifying and treating eating disorders. *Family Practice Recertification, 29*(8), 16–23.

Williamson, D. A., Martin, C. K., Anton, S. D., York-Crowe, E., Han, H., Redman, L., et al. (2008). Is caloric restriction associated with development of eating-disorder symptoms? Results from the CALERIE trial. *Health Psychology, 27*(1), S32–S42.

CHAPTER 17

Cognitive Disorders

Jane Stein-Parbury, Charlotte Eliopoulos, and Elizabeth M. Varcarolis

Key Terms and Concepts

agnosia, 381
agraphia, 384
Alzheimer's disease (AD), 379
aphasia, 381
apraxia, 381
cognitive disorders, 370
confabulation, 380
delirium, 370
dementia, 378
hallucinations, 373

hypermetamorphosis, 384
hyperorality, 384
hypervigilance, 374
illusions, 373
perseveration, 381
primary dementia, 379
pseudodementia, 381
secondary dementia, 379
sundowning, 373

Objectives

1. Compare and contrast the clinical picture of delirium with that of dementia.
2. Discuss three critical needs of a person with delirium, stated in terms of nursing diagnoses.
3. Identify three outcomes for patients with delirium.
4. Summarize the essential nursing interventions for a patient with delirium.
5. Recognize the signs and symptoms occurring in the four stages of Alzheimer's disease.
6. Give an example of the following symptoms assessed during the progression of Alzheimer's disease: (a) amnesia, (b) apraxia, (c) agnosia, and (d) aphasia.

7. Formulate three nursing diagnoses suitable for a patient with Alzheimer's disease, and define two outcomes for each.
8. Formulate a teaching plan for a caregiver of a patient with Alzheimer's disease, including interventions for (a) communication, (b) health maintenance, and (c) safe environment.
9. Compose a list of appropriate referrals in the community—including a support group, hotline for information, and respite services—for persons with dementia and their caregivers.

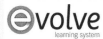 Visit the Evolve website for an **Audio Glossary & Flashcards, Concept Map Creator**, and additional resources related to the content in this chapter: **http://evolve.elsevier.com/Varcarolis/foundations**

The clarity and purpose of an individual's personal journey through life depend on the ability to reflect on its meaning. Cognition represents a fundamental human feature that distinguishes living from existing. This mental capacity has a distinctive, personalized impact on the individual's physical, psychological, social, and spiritual conduct of life. For example, the ability to remember the connections between related actions and how to initiate them depends on cognitive processing. Moreover, this cognitive processing has a direct relationship to activities of daily living.

Although primarily an intellectual and perceptual process, cognition is closely integrated with an individual's emotional and spiritual values. When human beings can no longer understand facts or connect the appropriate feelings to events, we have trouble responding to the complexity of life's challenges. Emotions take a back seat to profound disturbances in cognitive processing that either cloud or destroy the meaning of the journey.

The labyrinth of current knowledge about cognitive disorders requires a compassionate understanding of the patient and family. Nursing interventions are focused on protecting patient dignity, preserving functional status, and promoting well-being for cognitively impaired patients.

There are three main cognitive disorders: delirium, dementia, and amnestic disorder. *Cognitive disorder not otherwise specified* is a category defined in the *Diagnostic and Statistical Manual of Mental Disorders,* fourth edition, text revision *(DSM-IV-TR)* that allows for the diagnosis of cognitive disorders that do not meet the criteria for delirium, dementia, or amnestic disorders (American Psychiatric Association [APA], 2000). Cognitive disorders not otherwise specified are presumed to be caused by a specific medical condition, a pharmacologically active agent, or possibly both (Sadock & Sadock, 2008).

Figure 17-1 identifies the three main cognitive disorders and gives the *DSM-IV-TR* criteria for each. This chapter addresses the broad categories of delirium and dementia because these are by far the most common conditions nurses encounter. Amnestic disorders are not discussed.

A delayed or missed diagnosis can have serious implications because the longer a condition goes untreated, the greater the risk it can cause permanent damage. Table 17-1 offers some guidelines for distinguishing between delirium and dementia (as well as depression, which may have similar symptoms or co-occur in older adults).

Delirium

CLINICAL PICTURE

Delirium "is characterized by a disturbance of consciousness and a change in cognition that develop over a short period of time" (APA, 2000, p. 135).

DSM-IV-TR CRITERIA FOR COGNITIVE DISORDERS

COGNITIVE DISORDERS

Delirium

A. Disturbance of consciousness (i.e., reduced clarity of awareness of the environment with reduced ability to focus, sustain, or shift attention).

B. A change in cognition (memory deficit, disorientation, language disturbance) or the development of a perceptual disturbance that is not better accounted for by a preexisting, established, or evolving dementia.

C. The disturbance develops over a short period of time (usually hours to days) and tends to fluctuate during the course of the day.

Due to:

1. A general medical condition
   or
2. Substance-induced (intoxication or withdrawal)
   or
3. Multiple etiologies (both 1 and 2 above)
   or
4. Not known (not otherwise specified)

Amnestic Disorder

A. The development of memory impairment as manifested by impairment in the ability to learn new information or the ability to recall previously learned information.

B. The memory disturbance causes significant impairment in social or occupational functioning and represents a significant decline from a previous level of functioning.

C. The memory disturbance does not occur exclusively during the course of a delirium or a dementia.

Dementia

A. The development of multiple cognitive deficits manifested by both:

1. **Memory impairment** (impaired ability to learn new information or to recall previously learned information).

2. One (or more) of the following cognitive disturbances:
   (a) **Aphasia** (language disturbance)
   (b) **Apraxia** (impaired ability to carry out motor activities despite intact motor function)
   (c) **Agnosia** (failure to recognize or identify objects despite intact sensory function)
   (d) Disturbance in executive functioning (i.e., planning, organizing, sequencing, abstracting)

B. The cognitive deficits in criteria A1 and A2 each cause significant impairment in social or occupational functioning and represent a significant decline from a previous level of functioning.

Figure 17-1 Diagnostic criteria for delirium, dementia, and amnestic disorder. (Adapted from American Psychiatric Association. [2000]. *Diagnostic and statistical manual of mental disorders* [4th ed., text rev.]. Washington, DC: Author.)

TABLE 17-1 Comparison of Delirium, Dementia, and Depression

	Delirium	Dementia	Depression
Onset	Sudden, over hours to days	Slowly, over months	May have been gradual, with exacerbation during crisis or stress
Cause or contributing factors	Hypoglycemia, fever, dehydration, hypotension; infection, other conditions that disrupt body's homeostasis; adverse drug reaction; head injury; change in environment (e.g., hospitalization); pain; emotional stress	Alzheimer's disease, vascular disease, human immunodeficiency virus infection, neurological disease, chronic alcoholism, head trauma	Lifelong history, losses, loneliness, crises, declining health, medical conditions
Cognition	Impaired memory, judgment, calculations, attention span; can fluctuate through the day	Impaired memory, judgment, calculations, attention span, abstract thinking; agnosia	Difficulty concentrating, forgetfulness, inattention
Level of consciousness	Altered	Not altered	Not altered
Activity level	Can be increased or reduced; restlessness, behaviors may worsen in evening (sundowning); sleep/wake cycle may be reversed	Not altered; behaviors may worsen in evening (sundowning)	Usually decreased; lethargy, fatigue, lack of motivation; may sleep poorly and awaken in early morning
Emotional state	Rapid swings; can be fearful, anxious, suspicious, aggressive, have hallucinations and/or delusions	Flat; delusions	Extreme sadness, apathy, irritability, anxiety, paranoid ideation
Speech and language	Rapid, inappropriate, incoherent, rambling	Incoherent, slow (sometimes due to effort to find the right word), inappropriate, rambling, repetitious	Slow, flat, low
Prognosis	Reversible with proper and timely treatment	Not reversible; progressive	Reversible with proper and timely treatment

It should be considered to be a priority problem, and immediate attention should be given to prevent irreversible and serious damage (Caplan et al., 2008).

EPIDEMIOLOGY

Delirium is common in hospitalized patients, especially older adults. Delirium can be present in 11% to 42% of general medical patients, and its prevalence is as high as 60% in the older adult population. Up to 40% of patients in intensive care units develop delirium. The rate has been reported as between 20% and 40% in patients with cancer and 46% in patients with AIDS who are unwell (Siddiqi et al., 2007).

COMORBIDITY AND ETIOLOGY

Delirium is always secondary to another physiological condition and is a transient disorder. If the underlying condition is corrected, complete recovery should occur. The major causes are nervous system disease, systemic disease (such as cardiac failure), and either intoxication or withdrawal from a chemical substance (see Chapter 18). Clinicians should assume that any drug taken could result in delirium (Sadock & Sadock, 2008). This chapter highlights delirium secondary to medical conditions; although frequently encountered, it is often overlooked or misdiagnosed.

Nurses frequently encounter delirium in the general hospital setting. During certain phases of a hospital stay, confusion may be noted. For older adults, the second or third hospital day may herald the onset of confusion and difficulty adjusting to an unfamiliar environment.

Although delirium is seen in children with fever and patients who are terminally ill, it occurs most frequently in older adult patients. Surgery, the introduction of medications, urinary tract infections, cerebrovascular disease, and congestive heart failure are some of the most common causes (Box 17-1). There are numerous causes that may precipitate delir-

ium, but certain factors predispose patients to delirium, thus putting them at higher risk. These factors include existing cognitive impairment (especially on admission to the hospital), low functional autonomy, polypharmacy (especially benzodiazepines, narcotic analgesics, and anticholinergics), and clinical severity of the primary illness (Voyer et al., 2007). Consequently, nurses should pay particular attention to those patients who are at greatest risk (Evidence-Based Practice box).

BOX 17-1 Common Causes of Delirium

Postoperative States
Drug Intoxications and Withdrawals
- Alcohol, anxiolytics, opioids, and central nervous system stimulants (e.g., cocaine and crack cocaine)

Infections
- Systemic: pneumonia, typhoid fever, malaria, urinary tract infection, and septicemia
- Intracranial: meningitis and encephalitis

Metabolic Disorders
- Dehydration
- Hypoxia (pulmonary disease, heart disease, and anemia)
- Hypoglycemia
- Sodium, potassium, calcium, magnesium, and acid-base imbalances
- Hepatic encephalopathy or uremic encephalopathy
- Thiamine (vitamin B_1) deficiency (Wernicke encephalopathy)
- Endocrine disorders (e.g., thyroid or parathyroid)
- Hypothermia or hyperthermia
- Diabetic acidosis

Drugs
- Digitalis, steroids, lithium, levodopa, anticholinergics, benzodiazepines, central nervous system depressants, tricyclic antidepressants
- Central anticholinergic syndrome due to use of multiple drugs with anticholinergic side effects

Neurological Diseases
- Seizures
- Head trauma
- Hypertensive encephalopathy

Tumor
- Primary cerebral

Psychosocial Stressors
- Relocation or other sudden changes
- Sensory deprivation or overload
- Sleep deprivation
- Immobilization
- Pain

EVIDENCE-BASED PRACTICE

Strategies for Managing Delirium in Hospitalized Older Patients

Siddiqi, N., Stockdale, R., Britton, A. M., & Holmes, J. (2007). Interventions for preventing delirium in hospitalized patients. *Cochrane Database of Systematic Reviews* 2007, Issue 2. Art. No.: CD005563. DOI:10.1002/14651858.CD005563.pub2.

Problem

Advancing age is associated with a higher incidence of delirium in hospitalized patients and is associated with increased mortality, morbidity, and length of stay, as well as long-term institutionalization and caregiver burden. Delirium is often misdiagnosed or not recognized by hospital staff. Nurses are in a prime position to recognize delirium. They also must manage the care of patients who become delirious, and multicomponent strategies are needed in order to do so.

Purpose of Study

The purpose was to establish the best available evidence for the prevention and detection of delirium in hospitalized patients and review its management once delirium was recognized.

Methods

The authors searched an extensive database for randomized controlled clinical trials that evaluated interventions to prevent delirium in hospitalized patients. Experts in the field of geriatrics were also contacted and unpublished results

Continued

were also included in this review. The data was collected by three reviewers. Six studies were eventually included in this review. The 833 participants were studied in surgical settings and orthopedic units.

Key Findings
- Consultation by geriatric specialists may reduce delirium incidence.
- Prophylactic (given before a problem begins) low dose haloperidol (Haldol) may reduce the severity and duration of symptoms for patients undergoing hip surgery.
- There are few studies that identify practices to detect and prevent delirium.

Implications for Nursing Practice
Nurses who work with patients at high risk of developing delirium should engage in ongoing education about its detection and management, and regular systems should be put into place to identify those patients most at risk of developing delirium. Consultation with specialist nurses and doctors should be routine when caring for patients at risk of developing delirium. Haloperidol, while it may be helpful, should be used in low dosage ranges, because it is associated with parkinsonism and akathisia, which can be confused with worsening of delirium.

APPLICATION OF THE NURSING PROCESS

ASSESSMENT
General Assessment

According to Wei and colleagues (2008), there are four cardinal features of delirium:

1. Acute onset and fluctuating course
2. Inattention
3. Disorganized thinking
4. Disturbance of consciousness

Patients with delirium may appear withdrawn, agitated, or psychotic. **Sundowning** (also known as *sundown syndrome*), in which symptoms and problem behaviors become more pronounced in the evening, may occur in both delirium and dementia.

Suspect the presence of delirium when a patient abruptly develops a disturbance in consciousness that manifests as reduced clarity of awareness of the environment. The ability to focus, sustain, or shift attention is impaired. Questions must be repeated because the individual's attention wanders, and the person might easily get off track and need to be refocused. Conversation is made more difficult because the person may be easily distracted by irrelevant stimuli. The person may have difficulty with orientation—first to time, then to place, and last to person. For example, a man with delirium may think that the year is 1972, that the hospital is home, and that the nurse is his wife. Orientation to person is usually intact to the extent that the person is aware of the self's identity.

Fluctuating levels of consciousness are unpredictable. Disorientation and confusion are usually markedly worse at night and during the early morning. In fact, some patients may be confused or delirious only at night and may remain lucid during the day.

As nurses, our frequent interaction with hospitalized patients places us in a prime position to detect delirium. Nursing assessment includes observation of (1) cognitive and perceptual disturbances, (2) physical needs, and (3) moods and physical behaviors.

Cognitive and Perceptual Disturbances

It may be difficult to engage patients experiencing delirium in conversation because they are easily distracted, display marked attention deficits, and exhibit memory impairment. In mild delirium, memory deficits are noted only on careful questioning. In more severe delirium, memory problems usually take the form of obvious difficulty in processing and remembering recent events. For example, the person might ask when a son is coming to visit, even though the son left only an hour earlier.

Perceptual disturbances are also common. Perception is the processing of information about one's internal and external environment. Various misinterpretations of reality may take the form of illusions or hallucinations.

Illusions are errors in perception of sensory stimuli. A person may mistake folds in the bedclothes for white rats or the cord of a window blind for a snake. The stimulus is a real object in the environment; however, it is misinterpreted and often becomes the object of the patient's projected fear. Illusions, unlike delusions or hallucinations, can be explained and clarified for the individual.

Hallucinations are false sensory stimuli (see Chapter 15). Visual hallucinations are common in delirium, and tactile hallucinations may also be present. For example, individuals experiencing delirium may become terrified when they "see" giant spiders crawling over the bedclothes or "feel" bugs crawling on or under their bodies. Auditory hallucinations occur more often in other psychiatric disorders such as schizophrenia.

The individual with delirium generally is aware that something is very wrong. Statements like "My thoughts are all jumbled" may signal cognitive problems. When perceptual disturbances are present, the emotional response is often one of fear and anxiety, which may be manifested by psychomotor agitation.

Physical Needs

A person with delirium becomes disoriented and may try to "go home." Alternatively, a person may think that he or she *is* home and jump out of a window in an attempt to get away from "invaders." Wandering, pulling out intravenous lines and Foley catheters, and falling out of bed are common dangers that require nursing vigilance.

An individual experiencing delirium has difficulty processing stimuli in the environment, and confusion magnifies the inability to recognize reality. The physical environment should be made as simple and clear as possible. Objects such as clocks and calendars can maximize orientation to time. Eyeglasses, hearing aids, and adequate lighting without glare can maximize the person's ability to interpret more accurately what is going on in the environment. The nurse should interact with the patient whenever the patient is awake. Short periods of social interaction help reduce anxiety and misperceptions.

Self-care deficits, injury, or hyperactivity or hypoactivity may lead to skin breakdown and possible infection. Often this is compounded by poor nutrition, forced bed rest, and possible incontinence. These areas require nursing assessment and intervention.

Autonomic signs, such as tachycardia, sweating, flushed face, dilated pupils, and elevated blood pressure, are often present in delirium. These changes must be monitored and documented carefully and may require immediate medical attention.

Changes in the sleep/wake cycle usually are noted, and in some cases, a complete reversal of the night/day, sleep/wake cycle can occur. The patient's level of consciousness may range from lethargy to stupor or from semi-coma to hypervigilance. In **hypervigilance**, patients are extraordinarily alert, and their eyes constantly scan the room; they may have difficulty falling asleep or may be actively disoriented and agitated throughout the night.

Medications should always be suspected as a potential cause of delirium (Sadock & Sadock, 2008). To recognize drug reactions or anticipate potential interactions before delirium actually occurs, it is important to assess all medications (prescription *and* over-the-counter) the patient is taking.

Moods and Physical Behaviors

The individual's moods and physical behaviors may change dramatically within a short period. Moods may swing back and forth among fear, anger, anxiety, euphoria, depression, and apathy. These labile moods are often accompanied by physical behaviors associated with feeling states. A person may strike out from fear or anger or may cry, call for help, curse, moan, and tear off clothing one minute and become apathetic or laugh uncontrollably the next. In short, behavior and emotions are erratic and fluctuating. Lack of concentration and disorientation complicate interventions. The following vignette illustrates the fear and confusion a patient may experience when admitted to an intensive care unit (ICU).

VIGNETTE

Peter Wright, aged 43, survived numerous, life-threatening complications following open-heart surgery to replace his mitral valve. As a result, he spent 3 weeks in an ICU. The night before he was to be transferred, the nurses moved his bed to accommodate another patient who needed observation closer to the nursing unit. During the transfer he heard a nurse saying, "I need to get a gas." Another nurse answered in a loud voice, "Can you get a large needle for the injection?" Peter began to get frightened and thought the nurses were going to gas and sedate him. He became suspicious about his bed being moved and thought he was being transported, against his will, to another country to have his organs removed and donated for transplantation. His fear mounted when he realized that his wife, who had been at his bedside the entire ICU stay, was not there. He wanted her to know that he was being taken away. His incoherent attempts to summon his wife back to his bedside confirmed what he suspected: the very people who had saved his life (although, at the time he could not appreciate this fact) were now out to get him.

Peter began to diligently watch the clock on the wall, recording every movement of the nurses to try to ascertain a pattern to their behavior. He was planning his escape from his captors. When he was sure nobody was looking, he climbed over the bedrails and attempted to leave the unit. The nurses responded by calling security personnel to escort him back to bed. Once he was safely back in bed, the nurses applied mechanical restraints and then sedated him.

Peter's confusion abated the next day, at which time he was transferred from the ICU to another part of the hospital. Because he could recall the details of his confused state, both in the short and long term, he realized how distorted his thinking had been during the episode. However, the anxiety, fear, and trepidation he had experienced remained with him for months after discharge from the hospital. ■

What are some more helpful interventions the nurses could have used? What could the nurses have done differently? What would you have done? For example, the nurses could have told Peter why they were moving his bed, and they could have recognized his need to have his wife return to his bedside. They could have noted signs of his fear and anxiety.

Self-Assessment

Because the behaviors exhibited by the patient with delirium can be directly attributed to temporary medical conditions, intense personal reactions in staff are less likely to arise. In fact, intense, conflicting emotions are less likely to occur in nurses working with a patient with delirium than in nurses working with a patient with dementia, which is discussed later in this chapter. Nonetheless, it can be frustrating to interact with these patients, especially given the fluctuating nature of the clinical picture.

Assessment Guidelines Delirium

1. Assess for acute onset and fluctuating levels of consciousness, which are key in delirium.
2. Assess the person's ability to attend to the immediate environment, including responses to nursing care.
3. Establish the person's normal level of consciousness and cognition by interviewing family or other caregivers.
4. Assess for past cognitive impairment—especially an existing dementia diagnosis—and other risk factors.
5. Identify disturbances in physiological status, especially infection, hypoxia, and pain.
6. Identify any physiological abnormalities documented in the patient's record.
7. Assess vital signs, level of consciousness, and neurological signs.
8. Assess potential for injury, especially in relation to potential for falls and wandering.
9. Maintain comfort measures, especially in relation to pain, cold, or positioning.
10. Monitor situational factors that worsen or improve symptoms.
11. Assess for availability of immediate medical interventions to help prevent irreversible brain damage.
12. Remain nonjudgmental. Confer with other staff readily when questions arise.

DIAGNOSIS

Safety needs play a substantial role in nursing care. Patients with delirium often perceive the environment in a distorted way, and objects are often misperceived (illusions and/or hallucinations). People and objects may be misinterpreted as threatening or harmful, and patients often act on these misinterpretations. For example, if feeling threatened or thinking that common medical equipment is harmful, the patient may pull off an oxygen mask, pull out an intravenous or nasogastric tube, or try to flee. In such a case, the person demonstrates a *Risk for injury* related to confusion, as evidenced by sensory deficits or perceptual deficits.

Hallucinations, distractibility, illusions, disorientation, agitation, restlessness, and/or misperception are major aspects of the clinical picture. When some of these symptoms are present, *Acute confusion* related to delirium is an appropriate nursing diagnosis.

If fever and dehydration are present, fluid and electrolyte balance will need to be managed. If the underlying cause of the patient's delirium results in fever, decreased skin turgor, decreased urinary output or fluid intake, and dry skin or mucous membranes, then the nursing diagnosis of *Deficient fluid volume* is appropriate. Fluid volume deficit may be related to fever, electrolyte imbalance, reduced intake, or infection.

Because disruption in the sleep/wake cycle may be present, the patient may be less responsive during the day and may become disruptively wakeful during the night. Restful sleep is not achieved, day or night; therefore, *Insomnia* or *Sleep deprivation* related to impaired cerebral oxygenation or disruption in consciousness is a likely diagnosis.

Sustaining communication with a delirious patient is difficult. *Impaired verbal communication* related to cerebral hypoxia or decreased cerebral blood flow, as evidenced by confusion or clouding of consciousness, may be diagnosed.

Fear is one of the most common of all nursing diagnoses and may be related to illusions, delusions, or hallucinations, as evidenced by verbal and nonverbal expressions of fearfulness. Other nursing concerns include *Self-care deficit*, *Disturbed thought processes*, and *Impaired social interaction*. Table 17-2 identifies nursing diagnoses for any confused patient with delirium or dementia.

OUTCOMES IDENTIFICATION

The overall outcome is that the delirious patient will return to the premorbid level of functioning. Table 17-3 includes outcomes for acute confusion from the *Nursing Outcomes Classification (NOC)* (Moorhead et al., 2008). However, for many of the diagnoses we would use for the patient experiencing delirium, *NOC* is not specific enough. Although the patient can demonstrate a wide variety of needs, *Risk for injury* is always present. Appropriate outcomes are:

- Patient will remain safe and free from injury while in the hospital.
- During periods of lucidity, patient will be oriented to time, place, and person with the aid of nursing interventions, such as the provision of clocks, calendars, maps, and other types of orienting information.
- Patient will remain free from falls and injury while confused, with the aid of nursing safety measures.

TABLE 17-2 Potential Nursing Diagnoses for the Confused Patient

Symptoms	Nursing Diagnoses
Wanders, has unsteady gait, acts out fear from hallucinations or illusions, forgets things (leaves stove on, doors open)	*Risk for injury*
Awake and disoriented during the night *(sundowning)*, frightened at night	*Insomnia* *Sleep deprivation* *Fear* *Acute confusion*
Unable to take care of basic needs	*Self-care deficit (bathing, dressing, feeding, toileting)* *Ineffective coping* *Functional urinary incontinence* *Imbalanced nutrition: less than body requirements* *Deficient fluid volume*
Sees frightening things that are not there *(hallucinations)*, mistakes everyday objects for something sinister and frightening *(illusions)*, may become paranoid and think that others are doing things to confuse him or her *(delusions)*	*Anxiety* *Disturbed sensory perception* *Impaired environmental interpretation syndrome* *Disturbed thought processes**
Does not recognize familiar people or places, has difficulty with short- and/or long-term memory, forgetful and confused	*Impaired memory* *Impaired environmental interpretation syndrome* *Acute/chronic confusion*
Has difficulty with communication, cannot find words, has difficulty in recognizing objects and/or people, incoherent	*Impaired verbal communication* *Impaired social interaction*
Devastated over losing place in life as known (during lucid moments), fearful and overwhelmed by what is happening to him or her	*Risk for compromised human dignity* *Spiritual distress* *Hopelessness* *Situational low self-esteem Grieving*
Family and loved ones overburdened and overwhelmed, unable to care for patient's needs	*Disabled family coping* *Interrupted family processes* *Impaired home maintenance* *Caregiver role strain*

Data from North American Nursing Diagnosis Association International (NANDA-I). (2009). *NANDA-I nursing diagnoses: Definitions and classification 2009–2011.* Oxford, United Kingdom: Author.
*Diagnosis retired from North American Nursing Diagnosis Association. (2007). *NANDA-I nursing diagnoses: Definitions and classification 2007–2008.* Philadelphia: Author.

Because level of consciousness can change throughout the day, the patient needs to be frequently checked for orientation.

IMPLEMENTATION

The priorities of treatment are to keep the patient safe while attempting to identify the cause. If the underlying disorder is corrected, complete recovery is possible. If, however, the underlying disorder is not corrected and persists, irreversible neuronal damage can occur. Nursing concerns therefore center on the following:

- Preventing physical harm due to confusion, aggression, or electrolyte and fluid imbalance

- Performing a comprehensive nursing assessment to aid in identifying the cause
- Assisting with proper health management to eradicate the underlying cause
- Using supportive measures to relieve distress

The *Nursing Interventions Classification (NIC)* (Bulechek et al., 2008) can be used as a guide to develop interventions for a patient with delirium (Box 17-2). Medical management of delirium involves treating the underlying organic causes. If the underlying cause of delirium is not treated, permanent brain damage may ensue. Judicious use of antipsychotic or antianxiety agents may also be useful in controlling behavioral symptoms.

TABLE 17-3 *NOC* Outcomes Related to Acute Confusion

Acute confusion: Abrupt onset of reversible disturbance of consciousness, attention, cognition, and perception that develop over a short period of time.

Nursing Outcome and Definition	Intermediate Indicators	Short-Term Indicators
Cognitive Orientation: Ability to identify person, place and time accurately	Identifies correct day Identifies correct month Identifies correct year Identifies correct season Identifies current place Identifies significant current events	Identifies self Identifies significant other
Neurological Status: *Consciousness:* Arousal, orientation, and attention to the environment	Cognitive orientation Communicates appropriately for situation Attends to environmental stimuli	Opens eyes to external stimuli Obeys commands Makes motor responses to noxious stimuli

Data from Moorhead, S., Johnson, M., Maas, M., & Swanson, E. (2008). *Nursing outcomes classification (NOC)* (4th ed.). St. Louis: Mosby.

BOX 17-2 *NIC* Interventions for Delirium Management

Definition: Provision of a safe and therapeutic environment for the patient who is experiencing an acute confusional state

Activities:

- Identify etiological factors causing delirium.
- Initiate therapies to reduce or eliminate factors causing delirium.
- Monitor neurological status on an ongoing basis.
- Provide unconditional positive regard.
- Verbally acknowledge patient's fears and feelings.
- Provide optimistic but realistic reassurance.
- Allow patient to maintain rituals that limit anxiety.
- Provide patient with information about what is happening and what can be expected to occur in the future.
- Avoid demands for abstract thinking, if patient can only think in concrete terms.
- Limit need for decision making, if frustrating or confusing to patient.
- Administer prn (as needed) medications for anxiety or agitation.
- Encourage visitation by significant others, as appropriate.
- Recognize and accept patient's perceptions or interpretation of reality (hallucinations or delusions).
- State your perception in a calm, reassuring, and nonargumentative manner.
- Respond to the theme or feeling tone, rather than the content, of the hallucination or delusion.
- When possible, remove stimuli that create misperception in a particular patient (e.g., pictures on the wall or television).
- Maintain a well-lit environment that reduces sharp contrasts and shadows.
- Assist with needs related to nutrition, elimination, hydration, and personal hygiene.
- Maintain a hazard-free environment.
- Place identification bracelet on patient.
- Provide appropriate level of supervision and surveillance to monitor patient and allow for therapeutic actions, as needed.
- Use physical restraints, as needed.
- Avoid frustrating patient by quizzing with orientation questions that cannot be answered.
- Inform patient of person, place, and time, as needed.
- Provide a consistent physical environment and daily routine.
- Provide caregivers who are familiar to the patient.
- Use environmental cues (e.g., signs, pictures, clocks, calendars, and color coding of environment) to stimulate memory, reorient, and promote appropriate behavior.
- Provide a low-stimulation environment for patient in whom disorientation is increased by overstimulation.
- Encourage use of aids that increase sensory input (e.g., eyeglasses, hearing aids, and dentures).
- Approach patient slowly and from the front.
- Address patient by name when initiating interaction.
- Reorient patient to health care provider with each contact.
- Communicate with simple, direct, descriptive statements.
- Prepare patient for upcoming changes in usual routine and environment before their occurrence.
- Provide new information slowly and in small doses, with frequent rest periods.
- Focus interpersonal interactions on what is familiar and meaningful to patient.

From Bulechek, G. M., Butcher, H. K., & Dochterman, J. M. (2008). *Nursing interventions classification (NIC)* (5th ed., pp. 252–257). St. Louis: Mosby.

A patient in acute delirium should never be left alone. Because most hospitals and health facilities are unable to provide one-to-one supervision of the patient, family members can be encouraged to stay with the patient.

EVALUATION

Long-term outcome criteria for a person experiencing delirium include:

- Patient will remain safe
- Patient will be oriented to time, place, and person by discharge
- Underlying cause will be treated and ameliorated

Dementia

Dementia is defined as progressive deterioration of cognitive functioning and global impairment of intellect with no change in consciousness. Dementia is manifested as difficulty with memory, thinking, and comprehension. While the majority of dementias are irreversible, approximately 15% are due to a reversible illness (Sadock & Sadock, 2008).

CLINICAL PICTURE

Dementia is the general term used to describe a decline in cognitive functioning that interferes with daily living. Alzheimer's disease (AD), the most common cause of dementia in older adults, is a progressive brain disorder marked by impaired memory and thinking skills (Alzheimer's Disease Education and Referral Center [ADEAR], 2008a). It is a devastating disease that not only affects the person who has it but also places an enormous burden on the families and caregivers of those affected. Nurses practicing in any setting will care for patients with AD and must be prepared to respond.

It is important to distinguish between normal forgetfulness and the memory deficit of AD and other dementias. Severe memory loss is *not* a normal part of growing older. Slight forgetfulness is a common phenomenon of the aging process (age-associated memory loss), but not memory loss that interferes with one's activities of daily living. Table 17-4 outlines memory changes in normal aging and memory changes seen in dementia.

Many people who live to a very old age never experience significant memory loss or any other symptom of dementia. Most of us know of people in their 80s and 90s who lead active lives with the intellect intact. Pablo Picasso, Duke Ellington, Ansel Adams, and George Burns are just a few examples of people who were still active in their careers when they died, and all were older than 75 years of age. (Picasso was 91, George Burns was 100.) The slow, mild cognitive changes associated with aging should not impede social or occupational functioning.

Dementia, on the other hand, is marked by progressive deterioration in intellectual functioning, memory, and the ability to solve problems and

CONSIDERING CULTURE

Caregiver Burden in Dementia

It has long been recognized that caregivers suffer a great deal of burden in relation to caring for a person with dementia. They are prone to emotional distress, depression, and decreased quality of life as they cope with caregiving. It also has been recognized that the experience of stress and coping varies among cultural groups. For example, Asian cultures have a long tradition of respecting older adult family members and fulfilling a perceived obligation to care for them. In addition, people from Asian cultures are likely to have a collective orientation, as opposed to a Western view of individuality and autonomy. It is for these reasons that nurses must come to understand cultural meanings and understandings.

A study by Chun, Knight, and Youn (2007) investigated stress and coping of caregivers in three cultural groups: Korean, Korean American, and Caucasian American. There were commonalities in stress and coping; all three groups found the patient's disruptive behavior to be burdensome and a source of anxiety and depression. The study also found cultural variation among the groups. Instrumental support, such as direct assistance and advice, was found to be important to Korean caregivers, whereas emotional support, such as affirmation and empathic understanding, was more important to Korean American caregivers. In addition, only the Korean caregivers found patient problems, disruptive behaviors, memory problems, and depression as burdensome.

This study highlights the importance of cultural awareness and sensitivity in that the need for social support and perceptions of problem behaviors varied across the cultural groups represented.

Chun, M., Knight, B. G., & Youn, G. (2007). Differences in stress and coping models of emotional distress among Korean, Korean-American and White-American caregivers. *Aging & Mental Health, 11*(1), 2–29.

TABLE 17-4 Memory Deficit: Normal Aging Versus Dementia

Parameter	Normal Aging	Dementia
Degree of change	Slowing	More severe and increasing
	Cautiousness	Variable
	Reduced ability to solve new problems	More severe and increasing
	Mildly impaired memory	More severe and increasing
	Mild decline in fluid intelligence	More severe and increasing intellectual impairment
Extent of damage	Difficulty in word finding, but no dysphasia, dyspraxia, agnosia	Dysphasia, dyspraxia, agnosia often found
Rate of change	Slow change over many years	More rapid though gradual changes

learn new skills; a decline in the ability to perform activities of daily living; and a progressive deterioration of personality accompanied by impairment in judgment. A person's declining intellect often leads to emotional changes such as mood lability, depression, and aggressive acting out, as well as to neurological changes that produce hallucinations and delusions. There are several types of dementia, including dementia of the Alzheimer's type, vascular dementia, Lewy body disease, Pick's disease, Huntington's chorea, alcohol-related dementias (including Korsakoff's syndrome), Creutzfeldt-Jakob disease, and the dementias associated with Parkinson's disease, acquired immunodeficiency syndrome (AIDS), and head trauma.

Dementias can be classified as primary or secondary. Primary dementia is irreversible, progressive, and not secondary to any other disorder. As mentioned, AD accounts for about 60% of all dementias, and vascular dementia accounts for about 20% of all dementias (Sadock & Sadock, 2008). Both Alzheimer's and vascular dementias are primary, progressive, and irreversible.

Secondary dementia occurs as a result of some other pathological process (e.g., metabolic, nutritional, or neurological). AIDS-related dementia is an example of a secondary dementia that is increasingly seen in health care settings. The exact prevalence of AIDS-related dementia is unknown. In a recent study involving 658 patients infected with AIDS, the researchers reported that that 11.7% were significantly cognitively impaired, 36.4% were depressed, and 19.7% had symptoms of sensory neuropathy (Wright et al., 2008). Cognitive impairment associated with HIV is referred to as *AIDS dementia complex*. Other secondary dementias can result from viral encephalitis, pernicious anemia, folic acid deficiency, and hypothyroidism.

Korsakoff's syndrome is an example of a secondary dementia caused by thiamine (vitamin B₁) deficiency, which may be associated with prolonged, heavy alcohol ingestion. Along with progressive mental deterioration, Korsakoff's syndrome is marked by peripheral neuropathy, cerebellar ataxia, confabulation, and myopathy (APA, 2000).

EPIDEMIOLOGY

Alzheimer's disease (AD) constitutes 50% to 60% of all dementias. The rate increases with age (Sadock & Sadock, 2008):

- At 65 years of age, the prevalence is 0.6% to 0.8%.
- At 85 years of age, the prevalence is 11% to 14%.
- At 90 years of age, the prevalence is 21% to 25%.
- At 95 years of age, the prevalence reaches 36% to 31%.

After age 65, the number of people with AD doubles for every 5-year interval (ADEAR, 2008a).

Alzheimer's disease attacks indiscriminately, striking men and women, people of various ethnicities, rich and poor, and individuals with varying degrees of intelligence. Although the disease can occur at a younger age (early onset), most of those with the disease are 65 years of age or older (late onset). It is estimated that 2.4 to 4.5 million Americans have AD (ADEAR, 2008a). Globally, it is estimated that 24.3 million people have dementia, and the number of people will double every 20 years to 81.1 million by 2040 (Ferri et al., 2005).

The second most common type of dementia is related to cerebrovascular disease. Vascular dementias account for 15% to 30% of all dementias. Other common causes of dementia are related to head trauma, alcohol abuse, and movement disorders such as Parkinson's disease; these account for 1% to 5% of all cases (Sadock & Sadock, 2008).

ETIOLOGY

Although the cause of AD is unknown, numerous hypotheses have been put forward.

Biological Factors

Alzheimer's Tangles

Using a silver-staining technique during autopsy, Alois Alzheimer first identified a buildup of neurofibrillary tangles and gray neuritic plaques consisting of beta-amyloid protein fragments in 1907 (Wright et al., 2008). This pathology begins in the hippocampus, the part of the brain responsible for recent memory. Gradually, it spreads into the cerebral cortex, the part of the brain responsible for problem-solving and other higher-order cognitive functioning (ADEAR, 2008a). Computed tomography (CT) scans and magnetic resonance imaging (MRI) reveal brain atrophy along with enlargement of cortical sulci and cerebral ventricles.

Scientists have questioned whether the amyloid plaques found in the brains of Alzheimer's patients are a cause or effect of the disease. Recent evidence (Shankar et al., 2008) has shown that a two-molecule aggregate of beta-amyloid protein may play a role in initiating the disease, but more research is required to determine the mechanisms responsible for AD.

Genetic

Family history has been shown to play a role in the development of AD. For example, early-onset AD, which occurs between the ages of 30 and 60, is inherited. Three genes that lead to the devastating, early-onset form of AD have been identified and probably account for half of the cases (Wright et al., 2008).

A susceptibility gene has been identified for late-onset AD as well. It is a gene that makes the protein apolipoprotein E (APOE), which helps carry cholesterol and is also implicated in cardiovascular disease. About 15% of the U.S. population has the gene that increases risk of AD. Other genes yet to be identified may also be implicated (ADEAR, 2008b).

Individuals who have or have had family members with AD are understandably concerned about their own risk for developing the disorder. For those who may carry the early-onset gene, genetic counseling, available through the Alzheimer's Disease Research Center, is recommended. Commercial testing is available for one of the three genes that can confirm the disease or predict its onset, but this testing raises significant ethical concerns (Wright et al., 2008). APOE testing is also available but has limited predictive value.

Environmental Factors

Until recently, the only risk factors that seemed to play a role in noninherited cases of AD were increasing age, Down syndrome, and head injury. Currently scientists are studying a variety of lifestyle factors—including education level, diet, and environment—

that might play a role in the development of AD. There is growing evidence that physical, mental, and social activities may serve as protective factors. In addition, there is increasing evidence that risk factors for cardiovascular disease and stroke (high blood pressure, high cholesterol, and low levels of the vitamin folate, for example) may increase the risk of AD (ADEAR, 2008b).

Many experts claim that primary prevention should focus on certain risk factors, including vascular disease, hypertension, smoking, type 2 diabetes, and hyperlipidemia (Ferri et al., 2005).

APPLICATION OF THE NURSING PROCESS

ASSESSMENT

General Assessment

Alzheimer's disease is commonly characterized by progressive deterioration of cognitive functioning. Initial deterioration may be so subtle and insidious that others may not notice. In the early stages of the disease, the affected person may be able to compensate for loss of memory. Some people may have superior social graces and charm that give them the ability to hide severe deficits in memory, even from experienced health care professionals. This hiding is actually a form of **denial**, which is an unconscious protective defense against the terrifying reality of losing one's place in the world. Family members may also unconsciously deny that anything is wrong as a defense against the painful awareness that a loved one is deteriorating. As time goes on, symptoms become more obvious, and other defense mechanisms become evident, including (1) denial, (2) confabulation, (3) perseveration, and (4) avoidance of questions.

Confabulation is the creation of stories or answers in place of actual memories to maintain self-esteem. For example, the nurse addresses a patient who has remained in a hospital bed all weekend:

Nurse: Good morning, Ms. Jones. How was your weekend?

Patient: Wonderful. I discussed politics with the President, and he took me out to dinner.

or

Patient: I spent the weekend with my daughter and her family.

Confabulation is not the same as lying. When people are lying, they are aware of making up an answer; confabulation is an **unconscious** attempt to maintain self-esteem.

Perseveration (the repetition of phrases or behavior) is eventually seen and is often intensified under stress. The avoidance of answering questions is another mechanism by which the person is able to maintain self-esteem unconsciously in the face of severe memory deficits.

Cardinal symptoms observed in AD include the following (APA, 2000):

- **Amnesia or memory impairment.** Initially the person has difficulty remembering recent events. Gradually, deterioration progresses to include both recent and remote memory.
- Aphasia (loss of language ability), which progresses with the disease. Initially the person has difficulty finding the correct word, then is reduced to a few words, and finally is reduced to babbling or mutism.
- Apraxia (loss of purposeful movement in the absence of motor or sensory impairment). The person is unable to perform once-familiar and purposeful tasks. For example, in apraxia of gait, the person loses the ability to walk. In apraxia of dressing, the person is unable to put clothes on properly (may put arms in trousers or put a jacket on upside down).
- Agnosia (loss of sensory ability to recognize objects). For example, the person may lose the ability to recognize familiar sounds (auditory agnosia), such as the ring of the telephone, a car horn, or the doorbell. Loss of this ability extends to the inability to recognize familiar objects (visual or tactile agnosia), such as a glass, magazine, pencil, or toothbrush. Eventually, people are unable to recognize loved ones or even parts of their own bodies.
- **Disturbances in executive functioning** (planning, organizing, abstract thinking). The degeneration of neurons in the brain results in the wasting away of the brain's working components. These cells contain memories, receive sights and sounds, cause hormones to secrete, produce emotions, and command muscles into motion.

A person with AD loses a personal history, a place in the world, and the ability to recognize the environment and, eventually, loved ones. AD robs family and friends, husbands and wives, and sons and daughters of valuable human relatedness and companionship, which results in a profound sense of grief. AD robs society of productive and active participants. Because of these devastating effects, it challenges mental health professionals and social agencies, the medical and nursing professions, and researchers looking for possible solutions.

Diagnostic Tests

A wide range of problems may be mistaken for dementia or AD. For example, in older adults, depression and dementia may have similar symptoms. It is important that nurses and other health care professionals be able to assess some of the important differences among depression, dementia, and delirium. Review Table 17-1 for important differences among these three phenomena.

Other disorders that often mimic dementia include drug toxicity, metabolic disorders, infections, and nutritional deficiencies. A disorder that mimics dementia is sometimes referred to as a pseudodementia. This reinforces the importance of performing a comprehensive assessment to identify nondementia causes when symptoms of dementia are present. Making a diagnosis of Alzheimer's disease includes ruling out all other pathophysiological conditions through the history and through physical and laboratory tests, many of which are identified in Box 17-3.

Brain imaging with CT, positron emission tomography (PET), and other developing scanning technologies have diagnostic capabilities because they reveal brain atrophy and rule out other conditions such as neoplasms. The use of mental status questionnaires, such as the Mini-Mental State Examination and various other tests to identify deterioration in mental status and brain damage, are important parts of the assessment.

In addition to performing a complete physical and neurological examination, it is important to obtain a complete medical and psychiatric history, description of recent symptoms, review of medications used, and nutritional evaluation. The observations and history provided by family members are invaluable to the assessment process.

As already mentioned, depression in the older adult is the disorder frequently confused with dementia. Medical and nursing personnel should be cautioned, however, that dementia and depression or dementia and delirium *can* coexist. In fact, studies indicate that many people diagnosed with Alzheimer's dementia also meet the *DSM-IV-TR* criteria for a depressive disorder.

BOX 17-3 Basic Medical Workup for Dementia

- Chest and skull radiographic studies
- Electroencephalography
- Electrocardiography
- Urinalysis
- Sequential multiple analyzer 12-test serum profile
- Thyroid function tests
- Folate level
- Venereal Disease Research Laboratories (VDRL), human immunodeficiency virus tests
- Serum creatinine assay
- Electrolyte assessment
- Vitamin B_{12} level
- Liver function tests
- Vision and hearing evaluation
- Neuroimaging (when diagnostic issues are not clear)

Stages of Alzheimer's Disease

Alzheimer's disease is classified according to the stage of the degenerative process. The number of stages defined ranges from three to seven, depending on the source. However, four stages, as discussed subsequently, are commonly used to categorize the progressive deterioration seen in those diagnosed with AD. Table 17-5 can be used as a guide as we review the four stages of AD and highlight the deficits associated with each stage.

Stage 1: Mild Alzheimer's Disease

The loss of intellectual ability is insidious. The person with mild AD loses energy, drive, and initiative and has difficulty learning new things. Because personality and social behavior remain intact, others tend to minimize and underestimate the loss of the individual's abilities. The individual may still continue to work, but the extent of the dementia becomes evident in new or demanding situations. Depression may occur early in the disease but usually lessens as the disease progresses. Activities such as shopping or managing finances are noticeably impaired during this phase.

VIGNETTE

Mr. Collins, 56 years of age, is a lineman for a telephone company. He feels that he is getting old. He keeps forgetting things and writes notes to himself on scraps of paper. One day on the job, he forgets momentarily which wires to connect and connects all the wrong ones, causing mass confusion for a few hours. At home, Mr. Collins flies off the handle when his wife suggests that they invite the new neighbors for dinner. It is hard for him to admit that anything new confuses him, and he often forgets names (aphasia) and sometimes loses the thread of conversations. Once, he even forgot his

---

TABLE 17-5 Stages of Alzheimer's Disease

Stage	Hallmarks
Stage 1 (Mild) *Forgetfulness*	Shows short-term memory losses; loses things, forgets Memory aids compensate: lists, routines, organization Aware of the problem; concerned about lost abilities Depression common—worsens symptoms Not diagnosable at this time
Stage 2 (Moderate) *Confusion*	Shows progressive memory loss; short-term memory impaired; memory difficulties interfere with all abilities Withdrawn from social activities Shows declines in instrumental activities of daily living (ADLs), such as money management, legal affairs, transportation, cooking, housekeeping Denial common; fears "losing his or her mind" Depression increasingly common; frightened because aware of deficits; covers up for memory loss through confabulation Problems intensified when stressed, fatigued, out of own environment, ill Commonly needs day care or in-home assistance
Stage 3 (Moderate to Severe) *Ambulatory dementia*	Shows ADL losses (in order): willingness and ability to bathe, grooming, choosing clothing, dressing, gait and mobility, toileting, communication, reading, and writing skills Shows loss of reasoning ability, safety planning, and verbal communication Frustration common; becomes more withdrawn and self-absorbed Depression resolves as awareness of losses diminishes Has difficulty communicating; shows increasing loss of language skills Shows evidence of reduced stress threshold; institutional care usually needed
Stage 4 (Late) *End stage*	Family recognition disappears; does not recognize self in mirror Nonambulatory; shows little purposeful activity; often mute; may scream spontaneously Forgets how to eat, swallow, chew; commonly loses weight; emaciation common Has problems associated with immobility (e.g., pneumonia, pressure ulcers, contractures) Incontinence common; seizures may develop Most certainly institutionalized at this point Return of primitive (infantile) reflexes

From Hall, G. R. (1994). Caring for people with Alzheimer's disease using the conceptual model of progressively lowered stress threshold in the clinical setting. *Nursing Clinics of North America, 29*(1), 129–141.

address when his car broke down on the highway. He is moody and depressed and becomes indignant when his wife finds 3 months' worth of unpaid bills stashed in his sock drawer. Mrs. Collins is bewildered, upset, and fearful that something is terribly wrong. ∎

The rate of progression varies from person to person. Some individuals in stage 1 AD decline quickly and may die within 3 years. Others, although their condition worsens, may still function in the community with support. Still others may remain at this level for 3 years or more. The duration of the disease from onset of symptoms to death averages 8 to 10 years but can range from 3 to 20 years (APA, 2000).

Stage 2: Moderate Alzheimer's Disease

Deterioration becomes evident during the moderate phase. Often the person with moderate AD cannot remember his or her address or the date. There are memory gaps in the person's history that may fluctuate from one moment to the next. Hygiene suffers, and the ability to dress appropriately is markedly affected. The person may put on clothes backward, button the buttons incorrectly, or not fasten zippers (apraxia). Often the person has to be coaxed to bathe.

Mood becomes labile, and the individual may have bursts of paranoia, anger, jealousy, and apathy. Activities such as driving are hazardous, and families are faced with the difficulty of taking away the car keys from their loved one. Care and supervision become a full-time job for family members. Denial mercifully protects people from the realization that they are losing control of not only their minds but also their lives. Along with denial, people begin to withdraw from activities and from others because they often feel overwhelmed and frustrated when they have difficulty doing things that once were easy. They may also have moments of becoming tearful and sad.

As important as it is to recognize all of the deficits that occur in stage 2, caretakers should realize that the person still retains abilities that influence care (Box 17-4).

BOX 17-4 Abilities in Stage 2 Alzheimer's Disease

- Initiate familiar activity if supplies are available and within reach
- Perform steps of self-care with verbal and tactile cues
- Tell stories from past
- Read words slowly out loud
- Follow simple instructions
- Speak in short sentences or phrases; able to make needs known
- Sort, stack objects, count
- Ambulate if no physical disability is present
- Feel and name objects

For a short period, Mr. Collins is transferred to a less complicated work position after his inability to function is recognized. His wife drives him to work and picks him up. Mr. Collins often forgets what he is doing and stares blankly. He accuses the supervisor of spying on him. Sometimes he disappears at lunch and is unable to find his way back to work. The transfer lasts only a few months, and Mr. Collins is forced to take an early retirement. At home, Mr. Collins sleeps in his clothes. He loses interest in reading and watching sports on television and often breaks into angry outbursts, seemingly over nothing. Often he becomes extremely restless and irritable and wanders around the house aimlessly. ∎

Stage 3: Moderate to Severe Alzheimer's Disease

At the moderate to severe stage of AD, the person is often unable to identify familiar objects or people, even a spouse (severe agnosia). The person needs repeated instructions and directions to perform the simplest tasks (advanced apraxia): "Here is the face cloth, pick up the soap. Now, put water on the face cloth and rub the face cloth with soap." Often the individual cannot remember where the toilet is and becomes incontinent. Total care is necessary at this point, and the burden on the family can be emotionally, financially, and physically devastating. The world is very frightening to the person with AD because nothing makes sense any longer. Agitation, violence, paranoia, and delusions are commonly seen. Another problem that is frightening to family members and caregivers is wandering behavior. An estimated 60% of people with AD wander and are at risk for becoming lost (ADEAR, 2008a).

Admission to a long-term care facility may be the most appropriate recourse at this time because the level of care is so demanding, and violent outbursts and incontinence may be burdens the family can no longer handle. The following are some criteria that indicate the need for placement in a skilled care facility:
- The person wanders.
- The person is a danger to self and others.
- The person is incontinent.
- The person's behavior affects the sleep and general health of others.
- The person is totally dependent on others for physical care.

Mr. Collins is terrified. Memories come and then slip away. People come and go, but they are strangers. Someone is masquerading as his wife, and it is hard to tell what is real. Things never stay in the same place. Sometimes people hide the bathroom where he cannot find it. He in turn hides things to keep them safe, but he forgets where he hides them. Buttons and belts are confusing, and he does not know what they are doing there, anyway. Sometimes he tries to walk away from the terrifying feelings and the strangers. He tries to find something he has lost long ago…if he could only remember what it is. ■

Stage 4: Late Alzheimer's Disease

Late in AD, the following symptoms may occur: agraphia (inability to read or write), hyperorality (the need to taste, chew, and put everything in one's mouth), blunting of emotions, visual agnosia (loss of ability to recognize familiar objects), and hypermetamorphosis (manifested by touching of everything in sight). At this stage, the ability to talk, and eventually the ability to walk, is lost. End-stage AD is characterized by stupor and coma. Death frequently is secondary to infection or choking.

VIGNETTE

Mrs. Collins and the children keep Mr. Collins at home until his outbursts become frightening. Once he is lost for 2 days after he somehow unlocks the front door. Finally Mrs. Collins admits her husband to a Veterans Administration (VA) hospital. When his wife comes to visit, Mr. Collins sometimes cries, but he never talks. He is usually restrained in his chair during her visits. The staff explain to her that although Mr. Collins can still walk, he keeps getting into other people's beds and scaring them. They explain that perhaps he wants comfort and misses human touch. They encourage her visits, even though Mr. Collins does not seem to recognize her. He does respond to music. His wife brings a radio, and when she plays the country and western music he has always loved, Mr. Collins nods and claps his hands.

Mrs. Collins is torn between guilt and love, anger and despair. She is confused and depressed. She is going through the painful process of mourning the loss of the man she has loved and shared a life with for 34 years. Three months after his admission to the VA hospital, and 8 years after the incident of the crossed wires at the telephone company, Mr. Collins chokes on some food, develops pneumonia, and dies. ■

Self-Assessment

Working with cognitively impaired people in any setting should make us aware of the tremendous responsibility placed on caregivers. The behavioral problems these patients may display can cause tremendous stress for professionals and family caregivers alike. Caring for people who are unable to communicate and have lost the ability to relate and respond to others is extremely difficult, especially for student nurses or nurses who do not understand dementia or AD.

Nurses working in facilities for residents who are cognitively impaired (e.g., nursing homes and extended care facilities) need special education and skills. Education must include information about the process of the disease and effective interventions, as well as knowledge regarding antipsychotic drugs. Support and educational opportunities should be readily available, not just to nurses but also to nurse aides, who are often directly responsible for administering basic care.

Because stress is a common occurrence when working with persons with cognitive impairments, staff need to be proactive in minimizing its effects, which can be facilitated by:

- Having a realistic understanding of the disease so that expectations for the person are realistic.
- Establishing realistic outcomes for the person and recognizing when they are achieved. These outcomes may be as minor as *patient feeds self with spoon*, yet remember that even the smallest achievement can be a significant accomplishment for the impaired individual.
- Maintaining good self-care. As nurses, we need to protect ourselves from the negative effects of stress by obtaining adequate sleep and rest, eating a nutritious diet, exercising, engaging in relaxing activities, and addressing our own emotional and spiritual needs.

Assessment Guidelines Dementia

1. Evaluate the person's current level of cognitive and daily functioning.
2. Identify any threats to the person's safety and security and arrange their reduction.
3. Evaluate the safety of the person's home environment (e.g., with regard to wandering, eating inedible objects, falling, engaging in provocative behaviors toward others).
4. Review the medications (including, herbs, complementary agents) the patient is currently taking.
5. Interview family to gain a complete picture of the person's background and personality.
6. Explore how well the family is prepared for and informed about the progress of the person's dementia, depending on cause (if known).
7. Discuss with the family members how they are coping with the patient and their main issues at this time.
8. Review the resources available to the family. Ask family members to describe the help they receive from other family members, friends, and community resources. Determine if caregivers are aware of community support groups and resources.
9. Identify the needs of the family for teaching and guidance (e.g., how to manage catastrophic reactions, lability of mood, aggressive behaviors, and nocturnal delirium and increased confusion and agitation at night [sundowning]).

DIAGNOSIS

Caring for a person with dementia requires a great deal of patience, creativity, and maturity. The needs of such a person can be enormous for nursing staff and for families who care for their loved ones in the home. As the disease progresses, so do the needs of the person and the demands on the caregivers, staff, and family.

One of the most important areas of concern identified by both staff and families is the patient's safety. Many people with AD wander and may be lost for hours or days. Wandering, along with behaviors such as rummaging, may be perceived as purposeful to the person with AD. Wandering may result from changes in the physical environment, fear caused by hallucinations or delusions, or lack of exercise.

Seizures are common in the later stages of this disease. Injuries from falls and accidents can occur during any stage as confusion and disorientation progress. The potential for burns exists if the person is a smoker or is unattended when using the stove. Prescription drugs can be taken incorrectly, or bottles of noxious fluids can be mistakenly ingested, which results in a medical crisis. Therefore, *Risk for injury* is always present.

As the person's ability to recognize or name objects is decreased, *Impaired verbal communication* becomes a problem. As memory diminishes and disorientation increases, *Impaired environmental interpretation syndrome, Impaired memory,* and *Confusion* occur.

During the course of the disease, people show personality changes, increased vulnerability, and (often) inappropriate behaviors. Common behaviors include hoarding, regression, and being overly demanding. Therefore, nurses and family members often intervene in behaviors that signal *Ineffective coping.* Family caregivers may experience compromised or even disabling family coping.

Additional family issues may emerge. Perhaps some of the most crucial aspects of the patient's care are support, education, and referrals for the family. The family loses an integral part of its unit. Family members lose the love, the function, the support, the companionship, and the warmth that this person once provided. *Caregiver role strain* is always present, and planning with the family and offering community support is an integral part of appropriate care. *Anticipatory grieving* is also an important phenomenon to assess and may be an important target for intervention. Helping the family grieve can make the task ahead somewhat clearer and at times less painful. Review Table 17-2 for potential nursing diagnoses for confused patients.

OUTCOMES IDENTIFICATION

Families who have a member with dementia are faced with an exhaustive list of issues that need to be addressed. Table 17-6 provides a checklist that may

TABLE 17-6 Problems That May Affect People with Dementia and Their Families

Problem	Examples	Problem	Examples
Memory impairment	Forgets appointments, visits, etc. Forgets to change cloths, wash, go to the toilet Forgets to eat, take medications Loses things	Risks outside the home	Competence, judgment, and risks at work Driving, road sense Getting lost
		Apathy	Little conversation Lack of interest Poor self-care
Disorientation	Time: mixes night and day, mixes days of appointments, wears summer clothes in winter, forgets age Place: loses way around house Person: has difficulty recognizing visitors, family, spouse	Poor communication	Dysphasia
		Repetitiveness	Repetition of questions or stories Repetition of actions
Need for physical help	Dressing Washing, bathing Toileting Eating Performing housework Maintaining mobility	Uncontrolled emotion	Distress Anger or aggression Demands for attention
		Uncontrolled behavior	Restlessness day or night Vulgar table or toilet habits Undressing Sexual disinhibition Shoplifting
Risks in the home	Falls Fire from cigarettes, cooking, heating Flooding Admission of strangers to home Wandering out	Incontinence	Urine Feces Urination or defecation in the wrong place

Continued

TABLE 17-6 Problems That May Affect People with Dementia and Their Families—cont'd

Problem	Examples	Problem	Examples
Emotional reactions	Depression Anxiety Frustration and anger Embarrassment and withdrawal	Decision making	Indecisive Easily influenced Refuses help Makes unwise decisions
Other reactions	Suspiciousness Hoarding and hiding	Burden on family	Disruption of social life Distress, guilt, rejection Family discord
Mistaken beliefs	Still at work Parents or spouse still alive Hallucinations		

BOX 17-5 *NOC* Outcomes Related to Dementia*

Injury
- Person will remain safe in the hospital or at home.
- With the aid of an identification bracelet and neighborhood or hospital alert, the person will be returned within 1 hour of wandering.
- With the aid of interventions, person will remain burn free.
- With the aid of guidance and environmental manipulation, person will not hurt himself or herself if a fall occurs.
- Person will ingest only correct doses of prescribed medications and appropriate food and fluids.

Communication
- Person will communicate needs.
- Person will state needs in alternative modes when he or she is aphasic (e.g., will signal correct word on hearing it or will refer to picture or label).
- Person will wear prescribed glasses or hearing aid each day.

Agitation Level
- Person will have rest periods if pacing and restless.
- Person will cooperate with caregiving activities.
- Person will experience minimal frustrating experiences.
- Person will express frustrations in an appropriate manner.

Caregiver Role Strain
- Family members will have the opportunity to express "unacceptable" feelings in a supportive environment.

- Family members will have access to professional counseling.
- Family members will name two organizations within their geographical area that can offer emotional support and help with legal and financial burdens.
- Family members will participate in ill member's plan of care, with encouragement from staff.
- Family members will state that they have outside help that allows them to take personal time for themselves each week or month.

Impaired Environmental Interpretation: Chronic Confusion
- Person will acknowledge the reality of an object or a sound that was misinterpreted (illusion), after it is pointed out.
- Person will state that he or she feels safe after experiencing delusions or illusions.
- Person will remain nonaggressive when experiencing paranoid ideation.

Self-Care Needs
- Person will participate in self-care at optimal level.
- Person will be able to follow step-by-step instructions for dressing, bathing, and grooming.
- Person will put on own clothes appropriately, with aid of fastening tape (Velcro) and nursing supervision.
- Person's skin will remain intact and free from signs of pressure.

*Partial list.

From Moorhead, S., Johnson, M., Maas, M. L., & Swanson, E. (2008). *Nursing outcomes classification (NOC)* (4th ed.). St. Louis: Mosby.

---

help nurses and families identify areas for intervention. Self-care needs, impaired environmental interpretation, chronic confusion, ineffective individual coping, and caregiver role strain are just a few of the areas nurses and other health care members will need to target (Box 17-5).

PLANNING

Planning care for a person with dementia is geared toward the person's immediate needs. Refer to Table 17-6 for help in identifying areas of care needed. The Functional Dementia Scale (Figure 17-2) can be used

FUNCTIONAL DEMENTIA SCALE

Circle one rating for each item:
1. None or little of the time
2. Some of the time
3. Good part of the time
4. Most or all of the time

Client: _____
Observer: _____
Position or relation to patient: _____
Facility: _____
Date: _____

1	2	3	4	1. Has difficulty in completing simple tasks on own (e.g., dressing, bathing, doing arithmetic).
1	2	3	4	2. Spends time either sitting or in apparently purposeless activity.
1	2	3	4	3. Wanders at night or needs to be restrained to prevent wandering.
1	2	3	4	4. Hears things that are not there.
1	2	3	4	5. Requires supervision or assistance in eating.
1	2	3	4	6. Loses things.
1	2	3	4	7. Appearance is disorderly if left to own devices.
1	2	3	4	8. Moans.
1	2	3	4	9. Cannot control bowel function.
1	2	3	4	10. Threatens to harm others.
1	2	3	4	11. Cannot control bladder function.
1	2	3	4	12. Needs to be watched so doesn't injure self (e.g., by careless smoking, leaving the stove on, falling).
1	2	3	4	13. Destructive of materials around him/her (e.g., breaks furniture, throws food trays, tears up magazines).
1	2	3	4	14. Shouts or yells.
1	2	3	4	15. Accuses others of doing bodily harm or stealing his or her possessions — when you are sure the accusations are not true.
1	2	3	4	16. Is unaware of limitations imposed by illness.
1	2	3	4	17. Becomes confused and does not know where he or she is.
1	2	3	4	18. Has trouble remembering.
1	2	3	4	19. Has sudden changes of mood (e.g., gets upset, angered, or cries easily).
1	2	3	4	20. If left alone, wanders aimlessly during the day or needs to be restrained to prevent wandering.

Figure 17-2 Functional Dementia Scale. (From Moore, J. T., Bobula, J. A., Short, T. B., & Mischel, M. [1983]. A functional dementia scale. *Journal of Family Practice, 16,* 498.)

by nurses and families to plan strategies for addressing immediate needs and to track progression of the dementia.

Identifying level of functioning and assessing caregivers' needs help focus planning and identify appropriate community resources. Does the person or family need the following?

- Transportation services
- Supervision and care when primary caregiver is out of the home
- Referrals to day care centers
- Information on support groups within the community
- Meals on Wheels
- Information on respite and residential services
- Telephone numbers for help lines
- Home health aides
- Home health services
- Additional psychopharmaceuticals to manage distressing or harmful behaviors

IMPLEMENTATION

The attitude of unconditional positive regard is the nurse's single most effective tool in caring for people with dementia. It induces people to cooperate with care, reduces catastrophic outbreaks, and increases family members' satisfaction with care. Box 17-6 lists *NIC* interventions related to the management of dementia.

A considerable number of individuals with dementia have secondary behavioral disturbances, including depression, hallucinations, delusions, agitation, insomnia, and wandering. Because these symptoms impair the person's ability to function, increase the need for supervision, and influence the need for institutionalization, the control of these symptoms is a priority in managing AD. Helping the individual achieve the highest possible level of independence and function is the foundation of care.

Intervention with family members is critical. The effects of losing a family member to dementia—that is, watching the deterioration of a person who has had an important role within the family unit and who is loved and is a vital part of his or her family's history—can be devastating. The following interventions are useful.

Counseling and Communication Techniques

How one chooses to communicate with a person with dementia affects that person's ability to maintain self-esteem and his or her ability to participate in care. People with dementia often find it difficult to express themselves because they:

BOX 17-6 *NIC* Interventions for Dementia Management

Definition: Provision of a modified environment for the patient who is experiencing a chronic confusional state

Activities:
- Include family members in planning, providing, and evaluating care, to the extent desired.
- Identify usual patterns of behavior for such activities as sleep, medication use, elimination, food intake, and self-care.
- Determine physical, social, and psychological history of patient, usual habits, and routines.
- Determine type and extent of cognitive deficit(s), using standardized assessment tool.
- Monitor cognitive functioning, using standardized assessment tool.
- Determine behavioral expectations appropriate for patient's cognitive status.
- Provide a low-stimulation environment (e.g., quiet, soothing music; nonvivid and simple, familiar patterns in décor; performance expectations that do not exceed cognitive processing ability; and dining in small groups).
- Provide adequate but nonglare lighting.
- Identify and remove potential dangers in environment for patient.
- Place identification bracelet on patient.
- Provide a consistent physical environment and daily routine.
- Prepare for interaction with eye contact and touch, as appropriate.
- Introduce self when initiating contact.
- Address patient distinctly by name when initiating interaction, and speak slowly.
- Give one simple direction at a time.
- Speak in a clear, low, warm, respectful tone of voice.
- Use distraction, rather than confrontation, to manage behavior.
- Provide unconditional positive regard.
- Avoid touch and proximity if this causes stress or anxiety.
- Provide caregivers who are familiar to the patient (e.g., avoid frequent rotations of staff assignments).
- Avoid unfamiliar situations when possible (e.g., room changes and appointments without familiar people present).
- Provide rest periods to prevent fatigue and reduce stress.
- Monitor nutrition and weight.
- Provide space for safe pacing and wandering.
- Avoid frustrating patient by quizzing with orientation questions that cannot be answered.
- Provide cues—such as current events, seasons, location, and names—to assist orientation.
- Seat patient at small table in groups of three to five for meals, as appropriate.
- Allow patient to eat alone if appropriate.
- Provide finger foods to maintain nutrition for patient who will not sit and eat.
- Provide patient a general orientation to the season of the year by using appropriate cues (e.g., holiday decorations, seasonal decorations and activities, and access to contained, out-of-doors area).
- Decrease noise levels by avoiding paging systems and call lights that ring or buzz.
- Select television or radio programs based on cognitive processing abilities and interests.
- Select one-to-one and group activities geared to patient's cognitive abilities and interests.
- Label familiar photos with names of the individuals in the photos.
- Select artwork for patient's rooms featuring landscapes, scenery, or other familiar images.
- Ask family members and friends to see patient one or two at a time, if needed, to reduce stimulation.
- Discuss with family members and friends how best to interact with patient.
- Assist family to understand that it may be impossible for patient to learn new material.
- Limit number of choices patient has to make, so as not to cause anxiety.
- Provide boundaries, such as red or yellow tape on the floor, when low-stimulus units are not available.
- Place patient's name in large block letters in room and on clothing, as needed.
- Use symbols, rather than written signs, to assist patient in locating room, bathroom, or other area.
- Monitor carefully for physiological causes of increased confusion that may be acute and reversible.
- Remove or cover mirrors if patient is frightened or agitated by them.
- Discuss home safety issues and interventions.

From Bulechek, G. M., Butcher, H. K., & Dochterman, J. M. (2008). *Nursing interventions classification (NIC)* (5th ed.). St. Louis: Mosby.

- Have difficulty finding the right words
- Use familiar words repeatedly
- Invent new words to describe things
- Frequently lose their train of thought
- Rely on nonverbal gestures

Table 17-7 provides special guidelines for nurses, family members, and other caregivers to use in communicating with a cognitively impaired person.

Health Teaching and Health Promotion

Educating families who have a cognitively impaired member is one of the most important health-teaching duties nurses encounter. Families who are caring for a member in the home need to know about strategies for communicating and for structuring self-care activities (Table 17-8).

TABLE 17-7 Guidelines for Communication with People with Dementia

Intervention	Rationale
Always identify yourself and call the person by name at each meeting.	The person's short term memory is impaired—requires frequent orientation to time and environment.
Speak slowly.	The person needs time to process information.
Use short, simple words and phrases.	The person may not be able to understand complex statements or abstract ideas.
Maintain face-to-face contact.	Verbal and nonverbal clues are maximized.
Be near the person when talking, one or two arm-lengths away.	This distance can help the person focus on speaker, as well as maintain personal space.
Focus on one piece of information at a time.	Attention span of the person is poor, and the person is easily distracted—helps the person focus. Too much data can be overwhelming and can increase anxiety.
Talk with the person about familiar and meaningful things.	Self-expression is promoted, and reality is reinforced.
Encourage reminiscing about happy times in life.	Remembering accomplishments and shared joys helps distract the person from deficit and gives meaning to existence.
When the person is delusional, acknowledge the person's feelings and reinforce reality. Do not argue or refute delusions.	Acknowledging feelings helps the person feel understood. Pointing out realities may help the person focus on realities. Arguing can enhance adherence to false beliefs.
If the person gets into an argument with another person, stop the argument and temporarily separate those involved. After a short while (5 minutes), explain to each person matter-of-factly why you had to intervene.	Escalation to physical acting out is prevented. The person's right to know is respected. Explaining in an adult manner helps maintain self-esteem.
When the person becomes verbally aggressive, acknowledge the person's feelings, and shift the topic to more familiar ground (e.g., "I know this is upsetting for you, because you always cared for others. Tell me about your children.")	Confusion and disorientation easily increase anxiety. Acknowledging feelings makes the person feel more understood and less alone. Topics the person has mastery over can remind him or her of areas of competent functioning and can increase self-esteem.
Have the person wear prescription eyeglasses or hearing aid.	Environmental awareness, orientation, and comprehension are increased, which in turn increases awareness of personal needs and the presence of others.
Keep the person's room well lit.	Environmental clues are maximized.
Have clocks, calendars, and personal items (e.g., family pictures or Bible) in clear view of the person while he or she is in bed.	These objects assist in maintaining personal identity.
Reinforce the person's pictures, nonverbal gestures, Xs on calendars, and other methods used to anchor the person in reality.	When aphasia starts to hinder communication, alternate methods of communication need to be instituted.

Data from Bulechek, G. M., Butcher, H. K., & Dochterman, J. M. (2008). *Nursing interventions classification (NIC)* (5th ed.). St. Louis: Mosby.

Most importantly, families need to know where to get help. Help includes professional counseling and education regarding the process and progression of the disease. Families especially need to know about and be referred to community-based groups that can help shoulder this tremendous burden (e.g., day care centers, senior citizen groups, organizations providing home visits and respite care, and family support groups). A list with definitions of some of the types of services available in the person's community, as well as the names and telephone numbers of the providers of these services, should be given to the family.

Referral to Community Supports

The Alzheimer's Association (formerly known as the Alzheimer's Disease and Related Disorders Association) is a national umbrella agency that provides

TABLE 17-8 Patient and Family Teaching: Guidelines for Self-Care in Dementia

Intervention	Rationale
DRESSING AND BATHING	
Always have the person perform all tasks within his or her present capacity.	Maintains the person's self-esteem and uses muscle groups; impedes staff burnout; minimizes further regression.
Always have the person wear own clothes, even if in the hospital.	Helps maintain the person's identity and dignity.
Use clothing with elastic, and substitute fastening tape (Velcro) for buttons and zippers.	Minimizes the person's confusion and eases independence of functioning.
Label clothing items with the person's name and name of item.	Helps identify the person if he or she wanders and gives the person additional clues when aphasia or agnosia occurs.
Give step-by-step instructions whenever necessary (e.g., "Take this blouse. Put in one arm…now the other arm. Pull it together in front. Now….")	The person can focus on small pieces of information more easily; allows the person to perform at optimal level.
Make sure that water in faucets is not too hot.	Judgment is lacking in the person; the person is unaware of many safety hazards.
If the person is resistant to performing self-care, come back later and ask again.	Moods may be labile, and the person may forget but often complies after short interval.
NUTRITION	
Monitor food and fluid intake.	The person may have anorexia or be too confused to eat.
Offer finger food that the person can take away from the dinner table.	Increases input throughout the day; the person may eat only small amounts at meals.
Weigh the person regularly (once a week).	Monitors fluid and nutritional status.
During periods of hyperorality, watch that the person does not eat nonfood items (e.g., ceramic fruit or food-shaped soaps).	The person puts everything into mouth; may be unable to differentiate inedible objects made in the shape and color of food.
BOWEL AND BLADDER FUNCTION	
Begin bowel and bladder program early; start with bladder control.	Establishing same time of day for bowel movements and toileting—in early morning, after meals and snacks, and before bedtime—can help prevent incontinence.
Evaluate use of disposable diapers.	Prevents embarrassment.
Label bathroom door, as well as doors to other rooms.	Additional environmental clues can maximize independent toileting.
SLEEP	
Because the person may awaken, be frightened, or cry out at night, keep area well lighted.	Reinforces orientation, minimizes possible illusions.
Maintain a calm atmosphere during the day.	Encourages a calming night's sleep.
Order nonbarbiturates (e.g., chloral hydrate) if necessary.	Barbiturates can have a paradoxical reaction, causing agitation.
If medications are indicated, consider neuroleptics with sedative properties, which may be the most helpful (e.g., haloperidol [Haldol]).	Helps clear thinking and sedates.
Avoid the use of restraints.	Can cause the person to become more terrified and fight against restraints until exhausted to a dangerous degree.

various forms of assistance to persons with the disease and their families. The Alzheimer's Association has launched Safe Return, the first nationwide program to help locate and return missing people with AD and other memory impairments. Wandering is a common behavior during the second and third stages of AD, and the Safe Return program offers peace of mind to families. Information regarding housekeeping, home health aides, and companions is also available through this organization. Such outside resources can help prevent the total emotional and physical fatigue of family members. Additional resources that might be available in some communities are found in Table 17-9.

Although many families manage the care of their loved one until death, other families eventually find that they can no longer deal with the labile and aggressive behavior, incontinence, wandering, unsafe habits, or disruptive nocturnal activity. Family members need to know where and how to place their loved one for care if this becomes necessary. Families need information, support, and legal and financial guidance at this time. When the nurse is unable to provide the relevant information, proper referrals by the social worker are needed. Information regarding advance directives, durable power of attorney, guardianship, and conservatorship should be included in the communication with the family. Useful guidelines for families in structuring a safe environment and planning appropriate activities are found in Table 17-10.

Pharmacological Interventions

Table 17-11 presents drugs used in the United States to treat AD.

TABLE 17-9 Types of Services That May Be Available to People with Dementia	
Type of Service	**Services Provided**
Family/caregiver (Some people may live by themselves in the community; active case management is vital.)	Caregivers have a right to: Easy access to services Respite care Full involvement in decision making Assessment of the needs of both the caregiver and the person with dementia Information and referral Case management: coordination of community resources and follow-up
Community services	Adult day care: provides activities, socialization, supervision Physician services Protective services: prevent, eliminate, and/or remedy effects of abuse or neglect Recreational services Transportation Mental health services Legal services
Home care	Meals on Wheels Home health aide services Homemaker services Hospice services Occupational therapy Paid companion or sitter services Physical therapy Skilled nursing Personal care services: assistance in basic self-care activities Social work services Telephone reassurance: regular telephone calls to individuals who are isolated and homebound* Personal emergency response systems: telephone-based systems to alert others that a person who is alone is in need of emergency assistance*

*Vital for those living alone.

TABLE 17-10 Patient and Family Teaching: Guidelines for Care at Home

Intervention	Rationale
SAFE ENVIRONMENT	
Gradually restrict use of the car.	As judgment becomes impaired, the person may be dangerous to self and others.
Remove throw rugs and other objects in person's path.	Minimizes tripping and falling.
Minimize sensory stimulation.	Decreases sensory overload, which can increase anxiety and confusion.
If the person becomes verbally upset, listen briefly, give support, then change the topic.	Goal is to prevent escalation of anger. When attention span is short, the person can be distracted to more productive topics and activities.
Label all rooms and drawers. Label often-used objects (e.g., hairbrushes and toothbrushes).	May keep the person from wandering into other persons' rooms. Increases environmental clues to familiar objects.
Install safety bars in bathroom.	Prevents falls.
Supervise the person when he or she smokes.	Danger of burns is always present.
If the person has history of seizures, keep padded tongue blades at beside. Educate family on how to deal with seizures.	Seizure activity is common in advanced Alzheimer's disease.
WANDERING	
If the person wanders during the night, put mattress on the floor.	Prevents falls when the person is confused.
Have the person wear medical alert bracelet that cannot be removed (with name, address, and telephone number). Provide police department with recent pictures.	The person can easily be identified by police, neighbors, or hospital personnel.
Alert local police and neighbors about wanderer.	May reduce time necessary to return the person to home or hospital.
If the person is in hospital, have him or her wear brightly colored vest with name, unit, and phone number printed on back.	Makes the person easily identifiable.
Put complex locks on door.	Reduces opportunity to wander.
Place locks at top of door.	In moderate and late Alzheimer's-type dementia, ability to look up and reach upward is lost.
Encourage physical activity during the day.	Physical activity may decrease wandering at night.
Explore the feasibility of installing sensor devices.	Provides warning if the person wanders.
USEFUL ACTIVITIES	
Provide picture magazines and children's books when the person's reading ability diminishes.	Allows continuation of usual activities that the person can still enjoy; provides focus.
Provide simple activities that allow exercise of large muscles.	Exercise groups, dance groups, and walking provide socialization, as well as increased circulation and maintenance of muscle tone.
Encourage group activities that are familiar and simple to perform.	Activities such as group singing, dancing, reminiscing, and working with clay and paint all help to increase socialization and minimize feelings of alienation.

TABLE 17-11 Drug Treatment of Patients with Alzheimer's Disease

Generic (Trade)	Action	Indications	Side Effects	Warnings
CHOLINESTERASE INHIBITORS				
Tacrine* (Cognex) Donepezil* (Aricept) Rivastigmine* (Exelon) Galantamine* (Razadyne)	Prevent the breakdown of acetylcholamine and thereby increase its availability at cholinergic synapses	Modestly improves cognition, behavior, function. Slows disease progression.	Nausea, vomiting, diarrhea, insomnia, fatigue, muscle cramps, incontinence, bradycardia, and syncope	Tacrine no longer used extensively, owing to hepatotoxicity. Donepezil is better tolerated; dosage is only once a day and is preferred. Rivastigmine available as a once-daily patch.
***N*-METHYL-D-ASPARTATE (NMDA) ANTAGONIST**				
Memantine* (Namenda)	Normalizes levels of glutamate, which in excessive quantities contributes to neurodegeneration	Treatment of moderate to severe Alzheimer's disease. No evidence that it modifies underlying disease.	Dizziness, agitation, headache, constipation, and confusion	Clearance is reduced with renal impairment. Use cautiously with moderate renal impairment. Do not use with severe renal impairment.
SELECTIVE SEROTONIN REUPTAKE INHIBITORS				
Citalopram (Celexa) Escitalopram (Lexapro) Fluoxetine (Prozac) Paroxetine (Paxil) Sertraline (Zoloft)	Blocks the reuptake of serotonin, thereby making more available and improving mood	Useful with depression, irritability, sleep disturbances, and anxiety	Agitation, insomnia, headache, nausea and vomiting, sexual dysfunction, and hyponatremia	Discontinuation syndrome—dizziness, insomnia, nervousness, irritability, nausea, and agitation—may occur with abrupt withdrawal (depending on half-life). Taper slowly.
ANTIANXIETY AGENTS				
Lorazepam (Ativan) Oxazepam (Serax)	Facilitates the action of the inhibitory neurotransmitter GABA	Anxiety, restlessness, verbally disruptive behavior, and resistance	Drowsiness, dizziness, headaches. Restlessness, insomnia, and increased anxiety possible	Use cautiously due to risk for further memory impairment, sedation, and falls.
ATYPICAL ANTIPSYCHOTICS				
Aripiprazole (Abilify) Olanzapine (Zyprexa) Quetiapine (Seroquel) Risperidone (Risperdal) Ziprasidone (Geodon)	Blockade of serotonin and dopamine receptors	**Used with extreme caution** for paranoid thinking, hallucinations, and agitation. Questionable efficacy in clinical trials.	Many; see Chapters 3 and 15. Weight gain, increased serum glucose, and hyperlipidemia	Lower dose used in older adults. Nighttime dose is preferred. FDA Alert for increased risk of CVA and death in dementia patients issued in 2005.
ANTICONVULSANTS				
Carbamazepine (Tegretol) Divalproex (Depakote)	Reduces the excitability of neurotransmission	Agitated and aggressive behavior and emotional lability	Ataxia, sedation, confusion, and (rarely) bone marrow suppression	Monitor the complete blood count and liver-associated enzymes.

* Approved by the U.S. FDA for treatment of Alzheimer's disease.

Data from Bourgeois, J. A., Seaman, J. S., & Servis, M. E. (2008). Delirium, dementia, and amnestic and other cognitive disorders. In R. E. Hales, S. C. Yudofsky, & G. O. Gabbard (Eds.). *Textbook of psychiatry*. Arlington, VA: American Psychiatric Publishing; Lehne, R. A. (2010). *Pharmacology for nursing care* (7th ed.). Philadelphia: Saunders; and Wright, C. I., Trinh, N., Blacker, D., & Falk, W. E. (2008). Dementia. In T. A. Stern, J. F. Rosenbaum, M. Fava, J. Biederman, & S. L. Rauch (Eds.), *Massachusetts General Hospital comprehensive clinical psychiatry* (pp. 231–246). St. Louis: Mosby.

Cognitive Impairment

There is currently no cure for Alzheimer's disease. There are, however, five AD drugs approved by the U.S. Food and Drug Administration (FDA) that slow the progression of the illness (Raina et al., 2008). Since a deficiency of acetylcholine has been linked to AD, medications aimed at preventing its breakdown (cholinesterase inhibitors) have been developed, including tacrine hydrochloride (Cognex), donepezil (Aricept), rivastigmine (Exelon), and galantamine (Razadyne, formerly marketed as Reminyl). Memantine (Namenda) normalizes levels of glutamate, a neurotransmitter that may contribute to neurodegeneration (Wright et al., 2008). Refer to Chapter 3 for a more detailed discussion of drugs used to treat AD.

Although these medications are used widely and have been shown to have statistically significant effects when compared to placebos, it seems that they produce only a clinically marginal effect on cognition, behavior, or quality of life (Raina et al., 2008). Nonetheless, they do delay the cognitive progression of dementia and assist with some of the behavioral symptoms.

Tacrine (Cognex) was the first cholinesterase inhibitor to be approved by the FDA for the treatment of mild to moderate symptoms of AD. It improves functioning and slows the progress of the disease, particularly in the areas of cognition and memory, in about 20% to 50% of patients. Unfortunately, tacrine is associated with a high frequency of side effects, including elevated liver transaminase levels, gastrointestinal effects, and liver toxicity (Healy, 2005). As a result, it is no longer actively marketed for use with dementia (Wright et al., 2008).

Donepezil (Aricept), approved by the FDA in 1996, inhibits acetylcholine breakdown. It also appears to slow down deterioration in cognitive functions but without the potentially serious liver toxicity attributed to tacrine. This is the drug of choice for AD because of its once per day dosing and fewer side effects (Lehne, 2010). In studies of donepezil, some individuals with AD did experience diarrhea and nausea while taking the drug.

Rivastigmine (Exelon), a brain selective acetylcholinesterase inhibitor, was approved in 2000. The most common side effects are nausea, vomiting, loss of appetite, and weight loss. In most cases, these side effects are temporary (ADEAR, 2007). Rivastigmine should always be taken with food to reduce gastrointestinal side effects.

Galantamine (Razadyne [formerly known as *Reminyl*]) is a reversible cholinesterase inhibitor approved for use in the United States in 2001 (Lehne, 2010). Galantamine also works to increase the concentration of acetylcholine by blocking the action of acetylcholinesterase, the enzyme that breaks down acetylcholine. Galantamine is prescribed in the first and second stages of AD.

All of the cholinesterase inhibitors have the potential to cause nausea, diarrhea, and vomiting. In addition, they should be used with caution when patients are taking nonsteroidal antiinflammatory drugs (NSAIDs) (ADEAR, 2007).

Memantine (Namenda) (approved for treatment of Alzheimer's disease in 2003) is the first drug to target symptoms during the moderate to severe stages of the disorder, but it is not approved by the FDA for mild symptoms (Alzheimer's Association, 2007). This drug works by regulating the activity of glutamate, a chemical involved in learning and memory (Alzheimer's Association, 2007).

Behavioral Symptoms

Other medications are often useful in managing the behavioral symptoms of individuals with dementia, but these need to be used with extreme caution. The rule of thumb for elderly people is **"start low and go slow."** In addition, because people with dementia are at high risk of developing delirium, adding medications should always be done with caution.

Some of the troubling behaviors exhibited by people with dementia, with which their caregivers must cope, are (1) psychotic symptoms (hallucinations, paranoia), (2) severe mood swings (depression is very common), (3) anxiety (agitation), and (4) verbal or physical aggression (combativeness).

In June of 2008, the FDA warned that the use of antipsychotics, both conventional and atypical, is no longer indicated for dementia-related psychosis, because they are associated with increased risk of death (USFDA, 2008).

Of clinical relevance to nurses is the evidence that suggests that personalized nursing care, in which the idiosyncratic needs of the person are recognized and met are effective as nonpharmacological treatment for the behavioral problems associated with dementia (Ayalon et al., 2006). With this evidence in mind, nurses should try to decipher patients' needs as expressed in their behavior; people with dementia do not always communicate their needs verbally.

The Future of Drug Therapy

Among the most exciting developments in the treatment of AD are clinical trials of an **amyloid vaccine (AN-1792)**, which—it is hoped—will clear the brain of amyloid plaques. Unfortunately, the latest research reports that although AN-1792 did clear the amyloid plaques of people with AD, it did not alleviate the progression of the disease (Holmes et al., 2008). This is disappointing news, but it should not rule out the potential for other therapies (Holtzman, 2008).

Additional research is ongoing, with focus on:
- The development of other cholinesterase inhibitors
- The use of cholesterol-lowering agents, which is being investigated through multicenter trials
- The use of antiinflammatory agents as a preventive measure
- The use of neurotrophic agents with the potential to regenerate brain cells
- The use of diabetic treatments that might decrease blood vessel inflammation in the brain

Additional information about current clinical studies can be found at the Alzheimer's Association website: www.alz.org.

Integrative Therapy

A number of herbal or all-natural drugs are currently under investigation. However, currently there is not enough scientific evidence concerning their effectiveness or harmfulness. Keep in mind that the designation *all-natural* or *herbal* does not mean that a substance is safe. Some alternative treatments being investigated are *Ginkgo biloba*, as discussed in the Integrative Therapy box. According to Kidd (2008), omega-3 fatty acids, other antioxidant nutrients, and vitamins—especially folate, B$_6$, B$_{12}$, C, and E—may also be helpful in the treatment of AD.

EVALUATION

The outcome criteria for people with cognitive impairments need to be measurable, within the capabilities of the individual person, and evaluated frequently. As the person's condition continues to deteriorate, outcomes must be altered to reflect the person's diminished functioning. Frequent evaluation and reformulation of outcome criteria and short-term indicators also help reduce staff and family frustration and minimize the patient's anxiety by ensuring that tasks are not more complicated than the person can accomplish.

The overall outcomes for treatment are to promote the person's optimal level of functioning and to delay further regression whenever possible. Working closely with family members and providing them with the names of available resources and support sources may help increase the quality of life for both the family and the patient with AD (Case Study and Nursing Care Plan 17-1).

INTEGRATIVE THERAPY

Ginkgo Biloba

Many Americans take *Ginkgo biloba*, believing it will improve their memory and possibly prevent progression in dementia. However, the evidence is inconsistent and unconvincing (Birks, 2008). In a recent randomized, controlled pilot study (Dodge, 2008), researchers found that *Ginkgo biloba* neither altered the progression of dementia nor protected against a decline in memory. However, there were some improvements on both counts when the researchers took adherence into consideration. Further, the group taking ginkgo had a greater incidence of ischemic strokes and transient ischemic attacks. Use of ginkgo could pose risks for people who are taking warfarin, heparin, aspirin, or other anticoagulants. Those who use this herbal product should inform their attending health care professionals.

Dodge, H. H., Zitzelbergerk T., Oken, B. S., Howieson, D., & Kaye, J. (2008). A randomized trial of *Ginkgo biloba* for the prevention of cognitive decline. *Neurology, 70*(19, part 2), 1809–1817.

Birks, J., Grimley-Evans, J. (2008). Ginkgo biloba for cognitive impairment and dementia. *Cochrane Database of Systematic Reviews* 2008, Issue 4. Chichester, UK: John Wiley and Sons. DOI: 10.1002/14651858.CD003120.pub2

Case Study and Nursing Plan 17-1   Cognitive Impairment

During the past 4 years, Mr. Ludwig has demonstrated rapidly progressive memory impairment, disorientation, and deterioration in his ability to function, related to Alzheimer's disease. He is a 67-year-old man who retired at age 62 to spend some of his remaining "youth" with his wife and to travel, garden, visit family, and finally to get to do the things they always wanted to do. At age 63 he was diagnosed with Alzheimer's disease.

Mr. Ludwig has been taken care of at home by his wife and his daughter, Kelly. Kelly is divorced and has returned home with her two young daughters.

The family members find themselves closer to physical and mental exhaustion. Mr. Ludwig is becoming increasingly incontinent when he cannot find the bathroom. He wanders away from home, despite close supervision. The police and neighbors bring him back home an average of

Continued

four times a week. Once, he was lost for 5 days after he had somehow boarded a bus for Pittsburgh, 1000 miles from home. He was robbed and beaten before being found by the police and returned home.

He frequently wanders into his granddaughters' rooms at night while they are sleeping and tries to get into bed with them. Too young to understand that their grandfather is lonely and confused, they fear that he is going to hurt them. Four times in the past two weeks, he has fallen while getting out of bed at night, thinking he is in a sleeping bag, camping out in the mountains. After a conflicted and painful two months, the family places him in a care facility for people with Alzheimer's disease.

Mrs. Ludwig tells the admitting nurse, Mr. Jackson, that her husband wanders almost all the time. He has difficulty finding the right words for things (aphasia) and becomes frustrated and angry when that happens. Sometimes he does not seem to recognize the family (agnosia). Once, he thought that Kelly was a thief breaking into the house and attacked her with a broom handle. Telling this story causes Kelly to break down into heavy sobs: "What's happened to my father? He was so kind and gentle. Oh, God…I've lost my father."

Mrs. Ludwig tells Mr. Jackson that her husband can sometimes participate in dressing himself; at other times, he needs total assistance. At this point, Mrs. Ludwig begins to cry uncontrollably, saying "I can't bear to part with him… but I can't do it anymore. I feel as if I've betrayed him."

Mr. Jackson then focuses his attention on Mrs. Ludwig and her experience. He states, "This is a difficult decision for you." Mr. Jackson suggests that Mrs. Ludwig talk to other families who have a cognitively impaired member. "It might help you to know that you are not alone, and having contact with others to share your grief can be healing." One of the groups he suggests is the Alzheimer's Association, a well-known self-help group.

ASSESSMENT

Self-Assessment

Mr. Jackson has worked on his particular unit for four years. It is a unit especially designed for cognitively impaired individuals, which makes nursing care easier than on a regular unit. He applied for this position shortly after his own father died of complications secondary to Alzheimer's disease. Mr. Jackson refers to the process of living and dying with this disease as horrifying; his goal is to help other people go through this with caring, dignity, and the highest level of functioning as possible.

Caring for Mr. Ludwig and his family is becoming especially personal. Mr. Jackson is struck by the similarity between this family's situation and his own. Mr. Ludwig is about the same age his father had been, looks similar to him, and has many of his mannerisms. Mrs. Ludwig and her daughter Kelly seem to be responding in much the same way his family did. He finds that he is having stronger than usual transference feelings with this family and even became teary when Mrs. Ludwig did.

The evening after he met the Ludwigs, Mr. Jackson went home utterly exhausted and continued to think about them and his own father. He shared these feelings with his wife, and the two of them spent some time talking about his father and all they had been through together, good and bad. In the end, Mr. Jackson sat back, breathed a long, deep sigh of relief, and thanked his wife for being there for him. He told his wife that he supposed he will never really get over the death of his father, but he is getting better every day.

When Mr. Jackson returned to work, he nearly walked right into Mr. Ludwig, who was standing at the doorway wearing two shirts, a pair of pajama bottoms, and a baseball cap. "Are you the man who's taking me to pick up my car?" he asks. Mr. Jackson smiles and says, "It looks like you have quite a day planned. Let's start with a cup of coffee" and redirects him to the day hall.

Objective Data

Patient wanders away from home about four times a week
Was lost for 5 days and was robbed and beaten
Often incontinent when he cannot find the bathroom
Has difficulty finding words
Has difficulty identifying members of the family at times
Has difficulty dressing himself at times
Falls out of bed at night
Has memory impairment

Is disoriented much of the time
Gets into bed with granddaughters at night when wandering
Family undergoing intense feelings of loss and guilt

Subjective Data

"I can't bear to part with him."
"I feel as if I've betrayed him."
"I've lost my father."

DIAGNOSIS

1. *Risk for injury* related to confusion, as evidenced by wandering

Supporting Data
- Wanders away from home about four times a week
- Wanders despite supervision
- Falls out of bed at night
- Gets into other people's beds
- Wanders at night

2. *Functional urinary incontinence* related to disturbed cognition, as evidenced by inability to find the toilet

Supporting Data
- Incontinent when he cannot find the bathroom

3. Self-care deficit (self-dressing deficits) related to impaired cognitive functioning, as evidenced by impaired ability to put on and take off clothing

Supporting Data
- Sometimes is able to dress with help of wife
- At other times is too confused to dress self at all

4. *Anticipatory grieving* related to loss and deterioration of family member

Supporting Data
- "I can't bear to part with him."
- "I feel as if I've betrayed him."
- "I've lost my father."
- Family undergoing intense feelings of loss and guilt

OUTCOMES IDENTIFICATION

Although Mr. Ludwig has many unmet needs that require nursing interventions, Mr. Jackson decides to focus on the four initial nursing diagnoses. As other problems arise, they will be addressed.

Nursing Diagnosis	Long-Term Goals	Short-Term Goals
1. *Risk for injury* related to confusion, as evidenced by wandering	1. Resident will remain safe in nursing home.	1a. Throughout nursing home stay, resident will not fall out of bed. 1b. Throughout nursing home stay, resident will wander only in protected area. 1c. Resident will be returned within 2 hours if he succeeds in escaping from the unit.
2. *Functional urinary incontinence* related to disturbed cognition, as evidenced by inability to find the toilet	2. Resident will experience less incontinence (fewer episodes) by fourth week of hospitalization.	2a. By the end of 4 weeks, resident will participate in toilet training. 2b. By the end of 4 weeks, resident will find the toilet most of the time.
3. *Self-care deficit* (self-dressing) related to impaired cognitive functioning, as evidenced by impaired ability to put on and take off clothes	3. Resident will participate in dressing himself 80% of the time.	3a. By the end of 4 weeks, resident will follow step-by-step instructions for dressing most of the time. 3b. By the end of 4 weeks, resident will dress in own clothes with aid of fastening tape.

Continued

Nursing Diagnosis	Long-Term Goals	Short-Term Goals
4. Anticipatory grieving related to loss and deterioration of family member	4. In 3 months' time, all family members will state that they feel they have more support and are able to talk about their grieving.	4a. After 3 months, family members will state that they have opportunity to express "unacceptable" feelings in supportive environment. 4b. After 3 months, family members will state that they have found support from others who have a family member with Alzheimer's disease.

PLANNING

Mr. Jackson plans care to ensure Mr. Ludwig's safety, provide for the maintenance of his hygiene needs and incontinence, and assist Mrs. Ludwig as she deals with her husband's deterioration.

IMPLEMENTATION

Using the concepts of *NIC*, Mr. Jackson's plan of care (Nursing diagnosis: *Risk for injury* related to confusion, as evidenced by wandering) was personalized as follows:

Short-Term Outcome	Intervention	Rationale	Evaluation
1. Throughout nursing home stay, resident will not fall out of bed.	1a. Spend time with resident on admission.	1a. Lowers anxiety, provides orientation to time and place. Resident's confusion is increased by change.	**GOAL MET** Mattress on floor prevents falls out of bed.
	1b. Label resident's room in big, colorful letters.	1b. Offers clues in new surroundings.	
	1c. Remove mattress from bed and place on floor.	1c. Prevents falling out of bed.	
	1d. Keep room well lit at all times.	1d. Provides important environmental clues; helps lower possibility of illusions.	
	1e. Show resident clock and calendar in room.	1e. Fosters orientation to time.	
	1f. Keep window shade up.	1f. Allows day-night variations.	
2. Throughout nursing home stay, resident will wander only in protected area.	2a. At night, take resident to large, protected, well-lit room.	2a. Resident is able to wander safely in protected environment.	**GOAL MET** Resident continues to wander at night; with supervision, keeps out of other residents' rooms most of the time. By fourth week, resident starts to nap on couch in large room after snacks during the night.
	2b. Alert physician to check resident for cardiac decompensation.	2b. Addresses possible underlying cause of nocturnal wakefulness and wandering.	
	2c. Offer snacks when resident is up—milk, decaffeinated tea, sandwich.	2c. Helps replace fluid and caloric expenditure.	
	2d. Allow soft music on radio.	2d. Helps induce relaxation.	
	2e. Spend short, frequent intervals with resident.	2e. Decreases resident's feelings of isolation and increases orientation.	
	2f. Take resident to bathroom after snacks.	2f. Helps prevent incontinence.	
	2g. During day, offer activities that include use of large muscle groups.	2g. For some residents, helps decrease wandering.	

Short-Term Outcome	Intervention	Rationale	Evaluation
3. Resident will be returned within 2 hours if he succeeds in escaping from the unit.	3a. Order MedicAlert bracelet for resident (with name, unit, hospital, and phone number). 3b. Place brightly colored vest on resident with name, unit, and phone number taped on back. 3c. Check resident's whereabouts periodically during the day and especially at night.	3a. If resident gets out of hospital, he can be identified. 3b. If resident wanders in hospital, he can be identified and returned. 3c. Helps monitor resident's activities.	**GOAL MET** By fourth week, resident wanders off unit only once; is found in lobby and returned by security guard within 45 minutes.

EVALUATION

Although Mr. Ludwig continues to display wandering behaviors, his wandering is contained to safe areas of the unit except for one instance when he wanders to the lobby. He is stopped by security and safely returned to the unit within 45 minutes. He has not fallen out of bed. Nursing interventions such as placing his mattress on the floor and ensuring adequate lighting increase his safety while at the same time acknowledging that he continues to exhibit wandering behaviors.

KEY POINTS TO REMEMBER

- *Cognitive disorder* is a term that refers to disorders resulting from changes in the brain and marked by disturbances in orientation, memory, intellect, judgment, and affect.
- Delirium and dementia are discussed in this chapter because they are the cognitive disorders most frequently seen by health care workers.
- Delirium is marked by acute onset, disturbance in consciousness, and symptoms of disorientation and confusion that fluctuate by the minute, hour, or time of day.
- Delirium is always secondary to an underlying condition; therefore, it is temporary, transient, and may last from hours to days once the underlying cause is treated. If the cause is not treated, permanent damage to neurons can result.
- Dementia usually has a more insidious onset than delirium. Global deterioration of cognitive functioning (e.g., memory, judgment, ability to think abstractly, and orientation) is often progressive and irreversible, depending on the underlying cause.
- Dementia may be primary (e.g., Alzheimer's disease [AD], vascular dementia, Pick's disease, Lewy body disease). In this case, the disease is irreversible.
- Alzheimer's disease accounts for up to 70% of all cases of dementia, and vascular dementia accounts for about 20%.
- There are various theories regarding the cause of AD, but none is definitive.
- Signs and symptoms change according to the four stages of AD: stage 1 (mild), stage 2 (moderate), stage 3 (moderate to severe), and stage 4 (late).
- The behavioral manifestations of AD include confabulation, perseveration, aphasia, apraxia, agnosia, and hyperorality.
- No known cause or cure exists for AD, although a number of drugs that increase the brain's supply of acetylcholine (a nerve-communication chemical) are helpful in slowing the progress of the disease.
- People with AD have many unmet needs and present numerous management challenges to both their families and health care workers.
- Specific nursing interventions for cognitively impaired individuals can increase communication, safety, and self-care and are described in the chapter. The need for family teaching and support is strong.

CRITICAL THINKING

1. Mrs. Kendel is an 82-year-old woman who has Alzheimer's disease. She lives with her husband, who has been trying to care for her in their home. Mrs. Kendel is having trouble dressing. She has put her blouse on backwards, and sometimes puts her bra on over her blouse. She often forgets where things are. She makes an effort to cook but has recently attempted to "put out" the electric burners of the stove with pitchers of water. Once in a while, she cannot find the bathroom in time, often mistaking it for a closet. At times, she cries because she is aware that she is losing her sense of her place in the world. She and her husband have always been close, loving companions, and he wants to keep her at home as long as possible.

   A. Assist Mr. Kendel by writing out a list of suggestions that he can try at home that might help facilitate (a) communication, (b) activities of daily living, and (c) maintenance of a safe home environment.

   B. Identify at least three interventions that are appropriate to this situation for each of the areas cited above.

C. Identify resources available for maintaining Mrs. Kendel in her home for as long as possible. Provide the name of a self-help group that you would urge Mr. Kendel to join.

2. Share with your class or clinical group the name and function of at least three community agencies in your area that could be an appropriate referral for a family with a member with dementia. (For one, you can contact the Alzheimer's Association to find a local chapter; www.alz.org.)

CHAPTER REVIEW

1. A 73-year-old woman with pneumonia becomes agitated after being admitted to the intensive care unit through the emergency department. She is placed in soft restraints when she continues to try to leave her bed despite being too weak to walk. Her vital signs are erratic, and her thinking seems disorganized. During her first 24 hours in ICU, the patient varies from somnolent to agitated, and from laughing to angry. Her daughter reports that the patient "was never like this at home." What is the most likely explanation for the situation?
   1. Pneumonia has worsened the patient's early-stage dementia.
   2. The patient is experiencing delirium secondary to the pneumonia.
   3. The patient is sundowning due to the decreased stimulation of the intensive care unit.
   4. The patient does not want to be in the hospital and is angry that staff will not let her leave.

2. Intervention(s) appropriate for a hospitalized patient experiencing delirium include which of the following? *Select all that apply.*
   1. Immediately placing the patient in restraints if she begins to hallucinate or act irrationally or unsafely
   2. Assuring that a clock and a sign indicating the day and date is displayed where the patient can see it easily
   3. Being prepared for possible hostile responses to efforts to take vital signs or provide direct physical care
   4. Preventing sensory deprivation by placing the patient near the nurses' station and leaving the television and multiple lights turned on 24 hours per day
   5. Speaking with the patient frequently for short periods for reassurance, assisting the patient in remaining oriented, and ensuring the patient's safety
   6. Anticipating that the patient may try to leave if agitated and providing for continuous direct observation to prevent wandering
   7. Promoting normalized sleep patterns by encouraging the patient to remain awake during the day and facilitating rest at night

3. Which statement about dementia is accurate?
   1. The majority of people over age 85 are affected by dementia.
   2. Disorientation is the dominant and most disruptive symptom of dementia.
   3. People with dementia tend to be distressed by it and complain about its symptoms.
   4. Hypertension, diminished activity levels, and head injury increase the risk of dementia.

4. Mrs. Smith dies at the age of 82. In the 2 months following her death, her husband, aged 84 and in good health, has begun to pay less attention to his hygiene and seems less alert to his surroundings. He complains of difficulty concentrating and sleeping and reports that he lacks energy. His family sometimes has to remind and encourage him to shower, take his medications, and eat, all of which he then does. Which response is most appropriate?
   1. Arrange for an appointment with a therapist for evaluation and treatment of suspected depression.
   2. Reorient Mr. Smith by pointing out the day and date each time you have occasion to interact with him.
   3. Meet with family and support persons to help them accept, anticipate, and prepare for the progression of his stage II dementia.
   4. Avoid touch and proximity; these are likely to be uncomfortable for Mr. Smith and may provoke aggression when he is disoriented.

5. Which of the following intervention(s) would be beneficial for those caring for a loved one with Alzheimer's disease? *Select all that apply.*
   1. Guide the family to restrict the patient's driving as soon as signs of forgetfulness are exhibited.
   2. Recommend switching to hospital-type gowns to facilitate bathing, dressing, and other ph ysical care of the patient.
   3. Discourage wandering by installing complex locks or locks placed at the tops of doors where the patient cannot readily reach them.
   4. For situations in which the patient becomes upset, teach loved ones to listen briefly, provide support, and then change the topic.
   5. Encourage caregivers to care for themselves, as well as the patient, via use of support resources such as adult day care or respite care.
   6. If the patient is prone to wander away, encourage family to notify police and neighbors of the patient's condition, wandering behavior, and description.

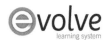

Visit the Evolve website for an **Audio Chapter Summary, Chapter Review Answers & Rationales, Critical Thinking Answer Guidelines,** and additional resources related to the content in this chapter: **http://evolve.elsevier.com/Varcarolis/foundations**

Companion CD Use the Companion CD to prepare for tests and the NCLEX® Examination with **Test-Taking Strategies** for psychiatric mental health nursing and hundreds of **Review Questions**.

References

Alzheimer's Association. (2007). *FDA-Approved Treatments for Alzheimer's*. Retrieved October 1, 2008, from http://alz.org.national/documents/topicsheet_treatments.pdf

Alzheimer's Disease Education and Referral Center (ADEAR). (2007). *Alzheimer's Disease Medication Fact Sheet*. Retrieved October 1, 2008 from http://www.nia.nih.gov/Alzheimers/Publications/medicationsfs.htm

Alzheimer's Disease Education and Referral Center (ADEAR). (2008a). *Alzheimer's disease fact sheet (NIH Publication No. 08-6423)*. Retrieved March 18, 2009, from http://www.nia.nih.gov/NR/rdonlyres/7DCA00DB-1362-4755-9E87-96DF669EAE20/11209/84206ADEARFactsheetAlzDiseaseFINAL08DEC23.pdf

Alzheimer's Disease Education and Referral Center (ADEAR). (2008b). *Scientists isolate a toxic key to Alzheimer's disease in human brains*. Retrieved March 18, 2009 from http://www.nia.nih.gov/NewsAndEvents/PressReleases/PR20080623beta-amyloid.htm

American Psychiatric Association. (2000). *Diagnostic and statistical manual of mental disorders (DSM-IV-TR)* (4th ed., text rev.). Washington, DC: Author.

Ayalon, L., Gunn, A. M., Feliciano, L., & Areân, P. A. (2006). Effectiveness of nonpharmacological interventions for the management of neuropsychiatric symptoms in patients with dementia. *Archives of Internal Medicine, 166,* 2182–2188.

Bulechek, G. M., Butcher, H. K., & Dochterman, J. M. (2008). *Nursing interventions classification (NIC)* (5th ed.). St. Louis: Mosby.

Caplan, J. P., Cassem, N. H., Murray, G. B., Park, J. M., & Stern, T. A. (2008). Delirium. In T. A. Stern, J. F. Rosenbaum, M. Fava, J. Biederman, & S. L. Rauch (Eds.), *Massachusetts General Hospital comprehensive clinical psychiatry* (pp. 217–229). Philadelphia: Saunders.

Ferri, C. P., Prince, M., Brayne, C., Brodaty, H., Fratiglioni, L., Ganguli, M., et al. (2005). Global prevalence of dementia: a Delphi consensus study. *The Lancet, 366*(9503), 2112–2117.

Healy, D. (2005). *Psychiatric drugs explained* (4th ed.). Edinburgh: Churchill Livingstone.

Holmes, C., Boche, D., Wilkinson, D., Yadegarfar, G., Hopkins, V., Bayer, A., et al. (2008). Long-term effects of A beta(42) immunisation in Alzheimer's disease: follow-up of a randomized, placebo-controlled phase I trial. *The Lancet, 372*(9634), 216–223.

Holtzman, D. M. (2008). Moving towards a vaccine. *Nature, 454,* 418–420.

Kidd, P. M. (2008). Alzheimer's disease, amnestic mild cognitive impairment, and age-associated memory impairment: current understanding and progress toward integrative prevention. *Alternative Medicine Review, 13*(2), 85–115.

Lehne, R. A. (2010). *Pharmacology for nursing care* (7th ed.). Philadelphia: Saunders.

Moorhead, S., Johnson, M., Maas, M., & Swanson, E. (2008). *Nursing outcomes classification (NOC)* (4th ed.). St. Louis: Mosby.

North American Nursing Diagnosis Association International (NANDA-I). (2009). *NANDA-I nursing diagnoses: definitions and classification 2009-2011*. Oxford, United Kingdom: Author.

Raina, P., Santaguida, P., Ismaila, A., Patterson, C., Cowan, D., Levine, M., et al. (2008). Effectiveness of cholinesterase inhibitors and memantine for treating dementia: evidence review for a clinical practice guideline. *Annals of Internal Medicine, 148*(5), 379–397.

Sadock, B. J., & Sadock, A. (2008). *Concise textbook of clinical psychiatry* (3rd ed.). Philadelphia: Lippincott Williams & Wilkins.

Shankar, G., Li, S., Mehta, T., Garcia-Munoz, A., Shepardson, N., Smith, I., et al. (2008). Amyloid-β protein dimers isolated directly from Alzheimer's brains impair synaptic plasticity and memory. *Nature Medicine, 14,* 837–842.

Siddiqi, N., Stockdale, R., Britton, A. M., & Holmes, J. (2007). Interventions for preventing delirium in hospitalized patients. *Cochrane Database of Systematic Reviews 2007,* Issue 2. Art. No.: CD005563. DOI: 10.1002/14651858.CD005563.pub2

U.S. Food and Drug Administration (USFDA). (2008). *Information for healthcare professionals: Antipsychotics; FDA ALERT [6/16/2008]*. Retrieved September 30, 2008, from http://www.fda.gov/CDER/drug/InfoSheets/HCP/antipsychotics_conventional.htm

Voyer, P., McCuskar, J., Cole, M. G., St-Jacques, S., & Khomenko, L. (2007). Factors associated with delirium severity among older patients. *Journal of Clinical Nursing, 16,* 819–831.

Wei, L. A., Fearing, M. A., Sternberg, E. J., & Inouye, S. K. (2008). The confusion assessment method: A systematic review of current usage. *Journal of the American Geriatrics Society, 56,* 823–830.

Wright, C. I., Trinh, N., Blacker, D., & Falk, W. E. (2008). Dementia. In T. A. Stern, J. F. Rosenbaum, M. Fava, J. Biederman, & S. L. Rauch (Eds.), *Massachusetts General Hospital comprehensive clinical psychiatry* (pp. 231–246). Philadelphia: Saunders.

Wright, E., Brew, B., Arayawichanont, A., Robertson, K., Samintharapanya, K., Kongsaengdao, S. et al. (2008). Neurologic disorders are prevalent in HIV-positive outpatients in the Asia-Pacific region. *Neurology, 71,* 50–56.

CHAPTER 18

Addictive Disorders

Joe Councill III, Margaret Jordan Halter, and Kathleen Smith-Dijulio

Key Terms and Concepts

Objectives

1. Compare and contrast the terms *substance abuse* and *substance dependence*, as defined by the *Diagnostic and Statistical Manual of Mental Disorders*, fourth edition, text revision *(DSM-IV-TR)*.
2. Discuss four components of the assessment process to be used with a person who is chemically dependent.
3. Describe the difference between the behaviors of a person with alcoholism and a nondrinker in relation to blood alcohol level.
4. Discuss the symptoms of alcohol withdrawal and alcohol delirium and the recommended treatments for each.
5. Describe the signs of alcohol poisoning and the appropriate treatment based on the individual's presentation.
6. List the appropriate steps to take if one observes an impaired co-worker.
7. Describe aspects of enabling behaviors and give examples.
8. Compare and contrast the signs and symptoms of intoxication, overdose, and withdrawal for cocaine and amphetamines.
9. Distinguish between the symptoms of narcotic intoxication and those of narcotic withdrawal.
10. Identify two short-term goals for a person who abuses alcohol in terms of (a) withdrawal, (b) active treatment, and (c) health maintenance.
11. Analyze the pros and cons of the following treatments for narcotic addictions: (a) methadone or levo-alpha-acetylmethadol, (b) therapeutic communities, and (c) abstinence-oriented self-help programs.
12. Recognize the phenomenon of relapse as it affects people who abuse substances during different phases of treatment.
13. Evaluate four indications that a person is successfully recovering from substance abuse.

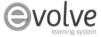 Visit the Evolve website for an **Audio Glossary & Flashcards, Concept Map Creator**, and additional resources related to the content in this chapter: **http://evolve.elsevier.com/Varcarolis/foundations**

The United States is a drug-oriented society in which people use a host of drugs for various purposes: to restore health, reduce pain and anxiety, increase energy, create a feeling of euphoria, induce sleep, and enhance alertness. Most of us have been personally affected by the maladaptive use of alcohol or substances by a relative, friend, or even ourselves.

The degree to which we have been affected can range from casual knowledge and frustration to profound family dysfunction and lasting emotional scars. In this chapter, we explore the clinical implications of addictive disorders and what psychiatric mental health nurses, as well as nurse generalists, should know about their care.

CLINICAL PICTURE

The *Diagnostic and Statistical Manual of Mental Disorders,* fourth edition, text revision *(DSM-IV-TR)* (American Psychiatric Association [APA], 2000a) focuses on the behavioral aspects and pathological patterns of substance use, emphasizing the physical symptoms of tolerance and withdrawal. An overview of *DSM-IV-TR* diagnostic criteria for substance abuse and dependence is provided in Figure 18-1.

Tolerance and Withdrawal

The diagnosis of substance dependence involves the concepts of tolerance and withdrawal. **Tolerance** occurs when a person's physiological reaction to a drug decreases with repeated administrations of the same dose. **Withdrawal** causes physiological changes to occur when blood and tissue concentrations of a drug decrease in individuals who have maintained heavy and prolonged use of a substance.

Because alcohol is still the most common drug of abuse in the United States and poses the greatest withdrawal danger, *DSM-IV-TR* diagnostic criteria for alcohol intoxication, withdrawal, and delirium are highlighted in Figure 18-2. Information on signs and symptoms of intoxication and withdrawal from other substances of abuse is given later in this chapter.

Other phenomena frequently encountered in substance abuse are flashbacks, synergistic effects, and antagonistic effects. These are discussed briefly here, although they are seen in many situations, not just in substance abuse.

Flashbacks

Flashbacks are transitory recurrences of perceptual disturbance caused by a person's earlier hallucinogenic drug use when he or she is in a drug-free state (APA, 2000a). Experiences such as visual distortions, time expansion, loss of ego boundaries, and intense emotions are reported. Often flashbacks are mild and perhaps pleasant, but at other times, individuals experience repeated recurrences of frightening images or thoughts.

DSM-IV-TR CRITERIA FOR SUBSTANCE ABUSE AND DEPENDENCE

SUBSTANCE ABUSE AND DEPENDENCE

Substance Abuse

Maladaptive pattern of substance use leading to clinically significant impairment or distress, manifested by one or more of the following within a 12-month period:

1. Inability to fulfill major role obligations at work, school, and home

2. Participation in physically hazardous situations while impaired (driving a car, operating a machine, exacerbating existing problem [e.g., ulcer])

3. Recurrent legal or interpersonal problems

4. Continued use despite recurrent social and interpersonal problems

Substance Dependence

Maladaptive pattern of substance use leading to clinically significant impairment or distress, manifested by three or more of the following within a 12-month period:

1. Presence of tolerance to the drug

2. Presence of withdrawal syndrome

3. Substance is taken in larger amounts/for longer period than intended

4. Unsuccessful or persistent desire to cut down or control use

5. Increased time spent in getting, taking, and recovering from the substance; may withdraw from family or friends

6. Reduction or absence of important social, occupational, or recreational activities

7. Substance used despite knowledge of recurrent physical or psychological problems or that problems were caused or exacerbated by one substance

Figure 18-1 Diagnostic criteria for substance abuse and dependence. (Adapted from American Psychiatric Association. [2000a]. *Diagnostic and statistical manual of mental disorders* [4th ed., text rev.] *[DSM-IV-TR]*. Washington, DC: Author.)

DSM-IV-TR CRITERIA FOR ALCOHOL-RELATED DISORDERS

ALCOHOL-RELATED DISORDERS

Alcohol Intoxication	**Alcohol Withdrawal**	**Substance-Induced Delirium**
1. Recent ingestion 2. Clinically significant, maladaptive behavior or psychological changes (sexual, aggressive, mood, and judgment) 3. At least one of the following: • Slurred speech • Incoordination • Unsteady gait • Nystagmus • Impairment in attention or memory • Stupor or coma 4. Symptoms not due to another medical/mental condition	1. Cessation (reduction) of alcohol use that has been heavy or prolonged 2. Two (or more) of the following: • Nausea or vomiting • Anxiety • Transient visual, tactile, or auditory hallucinations or illusions • Autonomic hyperactivity (e.g., sweating, increased pulse over 100 beats/min) • Psychomotor agitation • Insomnia • Grand mal seizures • Increased hand tremor	1. Impaired consciousness (reduced awareness of environment) 2. Changes in cognition (memory impairment, disorientation, language impairment, visual or tactile hallucinations, illusions) 3. Develops over short period of time — hours to days — and fluctuates over a day 4. Evidence of substance use (history, physical, laboratory findings) and symptoms developed during withdrawal

Figure 18-2 Diagnostic criteria for alcohol-related disorders. (Adapted from American Psychiatric Association. [2000a]. *Diagnostic and statistical manual of mental disorders* [4th ed., text rev.] [DSM-IV-TR]. Washington, DC: Author.)

Synergistic Effects

When some drugs are taken together, the effect of either or both of the drugs is intensified or prolonged. For example, combinations of alcohol plus a benzodiazepine, alcohol plus an opiate, and alcohol plus a barbiturate all produce **synergistic effects**. All these drugs are central nervous system (CNS) depressants. When people take two of these drugs together, it results in far greater CNS depression than the simple sum of the effects of each drug. Many unintentional deaths have resulted from lethal combinations of drugs.

Antagonistic Effects

Many people combine drugs to weaken or inhibit the effect of one of the drugs (i.e., for **antagonistic effect**). For example, cocaine is often mixed with heroin (speedball). The heroin (CNS depressant) is meant to soften the intense letdown of withdrawal from cocaine (CNS stimulant). **Naloxone (Narcan)**, an opiate antagonist, is often given to people who have overdosed on an opiate (usually heroin) to reverse respiratory and CNS depression. Because the duration of action of naloxone may be less than that of the narcotic that was taken, further monitoring and possible additional doses of naloxone may be needed.

Codependence

Codependence is a cluster of behaviors originally identified through research involving the families of alcoholic patients. Living with an individual who abuses alcohol or other substances is a source of stress and requires family system adjustments. People who are codependent often exhibit over-responsible behavior—doing for others what others could just as well do for themselves. They have a constellation of maladaptive thoughts, feelings, behaviors, and attitudes that effectively prevent them from living full and satisfying lives. Symptomatic of codependence is valuing oneself by what one does, what one looks like, and what one has, rather than by who one is (Box 18-1).

People who are codependent often define their self-worth in terms of caring for others to the exclusion of their own needs. The nursing profession is extremely attractive to people who are codependent since it involves caring for the most fundamental needs of others. A study conducted by Baldwin and colleagues (2006) surveyed 2646 Midwestern nursing and allied health professions students and found that 48% had a parent, sibling, or grandparent who was affected by addiction. These results suggest that nurses are at higher risk for relationship difficulties related to codependence and having grown up in environments which may have been dysfunctional due to one or more family members being addicted.

BOX 18-1 Codependent Behaviors

- Attempting to control someone else's drug use
- Spending an inordinate amount of time thinking about the person with the addiction
- Finding excuses for the person's substance abuse
- Covering up the person's drinking/drug taking or lying
- Feeling responsible for the person's drinking/drug use
- Feeling guilty for the person's behavior
- Avoiding family and social events because of concerns or shame about the behavior of the member with an addiction
- Making threats regarding the consequences of the behavior of the person with the substance-abuse problem and failing to follow through

- Eliciting promises for change
- Feeling like they are "walking on eggshells" on a routine basis to avoid causing problems, especially in relation to alcohol or drug use
- Allowing moods to be influenced by those of the person with the addiction
- Searching for, hiding, and destroying the person's drug or alcohol supply
- Assuming the duties and responsibilities of the person with the substance-abuse problem
- Feeling forced to increase control over the family's finances
- Often bailing the person with the addiction out of financial or legal problems

EPIDEMIOLOGY

Two thirds of the adult population in the United States consumes alcohol regularly (Hasin et al., 2007). At some point in their lives, about 18% of the population will abuse alcohol, and nearly 13% will become dependent on alcohol. Alcohol abuse is more common in men, young people, whites, and those who are unmarried. During any 12-month period, nearly 5% of adults will abuse alcohol, and nearly 4% will be alcohol dependent. Alcohol dependence is highest in men, young people, whites, Native Americans, people with low incomes, and those who are unmarried.

CONSIDERING CULTURE

A Culture of Alcohol and Substance Abuse

The college and university culture of alcohol and substance abuse has been blamed for the alarming increase in binge drinking at campuses across the United States. According to the National Center on Addiction and Substance Abuse (CASA) at Columbia University (2007), a variety of societal influences are the source for this epidemic. However, it emphasizes the responsibility of academic administrators for not providing evidence-based approaches to reduce and prevent this problem.

Some statistics about campus drinking include the following:

- About 50% of full-time students binge drink or use substances on a monthly basis.
- The percentage of students who abuse alcohol or are alcohol dependent may be as high as 25%—triple that of the general population.
- The average number of alcohol-related arrests jumped 21% during the first 5 years of the 21st century.

- More students drink to get drunk than they did a decade ago.

The report also suggests that administrators tend to take a "look-the-other-way" approach when it comes to students' alcohol consumption. Most administrators believe that the issue of drinking is a personal responsibility of the students, and it is not the role of the institution to police these young adults. The authors of the report disagree and recommend that colleges and universities take the "high" out of higher education.

Other issues that maintain this abusing culture relate to partying being viewed as a rite of passage, student resistance to intervention strategies despite knowing the risks, and parents' lack of involvement in addressing the issue. The stigma involved with admitting an alcohol abuse/dependence or substance abuse is also a barrier to changing this culture.

The National Center on Addiction and Substance Abuse at Columbia University. (2007). *Wasting the best and brightest: Substance abuse at America's colleges and universities.* <http://www.casacolumbia.org/absolutenm/articlefiles/380-Wasting%20the%20Best%20and%20the%20Brightest.pdf> Accessed 18.11.08.

Drug abuse is more common than drug dependence. The lifetime prevalence for drug abuse is nearly 8%, and the lifetime prevalence for drug dependence is about 3% (Compton et al., 2007). The 12-month prevalence of drug abuse is 1.4%, and the 12-month prevalence of drug dependence is 0.6%. Drug abuse and dependence are highest among men, people between the ages of 18 and 44, Native Americans, people with low incomes, those who are unmarried, and people who live in the western United States.

COMORBIDITY

Psychiatric Comorbidity

Approximately 6 out of every 10 people affected by a substance-abuse disorder are also affected by a mental health disorder (National Institute on Drug Abuse [NIDA], 2007). Individuals who abuse alcohol are more likely to abuse other substances and vice versa. Alcohol dependence is associated with abuse of other substances, mood and anxiety disorders, and paranoid, histrionic, and antisocial personality disorders (Hasin et al., 2007). Only 25% of people with alcohol dependence ever get treatment.

Antisocial personality disorders are also associated with drug use (Compton et al., 2007). Drug dependence is significantly associated with generalized anxiety disorders and mood disorders. Treatment for drug-use disorders is not common. About 8% of drug abusers and 38% of drug-dependent people will seek help for their problems.

Patients with comorbid mental illness and substance-abuse problems often experience more severe and chronic medical, social, and emotional problems. Because they have two or more disorders, they are vulnerable to both substance-abuse relapse and worsening of the psychiatric disorder. In addition, substance-abuse relapse often leads to psychiatric decompensation, and worsening of psychiatric problems often leads to substance-abuse relapse (Mancini et al., 2008).

Compared with patients who have a single disorder, patients with co-occurring disorders often require longer treatment, experience more crises, and progress more gradually in treatment. Common examples of co-occurring disorders include the combination of major depression with cocaine addiction, alcoholism with generalized anxiety disorder, alcoholism and polydrug addiction with schizophrenia, and borderline personality disorder with episodic polydrug abuse (Mancini et al., 2008).

Medical Comorbidity

Alcohol abuse is the most prevalent of the substance abuse disorders. Therefore, alcohol-related medical problems are the comorbidities most commonly seen in medical settings. Alcohol can affect all organ systems, in particular the CNS (resulting in disorders such as Wernicke's encephalopathy and Korsakoff's psychosis) and the gastrointestinal system (resulting in disorders such as esophagitis, gastritis, pancreatitis, alcoholic hepatitis, and cirrhosis of the liver). Also commonly associated with long-term alcohol use or abuse are tuberculosis, all types of accidents, suicide, and homicide. Alcohol use during pregnancy can have negative consequences for the fetus and result in fetal alcohol syndrome.

The route of drug administration influences medical complications. **Intravenous** drug users have a higher incidence of infections and sclerosing of veins. **Intranasal** users may have sinusitis and a perforated nasal septum. **Smoking** a substance increases the likelihood of respiratory problems. Table 18-1 lists physical complications associated with various classes of drugs and their routes of administration.

TABLE 18-1 Physical Complications Related to Drug Abuse

Drug	Route(s)	Physical Complications
Narcotics (e.g., heroin) Phencyclidine piperidine (PCP) Cocaine or crack	Intravenous*	Acquired immunodeficiency syndrome Hepatitis Bacterial endocarditis Renal failure Cardiac arrest Coma Seizures Respiratory arrest Dermatitis Pulmonary emboli Tetanus Abscesses—osteomyelitis Septicemia

TABLE 18-1 Physical Complications Related to Drug Abuse—cont'd

Drug	Route(s)	Physical Complications
Cocaine	Intravenous* Intranasal Smoking	Perforation of nasal septum (when taken intranasally) Respiratory paralysis Cardiovascular collapse Hyperpyrexia
Caffeine	Ingestion	Gastroesophageal reflux Peptic ulcer Increased intraocular pressure in unregulated glaucoma Tachycardia Increased plasma glucose and lipid levels
PCP	Ingestion	Respiratory arrest
Marijuana	Smoking Ingestion	Impaired lung structure Chromosomal mutation—increased incidence of birth defects Micronucleic white blood cells—increased risk of disease due to decreased resistance to infection Possible long-term effects on short-term memory
Nicotine	Smoking Chewing	Heavy chronic use associated with: Emphysema Cancer of the larynx and esophagus Lung cancer Peripheral vascular diseases Cancer of the mouth Cardiovascular disease Hypertension
Heroin	Intravenous* Smoking	Constipation Dermatitis Malnutrition Hypoglycemia Dental caries Amenorrhea
Inhalants	Sniffing Snorting Bagging (inhalation of fumes from a plastic bag) Huffing (placement of inhalant-soaked rag in the mouth)	Respiratory arrest Tachycardia Arrhythmias Nervous system damage

*Complications listed can result from any drug taken intravenously.

ETIOLOGY

Addiction is characterized by (1) loss of control of substance consumption, (2) substance use despite associated problems, and (3) tendency to relapse. The reason one person becomes addicted and another does not seems to relate to physical, developmental, psychosocial, and environmental factors, as well as genetic predisposition (Bailey et al., 2006). The difficulty in determining cause and effect is that the diagnosis of addiction generally occurs many years after the onset of use, and various factors are involved over the course of those years. Biological, psychological, and sociocultural theories are examined here briefly.

Biological Factors

In recent years, scientists have discovered that alcohol and drug use affects specific neurotransmitters and areas of the brain. The main systems that seem to be involved in substance abuse are the opioid, catecholamine (especially dopamine), and gamma-aminobutyric acid (GABA) systems (Sadock & Sadock, 2008). Opioid drugs act on opioid receptors. Alcohol and other CNS depressants act on GABA receptors and increase bioavailability of glutamate, norepinephrine, and dopamine. This helps explain the addictive and cross-tolerance effects that occur when alcohol is combined with barbiturates and benzodiazepines. Cocaine and amphetamines increase levels of norepinephrine, serotonin, and dopamine.

Berridge (2007) posits that dopamine is responsible for a phenomenon termed *incentive salience*, which is responsible for the craving of a substance many users experience when not currently using the substance. Addictive substances that directly activate dopamine transmission or induce neural sensitization cause persons who are addicted to become cue-sensitive. This means that when a person is presented with a stimulus previously associated with use of the addictive drug, the person will experience an overwhelming urge to use the drug. Incentive salience explains the high rate of first-year relapse for people who abuse substances.

Psychological Factors

Although an addictive personality type has not been proven to exist, associated psychodynamic factors have been identified, including the following:
- Lack of tolerance for frustration and pain
- Lack of success in life
- Lack of affectionate and meaningful relationships
- Low self-esteem, lack of self-regard
- Risk-taking propensity

Psychodynamic theories view substance use as a defense against anxious impulses, a form of oral regression (dependency), or self-medication for depression (Sadock & Sadock, 2008). Persons who abuse many substances are more likely to report an unstable childhood and self-medication than are persons who abuse only alcohol. Multiple studies link personality disorders and substance abuse. Behavioral theory focuses on the positive reinforcing effects of drug-seeking behavior.

Sociocultural Factors

Sociocultural theories attempt to explain differences in the incidence of substance use in various groups. Social and cultural norms influence when, what, and how a person uses substances. For example, in Asian cultures, the prevalence rate for alcohol abuse is relatively low. This is due in part to a deficiency in about 50% of the population of aldehyde dehydrogenase, the chemical that breaks down alcohol acetaldehyde. As the level of alcohol acetaldehyde increases in the blood, a severe flush and palpitations may occur and essentially keeps many people from drinking (APA, 2000a).

Another theory correlates substance use with the degree of socioeconomic stress. Being a drug addict can give a person a feeling of acceptance in his or her subculture. This is most true in economically deprived and unstable environments in which drugs may be taken to provide a person with a sense of belonging and identity.

Women in general are diagnosed with substance use at lower rates than men (APA, 2006a). One reason may be that women who use and abuse substances are viewed much more negatively than men in many cultural groups. This may lead to decreased substance use and abuse in women. It may also artificially deflate the statistics since women will hide these behaviors, which prevents them from receiving necessary treatment and services.

APPLICATION OF THE NURSING PROCESS

ASSESSMENT

Assessment of chemical impairment is becoming more complex because of the increase in **polydrug abuse, co-occurring psychiatric disorders**, and co-morbid physical illnesses, including human immunodeficiency virus (HIV) infection, acquired immunodeficiency syndrome (AIDS), dementia, and encephalopathy.

Sensitivity to cultural and racial issues is important in interpreting symptoms, making diagnoses, providing clinical care, and designing prevention strategies. Box 18-2 offers guidelines for areas to be covered in overall assessment of patients who use substances.

General Assessment

Current alcohol and other drug problems can be detected by asking two questions that are easily integrated into a clinical interview:

1. In the last year, have you ever drunk or used drugs more than you meant to?
2. Have you felt you wanted or needed to cut down on your drinking or drug use in the last year?

From that initial questioning, the nurse can then pinpoint specific drugs, depending on the particular clinical situation. The nurse should ask questions in a matter-of-fact, nonjudgmental fashion. Specific details include name(s) of drug(s) used, route, quantity, time of last use, and usual pattern of use.

Responses that serve as red flags indicating the need for further assessment are rationalizations ("You'd smoke dope too if…."); automatic responses, as if the question were predicted ("I figured you'd ask me that."); and slow, prolonged responses (as if the

---

BOX 18-2 General Assessment Guidelines for Patients Who Use Substances

History of Patient's Past Substance Use

- What are the date of first use, number of substances being taken, pattern of use, amount, frequency, periods of sobriety, time last taken?
- Was patient treated previously for substance abuse? What was the outcome?
- Is there a history of blackouts, delirium, or seizures?
- Is there a history of withdrawal symptoms, overdoses, and complications from past substance use?
- Is there a family history of drug or alcohol problems?

Medical History

- Does the patient have any coexisting physical conditions (e.g., human immunodeficiency virus infection)?
- What medications does the patient presently take?
- What is the patient's current medical status?
- What is the patient's present mental status?

Psychiatric History

- Is there a history of comorbid psychiatric problems (dual diagnosis)? Depression? Personality disorder? Conduct disorder? Schizophrenia?
- Has the patient undergone treatment for a specific disorder? What medications were given, and what was the outcome?

- Is there a history of abuse (physical, sexual)? Family violence?
- Is there a history of suicide? Violence toward others?
- Is the patient presently having suicidal thoughts?

Psychosocial Issues

- Does the patient have a poor work record related to substance use?
- How has the patient's substance use affected his or her relationships with others?
  - Family
  - Friends
  - Professional relationships
  - Community involvement
- How has the substance use affected the patient's ability to meet usual role expectations (e.g., parent, spouse, friend, employee)?
- Is there a police or criminal record, or have there been legal problems related to substance use (e.g., vehicle accidents, driving while intoxicated, physical violence)?
- Whom does the patient identify as his or her support system? Whom does the patient trust? Who cares for the patient? Who will help the patient if the patient asks for help?
- Does the patient use coping styles that contribute to the maintenance of his or her drug/alcohol lifestyle?

---

person were being careful about what to say). If the person is not able to provide a drug history, the nurse should assess for indications of substance abuse, such as dilated or constricted pupils, abnormal vital signs, needle marks, tremors, and alcohol on the breath and obtain history information from family and friends. The clothing should be checked for drug paraphernalia, such as used syringes, crack vials, white powder, razor blades, bent spoons, and pipes.

Intracranial hematomas, subdural hematomas, and other conditions can go unnoticed if symptoms of acute alcohol intoxication and withdrawal are not distinguished from the symptoms of a brain injury. Therefore, neurological signs (pupil size, equality, and reaction to light) should be assessed, especially in comatose patients suspected of having traumatic injuries. In addition, questions about alcohol abuse should be asked as part of the assessment of any trauma. A urine **toxicology screen** and **blood alcohol level (BAL)** can be useful for assessment purposes.

Assessment strategies must include collection of data pertaining to both substance dependence and psychiatric impairment. Unexplained exacerbations of psychiatric disorders may be due to substance abuse or dependence. Substance abuse can go undetected in patients with depression, anxiety, or suicidal ideation unless a thorough history is taken. Similarly, the understanding and treatment of people with substance dependencies are enhanced by inquiries about symptoms of depression and anxiety.

Once specific data are obtained, it is helpful to know if the person is abusing or is actively dependent on the substance. Review Figure 18-1 for guidance in making this distinction.

Psychological Changes

Certain psychological characteristics are associated with substance abuse, including denial, depression, anxiety, dependency, hopelessness, low self-esteem, and various psychiatric disorders. It is often difficult to determine which comes first, psychological changes or substance abuse. Some people self-medicate to cope with psychiatric symptoms. Some people develop psychiatric symptoms due to substance abuse.

People who abuse substances are threatened on many levels in their interactions with nurses. First, they are concerned about being rejected because not all nurses are willing to care for people with addictions. In fact, many patients have experienced instances of rejection in past encounters with nursing personnel. Second, people who abuse substances may be anxious about giving up the substance they think they need to survive. Third, people addicted to substances often are concerned about failing at recovering. Addiction is a chronic, relapsing condition. In fact, relapse is one of the criteria for diagnosing addiction. Most addicts have tried recovery at least once before and have experienced relapse. As a result, many become discouraged about their chances of ever succeeding. Discouragement and a high level of hopelessness can act as barriers to recovery.

These concerns can threaten the person's sense of security and sense of self, increasing anxiety levels. To protect against these feelings, the person with an addiction establishes a **predictable defensive style**.

The elements of this style include various defense mechanisms (e.g., denial, projection, rationalization), as well as characteristic thought processes (e.g., all-or-none thinking, selective attention) and behaviors (e.g., conflict minimization and avoidance, passivity, and manipulation). The person is unable to give up these maladaptive coping styles until more positive and functional skills are learned.

Signs of Intoxication and Withdrawal

Central Nervous System Depressants

CNS depressant drugs include alcohol, benzodiazepines, and barbiturates. Symptoms of intoxication, overdose, and withdrawal and possible treatments are presented in Table 18-2.

TABLE 18-2 Central Nervous System Depressants

Drug	Intoxication	Effects of Overdose	Possible Treatments for Overdose	Effects of Withdrawal	Possible Treatments for Withdrawal
Barbiturates Benzodiazepines Chloral hydrate Glutethimide Meprobamate Alcohol (ETOH)	*Physical:* Slurred speech Incoordination Unsteady gait Drowsiness Decreased blood pressure *Psychological-perceptual:* Disinhibition of sexual or aggressive drives Impaired judgment Impaired social or occupational function Impaired attention or memory Irritability	Cardiovascular or respiratory depression or arrest (mostly with barbiturates) Coma Shock Convulsions Death	*If awake:* Keep awake. Induce vomiting. Give activated charcoal to aid absorption of drug. Every 15 minutes, check vital signs (VS). *Coma:* Clear airway; insert endotracheal tube. Give intravenous (IV) fluids. Perform gastric lavage with activated charcoal. Check VS frequently for shock and cardiac arrest after patient is stable. Initiate seizure precautions. Possibly perform hemodialysis or peritoneal dialysis. Administer flumazenil (Romazicon) IV.	*Cessation of prolonged-heavy use:* Nausea and vomiting Tachycardia Diaphoresis Anxiety or irritability Tremors in hands, fingers, eyelids Marked insomnia Grand mal seizures *After 5–15 years of heavy use:* Delirium	Perform carefully titrated detoxification with similar drug. *Note:* Abrupt withdrawal can lead to death.

Data from American Psychiatric Association. (2000a). *Diagnostic and statistical manual of mental disorders* (4th ed., text rev.). Washington, DC: Author; and Bohn, M. J. (2000). Alcoholism. *Psychiatric Clinics of North America, 16*(4), 679.

Alcohol poisoning can result when an individual has consumed large amounts of alcohol quickly or over time. Alcohol poisoning can result in death from aspiration of emesis or a shutdown of body systems caused by severe CNS depression. Signs of alcohol poisoning include an inability to arouse the individual, cool or clammy skin, respirations less than 10 per minute, cyanosis under the fingernails or gums, and emesis while semiconscious or unconscious. Treatment for alcohol poisoning is outlined in Table 18-2.

Withdrawal reactions to alcohol and other CNS depressants are associated with severe morbidity and mortality, unlike withdrawal from other drugs (McKeon et al., 2007). The syndrome for alcohol withdrawal is the same as that for the entire class of CNS depressant drugs; therefore, alcohol is used here as the prototype. The time intervals are delayed when other CNS depressants are the main drugs of choice or are used in combination with alcohol. In addition, as patients age, their symptoms of withdrawal continue for longer periods and are more severe than in younger patients.

Multiple drug and alcohol dependencies can result in simultaneous withdrawal syndromes that present a bizarre clinical picture and may pose problems for safe withdrawal. Family and friends may help provide important information that can assist in care planning. The *DSM-IV-TR* identifies two alcohol withdrawal syndromes: *alcohol withdrawal* and the more severe *alcohol withdrawal delirium* (see Figure 18-2).

Alcohol Withdrawal. The early signs of withdrawal develop within a few hours after cessation or reduction of alcohol (ethanol) intake. They peak after 24 to 48 hours and then rapidly and dramatically disappear unless the withdrawal progresses to alcohol withdrawal delirium. The person may appear hyperalert, manifest jerky movements and irritability, startle easily, and experience subjective distress often described as "shaking inside." Grand mal seizures may appear 7 to 48 hours after cessation of alcohol intake, particularly in people with a history of seizures. Careful assessment followed by appropriate medical and nursing interventions can prevent the more serious withdrawal reaction of delirium.

A kind, warm, and supportive manner on the part of the nurse can allay anxiety and provide a sense of security. Consistent and frequent orientation to time and place may be necessary. Encouraging the family or close friends (one at a time) to stay with the patient in quiet surroundings can also help increase orientation and minimize confusion and anxiety.

Illusions are usually terrifying for the patient. Illusions are misinterpretations, usually of a threatening nature, of objects in the environment. For example, a person may think spots on the wallpaper are bloodsucking ants. However, illusions can be clarified, which

reduces the patient's terror: "See, they are not ants, they are just part of the wallpaper pattern." If a person experiencing withdrawal is argumentative, hostile, or demanding, it is often because of deep-seated anxiety and feelings of guilt and shame. The nurse can relieve some of these feelings and instill hope by demonstrating an accepting attitude and showing strong support for efforts at recovery.

Alcohol Withdrawal Delirium. Alcohol withdrawal delirium is considered a medical emergency and can result in death even if treated (Sadock & Sadock, 2008). Death is usually due to sepsis, myocardial infarction, fat embolism, peripheral vascular collapse, electrolyte imbalance, aspiration pneumonia, or suicide (McKeon et al., 2007). The state of delirium usually peaks 2 to 3 days (48 to 72 hours) after cessation or reduction of intake (although it can occur later) and lasts 2 to 3 days.

In addition to anxiety, insomnia, anorexia, and delirium, features of alcohol withdrawal delirium include:
- Autonomic hyperactivity (e.g., tachycardia, diaphoresis, elevated blood pressure)
- Severe disturbance in sensorium (e.g., disorientation, clouding of consciousness)
- Perceptual disturbances (e.g., visual or tactile hallucinations)
- Fluctuating levels of consciousness (e.g., ranging from hyperexcitability to lethargy)
- Delusions (paranoid), agitated behaviors, and fever (100° F to 103° F)

Immediate medical attention is warranted. The Pharmacological Interventions section later in this chapter has a full discussion of medical treatments.

Alcohol is the only drug for which objective measures of intoxication exist. The relationship between BAL and behavior in a nontolerant individual is shown in Table 18-3. Knowledge of the BAL assists the nurse in determining the levels of intoxication and tolerance and in ascertaining whether the person accurately reported recent drinking during the nursing history. These factors are also assessed by means of behavioral cues. As tolerance develops, a discrepancy is seen between BAL and expected behavior. A person with tolerance to alcohol may have a high BAL but minimal signs of impairment, as indicated in the following vignette.

VIGNETTE

Jordan comes to the emergency department with a BAL of 0.51 mg%. He is stuporous and ataxic and has slurred speech. The fact that he is still alive indicates a high tolerance for alcohol. A nursing history conducted as the patient sobers up reveals an extensive drinking history. When the BAL is this high, assessing for withdrawal symptoms is important. ∎

TABLE 18-3 Relationship Between Blood Alcohol Level and Effects in a Nontolerant Drinker		
Blood Alcohol Level	Blood Alcohol Accumulation	Effects
0.05 mg%	1-2 drinks	Changes in mood and behavior; impaired judgment
0.10 mg%	5-6 drinks	Clumsiness in voluntary motor activity; *legal level of intoxication in most states*
0.20 mg%	10-12 drinks	Depressed function of entire motor area of the brain, causing staggering and ataxia; emotional lability
0.30 mg%	15-18 drinks	Confusion, stupor
0.40 mg%	20-24 drinks	Coma
0.50 mg%	25-30 drinks	Death due to respiratory depression

The nursing history, physical examination, and laboratory tests are methods used to gather data about drug-related physical problems (McKeon et al., 2007). The extent of impairment depends on individual susceptibility, the amount of drug used, and the route of administration. Each class of drugs has its own physiological signs and symptoms of intoxication, which are summarized in the tables for each substance class.

Central Nervous System Stimulants

Table 18-4 outlines the physical and psychological effects of intoxication from amphetamines and other psychostimulants, possible life-threatening results of overdose, and emergency measures for both overdose and withdrawal. All stimulants accelerate the normal functioning of the body and affect the CNS. Common signs of stimulant abuse include dilation of the pupils, dryness of the oronasal cavity, and excessive motor activity.

When someone who has ingested a stimulant experiences chest pain, has an irregular pulse, or has a history of heart trouble, the person should be immediately taken to an emergency department.

Cocaine and Crack. Cocaine is a naturally occurring stimulant extracted from the leaf of the coca bush, and crack is a cheap, widely available, alkalinized form of cocaine. When crack is smoked, it takes effect in 4 to 6 seconds, producing a fleeting high (5 to 7 minutes) followed by a period of deep depression that reinforces

addictive behavior patterns and nearly guarantees continued use of the drug.

Cocaine is classified as a schedule II substance with high abuse potential; it has some recognized medical uses. Cocaine exerts two main effects on the body: anesthetic and stimulant. As an anesthetic, it blocks the conduction of electrical impulses within the nerve cells involved in sensory transmission, primarily pain transmission. It also acts as a stimulant for both sexual arousal and violent behavior.

Cocaine blocks the reuptake of norepinephrine, dopamine, and serotonin, and this imbalance of neurotransmitters (dopamine and norepinephrine) may be responsible for many of the physical withdrawal symptoms reported by heavy, chronic cocaine users: depression, paranoia, lethargy, anxiety, insomnia, nausea and vomiting, sweating and chills, and an intense craving for the drug. These are all signs of the body's struggle to regain its normal chemical balance.

Withdrawal has been classified as having three distinct phases. Phase one, the *crash phase*, can last up to 4 days. Users report depression, anergia, and an acute onset of agitated depression. Craving for the drug peaks during this phase, along with anxiety and paranoia. Inpatient care to prevent access to further doses of the drug is helpful during the first and second phase of withdrawal. The *second phase* is described as a prolonged sense of dysphoria, anhedonia, and a lack of motivation, along with intense cravings that can last up to 10 weeks. Relapse is most likely during the second phase of withdrawal. The *third phase* is characterized by intermittent craving and can last indefinitely (Koob & Le Moal, 2006).

Caffeine and Nicotine. Most people consume caffeine by way of coffee, tea, or soft drinks. People ingest coffee as a drug ("I've got to have two cups in the morning to function."), for social reasons ("Let's get together for coffee."), or as a reward ("After I finish this job, I'm going to take a coffee break.").

About one out of four Americans is an active smoker, with 20% of the population meeting the criteria for nicotine dependence (Centers for Disease Control and Prevention [CDC], 2007). A high proportion of psychiatric outpatients are nicotine dependent: up to 90% of patients with schizophrenia and about 70% of patients with bipolar I disorder or another substance-abuse disorder (Sadock & Sadock, 2008). Wellbutrin (Zyban) and nicotine-replacement therapy are successful treatments for many individuals during smoking cessation.

Opiates

The opiate drug class includes opium, morphine, heroin, codeine, fentanyl and its analogues, methadone, and meperidine. Table 18-5 lists signs and symptoms of intoxication, overdose, withdrawal, and possible treatments.

TABLE 18-4 Central Nervous System Stimulants

Drug	Intoxication	Effects of Overdose	Possible Treatments for Overdose	Effects of Withdrawal	Possible Treatments for Withdrawal
Cocaine, crack (short acting) Note: High obtained in: snorted, 3 minutes; injected, 30 seconds; smoked, 4-6 seconds (crack) Average high lasts 15-30 minutes for cocaine; 5-7 minutes for crack	Physical: Tachycardia Dilated pupils Elevated blood pressure Nausea and vomiting Insomnia Psychological-perceptual: Assaultiveness Grandiosity Impaired judgment Impaired social and occupational functioning Euphoria	Respiratory distress Ataxia Hyperpyrexia Convulsions Coma Stroke Myocardial infarction Death	Antipsychotics Medical and nursing management for: Hyperpyrexia (ambient cooling) Convulsions (diazepam) Respiratory distress Cardiovascular shock Acidification of urine (ammonium chloride for amphetamine)	Fatigue Depression Agitation Apathy Anxiety Sleepiness Disorientation Lethargy Craving	Antidepressants (desipramine) Dopamine agonist Bromocriptine
Amphetamines (long-acting) Dextroamphetamine Methamphetamine Ice (synthesized for street use)	Increased energy Severe effects: State resembling paranoid schizophrenia Paranoia with delusions Psychosis Visual, auditory, and tactile hallucinations Severe to panic levels of anxiety Potential for violence Note: Paranoia and ideas of reference may persist for months afterward.	Same as above	Same as above	Same as above	Same as above

Data from American Psychiatric Association. (2000). *Diagnostic and statistical manual of mental disorders* (4th ed., text rev.). Washington, DC: Author; O'Connor, P. G., Samet, J. H., & Stein, M. D. (1994). Management of hospitalized drug users: Role of the internist. *American Journal of Medicine, 96,* 551; and Bell, K. (1992). Identifying the substance abuser in clinical practice. *Orthopedic Nursing, 11*(2), 29.

Heroin is one of the most widely abused opiates. Heroin intoxication can be classified into four distinct phases. The *first phase* is a euphoria or rush that occurs almost immediately after injection of the drug. Users frequently characterize this euphoria in sexual terms. The euphoric phase is characterized physiologically by facial flushing and a deepening of the voice. The *second phase* is classified as "the high" and has been described as a sense of well being. This phase can extend for several hours. The *third phase*, which is often termed *the nod*, is an escape from reality that can range from lethargy to virtual unconsciousness. The *fourth phase* is the period before withdrawal occurs. During the fourth phase, users often seek more of the drug in order to avoid withdrawal.

TABLE 18-5 Opiates

Note: An opiate is a derivative or synthetic that affects the central nervous system and the autonomic nervous system. Medically used primarily as an analgesic (pain killer). Consistent use causes tolerance and distressing withdrawal symptoms.

Drug	Intoxication	Effects of Overdose	Possible Treatments for Overdose	Effects of Withdrawal	Possible Treatments for Withdrawal
Opium (paregoric) Heroin Meperidine (Demerol) Morphine Codeine Methadone (Dolophine) Hydromorphone (Dilaudid) Fentanyl (Sublimaze) Fentanyl analogues	*Physical:* Constricted pupils Decreased respiration Drowsiness Decreased blood pressure Slurred speech Psychomotor retardation *Psychological-perceptual:* Initial euphoria followed by dysphoria and impairment of attention, judgment, and memory	Possible dilation of pupils due to anoxia Respiratory depression or arrest Coma Shock Convulsions Death	Narcotic antagonist (e.g., naloxone [Narcan]) to quickly reverse central nervous system depression	Yawning Insomnia Irritability Runny nose (rhinorrhea) Panic Diaphoresis Cramps Nausea and vomiting Muscle aches ("bone pain") Chills Fever Lacrimation Diarrhea	Methadone tapering Clonidine-naltrexone detoxification Buprenorphine substitution

Data from American Psychiatric Association. (2000a). *Diagnostic and statistical manual of mental disorders* (4th ed., text rev.). Washington, DC: Author; O'Connor, P. G., Samet, J. H., & Stein, M. D. (1994). Management of hospitalized drug users: Role of the internist. *American Journal of Medicine, 96*, 551; and Bell, K. (1992). Identifying the substance abuser in clinical practice. *Orthopedic Nursing, 11*(2), 29.

Marijuana

Marijuana (*Cannabis sativa*) is an Indian hemp plant. **Tetrahydrocannabinol (THC)** is the active ingredient found in the resin secreted from the flowering tops and leaves of the cannabis plant. THC has mixed depressant and hallucinogenic properties. Marijuana, the leaves of the cannabis plant, is generally smoked, but it also can be ingested. It is the most widely used illicit drug in the United States. Desired effects include euphoria, detachment, and relaxation. Other effects include talkativeness, slowed perception of time, inappropriate hilarity, heightened sensitivity to external stimuli, and anxiety or paranoia. Long-term use of cannabis can result in lethargy, anhedonia, difficulty concentrating, and loss of memory for some people.

Overdose and withdrawal symptoms (other than cravings) rarely occur. Medical indications exist for the use of THC (e.g., control of chemotherapy-induced nausea, reduction of intraocular pressure in glaucoma, and appetite stimulation in AIDS wasting syndrome).

Hallucinogens

Table 18-6 gives the signs and symptoms of hallucinogen intoxication and overdose.

Lysergic Acid Diethylamide (LSD) and LSD-Like Drugs. **LSD** (also known as *acid*), **mescaline** (peyote), and **psilocybin** (mushrooms) are hallucinogens. Mescaline and the mushroom *Psilocybe mexicana* (from which psilocybin is isolated) have been used for centuries in religious rites by Native Americans living in the southwestern United States and northern Mexico. The hallucinogenic experience produced by LSD is called a "trip."

Phencyclidine Piperidine (PCP). **PCP** is also known as *angel dust*, *horse tranquilizer*, and *peace pill*. When taken orally, the onset of symptoms occurs about 1 hour after ingestion. When the drug is taken intravenously, intranasally, or smoked, the onset of symptoms may occur within 5 minutes. The signs and symptoms of PCP intoxication range from acute

TABLE 18-6 Hallucinogens

Note: A hallucinogen produces abnormal mental phenomena in the cognitive and perceptual spheres; for example, distortion in space and time, hallucinations, delusions (paranoid or grandiose), and synesthesia may occur.

Drug	Physical Effects of Intoxication	Psychological-Perceptual Effects of Intoxication	Effects of Overdose	Possible Treatments for Overdose
Lysergic acid diethylamide (LSD) Mescaline (peyote) Psilocybin	Pupil dilation Tachycardia Diaphoresis Palpitations Tremors Incoordination Elevated temperature, pulse, respiration	Fear of going crazy Paranoid ideas Marked anxiety, depression Synesthesia (e.g., colors are heard; sounds are seen) Depersonalization Hallucinations, although sensorium is clear Grandiosity (e.g., thinking one can fly)	Psychosis Brain damage Death	Keep patient in room with low stimuli—minimal light, sound, activity. Have one person stay with patient; reassure patient, "talk down" patient. Speak slowly and clearly in low voice. Give diazepam or chloral hydrate for extreme anxiety or tension.
Phencyclidine piperidine (PCP)	Vertical or horizontal nystagmus Increased blood pressure, pulse, and temperature Ataxia Muscle rigidity Seizures Blank stare Chronic jerking Agitated, repetitive movements Belligerence, assaultiveness, impulsiveness Impaired judgment, impaired social and occupational functioning	*Severe effects:* Hallucinations, paranoia Bizarre behavior (e.g., barking like a dog, grimacing, repetitive chanting speech) Regressive behavior Violent bizarre behaviors Very labile behaviors	Psychosis Possible hypertensive crisis or cardiovascular accident Respiratory arrest Hyperthermia Seizures	*If alert:* *Caution:* Gastric lavage can lead to laryngeal spasms or aspiration. Acidify urine (cranberry juice, ascorbic acid); in acute stage, ammonium chloride acidifies urine to help excrete drug from body—may continue for 10-14 days. Put in room with minimal stimuli. Do not attempt to talk down! Speak slowly, clearly, and in a low voice. Administer diazepam. Haloperidol may be used for severe behavioral disturbance (*not* a phenothiazine). Institute medical intervention for: Hyperthermia High blood pressure Respiratory distress Hypertension

Data from American Psychiatric Association. (2000a). *Diagnostic and statistical manual of mental disorders* (4th ed., text rev.). Washington, DC: Author; and Bell, K. (1992). Identifying the substance abuser in clinical practice. *Orthopedic Nursing, 11*(2), 29.

anxiety to acute psychosis. The drug produces a generalized anesthesia that lessens the sensations of touch and pain. Chronic use of PCP can result in long-term effects such as dulled thinking, lethargy, loss of impulse control, poor memory, and depression.

Suicidal risk is always assessed, especially in cases of toxicity or coma. If the patient awakens and appears to be suicidal, the nurse should determine whether previous suicide attempts have occurred. Information regarding suicide history of family members is also elicited. Additional history may be obtained through family and a review of medical records. Refer to Chapter 24 for more information on suicide assessment.

Inhalants

About 19% of adolescents in the United States say they have sniffed inhalants—usually volatile solvents such as spray paint, glue, cigarette lighter fluid, and propellant gases used in aerosols—at least once in their lives (SAMHSA, 2006). Types of inhalants, signs of intoxication, and side effects are given in Table 18-7. Inhalant use may be an early marker of substance abuse and should be the focus of increased preventive efforts and early diagnosis and treatment (Wu et al., 2006).

Club Drugs

Ecstasy (3,4-methylenedioxy-methamphetamine), also called *MDMA*, *Adam*, *yaba*, and *XTC*, is a prototype of a class of substituted amphetamines that also includes MDA (methylenedioxyamphetamine, or "love") and MDE (3,4-methylenedioxy-ethylamphetamine, or "Eve"). These recreational drugs produce subjective effects resembling those of stimulants and hallucinogens. MDMA causes a significant release of the neurochemicals serotonin, dopamine, and norepinephrine.

TABLE 18-7 Inhalants

Drug	Intoxication	Side Effects/Overdose	Treatment
Organic solvents (gases or liquids that vaporize at room temperature): Toluene Gasoline Lighter fluid Paint thinner Nail-polish remover Benzene Acetone Chloroform Model-airplane glue	Alcohol-like effects: euphoria, impaired judgment, slurred speech, flushing, CNS depression Visual hallucinations and disorientation	Chronic use is toxic to heart, liver, and kidneys. Toxicity may result in sudden death from anoxia, vagal stimulation, respiratory depression, and dysthythmias.	Support affected systems; no antidotes
Volatile nitrites: Room deodorizers Products sold for recreational use	Enhancement of sexual pleasure	Venodilation causes profound systolic blood pressure drop (dizziness, lightheadedness, palpitations, pulsate headache). Toxic dose may result in methemoglobinemia.	Toxicity may be treated with methylene blue and oxygen.
Anesthetics: Gas—especially nitrous oxide (used in dental procedures and as a propellant for whipped cream) Liquid Local	Giggling, laughter Euphoria	Numbness, weakness, sensory loss, loss of balance. May cause physical dependence. Possible polyneuropathy and myelopathy occurring in chronic users.	Neuropathy may be treated with B_{12}.

Data from Lehne, R. E. (2010). *Pharmacology for nursing care* (7th ed.). Philadelphia: Saunders; Ruiz, P., Strain, E. C., & Langrod, J. G. (2007). *The substance abuse handbook*. Philadelphia: Lippincott, Williams & Wilkins.

The brain's saturation of these neurotransmitters causes users to exhibit major empathy towards others, reduced inhibitions, and an outpouring of good feelings about others and the world around them. It also causes introspection about oneself. The release of serotonin also causes all of a user's senses to be extremely sensitive.

Users will be hyperactive and have inexhaustible energy (dancing all night long), dilated pupils with impaired reaction to light, elevated temperature, elevated pulse, elevated blood pressure, diaphoresis, dystonia, bruxism (grinding of the teeth), and other symptoms of stimulant use, such as tachycardia, mydriasis, tremors, arrhythmias, parkinsonism, esophoria (eyes turn inward), central serotonin syndrome, and severe hyponatremia. Users must drink a large quantity of water during MDMA use to prevent dehydration and hyperthermia.

After the effects of MDMA wear off, the user commonly goes through a period of depression. This depression is caused by a depletion of serotonin, levels of which do not return to normal within the CNS for at least 3 to 4 days. Many users describe the period after use with the term *blue Tuesdays*. Use of additional MDMA after serotonin stores have been depleted does not produce the same effects as the initial use, causing users to only experience the symptoms associated with the use of a stimulant amphetamine.

Date Rape Drugs

The drugs most frequently used to facilitate a sexual assault (rape) are flunitrazepam (Rohypnol or "roofies," a fast-acting benzodiazepine) and γ-hydroxybutyric acid (GHB) and its congeners (Crawford et al., 2008). They are odorless, tasteless, and colorless, mix easily with drinks, and can render a person unconscious in a matter of minutes. Perpetrators use these drugs because they rapidly produce disinhibition and relaxation of voluntary muscles; they also cause the victim to have lasting anterograde amnesia for events that occur. Alcohol potentiates their effects. Refer to Chapter 27 for additional discussion of the use of these drugs in sexual assault.

Self-Assessment

Although you may identify with (and have empathy for) patients addicted to caffeine or tobacco, your responses to patients who abuse other substances may not be so empathetic. A patient who has overdosed on heroin or cocaine or comes in with complications of ecstasy or other "techno drug" use may be met with disapproval, intolerance, and condemnation or may be considered morally weak. Also, the manipulative behaviors often seen in these patients may lead you to feel angry and exploited. You may want to help but

perceive the patient who abuses drugs to be willful, uncooperative, and impossible to work with.

In some areas of the United States, the recreational use of cocaine, marijuana, and amphetamine is so common the nurse may not have much emotional reaction. Becoming inured, or hardened, is as detrimental as strong emotional disapproval, because you may underestimate the importance of supportive measures, patient education, and the need for follow-up psychotherapeutic intervention.

To come to a true personal understanding means that you must examine your own attitudes, feelings, and beliefs about addicts and addiction. It often means you must examine your own substance use and that of others you know, and this is not always pleasant work. A history of substance abuse in a nurse's own family can overshadow that nurse's interactions with addicts. The negative or positive experiences a nurse has had with addicted family members can influence interpersonal interactions with present or future patients.

Therefore, it is vitally important to attend to personal feelings that arise when working with addicts. All health care professionals require supervision if they are not experienced in this area. Those who do not attend to—and work through—expected negative feelings that arise during treatment have power struggles with patients, and the therapeutic process is generally ineffective. These issues can become evident when it is a fellow nurse who has a substance-abuse problem.

Chemically Impaired Nurse

About 10% of nurses abuse alcohol and/or drugs, and 6% may have a problem that seriously interferes with their ability to provide safe nursing care (Dunn, 2005). Rehabilitating the chemically impaired nurse is difficult but not impossible. The choices for action are varied, and the only choice that is clearly wrong is to do nothing. Without intervention or treatment, the problems associated with chemical dependency escalate, and the potential for patient harm increases.

Often the impaired nurse volunteers to work additional shifts to be nearer to the source of the drug. The nurse may leave the unit frequently or spend a lot of time in the bathroom. When the impaired nurse is on duty, more patients may complain that their pain is unrelieved by their narcotic analgesic or that they are unable to sleep, despite receiving sedative medications. Increases in inaccurate drug counts and reports of vial breakage may occur.

If indicators of impaired practice are observed, the observations should be reported to the nurse manager. Intervention is the responsibility of the nurse manager and other nursing administrators. However, clear documentation by co-workers (specific dates, times, events, consequences) is crucial. The nurse manager's major concerns are with job performance and patient safety. Once the nurse manager has been informed, the legal and ethical responsibilities for in-house reporting have been met. If the impaired nurse remains in the situation, and no action is taken by the nurse manager, then the information must be taken to the next level in the chain of command. These measures can prevent harm to patients under the impaired nurse's care and can save a colleague's professional career or even life.

Reporting an impaired colleague is not easy, even though it is our responsibility. In efforts to not see what is going on, nurses may deny or rationalize, thus enabling the impaired nurse to potentially endanger lives while becoming sicker and more isolated. Box 18-3 can be used as a checklist to discern enabling behaviors with regard to a nurse colleague.

Referral to a treatment program should always be an option. Programs for chemically dependent nurses have been developed in some states in response to a policy statement issued by the American Nurses Association. Some state boards of nursing allow impaired nurses to avoid disciplinary action if they seek treatment. The aim of these programs is to protect patients and keep the nurse in active practice (perhaps with limitations) or return the nurse to practice after suspension and professional help. Nurses who continue to show signs of impaired practice should not be returned to direct patient care.

BOX 18-3   Have I Enabled?

Have I:

Excused or ignored behaviors that may be suggestive of impairment in a peer and justified those behaviors as the peer's "just having a bad day" or "stress"?

Never told the supervisor about behaviors I observed that were possibly indicative of impairment, because I was afraid of being wrong and did not want anyone to get angry at me?

Accepted responsibility for my colleague's unfinished work and at times attempted to counsel and solve his or her problem?

Believed that nurses do not use drugs or alcohol to the point of practice impairment and that substance use can be stopped at any time unless the person is morally weak?

Liked to use drugs or alcohol myself to relax or enjoy with friends? I do not want anyone to look at me. In fact, I have used a few discontinued drugs from work myself. Doesn't everyone?

Exonerated a peer's irresponsible actions by covering for attendance or tardiness? Have I cosigned controlled-substance "wastes" I have not truly witnessed; have I corrected the narcotic count to account for a discrepancy?

Defended a colleague when it was suggested there may be a problem with impairment?

Modified from Smith, L., Taylor, B. B., & Hughes, T. L. (1998). Effective peer response to impaired nursing practice. *Nursing Clinics of North America, 33* (1), 105–118.

Assessment Guidelines   Chemically Impaired Patients

1. Assess for a severe or major withdrawal syndrome.
2. Assess for an overdose to a drug or alcohol that warrants immediate medical attention.
3. Assess the patient for suicidal thoughts or other self-destructive behaviors.
4. Evaluate the patient for any physical complications related to drug abuse.
5. Explore the patient's interests in doing something about his or her drug or alcohol problem.
6. Assess the patient and family for knowledge of community resources for alcohol and drug treatment.

DIAGNOSIS

Formulation of appropriate nursing diagnoses depends on accurate assessment. Whereas the *DSM-IV-TR* criteria emphasize patterns of use and physical symptoms, nursing diagnoses identify how dependence on substances of abuse interferes with a person's ability to deal with the activities and demands of daily living.

Nursing diagnoses for patients with psychoactive substance use disorders are many and varied because of the large range of physical and psychological effects of drug abuse or dependence on the user and his or her family. Comorbid psychiatric problems also must be addressed. Potential nursing diagnoses for people with substance use disorders are listed in Table 18-8.

OUTCOMES IDENTIFICATION

Nursing Outcomes Classification (NOC) categories (Moorhead et al., 2008) for outcome criteria for patients with substance use disorders can be divided into withdrawal, initial and active drug treatment, and health maintenance. When the patient has a dual diagnosis, outcomes for the psychiatric disorder are also developed. *NOC* outcomes and examples of patient goals follow.

EVIDENCE-BASED PRACTICE

Web-Based Treatment for Alcohol Problems

Finfgeld-Connett, D., & Madsen, R. (2008). Web-based treatment of alcohol problems among rural women. *Journal of Psychosocial Nursing, 46*(9), 46–53.

Problem

Six million women in the United States have patterns of alcohol misuse. While all women with substance-abuse problems are underserved, women in rural communities have fewer options still. Local economies cannot support treatment programs, and facilities tend to be quite a distance from these women who may lack transportation.

Purpose of Study

The purpose of this study was to assess the effectiveness of a Web-based, personally-guided alcohol treatment program.

Methods

Participants were recruited through the newspaper and radio from Midwest counties that were considered 25% to 100% rural. Inclusion criteria were that participants had a connection to the Internet, that they were 18 and older, and that they drank at least three drinks a day or seven drinks a week for a year.

Forty-four women were randomly assigned to a Web-based treatment or a standard literature-based treatment. Web-based participants had access to an online bulletin board and also to a synchronous chat room where they could

interact with each other and the researcher. Standard care participants did not have interaction with one another but did have access to the researcher by telephone. Participants completed baseline assessments before the treatment and follow-up assessments 3 months after the treatment.

Key Findings

- Participants in both groups demonstrated an increase in self-efficacy.
- Mean levels of drinking were reduced in the Web-based group and the standard care group.

Implications for Nursing Practice

Both groups demonstrated improved drinking patterns after treatment. This indicates that Web-based therapy may be a viable alternative for people who are unable to make use of more traditional approaches. The privacy of Web-based treatment for a stigmatized condition such as alcohol abuse is attractive. Also, the expense factor is important—besides the use of computers and the researcher's time, there was little cost associated with the treatment. Larger-scale studies will be necessary to substantiate the findings in this study.

TABLE 18-8 Potential Nursing Diagnoses for Substance Abuse

Signs and Symptoms	Nursing Diagnoses
Vomiting, diarrhea, poor nutritional and fluid intake	*Imbalanced nutrition: less than body requirements* *Deficient fluid volume*
Audiovisual hallucinations, impaired judgment, memory deficits, cognitive impairments related to substance intoxication or withdrawal (deficits in problem solving, ability to attend to tasks and grasp ideas)	*Disturbed thought processes** *Disturbed sensory perception*
Changes in sleep/wake cycle, interference with stage 4 sleep, inability to sleep or long periods of sleeping related to effects of or withdrawal from substance	*Disturbed sleep pattern*
Lack of self-care (hygiene, grooming), failure to care for basic health needs	*Ineffective health maintenance* *Self-care deficit* *Noncompliance to health care regimen*
Feelings of hopelessness, inability to change, feelings of worthlessness, feeling that life has no meaning or future	*Hopelessness* *Spiritual distress* *Situational low self-esteem* *Chronic low self-esteem* *Risk for self-directed violence* *Risk for suicide*

TABLE 18-8 Potential Nursing Diagnoses for Substance Abuse—cont'd

Signs and Symptoms	Nursing Diagnoses
Family crises and family pain, ineffective parenting, emotional neglect of others, increased incidence of physical and sexual abuse of others, increased self-hate projected to others	*Interrupted family processes* *Impaired parenting* *Risk for other-directed violence*
Excessive substance abuse affecting all areas of a person's life: loss of friends, poor job performance, increased illness rates, proneness to accidents and overdoses	*Ineffective coping* *Impaired verbal communication* *Social isolation* *Risk for loneliness* *Anxiety* *Risk for suicide*
Increased health problems related to substance used and route of use, as well as overdose	*Activity intolerance* *Ineffective airway clearance* *Ineffective breathing pattern* *Impaired oral mucous membrane* *Risk for infection* *Decreased cardiac output* *Sexual dysfunction*
Total preoccupation with and majority of time consumed by taking and withdrawing from drug	*Delayed growth and development* *Ineffective coping* *Impaired social interaction* *Dysfunctional family processes*

Data from North American Nursing Diagnosis Association International. (2009). *NANDA-I nursing diagnoses: Definitions and classification 2009–2011*. Oxford, United Kingdom: Author.
*Diagnosis retired from North American Nursing Diagnosis Association. (2007). *NANDA-I nursing diagnoses: Definitions and classification 2007–2008*. Philadelphia: Author.

Withdrawal

Fluid Balance: Patient's blood pressure will not be compromised.
Neurological Status: Consciousness: Patient will have no seizure activity.
Distorted Thought Self-Control: Patient will consistently describe content of hallucinations.

Initial and Active Drug Treatment

Risk Control: Alcohol Use: Patient will consistently demonstrate a commitment to alcohol use control strategies.
Risk Control: Drug Use: Patient will consistently demonstrate acknowledgment of personal consequences associated with drug misuse.
Substance Addiction Consequences: Patient will demonstrate no difficulty supporting self financially.

Health Maintenance

Knowledge: Substance Abuse Control: Patient will describe actions to prevent and manage relapses in substance use.

Family Coping: Family will consistently demonstrate care for needs of all family members.

PLANNING

Planning care requires attention to the patient's social status, income, ethnic background, gender, age, substance use history, and current condition. It is safest to propose abstinence as a treatment goal for all addicts. Abstinence is strongly related to good work adjustment, positive health status, comfortable interpersonal relationships, and general social stability. Planning must also address the patient's major psychological, social, and medical problems, as well as the substance-using behavior. Involvement of appropriate family members is essential.

Unfortunately a person's social status and social relations often deteriorate as a result of addiction. Job demotion or loss of job, with resultant reduced or nonexistent income, may occur. Meeting basic needs for food, shelter, and clothing is thereby hampered. Marriage and other close relationships often deteriorate and fail, and the person is often left alone and isolated. The lack of interpersonal and social supports is a complicating factor in treatment planning for the addict. Case Study and Nursing Care Plan 18-1 on pages 427-430 presents a discussion of a dual-diagnosis patient who has alcohol dependence and depression.

IMPLEMENTATION

The aim of treatment is self-responsibility, not compliance. A major challenge is improving treatment effectiveness by matching subtypes of patients to specific types of treatment. Although addicts share some characteristics and dynamics, significant differences exist within the addict population with regard to physiological, psychological, and sociocultural processes. These differences influence the recovery process either positively or negatively.

Often the choice of inpatient or outpatient care depends on cost and the availability of insurance coverage. Outpatient programs work best for people with substance abuse disorders who are employed and have an involved social support system. People who have no support and structure in their day may do better in inpatient programs when these programs are available.

In addition, neuropsychological deficits have been associated with long-term alcohol abuse. Impairment has been found in abstract reasoning ability, ability to use feedback in learning new concepts, attention and concentration spans, cognitive flexibility, and subtle memory functions. These deficits undoubtedly have an impact on the process of alcoholism treatment.

At all levels of practice, the nurse can play an important role in the intervention process by recognizing the signs of substance abuse in both the patient and the family and by being familiar with the resources available to help with the problem.

Counseling and Communication Techniques

Communication strategies are designed to address behaviors that almost all people with substance abuse disorders have in common, including dysfunctional anger, manipulation, impulsiveness, and grandiosity. The nurse's ability to develop a warm, accepting relationship with a patient with an addiction can help the patient feel safe enough to start looking at problems with some degree of openness and honesty. The following is a portion of an intake

Dialogue	Therapeutic Tool/ Comment
Nurse: Elyse, I get the impression that life must have been getting very difficult for you lately.	Validating and empathizing
Elyse: *(Long pause)* I don't think you would understand.	
Nurse: I guess sometimes it feels as if no one understands, but I would like to try.	Reflecting and empathizing
Elyse: At times...I feel I can't go on any more...so many losses.	
Nurse: Loss is difficult. Elyse, tell me about your losses.	Encouraging the patient to share her painful feelings
Elyse: My brother's sudden death.... We were so close...I depended on him so much.	
Nurse: It must have been difficult for you to lose him so suddenly.	Empathizing
Elyse: *(Long pause)* No one knows.... Then Joseph, he left...*(Elyse starts to cry.)*	
Nurse: Tell me what you are feeling right now.	Encouraging the expression of feelings while feelings are close to the surface
Elyse: I don't know...angry maybe.... Why does everyone leave me? Oh, I hate them.... Oh, I wish I had a Valium now.	
Nurse: And what does the Valium do to help you?	Beginning to explore the drug dependence in a gentle, nonthreatening manner

interview with a patient upon admission to a treatment program.

The next example demonstrates the use of therapeutic leverage (i.e., making abstinence and sobriety worthwhile for the substance abuser). It is presented as a dialogue between a nurse and a 17-year-old young man whose parents are divorced and whose father abuses him when drinking. He was picked up three times during the preceding 7 months for possession of cocaine.

Dialogue	Therapeutic Tool/ Comment
Nurse: I understand you entered the treatment program yesterday afternoon following your court appearance.	Placing the event in time and sequence, validating the precipitating event
Kevin: Yeah—it was my dad's idea.	
Nurse: Well, what do you think of the idea?	Encouraging evaluation (actions first, thoughts, then feelings)
Kevin: I don't like it. I don't need this place. I'm not a junkie—I just use cocaine, that's all. I can handle it.	
Nurse: From what I've heard, your involvement with cocaine has gotten you into trouble.	Pointing out realities
Kevin: Yeah, well, I guess I can't deny that...but I still don't think I need this place.	
Nurse: Are you saying that you don't think you need a treatment program?	Validating the patient's perception
Kevin: Well, I don't know, I guess maybe I am a little messed up.	
Nurse: "Messed up."	Restating
Kevin: Yeah.	
Nurse: What is one thing about you that's messed up?	Encouraging the patient to be specific rather than global
Kevin: (Silence) I guess I feel like I don't belong anywhere.	
Nurse: Talk more about that.	Clarifying

It is also important to communicate in culturally appropriate ways.

A useful tool for helping the resistant addict develop a willingness to engage in treatment is known as **substance-abuse intervention**. The concept behind this approach is that addiction is a progressive illness and rarely goes into remission without outside help. Significant others arrange for a meeting with the addict to point out current problems and offer treatment alternatives. The steps or elements are outlined in Box 18-4 and can be applied to abuse of not only alcohol but also other substances.

Health Teaching and Health Promotion
Primary Prevention

Primary prevention through health teaching can have an important impact on how children and adolescents choose to solve problems and relate interpersonally. Young people who participate in groups such as scouting, 4-H clubs, school clubs, and organized church activities are at a lower risk for substance abuse. Activities help develop self-confidence and self-esteem. Older adults experiencing stressful life events are also at risk for substance abuse. This population may be reached through senior citizen centers and other community social or spiritual groups and organizations.

Brief Interventions

Use of brief interventions based on the FRAMES model to effect behavior change allow the nurse to take advantage of any interaction with a substance-abusing patient and use it as an opportunity for managing associated behaviors. Key interventions can be remembered by using the acronym *FRAMES*. The elements are the following (Becker & Walton-Moss, 2001):
Feedback of personal risk
Responsibility of the patient (personal control)
Advice to change
Menu of ways to reduce substance use (options)
Empathetic counseling
Self-efficacy or optimism of the patient

A case manager focuses on these elements when conducting a comprehensive needs assessment to (1) identify presenting problems; (2) develop an individualized plan, including patient goals and a plan to reach those goals; (3) link patients with various treatment providers; (4) monitor the treatment process and its progress; and (5) serve as the patient's advocate when needed.

Nursing Interventions Classification (NIC) categories applicable to patients with substance use disorders include *Substance Use Treatment, Family Support, Health Education, Coping Enhancement,* and *Self-Esteem Enhancement* (Bulechek et al., 2008).

Relapse Prevention

Relapses are common during a person's recovery. The goal of **relapse prevention** is to help the individual learn from these situations so that periods of sobriety can be lengthened over time, and lapses and relapses are not viewed as total failure. Relapse can result in a renewed and refined effort toward change.

VIGNETTE
Bill, a 20-year-old single man, is brought to the emergency department in a coma. He is accompanied by his mother, with whom he lives in a small apartment. Bill had been found unconscious in his room at home.

BOX 18-4 Steps in Substance-Abuse Intervention (for the Resistant Person with an Addiction)

1. All the people concerned about and affected by the person's substance abuse are gathered together to present their case. The intervention must be rehearsed before it is actually carried out, usually with the support and guidance of a counselor.
2. Specific evidence related to the substance abuse is presented by each person, and it is written down so that each person does not have to rely on memory in a tense situation.
3. Timing must be right:
   - There must be current evidence available.
   - The intervention must take place after a crisis is precipitated by substance use and *not* when the person is under the influence of the substance or in severe withdrawal.
4. The intervention requires privacy. It is held in a place where no interruptions can occur.

5. The use of defenses is anticipated. No reaction is made to them.
6. Genuine but firm concern is demonstrated.
7. Substance abuse is understood as a disease.
8. Treatment alternatives are presented.
9. Responses to possible outcomes are prepared. The goal is to get the affected person into treatment. If the substance-abusing person agrees to accept treatment, then he or she is taken immediately to a detoxification unit, where arrangements have been made previously. If the person refuses, then family members state that his or her decision must force them to make decisions of their own because they are no longer willing to live with the addicted person's behavior.

Adapted from Johnson, V. E. (1986). *Intervention: How to help someone who doesn't want help.* Reprinted with permission of Hazelden Foundation, Center City, MN.

When his mother was not able to rouse him, she dialed 911 for an ambulance. A syringe and some white powder were found next to Bill. On admission, his breathing is labored, and his pupils are constricted. Vital signs are taken; his blood pressure is 60/40 mmHg, and his pulse is 132 beats per minute. Bill's situation is determined to be life threatening. Bill's mother is extremely distressed, but she is able to report to the staff that Bill has a substance-abuse problem and had been taking heroin for 6 months before entering a methadone maintenance program. It is decided at this point to administer a narcotic antagonist, and naloxone is given intramuscularly. After this, Bill's breathing improves, and he responds to verbal stimuli. Bill's mother later tells staff that Bill has been in the methadone maintenance program for the past year but has not attended the program or received his methadone for the past week. At their urging, she calls the program, and arrangements are made to send an outreach worker, Mr. Rodriguez, to talk to her and Bill. Bill makes an appointment with Mr. Rodriguez for the following Monday. Mr. Rodriguez knows that Bill's future ultimately rests with Bill. On Monday, Mr. Rodriguez talks to Bill regarding how Bill perceives his situation, where Bill wants to go, and what Bill thinks he needs to get there.

After reviewing Bill's history, the health care team decides that a self-help, abstinence-oriented recovery program might be the most helpful treatment. Bill has not been taking drugs a long time, he has a job, and he appears motivated. Naltrexone (Trexan) will be given in conjunction with relapse prevention training, and Bill will regularly attend Narcotics Anonymous meetings. ▪

Dialogue	Therapeutic Tool/ Comment
Mr. Rodriguez: I was in the emergency department Friday afternoon when you were brought in by ambulance. **Bill:** Were you? I guess a lot of people thought it was over for me.	Placing the event in time and sequence, validating the precipitating event
Mr. Rodriguez: It certainly looked quite serious. **Bill:** Yeah. I should never have left the program. I was doing better, and I just didn't think I needed it anymore.	Emphasizing the reality—prevents minimizing the situation
Mr. Rodriguez: You said you were doing well. **Bill:** Yeah. I had a job, and I was beginning to save some money. Wow! I can't believe I blew this whole thing.	Reflecting
Mr. Rodriguez: I don't know that you really did. Your counselor for the program phoned your doctor this morning to find out how you were doing.	Pointing out reality

Dialogue	Therapeutic Tool/ Comment
Bill: Do you think they'll take me back?	
Mr. Rodriguez: Why don't we talk some more, and after we finish, I'll speak with the other staff about your situation. If you would like to get back into the program, you can call your counselor and we'll support your decision.	Gathering information

General strategies for relapse prevention are cognitive and behavioral: recognizing and learning how to avoid or cope with threats to recovery; changing lifestyle; learning how to participate fully in society without drugs; and securing help from other people, or social support. Box 18-5 and the Integrative Therapy box identify relapse prevention strategies.

INTEGRATIVE THERAPY

Alternative Treatment Approaches for Alcohol Abuse

Getting standard treatment through Alcoholics Anonymous for alcohol abuse is something that most people (75%) are not likely to do. Nonstandard treatment approaches could be more attractive. One study evaluated the likelihood of whether alternative approaches such as meditation and acupuncture might appeal to a certain segment of society, particularly based on sexual identity and those people who did not identify with mainstream society.

Not surprisingly, they found that the idea of alternative treatments were more acceptable to people who less strongly identified with mainstream thinking. However, sexual identity did not seem to have much to do with accepting alternative treatments. This study highlights the interest that a certain subgroup of society may have for nontraditional approaches for alcohol abuse treatment and the need for continued research into their viability.

Dillworth, T. M., Kaysen, D., Montoya, H. D., & Larimer, M. E. (2008). Identification with mainstream culture and preference for alternative alcohol treatment approaches in a community sample. *Behavior Therapy, 40*(1), 72–81.

Self-Help Groups for Patient and Family

Counseling and support should be encouraged for all family members of a person with a chemical dependency. Al-Anon and Alateen are self-help

---

groups that offer support and guidance for adults and teenagers, respectively. Self-help groups assist family members in dealing with many common issues. Their work is based on a combination of educational and operational principles centered around acceptance of the disease model of addiction, including pragmatic methods for avoiding enabling behaviors.

Twelve-Step Programs

One of the most effective treatment modalities for all addictions has been the 12-step program. Alcoholics Anonymous (AA) is the prototype for all the 12-step programs that were subsequently developed for many types of addiction. These programs offer the behavioral, cognitive, and dynamic structure needed in recovery. Three basic concepts are fundamental to all 12-step programs:

1. Individuals with addictive disorders are powerless over their addiction, and their lives are unmanageable.
2. Although individuals with addictive disorders are not responsible for their disease, they are responsible for their recovery.
3. Individuals can no longer blame people, places, and things for their addiction; they must face their problems and their feelings.

Using the 12 steps is often referred to as "working the steps" and helps a person refrain from addictive behaviors while fostering individual change and growth. In addition to AA, other 12-step programs include Pills Anonymous (PA), Narcotics Anonymous (NA), Cocaine Anonymous (CA), and Valium Anonymous.

A referral to the 12-step program that best fits the patient's addiction is recommended at discharge. Obtaining a sponsor prior to discharge can increase the likelihood of attendance at 12-step meetings. Sponsors are individuals who are recovering from addiction and can provide addicted persons with ideas and methods to help deal with cravings and coping deficits that may arise after prolonged substance use and abuse. Most programs offer assistance in facilitating sponsorship.

Residential Programs

Residential treatment programs are best suited for individuals who have a long history of antisocial behavior. The goal of treatment is to effect a change in lifestyle, including abstinence, development of social skills, and elimination of antisocial behavior. Follow-up studies suggest that patients who stay in such programs 90 days or longer exhibit a significant decrease in illicit drug use and recorded arrests and an increase in legitimate employment. Synanon, Phoenix House, and Odyssey House are three of the more familiar names among the 300-plus therapeutic communities in the United States.

Intensive Outpatient Programs

Most treatment for substance-abusing patients takes place in the community. Intensive outpatient treatment programs are becoming more popular because they are viewed as flexible, diverse, cost effective, and responsive to the specific needs of the individual.

Outpatient Drug-Free Programs and Employee Assistance Programs

These centers may offer vocational education and placement, counseling, and individual or group psychotherapy. Employee assistance programs have been developed to provide the delivery of mental health services in occupational settings. Many hospitals and corporations offer their employees counseling and support as an alternative to job termination when the employee's work performance is negatively affected by his or her impairment.

Pharmacological Interventions

The predominant somatic therapies are intended to support detoxification (management of withdrawal) or to alter drug use (e.g., disulfiram [Antabuse], methadone, and naltrexone) (Sadock & Sadock, 2008).

Alcohol Withdrawal Treatment

Not all people who stop drinking require management of withdrawal. This decision depends on the length of time and the amount the patient has been drinking, the prior history of withdrawal complications, and overall health status. Medication should not be given until the symptoms of withdrawal are seen. Drugs that are useful in treating patients with alcohol withdrawal delirium are listed in Table 18-9.

Treatment of Alcoholism

Naltrexone. **Naltrexone (Trexan, Revia)**—an agent used for narcotic addiction—is sometimes used in the treatment of alcoholism, especially for those with high levels of craving and somatic symptoms. Naltrexone works by blocking opiate receptors, thereby interfering with the mechanism of reinforcement and reducing or eliminating the alcohol craving (Srisurapanont & Jarusuraisin, 2005). Long-acting injectable forms with the brand names Vivitrex/Vivitrol, Naltrel, and Depotrex are being tested and show promise as having relatively level plasma levels; these drugs may have fewer side effects than naltrexone (Johnson, 2007).

Acamprosate. **Acamprosate (Campral)** is a second medication used to treat alcoholism. It was approved by the Food and Drug Administration in 2004. Acamprosate is used by people who have quit drinking and wish to remain abstinent; its helpfulness for people who have not undergone detoxification has not been demonstrated (Sadock & Sadock, 2008). Acamprosate probably works to reduce intake of alcohol by suppressing excitatory neurotranmission and enhancing inhibitory transmission (Lehne, 2010).

Topiramate. **Topiramate (Topamax)** works to decrease alcohol cravings by inhibiting the release of mesocorticolimbic dopamine, which has been associated with alcohol craving (Wellbery, 2008).

Disulfiram. **Disulfiram (Antabuse)** is used with motivated patients who have shown the ability to stay

TABLE 18-9 Drug Treatment of Patients with Alcohol Withdrawal Delirium

Drug Class	Specific Drugs	Purpose
Benzodiazepines	Chlordiazepoxide Diazepam (usually not recommended due to its short half-life and frequent dosing schedule) Lorazepam	Decrease withdrawal symptoms, stabilize vital signs, and prevent seizures and delirium tremens
Beta-adrenergic blockers	Atenolol Propranolol	Stabilize vital signs, decrease craving, reduce autonomic withdrawal symptoms
Alpha-adrenergic blockers	Clonidine	Reduce autonomic withdrawal symptoms
Antiepileptics	Carbamazepine	Decrease withdrawal symptoms, prevent seizures

Data from Lehne, R. E. (2010). *Pharmacology for nursing care* (7th ed.). Philadelphia: Saunders.

sober. Disulfiram works on the classical conditioning principle of inhibiting impulsive drinking because the patient tries to avoid the unpleasant physical effects caused by the alcohol-disulfiram reaction. These effects consist of facial flushing, sweating, throbbing headache, neck pain, tachycardia, respiratory distress, a potentially serious decrease in blood pressure, and nausea and vomiting. The adverse reaction usually begins within minutes to a half hour after drinking and may last 30 to 120 minutes. These symptoms are usually followed by drowsiness and are gone after the person naps (Lehne, 2010).

Disulfiram must be taken daily. The action of the drug can last from 5 days to 2 weeks after the last dose. It is most effectively used early in the recovery process while the individual is making the major life changes associated with long-term recovery from alcoholism. Disulfiram should always be prescribed with the full knowledge and consent of the patient. The patient needs to be told about the side effects and must be well aware that any substances that contain alcohol can trigger an adverse reaction. Three primary sources of hidden alcohol exist—food, medicines, and preparations that are applied to the skin. People also need to be careful to avoid inhaling fumes from substances that might contain alcohol, such as paints, wood stains, and stripping compounds. Voluntary compliance with the disulfiram regimen is often poor, but it may work best as a "psychological threat" and an adjunct to other pharmacological treatments (Suh et al., 2006).

Treatment of Opioid Addiction

Methadone. **Methadone (Dolophine)** is a synthetic opiate that blocks the craving for and effects of heroin. It has to be taken every day, is highly addicting, and when stopped produces withdrawal. For methadone to be effective, the patient must take a dose that will prevent withdrawal symptoms, block drug craving, and block any effects of illicit use of short-acting narcotics.

Methadone is the only medication currently approved for the treatment of the pregnant opioid addict. The clinical studies available demonstrate that methadone maintenance at the appropriate dosage, when combined with prenatal care and a comprehensive program of support, can significantly improve fetal and neonatal outcome.

Levo-alpha-acetylmethadol. As an alternative to methadone, **levo-alpha-acetylmethadol (LAAM)** is effective for up to 3 days (72 to 96 hours), so patients need to come to an outpatient facility for their medication only three times a week. This regimen makes it easier for patients to keep jobs and gives them more freedom than is available with methadone maintenance. LAAM is also an addictive narcotic: its therapeutic effects and side effects are the same as those of morphine. Its use has been found to be more effective in retaining patients in treatment than methadone (Douglas et al., 2007).

Naltrexone. **Naltrexone (Trexan, Revia)** is a relatively pure antagonist that blocks the euphoric effects of opioids. It has low toxicity and few side effects. A single dose provides an effective opiate blockade for up to 72 hours. Taking naltrexone three times a week is sufficient to maintain a fairly high level of opiate blockade. For many patients, long-term use results in gradual extinction of drug-seeking behaviors. Naltrexone does not produce dependence. As previously mentioned, it has also been approved for the treatment of alcoholism because it decreases the pleasant, reinforcing effects of alcohol.

Clonidine. **Clonidine (Catapres)** was initially marketed for high blood pressure, but it is also an effective somatic treatment for some chemically dependent individuals when combined with naltrexone. Clonidine is a nonopioid suppresser of opioid withdrawal symptoms. It is also nonaddicting.

Buprenorphine. **Buprenorphine (Subutex)** is a partial opioid agonist. At low doses (2 to 4 mg/day sublingually), the drug blocks signs and symptoms of opioid withdrawal. In experimental studies, buprenorphine has been shown to suppress heroin use in both inpatient and outpatient settings (Lanier et al., 2008).

Treatment of Nicotine Addiction

Transdermal administration of nicotine doubles long-term tobacco abstinence rates. The nicotine patch is preferred over nicotine gum because compliance with the treatment regimen is better, blood levels are steadier, little long-term dependence occurs, and instructions are less complicated. Antinicotine vaccines are being developed and tested and show promise in the treatment of nicotine addiction (Cerny & Cerny, 2008).

Advanced Practice Interventions

Psychotherapy

Nurses with advanced training may be involved in psychotherapy with substance-using patients. Psychotherapy assists patients in identifying and using alternative coping mechanisms to reduce reliance on substances. Eventually, psychotherapy can assist recovering addicts to become increasingly comfortable with sobriety.

Evidence-based practice and data indicate that cognitive-behavioral, motivational enhancement, behavioral, psychodynamic, interpersonal, family therapies are all effective for selected substance use disorders (APA, 2006b). See Chapters 34 and 35 for discussion of group and family therapy.

Confidentiality must be maintained throughout therapy *except* when this conflicts with requirements for mandatory reporting in certain circumstances (e.g., child abuse, danger to self or others).

Many critical issues arise during the first 6 months of sobriety:

- Physical changes take place as the body adapts to functioning without substances.
- Numerous signals occur in the patient's internal and external world that previously were cues to drinking and drug use. Different responses to these cues need to be learned.
- Emotional responses (feelings that were formerly diluted by substance use) are now experienced full strength. Because they are so unfamiliar, they can produce anxiety.
- Responses of family and co-workers to the patient's new behavior must be addressed. Sobriety disrupts a system, and everyone in that system needs to adjust to the change.
- New coping skills must be developed to prevent relapse and ensure prolonged sobriety.

Psychotherapy needs to be directive, open and honest, and caring. The therapeutic process involves teaching the patient to identify the physical and emotional changes that are occurring in the here and now. The nurse therapist can then assist in the problem-solving process.

EVALUATION

Favorable treatment outcome is judged by increased lengths of time in abstinence, decreased denial, acceptable occupational functioning, improved family relationships, and—ultimately—ability to relate normally and comfortably to other human beings.

The ability to use existing supports and skills learned in treatment is important for ongoing recovery. For example, recovery is actively viable if, in response to cues to use the substance, the patient calls his or her sponsor or other recovering persons; increases attendance at 12-step meetings, aftercare, or other group meetings; or writes feelings in a log and considers alternative action. Continuous monitoring and evaluation increase the chances for prolonged recovery.

Case Study and Nursing Care Plan **18-1** Alcohol Dependence with Depression

Mr. Stewart, aged 49 years, and his wife arrive in the emergency department one evening, fearful that he has had a stroke. His right hand is limp, and he is unable to hyperextend his right wrist. Sensation to the fingertips in his right hand is impaired.

Mr. Stewart looks much older than his stated age; in fact, he looks about 65. His complexion is ruddy and flushed. History taking is difficult. Mr. Stewart answers only what

is asked of him, volunteering no additional information. He states that he took a nap that afternoon, and when he awakened he noticed the problems with his right arm.

Ms. Winkler, the admitting nurse, begins the assessment. Mr. Stewart reveals that he has been unemployed for 4 years because the company he worked for went bankrupt. He has been unable to find a new job but has a job interview in 10 days. His wife is now working full time, so the family finances are okay. They have two grown children who no longer live at home. As he relates this, momentarily his lips start to tremble and his eyes fill with tears.

He denies any significant medical illness except for high blood pressure, just diagnosed last year. His father has a history of depression, and his mother is a recovering alcoholic. Ms. Winkler shares with him the fact that depression and alcoholism run in families. She asks Mr. Stewart (1) whether he knows this and (2) whether it concerns him with regard to his own drinking. He says that he knows and that he does not want to think about it.

Ms. Winkler speaks separately with Mr. Stewart's wife and asks if there is anything she would like to add. Mrs. Stewart's shoulders slump; she sighs and says, "I have spent the entire day talking to a counselor at the local treatment center to see if I can get him in. He won't admit that he has a problem." Mrs. Stewart recounts a 6-year history of steadily increasing alcohol use. She says that she could not admit to herself that her husband was an excessive drinker. "He tried to hide it, but gradually I knew. I could tell from little changes that he was intoxicated. I couldn't believe it was happening because he had been through the same thing with his mother. I thought I knew him. Actually, I guess I did when he was working. Being unemployed and

unable to find a job has really devastated him. And now he's going to job interviews intoxicated."

She describes her feelings, which are like an emotional roller coaster—elated and hopeful when he seems to be doing okay; dejected and desperate when he loses control. Mrs. Stewart hates going to work for fear of what her husband might do while she is gone. She says she is terrified that one day he will get into a car wreck and kill himself, because he often drives when intoxicated. He tells her not to worry, because the life insurance policy is paid up.

Meanwhile, the physician in the emergency department has examined Mr. Stewart. The diagnosis is radial nerve palsy. Mr. Stewart most likely passed out while lying on his arm. Because Mr. Stewart was intoxicated, he did not feel the signals that his nerves sent out to warn him to move (numbness, tingling). He was in this position for so long that the resultant cutoff of circulation was sufficient to cause some temporary nerve damage.

Mr. Stewart's BAL is 0.31 mg%. This is three times the legal limit for intoxication in many states (0.1 mg%). Even though he has a BAL of 0.31 mg%, Mr. Stewart is alert and oriented, not slurring his speech or giving any other outward signs of intoxication. The difference between Mr. Stewart's BAL and his behavior indicates the development of tolerance, a symptom of physical dependence.

ASSESSMENT

Self-Assessment

Ms. Winkler has come a long way in working with people who abuse alcohol. She grew up in a home in which alcohol transformed her father from a caring and responsible parent to one who was physically and verbally abusive to his wife and children. He eventually lost his job and left home. Ms. Winkler was determined to be everything he was not and firmly resolved never to drink or use drugs.

As a new nurse, Ms. Winkler became extremely frustrated and angry with patients like Mr. Stewart and found herself being overly protective of the family. At the end of a particular day in which she had to work with yet another intoxicated patient, she felt drained, depressed, and despondent. It became such a problem that she knew she needed to either leave her job or deal with the dynamics underlying her responses. She began to attend the support group, Al-Anon. There she was able to talk about her feelings with others who had similar backgrounds. Ms. Winkler was also provided with tools for dealing with her feelings and gained a greater understanding for the pathology behind alcohol abuse.

As Ms. Winkler approaches her work with the Stewart family, she does so with new confidence. She feels empathy and understanding for Mrs. Stewart, but she is able to maintain emotional boundaries and does not feel drained by their interactions. While she still feels a little frustration with Mr. Stewart, she recognizes these feelings and focuses on him as a person with a serious disorder.

Ms. Winkler organizes her data into objective and subjective components.

Objective Data

Driving when intoxicated

Covert references to death

Nerve damage from passing out while lying on arm

Increased alcohol use since becoming unemployed

Ability to find employment impaired by alcohol use

Disruption in marital relationship because of alcohol use

Inability to see effects of his drinking

Family history of alcoholism and depression

BAL three times the legal limit of intoxication; has developed tolerance

Subjective Data

Denies he has an alcohol problem

Denies he has depression

Continued

DIAGNOSIS

From the data, the nurse formulates the following nursing diagnoses:

1. *Risk for suicide* related to depressed mood

Supporting Data
- Dangerous behavior: driving when drinking
- Full payment of life insurance policy

2. *Ineffective coping* related to alcohol use

Supporting Data
- Increased alcohol use during stressful period of unemployment
- Impairment in capacity to obtain employment caused by alcohol use
- Disruption in marital relationship because of alcohol use
- Inability to see effect of his drinking on his life functioning

OUTCOMES IDENTIFICATION

Long-term outcomes:
The patient will refrain from attempting suicide.
The patient will report increase in psychological comfort.

PLANNING

The initial plan is to allow Mr. Stewart to sober up in the emergency department before discussing goals. After he is sober, the nurse establishes realistic outcomes with him.

IMPLEMENTATION

Mr. Stewart's plan of care is personalized as follows.
Nursing diagnosis: *Risk for suicide* related to depressed mood, as evidenced by dangerous behavior and full payment of life insurance policy
Outcome criteria: Patient will consistently demonstrate suicide self-restraint.

Short-Term Goal	Intervention	Rationale	Evaluation
1. Patient will seek treatment for depression.	1a. Determine presence and degree of suicidal risk.	1a. Risk of suicide is increased in substance-using patients.	**GOAL MET** After 3 weeks, patient attends appointment at local clinic and has started taking an antidepressant.
	1b. Refer patient to mental health care provider for evaluation and treatment.	1b. Addressing both substance use and mental health treatment needs improves outcomes.	

Nursing diagnosis: *Ineffective coping* related to alcohol use, as evidenced by increased alcohol use and impairment in life functioning
Outcome criteria: Patient will demonstrate mild to no change in health status and social functioning due to substance addiction.

Short-Term Goal	Intervention	Rationale	Evaluation
1. Patient will consistently acknowledge personal consequences associated with alcohol misuse.	1a. Identify with patient those factors (genetics, stress) that contribute to chemical dependence. 1b. Assist patient to identify negative effects of chemical dependency.	1a. Emphasis on alcoholism as a disease can lower guilt and increase self-esteem. 1b. Begins to decrease denial and increase problem-solving.	**GOAL MET** Patient admits that he cannot find a new job when he is intoxicated.

Short-Term Goal	Intervention	Rationale	Evaluation
2. Patient will commit to alcohol-use control strategies.	2a. Determine history of alcohol use. 2b. Identify support groups in community for long-term substance use treatment (for wife also).	2a. Identifies high-risk situations. 2b. Alcohol dependence requires long-term treatment; AA is effective.	**GOAL MET** After 3 weeks, patient states that he attends AA every day. He is learning about his triggers and new coping skills. His wife attends Al-Anon.

EVALUATION

See individual outcomes and evaluation in the care plan.

KEY POINTS TO REMEMBER

- Substance use and dependence occur on a continuum, and addiction develops over a period of time.
- The cause of substance use disorders is a combination of genetic, biological, and environmental factors.
- Assessment of patients with substance use disorders needs to be comprehensive, aimed at identifying common medical and psychiatric comorbidities.
- Patients with a dual diagnosis have more severe symptoms, experience more crises, and require longer treatment for successful outcomes.
- Substance use disorders affect the family system of the patient and may lead to codependent behavior in family members.
- Relapse is an expected complication of substance use disorders, and treatment includes a significant focus on teaching relapse prevention.
- Successful treatments include a dual-diagnosis approach, self-help groups, psychotherapy, therapeutic communities, and psychopharmacotherapy.
- Nurses need to be aware of their own feelings about substance use so they can provide empathy and hope to patients.
- Nurses themselves are at higher risk for substance use disorders and should be vigilant for signs of impairment in colleagues to assure patient safety and referral to treatment for the chemically dependent nurse.

CRITICAL THINKING

1. Write a paragraph describing reactions you might have to a drug-dependent patient to whom you are assigned.
   A. Would your response be different depending on the substance (for example, alcohol versus heroin or marijuana versus cocaine)? Give reasons for your answers.
   B. Would your response be different if the substance-dependent person were a professional colleague? How?

2. Casey is a 15-year-old girl who has started using heroin.
   A. When Casey asks you why she needs to take more and more to get "high," how would you explain to her the concept of tolerance?
   B. If she had recently used heroin, what would you find on assessment of physical and behavioral-psychological signs and symptoms?
   C. If she came into the emergency department with an overdose of heroin, what would be the emergency care? What might be effective long-term care?

3. Robert is a 45-year-old mechanic. He has a 20-year history of heavy drinking and he says he wants to quit drinking.
   A. Role-play with a classmate an initial assessment. Identify the kinds of information you would need to have in order to plan holistic care.
   B. Robert decided to stop drinking abruptly. He is now in the emergency department with delirium tremens. What are the dangers for him? What are the appropriate medical interventions?
   C. What are some possible treatment alternatives for Robert when he is safely detoxified? How would you explain to him the usefulness and function of AA? What are some additional treatment options that might be useful to Robert? What are available as referrals for him in your community?

CHAPTER REVIEW

1. The nurse is caring for a patient with an addictive disorder who is currently drug-free. The patient is experiencing repeated occurrences of vivid, frightening images and thoughts. Which term would the nurse use to document this finding?
   1. Tolerance
   2. Flashbacks
   3. Withdrawal
   4. Synergistic effect

2. Which condition would the nurse be most concerned about when caring for a patient who abuses alcohol?
   1. Cirrhosis of the liver
   2. Suicidal potential
   3. Wernicke's encephalopathy
   4. Korsakoff's psychosis

3. The nurse is caring for four patients. Which patient should be seen first, based upon substance-abuse risk potential?
   1. Female patient of Caucasian descent
   2. Female patient of Japanese descent
   3. Male patient of Native American descent
   4. Male patient of African American descent

4. Which patient response to the question, "Have you ever drunk more alcohol or used more drugs than you meant to?" should immediately cause the nurse to assess further?
   1. "No, I have never used drugs or alcohol."
   2. "I have drunk alcohol before but have never let myself get drunk."
   3. "I figured you'd ask me about that."
   4. "Yes, I did that once and will never do it again."

5. Which patient behaviors should the nurse suspect as related to alcohol withdrawal?
   1. Hyperalert state, jerky movements, easily startled
   2. Tachycardia, diaphoresis, elevated blood pressure
   3. Peripheral vascular collapse, electrolyte imbalance
   4. Paranoid delusions, fever, fluctuating levels of consciousness

---

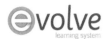

Visit the Evolve website for an **Audio Chapter Summary, Chapter Review Answers & Rationales, Critical Thinking Answer Guidelines**, and additional resources related to the content in this chapter: **http://evolve.elsevier.com/Varcarolis/foundations**

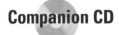

Companion CD   Use the Companion CD to prepare for tests and the NCLEX® Examination with **Test-Taking Strategies** for psychiatric mental health nursing and hundreds of **Review Questions**.

References

American Psychiatric Association. (2000a). *Diagnostic and statistical manual of mental disorders* (4th ed., text rev.) *(DSM-IV-TR)*. Washington, DC: Author.

American Psychiatric Association. (2006a). *Practice guidelines for the treatment of psychiatric disorders: Compendium 2006.* Washington, DC: Author.

American Psychiatric Association. (2006b). *Practice guidelines for the treatment of patients with substance abuse disorders* (2nd ed.). Retrieved March 26, 2009 from http://www.psychiatryonline.com/content.aspx?aID=141216

Bailey, J. A., Hill, K. G., Oesterle, S., & Hawkins, D. J. (2006). Linking substance use and problem behavior across three generations. *Journal of Abnormal Child Psychology, 34*(3), 273–292.

Baldwin, J. N., Scott, D. M., Agrawal, S., Bartek, J. K., Davis-Hall, R. L., Reardon, P. T., et al. (2006). Assessment of alcohol and other drug-use behaviors in health professions students. *Substance Abuse, 27*(3), 27–37.

Becker, K. L., & Walton-Moss, B. (2001). Detecting and addressing alcohol abuse in women. *Nurse Practitioner, 26*(10), 13–16, 19–23; quiz, 24–25.

Berridge, K. C. (2007). The debate over dopamine's role in reward: the case for incentive salience. *Psychopharmacology, 191,* 391–431.

Bulechek, G. M., Butcher, H. K., & Dochterman, J. M. (Eds.). (2008). *Nursing interventions classification (NIC)* (5th ed.). St. Louis: Mosby.

Centers for Disease Control and Prevention (CDC). (2007). State-specific prevalence of cigarette smoking among adults and quitting among persons aged 18-35 years: United States 2006. *Morbidity and Mortality Weekly Report,* Retrieved November 12, 2008, from http://www.cdc.gov/mmwr/preview/mmwrhtml/mm5638a2.htm

Cerny, E. H., & Cerny, T. (2008). Anti-nicotine abuse vaccines in the pipeline: an update. *Expert Opinion on Investigational Drugs, 17,* 691–696.

Compton, W. M., Thomas, Y. F., Stinson, F. S., & Grant, B. F. (2007). Prevalence, correlates, disability and comorbidity of *DSM-IV* drug abuse and dependence in the United States. *Archives of General Psychiatry, 64,* 566–576.

Crawford, E., O'Dougherty-Wright, M., & Bircheimer, Z. (2008). Drug-facilitated sexual assault: College women's risk perception and behavioral choices. *Journal of American College Health, 57,* 261–272.

Douglas, A. M., Conner, B. T., Annon, J., & Longshore, D. (2007). Levo-alpha-acetylmethadol (LAAM) versus methadone maintenance: 1-year treatment retention, outcomes, and status. *Addiction, 102,* 1432–1442.

Dunn, D. (2005). Substance abuse among nurses—defining the issue. *Association of Perioperative Registered Nurses Journal, 82,* 572–602.

Hasin, D. S., Stinson, F. S., Ogburn, E., Grant, B. F. (2007). Prevalence, correlates, disability, and comorbidity of *DSM-IV* alcohol abuse and dependence in the United States. *Archives of General Psychiatry, 64,* 830–842.

Johnson, B. A. (2007). Naltrexone long-acting formulation in the treatment of alcohol dependence. *Therapeutics and Clinical Risk Management, 3,* 741–749.

Koob, G. F., & Le Moal, M. (2006). *Neurobiology of addiction.* London: Elsevier.

Lanier, R. K., Umbricht, A., Harrison, J. A., Nuwayser, E. S., & Bigelow, G. E. (2008). Opioid detoxification via single 7-day application of a buprenorphine transdermal patch: an open-label evaluation. *Psychopharmacology, 198*(2), 149–159.

Lehne, R. A. (2010). *Pharmacology for nursing care* (7th ed.). Philadelphia: Saunders.

Mancini, M. A., Hardiman, E. R., & Eversman, M. H. (2008). A review of the compatibility of harm re-education and recovery-oriented best practices for dual disorders. *Best Practices in Mental Health, 4*(2), 99–113.

McKeon, A., Frye, M. A., & Delanty, N. (2007). The alcohol withdrawal syndrome. *Journal of Neurology, Neurosurgery, and Psychiatry, 79,* 854–862.

Moorhead, S., Johnson, M., Maas, M. L., & Swanson, E. (2008). *Nursing outcomes classification (NOC)* (4th ed.). St. Louis: Mosby.

National Institute on Drug Abuse. (2007). *Comorbid drug abuse and mental illness: A research update from the national institute on drug abuse.* Retrieved May, 30, 2008 from http://www.nida.nih.gov/pdf/tib/comorbid.pdf

North American Nursing Diagnosis Association International. (2009). *NANDA-I nursing diagnoses: definitions and classification 2009–2011.* Oxford, United Kingdom: Author.

Sadock, B. J., & Sadock, V. A. (2008). *Concise textbook of clinical psychiatry* (3rd ed.). Philadelphia: Lippincott Williams & Wilkins.

Substance Abuse and Mental Health Services Administration (SAMHSA). (2006). *Results from the 2006 national survey on drug use and health: National findings.* Retrieved November, 14, 2008, from http://www.oas.samhsa.gov/nsduh/2k6nsduh/2k6Results.pdf

Srisurapanont, M., & Jarusuraisin, N. (2005). Opioid antagonists for alcohol dependence. *Cochrane Database of Systematic Reviews 2005,* Issue 1. Art No.:CD001867. DOI: 10.1002/14651858.CD001867.pub2.

Suh, J. J., Pettinati, H. M., Kampman, K. M., & O'Brien, C. (2006). The status of disulfiram: A half of a century later. *Journal of Clinical Psychopharmacology, 26,* 290–302.

Wellbery, C. (2008). Topiramate is an effective treatment for alcohol dependence. *American Family Physician, 77,* 1160–1162.

Wu, L. T., Pilowsky, D. J., & Schlenger, W. E. (2006). High prevalence of substance use disorders among adolescents who use marijuana and inhalants. *Drug and Alcohol Dependence, 78*(1), 23–32.

CHAPTER 19

Personality Disorders

Claudia A. Cihlar and Nancy Christine Shoemaker

Key Terms and Concepts

antisocial personality disorder, 437
avoidant personality disorder, 440
borderline personality disorder, 437
dependent personality disorder, 440
diathesis-stress model, 444
dialectical behavior therapy (DBT), 455
histrionic personality disorder, 439
narcissistic personality disorder, 439

obsessive-compulsive personality disorder, 440
paranoid personality disorder, 436
personality, 434
personality disorder, 434
schizoid personality disorder, 436
schizotypal personality disorder, 436
splitting, 437

Objectives

1. Analyze the interaction of biological determinants and psychosocial stress factors in the etiology of personality disorders.
2. Identify the three clusters of personality disorders as currently defined.
3. Describe the major characteristic of one personality disorder from each cluster and give an example.
4. Formulate two nursing diagnoses for cluster B personality disorders.
5. Describe the emotional and clinical needs of nurses and other staff when working with patients who meet criteria for personality disorders.

6. Discuss two nursing outcomes for patients with borderline personality disorder.
7. Plan basic interventions for a patient with impulsive, aggressive, or manipulative behaviors.
8. Identify interventions the advanced practice nurse can employ when working with nursing staff caring for patients with personality disorders.

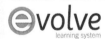

Visit the Evolve website for an **Audio Glossary & Flashcards, Concept Map Creator**, and additional resources related to the content in this chapter: **http://evolve.elsevier.com/Varcarolis/foundations**

How often do we come away from an encounter with someone and think to ourselves, "She's got a fantastic personality!" or "What an odd character he is!"? When we make evaluations such as these about other people, we are reacting to their personalities. What is a personality? Categorizing personalities has been attempted since at least the 5th century. Evidence from early Western and Eastern scholars reveal our interest in understanding the basis for personality and its various dimensions, including the characteristics of disordered personality.

The early Chinese culture characterized personality in the language of energy balance. Western scholars spoke of disordered personality as an imbalance of the "humors" of phlegm, blood, and bile. The scientist Galen proposed that these humors produced psychological profiles of personality identified as *phlegmatic* (calm and unemotional), *sanguine* (light-hearted and unemotional), *melancholic* (creative and depressive), and *choleric* (energetic and passionate) (Kagan, 2005).

In the 19th century, Sigmund Freud proposed a construct of personality that caused a paradigm shift from a biological imbalance to a psychological perspective for both healthy and disordered personality. Freud's hypothesis that personality emerged from childhood experiences rather than one's chemistry gave birth to the psychoanalytic movement.

Personality can be described operationally in terms of functioning. Personality, then, determines the quality of experiences among people and serves as a guide for one-to-one interaction and in social groups. Based on this description, we can tell when a personality is unhealthy, that is, "when it interferes with, or complicates, social and interpersonal function" (Blais et al., 2008, p. 527). The *Diagnostic and Statistical Manual of Mental Disorders*, fourth edition, text revision *(DSM-IV-TR)* formally defines a personality disorder as an enduring pattern of experience and behavior that deviates significantly from the expectations within the individual's culture (American Psychiatric Association [APA], 2000).

CLINICAL PICTURE

Previous chapters have focused on clinical disorders that are categorized on Axis I (e.g., major depression, schizophrenia, and bipolar disorder). (Refer to Chapter 1 for a detailed discussion of the *DSM-IV-TR* multiaxial system.) Personality disorders are categorized as Axis II diagnoses along with mental retardation. According to the APA (2000), the reason for this separation is not to imply that pathology and treatment of Axis II is fundamentally different but to (1) ensure that proper attention is given to these disorders and (2) they are not overlooked in the presence of Axis I disorders.

Personality disorders are among the most challenging and complex groups of disorders for mental health care workers. Individuals who meet criteria for personality disorders exhibit consistent difficulty in three areas of day-to-day functioning: thoughts and emotions, participation in interpersonal relationships, and managing impulses. These areas of difficulty create significant problems in living and disrupt the quality of life for the person and their family, friends, and others with whom the person interacts.

Some people who have a personality disorder do not view these areas of difficulty as problem behaviors attributable to themselves. They believe the problems originate from the behavior of other people. Still others may be unaware that they relate to others in an unusual way and are not distressed (Skodol & Gunderson, 2008). For example, a man with schizoid personality disorder who lives an isolated life is seemingly satisfied by his lifestyle. Compare this to a man with avoidant personality disorder who is quite unhappy about not having friends or close relationships with other people.

Judgments about an individual's personality functioning must take into account the person's ethnic, cultural, and social background. Patients who are of a different ethnicity or culture from their clinicians may be at risk for overdiagnosis of a personality disorder. It is important for clinicians to obtain additional information from others knowledgeable of the particular cultural or ethnic norms before determining the presence of a personality disorder (APA, 2000).

Ten basic personality disorders are presented in the *DSM-IV-TR* (APA, 2000). They are organized into three clusters, which are based on shared diagnostic criteria (Box 19-1). Personality disorder not otherwise specified, the fourth diagnosis, will not be discussed in this chapter. It is important to note that most patients who have a personality disorder often display traits of another personality disorder and can be diagnosed with more than one (Blais et al., 2008).

Cluster A Personality Disorders

Cluster A personality disorders include paranoid personality disorder, schizoid personality disorder, and schizotypal personality disorder. Persons diagnosed with these disorders share characteristics of eccentric and odd behaviors, such as social isolation and detachment. There may also be perception

---

BOX 19-1 *DSM-IV-TR* Criteria for Personality Disorders

A. An enduring pattern of inner experience and behavior that deviates markedly from the expectations of the individual's culture. This pattern is manifested in two (or more) of the following areas:
  1. Cognition (i.e., ways of perceiving and interpreting self, other people, and events)
  2. Affectivity (i.e., range, intensity, lability, and appropriateness of emotional response)
  3. Interpersonal functioning
  4. Impulse control
B. The enduring pattern is inflexible and pervasive across a broad range of personal and social situations.
C. The enduring pattern leads to clinically significant distress or impairment in social, occupational, or other important areas of functioning.
D. The pattern is stable and of long duration, and its onset can be traced back at least to adolescence or early adulthood.
E. The enduring pattern is not better accounted for as a manifestation or consequence of another mental disorder.
F. The enduring pattern is not due to the direct physiological effects of a substance (e.g., a drug of abuse, a medication) or a general medical condition (e.g., head trauma).

From American Psychiatric Association. (2000). *Diagnostic and statistical manual of mental disorders* (4th ed., text rev.). Washington, DC: Author.

distortions, unusual levels of suspiciousness, magical thinking, and cognitive impairment. The focus of biological research has been primarily on the deficits in cognition.

Persons who meet diagnostic criteria for cluster A personality disorders experience severe illness effects and are generally resistant to treatment (Figure 19-1). They firmly believe in their interpretation of events. These individuals may be seen in acute care settings and may require case management when their impairments interfere with day-to-day functioning.

DSM-IV-TR CRITERIA FOR CLUSTER A PERSONALITY DISORDERS

CLUSTER A (Odd or Eccentric)

Paranoid Personality Disorder	Schizoid Personality Disorder	Schizotypal Personality Disorder
A. A pervasive distrust and suspiciousness of others such that their motives are interpreted as malevolent, beginning by early adulthood and present in a variety of contexts, as indicated by four or more of the following: (1) Suspects, without sufficient basis, that others are exploiting, harming, or deceiving self (2) Is preoccupied with unjustified doubts about the loyalty or trustworthiness of friends or associates (3) Is reluctant to confide in others because of unwarranted fear that the information will be used maliciously against self (4) Reads hidden demeaning or threatening meanings into benign remarks or events (5) Persistently bears grudges (i.e., is unforgiving of insults, injuries, or slights) (6) Perceives attacks on his or her character or reputation that are not apparent to others and is quick to react angrily or to counterattack (7) Has recurrent suspicions, without justification, regarding fidelity of spouse or sexual partner	A. A pervasive pattern of detachment from social relationships and a restricted range of expression in interpersonal settings, beginning by early adulthood and present in a variety of contexts, as indicated by four or more of the following: (1) Neither desires nor enjoys close relationships, including being part of a family (2) Almost always chooses solitary activities (3) Has little, if any, interest in having sexual experiences with another person (4) Takes pleasure in few, if any, activities (5) Lacks close friends or confidants other than first-degree relatives (6) Appears indifferent to the praise or criticism of others (7) Shows emotional coldness, detachment, or flattened affect	A. A pervasive pattern of social and interpersonal deficits marked by acute discomfort with, and reduced capacity for, close relationships as well as by cognitive or perceptual distortions and eccentricities of behavior, beginning by early adulthood and present in a variety of contexts, as indicated by five or more of the following: (1) Ideas of reference (excluding delusions of reference) (2) Odd beliefs or magical thinking that influence behavior and are inconsistent with subcultural norms (e.g., superstitiousness, belief in clairvoyance, telepathy, or "sixth sense"; in children or adolescents, bizarre fantasies or preoccupations) (3) Unusual perceptual experiences, including bodily illusions (4) Odd thinking and speech (e.g., vague, circumstantial, metaphorical, overelaborate, or stereotyped) (5) Suspiciousness or paranoid ideation (6) Inappropriate or constricted affect (7) Behavior or appearance that is odd, eccentric, or peculiar (8) Lack of close friends or confidants other than first-degree relatives (9) Excessive social anxiety that does not diminish with familiarity and tends to be associated with paranoid fears rather than negative judgments about self

Figure 19-1 Diagnostic criteria for cluster A personality disorders. (Adapted from American Psychiatric Association. [2000]. *Diagnostic and statistical manual of mental disorders* [4th ed., text rev.]. Washington DC: Author.)

Paranoid Personality Disorder

Paranoid personality disorder is characterized by distrust and suspiciousness toward others based on the belief (unsupported by evidence) that others want to exploit, harm, or deceive the person. These individuals are hypervigilant, anticipate hostility, and may provoke hostile responses by initiating a "counterattack." They demonstrate jealousy, controlling behaviors, and unwillingness to forgive. Paranoid persons are difficult to interview because they are reluctant to share information about themselves. Underneath the guarded surface, they are actually quite anxious about being harmed.

VIGNETTE

Mrs. Alonzo is a 54-year-old unemployed female who comes to a mental health clinic complaining of depression and pain. She walks stiffly and uses two old, broken canes. She provides elaborate details about "nerve pain" all over her body resulting from an accident 5 years earlier. She states that multiple doctors refused to help her because of instructions from her insurance company. She believes that her health maintenance organization has circulated her medical record to all health care providers in the region to prevent her from being treated. She refuses to give any social history and is reluctant to share her telephone number. When the nurse indicates that the psychiatrist will not prescribe pain medications, she smiles bitterly and says, "So they already got to you." ■

Schizoid Personality Disorder

Schizoid personality disorder has the primary feature of emotional detachment. The person with this disorder does not seek out or enjoy close relationships. This individual may be able to function in a solitary occupation but shows indifference to praise or criticism from others. Depersonalization may occur as a result of the person's limited interactions with others. Schizoid personality disorder can be a precursor to schizophrenia or delusional disorder, and there is increased prevalence of the disorder in families with a history of schizophrenia or schizotypal personality disorder.

VIGNETTE

Mr. Gray is a 30-year-old single male who is a graduate student in mathematics at a large state university. He lives alone and has never been married. He works as an assistant in a math classroom in which the professor teaches the course via television. He wears thick eyeglasses, and his clothing is inconspicuous. He rarely smiles and seldom looks directly at the students, even when answering questions. He does get somewhat animated when he writes lengthy solutions to math problems on the blackboard. He is content with his low-paying job and has never been in psychiatric treatment. ■

Schizotypal Personality Disorder

Schizotypal personality disorder is expressed in strikingly odd characteristics, including magical thinking, derealization, perceptual distortions, and rigid, peculiar ideas. Responding inappropriately to cultural social cues is common for these individuals. Speech patterns may be distinctive and bizarre. These persons usually seek out help during episodes of depression or for anxiety they experience in social relationships.

It has been found that family members of persons diagnosed with schizophrenia are more likely to exhibit traits of schizotypal personality disorder, suggesting that there may be biological influences of the dopamine system as a primary neurotransmitter involved in its expression (Coccaro & Siever, 2005). Also, positive and negative symptoms observed in persons with schizophrenia are similar to the behaviors observed in persons with cluster A personality disorders. While it has been argued that persons with schizotypal personality disorders may represent a less severe form of schizophrenia, it has been difficult to draw any specific conclusions.

Neuroimaging studies using positive emission tomography (PET) scans show that persons with schizotypal personality disorders have structural abnormalities of the brain (Nahas et al., 2005). Ventricular enlargement and volume reduction in several regions of the brain have been documented in over twenty studies.

VIGNETTE

Raymond is a 55-year-old single male who lives with his mother. He is the youngest of seven children raised in a farming community. Three of his siblings are deaf, and Raymond also has some hearing loss. Raymond started therapy with Jenny, an advanced practice registered nurse in psychiatric mental health (APRN-PMH), after he suffered a career-ending injury from which he is completely disabled. Jenny and Raymond have been working together for several years on quality-of-life issues and depression. Raymond is frequently distressed by his unwavering belief that everyone in his hometown greets him with sexual gestures and believes he is gay. This belief extends to truck drivers who come through the town; he believes they talk about his sexuality on their CB radios. These beliefs create great distress and anxiety for him. He occasionally yells at people or gestures back. Jenny has been helping Raymond to understand how his perceptions may be faulty and how his hearing loss may contribute to his perceptual difficulties and anxiety. Raymond and Jenny have invited his mother into the discussion so she can support him at home. ■

Cluster B Personality Disorders

Cluster B personality disorders include antisocial personality disorder, borderline personality disorder, histrionic personality disorder, and narcissistic personality disorder. Persons diagnosed with cluster B personality disorders show patterns of responding to life demands with dramatic, emotional, or erratic behavior (Figure 19-2). Problems with impulse control, emotion processing and regulation, and interpersonal difficulties characterize this cluster of disorders.

Insight into these issues is generally limited. To get their needs met, these individuals may resort to behaviors that are desperate or entitled, including acting out, antisocial acts, or manipulating people and circumstances. Persons with cluster B personality disorders come into contact with health care providers both directly (usually for depression, substance abuse, acts of self-harm, or suicide) and indirectly (usually for acting out that leads to interaction with the legal system).

The focus of biological research for Cluster B disorders has primarily focused on altered processing of emotion, impulsivity, and social disruption in persons with borderline personality disorder and antisocial personality disorder. Reduced metabolism in the prefrontal cortex has been suggested for persons with borderline personality disorder, whereas persons with antisocial personality disorder have been found to have frontal-lobe dysfunction that may be related to problems with aggression (Nahas et al., 2005). Slow-wave activity has been detected by electroencephalogram (EEG) in studies of persons with borderline and antisocial personality disorders (Sadock & Sadock, 2008).

Antisocial Personality Disorder

Antisocial personality disorder has the main features of consistent disregard for others through exploitation and repeated unlawful actions. In the past, persons with antisocial personality disorder have been called *psychopaths* or *sociopaths*. There is a clear history of conduct disorder in childhood, and the individuals show no remorse for hurting others. They repeatedly neglect responsibilities, tell lies, and perform destructive or illegal acts without developing any insight into predictable consequences.

This disorder may be underdiagnosed in women and overdiagnosed in patients of lower socioeconomic status. These individuals do not voluntarily seek psychiatric care for symptoms of the personality disorder, but they are often seen for court-referred evaluation or treatment. See the Case Study and Care Plan for Antisocial Personality Disorder on the Evolve website.

VIGNETTE

Mr. Rouse is a 25-year-old divorced cab driver who is referred to the hospital by the court for competency evaluation after an assault charge. He told the arresting officer that he has bipolar disorder. He has a history of substance abuse and multiple arrests for disorderly conduct or assault. During his intake interview, he is polite and even flirtatious with the female RN. He insists that he is not responsible for his behavior, because he is manic. The only symptom he describes is irritability. He points out that he cannot tolerate any psychotropic medications because of the side effects. He also notes that he has dropped out of three clinics after several visits because "the staff don't understand me." ■

Borderline Personality Disorder

Borderline personality disorder is the most well-known and dramatic of the personality disorders and is characterized by severe impairments in functioning, a high mortality rate of nearly 10%, and extensive utilization of services from the health care system (Soeteman et al., 2008). The major features of this disorder are patterns of marked instability in emotion regulation, interpersonal relationships, impulsivity, identity or self-image distortions, and unstable mood.

Ineffective and harmful self-soothing habits, such as cutting, promiscuous sexual behavior, and numbing with substances are common and may result in unintentional death. Co-occurring mood, anxiety, or substance disorders complicate the treatment and prognosis of the condition.

Splitting, the primary defense or coping style used by persons with borderline personality disorder, is the inability to incorporate positive and negative aspects of oneself or others into a whole image. This kind of dichotomous thinking and coping behavior is believed to be partly a result of the person's failed experiences with adult personality integration and likely is influenced by exposure to earlier psychological, sexual, or physical trauma. For example, the individual may tend to idealize another person (friend, lover, health care professional) at the start of a new relationship, hoping that this person will meet all of his or her needs. But at the first disappointment or frustration, the individual quickly shifts to devaluation, despising the other person.

VIGNETTE

Shaina is a 38-year-old married woman with one young son. She works full time as a dietician at a large medical center. Shaina was diagnosed with fibromyalgia 2 years ago and is in treatment at a pain clinic. Most days, she comes home from work fatigued and goes to bed, leaving her son to play by himself after school or with friends until her husband gets home from work. Shaina also has struggled with an eating disorder since she was a teenager. When she feels guilty for ignoring her son's needs, she binges and then purges to relieve her negative emotions. Shaina recognizes that it helps only

DSM-IV-TR CRITERIA FOR CLUSTER B PERSONALITY DISORDERS

CLUSTER B (Dramatic, Emotional, or Erratic)

Antisocial Personality Disorder

A. A pervasive pattern of disregard for and violation of the rights of others occurring since age 15, as indicated by three or more of the following:

(1) Failure to conform to social norms with respect to lawful behaviors as indicated by repeatedly performing acts that are grounds for arrest
(2) Deceitfulness, as indicated by repeatedly lying, using aliases, or conning others for personal profit or pleasure
(3) Impulsivity or failure to plan ahead
(4) Irritability and aggressiveness, as indicated by repeated physical fights or assaults
(5) Reckless disregard for safety of self or others
(6) Consistent irresponsibility, as indicated by repeated failure to sustain consistent work behavior or honor financial obligations
(7) Lack of remorse, as indicated by being indifferent to, or rationalizing, having hurt, mistreated, or stolen from another

B. The individual is at least 18 years of age.

C. There is evidence of conduct disorder with onset before age 15 years.

Borderline Personality Disorder

A. A pervasive pattern of instability of interpersonal relationships, self-image, and affects, and marked impulsivity beginning in early adulthood and present in a variety of contexts, as indicated by five or more of the following:

(1) Frantic efforts to avoid real or imagined abandonment. *Note:* Do not include suicidal or self-mutilating behavior covered in criterion 5.
(2) A pattern of unstable and intense interpersonal relationships characterized by alternating between extremes of idealization and devaluation
(3) Identity disturbance: markedly and persistently unstable self-image or sense of self
(4) Impulsivity in at least two areas that are potentially self-damaging (e.g., spending, sex, substance abuse, reckless driving, binge eating). *Note:* Do not include suicidal or self-mutilating behavior covered in criterion 5.
(5) Recurrent suicidal behavior, gestures, or threats, or self-mutilating behavior
(6) Affective instability due to a marked reactivity of mood (e.g., intense episodic dysphoria, irritability, or anxiety, usually lasting a few hours and rarely more than a few days)
(7) Chronic feelings of emptiness
(8) Inappropriate intense anger or difficulty controlling anger (e.g., frequent displays of temper, constant anger, recurrent physical fights)
(9) Transient, stress-related paranoid ideation or severe dissociative symptoms

Narcissistic Personality Disorder

A. A pervasive pattern of grandiosity (in fantasy and behavior), need for admiration, and lack of empathy, beginning in early adulthood and present in a variety of contexts, as indicated by five or more of the following:

(1) Has a grandiose sense of self-importance (e.g., exaggerates achievements and talents, expects to be recognized as superior without commensurate achievements)
(2) Is preoccupied with fantasies of unlimited success, power, brilliance, beauty, or ideal love
(3) Believes that he or she is "special" and unique and can only be understood by, or should associate with, other special or high-status people (or institutions)
(4) Requires excessive admiration
(5) Has sense of entitlement (i.e., unreasonable expectations of especially favorable treatment or automatic compliance with personal expectations)
(6) Is interpersonally exploitative (i.e., takes advantage of others to achieve personal ends)
(7) Lacks empathy: is unwilling to recognize or identify with the feelings and needs of others
(8) Is often envious of others or believes that others are envious of self
(9) Shows arrogant, haughty behaviors or attitudes

Histrionic Personality Disorder

A. A pervasive pattern of excessive emotionality and attention seeking, beginning in early adulthood and present in a variety of contexts, as indicated by five or more of the following:

(1) Is uncomfortable in situations in which self is not the center of attention
(2) Interaction with others is often characterized by inappropriate sexually seductive or provocative behavior
(3) Displays rapidly shifting and shallow expression of emotions
(4) Consistently uses physical appearance to draw attention to self
(5) Has a style of speech that is excessively impressionistic and lacking in detail
(6) Shows self-dramatization, theatricality, and exaggerated expression of emotion
(7) Is suggestible (i.e., easily influenced by others or circumstances)
(8) Considers relationships to be more intimate than they actually are

Figure 19-2 Diagnostic criteria for cluster B personality disorders. (Adapted from American Psychiatric Association. [2000]. *Diagnostic and statistical manual of mental disorders* [4th ed., text rev.]. Washington DC: Author.)

temporarily and adds to her fatigue, but she still feels helpless to stop it. When her son asks her to play with him or take him to an activity, she becomes angry with him, and then feels angry at herself. Shaina has been referred by the palliative care nurse at the pain clinic to a dialectical behavior therapy group (discussed later in this chapter) to learn skills to deal with her chronic pain and discover alternative self-soothing strategies for her bingeing and purging behaviors. ■

Histrionic Personality Disorder

Histrionic personality disorder is marked by emotional attention-seeking behavior in which the person needs to be the center of attention. The person with histrionic personality disorder is impulsive and melodramatic and may act flirtatious or provocative. Relationships do not last, because the partner often feels smothered or reacts to the insensitivity of the histrionic person. The individual with histrionic personality disorder does not have insight into his or her role in breaking up relationships and may seek treatment for depression or another comorbid condition. In the treatment setting, the person demands "the best of everything" and can be very critical.

VIGNETTE

Ms. Lombard is a 35-year-old twice-divorced female admitted to an inpatient unit after an overdose of asthma medications and antibiotics. She took all of her pills after her primary care doctor refused to order a sleeping pill for her. On the first night, she is withdrawn and tearful in her room. But the next morning, she is neatly groomed, even wearing makeup, and socializes with everyone. She denies thoughts of self-harm. Over the next 2 days, she monopolizes the community meetings by talking about how unappreciated she is by her family and physician. She seeks special attention from an evening-shift male RN, asking if he can stay late after his shift to sit with her. When he refuses, she demands to be placed back on one-to-one precautions because she suddenly feels suicidal again. ■

Narcissistic Personality Disorder

Narcissistic personality disorder has the primary feature of arrogance with a grandiose view of self-importance. The individual with this disorder has a need for constant admiration, along with a lack of empathy for others, which strains most relationships. These individuals experience a feeling of personal entitlement; when paired with their lack of social empathy, it may result in the exploitation of other people, particularly vulnerable individuals (Cuzchta-Romano, 2004). Underneath the surface of arrogance, persons with narcissistic personality disorder feel intense shame and fear of abandonment. They are afraid of their own mistakes, as well as the mistakes of others. Narcissistic individuals may seek help for depression, feeling that loved ones do not show enough appreciation of their special qualities.

CONSIDERING CULTURE

Gender Bias in Diagnosing Personality Disorders

There may be a culture-bound gender bias in the diagnosing of personality disorders. Histrionic disorder is an example of such a bias. The word comes from the Latin word for "actor" and is defined by a pervasive attention-seeking behavior, including inappropriate sexual seductiveness and shallow or exaggerated emotions. Theoretically it should be diagnosed with equal prevalence in men as in women (Lynam & Widiger, 2007); yet it is diagnosed twice as often in women than in men and is among the most sex-linked personality disorders.

Consider a 28-year-old man who compulsively seeks attention, thinks about sex constantly, behaves seductively around women, is known as the life of the party, dominates conversation, and expresses his convictions in no uncertain terms. According to Vaknin (2007), such a man might likely be called "macho" and strong at the least and an overblown womanizer at worst. However, women who exhibit a sexual appetite and constantly draw attention to themselves are the objects of social disapproval, ridicule, and scorn.

It could be that the *DSM-IV-TR* weights the "feminine" characteristics—seductive appearance, overconcern with appearance, and dramatic speech—rather than the "male" characteristics—excitement seeking and low self-consciousness (Lynam & Widiger, 2007). Future diagnostic classifications may be made more gender neutral to correct bias; separate sets of criteria for men and women could even be developed.

Lynam, D. R., & Widiger, T. A. (2007). Using a general model of personality to understand sex differences in the personality disorders. *Journal of Personality Disorders, 21*, 583–602.
Vaknin, S. (2007). *Malignant self-love: Narcissism revisited* (8th Revised Printing). Republic of Macedonia: Narcissus Publications.

Dr. McLaughlin is a 40-year-old female attending psychiatrist at a university outpatient center. She is twice-divorced and has no children. Her grooming and makeup are impeccable, and she likes to chat about her expensive shopping habits. She is quite intelligent and is the only doctor on the staff trained in psychoanalysis. In clinical team meetings, she often discusses this fact, repeatedly telling others that psychoanalysis is the best treatment for mental illness. She frequently makes derogatory remarks to psychiatric residents if they suggest alternative treatment approaches for new cases. She is usually late to staff meetings, and when she is not speaking, she yawns and shifts noisily in her seat. She has a reputation for exhibiting angry outbursts at therapists in the hallway for minor mistakes, such as a scheduling error for a patient. She underwent 7 years of psychoanalysis but does not consider it to have been therapy—it "was only for training purposes." ∎

Cluster C Personality Disorders

Persons with cluster C personality disorders show patterns of anxious and fearful behaviors, rigid patterns of social shyness, hypersensitivity, need for orderliness, and relationship dependency. Biological research on cluster C disorders is more limited.

Persons with avoidant personality disorder tend to have relatives with social anxiety and panic disorders (Coccaro & Siever, 2005). Obsessive-compulsive traits are more common among monozygotic twins and occur more frequently in first-degree relatives who also have the disorder (Sadock & Sadock, 2008).

They often come into psychiatric care for treatment of anxiety related to fear of relationships or the loss of a relationship. Refer to Figure 19-3 for the diagnostic criteria for each disorder in this group.

Avoidant Personality Disorder

Avoidant personality disorder is fairly common and is believed to occur in about 2% of the U.S. population and about 15% of patients seen in treatment. The central characteristics are an extreme sensitivity to rejection and robust avoidance of interpersonal situations. A timid temperament in infancy and childhood may be associated with this disorder. These individuals demonstrate poor self-confidence and are prone to misinterpreting others' feedback because they are overly sensitive to rejection. Although they strongly desire close interpersonal relationships, they avoid them.

Ms. Lowell is a 35-year-old single female who works for a computer repair company. As a child, she had few friends and never participated in extracurricular activities. She lives alone in her own apartment and has never had an adult intimate relationship. On the job, she rarely talks to co-workers and prefers to work alone. If she has any questions, she asks the supervisor and carefully follows directions. Although she has 7 years of experience and a good work record, she refuses the offer of a promotion because it would require her to interact with customers. ∎

Dependent Personality Disorder

Persons with dependent personality disorder have a pattern of establishing relationships in which they are submissive, passive, self-doubting, and avoid self-responsibility. These individuals find it difficult to sustain autonomy and often seek out relationships in which they can be taken care of, whether the relationship is personal, professional, or therapeutic. In this context, they may look for ways to fuse themselves with the identity of the other individual, sometimes leading to an experience referred to as *folie à deux* ("madness between two"), which is a shared delusional belief by two persons (Sadock & Sadock, 2008).

Ashley is a 32-year-old married, former engineer and mother to two young children, ages 3 years and 11 months. Her therapist, an APRN-PMH, recommended that she come for brief treatment of depression and anxiety at the partial hospitalization program. Ashley's depression and anxiety have been more severe since she stopped working. She feels inadequate and overwhelmed by her responsibilities, so her mother moved in with the young family at her daughter's request. Ashley bonded quickly with her case manager and psychiatrist, both older women. She frequently asks them for reassurance that she is doing the "right thing" by coming to treatment. She seeks them out frequently for extra individual sessions. During her group therapies over the course of treatment, Ashley begins to realize that excessive dependence on her mother contributes to longstanding feelings of ineffectiveness, helplessness, and invalidation of her own parenting skills. ∎

Obsessive-Compulsive Personality Disorder

Obsessive-compulsive personality disorder has the key characteristic of perfectionism with a focus on orderliness and control. Individuals with this disorder become so preoccupied with details and rules that they may not be able to accomplish a given task.

DSM-IV-TR CRITERIA FOR CLUSTER C PERSONALITY DISORDERS

CLUSTER C (Anxious or Fearful)

Dependent Personality Disorder	Obsessive-Compulsive Personality Disorder	Avoidant Personality Disorder
A. A pervasive and excessive need to be taken care of that leads to submissive and clinging behavior and fear of separation, beginning by early adulthood and present in a variety of contexts, as indicated by five or more of the following:	A. A pervasive pattern of preoccupation with orderliness, perfectionism, and mental and interpersonal control, at the expense of flexibility, openness, and efficiency, beginning by early adulthood and present in a variety of contexts, as indicated by four or more of the following:	A. A pervasive pattern of social inhibition, feelings of inadequacy, and hypersensitivity to negative evaluation, beginning by early adulthood and present in a variety of contexts, as indicated by four or more of the following:
(1) Has difficulty making everyday decisions without an excessive amount of advice and reassurance from others (2) Needs others to assume responsibility for most major areas of life (3) Has difficulty expressing disagreement with others because of fear of loss of support or approval. *Note:* Does not include realistic fears of retribution (4) Has difficulty initiating projects or doing things on own (because of a lack of self-confidence in judgment or abilities rather than a lack of motivation or energy) (5) Goes to excessive lengths to obtain nurturance and support from others, to the point of volunteering to do things that are unpleasant (6) Feels uncomfortable or helpless when alone because of exaggerated fears of being unable to care for self (7) Urgently seeks another relationship as a source of care and support when a close relationship ends (8) Is unrealistically preoccupied with fears of being left to take care of self	(1) Is preoccupied with details, rules, lists, order, organization, or schedules to the extent that the major point of the activity is lost (2) Shows perfectionism that interferes with task completion (e.g., is unable to complete a project because overly strict personal standards are not met) (3) Is excessively devoted to work and productivity to the exclusion of leisure activities and friendships (not accounted for by obvious economic necessity) (4) Is overconscientious, scrupulous, and inflexible about matters of morality, ethics, or values (not accounted for by cultural or religious identification) (5) Is unable to discard worn-out or worthless objects even when they have no sentimental value (6) Is reluctant to delegate tasks or to work with others unless they submit exactly to own way of doing things (7) Adopts a miserly spending style toward both self and others; money is viewed as something to be hoarded for future catastrophes (8) Shows rigidity and stubbornness	(1) Avoids occupational activities that involve significant interpersonal contact, because of fears of criticism, disapproval, or rejection (2) Is unwilling to get involved with people unless certain of being liked (3) Shows restraint within intimate relationships because of fear of being shamed or ridiculed (4) Is preoccupied with being criticized or rejected in social situations (5) Is inhibited in new interpersonal situations because of feelings of inadequacy (6) Views self as socially inept, personally unappealing, or inferior to others (7) Is unusually reluctant to take personal risks or to engage in any new activities because they may prove embarrassing

Figure 19-3 Diagnostic criteria for cluster C personality disorders. (Adapted from American Psychiatric Association. [2000]. *Diagnostic and statistical manual of mental disorders* [4th ed., text rev.]. Washington DC: Author.)

Although a degree of obsessive-compulsive behavior can be productive in some occupations, it creates tension in close relationships, in which the person tries to control the partner.

Persons with obsessive-compulsive personality disorder feel genuine affection for friends and family but do not have insight about their own difficult behavior. Internally, they are fearful of imminent catastrophe. They rehearse over and over how they will respond in social situations. These individuals do not have full-blown obsessions or compulsions but may seek treatment for anxiety or mood disorders. The distinctions between this personality disorder and the Axis I obsessive-compulsive disorder (OCD) involve three symptoms that occur with less frequency or intensity in persons with obsessive-compulsive personality disorder: hoarding behaviors, perfectionism, and preoccupation with details (Eisen et al., 2006).

Mr. Wright is a 45-year-old single male postal worker in a small town. He lives alone and has never married. He is well groomed and wears a clean, neatly ironed uniform every day. He carefully follows all policies and procedures and is quite resistant whenever there is any update or change. He frequently challenges the supervisor about policy details and has been referred to the regional personnel office countless times for resolution of these conflicts. In staff meetings, he gives excessive circumstantial details and writes extra material on the back of any required report form. When dealing with the public, he sometimes gets into arguments with customers about postal rules or the schedule. The other staff do not consider him to be a team player, because he seldom volunteers to help others. Even if he is asked to help someone, he is quick to criticize his peer's performance. Although he has worked in the same office for 10 years, he has never advanced beyond the front-line position. He is fairly content with his work and has never been in psychiatric treatment. ▪

Personality Disorder Not Otherwise Specified

The category of *personality disorder not otherwise specified* (NOS) is for individuals who meet the general diagnostic criteria for a personality disorder but fail to meet the specific criteria for the other clusters. The NOS category is useful for clinicians diagnosing and treating enduring patterns of difficulty for persons seen across health care settings. This category is the most frequently selected description for patients with personality disorders (Widiger & Mullins-Sweatt, 2008). Two research categories currently being studied for future editions of the *DSM* are passive-aggressive and depressive personality disorders (Sadock & Sadock, 2008).

EPIDEMIOLOGY

While the prevalence of Axis I disorders have generally been established, the prevalence of personality disorders is less clear. Meta-analyses (pulling together the best and most relevant research) of studies suggest that the median prevalence rate for personality disorders combined for all clusters occurs at a rate of around 13% in community-based samples (Torgersen, 2005). Studies also suggest that between 20% and 40% of persons treated in psychiatric outpatient programs and around 50% of persons treated on psychiatric inpatient units meet the criteria for personality disorders (Davison, 2002).

Among the general U.S. population, about one in ten persons meet criteria for a personality disorder, which suggests that it is a common occurrence (Sadock & Sadock, 2008). Individuals with schizotypal (cluster A), borderline (cluster B), and avoidant (cluster C) personality disorders experience the most disruption in quality of life, dysfunction, and disability, because their symptoms create significant impairment in relationships, impulse control, and regulation of emotions (Torgersen, 2005). Persons with symptoms meeting criteria for histrionic (cluster B), obsessive-compulsive (cluster C), and passive-aggressive traits (NOS) tend to have less disruption in functioning and quality of life.

Table 19-1 summarizes the prevalence of each personality disorder within the major clusters according to total population, gender, and common Axis I comorbidities.

COMORBIDITY

Normal personality traits are amplified during the experience of any illness; therefore, it is premature and inappropriate to diagnose a personality disorder during the active phase of another illness, especially psychiatric disorders. Evidenced-based studies confirm that personality disorders frequently co-occur with disorders of mood, anxiety, eating, and substance abuse (Widiger & Samuel, 2005). Co-morbid personality disorders influence the expression of primary mental health symptoms. The *DSM-IV-TR* criteria emphasize that a personality disorder cannot be diagnosed until the primary mental health condition is resolved (APA, 2000).

ETIOLOGY

Personality disorders are the result of complex biological and psychosocial phenomena that are influenced by multifaceted variables involving genetics, neurobiology, chemistry, and environmental factors.

Biological Factors

Genetic

While genetics are thought to influence the development of personality disorders, individual genes are not believed to be associated with particular personality traits; thus, the relationship among genes and traits is a complex one (Skodol & Gunderson, 2008).

Several possible hypotheses attempt to account for the personality differences among persons in the

TABLE 19-1 Prevalence of Personality Disorders by Total Population, Gender, and Common Axis I Comorbidities

Personality Disorder	Total Population	Gender	Axis I Comorbidity
CLUSTER A PERSONALITY DISORDERS			
Paranoid	0.5%-2.5%	More men	Major depressive disorder Agoraphobia Obsessive-compulsive disorders Substance abuse disorders
Schizoid	0.4%-4.1%	More men	Major depressive disorder
Schizotypal	3%	More men	Major depressive disorder
Antisocial	Males, 3%; females, 1%	More men	Anxiety disorders Depressive disorders Substance use disorders Somatization disorders
Borderline	2%	More women	Mood disorders Substance use disorders Eating disorders Posttraumatic stress disorders Attention deficit hyperactivity disorder
Histrionic	2-3%	More women	Major depressive disorder Somatization disorder Conversion disorder
Narcissistic	1%	More women	Depressive disorders Substance use disorders Anorexia nervosa
CLUSTER C PERSONALITY DISORDERS			
Avoidant	0.5-1%	Equal in men and women	Mood disorders Anxiety disorders
Dependent	0.1-10%	More women	Mood disorders Anxiety disorders Adjustment disorders
Obsessive-compulsive	1%	More men	Anxiety disorders Mood disorders Eating disorders
PERSONALITY DISORDERS NOT OTHERWISE SPECIFIED			
Not otherwise specified	11.5%	Not adequately studied	Alcohol Abuse Major Depression

Data from American Psychiatric Association. (2000). *Diagnostic and statistical manual of mental disorders* (4th ed., text rev.). Washington, DC: Author; and Torgersen, S. (2005). Epidemiology. In J. M. Oldham, A. E. Skodol, & D. S. Bender (Eds.), *Textbook of personality disorders* (pp.129-142). Washington DC: American Psychiatric Publishing.

same family. One may be that a child's temperament can elicit different responses from family members. Individual children may perceive family experiences in unique ways and therefore respond differently from other family members. Children are also affected by forces outside the family that influence personality development. It may be that personality is even influenced by the intrauterine environment, although there is less data to support this hypothesis.

Neurobiological

Biological influences on personality expression are a promising area of research in understanding these disorders. Influences on the development of personality disorders likely incorporate a complex interaction of genetics, neurobiology, and neurochemistry. The chemical neurotransmitter theory proposes that certain neurotransmitters may regulate and influence temperament. Research in brain imaging has also revealed some differences in the size and function of specific structures of the brain in persons with some personality disorders (Coccaro & Siever, 2005).

Psychological Factors

Several psychological theories may help to explain the development of personality disorders. Learning theory emphasizes that the child developed maladaptive responses based on modeling of or reinforcement by important people in the child's life. Cognitive theories emphasize the role of beliefs and assumptions in creating emotional and behavioral responses that influence one's experiences within the family environment.

Psychoanalytic theory focuses on the use of primitive defense mechanisms by individuals with personality disorders. Defense mechanisms such as repression, suppression, regression, undoing, and splitting have been identified as dominant (Kernberg, 1985).

Environmental Factors

Behavioral genetics research has shown that about half of the variance accounting for personality traits emerges from the environment (Paris, 2005). These findings suggest that while the family environment is influential on development, there are other environmental factors besides family upbringing that shape an individual's personality. One need only think about the individual differences among siblings raised together to illustrate this point.

Diathesis-Stress Model

The diathesis-stress model is a general theory that explains psychopathology using a systems approach. This theory helps us understand how personality disorders emerge from the multifaceted factors of biology and environment (Paris, 2005). *Diathesis* refers to genetic and biological vulnerabilities and includes personality traits and temperament. *Temperament* is our tendency to respond to challenges in predictable ways. Descriptors of temperament may be "laid back," referring to a calm temperament, or "uptight" as an example of an anxious temperament. These characteristics remain stable throughout a person's life.

In this model, *stress* refers to immediate influences on personality such as the physical, social, psychological, and emotional environment. Stress also includes what happened in the past, such as growing up in one's family with exposure to unique experiences and patterns of interaction. Under conditions of stress, the diathesis-stress model proposes that personality development becomes maladaptive for some people, resulting in the emergence of a personality disorder (Paris, 2005).

There is a two-way directionality among stressors and diatheses. Genetic and biological traits are believed to influence the way an individual responds to the environment, while at the same time, the environment is thought to influence the expression of inherited traits. Many studies have suggested a strong correlation between trauma, neglect, and other dysfunctional family or social patterns of interaction on the development of personality disorders among individuals with certain personality traits and temperament.

The following is a summary of factors that are theorized to influence the development of each disorder (Skodol & Gunderson, 2008):

- **Paranoid personality disorder** may be found in people who grew up in households where they were the objects of excessive rage and humiliation, which resulted in feelings of inadequacy. Projection is the dominant defense mechanism; they blame others for their shortcomings. This personality disorder is thought to be related on a continuum with psychotic disorders such as schizophrenia.
- **Schizoid personality disorder** may be based on a genetic predisposition to shyness. People with this disorder are often raised in a cold and neglectful atmosphere in which they may conclude that relationships are unsatisfying and unnecessary.
- **Schizotypal personality disorder** is a schizophrenia spectrum disorder and genetically linked. There is a higher incidence of schizophrenia-related disorders in family members of people with schizotypal personality disorder.
- **Antisocial personality disorder** is genetically linked, and twin studies indicate a predisposition to this disorder. This predisposition is set into motion by a childhood environment of inconsistent parenting, significant abuse, and extreme neglect.
- **Borderline personality disorders** traditionally have been thought to develop as a result of early abandonment, which results in an unstable view of self and others. This abandonment is made more intense by a biological predisposition, and twin studies identify a heritability of 69%.

- **Histrionic personality disorder** has been explained psychodynamically as beginning at 3 to 5 years of age with an overly intense attachment to the opposite sex parent, which results in fear of retaliation by the same sex parent. Inborn character traits such as emotional expressiveness and egocentricity have also been identified as predisposing an individual to this disorder.
- **Narcissistic personality disorder** may be the result of childhood neglect and criticism. The child does not learn that other people can be the sources of comfort and support. As adults, they hide feelings of emptiness with an exterior of invulnerability and self-sufficiency. Little is known about inborn traits or heritability for this disorder.
- **Avoidant personality disorder** has been linked with parental and peer rejection and criticism. A biological predisposition to anxiety and physiological arousal in social situations has also been suggested. Genetically, this disorder may be part of a continuum of disorders related to social phobia (social anxiety disorder).
- **Dependent personality disorder** may be the result of chronic physical illness or punishment of independent behavior in childhood. The inherited trait of submissiveness may also be a factor, which has been found to be 45% heritable.
- Excessive parental criticism, control, and shame may be related to **obsessive-compulsive personality disorder**. The child responds to this negativity by trying to control his environment through perfectionism and orderliness. Heritable traits such as compulsivity, oppositionality, lack of emotional expressiveness, and perfectionism have all been implicated in this disorder.

APPLICATION OF THE NURSING PROCESS

ASSESSMENT

Assessment Tools

The preferred method for determining a diagnosis of personality disorder is the semi-structured interview obtained by clinicians. Open-ended or subjective interviews are more likely to result in biased and culturally-based decisions about diagnosis (Widiger & Mullins-Sweatt, 2008; Widiger & Samuel, 2005). A frequently used semi-structured interview tool is the Structured Clinical Interview for *DSM-IV-TR* Axis II Personality Disorders (SCID-II). Self-report inventories, such as the well-known Minnesota Multiphasic Personality Inventory (MMPI) are useful because they have built in validity and reliability scales for

the clinician to refer to when interpreting test results. However, these inventories may show higher false positive scores that result in over-diagnosing a person for a personality disorder (Widiger & Samuel, 2005).

Asking the patient questions may not always result in accurate responses, which may be due to lack of clarity about themselves, defensiveness, or simply not telling the truth. One way to elicit more objective information is to ask patients if family members and/or colleagues perceive them in a certain way. For example, "You said that you don't think you're emotionally distant. How would your wife describe you?"

Patient History

Taking a full medical history can help determine if the problem is a psychiatric one, a medical one, or both. Medical illness should never be ruled out as the cause for problem behavior until the data support this conclusion. Important issues in assessment for personality disorders include a history of suicidal or aggressive ideation or actions, current use of medicines and illegal substances, ability to handle money, and legal history.

Significant areas about which further details must be obtained include current or past physical, sexual, or emotional abuse and level of current risk of harm from self or others. At times, immediate interventions may be needed to ensure the safety of the patient or others. Information regarding prior use of any medication, including psychopharmacological agents, is important. This information gives evidence of other contacts the patient has made for help and indicates how the health care provider found the patient at that time.

Self-Assessment

Because enduring patterns of interpersonal difficulties are central to the problems faced by persons diagnosed with personality disorders, it is understandable that these problems surface in the treatment milieu and within the relationships between patients and caregivers. Anticipating that persons with personality disorders will likely have a disrupted, intense interpersonal experience with caregivers is helpful in monitoring personal stress responses when working with these individuals. Keep in mind that without the necessary skills to be effective in their lives, these dysfunctional behaviors may really represent the person's best effort to cope.

With borderline personality disorder, the therapeutic alliance often follows an initial upward curve of idealization (sometimes preceded by a brief

EVIDENCE-BASED PRACTICE

Self-Injurious Behaviors Among the General Population

Gollust, S. E., Eisenberg, D., & Golberstein, E. (2008). Prevalence and correlates of self-injury among university students. *Journal of American College of Health, 56,* 491–498.

Problem

Self-injury such as deliberately burning or cutting skin, irritating open wounds, and scratching results in social alienation, impaired relationships, shame, physical harm, and even disfigurement. While we have a good idea of how common this problem is among people who receive treatment for psychiatric disorders, there is little reliable information regarding the extent of these behaviors in the general population.

Purpose of Study

The purpose of this study was to determine the prevalence of self-injury without suicidal intent among university students.

Methods

With a $2 incentive, 5021 students were recruited from a Midwestern university to participate in the study. Participants completed an online survey that asked them about self-injury and asked them to identify other risk factors, including depression, eating disorders, anxiety, suicidal thinking, and other behaviors which may impair health.

Key Findings

- During the previous 4 weeks, 7% of the students engaged in self-injury.
- Self-injury was associated with depression, anxiety, and cigarette smoking.
- For men, self-injury was also associated with low socioeconomic status in childhood and eating disorders.
- About 75% of the students who engaged in self-injury received no mental health care or medication in the past year.

Implications for Nursing Practice

This study suggests that self-injury is a significant problem among young people and that they usually do not seek help for it. Nurses come into contact with young people in a variety of contexts and settings, especially those nurses who are employed in student health centers. During these times of contact, nurses have the opportunity to assess for self-injury, both by its physical manifestations and by its accompanying high level of anxiety and distress.

initial rejection) by the patient towards the caregiver, followed by a devaluation of the staff member when the patient is disappointed by their own unrealistic expectations not met by members of the treatment team. This process is often acted out in the treatment milieu and can interrupt the delivery of care. For example, a female patient may briefly idealize her male nurse on the inpatient unit, telling staff and patients alike that she is "the luckiest patient because she has the best nurse in the hospital." The rest of the team understands that this comment is an exaggeration. After days of constant dramatic praise for the nurse, with subtle insults to the rest of the staff, some members of the team may start to feel inadequate and resentful of the nurse. They begin to make critical remarks about minor events to prove that the nurse is not perfect. A similar scenario can occur if the patient constantly complains about one staff member; some staff are torn between defending and criticizing the targeted staff member.

Inexperience working with this heterogeneous population of patients, lack of appropriate education or supervision, and limited clinical support contribute to factors that maintain patient defense mechanisms. Clinical supervision and additional education is helpful and supportive to staff on the front lines of care (Bland et al., 2007). Awareness and monitoring of one's own stress responses to patient behaviors facilitates more effective and therapeutic intervention, regardless of the specific approach to their care.

Finding an approach that works with patients in the setting in which they are treated is important. Treatment approaches whose steps are listed one-by-one in a manual (manualized treatment), such as dialectical behavior therapy and mindfulness-based therapies, offer staff evidence-based interventions, clinical structure, and formalized support for identifying best practices (Gunderson & Hoffman, 2005).

Assessment Guidelines Personality Disorders

1. Assess for suicidal or homicidal thoughts. If these are present, the patient will need immediate attention.
2. Determine whether the patient has a medical disorder or another psychiatric disorder that may be responsible for the symptoms (especially a substance use disorder).
3. View the assessment about personality functioning from within the person's ethnic, cultural, and social background.
4. Ascertain whether the patient experienced a recent important loss. Personality disorders are often exacerbated after the loss of significant supporting people or in a disruptive social situation.
5. Evaluate for a change in personality in middle adulthood or later, which signals the need for a thorough medical workup or assessment for unrecognized substance use disorder.

DIAGNOSIS

People with personality disorders are usually admitted to psychiatric institutions because of symptoms of comorbid disorders, dangerous behavior, or court-ordered treatment. Borderline personality disorder and antisocial personality disorder both present a challenge for health care providers because the behaviors central to these disorders often cause disruption in psychiatric and medical-surgical settings. Emotions such as anxiety, rage, and depression and behaviors such as withdrawal, paranoia, and manipulation are among the most frequent that health care workers must address. Table 19-2 lists common potential nursing diagnoses related to personality disorders.

OUTCOMES IDENTIFICATION

Realistic outcomes are established for individuals with personality disorders based on the perspective that personality change occurs with one behavioral solution and one learned skill at a time. This can be expected to take much time and repetition. In the acute care setting, the focus is on the presenting problem, which may be depression or severe anxiety. During the hospital stay, the chronic behavior problems of patients with personality disorders are not expected to be resolved but rather to be met with appropriate therapeutic feedback.

Pertinent categories of nursing outcomes based on the *Nursing Outcomes Classification (NOC)* include *Aggression Self-Control, Impulse Self-Control, Social Interaction Skills, Fear Level, Abusive Behavior Self-Restraint,* and *Self-Mutilation Restraint* (Moorhead et al., 2008). Table 19-3 gives examples of other potential nursing outcomes for manipulative, aggressive, and impulsive behaviors.

TABLE 19-2 Potential Nursing Diagnoses for Personality Disorders

Signs and Symptoms	Nursing Diagnoses
Crisis, high levels of anxiety	Ineffective coping Anxiety Self-mutilation
Anger and aggression; child, elder, or spouse abuse	Risk for other-directed violence Ineffective coping Impaired parenting Disabled family coping
Withdrawal	Social isolation
Paranoia	Fear Disturbed sensory perception Disturbed thought processes* Defensive coping
Depression	Hopelessness Risk for suicide Self-mutilation Chronic low self-esteem Spiritual distress
Difficulty in relationships, manipulation	Ineffective coping Impaired social interaction Defensive coping Interrupted family processes Risk for loneliness
Failure to keep medical appointments, late arrival for appointments, failure to follow prescribed medical procedure or medication regimen	Ineffective therapeutic regimen management Nonadherence

Data from North American Nursing Diagnosis Association. (2009). *NANDA-I nursing diagnoses: Definitions and classification 2009-2011.* Oxford, United Kingdom: Author.
*Diagnosis retired from North American Nursing Diagnosis Association. (2007). *NANDA-I nursing diagnoses: Definitions and classification 2007-2008.* Philadelphia: Author.

PLANNING

It is often difficult to create a therapeutic relationship with patients who have antisocial or borderline personality disorders, because most of them have experienced failed relationships, including therapeutic alliances. Their distrust and hostility can be a setup for failure. When patients blame and attack others, the nurse needs to understand the context of their complaints; that is, these attacks spring from the feeling of being threatened. The more intense their complaints are, the greater

TABLE 19-3 *NOC* Outcomes for Manipulative, Aggressive, and Impulsive Behaviors

Nursing Outcome and Definition	Intermediate Indicators	Short-Term Indicators
Social Interaction Skills: Personal behaviors that promote effective relationships	Uses conflict resolution methods	Exhibits receptiveness Exhibits sensitivity to others Cooperates with others Uses assertive behaviors as appropriate Uses confrontation as appropriate
Personal Resiliency: Positive adaptation and function of an individual following significant adversity or crisis	Uses effective coping strategies	Expresses emotion Seeks emotional support Uses strategies to promote safety Takes responsibility for own actions Uses strategies to avoid violent situations Identifies available community resources Obtains needed support Self-initiates goal-directed behavior Expresses belief in ability to perform action Expresses that performance will lead to desired outcome
Aggression Self-Control: Self-restraint of assaultive, combative, or destructive behaviors toward others	Communicates needs appropriately	Identifies when frustrated Identifies when angry Identifies responsibility to maintain control Identifies alternatives to aggression Identifies alternatives to verbal outbursts Vents negative feelings appropriately Refrains from striking others Refrains from harming others
Impulse Self-Control: Self-restraint of compulsive or impulsive behaviors	Controls impulses	Identifies harmful impulsive behaviors Identifies feelings that lead to impulsive actions Identifies consequences of impulsive actions to self or others Avoids high-risk environments and situations Seeks help when experiencing impulses

Data from Moorhead, S., Johnson, M., Maas, M. L, and Swanson, E. (2008). *Nursing outcomes classification (NOC)* (4th ed.). St. Louis: Mosby.

their fear of potential harm or loss is. Lacking the ability to trust, patients with personality disorders require a sense of control over what is happening to them. Giving them realistic choices (e.g., selection of a particular group activity) may enhance adherence to treatment. Refer to Tables 19-4, 19-5, and 19-6 for guidelines for nursing care for each personality disorder cluster. Case Study and Nursing Care Plan 19-1 on pages 456-457 presents a patient with borderline personality disorder.

IMPLEMENTATION

People with borderline personality disorder are impulsive (e.g., suicidal, self-mutilating), aggressive, manipulative, and even psychotic during periods of stress. Persons with antisocial personality disorder are often involuntarily admitted and are manipulative, aggressive, and impulsive. Refer to Boxes 19-2, 19-3, and 19-4 on pages 452-453 for interventions to address these behaviors, based on the *Nursing Interventions Classification (NIC)* (Bulechek et al., 2008).

Milieu Management

When individuals with personality disorders are admitted to the hospital, partially hospitalized, or in day treatment settings, milieu management is a significant part of treatment. The primary goal is management of the patient's affect in a group context. Community meetings, coping skills groups, and socializing groups are all helpful for these patients. They have the opportunity to interact with peers and staff to discuss goals and learn problem-solving skills. Dealing with emotional issues that arise in the milieu requires a calm, united approach by the staff to maintain safety and to enhance self-control.

TABLE 19-4 Nursing and Therapy Guidelines for Cluster A Personality Disorders

Personality Disorder	Characteristics	Nursing Guidelines	Suggested Therapies
Schizotypal	Manifests ideas of reference Shows cognitive and perceptual distortions Socially inept Anxious	1. Respect patient's need for social isolation. 2. Be aware of patient's suspiciousness, and employ appropriate interventions. 3. As with schizoid patient, perform careful diagnostic assessment as needed to uncover any other medical or psychological symptoms that may need intervention (e.g., suicidal thoughts).	1. Supportive psychotherapy 2. Cognitive and behavioral measures 3. Group therapy may improve social skills 4. Low-dose antipsychotics and antidepressants
Paranoid	Projects blame Suspicious and mistrustful Hostile and violent Shows cognitive and perceptual distortions	1. Avoid being too "nice" or "friendly." 2. Give clear and straightforward explanations of tests and procedures beforehand. 3. Use simple, clear language; avoid ambiguity. 4. Project a neutral but kind affect. 5. Warn about any changes, side effects of medication, and reasons for delay. Such interventions may help allay anxiety and minimize suspiciousness. A written plan may help encourage cooperation.	1. Psychotherapy is treatment of choice; later cognitive-behavioral techniques 2. Group therapy may help with social skills 3. Antidepressant or antianxiety agents as needed; antipsychotics may be of use, especially if they become acutely psychotic
Schizoid	Reclusive Avoidant Uncooperative	1. Avoid being too "nice" or "friendly." 2. Do not try to increase socialization. 3. Perform thorough diagnostic assessment as needed to identify symptoms or disorders the patient is reluctant to discuss.	1. Supportive psychotherapy 2. Group therapy 3. Antipsychotics, antidepressants, antianxiety agents as needed

Data from American Psychiatric Association. (2000). *Diagnostic and statistical manual of mental disorders* (4th ed., text rev.). Washington, DC: Author; and Sadock, B. J., & Sadock, V. A. (2008). *Concise textbook of clinical psychiatry* (3rd ed.). Philadelphia: Lippincott Williams & Wilkins.

Common problems resulting from staff splitting can be minimized if the unit leaders hold weekly staff meetings in which staff members are allowed to ventilate their feelings about conflicts with patients and each other.

Patients take more responsibility for themselves if they are actively involved in treatment plans—for example, by being included in daily staff rounds to set goals and evaluate progress. Limit setting and confrontation about negative behavior is better accepted by the patient if the staff first employ empathic mirroring (i.e., reflecting back to the patient an understanding of the patient's distress without a value judgment). For example, the nurse can listen to a patient's emotional complaints about the staff and the hospital without

text continued on page 452

TABLE 19-5 Nursing and Therapy Guidelines for Cluster B Personality Disorders

Personality Disorder	Characteristics	Nursing Guidelines	Suggested Therapies
Borderline	Shows separation anxiety Manifests ideas of reference Impulsive (suicide, self-mutilation) Engages in splitting (adoring then devaluing persons)	1. Set realistic goals, use clear action words. 2. Be aware of manipulative behaviors (flattery, seductiveness, instilling of guilt). 3. Provide clear and consistent boundaries and limits. 4. Use clear and straightforward communication. 5. When behavioral problems emerge, calmly review the therapeutic goals and boundaries of treatment. 6. Avoid rejecting or rescuing. 7. Assess for suicidal and self-mutilating behaviors, especially during times of stress.	1. Individual psychotherapy 2. Dialectical behavior therapy 3. Group therapy 4. Antipsychotics may control anger and brief psychosis 5. Antidepressants such as SSRIs and MAOIs 6. Benzodiazepines help anxiety

Antisocial	Can seem normal
	Exhibits no anxiety or depression
	Manipulative
	Exploitive of others
	Aggressive
	Seductive
	Callous towards others
		1. Try to prevent or reduce untoward effects of manipulation (flattery, seductiveness, instilling of guilt):
		  • Set clear and realistic limits on specific behavior.
		  • Ensure that limits are adhered to by all staff.
		  • Carefully document signs of manipulation or aggression.
		  • Document behaviors (give times, dates, circumstances). Provide clear boundaries and consequences.
		2. Be aware that antisocial patients can instill guilt when they are not getting what they want. Guard against being manipulated through feelings of guilt.
		3. Substance abuse is best handled through a well-organized treatment program before counseling and other forms of therapy are started.
			1. More responsive to psychotherapy when hospitalized than when jailed
			2. Pharmacotherapy for anxiety, rage, and depression
			3. Careful use of addictive agents (e.g. benzodiazepines)
			4. Ritalin may help ADHD
			5. Anticonvulsants may help impulsive behavior

Narcissistic	Exploitive Grandiose Disparaging Filled with rage Very sensitive to rejection, criticism Cannot show empathy Handles aging poorly	1. Remain neutral; avoid engaging in power struggles or becoming defensive in response to the patient's disparaging remarks. 2. Convey unassuming self-confidence.	1. Psychotherapy only works after patient acknowledges narcissism 2. Group therapy may help empathy 3. Lithium may help those with mood swings, antidepressants also used

TABLE 19-5 Nursing and Therapy Guidelines for Cluster B Personality Disorders—cont'd

Personality Disorder	Characteristics	Nursing Guidelines	Suggested Therapies
Histrionic	Seductive Flamboyant Attention seeking Shallow Depressive and suicidal when admiration withdrawn	1. Understand seductive behavior as a response to distress. 2. Keep communication and interactions professional, despite temptation to collude with the patient in a flirtatious and misleading manner. 3. Encourage and model the use of concrete and descriptive rather than vague and impressionistic language. 4. Teach and role-model assertiveness.	1. Group therapy 2. Treatment of comorbid personality disorders 3. Antidepressants as needed

Data from American Psychiatric Association. (2000). *Diagnostic and statistical manual of mental disorders* (4th ed., text rev.). Washington, DC: Author; and Sadock, B. J., & Sadock, V. A. (2008). *Concise textbook of clinical psychiatry* (3rd ed.). Philadelphia: Lippincott Williams & Wilkins.

TABLE 19-6 Nursing and Therapy Guidelines for Cluster C Personality Disorders

Personality Disorder	Characteristics	Nursing Guidelines	Suggested Therapies
Dependent	Excessively clinging Self-sacrificing, submissive Needy, gets others to care for him or her	1. Identify and help address current stresses. 2. Try to satisfy patient's needs at the same time that limits are set up in such a manner that patient does not feel punished and withdraw. 3. Be aware that strong countertransference often develops in clinicians because of patient's excessive clinging (demands of extra time, nighttime calls, crisis before vacations); therefore, supervision is well advised. 4. Teach and role-model assertiveness.	1. Insight-oriented psychotherapy, behavioral therapy, assertiveness training. 2. Family and group therapy 3. Antianxiety agents and antidepressants used for specific symptoms. Panic attacks can be helped with imipramine.
Obsessive-compulsive	Perfectionistic Has need for control Inflexible, rigid Preoccupied with details Highly critical of self and others	1. Guard against power struggles with patient. Need for control is very high. 2. Intellectualization, rationalization, reaction formation, isolation, and undoing are the most common defense mechanisms.	1. Supportive or insightful psychotherapy 2. Clomipramine and SSRIs for obsessional thinking and depression

Continued

TABLE 19-6 Nursing and Therapy Guidelines for Cluster C Personality Disorders—cont'd

Personality Disorder	Characteristics	Nursing Guidelines	Suggested Therapies
Avoidant	Excessively anxious in social situations Hypersensitive to negative evaluation Desire social interaction	1. A friendly, accepting, reassuring approach is the best way to treat patients. 2. Being pushed into social situations can cause extreme and severe anxiety.	1. Psychotherapy focuses on trust 2. Group therapy 3. Assertiveness training 4. Antidepressants and antianxiety agents helpful; β-adrenergic receptor antagonists (e.g., atenolol) help reduce autonomic nervous system hyperactivity

Data from American Psychiatric Association. (2000). *Diagnostic and statistical manual of mental disorders* (4th ed., text rev.). Washington, DC: Author; and Sadock, B. J., & Sadock, V. A. (2008). *Concise textbook of clinical psychiatry* (3rd ed.). Philadelphia: Lippincott Williams & Wilkins.

BOX 19-2 *NIC* Interventions for Manipulative Behavior

Limit Setting

Definition: Establishing the parameters of desirable and acceptable patient behavior

Activities*:

- Discuss concerns about behavior with patient.
- Identify (with patient input when appropriate) undesirable patient behavior.
- Discuss with patient, when appropriate, what is desirable behavior in a given situation or setting.
- Establish consequences (with patient input when appropriate) for occurrence or nonoccurrence of desired behaviors.
- Communicate established behavioral expectations and consequences to patient in language that is easily understood and nonpunitive.
- Refrain from arguing or bargaining with patient about established behavioral expectations and consequences.
- Monitor patient for occurrence or nonoccurrence of desired behaviors.
- Modify behavioral expectations and consequences, as needed, to accommodate reasonable changes in patient's situation.

*Partial list.
Data from Bulechek, G. M., Butcher, H. K., & Dochterman, J. M. (Eds.). (2008). *Nursing interventions classification (NIC)* (5th ed.). St. Louis: Mosby.

BOX 19-3 *NIC* Interventions for Aggressive Behavior

Anger Control Assistance

Definition: Facilitation of the expression of anger in an adaptive, nonviolent manner

Activities*:

- Determine appropriate behavioral expectations for expression of anger, given patient's level of cognitive and physical functioning.
- Limit access to frustrating situations until patient is able to express anger in an adaptive manner.
- Encourage patient to seek assistance from nursing staff during periods of increasing tension.
- Monitor potential for inappropriate aggression, and intervene before its expression.
- Prevent physical harm if anger is directed at self or others (e.g., restraint and removal of potential weapons).
- Provide physical outlets for expression of anger or tension (e.g., punching bag, sports, clay, journal writing).
- Provide reassurance to patient that nursing staff will intervene to prevent patient from losing control.
- Assist patient in identifying source of anger.
- Identify function that anger, frustration, and rage serve for patient.
- Identify consequences of inappropriate expression of anger.

*Partial list.
Data from Bulechek, G. M., Butcher, H. K., & Dochterman, J. M. (Eds.). (2008). *Nursing interventions classification (NIC)* (5th ed.). St. Louis: Mosby.

---

correcting any errors, simply noting that the patient truly feels hurt. Showing empathy may also decrease aggressive outbursts if the patient feels that staff are trying to understand feelings of frustration. Table 19-7 depicts a therapeutic nurse-patient interaction after an antisocial patient initiates a fight with a peer in an inpatient unit.

A final approach that is useful for patients with borderline personality disorder relates to the response to superficial self-destructive behaviors. Acting in accordance with unit policies, the nurse remains neutral and dresses the wound in a matter-of-fact manner. Then the patient is instructed to

BOX 19-4 *NIC* Interventions for Impulsive Behavior

Impulse Control Training

Definition: Assisting the patient to mediate impulsive behavior through application of problem-solving strategies to social and interpersonal situations

Activities*:

- Assist patient to identify the problem or situation that requires thoughtful action.
- Assist patient to identify courses of possible action and their costs and benefits.
- Teach patient to cue himself or herself to "stop and think" before acting impulsively.
- Assist patient to evaluate the outcome of the chosen course of action.
- Provide positive reinforcement (e.g., praise and rewards) for successful outcomes.
- Encourage patient to self-reward for successful outcomes.
- Provide opportunities for patient to practice problem solving (role playing) within the therapeutic environment.
- Encourage patient to practice problem solving in social and interpersonal situations outside the therapeutic environment, followed by evaluation of outcome.

*Partial list.
Data from Bulechek, G. M., Butcher, H. K., & Dochterman, J. M. (Eds.). (2008). *Nursing interventions classification (NIC)* (5th ed.). St. Louis: Mosby.

write down the sequence of events leading up to the injury, as well as the consequences, before staff will discuss the event. This cognitive exercise encourages the patient to think independently about his or her own behavior instead of merely ventilating feelings. It facilitates the discussion with staff about alternative actions.

Pharmacological Interventions

Patients with personality disorders may be helped by a broad array of psychotropic agents, all geared toward maintaining cognitive function and relieving symptoms. Depending on the chief complaint, antidepressant, anxiolytic, or antipsychotic medication may be ordered. Patients with personality disorders usually do not like taking medicine unless it calms them down; they are fearful about taking something over which they have no control. They worry about not having an adequate supply but have difficulty organizing themselves to fill a prescription. Sometimes they panic and get preoccupied with side effects, then stop taking the medication. See Tables 19-4, 19-5, and 19-6 for recommended pharmacological treatments.

Case Management

Many patients with personality disorders function at a high level, but a significant number need assistance to maintain their independence. Case management is

TABLE 19-7 Dialogue With a Patient With Manipulative, Aggressive, and Impulsive Traits

Dialogue	Therapeutic Tool/Comment
Nurse: Donald, I would like to talk with you about what happened this morning.	Be clear as to purpose of interview.
Donald: OK, shoot.	
Nurse: Tell me what started the incident.	Use open-ended statements. Maintain a nonjudgmental attitude.
Donald: Well, as I told you before, I always had to fight to get what I wanted in life. My father and mother abandoned me emotionally when I was a child.	
Nurse: Yes, but tell me about this morning.	Redirect patient to present problem or situation.
Donald: OK. I disliked Richard from the first. He has it in for me, I just know it. He doesn't get along with anyone here. Just 2 days ago, he almost had a fight.	
Nurse: Donald, what do you mean, Richard has it in for you?	Explore situation.
Donald: When I'm talking to one of the nurses, he stares and makes comments under his breath.	
Nurse: What does he say?	Encourage description.

Continued

TABLE 19-7   Dialogue with a Patient with Manipulative, Aggressive, and Impulsive Traits—cont'd

Dialogue	Therapeutic Tool/Comment
Donald: How I'm "in" with the nurses. I'm just trying to do what's expected of me here.	
Nurse: You mean that Richard is envious of your relationship with the nurses?	Validate patient's meaning.
Donald: Right. He really doesn't want to be here. He doesn't care about all that therapeutic junk.	
Nurse: You seem to know a lot about how Richard thinks. I wonder how that is.	Assist patient to make association to present situation.
Donald: He reminds me of someone I knew when I was young. His name was Joe. We called him "Bones."	
Nurse: Tell me more about Bones.	Explore situation further.
Donald: We called him Bones because he was skinny. He was into drugs and never ate. He was also called Bones because he was selfish. He never shared anything. He never even had a girl that I knew about.	
Nurse: So Richard reminds you of someone who is selfish and lonely?	Make interpretation of information. Note increasing anxiety.
Donald: That's right. I've had three marriages and girlfriends on the side. No one can take them away from me. (Angrily.) Just let them try!	
Nurse: What makes you so angry now?	Identify feelings and explore threat or anxiety.
Donald: Richard! I know he wants to be like me, but he can't. I'll hurt him if he makes any more comments about me.	
Nurse: Donald, you will not hurt anyone here on the unit.	Set limits on, and expectations of, patient's behavior.
Donald: I'm sorry, I didn't mean that.	
Nurse: It's important that we examine your part in the incident this morning and ways to cope without threats or violence.	Focus on patient's responsibility and suggest alternative methods of coping with situation.
Donald: Listen, I know I've gotten into trouble because I can't control my temper, but that's because I won't get any respect until I can show them I don't fear them.	Patient exhibits rationalization.
Nurse: Who are "they"?	Clarify pronoun.
Donald: People like Richard.	
Nurse: You've told me that fighting was a way of survival as a child, but as an adult, there are other ways of handling situations that make you angry.	Show understanding and suggest other means of coping.
Donald: You're right. I've thought about this. Do you think it would help if you give me some meds to control my anger?	Patient exhibits superficial and concrete thinking—possible manipulation.
Nurse: I wasn't thinking of medications but of a plan for being aware of your anger and talking it out instead of fighting it out.	Clarify meaning toward behavior change. Start to explore alternatives Donald can use when angry instead of fighting.
Donald: I told you before, I *have* to fight.	
Nurse: Have you thought about the consequences of your fighting?	Identify results of impulsive behavior.
Donald: I feel bad afterwards. Sometimes I wish it hadn't happened.	Patient continues to explore.

helpful for patients with personality disorders who are persistently and severely impaired. These patients often have had multiple hospitalizations, have been unable to maintain work or personal relationships, and are relatively alone in their attempts to care for themselves. In the acute care setting, case management focuses on three goals: to gather pertinent history from current or previous providers; to support reintegration with family or loved ones as appropriate; and to ensure appropriate referrals to outpatient care, including substance disorder treatment, if needed. In the long-term outpatient setting, case-management objectives include reducing hospitalization by providing resources for crisis services and enhancing the social support system.

Advanced Practice Interventions

The APRN-PMH treats patients with personality disorders in a variety of inpatient and community settings. Research shows that treatment can be effective for many of these persons, especially when a comorbid major mental disorder is targeted. See Tables 19-4, 19-5, and 19-6 for a summary of nursing and therapy guidelines for personality disorders.

Advanced practice nurses are likely to interact with staff members regarding the treatment of individuals with personality disorders as part of their practice and clinical supervision responsibilities. The APRN can assist staff members in engaging these patients in a therapeutic alliance. One strategy is supporting staff as they develop rapport and trust with patients diagnosed with cluster A personality disorders when these patients are experiencing heightened anxiety from being hospitalized. Staff should understand that the patient's ability to interpret subtle, affective cues from the caregiver is limited, and straightforward communication is necessary (Hayward, 2007).

Psychotherapy

APRNs are increasingly involved in providing individual and group psychotherapy using **dialectical behavior therapy (DBT)**. DBT is an evidenced-based therapy developed by Dr. Marsha Linehan to successfully treat chronically suicidal persons with borderline personality disorder (Linehan, 1993). Data on the use of DBT with individuals experiencing comorbid personality disorders (such as obsessive-compulsive personality disorder) and Axis I disorders (such as depression) have recently received favorable research and clinical attention (Miller & Kraus, 2007).

DBT combines cognitive and behavioral techniques with *mindfulness*, which emphasizes being aware of thoughts and actively shaping them. The goals of DBT are to increase the patient's ability to manage distress, improve interpersonal effectiveness skills, and enhance the therapist's effectiveness in working with

this population. Treatment focuses on behavior targets, beginning with identification and interventions for suicidal behaviors and then progressing to a focus on interrupting destructive behaviors (Figure 19-4). Finally, DBT addresses quality-of-life behaviors across a hierarchy of care (Figure 19-5).

EVALUATION

Evaluating treatment effectiveness in this patient population is difficult. Nurses may never know the real results of their interventions, particularly in acute care settings. Even in long-term outpatient treatment, many personality disorder patients find the relationship too intimate an experience to remain long enough for successful treatment. As noted earlier, however, some motivated patients may be able to learn to change their behavior, especially if positive experiences are repeated.

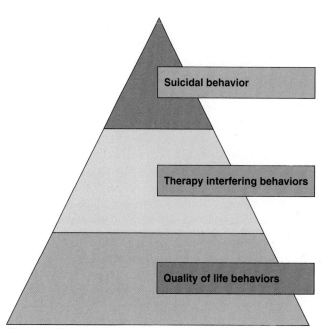

Figure 19-4 Dialectical behavior therapy treatment targets.

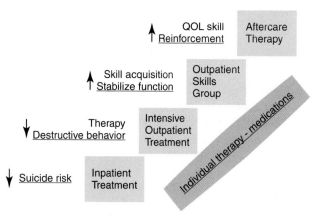

Figure 19-5 Dialectical behavior therapy treatment hierarchy. *QOL,* Quality of life.

Each therapeutic experience offers an opportunity for the patient to observe himself or herself interacting with caregivers who consistently try to teach positive coping skills. Perhaps effectiveness can be measured by how successfully the nurse is able to be genuine with the patient, maintain a helpful posture, offer substantial instruction, and still care for himself or herself. Specific short-term outcomes may be accomplished, and overall, the patient can be given the message of hope that quality of life can always be improved.

Case Study and Nursing Care Plan 19-1 Borderline Personality Disorder

Mary Drake is a 24-year-old single administrative assistant who lives alone. She has been seen in the emergency department several times for superficial suicide attempts. She is admitted because she has cut her wrists, ankles, and vagina with glass and has lost a lot of blood. This event is precipitated by her graduation from a community college.

Upon admission she is sweet, serene, and grateful to all the nurses, calling them "angels of mercy." Within a week, she is angry at half of the nurses and demands a new primary nurse, saying that the one she has (to whom she had grown attached) hates her. She has a history of heavy drinking and has managed to sneak alcohol onto the unit. She has been found in bed with a young male patient. She continually breaks unit rules and then pleads to have this behavior forgiven and forgotten. When angry, she threatens to cut herself again. When asked why she cut herself, Ms. Drake states, "I was tired." She appears restless and tense and frequently asks for antianxiety medication. When asked what she is anxious about, she says, "Uh...I don't know...I feel so empty inside." Ms. Drake frequently paces up and down the halls looking both angry and bored. Her admitting diagnoses include substance abuse disorder and borderline personality disorder.

ASSESSMENT

Self-Assessment

Ms. McCarthy, a recent graduate and Ms. Drake's primary nurse, talks to Ms. Drake's therapist twice a week in staff meetings. The therapist impresses upon Ms. McCarthy the difficulty health care workers have in dealing effectively with people with borderline personality disorders. These patients constantly act out their feelings in self-destructive and maladaptive ways. They usually are not aware of their feelings or what triggered their actions.

The most difficult area for many health care workers is dealing with the intense feelings and reactions these patients can provoke in others. Ms. McCarthy sets a time twice a week for supervision with Ms. Drake's therapist. At the next meeting, common goals and intervention strategies are discussed.

Objective Data

Makes frequent, superficial suicide attempts
Requests antianxiety medication frequently
Paces up and down the hall much of the day
Threatens self-mutilation when anxious
Brings alcohol onto the unit after pass
Is found in bed with male patient

Subjective Data

Initially "loved" her primary nurse, now "hates" her and wants another nurse
States she is restless and tense
Complains of feeling empty inside
Describes self as angry and bored much of the time

DIAGNOSIS

Ms. McCarthy formulates two initial nursing diagnoses that have the highest priority during this time:

1. *Ineffective coping* related to inadequate psychological resources, as evidenced by self-destructive behaviors

Supporting Data

- After stating that she feels frustrated, patient goes on pass and comes back with alcohol.
- After stating that she is in love with her therapist, patient is found in bed with a male patient.
- After stating that she hates her primary nurse, patient demands a new primary nurse.

2. *Self-mutilation* related to borderline personality disorder, as evidenced by suicidal gestures and poor impulse control

Supporting Data

- Is admitted following self-mutilation
- Threatens self-mutilation when anxious
- Threatens self-mutilation on unit

OUTCOMES IDENTIFICATION

1. Patient will consistently demonstrate the use of effective coping strategies.
2. Patient will refrain from injuring self.

PLANNING

The initial plan is to maintain patient safety and to encourage verbalization of feelings and impulses instead of action.

IMPLEMENTATION

Ms. Drake's plan of care is personalized as follows.

Nursing diagnosis: *Ineffective coping* related to inadequate psychological resources, as evidenced by self-destructive behaviors

Outcome criteria: Patient will consistently demonstrate the use of effective coping strategies.

Short-Term Goal	Intervention	Rationale	Evaluation
Ms. Drake will consistently demonstrate a decrease in stress as evidenced by talking about feelings with staff every day and an absence of acting-out behaviors	1. Encourage verbalization of feelings, perceptions, and fears.	1. Discussing and understanding the dynamics of frustration help reduce the frustration by helping patient take positive action.	**GOAL MET** Ms. Drake was able to experience problems and deal with them appropriately. Acting out was minimal or absent. *Example:* Patient had an appointment for a job interview. She wanted to stay in bed and avoid the interview, but instead she talked with the nurse about her fear of "growing up" and was able to get up and go to the interview.
	2. Support the use of appropriate defense mechanisms.	2. Discussing and understanding the meaning of defenses help reduce the potential for acting out.	

Nursing diagnosis: *Self-mutilation* related to borderline personality disorder, as evidenced by suicidal gestures and poor impulse control

Outcome criteria: Patient will refrain from injuring self.

Short-Term Goal	Intervention	Rationale	Evaluation
Ms. Drake will consistently demonstrate that she will seek help when feeling urge to injure self as evidenced by the absence of self-injurious behaviors and talking to staff about her troubling feelings on a daily basis.	1. Assist patient to identify situations and/or feelings that may prompt self-harm.	1. Observing, describing, and analyzing thoughts and feelings reduce the potential for acting them out destructively.	**GOAL MET** Ms. Drake was able to experience troubling thoughts and feelings without self-mutilation. Stated, "I was mad at my therapist today and decided to cut my arms after the session. Instead, I told her I was angry, and together we figured out why."
	2. Instruct patient in coping strategies.	2. Alternative behaviors are offered that can be more satisfying and growth promoting.	
	3. Provide ongoing surveillance of patient and environment.	3. Times of increased anxiety, frustration, or anger without external controls could increase probability of patient using self-mutilating behaviors.	

Evaluation

See individual outcomes and evaluation in the care plan.

KEY POINTS TO REMEMBER

- All personality disorders share characteristics of inflexibility and difficulties in interpersonal relationships that impair social or occupational functioning.
- Personality disorders are most likely caused by a combination of biological and psychosocial factors.
- The *DSM-IV-TR* organizes personality disorders into three clusters (A, B, C) based on similarities in behavior patterns.
- Patients with personality disorders often enter psychiatric treatment because of distress from a comorbid major mental illness.
- Nurses may experience intense emotional reactions to patients with personality disorders and need to make use of clinical supervision to maintain objectivity.
- Despite the relatively fixed patterns of maladaptive behavior, some patients with personality disorders are able to change their behavior over time as a result of treatment.

CRITICAL THINKING

1. Mr. Beach is undergoing surgery for a broken leg. He is very suspicious of the staff and believes that everyone is trying to harm him and "do him in." He scans his environment constantly for danger (hypervigilance) and speaks very little to the nurses or the other patients. He has a paranoid personality disorder.
   A. Explain how being friendly and outgoing may be threatening to Mr. Beach.
   B. Explain how being matter-of-fact and neutral and sticking to the facts would be effective to Mr. Beach.
   C. What could be done to give Mr. Beach some control over his situation as a hospitalized patient?
   D. How could you best handle his sarcasm and hostility so both you and he would feel most comfortable?

2. Cherie is brought to the emergency department after slashing her wrist with a razor. She has previously been in the emergency department for drug overdose and has a history of addictions. Cherie can be sarcastic, belittling, and aggressive to those who try to care for her. She has a history of difficulty with interpersonal relationships at her job. When the psychiatric triage nurse comes in to see her, Cherie is initially adoring and compliant, telling him, "You are the best nurse I've ever had, and I truly want to change." But when he refuses to support her request for diazepam (Valium) and meperidine (Demerol) for "pain," she yells at him, "You are a stupid excuse for a nurse. I want to see the doctor immediately." Cherie has borderline personality disorder.
   A. What defense mechanisms is Cherie using?
   B. How could the nurse handle this situation while setting limits and demonstrating concern?

CHAPTER REVIEW

1. A patient complains that most staff do not like her or care what happens to her, but you are special and she can tell that you are a caring person. She talks with you about being unsure of what she wants to do with her life and her "mixed-up feelings" about relationships. When you tell her that you will be on vacation next week, she becomes very angry. Two hours later, she is found using a curling iron to burn her underarms and explains that it "makes the numbness stop." Given this presentation, you would deduce that this patient most likely has which personality disorder?
   1. Histrionic
   2. Borderline
   3. Dependent
   4. Schizotypal

2. Which statement about persons with personality disorders is accurate?
   1. They, unlike those with mood or psychotic disorders, are at very low risk of suicide.
   2. They tend not to perceive themselves as having a problem but instead believe their problems are caused by how others behave toward them.
   3. They are believed to be purely psychological disorders, that is, disorders arising from psychological rather than neurological or other physiological abnormalities.
   4. Their symptoms are not as disabling as most other mental disorders; therefore, their care tends to be less challenging and complicated for staff.

3. A patient shows the nurse multiple fresh, serious (but non-life-threatening) self-inflicted cuts on her forearm. Which response would be most therapeutic?
   1. Convey empathy and explore issues that led to the self-injury as you administer first-aid to the wounds.
   2. Care for the wounds, then search the patient for sharp objects, and place the patient on one-to-one observation or in seclusion for her own safety.
   3. Recognizing that the self-injury is, at its heart, a maladaptive attempt to obtain attention, extinguish the behavior by minimizing the attention paid to it.
   4. Maintain a neutral demeanor while dressing the wounds, and then assign the patient to write a list of circumstances that led to the injury before discussing it further.

4. A patient is flirting with a peer and is overheard asking him to intercede with staff so that she will be given privileges to leave the inpatient mental health unit. Later she offers a backrub to a nurse if that nurse will give her the prn sedation at 9:00 pm that is not ordered until 10:00 pm. Which response(s) to such behaviors would be most therapeutic? *Select all that apply.*
   1. Label the behavior as undesirable, and explore with the patient more effective ways to meet her needs.

2. By role-playing, demonstrate other approaches the patient could use to meet her needs.
3. Advise the other patients that this patient is being manipulative and that they should ignore the patient when she behaves this way.
4. Bargain with the patient to determine a reasonable compromise regarding how much of such behavior is acceptable before the patient crosses the line.
5. Explain that such behavior is unacceptable, and give the patient specific examples of consequences that will be enacted if the behavior continues.
6. Ignore the behavior for the time being so the patient will find it unrewarding and in turn seek other, and hopefully more adaptive, ways to meet her needs.

5. A patient becomes frustrated and angry when trying to get his MP3 player and headset to function properly and angrily throws it across the room, nearly hitting a peer with it. Which intervention(s) would be the most therapeutic? *Select all that apply.*

1. Place the patient in seclusion for 1 hour to allow him to de-escalate.
2. Tell the patient that any further outbursts will result in a loss of privileges.
3. Offer to help the patient learn how to operate his music player and headset.
4. Explore with the patient how he was feeling as he worked with the music player.
5. Point out the consequences of such behavior, and note that it cannot be tolerated.
6. Limit the patient's exposure to frustrating experiences until he attains improved coping skills.
7. Encourage the patient to recognize signs of mounting tension and seek assistance.

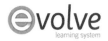 Visit the Evolve website for an **Audio Chapter Summary, Chapter Review Answers & Rationales, Critical Thinking Answer Guidelines,** and additional resources related to the content in this chapter: **http://evolve.elsevier.com/Varcarolis/foundations**

Companion CD Use the Companion CD to prepare for tests and the NCLEX® Examination with **Test-Taking Strategies** for psychiatric mental health nursing and hundreds of **Review Questions**.

References

American Psychiatric Association. (2000). *Diagnostic and statistical manual of mental disorders* (4th ed., text rev.) *(DSM-IV-TR)*. Washington DC: Author.

Blais, M. A., Smallwood, P., Groves, J. E., & Rivas-Vazquez, R. A. (2008). Personality and personality disorders. In T. A. Stern, J. F. Rosenbaum, M. Fava, J. Biederman, & S. L. Rauch (Eds.), *Massachusetts General Hospital comprehensive clinical psychiatry* (pp. 527–540). Philadelphia: Saunders.

Bland, A. R., Tudor, G., & McNeil-Whitehouse, D. (2007). Nursing care of inpatients with borderline personality disorder. *Perspectives in Psychiatric Care, 43*(4), 204–212.

Bland, A. R., Williams, D., Scharer, K., & Manning, S. (2004). Emotion processing in borderline personality disorders. *Issues in Mental Health Nursing, 25,* 655–672.

Bulechek, G. M., Butcher, H. K., & Dochterman, J. M. (2008). *Nursing interventions classification (NIC).* (5th ed.). St. Louis: Mosby.

Coccaro, E. F., & Siever, L. J. (2005). Neurobiology. In J. M. Oldham, A. E. Skodol, & D. S. Bender (Eds.), *Textbook of personality disorders* (pp. 155–169). Washington DC: American Psychiatric Publishing.

Cuzchta-Romano, D. (2004). A self-psychology approach to narcissistic personality disorder: A nursing reflection. *Perspectives in Psychiatric Care, 40*(1), 20–28.

Davison, S. (2002). Principles of managing patients with personality disorder. *Advances in Psychiatric Treatment, 8,* 1–9.

Eisen, J., Coles, M., Shea, T., Pagano, M., Stout, R., Yen, S., et al. (2006). Clarifying the convergence between obsessive compulsive personality disorder criteria and obsessive compulsive disorder. *Journal of Personality Disorders, 20*(3), 294–305.

Gunderson, J. G., & Hoffman, P. D. (2005). *Understanding and treating borderline personality disorder: A guide for professionals and families.* Washington DC: American Psychiatric Publishing.

Hayward, B. A. (2007). Cluster A personality disorders: Considering the "odd-eccentric" in psychiatric nursing. *International Journal of Mental Health Nursing, 16,* 15–21.

Kagan, J. (2005). Personality and temperament. In M. Rosenbluth, S. H. Kennedy, & R. M. Bagby (Eds.), *Depression and personality: Conceptual and clinical challenges* (pp. 3–18). Washington DC: American Psychiatric Publishing.

Kernberg, O. (1985). *Internal world and external reality.* London: Aronson.

Linehan, M. M. (1993). *Cognitive behavioral treatment of borderline personality disorder.* New York: Guilford.

Miller, T. W., & Kraus, R. F. (2007). Modified dialectical behavior therapy and problem solving for obsessive-compulsive personality disorder. *Journal of Contemporary Psychotherapy, 37,* 79–85.

Moorhead, S., Johnson, M., Maas, M. L., & Swanson, E. (2008). *Nursing outcomes classification (NOC)* (4th ed.). St. Louis: Mosby.

Nahas, Z., Molnar, D., & George, M. (2005). Brain imaging. In J. M. Oldham, A. E. Skodol, & D. S. Bender (Eds.), *Textbook of personality disorders* (pp. 623–639). Washington DC: American Psychiatric Publishing.

Paris, J. (2005). A current integrative perspective on personality disorders. In J. M. Oldham, A. E. Skodol, & D. S. Bender (Eds.), *Textbook of personality disorders* (pp. 119–128). Washington DC: American Psychiatric Publishing.

Sadock, B. J., & Sadock, V. A. (2008). *Kaplan & Sadock's concise textbook of clinical psychiatry* (3rd ed.). Philadelphia: Lippincott Williams & Wilkins.

Soeteman, D. I., Hakkaart-VanRoijen, L., Verheul, R., & Busschbach, J. J. (2008). The economic burden of personality disorders in mental health care. *The Journal of Clinical Psychiatry*, 69(2), 259–265.

Skodol, A. E., & Gunderson, J. G. (2008). Personality disorders. In R. E. Hales, S. C. Yudofsky, & G. O. Gabbard (Eds.), *Textbook of psychiatry* (pp. 821–860). Washington DC: American Psychiatric Publishing.

Torgersen, S. (2005). Epidemiology. In J. M. Oldham, A. E. Skodol, & D. S. Bender (Eds.), *Textbook of personality disorders* (pp. 129–142). Washington DC: American Psychiatric Publishing.

Widiger, T., & Mullins-Sweatt, S. (2008). Personality disorders. In A. Tassman, J. Kay, J. Lieberman, M. B. First, & M. Maj (Eds.), *Psychiatry* (3rd ed.) (pp. 1718–1753). London: John Wiley & Sons.

Widiger, T., & Samuel, D. (2005). Evidence-based assessments of personality disorders. *Psychological Assessment*, 17, 278–287.

CHAPTER **20**

Sleep Disorders

Margaret Trussler

Key Terms and Concepts

dyssomnias, 466
excessive sleepiness (ES), 462
parasomnias, 470
sleep architecture, 463
sleep continuity, 463
sleep deprivation, 462

sleep efficiency, 465
sleep fragmentation, 464
sleep hygiene, 467
sleep latency, 462
sleep restriction, 470
stimulus control, 470

Objectives

1. Discuss the impact of inadequate sleep on overall health and well-being.
2. Describe the social and economic impact of sleep disturbance and chronic sleep deprivation.
3. Recognize the risks to personal and community safety imposed by sleep disturbance and chronic sleep deprivation.
4. Describe normal sleep physiology, and explain the variations in normal sleep.
5. Differentiate between dyssomnias and parasomnias, and identify at least two examples of each.
6. Identify the predisposing, precipitating, and perpetuating factors for patients with insomnia.

7. Identify and describe the use of two assessment tools in the evaluation of patients experiencing sleep disturbance.
8. Develop a teaching plan for a patient with primary insomnia, incorporating principles of sleep restriction, stimulus control, and cognitive-behavioral therapy.
9. Formulate three nursing diagnoses for patients experiencing a sleep disturbance.
10. Develop a care plan for the patient experiencing sleep disturbance incorporating basic sleep hygiene principles.

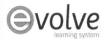 Visit the Evolve website for an **Audio Glossary & Flashcards, Concept Map Creator**, and additional resources related to the content in this chapter: **http://evolve.elsevier.com/Varcarolis/foundations**

Sleep and sleep disorders are receiving increased attention in the medical, nursing, research, and social science literature. The National Center on Sleep Disorders Research (NCSDR) was established in 1996 to facilitate research, training, health information dissemination, and other activities with respect to the basic understanding of sleep and sleep disorders. Under the guidance of the NCSDR, there has been exponential growth in the scientific understanding of sleep over the last 15 years. Despite the investment in sleep-related research and tremendous growth in our understanding of sleep physiology and pathology, application of the findings has been slow.

Sleep

In a fast-paced society sleep is often forfeited and people subject themselves to schedules that disrupt normal sleep physiology. The National Sleep Foundation (2008) recommends that the average adult get 7 to 9 hours of sleep each night, yet epidemiological surveys suggest that mean sleep duration among U.S. adults has decreased during the last century (Centers for Disease Control and Prevention, 2008).

Sleep has become an expendable commodity. People frequently cut back on sleep to meet other social

461

demands, with compensated work time and travel time being the most potent determinants of total sleep time (Basner et al., 2007). The 2008 NSF Sleep in America Poll indicates that more than half (54%) of respondents are working more than 40 hours a week, and 13% are working 60 hours a week or more.

CONSEQUENCES OF SLEEP LOSS

The major consequence of acute or chronic sleep curtailment is **excessive sleepiness (ES)**. ES is a subjective report of difficulty staying awake that is serious enough to impact social and vocational functioning and increase the risk for accident or injury. While self-imposed sleep restriction is a common cause of ES, disruption of the normal sleep cycle (as seen in shift work), underlying sleep disorders, medications, alcohol, and many medical disorders are important causes of excessive sleepiness.

We need only look to our own experiences with acute or total sleep loss to recognize its consequences. After a poor night's sleep, we feel tired, lethargic, and out of synch. The effects of chronic sleep deprivation may be less obvious but may have a greater overall impact on health and well-being. A discrepancy between hours of sleep obtained and hours of sleep required for optimal functioning is responsible for a state of **sleep deprivation**, which has widespread implications for health, safety, and quality of life. Adults who sleep less than 6 hours a night are more likely to report fair to poor general health, frequent physical distress, frequent mental distress, limitations in activities of daily living, depressive symptoms, anxiety, and pain (Strine & Chapman, 2005).

Sleep loss diminishes safety and results in the loss of lives and property. Some of the most devastating environmental and human tragedies of our time can be linked to human error due to sleep loss and fatigue. The grounding of the Exxon Valdez, the nuclear meltdown at Three Mile Island, and the explosion of the Union Carbide chemical plant in India are prime examples (Institute of Medicine [IOM], 2006). Sleepiness while driving has become a national epidemic, with almost 20% of all serious car accidents being associated with driver sleepiness (IOM, 2006). The National Highway Traffic and Safety Administration estimates approximately 40,000 nonfatal injuries and 1,550 fatalities a year are the result of driver drowsiness and fatigue (2008).

Sleep deprivation can produce psychomotor impairments equivalent to those induced by alcohol consumption at or above the legal limit. Daytime wakefulness in excess of 17 to 19 hours can produce psychomotor deficits equivalent to blood alcohol concentrations (BACs) between 0.05% and 0.1% (the legal limit in most states is 0.08%) (Williamson & Feyer, 2007).

There is relatively little comprehensive data available on the economic burden of sleep disruption. However, considering the prevalence, impact on overall health and quality of life, and the indirect costs associated with property loss and damage, the economic burden is likely in the billions of dollars. For example, it has been estimated that chronic insomnia results in nearly $14 billion dollars in direct expenses annually (Walsh, 2004) and that sleep related fatigue costs businesses $150 billion dollars a year in absenteeism, accidents, property damage, and decreased or lost productivity (Health Care Strategic Management, 2001).

Formal training in sleep or sleep disorders within medical and nursing education is limited, and the number of trained clinicians and scientists is insufficient (IOM, 2006). Awareness among health care providers regarding the prevalence and burden of sleep disruption and the problem of inadequate sleep is underappreciated, and providers do not routinely screen for sleep disturbance or inquire about overall sleep quality (Sorscher, 2008). Consequently, there is inadequate recognition, diagnosis, management, and treatment of sleep disturbance.

In this chapter, we briefly review the components of normal sleep, sleep regulation, and functions of sleep; give an overview of the most common sleep disturbances encountered in the clinical environment, with a focus on their relationship to psychiatric illness; and discuss the nurse's role in the assessment and management of a patient presenting with sleep disturbance.

NORMAL SLEEP CYCLE

Sleep is a dynamic neurological process that involves complex interaction between the central nervous system and the environment. Behaviorally, sleep is associated with low or absent motor activity, a reduced response to environmental stimuli, and closed eyes. Neurophysiologically, sleep is categorized according to specific brain wave patterns, eye movements, and general muscle tone. Sleep is measured electrophysiologically through an electroencephalogram (EEG) and consists of two distinct physiological states: non–rapid eye movement (NREM) sleep and rapid eye movement (REM) sleep. Figure 20-1 shows the EEG patterns characteristic of these sleep stages.

NREM sleep is divided into four stages characterized by progressive or deeper sleep. Stage 1 is a brief transition between wakefulness and sleep and comprises between 2% and 5% of sleep time. The time it takes to go to sleep is referred to as **sleep latency**. During stage 1 sleep, body temperature declines and muscles relax. Slow, rolling eye movements are common. People lose awareness of their environment but are generally easily aroused. Stage 2 sleep occupies 45% to 55% of total sleep time. Heart rate and respiratory rate decline. Arousal from stage 2 sleep requires more intense stimuli than stage 1.

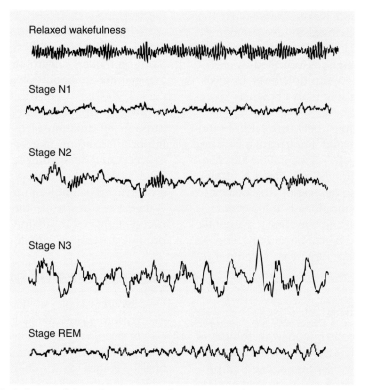

Figure 20-1 Stages of sleep. (Reprinted with permission of Sleep HealthCenters, Boston, MA.)

Stages 3 and 4 are collectively known as *slow wave sleep* or *delta sleep*. Stage 3 is relatively short and constitutes only about 3% to 8% of sleep time; stage 4 is longer and represents 10% to 15% of sleep time. Slow wave sleep is characterized by further reduction in heart rate, respiratory rate, blood pressure, and response to external stimuli. The four stages of NREM sleep make up 75% to 80% of total sleep time (Carskadon & Dement, 2005).

REM sleep comprises 20% to 25% of total sleep time and is characterized by reduction and absence of skeletal muscle tone (muscle atonia), bursts of rapid eye movement, myoclonic twitches of the facial and limb muscles, reports of dreaming, and autonomic nervous system variability. The atonia in REM sleep is thought to prevent the acting out of nightmares and dreams (Carskadon & Dement, 2005).

Sleep normally begins with NREM sleep. Continuous EEG recordings of sleep demonstrate an alternating cycling between NREM and REM sleep. There are typically 4 to 6 cycles of NREM and REM sleep occurring over 90- to 120-minute intervals across the sleep period. There is also a distinct organization to sleep, with NREM predominating during the first half of the sleep period and REM sleep predominating during the second half. The shortest REM period occurs 60 to 90 minutes after sleep onset and only last for several minutes. The longest REM period occurs at the end of the sleep period and can last up to an hour. This is the reason why many people remember dreaming upon awakening in the morning (Carskadon & Dement, 2005).

The structural organization of NREM and REM sleep is known as **sleep architecture** and is often displayed graphically as a *hypnogram*. Figure 20-2 is a hypnogram depicting the progression of the stages of sleep in a young adult and an older adult. The visual depiction of sleep is helpful in identifying **sleep continuity**

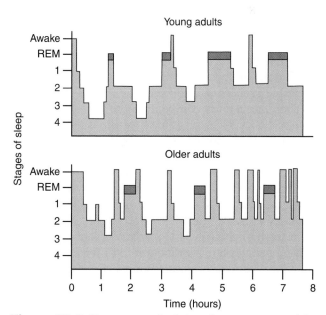

Figure 20-2 Hypnogram depicting the progression of the stages of sleep in a young adult and an older adult (From Duthie, E. H., Katz, P. R., & Malone, M. *Practice of geriatrics* [4th ed.]. [2007]. Philadelphia: Saunders.)

(the distribution of sleep and wakefulness across the sleep period), as well as changes in sleep that may occur as a result of aging, illness, or certain medications. Disruption of sleep stages as indicated by excessive amounts of stage 1 sleep, multiple brief arousals, and frequent shifts in sleep staging is known as **sleep fragmentation**.

The function of alterations between NREM and REM sleep is not yet understood, but irregular cycling, absent sleep stages, and sleep fragmentation are associated with many sleep disorders (Zepelin et al., 2005). For example, in patients with depression, the latency to REM sleep is frequently reduced, as is the percentage of slow wave sleep. Patients with narcolepsy frequently enter sleep through REM. Benzodiazepines tend to suppress slow wave sleep, whereas serotonergic drugs suppress REM sleep.

REGULATION OF SLEEP

Although the regulation of sleep and wakefulness is not completely understood, it is believed to be a complex interaction between two processes, one that promotes sleep—known as the *homeostatic process* or *sleep drive*—and one that promotes wakefulness—known as the *circadian process* or *circadian drive*. The homeostatic process is dependent on the number of hours a person is awake. The longer the period of wakefulness, the stronger the sleep drive. During sleep, the sleep drive gradually dissipates.

Circadian drives are near-24-hour cycles of behavior and physiology generated and influenced by endogenous and exogenous factors and are wake-promoting. The exogenous factors are various clues from the environment known as *zeitgebers* (time-givers) that help set our internal clock to a 24-hour cycle. The strongest external cue for wakefulness is light, whereas darkness is the cue for sleep. Other environmental cues include the timing of social events, such as meals, work, or exercise (Czeisler et al., 2005).

The endogenous component known as the *master biological clock* is located in the suprachiasmatic nucleus (SCN) of the hypothalamus. This clock regulates not only sleep but a host of other biological and physiological functions within the body. Information about the lighting conditions of the external environment is relayed to the SCN from the retina via the retinohypothalamic tract. The SCN also receives information from the thalamus and the midbrain. These two pathways transmit photic and nonphotic information to the circadian clock through an expansive network. They also exert control over endocrine regulation, body temperature, sleep/wake cycles, metabolism, autonomic regulation, psychomotor and cognitive performance, attention, memory, and emotion (Czeisler et al., 2005).

In addition to the circadian and homeostatic processes, several neurotransmitter systems are responsible for sleep and wakefulness. The neurotransmitters responsible for wakefulness are dopamine, norepinephrine, acetylcholine, histamine, glutamate, and hypocretin. Sleep-promoting neurotransmitters include adenosine, **gamma**-aminobutyric acid (GABA), and serotonin (Siegel, 2004). Any medication that crosses the blood-brain barrier may have effects on sleep and wakefulness through modulation of these neurotransmitters. It is important to appreciate the neurotransmitters involved in sleep and wakefulness; many of the medications used in psychiatry manipulate these neurotransmitter systems. For example, amphetamines—which promote wakefulness—increase the release of dopamine and norepinephrine. Caffeine (methylxanthine)—which promotes alertness—functions by blocking adenosine.

FUNCTIONS OF SLEEP

Despite remarkable advances in the understanding of sleep disorders and the biological and physiological process of sleep, very little is known about the true function of sleep. Most of the information regarding the function of sleep comes to us from animal models of sleep deprivation and human models of partial sleep deprivation. Based on these models, several theories are proposed and include brain tissue restoration, body restoration (NREM sleep), energy conservation, memory reinforcement and consolidation (REM sleep), regulation of immune function, metabolism and regulation of certain hormones, and thermoregulation (Bonnet, 2005; Dinges et al., 2005).

SLEEP REQUIREMENTS

Sleep architecture and efficiency may change over time, but there is little change in the amount of sleep required once we reach adulthood. Sleep requirement varies considerably from individual to individual and to some degree is probably genetically mediated. While most adults require 7 to 8 hours of sleep for optimal functioning, there is a small percentage of individuals who are defined as *long sleepers* (requiring 10 or more hours per night) and *short sleepers* (requiring less than 5 hours per night) (American Academy of Sleep Medicine [AASM], 2005). The amount of sleep required is the amount necessary to feel fully awake and able to sustain normal levels of performance during the periods of wakefulness.

For many people, there is a misconception regarding sleep need and a tendency to allow circumstances to dictate the amount of sleep obtained. The most accurate way to determine sleep requirements is to establish a routine bedtime and allow oneself to sleep undisturbed without an alarm for several days. This is usually best accomplished during an extended period of leisure time, such as during a vacation. The average of several nights' sleep undisturbed is probably a good estimate of total sleep requirement (Epstein, 2007).

CONSIDERING CULTURE

The Role of Sleep in U.S. Culture

Jane is a busy, full-time professional and mother of three teenage girls. It is not unusual for her to leave the house by 6 AM and return home at 6 or 7 PM. She is active in the PTA and Girl Scouts and coaches the girls' soccer team during the spring. Her 86-year-old mother's health is failing, and Jane spends weekends helping her to shop and running errands. She estimates that between her "real job" and her "second shift" domestic and community responsibilities, she works 16 to 18 hours a day, 7 days a week. How does she do it? Jane only sleeps 4 or 5 hours a night, some nights less. If she feels tired or fatigued, she reaches for a double latte and is on her way again. Sleep just isn't a priority for her.

In the United States, the individual who seems to be able to do it all is held in high regard. Employers have come to expect near-24-hour access to their employees, making sleeplessness a cultural phenomenon. What some individuals are describing as insomnia may in actuality be symptomatic of inadequate sleep opportunity and lack of leisure time to recharge and rejuvenate. Have you ever wondered what toll this may be having on health, functioning, relationships, and quality of life?

Nurses can play a key role in educating patients and the public about the health and societal consequences of inadequate sleep. Helping patients strike a healthy balance between work and home may have significant implications for primary prevention.

Henry, D., McClellen, D., Rosenthal, D., and Gosdin, M. (2008). Is sleep really for sissies? Understanding the roll of work in insomnia in the US. *Social Science and Medicine, 66*(3), 715–726.

SLEEP PATTERNS

Sleep architecture changes over the lifespan. The percentage in each stage of sleep, as well as the overall sleep efficiency, or ratio of sleep duration to time spent in bed, varies according to age. For example, infants sleep 16 to 18 hours a day, enter sleep through REM (not NREM) sleep, and spend up to 50% of sleep time in REM sleep. The percentage of REM sleep decreases to 20% to 25% by age 3 and stays relatively constant throughout old age. The amount of slow wave sleep is maximal in young children and declines with age to almost none, particularly in men. This results in a tendency for middle-of-the-night awakenings and reduced sleep efficiency with age (Bliwise, 2005).

Sleep Disorders

Sleep testing is often indicated for patients complaining of sleep disturbance or ES that impairs social and vocational functioning. There are four common diagnostic procedures used in the evaluation of sleep disorders: polysomnography (PSG), the multiple sleep latency test (MSLT), the maintenance of wakefulness test (MWT), and actigraphy.

PSG is the most common sleep test and is used to diagnose and evaluate patients with sleep-related breathing disorders, nocturnal seizure disorders, and various parasomnias (unusual behaviors of sleep) (Kushida et al., 2005). The **MSLT** is a daytime nap test used to objectively measure sleepiness in a sleep-conducive setting. PSG and MSLT performed on the day following PSG evaluation are routinely indicated in patients suspected of having narcolepsy. **MWT** evaluates a patient's ability to remain awake in a situation conducive to sleep and is used to document adequate alertness in individuals with careers for which sleepiness would pose a risk to public safety (Littner et al., 2005). **Actigraphy** involves using a wristwatch-type device that records body movement over a period of time and is helpful in evaluating sleep patterns and sleep duration. It is used in patients with circadian rhythm disorders and insomnia (Morgenthaler et al., 2007).

CLINICAL PICTURE

The *Diagnostic and Statistical Manual of Mental Disorders,* fourth edition, text revision *(DSM-IV-TR)* (APA, 2000) classifies **sleep disorders** into four major categories: primary sleep disorders, sleep disorders related to another mental disorder, sleep disorders related to a general medical condition, and substance-induced sleep disorders. Figure 20-3 presents the diagnostic criteria for various sleep disorders.

Primary Sleep Disorders

The primary sleep disorders are those not directly attributable to another medical, psychiatric, or substance abuse disorder. They are further subdivided into dyssomnias and parasomnias.

DSM-IV-TR Criteria for Primary Insomnia

A The predominant complaint is difficulty initiating or maintaining sleep, or nonrestorative sleep, for at least one month.

B The sleep disturbance (or associated daytime fatigue) causes clinically significant distress or impairment in social, occupational, or other important areas of functioning.

C The sleep disturbance does not occur exclusively during the course of narcolepsy, breathing-related sleep disorder, circadian rhythm sleep disorder, or parasomnia.

D The disturbance does not occur exclusively during the course of another mental disorder (e.g., major depressive disorder, generalized anxiety disorder, a delirium).

E The disturbance is not due to the direct physiological effects of a substance (e.g., a drug of abuse, a medication) or a general medical condition.

Figure 20-3 Diagnostic criteria for primary insomnia (Adapted from American Psychiatric Association. [2000]. *Diagnostic and statistical manual of mental disorders* [4th ed., text rev.]. Washington, DC: Author.)

Dyssomnias

Dyssomnias are sleep disturbances associated with the initiation and maintenance of sleep or of excessive sleepiness. Dyssomnias include primary insomnia, primary hypersomnia, narcolepsy, breathing-related sleep disorders such as obstructive sleep apnea, circadian rhythm disorders, and dyssomnias not otherwise specified (such as restless legs syndrome [RLS]). Because of its significant relationship to other psychiatric disorders, the focus here is on primary insomnia; however, a brief discussion of each of the other major dyssomnias is presented in Box 20-1, because there can be considerable overlap among these disorders and other psychiatric symptoms.

VIGNETTE

Kathy is a 32-year-old woman who was referred by her primary care provider for a psychiatric evaluation for

---

BOX 20-1 Dyssomnias

Primary Hypersomnia

Excessive sleepiness for at least 1 month, evidenced by either prolonged sleep episodes or daytime sleep episodes that occur almost daily and cause significant distress and social and vocational impairment. Key diagnostic features to this diagnosis are a report of continuous yet unrefreshing and non-restorative sleep and difficulty waking up, either in the morning or at the end of a nap. Some patients with this disorder can sleep up to 20 hours a day. Diagnosis is determined by clinical evaluation and PSG and MSLT. Treatment is through lifestyle modification and stimulant medication.

Narcolepsy

The classic tetrad of narcolepsy includes episodes of irresistible attacks of refreshing sleep, cataplexy (muscle weakness), sleep paralysis, and hypnagogic hallucinations. While all patients with narcolepsy report impairing degrees of excessive sleepiness, not all patients experience cataplexy, sleep paralysis, and hypnagogic hallucinations, making diagnosis sometimes difficult. Narcolepsy is distinguished from primary hypersomnia in that patients with narcolepsy generally feel refreshed upon awakening. Associated symptoms include disturbed nighttime sleep with multiple middle-of-the-night awakenings and automatic behaviors characterized by memory lapses. Diagnosis is determined by clinical evaluation and PSG and MSLT. Treatment is through lifestyle modifications and stimulant medication.

Breathing-Related Sleep Disorder

The most common disorder of breathing and sleeping is obstructive sleep apnea, which is characterized by repeated episodes of upper airway collapse and obstruction that result in sleep fragmentation. Essentially, patients with obstructive

sleep apnea are not able to sleep and breathe at the same time. Typical symptoms include loud, disruptive snoring, witnessed apnea episodes, and excessive daytime sleepiness. Obesity is an important risk factor for obstructive sleep apnea. Diagnosis is determined by clinical evaluation and PSG. Treatment is with continuous positive airway pressure (CPAP) therapy.

Circadian Rhythm Sleep Disorder

Persistent or recurrent pattern-of-sleep disruption resulting from altered function of the circadian timing system or from a mismatch between the individual's natural circadian sleep/wake cycle and external demands regarding the timing and duration of sleep, such as in those who do shift work or experience jet lag. Diagnosis is determined by clinical evaluation, sleep diaries, and actigraphy. Treatment is with aggressive lifestyle management strategies aimed at adapting to or modifying the required sleep schedule.

Restless Legs Syndrome (RLS)

A sensory and movement disorder characterized by an unpleasant, uncomfortable sensation in the legs (occasionally the arms and trunk are affected) accompanied by an urge to move. Symptoms begin or worsen during periods of inactivity and are relieved or reduced by physical activity such as walking, stretching, or flexing. Symptoms are worse in the evening and at bedtime and can have a significant impact on the individual's ability to fall asleep and stay asleep. Symptoms may be induced or exacerbated by serotonergic agents such as SSRIs or SNRIs. Diagnosis is determined by clinical evaluation. Many patients with RLS also have periodic limb movements of sleep that are observed during PSG. Treatment is through lifestyle modification and dopamine agonist therapy, such as pramipexole and ropinirole.

Adapted from American Psychiatric Association. (2000). *Diagnostic and statistical manual of mental disorders* (4th ed., text rev.). Washington, DC: Author.

complaints of anxiety and restlessness. She reported feeling fine during the day, but in the evening, she felt nervous and anxious. The symptoms always started at the same time. As soon as she would settle down for the evening to watch some television she would begin to have a restless sensation in her legs that would make her jump up and pace up and down. She described the sensation as having "soda pop fizzing through my veins." Sometimes she would go out for a walk at night even if it was very late in order to "calm down." These episodes began to occur almost nightly, and as a result, she was having difficulty getting a good night's sleep. She began to dread the approach of nightfall. A full clinical evaluation suggested the diagnosis of RLS, and a course of the dopamine agonist pramipexole was initiated in the evening, with dramatic improvement in her symptoms and total resolution of her sleep complaint. ▪

Primary Insomnia. Individuals who experience primary insomnia complain that they have difficulty with sleep initiation, sleep maintenance, early awakening, or non-refreshing non-restorative sleep. It is not usual for a patient to have a combination of complaints. According to the *DSM-IV-TR*, this condition must persist for 1 month and must not be related to any known physical or medical condition (see Figure 20-3). Key to the diagnosis is a report of some type of daytime consequence associated with the sleep disturbance, such as impaired social or vocational functioning, decreased concentration or memory impairment, somatic complaints, or mood disturbance.

Insomnia is best understood as a state of constant hyperarousal that involves biological, psychological, and social factors (IOM, 2006). In addition to a thorough medical, psychiatric, and substance use history, it is helpful to use Spielman's **3P model of insomnia** to comprehensively assess the causes of insomnia, suggest appropriate interventions, and provide rationales for treatment (Spielman & Glovinsky, 2004). This model suggests that there are three factors that contribute to the insomnia complaint: **predisposing, precipitating,** and **perpetuating factors**.

Predisposing factors are individual factors that create a vulnerability to insomnia. These may include a prior history of poor-quality sleep, history of depression and anxiety, or a state of hyperarousal. Patients at risk to develop insomnia may describe themselves as light sleepers and night owls. **Precipitating** factors are external events that trigger insomnia. Personal and vocational difficulties, medical and psychiatric disorders, grief, and changes in role or identity (as seen with retirement) are examples. **Perpetuating** factors are sleep practices and attributes that maintain the sleep complaint, such as excessive caffeine or alcohol use, spending excessive amounts of time in bed or napping, and worry about the consequences of insomnia (Spielman & Glovinsky, 2004).

Successful treatment of insomnia involves an integration of the basic principles of sleep hygiene

---

BOX 20-2 Sleep Hygiene

- Maintain a regular sleep/wake schedule.
- Develop a pre-sleep routine that signals the end of the day.
- Reserve the bedroom for sleep and a place for intimacy.
- Create an environment that is conducive to sleep (taking into consideration light, temperature, and clothing).
- Avoid clock watching.
- Limit caffeinated beverages to 1 or 2 a day and none in the evening.
- Avoid heavy meals before bedtime.
- Use alcohol cautiously, and avoid use for several hours before bed.
- Avoid daytime napping.
- Exercise daily but not right before bed.

Data from Epstein, L. (2007). *The Harvard Medical School guide to a good night's sleep.* New York: McGraw-Hill.

(conditions and practices that promote continuous and effective sleep) (Box 20-2), behavioral therapies, and in some instances, the use of hypnotic medication. Hypnotic medication is always used with caution, and over-the-counter sleeping aids have limited effectiveness. Melatonin, a naturally occurring hormone, is a popular over-the-counter nutraceutical, but there is little data to support its use in the management of insomnia (Integrative Therapy box).

Generally, long-term hypnotic use is discouraged because nonpharmacological treatments have shown efficacy in reducing insomnia. Table 20-1 provides information about hypnotics approved by the U.S. Food and Drug Administration (FDA) for treatment of insomnia. Many antidepressants and atypical antipsychotics are also used off-label (without specific approval from the FDA) for their sedative properties in the treatment of sleep disorders.

Cognitive-behavioral therapy for insomnia (CBT-I) includes educational, behavioral, and cognitive components; it targets factors that perpetuate insomnia over time (Morin, 2004). The first objectives are to provide education regarding sleep and sleep needs and help the patient to set realistic expectations regarding sleep. Patients should be asked what they believe constitutes healthy sleep and have any misconceptions clarified. Eliciting information about the total number of hours spent sleeping typically has little value. Many patients are stuck on a set number of sleep hours rather than on the quality of sleep obtained. Focusing on the number of hours slept rather than the quality of sleep and daytime functioning increases the insomnia experience.

The next approach involves modifying poor sleep habits and establishing a regular sleep/wake schedule. Sleep diaries (Figure 20-4) for a period of 2 weeks are helpful in establishing overall sleep patterns and

INTEGRATIVE THERAPY

Melatonin for Insomnia

Individuals with insomnia routinely turn to over-the-counter solutions. Melatonin is a hormone secreted by the pineal gland in response to information it receives from the suprachiasmatic nucleus regarding light and dark. It is available as a synthetic product at most health food stores and pharmacies. Normally, as night approaches, melatonin is secreted, and blood levels rise, producing a sensation of sleepiness. Melatonin levels stay elevated throughout the night but begin to decline in the early morning hours and are essentially undetectable during the day. It would stand to reason then that melatonin supplementation would be a safe and effective soporific.

Unfortunately, research into the role of melatonin in the management of insomnia has been disappointing, with most data pointing to little to no benefit at all. It does seem, however, that melatonin may be effective in the management of circadian rhythm disorders such as jet lag, shift work disorder, and advances and delays in the sleep cycle.

Although there have been no documented reports of toxicity or overdose of synthetic melatonin, it is important to tell patients that (1) there is no identified effective dosage range; and (2) because melatonin is available over the counter and unregulated by the FDA, there is no standardization of nutraceutical ingredients. Reported side effects include nausea, headache, and orthostatic blood pressure changes.

Passarell, S. and Duong, M. (2008). Diagnosis and treatment of insomnia. *American Journal of Health-Systems Pharmacy, 65*(10), 927–934; and U.S. Department of Health & Human Services, Agency for Healthcare Research and Quality. (2004). *Melatonin for treatment of sleep disorders*, Structured abstract. (AHRQ Publication No. 05-E002-1). Rockville, MD: Author. <http://www.ahrq.gov/clinic/tp/melatntp.htm>

TABLE 20-1 Drug Treatment of Patients With Insomnia

Generic (Brand) Name	Onset of Action (min)	Duration of Action	FDA-Approved for Insomnia	Habit Forming
BENZODIAZEPINES				
Estazolam	15-60	Intermediate	Yes	Yes, all drugs in this class are Schedule IV
Flurazepam	30-60	Long	Yes	
Quazepam (Doral)	20-45	Long	Yes	
Temazepam (Restoril)	45-60	Intermediate	Yes	
Triazolam (Halcion)	15-30	Short	Yes	
BENZODIAZEPINE-LIKE DRUGS				
Eszopiclone (Lunesta)	60	Intermediate	Yes	Yes, all drugs in this class are Schedule IV
Zaleplon (Sonata)	15-30	Ultra Short	Yes	
Zolpidem (Ambien)	30	Short	Yes	
MELATONIN RECEPTOR AGONIST				
Ramelteon (Rozerem)	30	Short	Yes	No
ANTIDEPRESSANT				
Trazodone (Desyrel)	60-120	Long	No	No
ANTIHISTAMINES				
Diphenhydramine (Nytol, Sominex)	60-180	Long	As a sleep aid	Tolerance to hypnotic effects develops in 1-2 weeks
Doxylamine (Unisom)	60-120	Long	As a sleep aid	

From Lehne, R. A. (2010) *Pharmacology for nursing care* (7th ed.). Philadelphia: Saunders; and Weilburg, J. B., Stakes, J. W., & Roth, T. (2008). Sleep disorders. In T. A. Stern, J. F. Rosenbaum, M. Fava, J. Biederman, & S. L. Rauch (Eds.), *Massachusetts General Hospital comprehensive clinical psychiatry* (pp. 285–301). St. Louis: Mosby.

Two-week sleep diary

INSTRUCTIONS:
1 Write the date, day of the week, and type of day: Work, School, Day off, or Vacation.
2 Put the letter "C" in the box when you have coffee, cola or tea. Put "M" when you take any medicine. Put "A" when you drink alcohol. Put "E" when you exercise.
3 Put a line (I) to show when you go to bed. Shade in the box that shows when you think you fell asleep.
4 Shade in all the boxes that show when you are asleep at night or when you take a nap during the day.
5 Leave boxes unshaded to show when you wake up at night and when you are awake during the day.

SAMPLE ENTRY BELOW: On a Monday when I worked, I jogged on my lunch break at 1 PM, had a glass of wine with dinner at 6 PM, fell asleep watching TV from 7 to 8 PM, went to bed at 10:30 PM, fell asleep around Midnight, woke up and couldn't get back to sleep at about 4 AM, went back to sleep from 5 to 7 AM, and had coffee and medicine at 7:00 in the morning.

Today's Date	Day of the week	Type of Day Work, School, Off, Vacation	Noon	1 PM	2	3	4	5	6 PM	7	8	9	10	11 PM	Midnight	1 AM	2	3	4	5	6 AM	7	8	9	10	11	
sample	Mon.	Work		E					A				I									C M					
																											Week 1
																											Week 2

Figure 20-4 Two-week sleep diary. (Modified from the American Academy of Sleep Medicine. <http://www.sleepeducation.com/pdf/sleepdiary.pdf>)

determining overall sleep efficiency ([total sleep time ÷ total time in bed] × 100). After reviewing sleep diaries, patients are sometimes surprised to discover that their sleep problems are not as bad as previously believed. **Sleep restriction** or limiting the total sleep time creates a temporary, mild state of sleep deprivation and strengthens the sleep homeostatic drive. This decreases sleep latency and improves sleep continuity and quality. If, for example, a patient's sleep diary indicates that they are in bed for 8 hours but only sleeping 6 hours, sleep is restricted to 6 hours, and the bed time and wake time are adjusted accordingly. The sleep time should not be reduced below 5 hours, regardless of sleep efficiency, and patients should be cautioned about the dangers of sleepiness with driving while undergoing a trial of sleep restriction. Once sleep efficiency is improved, total sleep time is gradually increased by 10- to 20-minute increments.

Stimulus control involves adherence to five basic principles that decrease the negative associations between the bed and bedroom and strengthen the stimulus for sleep. Patients should be instructed to:

1. Go to bed only when sleepy.
2. Use the bed or bedroom only for sleep and intimacy (no television, reading, or other activities in the bedroom).
3. Get out of bed if unable to sleep and engage in a quiet-time activity such as reading or crossword puzzles (no television, work, or computer).
4. Maintain a regular sleep/wake schedule, with getting up at the same time each day being the most important factor.
5. Avoid daytime napping (if napping is necessary to avoid accident or injury, it should be limited to 20 to 30 minutes maximum).

Other objectives of CBT-I are aimed at identifying and correcting maladaptive attitudes and beliefs about sleep that perpetuate insomnia. For example, patients frequently amplify the consequences of their insomnia and attribute most daytime experiences to their sleep complaint. They may rationalize maladaptive coping behaviors such as excessive time in bed to "catch up" on lost sleep and may exhibit unrealistic expectations about sleep. The practitioner offers alternative interpretations regarding the sleep complaint to assist the patient to think about his or her insomnia in a different way, empowering the patient to be in control of their sleep (Morin, 2004). Because CBT-I approaches are not immediately effective and may take several weeks of practice before improvement is seen, success is dependent on both a high degree of motivation in patients and a commitment on the part of the practitioner.

VIGNETTE

Josie Harris is a 52-year-old woman who complains of difficulty falling asleep and staying asleep every night. It is not unusual for Josie to take several hours to fall asleep, and once she does fall asleep she is only able to sleep for 2 to 3 hours at a time. She tosses and turns and lies in bed "hoping to fall asleep." She estimates that she is only sleeping about 4 or 5 hours a night. Josie reports that this has been going on for at least a year but it seems to be getting progressively worse over the last several months. Because she sleeps poorly at night, she has been staying in bed until 9 or 10 AM and has been late for work several times during the last month. She feels tired during her waking hours and has difficulty focusing on the task at hand in her accounting job. To improve her work performance, she has been drinking 5 or 6 cups of coffee during the day. Even though she feels tired, she is unable to nap. Family members complain that she is irritable and short-tempered with them. Interestingly, she reports that she was able to sleep fairly well while on vacation recently. Josie completes a sleep diary for a 2-week period and undergoes a complete assessment. Since there seems to be no underlying medical or psychiatric disorder associated with her sleep complaint, she is diagnosed with primary insomnia and begins a cognitive-behavioral therapy program. ■

Parasomnias

The **parasomnias** are characterized by unusual or undesirable behaviors or events that occur during sleep/wake transitions, certain stages of sleep, or during arousal from sleep (APA, 2000). Patients with parasomnia usually do not have a specific sleep-related complaint such as insomnia or daytime sleepiness. Frequently it is the sleep partner that reports the behavioral disturbance, highlighting the importance of obtaining independent verification of the nighttime behavior. A brief discussion of the most frequently encountered parasomnias is provided in Box 20-3.

VIGNETTE

An 80-year-old man with Parkinson's disease is referred to a sleep clinic by his primary care physician. The patient's wife became concerned when on several occasions, she awoke to find him shouting and thrashing in the bed. It appeared that he was acting out his dreams. The patient reported no memory of these events and had no particular sleep complaint. During one of these episodes, he knocked over the bedside lamp and struck her. When he was awoken, he reported that he was dreaming there was an intruder in the house, and he was attempting to save her. A PSG examination demonstrated an absence of the muscle atonia normally seen in REM sleep, confirming a diagnosis of REM sleep behavior disorder. He was treated with a low dose of a benzodiazepine and given instructions regarding personal and sleep partner safety. ■

BOX 20-3 Parasomnias

Nightmare Disorder

Characterized by long, frightening dreams from which people awaken scared. They almost always occur during rapid eye movement (REM) sleep and usually after a long REM period late in the night. For some people, this is a lifetime condition; for others nightmares occur at times of stress and illness. Diagnosis is determined by clinical evaluation. PSG is sometimes necessary to rule out the possibility of an underlying disorder of sleep fragmentation such as obstructive sleep apnea. Treatment is dependent on the frequency and severity of the symptoms, as well as the underlying cause. Treatment with hypnotic therapy is sometimes indicated. Many patients do well with lifestyle modification measures, attention to sleep hygiene, and stress reduction.

Sleepwalking

Also referred to as *somnambulism*. Consists of a sequence of complex behaviors that begin in the first third of the night during deep NREM sleep (stages 3 and 4) and usually progress (without full consciousness or later memory) to leaving bed and walking about (may include dressing, going to the bathroom, screaming, and even driving). Because of the possibility of accident or injury, somnambulism in adults should be evaluated by a sleep specialist. PSG is sometimes indicated to rule out the possibility of an underlying disorder of sleep fragmentation. Treatment consists of instructing the patient and family regarding safety measures such as alarms or locks on windows and doors and gating stairways. Attention to sleep hygiene, limiting alcohol prior to bed, obtaining adequate amounts of sleep, and stress reduction is helpful.

REM Sleep Behavior Disorder (RSBD)

Characterized by absence of muscle atonia during sleep. Patients with this disorder display elaborate motor activity associated with dream mentation. These patients are actually acting out their dreams. RSBD is most frequently seen in elderly men but can be seen as the heralding symptom of neurological pathology such as Parkinson's disease. Serotonergic medications (such as SSRIs or SNRIs) can induce or exacerbate episodes. Diagnosis is determined by clinical evaluation and PSG with video recording. Treatment focuses on patient and sleep partner safety. Placing the mattress on the floor is sometimes necessary to prevent injury as a result of falling out of bed. The use of intermediate-acting benzodiazepine can be helpful, especially in cases of severe disruption to the sleep partner and concerns about safety.

Sleep Paralysis

The sensation of paralysis at sleep onset or upon awakening. The patient describes a complete awareness of their surroundings but is unable to move. For many patients, sleep paralysis is associated with extreme anxiety and even panic. For a number of patients, these events are rare or isolated and do not require any long-term treatment. Reassurance that the sensation is harmless and temporary is helpful. For those individuals with more frequent or severe episodes, further evaluation and treatment by a sleep specialist is warranted. Because sleep paralysis can be seen in patients with narcolepsy, screening for this sleep disorder is indicated.

Data from American Psychiatric Association. (2000). *Diagnostic and statistical manual of mental disorders* (4th ed., text rev.). Washington, DC: Author.

Sleep Disorders Related to Other Mental Disorders

There are two distinct classifications of sleep disorders associated with major mental disorders: *insomnia related to another mental disorder* (axis I or axis II) and *hypersomnia related to another mental disorder* (axis 1 or axis II). An additional diagnosis of a sleep disorder is made when the sleep disturbance is sufficiently severe to warrant independent clinical attention (APA, 2000). Patients with this type of insomnia or hypersomnia tend to focus on their sleep and ignore the symptoms of the related mental disorder, even to the point of denying that they have a mental disorder. It is not unusual for patients to present to a sleep disorders center for a sleep evaluation and later be diagnosed with a primary psychiatric disorder. For example, patients with major depressive disorder frequently experience insomnia that involves relatively normal sleep onset followed by repeated awakenings during the second half of the night and early-morning awakening. This is usually followed by a difficult mood in the morning. Patients point to the sleep disruption as the cause of the mood disturbance and report that if they could just get a good night's sleep, the mood symptoms would improve.

Difficulty with sleep latency is common with all anxiety disorders, and it is not usual for patients with a previously undiagnosed anxiety disorder to present for treatment of an insomnia complaint of lifelong duration. Management of the underlying anxiety diagnosis in conjunction with the insomnia complaint results in the best clinical outcome. Finally, patients with schizophrenia have prolonged sleep latencies, sleep fragmentation, and multiple middle-of-the-night awakenings. Poor health habits such as excessive caffeine use, smoking, and inattention to a regular sleep schedule contribute to sleep complaints. As a result of many of the medications used to treat schizophrenia, these patients are at increased risk for the development of obstructive sleep apnea due to weight gain.

VIGNETTE

Sarah had been living with treatment-resistant schizophrenia for many years. Despite multiple medication trials, she had poor control of her symptoms and was frequently hospitalized. Last year she was started on clozapine; within a few months, she had a dramatic reduction in her command hallucinations and total resolution of paranoid delusions. Her family was thrilled. She was finally working and living in a group home. Over the last few months, however, the group home staff have noticed a change in Sarah's sleep patterns. She frequently wakes during the night and in the morning complains of a headache and a sore throat. When she returns home from work in the afternoon, it is not unusual for her to take a nap for 60 minutes or longer. In addition, the group home staff express concern that she has gained over 40 lbs in the last year and feel she is out of shape. They have been trying to get her motivated to exercise, but she complains of feeling too tired. While home on a family visit, her mother noted loud snoring and discussed this with the psychiatrist. A PSG was performed, which demonstrated a severe degree of obstructive sleep apnea, most likely related to her recent weight gain. Continuous positive airway pressure (CPAP) therapy was initiated, and she was able to return to her baseline level of functioning. ◼

Hypersomnia related to another mental disorder is seen in many mental conditions, including mood disorders. Many patients report excessive daytime sleepiness in the beginning stages of a mild depressive disorder. A similar complaint is characteristic of the depressed phase of bipolar I disorder. Uncomplicated grief may temporarily be associated with hypersomnia. Personality disorders, dissociative disorders, somatoform disorders, and dissociative fugue are all associated with hypersomnia. Generally speaking, treatment is directed at the primary disorder (APA, 2000; Sadock & Sadock, 2008).

Other Sleep Disorders

The last two categories of sleep disorders include *sleep disorders due to a general medical condition* and *substance-induced sleep disorders*. In both of these disorders, the sleep disturbance may be insomnia, hypersomnia, parasomnia, or a combination.

Many medical conditions are associated with insomnia. For instance, conditions accompanied by pain and discomfort, such as arthritis and cardiovascular and pulmonary disease, are frequently associated with insomnia. Insomnia is also associated with neoplasms, vascular lesions, infections, and degenerative

and traumatic conditions. Chronic fatigue syndrome and hypothyroidism have been associated with hypersomnia. The relationship between chronic medical disorders and sleep disturbance highlights the importance of screening patients with medical disorders for sleep complaints. The treatment is directed at the underlying medical condition (APA, 2000; Sadock & Sadock, 2008).

VIGNETTE

Robbie Carson is a student nurse assigned to Mrs. Viatelli in a nursing home. Robbie is in his psychiatric nursing rotation, part of which is spent in a skilled nursing facility taking care of patients with dementia. When Robbie receives the report in the morning, he learns that Mrs. Viatelli has been experiencing significant sleep disturbance. She seems to have difficulty falling asleep and frequently wakes up groaning during the night. Robbie notes that Mrs. Viatelli is very confused, as well as agitated. She grimaces whenever she moves. Robbie believes Mrs. Viatelli is in pain. He checks the patient's history to find that she has had arthritis for many years. He then checks her medication profile and discovers that Mrs. Viatelli is not on any pain medication for her arthritis. He speaks to the charge nurse, who calls the physician. Immediately, the physician orders acetaminophen at bedtime for Mrs. Viatelli. Over the next few days, not only is there a dramatic improvement in Mrs. Viatelli's sleep, but her confusion abates, and the agitation disappears. ◼

A substance-induced sleep disorder can result from the use or recent discontinuance of a substance or medication. While it is quite obvious that many prescriptions and over the counter medications may affect sleep, there is less appreciation for the effects of commonly used substances on sleep. Alcohol, nicotine, and caffeine all have an impact on sleep quantity and quality. **Alcohol**—despite its great soporific effects—decreases deep sleep (stage 3 and 4) and REM sleep and is responsible for middle-of-the-night awakenings with difficulty returning to sleep. **Nicotine** is a central nervous system stimulant, increasing heart rate, blood pressure, and respiratory rate. As nicotine levels decline through the night, patients wake in response to mild withdrawal symptoms. **Caffeine** blocks the neurotransmitter adenosine, promoting wakefulness. It increases sleep latency, reduces slow wave sleep, and acts as a diuretic, causing middle-of-the-night awakening for urination (Epstein, 2007).

EPIDEMIOLOGY

Sleep-related problems are highly prevalent and occur across all age groups, cultures, and genders. An estimated 50 to 70 million Americans suffer from a chronic disorder of sleep and wakefulness (National Heart,

Lung, and Blood Institute, 2003). Obstructive sleep apnea, a disorder of breathing and sleeping, affects 4% of middle-aged men and 2% of middle-aged women (Young et al., 1993). Shift work disorder, a misalignment of the normal sleep/wake pattern to accommodate vocational demands, affects up to 32% of night workers and 26% of rotating workers (Sack et al., 2007). Chronic insomnia, the most common sleep disturbance, affects 10% to 15% of the population, with 85% to 90% of chronic insomnia being attributable to comorbid psychiatric and medical disorders, substance use, or medication effect (Ohayon, 2002).

COMORBIDITY

Multiple studies suggest that sleeping less than 7 hours per night may have a significant impact on cardiovascular, endocrine, immune, and neurological function (IOM, 2006). Short sleep duration has been associated with obesity, cardiovascular disease and hypertension, and impaired glucose tolerance and diabetes (Hasler et al., 2004; Gottlieb et al., 2005; Gottlieb et al., 2006).

Many sleep disorders increase the risk for the development of certain medical conditions. For example, obstructive sleep apnea has been associated with hypertension, diabetes, cardiovascular disease, and stroke (Tracova et al., 2008). Individuals with neurological disease, such as Alzheimer's and Parkinson's disease, frequently experience sleep disturbance that worsens with the progression of the illness. Sleep disturbance is a major factor contributing to nursing-home placement in patients with dementia.

Most psychiatric disorders are associated with sleep disturbance. Insomnia is the most frequent complaint, but reports of hypersomnia are also common. About 85% of patients with a major mood disorder will report some type of a sleep disturbance over the course of the illness. In addition, there is evidence to demonstrate that sleep disruption itself may be a precipitating factor in triggering mood and other psychiatric disorders and increases the risk to relapse, making the identification and management of sleep disturbance in patients with affective disorders critical (Ohayon & Roth, 2003). Of special concern is that

EVIDENCE-BASED PRACTICE

Sleep and Sociocultural Factors

Lauderdale, D., Knutson, K., Yan, L., Rathouz, P., Hulley, S., Sidney, S., & Liu, K. (2006). Objectively measured sleep characteristics among early-middle-aged adults: The CARDIA study. *American Journal of Epidemiology, 164*(1), 5–16.

Problem
Little is known about the associations among sleep and socioeconomic status, gender, race, and health.

Purpose of Study
The authors of this study proposed to examine whether time in bed, sleep latency, total sleep duration, and sleep efficiency vary by gender, race, demographic, socioeconomic, employment, household, and lifestyle (smoking, alcohol, physical activity) factors.

Methods
The authors use wrist actigraphy and sleep logs over 3 nights to measure time in bed, sleep latency, total sleep duration, and sleep efficiency in 669 middle age adults (ages 38 to 50) who were participating at one of the four Coronary Artery Risk Development in Young Adults (CARDIA) study sites. Of the participants, 30% were Caucasian women, 26% Caucasian men, 28% African American women, and 16% African American men.

Key Findings
- Self-reported sleep duration was greater than actigraphic determined sleep.

- African American men had significantly less total sleep time (5.1 hours a night) than Caucasian women (6.7 hours per night).
- Increased levels of income were associated with shorter sleep latency, longer sleep duration, and greater sleep efficiency.
- Not unexpectedly, alcohol and smoking were associated with longer sleep latency and less sleep efficiency.

Implications for Nursing Practice
Nurses play a key role in identifying individuals at increased risk for illness, accident, and injury. Self-reported sleep may be underestimated, so nurses should use available clinical tools such as sleep diaries to help patients accurately estimate total sleep time. In addition, recognition that gender, race, and socioeconomic status may play a role in sleep quality and quantity has important implications for both nursing assessment and treatment planning. Interventions aimed at identifying and intervening with vulnerable populations may improve long-term health outcomes. The need to identify patients at risk for sleep disturbance secondary to alcohol and tobacco use is clear.

depressed patients who experience a sleep disturbance demonstrate greater degrees of suicidal ideation (Chellappa & Araujo, 2007). Sleep disturbance is common in patients with alcoholism, and insomnia occurs in 36% to 72% of patients in early recovery and persists for months or even years. Sleep disturbance increases the risk for relapse to alcohol abuse. Targeting sleep disturbance during recovery may support continued abstinence (Arnedt et al., 2007).

APPLICATION OF THE NURSING PROCESS

Regardless of the clinical environment or the presenting complaint, all patients can benefit from an evaluation of their sleep. Assessment of the patient's sleep allows the nurse to identify short- and long-term health risks associated with sleep disorders and sleep deprivation, provide health teaching and counseling regarding sleep needs, and improve clinical outcomes in patients experiencing a sleep disturbance.

ASSESSMENT

General Assessment

Sleep Patterns

Patients frequently do not report sleep difficulties or discuss their sleep-related concerns with care providers. People tend to minimize or adapt to the consequences of sleep disturbance. Furthermore, there is a lack of appreciation about the impact sleep disturbance and sleep deprivation has on overall functioning and health. Many patients do not complain of sleep disturbance directly, but rather complain of associated symptoms such as fatigue, decreased concentration, mood disturbance, or physical ailments.

In assessing the patient with a sleep complaint, it is important to recognize the 24-hour nature of the sleep disturbance. Sleep disturbance is not confined to the 7 or 8 hours devoted to sleep. Sleep diaries (see Figure 20-4) are helpful in identifying sleep patterns and behaviors that may be contributing to the sleep complaint. Assigning the patient the homework of completing a sleep diary for 2 weeks will help guide the assessment and direct the plan of care. The following questions and comments provide direction for the assessment:

- When did you begin having trouble with sleep? Have you had trouble with sleep in the past?
- Describe your pre-bedtime routine. What are the activities you customarily engage in before sleep?
- Describe your sleeping environment. Are there things in your sleep environment that are ham-

pering your sleep (such as noise, light, temperature, overall comfort)?
- Do you use your bedroom for things other than sleep or sexual activity (such as working, eating, or watching television)?
- What time do you go to bed? How long does it take to fall asleep?
- Once asleep, are you disturbed by middle-of-the-night awakening? If so, what wakes you up? Are you able to return to sleep?
- If you are unable to sleep, what do you do?
- What time do you wake up? What time do you get out of bed?
- How much time do you actually think you sleep?
- Do you sleep longer on weekends or days off?
- Do you nap? Is so, for how long? Do you feel refreshed after napping?
- Can you identify any stress or problem that may have initially contributed to your sleep difficulties? Is there any particular issue or problem troubling you now?
- How have you dealt with that stress or problem?
- Tell me about your daily habits. I am interested in your diet, exercise, and medications you take. I am interested in whether or not you smoke or drink caffeinated or alcoholic beverages.
- Can you describe for me the thoughts you experience when you are lying in bed unable to get to sleep?
- What changes if any have you made to improve your sleep? What were the results?

Identifying Sleep Disorders

It is helpful to think about sleep disorders according to the predominant symptoms of insomnia, hypersomnia, parasomnia, and circadian rhythm disturbance (see Boxes 20-1 and 20-3). Box 20-4 provides pertinent screening questions for each diagnosis. An affirmative answer to any of these questions demands further investigation and evaluation.

Functioning and Safety

As previously described, sleep disturbance can result in increased risk for accident and injury and impose serious limitations on quality of life. Several screening tools are available to assist the clinician in evaluating sleep quality and the safety risk associated with ES. The Pittsburgh Sleep Quality Index (PSQI) is a subjective measure of sleep quality. A global sum of 5 or greater indicates poor quality and patterns of sleep (Buysse et al., 1989). The Epworth Sleepiness Scale (ESS) is a validated psychometric tool used to measure subject reports of sleepiness and has been validated by objective measures using the MSLT. Scores of less than 10 are considered normal, 10 to 15 is moderately sleepy, and greater than 15 is excessively sleepy. In addition to

BOX 20-4 Primary Symptoms of Sleep Disorders Screening Questions

Insomnia

- Do you have difficulty falling asleep, staying asleep, or early-morning awakenings?
- Do you feel unrefreshed and unrestored in the morning?
- Have you noticed any problems with your energy, mood, concentration, or work quality as a result of your sleep problem?

Hypersomnia

- Have you ever been told that you snore or that it looks like you stop breathing in your sleep? (Obstructive sleep apnea)
- Do you have an unpleasant or uncomfortable sensation in your legs (or arms) that prevents you from sleeping or wakes you up from sleep and makes you want to move? (RLS)
- Do you have episodes of sleepiness you cannot control? (Narcolepsy)
- Do you ever feel unrested even after an extended sleep period? (Primary hypersomnia)

Parasomnia

- Have you ever been told that you have done anything unusual in your sleep, such as walking or talking? (Somnambulism/somliquoly)
- Have you ever been told that you act out your dreams? (REM sleep behavior disorder)
- Have you ever had an unusual experience associated with sleep, such as the inability to move upon awakening or falling asleep? (Sleep paralysis)

Sleep/Wake Schedule Disturbance

- Is your desired sleep schedule in conflict with your social and vocational goals? What is your preferred sleep schedule? (Circadian rhythm disturbance)

these screening tools, the following questions provide direction for further assessment:

- Have you had an accident or injury as a result of sleepiness?
- Are you sleepy when you drive a car? What do you do if you are sleepy while driving?
- What kind of work do you do? Do you operate heavy equipment or machinery? How many hours a week do you work? How long is your commute?
- How does your sleep disturbance affect your work performance?
- Do you avoid social obligations as a result of your sleep problems?
- Do you feel like your sleep disturbance is affecting your physical health? How so?

Self-Assessment

Nurses are especially venerable to the effects of sleep deprivation and sleep disruption. Rotating shifts and night work result in circadian rhythm disruption that can cause problems with insomnia and excessive sleepiness. Long shifts and working overtime may lead to a decrease in total available sleep time. Inadequate sleep time and sleep quality have been shown to impair performance and judgment, both of which may affect patient safety and quality of care. In addition, nurses who work rotating or night shifts may pose an increased risk for accident or injury to self and the community as a result of excessive sleepiness while driving.

Nurses need to be able to recognize the effects of chronic partial sleep deprivation on their performance and functioning and take measures to assure that they are well rested and able to provide safe and competent care. Self-evaluation for a possible sleep disorder and ability to cope with the rigors of shift work is warranted. Consultation with a sleep professional is indicated if there is significant disruption to sleep, physical and mental health, job performance, job satisfaction, and social functioning. Attention to issues of sleep hygiene, limiting overtime, limiting shift work to 8 hours, and obtaining 7 to 8 hours of sleep within a 24-hour period are essential for personal, patient, and community safety.

DIAGNOSIS

There are three specific North American Nursing Diagnosis Association International (NANDA-I) nursing diagnoses for sleep disturbance (2009):

1. *Sleep deprivation*—prolonged periods of time without sleep
2. *Insomnia*—a disruption in amount and quality of sleep that impairs functioning
3. *Readiness for enhanced sleep*—a pattern of natural, periodic suspension of consciousness that provides adequate rest, sustains a desired lifestyle, and can be strengthened

OUTCOMES IDENTIFICATION

The *Nursing Outcomes Classification (NOC)* (Moorhead et al., 2008) identifies several appropriate outcomes for the patient experiencing sleep disruption, including *Sleep, Rest, Risk control,* and *Personal well-being.* Table 20-2 provides selected intermediate and short-term indicators for these categories.

PLANNING

The majority of patients with sleep disorders are treated in the community. The exceptions are cases in which the patient has a primary psychiatric disorder or a medical

TABLE 20-2 *NOC* Outcomes for Sleep Disturbances

Nursing Outcome and Definition	Intermediate Indicators	Short-Term Indicators
Sleep: Natural periodic suspension of consciousness during which the body is restored	Sleeps through the night consistently Sleep pattern Sleep quality	Hours of sleep Sleep routine Wakefulness at appropriate times
Rest: Quantity and pattern of diminished activity for mental and physical rejuvenation	Physically rested Emotionally rested Mentally rested Energy restored after rest	Amount of rest Rest pattern Rest quality Rested appearance
Risk Control: Personal actions to prevent, eliminate or reduce modifiable health risks	Acknowledges risk factors Modifies lifestyle to reduce risk factors	Develops effect risk control strategies Commits to risk control strategies
Personal Well-Being: Extent of positive perception of one's health status and life circumstances	Spiritual life Physical health Cognitive function	Performance of activities of daily living Performance of usual roles

Data from Moorhead, S., Johnson, M., Maas, M., & Swanson, E. (2008). *Nursing outcomes classification (NOC)* (4th ed.). St. Louis: Mosby.

condition that requires hospitalization. Because long-standing sleep problems are associated with a host of occupational, social, interpersonal, psychiatric, and medical conditions, the treatment is multifaceted and frequently requires a team approach under the leadership of a sleep disorder specialist. The role of the nurse is generally to conduct a full assessment, provide support to the patient and family while the appropriate interventions are determined, and teach the patient and family strategies that may improve sleep.

IMPLEMENTATION

Counseling

The nurse's counseling role begins with the assessment of the sleep disorder. The nurse's questions and responses provide support to the patient and family, as well as assurance that the sleep problems are amenable to treatment. For many patients, the distress caused by chronic sleep difficulties sets up a conditioned barrier of hopelessness. Through the nurse's counseling approach, this hopelessness is identified and countered with encouragement, positive suggestions, and the belief that the patient will be able to manage sleep difficulties.

Health Teaching and Health Promotion

The nurse's role in health teaching cannot be overemphasized. Most individuals do not think about their sleep. This means that they also do not recognize the importance of a sleep routine or consider factors that influence good sleep. In addition, there are many myths regarding what constitutes "good sleep" and what factors contribute to sleep quality (see Box 20-2). The nurse may also be involved in teaching relaxation techniques such as meditation, guided imagery, progressive muscle relaxation, or controlled breathing exercises. Use of these techniques has been linked to sustained benefits for patients with primary insomnia (Sadock & Sadock, 2008).

Pharmacological Interventions

Many patients use medication to address their sleep problems. Nurses frequently provide education about the benefits of a particular drug, the side effects, untoward effects, and the fact that medications are usually prescribed for no more than 2 weeks, because tolerance and withdrawal may result (Sadock & Sadock, 2008). In many settings, the nurse also monitors the effectiveness of the medication.

Advanced Practice Interventions

Although psychotherapy offers little value in the treatment of primary insomnia, there is a component of primary insomnia that involves a conditioned response. The initial episode of insomnia is frequently associated with a stressful event or crisis that produces anxiety. This anxiety becomes associated with worry about not being able to get to sleep and leads to preoccupation with getting enough sleep. The more the patient tries to sleep, the more elusive sleep becomes and the greater the patient's experienced anxiety. The advanced practice nurse may be closely involved in the use of cognitive-behavioral therapy to manage insomnia.

EVALUATION

Evaluation is based on whether or not the patient experiences improved sleep quality as evidenced by decreased sleep latency, fewer nighttime awakenings, and a shorter time to get back to sleep after awakening. This evaluation is accomplished through patient report and patient maintenance of a sleep diary. Just as important as objective changes in the patient's sleep pattern is the patient's perception that there has been an improvement. Objectively, the improvement may be quite modest, but the patient may perceive that he or she is no longer *controlled by* sleep (or the lack of it) but exerting *control over* sleep through lifestyle changes and a better sleep routine.

KEY POINTS TO REMEMBER

- Sleep disturbance has major implications for overall health, quality of life, and personal and community safety.
- Research into the physiology of normal sleep, as well as sleep disorders, is expanding.
- Most patients with a mood disorder will report sleep disturbance; recognition and treatment of sleep disturbance in patients with psychiatric disorders improves clinical outcomes.
- Regardless of the clinical environment or the presenting complaint, all patients can benefit from an evaluation of their sleep needs.
- It is helpful to categorize sleep disturbance according to the four major symptom categories of insomnia, hypersomnia, circadian rhythm disturbance, and parasomnia.
- Primary insomnia can be effectively treated with nonpharmacological interventions such as CBT-I, sleep restriction, stimulus control and attention to issues of sleep hygiene. Long-term pharmacological management is generally not indicated.

CRITICAL THINKING

1. Anthony is a 46-year-old who complains of waking frequently at night. Consequently, he is tired all day and knows that he has not been functioning as well as he should. Whenever he can manage it, he goes out to his car at lunchtime to take a 60-minute nap, because he has fallen asleep at his desk and been given a disciplinary warning. He is drinking 2 to 3 cups of coffee in the afternoon so that he does not feel sleepy while driving home.
   A. What questions would you ask to determine if Anthony might have a sleep disorder?
   B. What recommendations will you make to improve his sleep hygiene?
   C. What instructions and education should you give this patient regarding personal and community safety?

2. Your patient, Vivian, has been using temazepam (Restoril) for several years to treat insomnia. She has been reading that long-term use of hypnotics is not healthy or productive and wants to quit taking them. However, she is focused on needing nine hours of sleep each night and is extremely worried about what will happen when she quits the temazepam.
   A. What instructions would you provide to Vivian regarding stimulus control, sleep restriction, and cognitive restructuring of her sleep complaint?
   B. Identify alternative pharmacological therapies.

3. Mrs. Levine is a 72-year-old woman with a history of major depression. She takes fluoxetine (Prozac) 10 mg every day and has experienced significant relief from depression. While reviewing her medications, she tells you she is using a variety of over-the-counter (OTC) sleep aids because she has been having some difficulty sleeping recently. These OTC products include diphenhydramine, melatonin, valerian, and something that her neighbor gave her to try.
   A. In light of the patient's age and history of depression, what are your concerns?
   B. What further assessment is required?
   C. What specific question would you need to ask concerning her use of Prozac?
   D. What instructions and education will you provide?

CHAPTER REVIEW

1. A patient states that he only needs 6 hours of sleep per night to feel rested. How should the nurse interpret this statement?
   1. The patient is not sleeping enough.
   2. The patient is sleeping too much.
   3. The patient is sleeping according to his own body's needs.
   4. The patient is not getting enough REM sleep.

2. The nurse is planning care for a patient with primary insomnia. What is an appropriate outcome?
   1. The patient will sleep 12 hours nightly.
   2. The patient will go to bed and wake up at consistent times daily.
   3. The patient will take one nap daily to restore energy.
   4. The patient will drink a warm cup of tea before bedtime.

3. The nurse is providing teaching for a patient who has been taking a hypnotic medication to sleep. What statement by the nurse is appropriate?
   1. "You can use this medication for as long as you would like."
   2. "It would be better to take an over-the-counter medication instead."
   3. "Melatonin has been shown to be just as effective as hypnotic medications."
   4. "Be certain to follow up with your doctor regularly while you take this medication."

4. Which condition should the nurse assess for in a patient with hypothyroidism?
   1. Hypersomnia
   2. Parasomnia
   3. Insomnia
   4. A combination of insomnia and parasomnia

5. Which patient behavior would alert the nurse to a circadian rhythm sleep disorder?

1. Excessive sleepiness for at least 1 month, accompanied by prolonged sleep episodes
2. Multiple episodes of brief daytime sleeping followed by disturbed nighttime sleep
3. Persistent patterns of sleep disruption after traveling for business
4. Repeated episodes of upper airway collapse and obstruction that results in sleep fragmentation

---

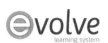

Visit the Evolve website for an **Audio Chapter Summary, Chapter Review Answers & Rationales, Critical Thinking Answer Guidelines**, and additional resources related to the content in this chapter: **http://evolve.elsevier.com/Varcarolis/foundations**

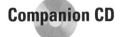

Use the Companion CD to prepare for tests and the NCLEX® Examination with **Test-Taking Strategies** for psychiatric mental health nursing and hundreds of **Review Questions**.

References

American Academy of Sleep Medicine (AASM). (2005). *The international classification of sleep disorders (ICSD)* (2nd ed.). Westchester, IL: American Academy of Sleep Medicine.

American Psychiatric Association. (2000). *Diagnostic and statistical manual of mental disorders* (4th ed., text rev.) *(DSM-IV-TR)*. Washington, DC: Author.

Arnedt, J. T., Conroy, D. A., & Bower, K. J. (2007). Treatment options for sleep disturbance during alcohol recovery. *Journal of Addictive Diseases, 26*(4), 41–54.

Basner, M., Fomberstein, K., Razavi, F., Banks, S., William, J., Rosa, R., et al. (2007). American Time Use Survey: Sleep time and its relationship to waking activities. *Sleep, 30,* 1085–1095.

Bliwise, D. (2005). Normal aging. In M. Kryger, T. Roth, & W. Dement (Eds.), *Principles and practice of sleep medicine* (4th ed.). Philadelphia: Saunders.

Bonnet, M. (2005). Acute sleep deprivation. In M. Kryger, T. Roth, & W. Dement (Eds.), *Principles and practice of sleep medicine* (4th ed.). Philadelphia: Saunders.

Buysse, D. J., Reynolds, C. F., 3rd, Monk, T. H., Berman, S. R., & Kupfer, D. J. (1989). The Pittsburgh Sleep Quality Index: A new instrument for psychiatric practice and research. *Psychiatry Research, 28*(2), 193–213.

Carskadon, M., & Dement, W. (2005). Normal human sleep: An overview. In M. Kryger, T. Roth, & W. Dement (Eds.), *Principles and practice of sleep medicine* (4th ed.) Philadelphia: Saunders.

Centers for Disease Control and Prevention. (2008). Perceived insufficient rest or sleep—four states, 2006. *Morbidity and Mortality Weekly Report, 57*(8), 200–203. Retrieved September 11, 2008 from http://www.cdc.gov/mmwr/preview/mmwrhtml/mm5708a2.htm

Chellappa, S. L., & Araujo, J. F. (2007). Sleep disorders and suicidal ideation in patients with depressive disorder. *Psychiatry Research, 153*(2), 131–136.

Czeisler, C., Buxton, O., & Khalsa, S. (2005). The human circadian system and sleep-wake regulation. In M. Kryger, T. Roth, & W. Dement (Eds.), *Principles and practice of sleep medicine* (4th ed., pp. 136–154). Philadelphia: Saunders.

Dinges, D., Borger, N., & Baynard, M. (2005). Chronic sleep restriction. In M. Kryger, T. Roth, & W. Dement (Eds.), *Principles and practice of sleep medicine* (4th ed.). Philadelphia: Saunders.

Epstein, L. (2007). *The Harvard Medical School guide to a good night's sleep.* New York: McGraw-Hill.

Gottlieb, D. J., Punjabi, N. M., Newman, A. B., Resnick, H. E., Redline, S., Baldwin, C. M., et al. (2005). Association of sleep time with diabetes mellitus and impaired glucose tolerance. *Archives of Internal Medicine, 165,* 863–867.

Gottlieb, D. J., Redline, S., Nieto, F. J., Baldwin, C. M., Newman, A. B., Resnick, H. E., et al. (2006). Association of usual sleep duration with hypertension: the sleep heart health study. *Sleep, 29,* 1009–1014.

Hasler, G., Buysse, D. J., Klaghoffer, R., Gamma, A., Ajdacic, V., Eich, D., et al. (2004). The association between short sleep duration and obesity in young adults: a 13-year prospective study. *Sleep, 27,* 661–666.

Health Care Strategic Management. (2001). Sleep disorders create growing opportunities for hospitals. *Health Care Strategic Management, 19*(2), 16–17.

Institute of Medicine. (2006). *Sleep disorders and sleep deprivation: An unmet public health problem.* Washington, DC: The National Academies Press.

Kushida, C., Littner, M., Morgenthaler, T., Alessi, C., Bailey, D., Coleman, J., et al. (2005). Practice parameters for the indications for polysomnography and related procedures. *Sleep, 28,* 499–521.

Littner, M., Kushida, C., Wise, M., Davila, D., Morgenthaler, T., Lee-Chiong, T., et al. (2005). Practice parameters for clinical use of the multiple sleep latency test and maintenance of wakefulness test. *Sleep, 28*(1), 113–121.

Moorhead, S., Johnson, M., Maas, M., & Swanson, E. (Eds.). (2008). *Nursing outcomes classification (NOC)* (4th ed.). St. Louis: Mosby.

Morgenthaler, T., Alessi, C., Friedman, L., Owens, J., Kapur, V., Boehlecke, B., et al. (2007). Practice parameters for the use of actigraphy in the assessment of sleep and sleep disorders: An update for 2007. *Sleep, 30,* 519–529.

Morin, C. (2004). Cognitive-behavioral approaches to the treatment of insomnia. *Journal of Clinical Psychiatry, 65*(Suppl. 16), 33–40.

National Heart Lung and Blood Institute. (2003). *National sleep disorders research plan, 2003.* Bethesda, MD: National Institutes of Health.

National Highway Traffic and Safety Administration. (2008). *Drowsy driving and automobile crashes: NCSDR and NHTSA expert panel on driver fatigue and sleepiness.* Retrieved September 12, 2008 from http://www.nhtsa.dot.gov/people/injury/drowsy_driving1/drowsy.html

National Sleep Foundation. (2008). *Sleep in America Poll: Summary of findings.* Retrieved September 11, 2008 from http://www.sleepfoundation.org/atf/cf/{f6bf2668-a1b4-4fe8-8d1a-a5d39340d9cb}/2008%20POLL%20SOF.PDF

North American Nursing Diagnosis Association International (NANDA-I). (2009). *NANDA-I nursing diagnoses: Definitions and classification 2009-2011.* Oxford, United Kingdom: Author.

Ohayon, M. (2002). Epidemiology of insomnia: What we know and what we still need to learn. *Sleep Medicine Reviews, 6*(2), 97–111.

Ohayon, M., & Roth, T. (2003). Place of chronic insomnia in the course of depression and anxiety disorders. *Journal of Psychiatric Research, 37*(1), 9–15.

Sack, R., Auckley, D., Auger, R., Carskadon, M., Wright, K., & Vitiello, M. (2007). Circadian rhythms sleep disorders: Part I, basic principles, shift work and jet lag disorders. *Sleep, 30*(11), 1460–1524.

Sadock, B. J., & Sadock, A. (2008). *Kaplan & Sadock's concise textbook of clinical psychiatry* (3rd ed.). Philadelphia: Lippincott Williams & Wilkins.

Siegel, J. (2004). The neurotransmitters of sleep. *Journal of Clinical Psychiatry, 65*(Suppl. 16), 4–7.

Sorscher, A. (2008). How is your sleep: A neglected topic for health care screening. *Journal of the American Board of Family Medicine, 21*(2), 141–148.

Strine, T. W., & Chapman, D. P. (2005). Association of frequent sleep insufficiency with health-related quality of life and health behaviors. *Sleep Medicine, 6*(1), 23–27.

Tracova, R., Dorkova, Z., Molcanyiova, A., Radikova, Z., Klimes, I., & Tkac, I. (2008). Cardiovascular risk and insulin resistance in patients with obstructive sleep apnea. *Medical Science Monitor, 14*(9), CR438–CR444.

Spielman, A., & Glovinsky, P. (2004). A conceptual framework of insomnia for primary care providers: Predisposing, precipitating, and perpetuating factors. *Sleep Medicine Alert, 9*(1), 1–6.

Walsh, J. K. (2004). Clinical and socioeconomic correlates of insomnia. *Journal of Clinical Psychiatry, 65*(Suppl. 8), 13–29.

Williamson, A. M., & Feyer, A. M. (2007). Moderate sleep deprivation produces impairments in cognitive and motor performance equivalent to legally prescribed levels of alcohol intoxication. *Occupational and Environmental Medicine, 57*, 649–655.

Young, T., Palta, M., Dempsey, J., Skatrud, J., Weber, S., & Badr, S. (1993). The occurrence of sleep-disordered breathing among middle-age adults. *The New England Journal of Medicine, 328*, 1230–1235.

Zepelin, H., Siegel, J. M., & Tober, I. (2005). Mammalian sleep. In M. Kryger, T. Roth, & W. Dement, (Eds.), *Principles and practice of sleep medicine* (4th ed.). Philadelphia: Saunders.

CHAPTER 21

Sexual Dysfunction and Sexual Disorders

Margaret Jordan Halter and Verna Benner Carson

Key Terms and Concepts

dyspareunia, 482
exhibitionism, 493
fetishism, 493
frotteurism, 494
gender dysphoria, 492
gender identity, 492
gender identity disorder, 492
hypoactive sexual desire, 483
paraphilias, 492

pedophilia, 493
premature ejaculation, 484
sex, 492
sex reassignment surgery, 498
sexual disorders, 492
sexual dysfunction, 482
transsexualism, 492
vaginismus, 482
voyeurism, 493

Objectives

1. Describe the four phases of the sexual response cycle.
2. Define at least three areas of sexual dysfunction, and describe the treatment of each.
3. Consider the impact of medical problems and treatments on normal sexual functioning.
4. Examine the importance of nurses being knowledgeable about and comfortable discussing topics pertaining to sexuality.
5. Describe treatments available for sexual dysfunction.
6. Apply assessment techniques by role playing with a classmate the taking of a sexual history. Discuss how you feel and how your feelings influence your ability to perform this assessment.
7. Identify sexual preoccupations considered to be sexual disorders.
8. Discuss personal values and biases regarding sexuality and sexual behaviors.
9. Develop a plan of care for individuals diagnosed with sexual disorders.

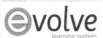 Visit the Evolve website for an **Audio Glossary & Flashcards, Concept Map Creator**, and additional resources related to the content in this chapter: **http://evolve.elsevier.com/Varcarolis/foundations**

Everyday professional nursing practice requires us to engage in matter-of-fact discussions with patients on topics generally considered to be extremely private and personal. We perform head-to-toe assessments in which we inquire about everything from headaches and sore throats to difficulties urinating and problems with constipation. The realities of providing physical care necessitate becoming comfortable with a number of skills that relate to privacy and modesty—performing breast examinations, initiating urinary catheters, and inserting rectal medications to name a few.

Despite a sort of learned fearlessness when it comes to addressing other intimate issues, the topic of sexuality is often a source of discomfort for not only nurses but also other health care providers. Although most recognize that addressing sexuality is part of holistic care, many do not routinely include the topic when doing assessments (Mick, 2007). Nursing curricula typically have a deficiency in training nurses in the fundamentals of sexuality and nursing care. Patients want to know how, for example, medications or treatments will affect their relationships and ability to have satisfying sex lives. Nurses can set the comfort level for discussing such issues and fostering opportunities to address feelings and fears.

Our views regarding sexuality are based on our individual beliefs about ourselves as women and men, mothers and fathers, and generative individuals who create and give to society in multiple ways. Multiple factors, including societal attitudes and traditions, parental views, cultural practices, spiritual and religious teaching, socioeconomic status, and education affect our sexual behaviors and our attitudes toward the sexual behaviors of others, including our patients.

Health promotion and disease prevention are key responsibilities for nurses. All nurses must assess a patient's sexuality and be prepared to educate, dispel myths, assist with values clarification, refer to appropriate care providers when indicated, and share resources. These actions alleviate or decrease patient illness and suffering and reduce health care costs through prevention. As a nursing student, you are introduced to complex aspects of sexual behavior that should help facilitate thoughtful discussion of the topic, make you aware of your personal belief systems, and help you consider the broader perspective of sexual issues as they exist in contemporary society.

This chapter addresses two general categories of concern related to sexuality. The first half of the chapter examines the normal sexual response cycle, clinical disorders related to the disruption or malfunction of this cycle, and guidelines for nursing care. The second half focuses on disorders related to sexual focus and preoccupation. These disorders may be sources of discomfort and distress to the person experiencing them (e.g., gender identity disorder) and may be a source of pain and trauma for others whose rights are violated (e.g., pedophilia).

Sexuality

PHASES OF THE SEXUAL RESPONSE CYCLE

Before looking more closely at the dysfunctions of sexual functioning, we will first review normal sexual functioning. The *Diagnostic and Statistical Manual of Mental Disorders,* fourth edition, text revision *(DSM-IV-TR)* describes a four-phase sexual response cycle (American Psychiatric Association [APA], 2000):

- Phase 1: Desire
- Phase 2: Excitement
- Phase 3: Orgasm
- Phase 4: Resolution

Desire

Many factors may affect interest in sexual activity, including age, physical and emotional health, availability of a sexual partner, and the context of an individual's life. In fact, for a number of individuals,

CONSIDERING CULTURE

Female Genital Mutilation and Sexual Functioning

Female genital mutilation is the surgical altering of female sexual organs for nonmedical reasons. The World Health Organization (2008) condemns this practice, as does the United Nations. One hundred million to 140 million females currently are living with the consequences of this surgery, which occurs between birth and 15 years of age. It is done to decrease libido (ensuring chastity and fidelity to spouses), prevent premarital sex, uphold a cultural tradition, or make the girl more feminine and beautiful by removing parts that are considered "male."

The actual practice varies and may include partial or total removal of the clitoris, the clitoral hood, and labia minora; cutting or fusing of the labia; and narrowing the vaginal opening. The surgery results in severe pain, infection, recurrent urinary tract infections, cysts, infertility, and childbirth complications and may deny women the ability to experience sexual pleasure.

The procedure occurs mainly in Africa, the Middle East, and Asia and is increasingly being protested and restricted by law. Clinicians in the United States are encountering females who have undergone this procedure. Developing a trusting relationship with patients who have been subjected to this custom includes understanding the types of mutilation, as well as the culture in which it occurs (Braddy & Files, 2007). According to Catania and colleagues (2007), these practices do not always result in an inability to experience orgasm, and sexual pleasure can be improved with appropriate sexual therapy.

Braddy, C., & Files, J. (2007). Female genital mutilation: Cultural awareness and clinical considerations. *Journal of Midwifery and Women's Health, 52*(2),158–163.
Catania, L., Abdulcadir, O., Puppo, V., Verde, J. B., Abdulcadir, J., & Abdulcadir, D. (2007). Pleasure and orgasm in women with female genital mutilation/cutting. *Journal of Sexual Medicine, 4,* 1666–1678.
World Health Organization. (2008). *Female genital mutilation.* Retrieved March 31, 2009 from http://www.who.int/mediacentre/factsheets/fs241/en/

the lack of sexual desire is not a source of distress either to the person or to his or her partner; in such a situation, decreased or absent sexual desire is not viewed as an illness. However, low sexual desire may be a source of frustration, both for the one experiencing it and also for partners. It is associated with other psychiatric or medical conditions. Conversely, excessive sexual desire becomes a problem when it creates difficulties for the individual's partner or when such excessive desire drives the person to demand sexual compliance from or force it upon unwilling partners.

Testosterone (normally present in the circulation of both males and females but in a much higher level in males) appears to be essential to sexual desire in both men and women. Men who, for one reason or another, have lost the ability to produce testosterone describe the change in their sexual feelings in terms such as "I still have the basic inclination for sex but do not seem to have the energy to put it into effect." In some of these men, testosterone replacement therapy appears to restore their sexual energy.

Estrogen does not seem to have a direct effect on sexual desire in women. A secondary effect, however, may be present in the requirement of estrogen for the maintenance of normal vaginal elasticity and lubrication. If these functions are lost due to estrogen deficiency, as may occur in some postmenopausal women or in younger women who have had their ovaries removed, **dyspareunia** (painful coitus) and **vaginismus** (spasm of the vagina) may be the result. In addition to estrogen deficiency, other physical conditions, such as vaginal infections and lesions, can lead to dyspareunia and vaginismus. Physical distress during sexual activities leads to psychological distress as anticipation of pain compounds the problem.

Excitement

The excitement phase of the normal human sexual response cycle is that period of time during which sexual tension continues to increase from the preceding level of sexual desire. Traditionally, penile erection and vaginal lubrication have been used as indicators of the presence of sexual excitement. If erection or lubrication does not occur in what, for that individual, is a sexually stimulating and appropriate situation, then there has been an inhibition of sexual excitement, regardless of the causative factors.

Orgasm

The orgasm phase of the human sexual response cycle is attained only at high levels of sexual tension in both women and men. Sexual tension (also described as sexual arousal) is produced by a combination of mental activity—including thoughts, fantasies, and dreams—

and erotic stimulation of erogenous areas, which may be more or less specific for each individual. Most men require some penile stimulation and most women some clitoral stimulation, either directly or indirectly, to produce the high levels of sexual tension necessary for orgasm to occur.

Most women who have experienced one orgasm may have repeated orgasms during the continuation of the same sexual activity. The occurrence of multiple orgasms depends on the maintenance of high levels of sexual tension through continued stimulation. On the other hand, once men ejaculate as a part of orgasm, they go through a refractory period. This is the time required to produce another ejaculate, which varies primarily with age. In a young man, this refractory period is measured in minutes, whereas in an older man, it may last several hours.

Resolution

During the resolution phase, sexual tension developed in prior phases subsides to baseline levels, provided sexual stimulation has ceased. The physiological changes that occurred during the earlier phases of the response cycle now tend to dissipate. This is a period of psychological vulnerability and can either be experienced as a period of pleasurable "afterglow" or described as being "uncomfortably emotionally exposed." With the restoration of normal physiological pulse, respiratory rate, and blood pressure, individuals frequently experience markedly increased perspiration.

Sexual Dysfunction

A **sexual dysfunction** is a disturbance in the desire, excitement, or orgasm phases of the sexual response cycle or pain during sexual intercourse (APA, 2000). It may prevent or reduce a person's ability to enjoy sex and can be classified according to the phase of the sexual response cycle in which it occurs. In evaluating a patient with a sexual dysfunction, a physical assessment—including laboratory studies—is performed before exploring psychological factors, such as emotional issues, life situation, and experiences.

CLINICAL PICTURE

Seven major classes of sexual dysfunction are listed in the *DSM-IV-TR: sexual desire disorders, sexual arousal disorders, orgasm disorders, sexual pain disorders, sexual dysfunction due to a general medical condition, substance-induced sexual dysfunction, and sexual dysfunction not otherwise specified.* Sexual dysfunctions can be the result of physiological problems, interpersonal conflicts, or a combination of both. Stress of any kind can adversely affect sexual function (Sadock & Sadock, 2008).

Sexual Desire Disorders

Sexual desire disorders are based on damage to biological sex drive, self-esteem, acceptance of personal sexuality, sexual experiences, and relationships (Sadock & Sadock, 2008). They are divided into two classes: *hypoactive sexual desire disorder*, characterized by a deficiency or absence of sexual fantasies or desire for sexual activity, and *sexual aversion disorder*, characterized by an aversion to and avoidance of genital sexual contact with a sexual partner or by masturbation.

An estimated 20% of the U.S. population has **hypoactive sexual desire**. A meta-analysis (summary of data) of all recent epidemiological studies ranks it as high as 24% to 34% (Segraves & Woodard, 2006). This disorder may be related to chronic stress and depression, prolonged suppression of sexual impulses, and a deteriorating relationship.

Although the incidence is unknown, sexual aversion disorder is thought to be a common disorder and happens more frequently in men (Shafer, 2008). About 25% of the time, it is comorbid with panic disorder.

Sexual Arousal Disorders

Female sexual arousal disorder is physiologically characterized by persistent or recurrent partial or complete failure to attain or maintain the lubrication and swelling response of sexual excitement until the completion of the sexual act. To receive this diagnosis, the lack of arousal must be distressing to the woman. This can be a lifelong problem, or it may be acquired (i.e., developed following normal functioning) (Becker & Stinson, 2008). The condition may be the result of hormonal alterations in testosterone, estrogen, prolactin, and thyroxin. Medications such as antihistamines and anticholinergics may result in decreased lubrication (Sadock & Sadock, 2008).

Male erectile disorder (also called *erectile dysfunction* and *impotence*) is characterized by the recurrent and persistent partial or complete failure to attain or maintain an erection to perform the sex act (Sadock & Sadock, 2008). This problem may be a rare, lifelong condition in which a man has never been able to obtain an erection sufficient for intercourse. It may also be an acquired condition in which a man has previously been able to have sexual intercourse but has lost the ability. Acquired erectile disorder occurs at a rate of 10% to 20% of all men and constitutes about half the complaints of sexual dysfunction in men. In young men, the disorder is uncommon, and the cause is usually psychological.

Orgasm Disorders

Female Orgasmic Disorder

Female orgasmic disorder is sometimes referred to as *inhibited female orgasm* or *anorgasmia* and is defined

---

INTEGRATIVE THERAPY

Nonhormonal Treatment of Menopausal Symptoms

Warnings about the risks of breast cancer and strokes have led increasing numbers of women to request non-hormonal treatments for perimenopausal and menopausal symptoms related to sexual arousal, but relatively few high-quality studies examine these treatments (Hickey et al., 2007). One herbal treatment that has received attention as possibly reducing these symptoms due to its estrogen-like effects is black cohosh *(Cimicifuga racemosa)*, which is sold as a dietary supplement in the United States.

Concerns have been expressed regarding both minor side effects, such as gastrointestinal problems, and more serious side effects, such as liver toxicity. Despite the fact that black cohosh is widely available on drugstore shelves and is touted as a treatment for sexual dysfunction related to menopause, a search of literature reveals little data as to its efficacy. The bottom line is that women do not have enough information about any herbal therapy, including black cohosh, that may promote sexual responsiveness.

Cumming, G. P., Herald, J., Moncur, R., Currie, H., & Lee, A. J. (2007). Women's attitudes to hormone replacement therapy, alternative therapy, and sexual health: A web-based survey. *Menopause International, 13,* 79–83; and Hickey, C., Saunders, B., & Stuckey, B. (2007). Non-hormonal treatments for menopausal symptoms. *Maturitas, 57*(1), 85–89.

---

as the recurrent or persistent inhibition of female orgasm, as manifested by the recurrent delay in, or absence of, orgasm after a normal sexual excitement phase (achieved by masturbation or coitus). It may be a lifelong disorder (never having achieved orgasm) or acquired (having had at least one orgasm and then having difficulties). The prevalence of either type of this disorder is estimated at 30% (Sadock & Sadock, 2008). Psychological factors (including fears of pregnancy, rejection, or loss of control), hostility toward men, and cultural/societal restrictions may be causative. There is some evidence to suggest that female orgasmic disorder may be inherited.

Male Orgasmic Disorder

In male orgasmic disorder, sometimes called *inhibited orgasm* or *retarded ejaculation*, a man achieves ejaculation during coitus only with great difficulty. A man with a *lifelong orgasmic disorder* has never been able to ejaculate during coitus; the condition may result from a rigid background in which sex is seen as a sin. This is an uncommon diagnosis. *Acquired orgasmic disorder* develops after previously normal functioning and is fairly common. Interpersonal problems may be the cause.

Physical conditions, substance abuse, and prescribed medication may also cause this problem and should be assessed. The prevalence of male orgasmic disorder has been reported at 5% (Sadock & Sadock, 2008).

Premature Ejaculation

In premature ejaculation, a man persistently or recurrently achieves orgasm and ejaculation before he wishes to. Diagnosis is made when a man regularly ejaculates before or immediately after the penis enters the vagina. Considerations as to age, newness of the relationship, and how often the man has intercourse should be assessed. About 35% to 40% of men who are treated for sexual disorders complain of premature ejaculation. Physical factors may be involved; some men may be more tactilely sensitive and respond more intensely to stimulation. Psychological factors include fear about performance and stressful relationships where the man feels hurried.

Sexual Pain Disorders

Dyspareunia

Recurrent or persistent genital pain can occur in either men or women during or after intercourse. Dyspareunia is more common in women and is frequently associated with vaginismus. Psychological factors include a history of childhood abuse or rape and anxiety about sex, but the pain is real and makes sex unpleasant at the least and unbearable in extreme cases.

Vaginismus

Vaginismus is an involuntary constriction response of the muscles that close the vagina. This condition interferes with penile insertion and intercourse and may even be elicited during a normal gynecological examination with a speculum.

Other Sexual Dysfunctions and Problems

Sexual dysfunction due to a general medical condition includes sexual desire disorders, orgasm disorders, and sexual pain disorders, but the cause of each is related to a medical condition, such as cardiovascular, neurological, or endocrine disease.

The diagnosis *substance-induced sexual dysfunction* is used when evidence of substance intoxication or withdrawal is apparent from the history, physical examination, or laboratory findings. Distressing sexual dysfunction occurs within a month of significant substance intoxication or withdrawal. Specified substances include alcohol, amphetamines or related substances, cocaine, opioids, sedatives, hypnotics, antianxiety agents, and other known and unknown substances. Abused recreational substances can have a variety of effects on sexual functioning. In small doses, many substances enhance sexual performance. With continued use, sexual difficulties become the norm.

Sexual dysfunction not otherwise specified is a category that covers sexual dysfunctions that cannot be classified under one of the other categories. Examples include the experience of physiological sexual excitement and orgasm with no erotic sensation or even with anesthesia. Women with a condition similar to premature ejaculation are classified as having this disorder. Disorders of excessive, rather than inhibited, sexual dysfunction (e.g., compulsive masturbation or coitus (sex addiction) or genital pain occurring during masturbation) may be classified in this category.

Sexual problems can also result from head trauma, chromosomal abnormalities, and psychosis. Patients who have experienced head trauma with damage to the frontal lobe of the brain may display symptoms of promiscuity, poor judgment, inability to recognize triggers that set off sexual desires, and poor impulse control.

In Klinefelter's syndrome, a condition identified through genetic analysis, the patient has at least one extra X chromosome; the karyotype is XXY instead of the normal XY genetic coding for the male. These patients frequently have immature genitalia, and gender identity disorder is a possibility.

The patient with schizophrenia may experience an alteration in sexual drive only during the acute phase of illness, or it may be ongoing. This could depend partly on the severity of the illness. In addition, patients with chronic schizophrenia have difficulty communicating their needs and concerns to others. For the patient with schizophrenia, self-concept and ego strength deteriorate over time, further decreasing the patient's ability to develop or maintain intimate relationships.

Schizophrenia is not necessarily associated with sexual dysfunction or deviant sexual behavior, but the symptoms of schizophrenia and even the treatment with antipsychotic medications may make the patient vulnerable to disturbances in sexual functioning and often cause the patient to be childlike and passive in relationships. The primary goal of the treatment team while the patient is hospitalized is the control of acute symptoms. Sometimes the acute symptoms present as delusions. These delusions can be sexual, or they can be of a paranoid type that drives the patient away from meaningful relationships and produces a sexual problem due to the resulting alienation. Delusions may also be of a grandiose nature, so that the patient believes himself or herself to be a great lover or have a "special mission" of a sexual nature.

EPIDEMIOLOGY

The prevalence of specific sexual dysfunctions was addressed in the previous discussion; however, some general statements may be made concerning these disorders as a category. Overall, they are more common in women than men (Shafer, 2008). Regardless of gender, these disorders become more prevalent as we age. In later life, 20% to 30% of men and 40% to 45% of women report difficulties (Becker & Stinson, 2008). Education seems to have a buffering effect, and people who have more education have fewer sexual problems and are less anxious about issues pertaining to sex (Shafer, 2008).

COMORBIDITY

Sexual functioning may be adversely affected any time there is a disturbance in an individual's ability to develop and maintain stable relationships. This is especially true for patients with schizophrenia, who show difficulty coping with stress, a decrease in reality-based orientation to the world, and defense mechanisms that lead to withdrawn behavior. Sexual dysfunction may also be associated with depression and personality disorders (Becker & Stinson, 2008). Several physical conditions are related to sexual dysfunction and are presented in Table 21-1.

ETIOLOGY

Pioneers in the study of human sexuality included Helen Singer Kaplan (1929-1995). According to Kaplan (1974), sexual dysfunctions are the result of a combination of factors, including:

- Misinformation or ignorance regarding sexual and social interaction
- Unconscious guilt and anxiety regarding sex
- Anxiety related to performance, especially with erectile and orgasmic dysfunction
- Poor communication between partners about feelings and what they desire sexually

TABLE 21-1   Medical Conditions and Surgical Procedures That Cause Sexual Dysfunction

System/State	Organic Disorders	Sexual Impairment
Endocrine	Hypothyroidism, adrenal dysfunction, hypogonadism, diabetes mellitus	Low libido, impotence, decreased vaginal lubrication, early impotence
Vascular	Hypertension, atherosclerosis, stroke, venous insufficiency, sickle cell disorder	Impotence, but ejaculation and libido intact
Neurological	Spinal cord damage, diabetic neuropathy, herniated disk, alcoholic neuropathy, multiple sclerosis, temporal lobe epilepsy	Sexual disorder—early signs: low or high libido, impotence, impaired orgasm
Genital	*Male*—Priapism, Peyronie's disease, urethritis, prostatitis, hydrocele *Female*—Imperforate hymen, vaginitis, pelvic inflammatory disease, endometriosis	Low libido, impotence Vaginismus, dyspareunia, low libido, decreased arousal
Systemic	Renal, pulmonary, hepatic, advanced malignancies, infections	Low libido, impotence, decreased arousal
Psychiatric	Depression Bipolar disorder (manic phase) Generalized anxiety disorder, panic disorder, posttraumatic stress disorder (PTSD), obsessive-compulsive disorder (OCD) Schizophrenia Personality disorders (passive-aggressive, obsessive-compulsive, histrionic)	Low libido, erectile dysfunction Increased libido Low libido, erectile dysfunction, reduced vaginal lubrication, anorgasmia, "anti-fantasies" focusing on partner's negative qualities (OCD only) Low desire, bizarre sexual fantasies Low libido, erectile dysfunction, premature ejaculation, anorgasmia
Surgical-postoperative	*Male*—Prostatectomy, abdominal-perineal bowel resection *Female*—Episiotomy, vaginal prolapse repair, oophorectomy *Male and female*—Leg amputation, colostomy, ileostomy	Impotence, no loss of libido, ejaculatory impairment Dyspareunia, vaginismus, decreased lubrication Mechanical difficulties in sex, low self-image, fear of odor

Data from Shafer, L. C. (2008). Sexual disorders and sexual dysfunction. In T. A. Stern, J. F. Rosenbaum, M. Fava, J. Biederman, & S. L. Rauch (Eds.), *Massachusetts General Hospital comprehensive clinical psychiatry* (pp. 487–497). St. Louis: Mosby.

Additional factors have been identified to explain sexual dysfunction. Unacknowledged sexual orientation may lead to poor performance with the opposite sex, or the presence of one sexual problem may lead to another. For example, difficulty maintaining an erection may lead to hypoactive sexual desire (Becker & Stinson, 2008). Sexual trauma is also frequently associated with sexual dysfunction.

APPLICATION OF THE NURSING PROCESS

ASSESSMENT

General Assessment

Sexual assessment includes both subjective and objective data. Many psychiatric hospitals use a nursing history tool that is biologically oriented but typically has few questions on sexual functioning. Health history questions pertaining to the reproductive system may be limited to menstrual history, parity, history of sexually transmitted diseases, method of contraception, and questions regarding "safer sex" practices. There may be some vague questions about sexual functioning or sexual concerns.

Self-Assessment

According to Dhalwani (2008), our discomfort in assessing sexual history is related to personal embarrassment, concerns about embarrassing the patient, poor training, inexperience, inadequate time, and beliefs that sexual history is not important. Indeed, you may experience discomfort exploring sexual issues with patients, fearing that this discussion will be personally embarrassing, as well as embarrassing to the patient. You may fear that you will not know what questions to ask or why the questions should be asked.

Concerns related to age and gender differences are understandable. If the patient is approximately your age and of the opposite sex, you might worry that talking about sexuality may not be appropriate or whether the patient might conclude that you are a little too interested. Discussing issues related to sexuality with people who are your parents' or grandparents' age may also create a level of discomfort, especially if you grew up in a home where such topics were avoided, and you had to rely on your friends for information (or misinformation) about sex.

Remembering your position as a professional and addressing the topics in a tone and manner appropriate of a professional will increase your comfort, along with the patient's. Also, letting the patient know *why*

you are asking such personal questions increases openness and cooperation. For example, "People who are depressed sometimes find that it affects their sexual desire. Since you have been depressed, have you noticed a change in your interest in sex?" Sometimes a more subtle approach that shifts the focus away from the patient is helpful. "Since you have been depressed, has your husband felt like you are less interested in him?"

Perhaps most the most helpful consideration is recognizing that assessing sexuality is part of holistic nursing care. Your role and responsibility is in assisting the patient in dealing with responses to illness and/or the treatment of the illness. Understanding your patient's concerns, acknowledging the patient's discomfort, and providing useful feedback will enhance your professional abilities to care for your patient and perhaps even improve self-understanding.

Patients may cue the nurse into the presence of sexual concerns without explicitly verbalizing them. Box 21-1 presents a discussion of these cues.

BOX 21-1 Patient Cues That May Indicate Concerns About Sexuality

Nonverbal Behaviors
- Showing discomfort by blushing, looking away, making tight fists, fidgeting, crying
- Openly engaging in overt sexual behaviors (e.g., touching own body parts, masturbating, exposing genitals, placing nurse's hand on genitals, making sexually suggestive sounds)

Verbal Behaviors
- Telling sexually explicit jokes
- Making sexual comments about the nurse
- Asking inappropriate questions about the nurse's sexual activity
- Discussing sexual exploits
- Expressing concern about relationship with partner:
  - "I don't feel the same about my partner."
  - "My partner doesn't feel the same about me."
  - "We're not as close."
  - "Our relationship has changed."
  - "My personal life has changed."
- Expressing concern that sexuality has been diminished (e.g., feeling less of a man, less of a woman):
  - "I've lost my manhood."
  - "I'm not as desirable as I once was."
- Expressing concern over lack of sexual desire:
  - "I'm not interested in sex anymore."
  - "My desire has changed."
  - "I'm not the man/woman I used to be."
  - "We don't click anymore."

Continued

<table>
<tr><td>

BOX 21-1 Patient Cues That May Indicate Concerns About Sexuality—cont'd

- Expressing concern over sexual performance:
  - "I don't get wet."
  - "I've lost my power."
  - "Will I still be able to get hard?"
  - "What will happen to my ability to perform?"
  - "I can't perform like I used to."
- Expressing concern about one's love life:
  - "My love life has changed."
  - "The spark is gone."
- Expressing concern over the sexual impact of drugs, surgery, or some other medical treatment:
  - "Will this drug interfere with my sex life?"
  - "Will I still be able to perform sexually after surgery?"

</td></tr>
</table>

to the patient's experience. For example: "Some people who are prescribed this medication find it difficult to achieve an erection. Have you had this problem?" This allows the patient to feel that he is not alone in what he is experiencing. Table 21-2 provides facilitative statements for the interviewer conducting a sexual assessment.

The sexual history includes the patient's perception of physiological functioning and behavioral, emotional, and spiritual aspects of sexuality. It also includes cultural and religious beliefs with regard to sexual behavior and sexual knowledge base. During the assessment, both the nurse and the patient are free to ask questions and clarify information. It is reasonable to defer lengthy sexual health assessment when acute psychiatric symptoms preclude a calm, thoughtful discussion. As symptoms subside and rapport is developed, the assessment may be resumed. With experience, the nurse is able to identify those patients who are at greater risk for difficulties in sexual functioning. This includes patients with a history of certain medical problems or surgical procedures (see Table 21-1) and patients taking some drugs (Table 21-3).

The nurse may ask the patient if there is discomfort in the area of sexual functioning. Generally, it is more comfortable for the patient if the nurse firsts asks questions in a general manner and then proceeds

TABLE 21-2 Facilitative Statements for the Interviewer Conducting a Sexual Assessment

Purpose	Facilitative Statement
To provide a rationale for a question	"As a nurse, I'm concerned about all aspects of your health. Many individuals have concern about sexual matters, especially when they are sick or having other health problems."
To give statements of generality or normality	"Most people are hesitant to discuss...." "Many people worry about feeling...." "Many people have concerns about...."
To identify sexual dysfunction	"Most people have difficulties sometime during their sexual relationships. What have yours been?"
To obtain information	"The degree to which unmarried persons have sexual outlets varies considerably. Some have sexual partners. Some relieve sexual tension through masturbation. Others need no outlet at all. What has been your pattern?"
To identify sexual myths	"While growing up, most of us have heard some sexual myths or half-truths that continue to puzzle us. Are there any that come to mind?"
To determine whether homosexuality is a source of conflict	"What is your attitude toward your homosexual orientation?"
To identify an older person's concerns about sexual function	"Many people, as they get older, believe or worry that this signals the end of their sex life. Much misinformation continues this myth. What is your understanding about sexuality during the later years? How has the passage of time affected your sexuality (sex life)?"
To obtain and give information (miscellaneous areas)	"Frequently people have questions about...." "What questions do you have about...." "What would you like to know about...."
To close the history	"Is there anything further in the area of sexuality that you would like to bring up now?"

Adapted from Green, R. (1975). *Human sexuality: A health practitioner's text.* Baltimore: Williams & Wilkins.

TABLE 21-3 Drugs That Can Cause Sexual Dysfunction

Category	Drug	Sexual Side Effect
Cardiovascular drugs	Methyldopa	Low libido, impotence, anorgasmia
	Thiazides	Low libido, impotence, decreased lubrication
	Clonidine	Impotence, anorgasmia
	Propranolol	Low libido
	Digoxin	Gynecomastia, low libido, impotence
	Clofibrate	Low libido, impotence
Gastrointestinal drugs	Cimetidine	Low libido, impotence
	Methantheline bromide	Impotence
Hormones	Estrogen	Low libido in men
	Progesterone	Low libido, impotence
Sedatives	Alcohol	Higher doses cause sexual problems
	Barbiturates	Impotence
Antianxiety drugs	Alprazolam	Low libido, delayed ejaculation
	Diazepam	
Antipsychotics	Thioridazine	Retarded or retrograde ejaculation
	Haloperidol	Low libido, impotence, anorgasmia
Antidepressants	MAOIs (Phenelzine)	Impotence, retarded ejaculation, anorgasmia
	Tricyclics (imipramine)	Low libido, impotence, retarded ejaculation
	SSRIs (fluoxetine, sertraline)	Low libido, impotence, retarded ejaculation
	Atypical (trazodone)	Priapism, retarded or retrograde ejaculation
Antimanic drugs	Lithium	Low libido, impotence
Anticonvulsants		Low libido, impotence, priapism
Opiates		Low libido, orgasmic dysfunction

MAOIs, monoamine oxidase inhibitors; *SSRIs*, selective serotonin reuptake inhibitors.
Data from Shafer, L. C. (2008). Sexual disorders and sexual dysfunction. In T. A. Stern, J. F. Rosenbaum, M. Fava, J. Biederman, & S. L. Rauch (Eds.), *Massachusetts General Hospital comprehensive clinical psychiatry* (pp. 487–497). St Louis: Mosby.

Assessment Guidelines   Sexual Dysfunction

1. A sexual assessment should be conducted in a setting that allows privacy and eliminates distractions.
2. Although note taking may be necessary for the beginner, it can be distracting to the patient and interrupt the flow of the interview. When note taking is necessary, it should be unobtrusive and kept to a minimum.
3. The interview should be free from personal biases and judgmental attitudes that could block open discussion of sexual issues.
4. Good eye contact, relaxed posture, and friendly facial expressions facilitate the patient's comfort and communicate openness and receptivity on the part of the nurse.

DIAGNOSIS

A comprehensive sexual assessment can reveal areas of sexual concern and dysfunction for the patient. These data are analyzed to determine the appropriate nursing diagnoses. Priority nursing diagnoses, their definitions, and possible etiology follow (NANDA-I, 2009):

Sexual dysfunction is the state in which an individual experiences a change in sexual function during the sexual response phases of desire, excitation, and/or orgasm. The change is viewed as unsatisfying, unrewarding, or inadequate and may be related to:

- Altered body function from medication
- Biopsychosocial alteration of sexuality
- Psychosocial abuse from significant other

Ineffective sexuality pattern is indicated by expressions of concern regarding one's own sexuality. It may be related to:

- Impaired relationship with significant other
- Knowledge deficit about alternative responses to illness

OUTCOMES IDENTIFICATION

Some sexual problems can be remedied by achieving short-term outcomes that use education as a nursing intervention. Frequently, sexual myths and misinformation can be corrected, giving the patient almost instant relief from perceived problems. Moorhead and colleagues' (2008) *Nursing Outcomes Classification (NOC)* identifies a number of outcomes related to sexual dysfunction or ineffective sexuality patterns. Included are *Abuse Recovery: Emotional/Physical/Sexual, Sexual Functioning, Sexual Identity, Role Performance, and Self-Esteem*. Table 21-4 provides selected intermediate and short-term indicators for *Sexual Functioning* and *Sexual Identity*.

PLANNING

Planning nursing care for the patient with a sexual dysfunction may occur as part of care for a coexisting disorder. Nurses prepared at the basic level may encounter such patients when they are being treated for a variety of conditions in any setting.

IMPLEMENTATION

An understanding of sexual function and dysfunction is essential for nurses who work in psychiatry, as well as most any specialty area in nursing, including oncology, cardiology, and neurology. All nurses need to be able to facilitate a discussion about sexuality with the patient. To be a facilitator, the nurse must be nonjudgmental, have basic knowledge of sexual functioning, and have the ability to conduct a basic sexual assessment. Once the assessment is completed, the nurse needs to know when and to whom to refer the patient with a sexual complaint. Depending on the nature of the problem, the patient may need a referral to a professional such as a marital counselor, psychiatrist, gynecologist, urologist, clinical nurse specialist, or pastoral counselor.

Box 21-2 provides sample interventions from *Nursing Interventions Classification (NIC)* (Bulechek et al., 2008) for *Sexual Counseling*.

BOX 21-2 *NIC* Interventions for Sexual Counseling

Definition: Use of an interactive helping process focusing on the need to make adjustments in sexual practice or to enhance coping with a sexual event or disorder

Activities*:

- Establish a therapeutic relationship based on trust and respect.
- Provide privacy and ensure confidentiality.
- Discuss the effect of the illness or health situation on sexuality.
- Discuss the effect of medications on sexuality, as appropriate.
- Avoid displaying aversion to an altered body part.
- Provide factual information about sexual myths and misinformation that patient may verbalize.
- Provide reassurance that current and new sexual practices are healthy, as appropriate.
- Include the spouse/sexual partner in the counseling as much as possible, as appropriate.
- Refer patient to a sex therapist, as appropriate.

---

*Partial list.
Data from Bulechek, G. M., Butcher, H. K., & Dochterman, J. M. (Eds.). (2008). *Nursing interventions classification (NIC)* (5th ed.). St. Louis: Mosby.

TABLE 21-4 *NOC* Outcomes for Sexual Dysfunction

Nursing Outcome and Definition	Intermediate Indicators	Short-Term Indicators
Sexual Functioning: Integration of physical, socioemotional, and intellectual aspects of sexual expression and performance	Expresses ability to perform sexually despite physical imperfections Expresses comfort with sexual expression	Attains sexual arousal Adapts sexual technique as needed Sustains penile or clitoral erection through orgasm
Sexual Identity: Acknowledgment and acceptance of own sexual identity	Challenges negative images of sexual self Reports healthy sexual functioning	Affirms self as a sexual being Exhibits clear sense of sexual orientation Seeks social support

Data from Moorhead, S., Johnson, M., Maas, M., & Swanson, E. (Eds.). (2008). *Nursing outcomes classification (NOC)* (4th ed.). St. Louis: Mosby.

Pharmacological Interventions

Treatments for sexual dysfunction increasingly are becoming the target of pharmaceutical industries. Despite the fact that there is an increased interest in treatment for hypoactive sexual desire disorder in women, there is a deficiency of approved treatments, and treatment guidelines are negligible—partly due to vague criteria for this disorder (Segraves & Woodard, 2006). Most of the available treatment for sexual dysfunction is targeted at male dysfunction, and there are no treatments approved by the U.S. Food and Drug Administration (FDA) for female sexual disorders (Evidence-Based Practice box). Table 21-5 summarizes treatments for sexual dysfunction.

Health Teaching and Health Promotion

Nurses should help patients weigh the pros and cons of any type of pharmacotherapy. Many drugs cause sexual side effects, and psychotropic medications used for psychiatric disorders are common offenders. Nurses tend to ignore the sexual side effects

TABLE 21-5 Pharmacological, Psychosocial, and Other Treatments for Sexual Dysfunction

Sexual Disorder	Pharmacological Treatment	Psychosocial Approaches	Other
Hypoactive sexual desire disorder	Menopausal women: LibiGel testosterone patch (in clinical trials)	Sensate focus exercises Masturbation training Erotic material	
Sexual aversion disorder	Tricyclic antidepressants Antianxiety drugs	Sensate focus exercises Masturbation training Erotic material Systematic desensitization Sex therapy	
Female sexual arousal disorder	Alprostadil cream (Femprox) (MUSE) (topical) Testosterone with estrogen Tibolone Lubrication (K-Y Jelly)	Sensate focus exercises	Eros clitoral suction device*
Male erectile disorder	Sildenafil citrate (Viagra)* Tadalafil (Cialis)* Vardenafil (Levitra)* Alprostadil (MUSE)* penile self-injection and intraurethral suppository Testosterone (for hypogonadism) Yohimbine (Yocon)* Phentolamine (Vasomax)	Sensate focus exercises Group therapy Hypnotherapy Systematic desensitization Psychodynamic therapy Couples therapy	Vacuum pump Penile prostheses
Female orgasmic disorder	Sildenafil (Viagra)	Masturbation training Couples therapy Kegel vaginal exercises	
Male orgasmic disorder	Sildenafil (Viagra)	Masturbatory training Systematic desensitization	
Premature ejaculation	(None with FDA approval) SSRIs to delay or retard ejaculation Topical anesthetics	Start-stop technique Squeeze technique Increased sexual frequency	

*FDA approved.
Data from Shafer, L. C. (2008). Sexual disorders and sexual function. In T. A. Stern, J. F. Rosenbaum, M. Fava, J. Biederman, & S. L. Rauch (Eds.), *Massachusetts General Hospital comprehensive clinical psychiatry* (pp. 487-497). Philadelphia: Mosby; and Becker, J. V., & Stinson, J. D. (2008). Human sexuality and sexual dysfunctions. In R. E. Hales, S. C. Yudofsky, & Gabbard, G. O. (Eds.), *Textbook of psychiatry* (5th ed.) (pp. 711-728). Washington, DC: American Psychiatric Publishing.

EVIDENCE-BASED PRACTICE

Testosterone for Postmenopausal Women With Low Libido

Davis, S., Moreau, M., Kroll, R., Bouchard, C., Panay, N., Gass, M., Braunstein, G., Hirschberg, A., Rodenberg, C., Pack, S., Koch, H., Moufarege, A., Studd, J., & the APHRODITE Study Team. (2008). Testosterone for low libido in postmenopausal women not taking estrogen. *New England Journal of Medicine, 359*(19), 2005–2017.

Problem

Nearly one third of women in the United States may experience lack of sexual interest, and about one fourth cannot achieve orgasm. Postmenopausal women in particular can be distressed by a loss of sexual interest. When taken along with estrogen and progesterone, testosterone has been demonstrated to increase sexual interest in postmenopausal women; however, many women are (understandably) reluctant to take estrogen and/or progesterone due to the increased risk of breast cancer, heart attacks, and strokes.

Purpose of Study

The purpose of this study was to determine if testosterone, a hormone that is actually more prevalent in the bloodstreams of premenopausal women than estrogen, would improve sexual well-being in postmenopausal women.

Methods

This international study included 814 naturally or surgically postmenopausal women. They were randomly selected to be in one of two groups. One group received a testosterone patch, and the other received a placebo patch. The length of the study was 52 weeks.

Key Findings

- Participants who received the testosterone patch reported an average increase of 2.1 satisfying sexual episodes per month versus a 0.7 increase among the placebo group.

- Of participants who reported benefits from the treatment, 85% said they would like to continue the treatment.
- A significant reduction in distress was also found in participants receiving treatment.
- Of women who had the testosterone patch, 30% reported adrenergic side effects such as unwanted hair growth.
- Breast cancer was diagnosed in four women in the treatment group but none in the placebo group. (One woman was diagnosed in the first 4 months of the study, and another had symptoms prior to the study.)

Implications for Nursing Practice

Testosterone is already being widely prescribed off-label (without formal FDA approval), primarily to postmenopausal women who are experiencing a decreased sex drive. The study supports this prescribing practice yet calls into question the risk/benefit ratio. The report of four cases of breast cancer in the treatment group may be coincidental, but certainly this type of therapy will be studied more.

Menopause is a mystery to many women, and its symptoms may be bewildering. Sexual interest and emotional distress are two symptoms relevant to psychiatric mental health nurses, professionals who are in positions to educate women about their options. Keeping current in research by reading studies such as these improves our ability to provide the best care possible for our patients.

---

associated with these medications, perhaps in an attempt to promote adherence. Helping patients to evaluate for themselves the benefits versus the risks of psychopharmacotherapy empowers patients to choose the best course of action and increases their ability to be informed consumers of mental health services (Higgins, 2007).

Advanced Practice Interventions

Advanced practice nurses can be qualified to treat sexual dysfunction through advanced training and certification. General therapies include psychoanalytic therapy, couples therapy, group therapy, and hypnotherapy.

Some specific therapies available for sexual dysfunction include:

- Sensate focus: a therapeutic treatment in which patients progress from general touching and cuddling without intercourse to more intimate forms of expression
- Systematic desensitization: involves combining relaxation exercises with sexually anxiety-producing stimuli
- Masturbation training: especially helpful in women who have never had an orgasm. This approach helps women learn about their bodies and their responses in order to understand their sexual responsiveness.

Maria is a 67-year-old woman, widowed many years, who has recently been approached by a 75-year-old widower with a marriage proposal. Maria is concerned about the sexual implications of a marriage so late in life. She confides in her nurse practitioner, "I really haven't even thought about sex for so many years. I know Joe is just an old goat. He's always after me to take my clothes off." After discussing the possibility of a physiological cause for her lack of interest in sex, Maria's nurse practitioner gives her small doses of testosterone. Within a remarkably short time, Maria stops talking about Joe as "an old goat" and begins talking again about "how great life can be if you have the right partner." ■

EVALUATION

Evaluation of expected outcomes relates to the level of control and personal satisfaction achieved. Acceptance of sexual dysfunction (e.g., impotence) as being part—but not necessarily the defining characteristic—of sexual behavior can result in greater satisfaction. The degree to which negative attitudes about sex are no longer problematic is also important.

Sexual Disorders

CLINICAL PICTURE

In the first part of this chapter, we examined normal sexual functioning and sexual dysfunction. We now turn our attention to sexual disorders—psychiatric disorders in which sexual problems are considered to be socially atypical, have the potential to disrupt meaningful relationships, and may result in insult or even significant injury to other people. The *DSM-IV-TR* classifies sexual disorders as either *gender identity disorder* or one of the following paraphilias: *fetishism, pedophilia, exhibitionism, voyeurism, transvestic fetishism, sexual sadism, frotteurism, and paraphilia not otherwise specified (NOS)*.

Gender Identity Disorder

When we inquire about the birth of a new infant, we want to know if it is a boy or a girl. Actually, we are asking about the sex of the child (i.e., whether its chromosomes are XX or XY). However, biological assignment does not determine whether individuals think of themselves as male or female. Gender identity, the sense of maleness or femaleness, is not inborn but usually is established by the time a child is 3 years old (Becker & Johnson, 2008). Although we may be predisposed to male or female gender orientation, gender identity is mainly a product of how we are raised.

Gender identity disorder is defined as strong and persistent cross-gender identification (Sadock & Sadock, 2008). Little is known about the origins of gender identity disorder, but childhood patterns seem to be fairly consistent. As early as 2 to 4 years of age, some children may have cross-gender interests and activities. However, only a small percentage of children who display gender identity disorder characteristics will continue to show these characteristics into adolescence or adulthood. Typically, children who later become transsexual as adults relate better to members of the sex opposite to their biological sex. Boys prefer female friends and activities and cross-dress whenever possible. Girls imitate what they consider masculine behavior and refuse to be involved in activities usually assigned to females.

People with gender identity disorder continue to prefer the opposite-sex behavioral style into adulthood. These individuals never consider themselves to be homosexual. The biological female who falls in love with a woman believes herself actually to be a man who loves that woman. Thus, a desire for congruity in gender identity and physiology becomes important for many individuals.

When biological sex differs from gender identity, the individual suffers from gender dysphoria, or feelings of unease about their maleness or femaleness. Such an individual might have a physically normal female reproductive tract and yet have a sense that she is male. She might describe herself by saying, "I am a man trapped in a woman's body." This is an example of the most extreme case of gender dysphoria, called transsexualism, in which a person wishes to change his or her anatomical sexual characteristics to those of the opposite sex.

Paraphilias

People do not consciously decide what arouses them sexually. Rather, during the maturation process they discover the nature of their own sexual orientation and interests. Individuals differ from one another in terms of the types of partners they find to be erotically appealing and the types of behaviors they find to be erotically stimulating. They also differ in the intensity of the sexual drive, in the degree of difficulty they experience in trying to resist sexual urges, and in their attitudes about whether or not such urges should be resisted.

The sexual disorders include many forms of paraphilias, also known as *sexual impulse disorders*. These terms refer to acts or sexual stimuli that are outside of what society considers normal but necessary for some individuals to experience desire, arousal, and orgasm (Sadock & Sadock, 2008). Criteria for being diagnosed with this category of disorders include that the symptoms occur for at least 6 months. Experimenting with paraphiliac behavior from time to time does not constitute a disorder. Paraphilias are "recurrent, intense sexually arousing fantasies, sexual urges, or behaviors" (APA, 2000, p. 566). Typically they involve nonhuman articles and nonconsenting partners.

Fetishism

Fetishism is characterized by a sexual focus on objects—such as shoes, gloves, pantyhose, and stockings—that are intimately associated with the human body. The particular fetish is linked to someone involved with the patient during childhood and thus is invested with a quality associated with this loved, needed, or even traumatizing person (APA, 2000; Sadock & Sadock, 2008). Preferred items are shoes, leather or latex items, and women's underclothing. This interest may replace sexual partners or may include a component of the fetish within a consenting relationship. Fetishes may become all-consuming and destructive. They occur in more men than women.

Pedophilia

Pedophilia is, unfortunately, the most common paraphilia. It involves sexual activity with a prepubescent child (generally 13 years or younger). This behavior is unacceptable in most cultures, including the United States, and represents a profound violation of the boundaries of the child. Because pedophilia is illegal, its exact incidence is unknown. For the definition of pedophilia to be met, the perpetrator must be at least 16 years of age and at least 5 years older than the victim (Sadock & Sadock, 2008). The nature of the child molestation ranges from undressing and looking at the child, to genital fondling or oral sex, to penetration, and even torture (Shafer, 2008).

Although most people believe that girls are more frequently molested, 60% of identified victims are boys. Pedophiles who are attracted to females tend to prefer 8- to 10-year-old children, whereas those who are attracted to males prefer older children and teens. A significant number of pedophiles have previous or current involvement in voyeurism, exhibitionism, or rape (Sadock & Sadock, 2008).

Exhibitionism

Exhibitionism is an illegal activity that involves the intentional display of the genitals in a public place. Almost 100% of cases of exhibitionism involve a man exposing himself to a woman. This may occur as a man walks around exposed in a busy shopping mall or exposes himself on a doorstep after ringing the doorbell. Excitement results from the anticipation of the act, and the individual masturbates during or after exposing himself. The exhibitionist becomes aroused by observers' responses of shock and even disgust, and some fantasize that the person will also be aroused by the experience and actually want to be with them sexually.

On the other hand, some people with exhibitionism may experience deep shame and judge themselves by the same standard that society does and consider themselves perverts. They may cover their actions and live in intense fear that they will be recognized and shame themselves and their families.

Although exhibitionism is illegal, it seems to be done more for shock value than as a precursor to sexual assault or rape. Actual contact is rarely sought. Since few people are arrested for this behavior after age 40, we can speculate that it resolves with age (Shafer, 2008).

Voyeurism

Voyeurism is another illegal activity that begins in adolescence or early adulthood. It is marked by seeking sexual arousal through viewing, usually secretly, other people in intimate situations (e.g., naked, in the process of disrobing, or engaging in sexual activity). In the language of the layperson, this behavior is called being a "peeping Tom." The disorder often begins in adolescence and may become a chronic condition and the only type of sexual activity for the person. Voyeurism may be driven by anger and a need to retaliate. Typically, people who engage in voyeurism also engage in other compulsive sexual behavior and are frequently addicted to pornography and going to strip clubs.

Like an exhibitionist, a person who engages in voyeurism may also be consumed by dissonance. The drive to engage in this activity does not make sense, considering the lengths to which the voyeur goes and the risks taken. "Why am I throwing away 2 or 3 hours staring through these binoculars on the off chance that I will see somebody naked, when I can rent a movie, buy a magazine, or even find a real relationship? I must be such a loser." As with all obsessions and compulsions, the shame and anxiety is temporarily relieved by engaging in the very activity that brings it about.

Transvestic Fetishism

In **transvestic fetishism**, sexual satisfaction is achieved by dressing in the clothing of the opposite gender. This behavior is related to fetishism but often goes beyond the use of one particular object. Generally this behavior develops early in life and is associated with someone with whom the person is closely associated, whether in a loving relationship or through abuse. Unlike in gender identity disorders, there are no sexual orientation issues, and people with transvestic fetishism do not desire a sex change. Transvestites are usually heterosexual; many cross-dress only in specific sexual situations, and they often receive the cooperation and support of their partners. This paraphilia is more common in men than in women. Over time some men, as well as some women, with transvestic fetishism desire to dress and live permanently as the opposite sex.

Sexual Sadism

Sexual sadism is a term derived from the Marquis de Sade (1740-1814), a well-known French writer who was obsessed with sexual violence. This disorder involves the achievement of sexual satisfaction from the physical or psychological suffering (including humiliation) of the victim. The sadist inflicts pain and suffering on (usually) nonconsenting persons. Most persons with this disorder are male, and the onset usually occurs prior to age 18 (Sadock & Sadock, 2008).

Consenting partners for sadists may be sexual masochists. **Sexual masochism** involves the achievement of sexual satisfaction by being humiliated, beaten, bound, or otherwise made to suffer. Sexual masochistic practices are more common among men than among women (Sadock & Sadock, 2008). In either case, participants tend to know this is a "game," and actual humiliation or pain is avoided.

Frotteurism

Frotteurism is characterized by rubbing or touching a nonconsenting person. In fact, the word *frotteurism* originates from the French word *frotter*, which means to "rub or scrape." The disorder is usually seen in men and typically occurs in busy public places, particularly in subways and buses, where the individual can escape after touching his victim (APA, 2000; Becker & Johnson, 2008). People with this disorder often have no close relationships, and this sort of aggressive contact is their only means of sexual gratification (Sadock & Sadock, 2008).

Paraphilia Not Otherwise Specified

The diagnosis of *paraphilia not otherwise specified* includes various paraphilias that do not meet the criteria for the other categories. Included in this grouping are:
- **Telephone and computer scatologia**—obscene phone calling to an unsuspecting person or sending obscene messages or video images by email
- **Necrophilia**—obsession with having a sexual encounter with a cadaver
- **Partialism**—a concentration of sexual activity on one part of the body to the exclusion of all other parts
- **Zoophilia**—incorporation of animals into sexual activity
- **Urophilia**—sexual activity that involves urinating on one's partner or being urinated on
- **Hypoxyphilia**—desire to achieve an altered state of consciousness secondary to hypoxia while experiencing orgasm; a drug such as nitrous oxide may be used to produce hypoxia

Many of the people involved in nonstandard sexual practices find no need for therapy because their sexual activities are carried out with a consenting adult partner, and they are neither illegal nor physically or emotionally harmful to either partner. If, however, the person is experiencing relationship difficulties, wishes to change the sexual behaviors, becomes involved in illegal activity, or is physically or emotionally harming others or being harmed, therapy is indicated.

EPIDEMIOLOGY

Some parents report symptoms of gender identity disturbances that were apparent before the age of 3 (Sadock & Sadock, 2008). This condition is extremely uncommon and affects 3 to 4 times as many males as females (Becker & Johnson, 2008).

Although the paraphilias are uncommon, the repetitive and consuming nature of the disorders make the occurrence highly frequent (Sadock & Sadock, 2008). Most people with paraphilias are Caucasian males, and in about 50% of these individuals, the onset of the paraphiliac arousal is before age 18 years (APA, 2000). The behaviors associated with the disorder tend to peak in the decade between 15 and 25 years of age and then become virtually nonexistent by age 50. Patients with paraphilias often have more than one paraphilia, which can occur simultaneously or at different points in their lives.

COMORBIDITY

Personality disorders are present in about 60% of people with gender identity disorder. The most common are borderline, antisocial, and narcissistic. Substance abuse and self-destructive behavior are also common. Attention deficit hyperactivity disorder (ADHD) in childhood, substance abuse, phobic disorders, and major depression/dysthymia are strongly associated with paraphilias (Shafer, 2008).

ETIOLOGY
Biological Factors

While biological factors are not thought to *cause* this disorder, they are believed to influence its development (Becker & Johnson, 2008). Hormones may play a role, since decreased levels of testosterone in males and increased levels in women are associated with transsexualism.

A variety of theories attempt to identify what predisposes an individual to the development of paraphilias, but these theories are far from conclusive, since they have focused primarily on violent offenders. Some people with paraphilias have temporal lobe diseases (Becker & Stinson, 2008). Inappropriate sexual arousal has been linked to abnormal levels of androgens.

Psychosocial Factors

Learning theorists suggest the absence of same-sex role models may contribute to gender identity disorder. In this scenario, caregivers provide either covert or overt approval for cross-gender identification and behaviors. Psychoanalytic theorists have posited that male children who are deprived of their mothers seek to internally meld or become one with their mothers. This melding prevents them from developing fully as a separate entity. Clinical studies indicate that boys who have gender identity disorders have overly close relationships with their mothers and are disconnected with their fathers.

Psychoanalytic theories also suggest that castration anxiety results in a safer substitution of a symbolic object for the mother, which results in fetishism and transvestism. The need for a safe substitute may result in extreme behaviors such as pedophilia, exhibitionism, and voyeurism (Shafer, 2008). Learning theorists explain paraphilias in terms of timing and reinforcement. During vulnerable periods, especially puberty, sexual exploration is common; if it is pleasurable and there are no negative consequences, the activity becomes reinforced and is repeated. For example, if an adolescent boy experiments sexually with a 7-year-old boy, does not get caught, and continues to fantasize, he may develop arousal to young boys.

Cognitive theorists identify paraphilias as being based on cognitive distortions. Errors in thought make it seem acceptable for deviant and destructive sexual behaviors to occur. For example, belief that there is agreement on the part of a child makes it okay in the individual's mind to have relations with her; or watching others engage in sexual relations is okay "as long as no one gets hurt." Perhaps the perpetrator of exhibitionistic behavior believes that young girls may get as excited as he does when he exposes himself.

APPLICATION OF THE NURSING PROCESS

ASSESSMENT
General Assessment

Patients with gender identity disorders and paraphilias rarely are hospitalized as a direct result of their condition. People with both gender identity disorder and paraphilias may be overrepresented in psychiatric care settings, owing to the frequency of comorbid psychiatric conditions that are undoubtedly exacerbated by the sexual disorder. Nurses who work in forensic settings such as prisons and jails may care for inmates who are imprisoned due to consequences of paraphilias (e.g., sexual impulse disorders). Depression with suicidal ideation and substance abuse are common comorbid conditions and should be assessed using principles outlined in Chapters 13 and 18.

During a thorough assessment for any psychiatric disorder (or medical condition as well), you may discover symptoms of gender identity disorder or one of the paraphilias. For example, you may ask a patient about his family, and he may remark that he and his wife "aren't getting along so great lately." As you explore this area of concern further, he reveals, "My wife wants to do the same old boring things…you know…sexually, all the time." As the assessment continues, you may learn that he is focused on sadistic sorts of activities, is obsessed with pornography, and no longer becomes aroused by his wife.

Self-Assessment

It is common for students to read descriptions of sexual disorders and respond with disgust to behaviors that seem objectionable or ridiculous. It is also common to respond with frustration, anger, and even hostility to people with disorders like sexual masochism and pedophilia. While it may be difficult, stop and consider that these deviations are not the sum total of who the person is. There are other aspects to their temperament, and they may well have traits of character more to your liking, such as kindness over cruelty, caring over noncaring, sensitivity over insensitivity, conscientiousness over lack of conscience, and so on. Furthermore, they can legitimately suffer from the full range of mental, emotional, and spiritual distress anyone can. You may even know individuals who, despite their carefully guarded secret obsessions, you care for on many levels.

It may be argued that people have control over their thoughts and deviant sexual behaviors. In fact, the notion of control is the basis for placing blame or stigmatizing anyone with a psychiatric disorder. While you may not blame a person with schizophrenia for exhibiting psychotic symptoms, it is easier to conclude that any sexual deviance could be stopped if the patient really wanted to and would simply make up his or her mind to do so. However, when it comes to appetites or drives such as hunger, thirst, pain, and the need for sleep or sex, biological regulatory systems may exert tremendous influence that overcomes willpower. A major issue in trying to understand human behavior is where to draw the line between considering a person to be the product of life experiences and biological makeup, and considering him or her (by virtue of having subjective consciousness) to be an active agent capable of transcending previous determinants.

Nurses may also experience some dissonance when they think about providing care for someone who engages in what they view as objectionable, or even reprehensible, acts. We may have known someone who was the victim of a voyeur or a pedophile, or we may personally have been victimized. Exploring sexual disorders, even in an academic context, may evoke significant distress. At this point, talking with a faculty member, a primary care provider, or someone at a mental health clinic can be helpful and important and may even result in better personal understanding and coping.

Assessment Guidelines Sexual Disorders

1. Assess the potential for self-harm, because patients with gender identity disorders and paraphilias may become despondent and be more of a suicide risk.
2. The main focus of the assessment should be on the presenting problem (e.g., depression with suicidal ideation).
3. Elicit the patient's perception of the impact of the sexual disorder upon the current illness.

DIAGNOSIS

Nursing diagnoses for individuals with gender identity disorder or a paraphilia are suggested in Table 21-6. Other diagnoses should be considered, depending upon the comorbid psychiatric condition that has precipitated the admission.

OUTCOMES IDENTIFICATION

NOC (Moorhead et al., 2008) identifies a number of outcomes for patients with either ineffective sexuality patterns or risk for other-directed violence. Included are *Sexual Identity* and *Impulse Self-Control*. Table 21-7 provides selected intermediate and short-term indicators for these outcomes.

TABLE 21-6 Potential Nursing Diagnoses for Sexual Disorders

Signs and Symptoms	Nursing Diagnoses
History of violating the boundaries of others	*Risk for other-directed violence*
Profound shame and worthlessness	*Risk for self-directed violence*
Uncomfortable with sexual obsessions	*Ineffective sexuality pattern*
Regret and shame related to sexual obsessions and behaviors; believes he is different and deviant; poor eye contact	*Self-esteem disturbance*
States, "I am a woman trapped in a man's body."	*Disturbed personal identity*
Responds to stress with deviant sexual behavior Abuse of substances	*Ineffective coping*
Isolates self from others; has difficulty and disinterest in connecting in a meaningful way with others	*Impaired social interaction*
Disorganization or dysfunction in usual patterns of behavior (absence from work, withdrawal from relationships, changes in role function)	*Ineffective role performance*
Feeling of being out of control, behaviors, and awareness	*Anxiety*
Inability to explain actions or behaviors	*Spiritual distress*

Data from North American Nursing Diagnosis Association International (NANDA-I). (2009). *NANDA-I nursing diagnoses: Definitions and classification 2009-2011.* Oxford, United Kingdom: Author.

TABLE 21-7 *NOC* Outcomes for Sexual Disorders

Nursing Outcome and Definition	Intermediate Indicators	Short-Term Indicators
Sexual Identity: Acknowledgment and acceptance of own sexual identity	Seeks social support	Uses healthy coping behaviors to resolve sexual identity issues Reports healthy sexual functioning
Impulse Self-Control: Self-restraint of compulsive or impulsive behaviors	Identifies harmful impulsive behaviors Identifies feelings that lead to impulsive actions Identifies consequences of impulsive actions	Avoids high-risk environments Avoids high-risk situations Upholds contract to control behavior Maintains self-control without supervision

Data from Moorhead, S., Johnson, M., Maas, M., & Swanson, E. (Eds.). (2008). *Nursing outcomes classification (NOC)* (4th ed.). St. Louis: Mosby.

PLANNING

Planning nursing care for the patient with a gender identity disorder or paraphilia is influenced by the setting and presenting problem. The basic level nurse may encounter such a patient during treatment for a comorbid condition, especially when the patient is admitted to the hospital for suicidal thoughts and behavior. Sometimes psychiatric care and treatment are mandated, such as when a voyeur or exhibitionist gets caught.

The care plan will focus on safety and crisis intervention. The patient may also be treated for comorbid depression or anxiety disorders in the community setting. Planning will address the major complaint, along with the sexual disorder.

IMPLEMENTATION

Interventions are aimed at offering a nonjudgmental emotional presence while exploring identity issues, self-esteem, and anxiety and encouraging an optimal level of functioning. Patients with a potential for violating the boundaries of others may require closer observation and firm limit setting. Box 21-3 lists examples of basic-level *NIC* interventions for gender identity disorders.

Health Teaching and Health Promotion

Education for the patient with a sexual disorder is typically geared toward reducing symptoms from the presenting problem, typically depression and anxiety. Patients with paraphilias can be taught to journal their feelings and begin to identify triggers for pathological behavior.

Milieu Management

When the patient who has a gender identity disorder or a paraphilia is in a crisis that requires hospitalization, providing a safe environment is fundamental. All patients on a psychiatric inpatient unit should be informed on admission about unit rules regarding personal contact between patients and between patients and staff. Limit setting is done consistently when it is needed.

Individuals with paraphilias tend to isolate themselves. The unit environment may be a challenge. Sharing meals with others may result in discomfort, and the patient might wonder what other people know about him or her. A particular challenge may be interacting in formal group settings and the expectation of participation. But the group setting may actually provide patients with the greatest opportunity for growth, in that they can experience others as

---

> ### BOX 21-3 *NIC* Interventions for Gender Identity Disorders and Paraphilias
>
> **Behavior Management: Sexual**
> *Definition:* Delineation and prevention of socially unacceptable sexual behaviors
> *Activities*:*
> - Discuss consequences of unacceptable behavior.
> - Discuss the negative impact that behavior has on others.
> - Encourage expression of feelings about past crises.
> - Provide opportunities for caregivers to process their feelings about the patient.
>
> **Self-Esteem Enhancement**
> *Definition:* Assisting a patient to increase his/her personal judgment of self-worth
> *Activities*:*
> - Encourage patient to identify strengths.
> - Assist in setting realistic goals to achieve higher self-esteem.
> - Assist patient to accept dependence on others, as appropriate.
> - Explore previous achievements of success.
> - Encourage patient to accept new challenges.
>
> **Social Skills Behavior Modification**
> *Definition:* Assisting the patient to develop or improve interpersonal social skills
> *Activities*:*
> - Assist in identifying problems resulting from social skill deficits.
> - Encourage verbalization of feelings regarding social interaction.
> - Identify a specific skill to improve.
> - Identify steps to reach skill and role-play the steps.
>
> ---
> *Partial list.
> Data from Bulechek, G. M., Butcher, H. K., & Dochterman, J. M. (Eds.). (2008). *Nursing interventions classification (NIC)* (5th ed.). St. Louis: Mosby.

---

humans with feelings, perhaps learning how much anguish and pain personal violations have caused them. The group milieu can mean having others present who empathize with one's background and current distress.

Pharmacological Interventions

While there is no single treatment for sexual disorders, two classes of pharmacological agents, antiandrogens and serotonergic antidepressants, are prescribed during treatment. Medication is not used independently as a treatment without other interventions. Drugs that reduce levels of testosterone may be used to treat sex offenders. The drugs that are frequently used are progestin derivatives, including medroxyprogesterone acetate (MPA) (an analog of progesterone) and cyproterone acetate (CPA) (an inhibitor of testosterone). Both of these drugs act to decrease libido and break the individual's pattern of compulsive deviant sexual behavior. They work best in patients with paraphilias and a high sexual drive, such as pedophiles and exhibitionists, and less well in those with a low sexual drive or an antisocial personality (Becker & Johnson, 2008).

Current research is focusing on the use of SSRIs in the treatment of sexual disorders. Fluoxetine (Prozac) has been used successfully to treat patients with exhibitionism, voyeurism, and pedophilia and persons who have committed rape. In addition to fluoxetine, other drugs, such as clomipramine (Anafranil) and fluvoxamine (Luvox), have been used in the treatment of sexual obsessions, addictions, and paraphilias. The role of the nurse in pharmacotherapy is to educate patients regarding the specific drug prescribed and to monitor the drug's effectiveness and watch for untoward side effects (Becker & Johnson, 2008).

Advanced Practice Interventions

Psychotherapy

Psychotherapy is recommended to address gender dysphoria and comorbid conditions (Shafer, 2008). However, patients with gender identity disorder tend to resist psychotherapy except as a means to reach the goal of sex reassignment surgery. When gender dysphoria is severe and intractable, this may be an option. If the patient is considered appropriate for sex reassignment, psychotherapy is usually initiated to prepare the patient for the cross-gender role. The patient is then instructed to live in the cross-gender role before surgery is performed—including going to work or attending school—to help the individual determine whether he or she can interact successfully with members of society in the cross-gender mode. Legal and social arrangements are made: the name is changed on various documents, and new employment is obtained if it is necessary to leave a former job because of discrimination. Relationship issues, such as what to tell parents, children, and former spouses, must be resolved. Males are instructed to have electrolysis and practice female behaviors. Females are instructed to cut their hair, bind or conceal their breasts, and similarly take on the identity of a man.

After 1 or 2 years, if these measures have been successful and the patient still wishes reassignment, hormone treatment is begun; males take estrogen, and females take androgen. After another 1 to 2 years of hormone therapy, the patient may be considered for surgical reassignment if it is still desired. In the male-to-female patient, the procedure consists of bilateral orchiectomy, penile amputation, and creation of an artificial vagina. Female-to-male patients undergo

bilateral mastectomy and optional hysterectomy with removal of the ovaries. Efforts to create an artificial penis have met with mixed results. Psychotherapy is indicated after surgery to help the patient adjust to the surgical changes and discuss sexual functioning and satisfaction (Becker & Johnson, 2008). Box 21-4 describes a case of sexual reassignment gone wrong.

The usual treatment plan for working with patients with paraphilias is cognitive-behavioral therapy. An attempt is made to help the person learn a new sexual response pattern that will eliminate the need for the activity that is causing the problem. Techniques range from positive reinforcement for appropriate object choices to aversion techniques, in which mild electric shocks may be applied for inappropriate choices. Other treatment modalities include psychodynamic techniques designed to help the patient understand the origin of the paraphilia.

Advanced practice nurses may seek specialized training to enable them to work effectively with patients with gender identity disorders and paraphilias. This preparation allows the advanced practice nurse to practice sex therapy and conduct sex research. The American Association of Sex Educators, Counselors, and Therapists (AASECT) provides credentialing

---

BOX 21-4 Nature or Nurture? A Case of Sex Reassignment Gone Wrong

Accidents in early infancy may result in sexual reassignment. One such fascinating case is that of David Reimer, a Canadian-born identical twin male whose penis was destroyed as the result of a botched circumcision. With the advice of health care professionals, the child underwent surgical reassignment and later received hormonal therapy in puberty to induce the development of breasts and secondary female sex characteristics.

While the family psychologist proclaimed the reassignment from male to female a success and concluded that gender identity was primarily based on socialization, David never felt comfortable. He rejected his female designation of Brenda, and began living his life as a male at age 14. Shortly after he learned of his biological sex, he had the reassignment surgically reversed, married a woman, and became stepfather to her three children.

However, David always felt uncomfortable and ultimately committed suicide. His case bolstered support for the biological influence of prenatal and early-life exposure to male hormones on gender identity. David Reimer's life is chronicled in the book *As Nature Made Him*, which raises questions about gender reassignment and the modification of an unconsenting minor's genitals.

From Colapinto, J. (2006). *As nature made him: The boy who was raised as a girl.* New York: Harper Collins.

based on academic preparation, clinical supervision, experience, and skills. Credentialing is a method by which consumers of mental health care services can be assured of the professional competency of the therapist treating them.

EVALUATION

Evaluation for patients with sexual disorders is partly based on determining whether the outcomes for the presenting problem were achieved. Outcomes specific to the sexual disorder are also evaluated. Long-term goals, such as "achieves healthy sexual functioning," can only be aimed at during a typical inpatient stay; realistically, such outcomes require continued outpatient therapy. People with sexual impulse disorders, especially those that generate victims, may be required to continue treatment, which has been demonstrated to reduce recidivism (relapse into the offending behavior) (Becker & Johnson, 2008).

In regards to gender identity disorder, the issues may have only been touched upon. Long-term therapy is required. In rare cases, psychotherapy results in the reversal of this disorder (Becker & Johnson, 2008). Ultimately, the patient may opt for sexual reassignment.

KEY POINTS TO REMEMBER

- A *sexual dysfunction* is defined as a disturbance in the normal sexual response cycle.
- There are seven different types of sexual dysfunction.
- Sexual problems are considered to be socially atypical, have the potential to disrupt meaningful relationships, and may result in insult or even significant injury to other people.
- Health care workers are often uncomfortable asking questions related to sexuality. Providing professional and holistic care requires that nurses include this vital area of assessment.
- Certain medical and surgical conditions and some drugs result in a variety of sexual dysfunctions, including low libido, impotence, erectile dysfunction, anorgasmia, and priapism.
- There are distinctions between biological sex and gender identity. Gender identity disorder is a strong and persistent cross-gender identification.
- *Paraphilia* is a term used to identify repetitive or preferred sexual fantasies or behaviors that involve preference for use of a nonhuman object, repetitive sexual activity with humans involving real or simulated suffering or humiliation, and repetitive sexual activity with nonconsenting partners.
- Paraphilias include fetishism, pedophilia, exhibitionism, voyeurism, transvestic fetishism, sexual sadism and masochism, frotteurism, and paraphilia not otherwise specified.

- In addition to conducting a sexual assessment, nurses are involved in milieu and behavioral therapy, counseling, education, and medication management.
- Nursing interventions for paraphilias involve administration of medications (e.g., medroxyprogesterone [Depo-Provera] and SSRIs) and therapy.
- Advanced practice nurses may specialize in the area of sexual counseling, treatment, and therapy.

CRITICAL THINKING

1. As a nurse on an adolescent psychiatric mental health nursing unit, you often encounter teenagers who are misinformed about growth and development as well as sexuality. What information would you include in a series of teaching sessions that would help these adolescents acquire a greater understanding of the developmental changes they are going through?

2. In order to understand your own beliefs, answer these questions:
   A. Are you comfortable with your own sexuality? With that of others?
   B. Are you judgmental?
   C. Could you be helpful to someone who has a sexual disorder?
   D. What factors have influenced your beliefs and values regarding sexuality?
   E. What do you think is the impact of sexually explicit television, music videos, and movies on your sexual attitudes, values, and beliefs?

3. During a one-to-one session, Mrs. Chase, a patient who was admitted to your inpatient unit with depression and anxiety confides concern about her 17-year-old son, Alex. She becomes tearful and says, "I don't know what I've done wrong. Alex was arrested for exposing himself to a girl at school. I'm worried that he may begin doing even worse things."
   A. Provide Mrs. Chase with information regarding Alex's condition.
   B. What sort of feelings in yourself about Alex would you need to be aware of in order to be the most helpful to Mrs. Chase?

CHAPTER REVIEW

1. A 27-year-old patient states that since her marriage ended 2 years ago, she has found herself lacking interest and motivation in sexual activity. Which response is most likely to be therapeutic?
   1. "What was your view of sex before your divorce?"
   2. "Tell me more about your life since your marriage ended."

3. "Often physical illness causes decreased desire in women."
4. "This is a common problem, what with all the stress women face."

2. A young, newly-married man with schizophrenia presents in the emergency department with a complaint of "demons sticking needles in my penis." Which initial response by the triage nurse would be appropriate?
   1. Arrange for the patient to be evaluated by the doctor or advanced practice registered nurse on duty, because the patient may be expressing real pain in a delusional manner.
   2. Request an order for labs to rule out a sexually transmitted disease, given that the patient has recently begun sexual relations with his new wife and may have been exposed.
   3. Complete the triage process, and refer the patient to the psychiatric liaison nurse for a mental health evaluation, since he appears to be psychotic and possibly having a relapse.
   4. Reassure the patient that it is not possible for demons to be in the emergency room and, with his permission, ask to speak with his wife to get a better understanding of his needs.

3. A young male patient tells you that somehow he feels that he should not be a man, that inside he is a woman. This is likely an example of:
   1. fetishism.
   2. frotteurism.
   3. transsexualism.
   4. transvestic fetishism.

4. Mary is the nurse assigned to work with Mr. Roberts, a transsexual male on a step-down unit. He is in counseling as part of the process of seeking sexual reassignment surgery and has female clothing in his hospital locker. Mary is anxious at the prospect of working with someone like Mr. Roberts and spends only the briefest amounts of time possible responding to his needs. What are the best descriptions of what is occurring here? *Select all that apply.*
   1. Mary may believe that Mr. Roberts has chosen to behave in a deviant fashion, rather than that he has a gender identity disorder.
   2. Mary is failing to maintain professional objectivity because of her values and beliefs about this particular patient's decisions and behavior.
   3. Mary is experiencing a common negative response to a situation about which she has limited knowledge and that she is unable to understand.
   4. Mary may be having difficulty looking beyond Mr. Robert's gender issues and as a result is failing to see or respond to him simply as a person.
   5. Nurses have a right to have personal feelings about social issues, and as long as Mr. Robert's minimal care needs are addressed, Mary is within her rights to respond this way.
   6. Mary may be disgusted with Mr. Roberts because she is confusing his disorder with the predatory behavior sometimes exhibited by patients with paraphilias such as pedophilia.

5. Ms. Thompson is the nurse working with Mr. Williams, a patient in his early 30s who is in good health overall and is being evaluated for erectile dysfunction. Mr. Williams is very embarrassed by his condition, distressed by the impact he feels it is having on his marriage, and reports that he "does not feel like a man" as a result of this disorder. What is a realistic short-term outcome to expect when caring for this patient? Mr. Williams:
   1. reports that he has begun to feel like a man.
   2. is able to maintain an erection through orgasm.
   3. reports that he has accepted his impaired erectile function.
   4. demonstrates an accurate understanding of the meaning of his disorder.

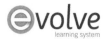

Visit the Evolve website for an **Audio Chapter Summary, Chapter Review Answers & Rationales, Critical Thinking Answer Guidelines,** and additional resources related to the content in this chapter: **http://evolve.elsevier.com/Varcarolis/foundations**

Companion CD Use the Companion CD to prepare for tests and the NCLEX® Examination with **Test-Taking Strategies** for psychiatric mental health nursing and hundreds of **Review Questions.**

References

American Psychiatric Association (APA). (2000). *Diagnostic and statistical manual of mental disorders* (4th ed., text rev.) *(DSM-IV-TR)*. Washington, DC: Author.

Becker, J. V., & Johnson, B. R. (2008). Gender identity disorders and paraphilias. In R. E. Hales, S. C. Yudofsky, & G. O. Gabbard (Eds.), *Textbook of psychiatry* (5th ed., pp. 729–753). Washington, DC: American Psychiatric Publishing.

Becker, J. V., & Stinson, J. D. (2008). Human sexuality and sexual dysfunctions. In R. E. Hales, S. C. Yudofsky, & G. O. Gabbard (Eds.), *Textbook of psychiatry* (5th ed., pp. 711–728). Washington, DC: American Psychiatric Publishing.

Bulechek, G. M., Butcher, H. K., & Dochterman, J. M. (Eds.). (2008). *Nursing interventions classification (NIC)* (5th ed.). St. Louis: Mosby.

Dhalwani, N. N. (2008). Barriers and facilitators in sexual history taking. From a presentation entitled *Health care challenges in diverse populations*. Retrieved November 14, 2008 from http://stti.confex.com/stti/congrs08/techprogram/paper_39904.htm

Hickey, C., Saunders, B., & Stuckey, B. (2007). Non-hormonal treatments for menopausal symptoms. *Maturitas, 57*(1), 85–89.

Higgins, A. (2007). Impact of psychotropic medication on sexuality: Literature review. *British Journal of Nursing, 16,* 545–550.

Kaplan, H. S. (1974). *The new sex therapy: Active treatment of sexual dysfunctions*. New York: Brunner/Mazel.

Mick, J. M. (2007). Sexuality assessment: 10 strategies for improvement. *Clinical Journal of Oncology Nursing, 11,* 671–675.

Moorhead, S., Johnson, M., Maas, M., & Swanson, E. (Eds.). (2008). *Nursing outcomes classification (NOC)* (4th ed.). St. Louis: Mosby.

North American Nursing Diagnosis Association International (NANDA-I). (2009). *NANDA-I nursing diagnoses: Definitions and classification 2009-2011*. Oxford, United Kingdom: Author.

Sadock, B. J., & Sadock, V. A. (2008). *Kaplan & Sadock's concise textbook of clinical psychiatry* (3rd ed.). Philadelphia: Lippincott Williams & Wilkins.

Segraves, R., & Woodard, T. (2006). Female hypoactive sexual desire disorder: History and current status. *The Journal of Sexual Medicine, 3,* 408–418.

Shafer, L. C. (2008). Sexual disorders and sexual dysfunction. In T. A. Stern, J. F. Rosenbaum, M. Fava, J. Biederman, & S. L. Rauch (Eds.), *Massachusetts General Hospital comprehensive clinical psychiatry* (pp. 487–497). St. Louis: Mosby.

CHAPTER **22**

Somatoform, Factitious, and Dissociative Disorders

Faye J. Grund and Nancy Christine Shoemaker

Key Terms and Concepts

Objectives

1. Compare and contrast essential characteristics of the somatoform, factitious, and dissociative disorders.
2. Identify a clinical example of what would be found in each of the somatoform disorders.
3. Describe five psychosocial interventions that would be appropriate for a patient with somatic complaints.
4. Plan interventions for a patient with conversion disorder who is receiving a great deal of secondary gain from his or her "blindness." Include self-care and family teaching.

5. Describe disorders that are conscious attempts to deceive health care professionals.
6. Explain the key symptoms of the four dissociative disorders.
7. Compare and contrast dissociative amnesia and dissociative fugue.
8. Identify three specialized elements in the assessment of a patient with a dissociative disorder.
9. Identify nursing interventions for patients with somatoform and dissociative disorders.

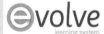 Visit the Evolve website for an **Audio Glossary & Flashcards, Concept Map Creator**, and additional resources related to the content in this chapter: **http://evolve.elsevier.com/Varcarolis/foundations**

Anxiety exerts a powerful influence on the mind and may lead to clinical conditions known as anxiety disorders. Although patients with anxiety disorders often have some somatic (physical) symptoms, the predominant complaint is mental or emotional distress. In somatoform and dissociative disorders, the primary focus of the patient is on physical manifestations of the disorders. These conditions are relatively rare in the psychiatric setting, but the nurse may encounter patients with such disorders in the general medical setting or in specialized units. This chapter presents an overview of the unconsciously motivated somatoform disorders and associated nursing care. We will also take a brief look at factitious disorders in which symptoms of illness are intentionally induced. The chapter concludes with a presentation of the dissociative disorders and a description of nursing care.

Somatoform Disorders

Somatoform disorders are defined in the *Diagnostic and Statistical Manual of Mental Disorders*, fourth edition, text revision *(DSM-IV-TR)* (American Psychiatric Association [APA], 2000) as a group in which:

- Physical symptoms suggest a physical disorder for which there is no demonstrable base.
- There is a strong presumption that the symptoms are linked to psychobiological factors.

Soma is the Greek word for "body," and **somatization** is the expression of psychological stress through physical symptoms. Somatoform disorders demonstrate complex mind-body interactions, and they cause real distress to the patient, with significant impairment in social and occupational functioning. These disorders are difficult to distinguish from physical disorders with organic causes, and the patient's history is extremely important for accurate diagnosis. Often the patient has a comorbid psychiatric disorder. (Refer to Chapter 3 to review the biology of the brain and better understand the varied symptoms of these disorders.)

CLINICAL PICTURE

The somatoform disorders currently recognized by the *DSM-IV-TR* include:

- Somatization disorder
- Undifferentiated somatoform disorder
- Conversion disorder
- Pain disorder
- Hypochondriasis
- Body dysmorphic disorder
- Somatoform disorder not otherwise specified

The five main somatoform disorders—diagnostic criteria for which are presented in Figure 22-1—are addressed in this chapter.

Somatization Disorder

Somatization disorder is the most common somatoform disorder (Yutzy & Parish, 2008). Diagnosis requires the presence of a certain number of symptoms accompanied by significant functional impairment. Pain, gastrointestinal symptoms, sexual symptoms, and pseudoneurological symptoms are hallmarks of this disorder. Patients report significant distress and seek out multiple providers for medical care. Anxiety and depression are common comorbid conditions. Patients often report being ill for prolonged periods of time and have a variety of symptoms. The course of the illness is chronic and relapsing, with most patients developing a new symptom at least once a year. Suicide threats and gestures are common, but attempts are rarely lethal. On average, patients with this disorder spend 7 days per month sick in bed.

People who meet the criteria for somatization disorder are more often female, nonwhite, poorly educated, of a low socioeconomic status, and from rural areas (Greenberg et al., 2008). Women with this disorder tend to come from chaotic and neglectful families and often have histories of physical and sexual abuse. Somatization can be viewed as an ineffective but drastic attempt to seek help and care.

Complaints are dramatic, shocking, and may be hard to believe (e.g., "I haven't been able to eat or drink for a week, and I've been in a coma for half that time"). It is difficult to clarify exactly what is going on, and details are vague and inconsistent (Greenberg et al., 2008). Attempts to point out the possibility of depression or anxiety often are met with indignation (e.g., "Who wouldn't be anxious when they're sick all the time and no one can seem to get to the bottom of this!").

Hypochondriasis

Hypochondriasis results in the misinterpretation of innocent physical sensations as evidence of a serious illness. Persons with this disorder exhibit an overconcern for their health and become preoccupied with symptoms they believe may be serious. The extreme worry and fear associated with the possibility of having a disease distinguishes hypochondriasis from other somatoform and anxiety disorders. Most patients refuse a referral to see a mental health professional. The course of the illness is chronic and relapsing, with symptoms becoming amplified during times of increased stress (Greenburg et al., 2008).

Pain Disorder

Pain is one of the most frequent reasons people seek medical attention. When testing rules out any organic cause for the pain, and the discomfort leads to significant impairment, **pain disorder** is diagnosed. Although most pain can be reduced, chronic pain results in significant disability and high costs for health care. Patients who have pain in multiple sites report poorer physical and mental well-being (Baune et al., 2008). More severe or chronic cases of pain are associated with higher prevalence rates of depression.

Pain is difficult to measure objectively, and individuals react differently to the same injury. Pain thresholds vary among individuals. Pain locations often identified include the back, head, lower limbs, temporomandibular joint, and pelvis. The course of the pain disorder varies according to the acuity of symptoms. Acute pain often can be reduced, especially with treatment of a comorbid psychiatric condition and family involvement. Chronic pain is more difficult to treat. Primary care providers should focus on ways of coping with pain, cognitive distortions, and dysfunctional pain behavior.

DSM-IV-TR CRITERIA FOR SOMATOFORM DISORDERS

SOMATOFORM DISORDERS

Somatization Disorder

1. History of many physical complaints beginning before 30 years of age, occurring over a period of years and resulting in impairment in social, occupational, or other important areas of functioning.

2. Complaints must include all of the following:
   - History of pain in at least **four** different sites or functions
   - History of at least **two** gastrointestinal symptoms other than pain
   - History of at least **one** sexual or reproduction symptom
   - History of at least **one** symptom defined as or suggesting a neurological disorder

Conversion Disorder

1. Development of one or more symptoms or deficits suggesting a neurological disorder (blindness, deafness, loss of touch) or general medical condition.

2. Psychological factors are associated with the symptom or deficit because the symptom is initiated or exacerbated by psychological stressors.

3. Not due to malingering or factitious disorder and not culturally sanctioned.

4. Cannot be explained by general medical condition or effects of a substance.

5. Causes impairment in social or occupational functioning, causes marked distress, or requires medical attention.

Hypochondriasis

For at least 6 months:

1. Preoccupation with fears of having, or the idea that one has, a serious disease.

2. Preoccupation persists despite appropriate medical tests and reassurances.

3. Other disorders are ruled out (e.g., somatic delusional disorders).

4. Preoccupation causes significant impairment in social or occupational functioning or causes marked distress.

Pain Disorder

1. Pain in one or more anatomical sites is a major part of the clinical picture.

2. Causes significant impairment in occupational or social functioning or causes marked distress.

3. Psychological factors thought to cause onset, severity, or exacerbation. **Pain associated with psychological factors.**

4. Symptoms not intentionally produced or feigned. If medical condition present, it plays minor role in accounting for pain.

5. **Pain may be associated with a psychological and/or medical condition.** Both factors are judged to be important in onset, severity, exacerbation, and maintenance of pain.

Body Dysmorphic Disorder (BDD)

1. Preoccupation with some imagined defect in appearance. If the defect is present, concern is excessive.

2. Preoccupation causes significant impairment in social or occupational functioning or causes marked distress.

3. Preoccupation not better accounted for by another mental disorder.

Figure 22-1 Diagnostic criteria for somatoform disorders. (Adapted from American Psychiatric Association. [2000]. *Diagnostic and statistical manual of mental disorders* [4th ed., text rev.]. Washington, DC: Author.)

Body Dysmorphic Disorder

Body dysmorphic disorder was first described over a century ago and continues to be a challenge to treat. Patients with body dysmorphic disorder are commonly seen in community, psychiatric, cosmetic surgery, and dermatological settings. Although patients usually have a normal appearance, their preoccupation with an imagined defective body part results in obsessional thinking and compulsive behavior, such as mirror checking and camouflaging.

Patients' false assumptions about the importance of appearance, fear of rejection by others, perfectionism, and conviction of being disfigured lead to overwhelming emotions of disgust, shame, and depression (Stangier et al., 2008). Patients frequently are concerned with their skin, hair, nose, stomach, teeth, weight, and breasts/chest. In one study, men were more likely to be concerned with the appearance of their genitals and body build (90% of men thought they were too small and/or inadequately muscular), and women were found to be more focused on the appearance of their skin, stomach, weight, breasts, buttocks, thighs, legs, hips, and toes (Phillips et al., 2006).

Often the patient keeps the disorder secret for many years and does not respond to reassurance. The disorder is chronic, and response to treatment is limited. The Evidence-Based Practice box describes research related to impairment of psychosocial functioning in patients with body dysmorphic disorder.

EVIDENCE-BASED PRACTICE

Psychosocial Functioning of Patients With Body Dysmorphic Disorder

Phillips, K. A., Quinn, G., Stout, R. L. (2008). Functional impairment in body dysmorphic disorder: A prospective, follow-up study. *Journal of Psychiatric Research, 42*, 701–707.

Problem

Individuals who struggle with body dysmorphic disorder often use avoidance to cope with their perceived bodily defect. This leads to difficulties for them in the work environment, as well as with interpersonal relationships. Results from earlier studies found that a high percentage of individuals with body dysmorphic disorder reported avoiding usual social or occupational activities due to embarrassment over perceived appearance defects. Additionally, individuals with this diagnosis also report impairment in psychosocial functioning. Health care professionals can assist these individuals to recognize their false perceptions, thereby promoting their social, occupational, and psychosocial functioning.

Purpose of Study

The purpose of this longitudinal 3-year study was to examine certain aspects of psychosocial functioning in individuals diagnosed with body dysmorphic disorder. Functional aspects included level of psychosocial functioning, stability of functional impairment, the probability of attaining "functional remission," and predictors of psychosocial functioning.

Methods

Study participants were 176 individuals who met *DSM-IV-TR* criteria for body dysmorphic disorder. By the end of the first year, there were 163 (92.6%) of the original subjects remaining, with 141 and 78 subjects remaining after 2 and 3 years, respectively. Subjects were interviewed at intake and reinterviewed annually. Three tools were used at each interview to determine overall functioning of the subjects. These tools were designed to measure current functioning at work, in interpersonal relations, and in recreation, as well as overall satisfaction.

Key Findings

- Individuals with body dysmorphic disorder had poor psychosocial functioning that remained poor over time.
- Few subjects achieved functional remission during the 3-year period.
- Individuals with more severe symptoms had poorer psychosocial functioning on all three functioning measures.
- Those individuals with more delusional body dysmorphic disorder beliefs had significantly poorer functioning on all three measures.
- Treatment with selective serotonin reuptake inhibitors or cognitive-behavioral therapy did not yield significant improvement in the subjects.
- Owing to the limitations of this study, further studies are needed to confirm the results.

Implications for Nursing Practice

The needs of patients with body dysmorphic disorder merit nursing attention and support. The majority of these patients will initially refuse a referral to psychiatric treatment because they believe their misperception is real. The nurse should develop a trusting therapeutic relationship with the patient and reduce fears about mental health treatment by demonstrating the belief that these interventions are just as acceptable as standard medical treatments. Additionally, nurses must recognize the concerns of family members and be actively engaged in education regarding the nature of the disorder.

Conversion Disorder

Conversion disorder is marked by the presence of deficits in voluntary motor or sensory functions, including paralysis, blindness, movement disorder, gait disorder, numbness, paresthesia, loss of vision or hearing, or episodes resembling epilepsy (Yutzy & Parish, 2008). Many patients show a lack of emotional concern about the symptoms (*la belle indifférence*), although others are quite distressed. Imagine someone casually discussing sudden blindness. Care providers should assume there is an organic cause to the symptoms until physical pathology has been ruled out. Patients truly believe in the presence of the symptoms; they are not fabricated or under voluntary control.

Conversion disorder is the most common somatoform disorder and is more common in females (particularly homemakers), lower socioeconomic groups, lower educational levels, rural areas, and veterans who have been exposed to combat (Sadock & Sadock, 2008). Childhood physical or sexual abuse is common in patients with conversion disorder, and comorbid psychiatric conditions include depression, anxiety, other somatoform disorders, and personality disorders. There are also cases in which a comorbid medical or neurological condition exists, and the conversion symptom is an exaggeration of the original problem.

The course of the disorder is related to its acuity. In cases with acute onset during stressful events, remission rate is high; in cases with a more gradual onset, the disorder is not readily treated. Cases generally remit by themselves 95% of the time (Sadock & Sadock, 2008). Recurrence is as high as 25%, often recurring within the first year.

EPIDEMIOLOGY

Prevalence rates for somatoform disorders in the general population are unknown. Instead, the literature describes their occurrence in the population of individuals who seek medical care. Differentiating somatoform disorders from physical disorders and identifying comorbid conditions are significant issues for the primary care provider. Research shows that half of all frequent users of medical care have psychological problems.

A comprehensive physical examination with appropriate diagnostic studies is necessary to rule out the following medical conditions, which can be confused with somatoform disorders:

- Multiple sclerosis
- Brain tumor
- Hyperthyroidism
- Hyperparathyroidism
- Lupus erythematosus
- Myasthenia gravis

A thorough psychosocial history is also required to clarify a somatoform diagnosis, as well as comorbid psychiatric disorders. Table 22-1 gives detailed information on the prevalence of somatoform disorders in the general medical population, the age of onset, gender predilection, and comorbidity with other psychiatric disorders.

ETIOLOGY

Somatoform disorders include a variety of related but quite different disorders. In the preceding sections of this chapter, you were presented with a brief clinical picture of each of the main somatoform disorders,

CONSIDERING CULTURE

Falling Out

Dante is a 22-year-old Jamaican immigrant who lives in New York City. He drives a cab during the day and attends school in the evening. He wants to become an accountant, and his goal is to attain the first college degree in his family. Life moves by quickly in a blur of passengers and fares, textbooks, teachers, and tests. He has made few friends and is isolated from his family, who are home in the Caribbean.

At the end of another long day, Dante hastily turns in the keys to his cab to the manager, exits the garage onto the rush-hour filled sidewalk, and begins a near-jog as he hurries to get to his first class. A wave of dizziness hits him and casts him into a slow-motion world, blackness surrounds

him, and he falls to the ground. Dante hears the sounds of the street, people walking, and horns blaring. A baby cries somewhere close by. A man's voice says, "What's wrong with you? Get up and out of the way." Dante tries to respond, but he cannot lift a finger, let alone stand up.

What Dante experienced is known as *falling out* (or blacking out). This is a culture-bound syndrome that occurs in people from the Caribbean and the southern part of the United States. It is characterized by a sudden collapse followed by an inability to see or move. The individual is aware of what is happening around him, and his eyes remain open. Falling out may be a variant of conversion or dissociative disorder (Hales et al., 2008).

Hales, R. E., Yudofsky, S. C., & Gabbard, G. O. (2008). *Textbook of psychiatry* (5th ed.). Washington, DC: American Psychiatric Publishing.

TABLE 22-1 Somatoform Disorders

Disorder	Prevalence	Age of Onset	Gender Prediction	Comorbidities
Somatization disorder	1%-2% in general population 5%-10% in doctors' offices	Adolescence to 30s	Women 80%, men 20%	Major depression Anxiety disorder Personality disorder
Conversion disorder	5%-15% of consults in general hospital	Any age	Twice as frequent in women	Major depression Anxiety disorder Schizophrenia
Hypochondriasis	4%-6% (maybe as high as 15%) in general medical population	20-30 years of age	Equal prevalence in women and men	Depressive disorder Anxiety disorder Other somatoform disorders
Pain disorder	12% lifetime prevalence in the general population	Any age	Gender ratio unknown	Depressive disorder Substance dependence
Body dysmorphic disorder	Unknown to 30s	15-30 years of age	Slightly more women than men	Major depression Anxiety disorder Psychotic disorder

Data from Sadock, B. J., & Sadock, V. A. (2008). *Kaplan & Sadock's concise textbook of clinical psychiatry* (3rd ed.). Philadelphia: Lippincott Williams & Wilkins.

along with possible etiologies. In the following sections, we will discuss the classification as a whole.

Biological Factors

Any abnormality in the structure of the brain or the function of the neurotransmitters can lead to a misinterpretation of ordinary events. For example, the brain may misunderstand (or amplify) a stimulus, identifying a minor gas pain as a serious abdominal injury (somatization); or the brain may overreact in its analysis of the stimulus, deciding that the same minor gas pain is a sign of colon cancer (hypochondriasis).

Remember that research into anxiety disorders has demonstrated structural changes in the brain that may result from prolonged stress or trauma, as well as imbalances in neurotransmitters. In the case of anxiety disorders, these abnormalities create altered feeling and thinking processes, whereas the processes of perception and interpretation of bodily sensations are fairly intact. It is not known why some patients develop an anxiety disorder, and others develop a somatoform disorder.

Neurochemistry may be altered in somatoform disorders. Han and colleagues (2008) studied patients meeting the diagnostic criteria for undifferentiated somatoform disorder, and from baseline to end of treatment, somatic symptoms were significantly decreased after treatment with a selective serotonin reuptake

inhibitor (SSRI). Although further research is warranted, treatment with antidepressants has been found to have beneficial effects in individuals with somatic symptoms.

Genetic

The *DSM-IV-TR* notes that somatoform disorders may have a genetic component. Somatization disorder tends to run in families, occurring in 10% to 20% of first-degree female relatives of women with somatization disorder (Sadock & Sadock, 2008). Twin studies show an increased risk of conversion disorder in monozygotic twin pairs. First-degree biological relatives of people with chronic pain disorder are more likely to have chronic pain, depressive disorder, and alcohol dependence.

Psychosocial Factors

Psychoanalytic Theory

Psychoanalytic theorists believe that psychogenic complaints of pain, illness, or loss of physical function are related to repression of a conflict (usually of an aggressive or sexual nature) and transformation of anxiety into a physical symptom that is symbolically related to the conflict. For example, in conversion disorder, conversion symptoms allow a forbidden wish or urge to be partly expressed but sufficiently disguised so that the individual does not have to face the unacceptable wish. The symptoms also permit the individual to communicate a need for special treatment or consideration from others.

Hypochondriasis is considered by many clinicians to have psychodynamic origins. These clinicians suggest that anger, aggression, or hostility that had its source in past losses or disappointments is expressed as a need for help and concern from others. Other clinicians suggest that hypochondriasis is a defense against guilt or low self-esteem. In the patient's view, the somatic symptoms serve as deserved punishment. In pain disorder, the individual's pain may serve an unconscious function, such as a means of obtaining the love and concern of others or a punishment for real or imagined wrongdoing.

According to the same theorists, an individual with body dysmorphic disorder invests a part of the body with special meaning that may be traceable to some event that occurred at an earlier stage of psychosexual development. The original event is repressed, and the attachment of special meaning to a part of the body comes about through symbolization. Projection is used when the individual makes statements such as "It makes everyone look at me with horror."

Behavioral Theory

Behaviorists suggest that people with somatoform symptoms learn methods of communicating helplessness and that these methods help the individuals to manipulate others to care for them. The symptoms become more intense when they are reinforced by attention from others. In the United States, primary care providers and nurses are taught to be attentive and responsive to a patient's reports of pain. Other reinforcers include avoiding activities the individual considers distasteful, obtaining financial benefit, or gaining some advantage in interpersonal relationships due to the symptom.

Cognitive Theory

Cognitive theorists believe that the patient with somatoform symptoms focuses on body sensations, misinterprets their meaning, and then becomes excessively alarmed by them.

Cultural Considerations

The *DSM-IV-TR* provides information about the role of culture in somatoform disorders and states that the type and frequency of somatic symptoms vary across cultures. Burning hands and feet or the sensation of worms in the head or ants under the skin is more common in Africa and southern Asia than in North America. Alteration of consciousness with falling is a symptom commonly associated with culture-specific religious and healing rituals. Somatization disorder, which is rarely seen in men in the United States, is

often reported in Greek and Puerto Rican men, which suggests that cultural customs may permit these men to use somatization as an acceptable approach to dealing with life stress.

In some cultures, certain physical symptoms are believed to result from the casting of spells. Spellbound individuals often seek the help of traditional healers in addition to modern medical staff. The medical provider may diagnose a non–life-threatening somatoform disorder, whereas the traditional healer may offer an entirely different explanation and prognosis. The individual may not show improvement until the traditional healer removes the spell.

APPLICATION OF THE NURSING PROCESS

ASSESSMENT

Assessment of patients with somatoform disorders is a complex process that requires careful and complete documentation. This section outlines several areas not normally included in a nursing assessment but of considerable importance in the assessment of a patient with suspected somatoform disorder.

General Assessment

Symptoms and Unmet Needs

Assessment should begin with collection of data about the nature, location, onset, character, and duration of the symptom or symptoms. Often patients with conversion disorder report having a sudden loss in function of a body part. "I woke up this morning and couldn't move my arm." Patients with somatization disorder, hypochondriasis, or somatoform pain disorder usually discuss their symptoms in dramatic terms. They may use colorful metaphors and exaggerations: "The pain was searing, like a hot sword drawn across my forehead." "My symptoms are so rare that I've stumped hundreds of doctors." Individuals with body dysmorphic disorder are concerned about only one part of the body and seek cosmetic surgery; they display disgust with the offending body part.

Information should be sought about patients' ability to meet their own basic needs. Common problems connected with the need for oxygen include tachypnea and tachycardia associated with anxiety. Nutrition, fluid balance, and elimination needs should be evaluated because patients with somatization disorders often complain of gastrointestinal distress, diarrhea, constipation, and anorexia. The physiological need for sex may be altered by patient experiences of painful intercourse, pain in another part of the body, or lack of interest in sex.

Rest, comfort, activity, and hygiene needs may be altered as a result of patient problems such as fatigue, weakness, insomnia, muscle tension, pain, and avoidance of diversional activity. Safety and security needs may be threatened by patient experiences of blindness, deafness, loss of balance and falling, and anesthesia of various parts of the body.

Voluntary Control of Symptoms

During assessment, it is important to determine whether symptoms are under the patient's voluntary control. *Somatoform symptoms are not under the individual's voluntary control.* Although the relationship between symptoms and interpersonal conflicts may be obvious to others, the patient cannot see it.

Secondary Gains

The nurse tries to identify secondary gains the patient may be receiving from the symptoms. **Secondary gains** are those benefits derived from the symptoms alone; for example, in the sick role, the patient is not able to perform the usual family, work, and social functions and receives extra attention from loved ones. If a patient derives personal benefit from the symptoms, giving up the symptoms is more difficult. The clinician works with the patient to achieve the same benefits through healthier avenues, such as learning to communicate more adaptively and connect with others. One approach to identifying the presence of secondary gains is to ask the patient questions such as:

- What are you unable to do now that you used to be able to do?
- How has this problem affected your life?

Cognitive Style

In general, patients with these disorders misinterpret physical stimuli and distort reality regarding their symptoms. Sensations a normal individual would interpret as a headache might suggest a brain tumor to a patient with hypochondriasis. Exploring the patient's cognitive style is helpful in distinguishing between hypochondriasis and somatization disorder. The patient with hypochondriasis exhibits more anxiety and an obsessive attention to detail, along with a preoccupation with the fear of serious illness. The patient with somatization disorder is often rambling and vague about the details of his or her many symptoms and gives a disorganized history.

Ability to Communicate Feelings and Emotional Needs

Patients with somatoform disorders have difficulty communicating their emotional needs. Although they are able to describe their physical symptoms, they cannot verbalize feelings, especially those related to anger, guilt, and dependence. The somatic symptom may be the patient's chief means of communicating emotional needs. Psychogenic blindness or hearing loss may represent the symbolic statement "I can't face this knowledge." For example, after a woman overheard friends discussing her husband's sexual infidelity, she developed total deafness.

Dependence on Medication

Individuals experiencing many somatic complaints often become dependent on medication to relieve pain or anxiety or to induce sleep. Primary care providers prescribe anxiolytic agents for patients who seem highly anxious and concerned about their symptoms. Patients often return to the primary care provider for prescription renewal or seek treatment from numerous primary care providers. It is important that the nurse assess the type and amount of medications being used.

Self-Assessment

Nurses and other health care workers often find working with patients with somatoform disorders to be difficult and unsatisfying. When a physiological basis for the patient's symptoms is absent, you may wonder why this patient is taking up valuable time that might better be spent on a "sick" patient. You may feel resentment or anger toward such a patient. Negative feelings occur whether the patient is being cared for in a medical setting—whose staff tend to feel more comfortable working with patients who have physical illnesses—or by psychiatric staff who tend to prefer working with disorders of emotion or thought. It is helpful to remember that the symptom the patient is experiencing feels *real* to him or her, even though the objective data do not support a physiological basis for it.

Anger may also arise when staff members find themselves dealing with a patient who uses somatic symptoms to manipulate the environment and people in the environment. Feelings of helplessness over being unable to make a patient realize his or her symptoms have no organic basis can be a source of frustration. Patients who use somatization exhibit remarkable resistance to change. They cling to unrealistic beliefs about the origin of the somatic symptoms, despite objective evidence to the contrary. As you plan the care of this patient, a useful strategy is to set goals with staged outcomes (i.e., small, attainable steps) to offset feelings of helplessness or ineffectuality.

It is helpful for health care workers, no matter the setting, to discuss responses to these patients in conferences with other health care members to allow for expression of feelings and, ultimately, to provide for consistent care.

Assessment Guidelines Somatoform Disorders

1. Assess for nature, location, onset, characteristics, and duration of the symptom(s).
2. Assess the patient's ability to meet basic needs.
3. Assess risks to safety and security needs of the patient as a result of the symptom(s).
4. Determine whether the symptoms are under the patient's voluntary control.
5. Identify any secondary gains the patient is experiencing from symptom(s).
6. Explore the patient's cognitive style and ability to communicate feelings and needs.
7. Assess type and amount of medication the patient is using.

DIAGNOSIS

Patients with somatoform disorders present various nursing problems. *Ineffective coping* is frequently diagnosed. Causal statements might include:

- Distorted perceptions of body functions and symptoms
- Chronic pain of psychological origin
- Dependence on pain relievers or anxiolytics

Table 22-2 identifies potential nursing diagnoses for patients with somatoform disorders.

OUTCOMES IDENTIFICATION

Because shared decision making promotes goal attainment, the patient should participate in identifying desired outcomes. Outcome criteria must be realistic and attainable. Structuring outcomes in small steps helps the patient see concrete evidence of progress. Pertinent *Nursing Outcomes Classification (NOC)* categories for outcomes for somatoform patients include *Body Image, Coping, Identity, Role Performance, Social Interaction Skills, Family Coping,* and *Self-Esteem* (Moorhead et al., 2008). The following are examples of possible indicators related to *NOC:*

- Patient will exhibit sensitivity to others.
- Patient will resume performance of work role behaviors.
- Patient will identify ineffective coping patterns.
- Patient will make realistic appraisal of strengths and weaknesses.
- Patient will verbalize feelings such as anger, shame, or guilt.
- Patient will allow family to be involved in decision making.

TABLE 22-2 Potential Nursing Diagnoses for Somatoform Disorders

Signs and Symptoms	Nursing Diagnoses
Inability to meet occupational, family, or social responsibilities because of symptoms	*Ineffective coping*
Inability to participate in usual community activities or friendships because of psychogenic symptoms	*Ineffective role performance* *Impaired social interaction*
Dependence on pain relievers	*Powerlessness*
Distortion of body functions and symptoms	*Disturbed body image*
Presence of secondary gains by adoption of sick role	*Pain, acute or chronic*
Inability to meet family role function and need for family to assume role function of the somatic individual	*Interrupted family processes* *Ineffective sexuality pattern*
Assumption of some of the roles of the somatic parent by the children	*Impaired parenting*
Shifting of the sexual partner's role to that of caregiver/parent and of the patient's role to that of recipient of care	*Risk for caregiver role strain*
Feeling of inability to control symptoms or understand why he or she cannot find help	*Chronic low self-esteem*
Development of negative self-evaluation related to losing body function, feeling useless, or not feeling valued by significant others	*Spiritual distress*
Inability to take care of basic self-care needs related to conversion symptom (paralysis, seizures, pain, fatigue) Inability to sleep due to psychogenic pain	*Self-care deficit* *Disturbed sleep pattern*

Data from North American Nursing Diagnosis Association International (NANDA-I). (2009). *NANDA-I nursing diagnoses: Definitions and classification 2009-2011.* Oxford, United Kingdom: Author.

PLANNING

Because patients are seldom admitted to psychiatric care settings specifically for treatment of somatoform disorders, long-term interventions usually take place on an outpatient basis or in the home. Short-term planning may be initiated if the patient is admitted to a medical-surgical unit. Such a stay is usually short, and discharge will occur as soon as diagnostic tests are completed and negative results are received.

Initially, nursing interventions should focus on establishing a helping relationship with the patient. The therapeutic relationship is vital to the success of the care plan, given (1) the patient's resistance to the concept that no physical cause for the symptom exists and (2) the patient's tendency to go from caregiver to caregiver.

To be successful, therapeutic interventions must address ways to help the patient get needs met without resorting to somatization. The secondary gains derived from illness behaviors become less important to the patient when underlying needs can be met directly. Collaboration with family or significant others is essential for success.

Case Study and Nursing Care Plan 22-1 on pages 523-524 gives the plan of care for a patient with conversion disorder.

IMPLEMENTATION

Nursing interventions for patients with somatoform disorders generally take place in the home or clinic setting and entail helping the patient improve overall functioning through the development of effective coping strategies. The *Nursing Interventions Classification (NIC)* offers several categories pertinent to caring for patients with somatoform disorders: *Assertiveness Training, Body Image Enhancement, Family Involvement Promotion, Limit Setting, Self-Awareness Enhancement,* and *Self-Esteem Enhancement* (Bulechek et al., 2008). Table 22-3 lists examples of basic-level interventions.

TABLE 22-3 Basic Level Interventions for Somatoform Disorders

Intervention	Rationale
Offer explanations and support during diagnostic testing.	Reduces anxiety while ruling out organic illness
After physical complaints have been investigated, avoid further reinforcement (e.g., do not take vital signs each time patient complains of palpitations).	Directs focus away from physical symptoms
Spend time with patient at times other than when patient summons nurse to voice physical complaint.	Rewards non–illness-related behaviors and encourages repetition of desired behavior
Observe and record frequency and intensity of somatic symptoms. (Patient or family can give information.)	Establishes a baseline and later enables evaluation of effectiveness of interventions
Do not imply that symptoms are not real.	Acknowledges that psychogenic symptoms are real to the patient
Shift focus from somatic complaints to feelings or to neutral topics.	Conveys interest in patient as a person rather than in patient's symptoms; reduces need to gain attention via symptoms
Assess secondary gains "physical illness" provides for patient (e.g., attention, increased dependency, and distraction from another problem).	Allows these needs to be met in healthier ways and thus minimizes secondary gains
Use matter-of-fact approach to patient exhibiting resistance or covert anger.	Avoids power struggles; demonstrates acceptance of anger and permits discussion of angry feelings
Have patient direct all requests to case manager.	Reduces manipulation
Help patient look at effect of illness behavior on others.	Encourages insight; can help improve intrafamily relationships
Show concern for patient while avoiding fostering dependency needs.	Shows respect for patient's feelings while minimizing secondary gains from "illness"
Reinforce patient's strengths and problem-solving abilities.	Contributes to positive self-esteem; helps patient realize that needs can be met without resorting to somatic symptoms
Teach assertive communication.	Provides patient with a positive means of getting needs met; reduces feelings of helplessness and need for manipulation
Teach patient stress reduction techniques, such as meditation, relaxation, and mild physical exercise.	Provides alternate coping strategies; reduces need for medication

Promotion of Self-Care Activities

When somatization is present, the patient's ability to perform self-care activities may be impaired, and nursing intervention is necessary. In general, interventions involve the use of a matter-of-fact approach to support the highest level of self-care the patient is capable of. For patients manifesting paralysis, blindness, or severe fatigue, an effective nursing approach is to support patients while expecting them to feed, bathe, or groom themselves (e.g., the patient who demonstrates paralysis of an arm can be expected to eat using the other arm). To encourage the patient experiencing blindness to feed himself, he can be told at what numbers on an imaginary clock the food is located on the plate. These strategies are effective in reducing secondary gain.

Health Teaching and Health Promotion

Some patients who use somatization as a way of coping with anxiety have little formal education. Therefore, teaching these patients basic information about body functions is often warranted. Pictures and charts can be helpful, and it is useful to review the same information with the family, because their knowledge may also be faulty.

Assertiveness training is often identified as appropriate teaching for patients with somatoform disorders. Use of assertiveness techniques gives patients a direct means of getting needs met and thereby decreases the need for somatic symptoms. Teaching an exercise regimen, such as doing range-of-motion exercises for 15 to 20 minutes daily, can help the patient feel in control, increases endorphin levels, and may help decrease anxiety.

Case Management

"Doctor shopping" is common among patients with somatoform disorders. They go from physician to physician, clinic to clinic, or hospital to hospital, hoping to establish a physical basis for their distress. Repeated computed tomographic scans, magnetic resonance images, and other diagnostic tests are often documented in the medical record. Case management can help limit health care costs associated with such visits. The case manager can recommend to the primary care provider that the patient be scheduled for brief appointments every 4 to 6 weeks at set times, rather than on demand, and that laboratory tests be avoided unless they are absolutely necessary. The patient who establishes a relationship with the case manager often feels less anxiety because the patient has someone to contact and knows that someone is "in charge."

Pharmacological Interventions

It is unclear whether medications are useful for treatment in all the somatoform disorders. Certainly if there are underlying psychiatric diagnoses, appropriate utilization of medication is indicated and may result in the somatoform symptoms decreasing. The decision to medicate patients with a somatization disorder should weigh the benefits against the possibility that these patients may misuse their medication, taking it erratically and irregularly (Sadock & Sadock, 2008).

Tricyclic antidepressants (TCAs) and SSRIs may be helpful in pain disorder, and SSRIs have been found to be useful in reducing symptoms in body dysmorphic disorder (Yates, 2008). Patients may also benefit from short-term use of antianxiety medication, which must be monitored carefully because of the risk of dependence. The nurse may administer these medications in certain settings, but teaching patients and families about the medication is helpful in all settings. Also, teaching relaxation techniques gives the patient a means of controlling symptoms.

Advanced Practice Interventions

Advanced practice nurses may use various types of psychotherapy or consultation with the primary care provider in the treatment of somatoform disorders. Refer to Table 22-4 for a summary of the somatoform disorders, along with a description of the illness course and specific therapeutic approaches.

EVALUATION

Evaluation of patients with somatoform disorders is a simple process when measurable behavioral outcomes have been written clearly and realistically. For these patients, you might often find that goals and outcomes are only partially met. This should be considered a positive finding, because these patients often exhibit remarkable resistance to change. Patients are likely to report the continuing presence of somatic symptoms, but they often say they are less concerned about the symptoms. Families are likely to report relatively high satisfaction with outcomes, even without total eradication of the patient's symptoms.

Factitious Disorders

Whereas somatoform disorders are not under conscious control, people with a factitious disorder consciously pretend to be ill to get emotional needs met and attain the status of "patient" (Sadock & Sadock,

TABLE 22-4 Advanced Practice Interventions for Somatoform Disorders

Disorder	Course	Interventions
Conversion disorder	Usually acute onset; resolves quickly	Suggest that the conversion symptom will gradually improve Behavioral therapy Insight-oriented therapy Hypnosis Antianxiety drugs
Somatization disorder	Chronic and relapsing	Consistent primary care provider with regular patient visits, limited tests Group therapy Cognitive-behavioral therapy
Hypochondriasis	Chronic and relapsing, but 50% of patients improve	Cognitive-behavioral therapy Insight-oriented therapy Group therapy Psychopharmacological management for comorbid conditions Stress management
Pain disorder	If acute onset, may improve; risk of suicide	Antidepressants Couples therapy Cognitive-behavioral therapy Biofeedback Hypnosis Antidepressants
Body dysmorphic disorder	Limited response to treatment	Cognitive-behavioral therapy Antidepressants

Data from Sadock, B. J., & Sadock, V. A. (2008). *Kaplan & Sadock's concise textbook of clinical psychiatry* (3rd ed.). Philadelphia: Lippincott Williams & Wilkins; and Greenberg, D. B., Braun, I. M., & Cassem, N. H. (2008). Functional somatic symptoms and somatoform disorders. In T. A. Stern, J. F. Rosenbaum, M. Fava, J. Biederman, & S. L. Rauch (Eds.), *Massachusetts General Hospital comprehensive clinical psychiatry* (pp. 319–330). St. Louis: Mosby.

2008). The term *factitious* is derived from the Latin word meaning "artificial or contrived." Patients with this disorder artificially, deliberately, and dramatically fabricate symptoms or self-inflict injury, with the goal of assuming a sick role (APA, 2000). Examples of contrived illnesses include bleeding, fever, hypoglycemia, seizures, and even cancer and human immunodeficiency virus (HIV) (Smith, 2008). Factitious disorder results in disability and immeasurable costs to the health care system.

People with this disorder do not usually doctor shop (i.e., go from one primary care provider to another). They visit the same person time and again and are known by the health care personnel. The patient may get admitted to the hospital through the emergency room, where he or she dramatically describes the illness, using proper medical terminology, and can be quite convincing. The patient is often reluctant for professionals to speak with family members, friends, or previous health care providers. Once admitted, the patient is frequently demanding and requests specific treatments and interventions. Negative test results are often followed by new or additional symptoms. If the health care team sets limits and does not follow through with requests, the patient may become angry and accuse the staff of incompetence and maltreatment.

CLINICAL PICTURE

Figure 22-2 presents the *DSM-IV-TR* criteria for factitious disorder. Three subtypes of factitious disorders are based on signs and symptoms: those that are predominantly physical, those that are predominantly psychological, and combinations of physical and psychological. Factitious disorder not otherwise specified is a category reserved for symptoms that do not meet the criteria for factitious disorder; this category includes Munchausen by proxy.

DSM-IV-TR CRITERIA FOR FACTITIOUS DISORDER

A. Intentional production or feigning of physical or psychological signs or symptoms.

B. The motivation for the behavior is to assume the sick role.

C. External incentives for the behavior (such as economic gain, avoiding legal responsibilities, or improving physical well-being, as in Malingering) are absent.

Figure 22-2 Diagnostic criteria for factitious disorder. (Adapted from American Psychiatric Association. [2000]. *Diagnostic and statistical manual of mental disorders* [4th ed., text rev.]. Washington, DC: Author.)

Factitious Disorder With Physical Symptoms

The most frequently seen factitious disorder is **common fictitious disorder**. Patients tend to see the same caregiver and are well known in the health care system (Smith, 2008). They prefer to use the emergency room at night, when people are less likely to know them. They use medical terminology, know which symptoms will get them admitted, and once admitted become increasingly demanding and attention-seeking until they ultimately elope or are discharged.

Munchausen Syndrome

Munchausen syndrome, the most severe and chronic form of factitious disorders, is named after Baron Karl Friedrich Hieronymus von Münchausen (1720-1797), an 18th-century German cavalry officer with a reputation for fabricating exaggerated tales. Munchausen syndrome is notable for the way patients go from one primary care provider or hospital to another, seeking attention. The severity of the symptoms is evident in the aggressiveness of treatments by clinicians. Serious complications and sepsis may result from self-injections of toxins such as *E. coli*. Patients may have "crisscrossed" or "railroad-track" abdomens due to scars from numerous exploratory surgeries to investigate unexplained symptoms. In the extreme, amputations may even result from this disorder.

Factitious Disorder With Psychological Symptoms

Although most cases of factitious disorder involve physical symptoms, some patients primarily report psychological symptoms (Smith, 2008). They may complain of hallucinations, depression, and suicidal thoughts and intense bereavement due to the loss of a loved one, including the dramatic loss of a child.

Factitious Disorder Not Otherwise Specified

Any factitious disorder that does not meet the above criteria is diagnosed as factitious disorder not otherwise specified.

Factitious Disorder by Proxy

The most insidious form of factitious disorders is **factitious disorder by proxy** (also known as *Munchausen syndrome by proxy*), in which a caregiver deliberately feigns illness in a vulnerable dependent, usually a child, for the purpose of the attention, excitement, and treatment by health care providers of that dependent. The caregiver frequently is a health care worker or someone with extensive knowledge of the health care system. The disorder results in unnecessary medical visits and sometimes harmful medical procedures. Examples of this disorder include inducing premature delivery by rupturing the amniotic sac with a fingernail, infant apnea and sudden infant death, and introducing microorganisms into a child's wound (DiMario, 2008; Vennemann et al., 2007; Feldman & Hamilton, 2006). Falsification of illnesses results in extreme pain, surgical procedures, and even death of dependents (Feldman et al., 2007).

Malingering

While not a specific mental disorder, **malingering** is mentioned here as a condition that is related to the factitious disorders. Malingering is a consciously motivated act to deceive based on the desire for material gain (Sadock & Sadock, 2008). It involves a conscious process of fabricating an illness or exaggerating symptoms in order to become eligible for disability compensation, commit fraud against insurance companies, obtain prescription medications, evade military service, or receive a reduced prison sentence. Reported pains are vague and hard for clinicians to prove or disprove (e.g., back pain, headache, or toothache).

This disorder is thought to be more common in men than in women and is often seen in people with antisocial personality disorder (Smith, 2008). Among the criminal population, the rates may be as high as 10% to 20% (Sadock & Sadock, 2008). Malingering is associated with antisocial, narcissistic, and borderline personality disorders.

EPIDEMIOLOGY

It is nearly impossible to determine the prevalence of this illness, owing to the concealment of its origins. Childhood neglect and abuse are thought to be causative for this disorder. A childhood history of frequent illnesses, especially those that result in hospitalization, may also be present in people who develop this disorder (McDermott et al., 2008).

COMORBIDITY

Although symptoms tend to be physiological, some patients may also try to convince clinicians that they have a psychiatric disorder. Patients may describe symptoms of depression, dissociation, conversion, and psychoses and seek treatment for these problems (Sadock & Sadock, 2008). The patient who pretends to have hallucinations often has a comorbid borderline personality disorder.

ETIOLOGY

Biological Factors

Brain dysfunction has been identified as a possible source of the symptoms of factitious disorders (Sadock & Sadock, 2008). Specifically, impaired information processing has been suggested as causative. No other biological abnormalities have been proposed at this time.

Psychological Factors

It is difficult to determine or understand the psychological basis of these disorders because of the patients' intention to skew the facts. There is some evidence that people with these disorders suffered abuse and neglect as children and may have been hospitalized more frequently than is typical (Sadock & Sadock, 2008). These hospitalizations may have been perceived as a refuge from a chaotic home life. It has also been suggested that patients with factitious disorders may have a masochistic side and feel a need to be punished through painful procedures.

APPLICATION OF THE NURSING PROCESS

ASSESSMENT AND DIAGNOSIS

Many of the principles of care for somatoform disorders apply to factitious disorders. Often, determining if a patient's signs and symptoms are conscious or unconscious (i.e., whether they are a somatoform disorder or a factious disorder) is a challenge for clinicians, particularly those in the position to diagnose psychiatric disorders. Your role as a nurse, whether you work in psychiatry and mental health or any other setting, is to carefully assess the patient and document your care. A general principle in treating people with a factitious disorder is to avoid confrontation, which may result in the patient's defensiveness, elusiveness, or leaving the treatment facility (Smith, 2008).

Self-Assessment

Nurses who work with patients with factitious disorders—patients who intentionally and consciously feign illnesses—are often angry and resentful. After all, there are patients who really need care and have no control over how sick they are, and then there are patients with factitious disorders who are probably causing their own problems. These countertransference reactions should be acknowledged and can be addressed through discussions with other members of the treatment team and careful treatment planning. It is important to consider that factitious disorders may cause real problems that can be overlooked.

PLANNING AND IMPLEMENTATION

In cases of Munchausen syndrome, and particularly factitious disorder by proxy, the nurse must consider safety. Patients who may purposefully inflect damage to themselves or others must be carefully monitored, and suspicious activities should be reported to and discussed by the health care team. It is essential that the nurse share any information that may prevent a person or a vulnerable and unsuspecting child from undergoing unnecessary surgery or treatments.

Dissociative Disorders

Dissociative disorders are another group of disorders in which altered mind-body connections are believed to be related to stress or anxiety. Patients with somatoform disorders complain of somatic distress and experience altered perception of physical sensation, but they retain normal patterns of thinking and feeling overall. Patients with dissociative disorders respond to unusually stressful experiences with a severe interruption of consciousness and awareness of themselves and their surroundings.

The *DSM-IV-TR* defines dissociative disorders as disturbances in the normally well-integrated continuum of consciousness, memory, identity, and perception. Dissociation is an unconscious defense mechanism that protects the individual against overwhelming anxiety. Patients with dissociative disorders have intact reality testing; that is, they are not delusional or hallucinating. Mild, fleeting dissociative experiences are relatively common to all of us; for example, we say we are on "automatic pilot" when we drive home from work and cannot recall the last 15 minutes before reaching the house. But these common experiences are distinctly different from the processes of pathological dissociation.

CLINICAL PICTURE

The *DSM-IV-TR* lists four major dissociative disorders: (1) depersonalization disorder, (2) dissociative amnesia, (3) dissociative fugue, and (4) dissociative identity disorder (DID). Figure 22-3 lists the diagnostic criteria for each disorder.

Depersonalization Disorder

The *DSM-IV-TR* describes depersonalization disorder as a persistent or recurrent alteration in the perception of the self while reality testing remains intact. The person experiencing depersonalization may feel mechanical, dreamy, or detached from the body. These experiences of feeling a sense of deadness of the body, of seeing oneself from a distance, or of perceiving the limbs to be larger or smaller than normal are described by patients as being very disturbing. Depersonalization disorder most often begins in adolescence and often does not respond to therapy or medication (Michal et al., 2005).

VIGNETTE

Margaret describes becoming very distressed at perceiving changes in her appearance when she looks in a mirror. She thinks that her image looks wavy and indistinct. Soon after, she describes feeling as though she is floating in a fog, with her feet not actually touching the ground. Questioning reveals that Margaret's son has recently confided to her that he tested positive for human immunodeficiency virus. ▨

Dissociative Amnesia

Dissociative amnesia is marked by the inability to recall important personal information, often of a traumatic or stressful nature; this lack of memory is too pervasive to be explained by ordinary forgetfulness. A patient with generalized amnesia is unable to recall information about his or her entire lifetime. The amnesia may also be localized (the patient is unable to remember all events in a certain period) or selective (the patient is able to recall some but not all events in a certain period).

DSM-IV-TR CRITERIA FOR DISSOCIATIVE DISORDERS

DISSOCIATIVE DISORDERS

Dissociative Amnesia*	Dissociative Fugue*	Dissociative Identity Disorder* (DID)	Depersonalization Disorder*
1. One or more episodes of inability to recall important information — usually of a traumatic or stressful nature. 2. Causes significant distress or impairment in social, occupational, or other important areas of functioning.	1. Sudden, unexpected travel away from home or one's place of work with inability to remember past. 2. Confusion about personal identity or assumption of new identity. 3. Symptoms cause significant distress or impairment in social, occupational, or other important areas of functioning.	1. Existence of two or more distinct subpersonalities, each with its own patterns of relating, perceiving, and thinking. 2. At least two of these subpersonalities take control of the person's behavior. 3. Inability to recall important information too extensive to be explained by ordinary forgetfulness.	1. Persistent or recurrent experience of feeling detached from and outside of one's mental processes or body. 2. Reality testing remains intact. 3. The experience causes significant impairment in social or occupational functioning or causes marked distress.
*Not due to substance, medical, neurological, or other psychiatric disorder.	*Not due to substance, medical, neurological, or other psychiatric disorder.	*Not due to substance, medical, neurological, or other psychiatric disorder.	*Not due to substance, medical, neurological, or other psychiatric disorder.

Figure 22-3 Diagnostic criteria for dissociative disorders. (Adapted from American Psychiatric Association. [2000]. *Diagnostic and statistical manual of mental disorders* [4th ed., text rev.]. Washington, DC: Author.)

A young woman found wandering in a Florida park is partly dressed and poorly nourished. She has no knowledge of who she is. Her parents identify her 2 weeks later when she appears in an interview on a national television show. She had just broken up with her boyfriend of 3 years. ■

Dissociative Fugue

Dissociative fugue is characterized by sudden, unexpected travel away from the customary locale and inability to recall one's identity and information about some or all of the past. In rare cases, an individual with dissociative fugue assumes a whole new identity. During a fugue state, individuals tend to lead rather simple lives, rarely calling attention to themselves. After a few weeks to a few months, they may remember their former identities and become amnesic for the time spent in the fugue state. Usually a dissociative fugue is precipitated by a traumatic event.

A middle-aged woman awakens one morning and notices snow outside the window, swirling around unfamiliar buildings and streets. The radio tells her it is December. She is perplexed to find herself in a residential hotel in Chicago with no idea of how she got there. She feels confused and shaken. As she leaves the hotel, she is surprised to find that strangers recognize her and say, "Good morning, Sally." The name Sally does not seem right, but she cannot remember her true identity. She finds her way to a hospital, where she is evaluated and referred to the psychiatric nurse in the emergency department. A day later, "Sally" is able to remember her true identity, Mary Hunt. She tells the nurse tearfully that she can now recall that her husband came home one day and "out of the blue" told her he wanted a divorce to marry a younger woman. Mary calls her sister in New York, who comes to Chicago to take her home. ■

Dissociative Identity Disorder

The essential feature of **dissociative identity disorder (DID)** is the presence of two or more distinct personality states that recurrently take control of behavior. Each **alternate personality (alter) or subpersonality** has its own pattern of perceiving, relating to, and thinking about the self and the environment. It is believed that severe sexual, physical, or psychological trauma in childhood predisposes an individual to the development of DID.

Dissociative identity disorder appears to be associated with two dissociative identity states: first,

a state in which the individual blocks access and responses to traumatic memories so they are able to function daily; and second, a state fixated on traumatic memories. Different regional cerebral blood flow patterns and autonomic and subjective reactions are displayed during each of these states when the individual is exposed to trauma-related stimuli (Reinders et al., 2006).

Each alternate personality or subpersonality is a complex unit with its own memories, behavior patterns, and social relationships that dictate how the person acts when that personality is dominant. Often the original or primary personality is religious and moralistic, and the subpersonalities are pleasure seeking and nonconforming. The alter personalities may behave as individuals of a different sex, race, or religion. The dominant hand and the voice may be different; intelligence and electroencephalographic findings may also be altered.

Typical cognitive distortions include the insistence that alternate personalities inhabit separate bodies and are unaffected by the actions of one another. The primary personality or host is usually not aware of the subpersonalities and is perplexed by lost time and unexplained events. Experiences such as finding unfamiliar clothing in the closet, being called a different name by a stranger, or not having childhood memories are characteristic of DID. Subpersonalities are often aware of the existence of each other to some degree. Transition from one personality to another occurs during times of stress and may range from a dramatic to a barely noticeable event. Some patients experience the transition when awakening. Shifts may last from minutes to months, although shorter periods are more common.

Several movies that demonstrate actual case studies of individuals diagnosed with DID have been produced, including *Sybil* (1976) and *The Three Faces of Eve* (1957).

Andrea, a conservative 28-year-old electrical engineer, is the primary personality. Three alternate personalities coexist and vie for supremacy.

Michele is a 5-year-old who is sometimes playful and sometimes angry. She speaks with a slight lisp and with the facial expressions, voice inflections, and vocabulary of a precocious child. She likes to play on swings, draw with a crayon, and eat ice cream. She likes to cuddle a teddy bear and occasionally sucks her thumb. Her favorite outfit is jeans and a Mickey Mouse sweatshirt.

Ann is an accomplished ballet dancer. She is shy but firm about needing time to practice. When she is dominant, she likes to wear white and fixes her hair in a severe, pulled-back style. She does little but dance when she is in control.

Bridget is near Andrea's age, although she says a lady never tells her age. She dresses seductively in bright colors, wears her hair tousled, and likes to frequent bars and stay out late. She often drinks to excess and has several male admirers. Bridget has many moods. She states that she would like to get rid of Ann and Andrea because they're such "goody-goodies."

Andrea does not drink, hates ice cream, and sees herself as somewhat awkward. She does not dance. She is a paid soloist in a church choir. Andrea takes public transportation, but Ann and Bridget have driver's licenses. Andrea goes to bed and arises early, but Bridget and Michele like to stay up late.

Andrea seeks treatment when she finds herself behind the wheel of a moving car and realizes that she does not know how to drive. She has been concerned for some time because she has found strange clothes in her closet. She has also received phone calls from men who insist that she has flirted with them in bars. She sometimes misses appointments and cannot account for periods of time. Although she goes to bed early, she is often unaccountably tired in the morning. ■

EPIDEMIOLOGY

The prevalence rate of dissociative disorders occurring at some time during a person's life in the United States is approximately 7% (Mayo Clinic Staff, 2007). Overall, these conditions are considered rare. Dissociative amnesia may occur in any age group from children to adults. The amnesia is often related to trauma, and memory returns spontaneously after the individual is removed from the stressful situation (APA, 2000). Dissociative fugue is also related to trauma and occurs mostly in adults. The occurrence of fugue is known to increase in times of stress, such as during war or natural disasters (APA, 2000). DID may occur at any age but is diagnosed three to nine times more frequently in adult females than in adult males. There is often a childhood history of severe physical or sexual abuse.

In the United States, about 50% of the population may experience a transient or temporary depersonalization, a problem that usually goes away on its own (Schlozman & Nonacs, 2008). An actual depersonalization disorder is more severe and is found in both adolescents and adults, often in response to acute stress. Patients with this disorder usually seek treatment for another problem such as anxiety or depression.

COMORBIDITY

Mood disorders and substance-related disorders commonly co-occur with all of the dissociative disorders. In addition, dissociative amnesia may be comorbid with conversion disorder or personality disorder.

Dissociative fugue may co-occur with posttraumatic stress disorder (PTSD). Patients with DID may also have PTSD, borderline personality disorder, or sexual, eating, or sleep disorders. Depersonalization disorder occurs with hypochondriasis, anxiety disorder, and personality disorder (APA, 2000).

ETIOLOGY

The actual cause of dissociative disorders is unknown, but essentially they are all believed to be related to trauma (Schlozman & Nonacs, 2008). Childhood physical, sexual, or emotional abuse and other traumatic life events are associated with adults experiencing dissociative symptoms.

Biological Factors

Current research suggests that the limbic system is involved in the development of dissociative disorders. Traumatic memories are processed in the limbic system, and the hippocampus stores this information. Animal studies show that early prolonged detachment from the caretaker negatively affects the development of the limbic system. Significant early trauma and lack of attachment have also been demonstrated to have effects on neurotransmitters, specifically irregular serotonin activity (Schlozman & Nonacs, 2008).

Genetic

Several studies suggest that DID is more common among first-degree biological relatives of individuals with the disorder than in the population at large.

Psychosocial Factors

Learning theory suggests that dissociative disorders can be explained as learned methods for avoiding stress and anxiety. The pattern of avoidance occurs when an individual deals with an unpleasant event by consciously deciding not to think about it. The more anxiety-provoking the event is; the greater the need to avoid thinking about it. As the individual increasingly utilizes this technique, the more likely it is to become automatically invoked as dissociation. When stress is intolerable—for example, in an abused child—the individual develops dissociation to defend against pain and the memory of it.

Cultural Considerations

Certain culture-bound disorders exist in which there is a high level of activity, a trancelike state, and running or fleeing, followed by exhaustion, sleep, and amnesia regarding the episode. These syndromes include *piblokto*, seen in native people of the Arctic,

Navajo *frenzy* witchcraft, and *amok* among Western Pacific natives. These syndromes, if observed in individuals native to the corresponding geographical areas, must be differentiated from dissociative disorders.

APPLICATION OF THE NURSING PROCESS

ASSESSMENT

For a diagnosis of dissociative disorder to be made, medical and neurological illnesses, substance use, and other coexisting psychiatric disorders must be ruled out as the cause of the patient's symptoms. The assessment should include objective data from physical examination, electroencephalography, imaging studies, and specific questions to identify dissociative symptoms. Scales have been developed to assess dissociation, including the Dissociative Experience Scale (DES) and the Structured Clinical Interview for Dissociative Disorders (SCID-D) (Schlozman & Nonacs, 2008).

Usually the patient with DID is treated in the community. However, a patient with DID is admitted to a psychiatric unit when they are suicidal or in need of crisis stabilization. At that time, the nurse gathers specific information about identity, memory, consciousness, life events, mood, suicide risk, and the impact of the disorder on the patient and the family.

General Assessment

Identity and Memory

Assessing patients' ability to identify themselves requires more than asking them to state their names. Changes in patient behavior, voice, and dress might signal the presence of an alternate personality. Referring to the self by another name or in the third person and using the word *we* instead of *I* are indications that the patient may have assumed a new identity. The nurse should consider the following when assessing memory:

- Can the patient remember recent and past events?
- Is the patient's memory clear and complete or partial and fuzzy?
- Is the patient aware of gaps in memory, such as lack of memory for events such as a graduation or a wedding?
- Do the patient's memories place the self with a family, in school, in an occupation?

Patients with amnesia and fugue may be disoriented with regard to time and place, as well as person. Relevant assessment questions include:

- Do you ever lose time or have blackouts?
- Do you find yourself in places with no idea how you got there?

History

The nurse must gather information about events in the person's life. Has the patient sustained a recent injury, such as a concussion? Does the patient have a history of epilepsy, especially temporal lobe epilepsy? Does the patient have a history of early trauma, such as physical, mental, or sexual abuse? If DID is suspected, pertinent questions include:

- Have you ever found yourself wearing clothes you cannot remember buying?
- Have you ever had strange people greet and talk to you as though they were old friends?
- Does your ability to engage in things such as athletics, artistic activities, or mechanical tasks seem to change?
- Do you have differing sets of memories about childhood?

Mood

Is the individual depressed, anxious, or unconcerned? Many patients with DID seek help when the primary personality is depressed. The nurse also observes for mood shifts. When subpersonalities of DID take control, their predominant moods may be different from that of the principal personality. If the subpersonalities shift frequently, marked mood swings may be noted.

Impact on Patient and Family

Has the patient's ability to function been impaired? Have disruptions in family functioning occurred? Is secondary gain evident? In fugue states, individuals often function adequately in their new identities by choosing simple, undemanding occupations and having few intimate social interactions. The families of patients in fugue states report being highly distressed over the patient's disappearance.

Patients with amnesia may be more dysfunctional. Their perplexity often renders them unable to work, and their memory loss impairs normal family relationships. Families often direct considerable attention toward the patient but may exhibit concern over having to assume roles that were once assigned to the patient.

Patients with DID often have both family and work problems. Families find it difficult to accept the seemingly erratic behaviors of the patient. Employers dislike the lost time that may occur when subpersonalities are in control. Patients with depersonalization disorder are often fearful that others may perceive their appearance as distorted and may avoid being seen in public. If they exhibit high anxiety, the family is likely to find it difficult to keep relationships stable.

Suicide Risk

Whenever a patient's life has been substantially disrupted, the patient may have thoughts of suicide. The nurse gathering data should be alert for expressions of hopelessness, helplessness, or worthlessness and for verbalization or other behavior of a subpersonality that indicates the intent to engage in self-destructive or self-mutilating behaviors.

Self-Assessment

It is natural to experience feelings of skepticism while caring for patients who are diagnosed with dissociative disorders. You may find it difficult to believe in the authenticity of the symptoms the patient is displaying.

Feeling confused and bewildered by the presence of multiple identities is not unusual. Anger is commonly experienced in reaction to a subpersonality of a patient with DID if one personality is perceived as immature, challenging, or unpleasant. Some nurses experience feelings of fascination and are caught up in the intrigue of caring for a patient with multiple identities. A sense of inadequacy may accompany the need to be ready to interact in a therapeutic way with whichever personality is in control at the moment.

Feelings of inadequacy can also arise when establishment of a trusting relationship occurs slowly. It is important to remember that the patient with a dissociative disorder has often experienced relationships in which trust was betrayed. When subpersonalities vie for control and attempt to embarrass or harm each other, crises are common, and nurses must be alert and ready to intervene. Preparing for the unexpected, including the possibility of a suicide attempt, means constant hypervigilance by staff, and such demands can eventually lead to great fatigue. Caring for a patient with dissociative disorder can generate anxiety in any of the following situations:

- When a patient who has regained memory develops panic-level anxiety related to guilt feelings
- When a patient becomes assaultive because of extreme confusion or panic-level anxiety
- When a patient attempts self-harm by acting out against the primary personality or other personalities

If the patient manifesting symptoms of a dissociative disorder has been involved in the commission of a crime, the medical record is likely to be a court exhibit. You may experience concern over that fact or be angry if you believe the patient is faking illness to avoid being found guilty of the crime.

Supervision should always be available for nursing staff and clinicians caring for a patient with a dissociative disorder. By discussing feelings and the plan of care with the treatment team or peers, the nurse can better ensure objective and appropriate care for the patient.

Assessment Guidelines Dissociative Disorders

1. Assess for a history of a similar episode in the past with benign outcomes.
2. Establish whether the person suffered abuse, trauma, or loss as a child.
3. Identify relevant psychosocial distress issues by performing a basic psychosocial assessment.

DIAGNOSIS

Potential nursing diagnoses for patients with dissociative disorders are suggested in Table 22-5.

OUTCOMES IDENTIFICATION

Outcomes must be established for each nursing diagnosis. General outcome goals for the patient include developing trust, disclosing multiplicity, and achieving acceptance of responsibility for behavior of any of the alter personalities (Stickley & Nickeas, 2006). *NOC* outcomes potentially appropriate for patients with dissociative disorders include *Identity, Role Performance, Coping, Anxiety Self-Control, Self-Mutilation Restraint,* and *Aggression Self-Control.* Specific examples of indicators that the outcomes are being achieved are:

- Patient will verbalize clear sense of personal identity.
- Patient will report decrease in stress.
- Patient will report comfort with role expectations.
- Patient will plan coping strategies for stressful situations.
- Patient will refrain from injuring self.

PLANNING

The planning of nursing care for the patient with a dissociative disorder is influenced by the setting and presenting problem. The nurse will encounter such a patient in times of crisis, when the patient is admitted to the hospital for suicidal or homicidal behavior. The care plan will focus on safety and crisis intervention. The patient may also come for treatment of a comorbid depression or anxiety disorder in the community setting. Planning will address the major complaint with appropriate referrals for treatment of the dissociative disorder.

TABLE 22-5 Potential Nursing Diagnoses for Dissociative Disorders

Signs and Symptoms	Nursing Diagnoses
Amnesia or fugue related to a traumatic event Symptoms of depersonalization; feelings of unreality and/or body image distortions	*Disturbed personal identity* *Disturbed body image*
Alterations in consciousness, memory, or identity Abuse of substances related to dissociation Disorganization or dysfunction in usual patterns of behavior (absence from work, withdrawal from relationships, changes in role function)	*Ineffective coping* *Ineffective role performance*
Disturbances in memory and identity Interrupted family processes related to amnesia or erratic and changing behavior	*Interrupted family processes* *Impaired parenting*
Feeling of being out of control of memory, behaviors, and awareness Inability to explain actions or behaviors when in altered state	*Anxiety* *Spiritual distress* *Risk for other-directed violence* *Risk for self-directed violence*

Data from North American Nursing Diagnosis Association International (NANDA-I). (2009). *NANDA-I nursing diagnoses: Definitions and classification 2009-2011.* Oxford, United Kingdom: Author.

IMPLEMENTATION

Basic level interventions are aimed at offering emotional presence during the recall of painful experiences, providing a sense of safety, and encouraging an optimal level of functioning. *NIC* topics that offer relevant interventions include *Anxiety Reduction, Coping Enhancement, Self-Awareness Enhancement, Self-Esteem Enhancement,* and *Emotional Support.* Refer to Table 22-6 for examples of basic level interventions.

Milieu Management

When the patient is in a crisis that requires hospitalization, providing a safe environment is fundamental. Other desirable characteristics of the environment are that it be quiet, simple, structured, and supportive. Confusion and noise increase anxiety and the potential for depersonalization, delayed memory return, or shifts among subpersonalities. Inpatient group therapy is not as helpful as task-oriented therapy, such as occupational and art therapy, which give an opportunity for self-expression. Attendance at community or unit milieu meetings relieves feelings of isolation.

Health Teaching and Health Promotion

Patients with dissociative disorders need teaching about the illness and instruction in coping skills and stress management. They may need to develop a plan to interrupt a dissociative episode, such as singing or doing a specific activity. Staff and significant others are made aware of the plan in order to foster their cooperation. Patients should also be taught to keep a daily journal to increase their awareness of feelings and to identify triggers to dissociation. If a patient has never written a journal, the nurse should suggest beginning with a 5- to 10-minute daily writing exercise.

Pharmacological Interventions

There are no specific medications for patients with dissociative disorders, but appropriate antidepressants or anxiolytic medications are given for comorbid conditions. Substance use disorders and suicidal risk, which are common, must be assessed carefully if medication is to be used. In the acute setting, the nurse may witness dramatic memory retrieval in patients with dissociative amnesia or fugue after treatment with intravenous benzodiazepines.

Advanced Practice Interventions

Advanced practice nurses may use cognitive-behavioral therapy or psychodynamic psychotherapy to treat patients with dissociative disorders. Cognitive-behavioral group therapy has also proven to decrease self-reported anxiety and increase self-reported self-esteem for female adolescent victims of sexual abuse (Avinger & Jones, 2007).

TABLE 22-6 Basic-Level Interventions for Dissociative Disorders

Intervention	Rationale
Ensure patient safety by providing safe, protected environment and frequent observation.	Sense of bewilderment may lead to inattention to safety needs; some subpersonalities may be thrill seeking, violent, or careless
Provide undemanding, simple routine.	Reduces anxiety
Confirm identity of patient and orientation to time and place.	Supports reality and promotes ego integrity
Encourage patient to do things for self and make decisions about routine tasks.	Enhances self-esteem by reducing sense of powerlessness and reduces secondary gain associated with dependence
Assist with other decision making until memory returns.	Lowers stress and prevents patient from having to live with the consequences of unwise decisions
Support patient during exploration of feelings surrounding the stressful event.	Helps lower the defense of dissociation used by patient to block awareness of the stressful event
Do not flood patient with data regarding past events.	Memory loss serves the purpose of preventing severe to panic levels of anxiety from overtaking and disorganizing the individual
Allow patient to progress at own pace as memory is recovered.	Prevents undue anxiety and resistance
Provide support during disclosure of painful experiences.	Can be healing, while minimizing feelings of isolation
Help patient see consequences of using dissociation to cope with stress.	Increases insight and helps patient understand own role in choosing behaviors
Accept patient's expression of negative feelings.	Conveys permission to have negative or unacceptable feelings
Teach stress-reduction methods.	Provides alternatives for anxiety relief
If patient does not remember significant others, work with involved parties to reestablish relationships.	Helps patient experience satisfaction and relieves sense of isolation

INTEGRATIVE THERAPY

Body-Mind Therapy

Dissociation causes people to experience a distressing fragmentation of consciousness and a sense of separation from themselves. Body-mind therapy may provide a useful treatment for these symptoms by helping people become more aware of bodily sensations, emotions, and behavior. This therapy is based on the premise that the body, mind, emotions, and spirit are interrelated, and a change at one level results in changes in the others. Awareness, focusing on the present, and recognizing touch as a means of communicating are some of the principles of this therapy.

Dissociative experiences include self-absorption, depersonalization, and amnesia. These may be reduced through body-mind therapy. Massage has been used to make patients aware of what and where they were feeling; patients are asked to describe their inner experiences (Price, 2006). This technique has been found to be particularly helpful in reducing dissociative symptoms. A specific body-mind therapy, sensorimotor psychotherapy, has been reported to be helpful in addressing these symptoms as well, especially for victims of trauma (Ogden, Minton, & Pain, 2006). This type of therapy combines psychological principles with body therapy. During psychotherapy sessions, the patient is asked to describe physical sensations they are experiencing. The goal is to safely disarm the pathological defense mechanism of dissociation and replace it with other resources, especially body awareness and mindfulness.

Ogden, P., Minton, K., & Pain, C. (2006). *Trauma and the body: A sensorimotor approach to psychotherapy.* New York: Norton.
Price, C. (2006). Dissociation reduction in body therapy during sexual abuse recovery. *Complementary Therapies in Clinical Practice, 13*(2), 116–128.

EVALUATION

Treatment is considered successful when outcomes are met. In the final analysis, the evaluation is positive when:

- Patient safety has been maintained.
- Anxiety has been reduced, and the patient has returned to a functional state.
- Conflicts have been explored.
- New coping strategies have permitted the patient to function at a better level.
- Stress is handled adaptively, without the use of dissociation.

Case Study and Nursing Care Plan 22-1 · Conversion Disorder

Ms. Andrews is a single female admitted to the neurological unit of a general hospital for evaluation of sudden onset of seizures. It is the eve of her 30th birthday, and she is an attractive fashion model who quickly begins to flirt with the male nursing staff and primary care providers. Her first seizure after admittance occurs during morning rounds just as the staff enters her room. She arches her back and begins pelvic thrusting motions while thrashing her arms and legs about in the bed. She has no loss of consciousness, and she is not incontinent. Similar seizures occur over the next 2 days, always witnessed by staff or visitors. Ms. Andrews does not seem concerned about the impact of her symptoms on her career (la belle indifférence). She remains calm and is playful with the male staff. When she is told that her diagnostic test results are negative, she agrees to transfer to the psychiatric unit for further evaluation.

On the psychiatric unit, Ms. Andrews is observed behaving in a more helpless, dependent manner. She will not come out of her room for fear of a seizure, and her father refers to her as his "little girl."

ASSESSMENT

Self-Assessment

Ms. D'Angelo is a registered nurse with an AA degree and 2 years of experience on the psychiatric unit. She recognizes mixed feelings toward Ms. Andrews. On the one hand, the patient is interesting and charming as she relates stories of her glamorous career. On the other hand, she is demanding and childish, expecting special privileges on the unit. Ms. Andrews quickly becomes a favorite topic during nursing report, with staff comparing notes on her attention-seeking behaviors. Ms. D'Angelo realizes that she has to carefully monitor her emotional reactions to Ms. Andrews. The nurse will need to adopt a matter-of-fact approach to reduce secondary gains and encourage the patient to resume her independence.

Objective Data

Results of all diagnostic tests for seizure disorder are negative.

Sudden onset of symptoms coincides with the patient's 30th birthday.

The symptoms interrupt the patient's career.

There is no prior history of somatoform or psychiatric disorders.

Subjective Data

"I don't know what I'm doing here with all of these mental patients."

"Can my daddy bring in my birthday cake? I never got to celebrate on the other unit."

DIAGNOSIS

Ineffective coping related to low self-esteem and unmet needs for recognition and attention, as evidenced by use of conversion symptoms (seizures)

Supporting Data

- No incontinence or injury; seizures vary and occur only in the presence of others
- Relates with seductive behavior toward men
- Bland affect regarding personal problems (la belle indifférence)

OUTCOMES IDENTIFICATION

Patient will consistently identify effective coping patterns without using conversion (long-term goal).

Continued

PLANNING

The initial plan is to maintain safety for Ms. Andrews while encouraging her to explore recent stressful events.

IMPLEMENTATION

The plan of care for Ms. Andrews is personalized as follows:

Short-Term Goal	Intervention	Rationale	Evaluation
1. Patient will perform all activities of daily living (ADLs) by the end of the second day.	1. Explain routine. Establish expectations regarding unit routines; do not allow special privileges. Expect patient to eat in dining room, perform ADLs, attend activities.	1. Reduces anxiety; reduces secondary gain and manipulation	**GOAL MET** Patient initially refuses to leave room for meals. Misses one meal. Goes to dining room thereafter. Performs all ADLs, with special attention to applying make-up.
2. Patient will remain free of injury throughout the hospitalization.	2. Provide safety measures during seizures, but limit attention and discussion about seizures afterward. Monitor physical condition unobtrusively.	2. Prevents harm; reduces secondary gain; minimizes secondary gain while condition is assessed	**GOAL MET** Patient remains free of injury during seizures. States, "I guess my seizures don't interest staff. No one will talk to me about them." Patient remains free of seizures after day 3 on the psychiatric unit.
3. Patient will express feelings about self-worth by the end of the second day.	3. Encourage exploration of feelings about life, work, loved ones.	3. Conveys interest and uncovers sources of stress	**GOAL MET** Patient states she is scared of losing her glamorous appearance and her job because of age. Demonstrates appropriate affect.
4. Patient will verbalize optimism about future by discharge.	4. Focus on alternatives available to patient to earn a living when modeling is no longer an option.	4. Encourages problem solving	**GOAL MET** Patient shows fashion sketches to nurse and reveals that she had once thought she might be a good designer. With encouragement, she decides to explore evening classes in illustration and design to prepare for second career.
5. Patient will allow family involvement in decision making by the end of the second day.	5. Identify family's perceptions of the situation, precipitating events, and patient's feelings and behaviors.	5. Encourages realistic feedback to patient; reduces secondary gain	**GOAL MET** Family supports plan to study fashion design.

EVALUATION

See individual outcomes and evaluation in the care plan.

KEY POINTS TO REMEMBER

- Somatoform disorders are characterized by the presence of multiple, real, physical symptoms for which there is no evidence of medical illness.
- Dissociative disorders involve a disruption in consciousness with a significant impairment in memory, identity, or perceptions of self.
- Somatoform and dissociative disorders are believed to be responses to psychological stress, although the patient shows no insight into the potential stressors.
- Patients with somatoform and dissociative disorders often have comorbid psychiatric illness, primarily depression, anxiety, or substance abuse.
- The course of these disorders may be brief, with acute onset and spontaneous remission, or chronic, with a gradual onset and prolonged impairment.
- Because these patients may not seek psychiatric treatment, the nurse does not usually see them in the acute psychiatric setting, except during a period of crisis such as suicidal risk.
- The nursing assessment is especially important to clarify the history and course of past symptoms, as well as to obtain a complete picture of the current physical and mental status.
- Although these patients do respond to crisis intervention, they usually require referral for psychotherapy to attain sustained improvement in level of functioning.

CRITICAL THINKING

1. A patient with suspected somatization disorder has been admitted to the medical-surgical unit after an episode of chest pain with possible electrocardiographic changes. She frequently complains of palpitations, asks the nurse to check her vital signs, and begs staff to stay with her. Some nurses take her pulse and blood pressure when she asks. Others evade her requests. Most staff tries to avoid spending time with her.
   A. How would you feel as a nurse in this situation? Consider why staff might wish to avoid her.
   B. Design interventions to cope with the patient's behaviors. Give rationales for your interventions.

2. A patient with body dysmorphic disorder talks incessantly about how big her nose is, how those around her are offended by her appearance, and how her appearance has negatively affected her employment and her social life. What interventions could you make to reduce her anxiety?

CHAPTER REVIEW

1. A patient states she has been ill for several months with stomach pain, headache, and dizziness. A review of records shows that she has been tested repeatedly for various conditions, yet no clinical diagnosis has been found. She states her pain is "10 out of 10" on a scale of 1 to 10. She has been treated in the past for anxiety and depression. Which condition should the nurse anticipate?
   1. Hypochondriasis
   2. Somatization
   3. Conversion disorder
   4. Body dysmorphic disorder

2. The nurse is caring for a patient who has experienced the onset of a headache and has no history of headaches. When talking with the nurse, the patient states, "I am sure this is a brain tumor." Which condition should the nurse anticipate?
   1. Hypochondriasis
   2. Somatization
   3. Conversion disorder
   4. Body dysmorphic disorder

3. A patient presents to the emergency department with a sudden onset of lower paralysis. Although the patient's wife is hysterical, the patient himself is calm and unemotional. All organic causes for the paralysis have been ruled out. Which condition should the nurse anticipate?
   1. Hypochondriasis
   2. Somatization
   3. Conversion disorder
   4. Body dysmorphic disorder

4. A patient has been diagnosed with Munchausen's syndrome. Which behavior should the nurse anticipate?
   1. Tendency to frequent the same caregiver and use the emergency department at night
   2. Exaggeration of symptoms with the intent of becoming eligible for disability compensation
   3. Inability to recall important information related to a recent rape attempt
   4. Attempts to make oneself ill and going from one hospital to another to call attention to oneself

5. The nurse is planning care for a patient with a somatoform disorder. Which intervention(s) would be appropriate? *Select all that apply.*
   1. Have patient direct requests to varying nurses so they will become familiar with the patient's needs.
   2. Objectively explain that the patient's symptoms are not real.
   3. Teach assertive communication.
   4. Shift focus from somatic concerns to feelings.
   5. Spend time with patient only when summoned.

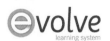

Visit the Evolve website for an **Audio Chapter Summary, Chapter Review Answers & Rationales, Critical Thinking Answer Guidelines,** and additional resources related to the content in this chapter: **http://evolve.elsevier.com/Varcarolis/foundations**

Companion CD Use the Companion CD to prepare for tests and the NCLEX® Examination with **Test-Taking Strategies** for psychiatric mental health nursing and hundreds of **Review Questions.**

References

American Psychiatric Association. (2000). *Diagnostic and statistical manual of mental disorders* (4th ed., text rev.) *(DSM-IV-TR)*. Washington, DC: Author.

Avinger, K. A., & Jones, R. A. (2007). Group treatment of sexually abused adolescent girls: A review of outcome studies. *American Journal of Family Therapy, 35,* 315–326.

Baune, B., Caniato, R., Garcia-Alcaraz, M., & Berger, K. (2008). Combined effects of major depression, pain and somatic disorders on general functioning in the general adult population. *Pain, 138,* 310–317.

Bulechek, G. M., Butcher, H. K., & Dochterman, J. M. (2008). *Nursing interventions classification (NIC)* (5th ed.). St. Louis: Mosby.

DiMario, F. J. (2008). Apparent life-threatening events: So what happens next? *Pediatrics, 122*(1), 190–191.

Feldman, K. W., Feldman, M. D., Grady, R., Burns, M., & McDonald, R. (2007). Renal and urologic manifestations of pediatric condition falsification/Munchausen by proxy. *Pediatric Nephrology, 22,* 849–856.

Feldman, M. D., & Hamilton, J. C. (2006). Serial factitious disorder and Munchausen by proxy in pregnancy. *International Journal of Clinical Practice, 60,* 1675–1678.

Greenberg, D. B., Braun, I. M., & Cassem, N. H. (2008). Functional somatic symptoms and somatoform disorders. In T. A. Stern, J. F. Rosenbaum, M. Fava, J. Biederman, & S. L. Rauch (Eds.), *Massachusetts General Hospital comprehensive clinical psychiatry* (pp. 319–330). St. Louis: Mosby.

Han, C., Marks, D., Pae, C., Lee, B., Ko, Y., Masand, P., et al. (2008). Paroxetine for patients with undifferentiated somatoform disorder: A prospective, open-label, 8-week pilot study. *Current Therapeutic Research, 69*(3), 221–231.

Mayo Clinic Staff. (2007). *Dissociative disorders.* Retrieved August 16, 2008 from Mayo Clinic.com website: http://www.mayoclinic.com/print/dissociative-disorders/DS00574?Method=print&DSE

McDermott, B. E., Leamon, M. H., Feldman, M. D., & Scott, C. L. (2008). Factitious disorder and malingering. In R. E. Hales, S. C. Yudofsky, & G. O. Gabbard (Eds.), *Textbook of psychiatry* (5th ed., pp. 643–664). Washington, DC: American Psychiatric Publishing.

Michal, M., Kaufhold, J., Grabhorn, R., Krakow, K., Overbeck, J., & Heidenreich, T. (2005). Depersonalization and social anxiety. *Journal of Nervous and Mental Disease, 193*(9), 629–632.

Moorhead, S., Johnson, M., Maas, M., & Swanson, E. (Eds.). (2008). *Nursing outcomes classification (NOC)* (4th ed.). St. Louis: Mosby.

Phillips, K. A., Menard, W., & Fay, C. (2006). Gender similarities and differences in 200 individuals with body dysmorphic disorder. *Comprehensive Psychiatry, 47,* 77–87.

Reinders, A., Nijenhuis, E., Quak, J., Korf, J., Haaksma, J., Paans, A., et al. (2006). Psychobiological characteristics of dissociative identity disorder: A symptom provocation study. *Biological Psychiatry, 60,* 730–740.

Sadock, B. J., & Sadock, V. A. (2008). *Kaplan & Sadock's concise textbook of clinical psychiatry* (3rd ed.). Philadelphia: Lippincott Williams & Wilkins.

Schlozman, S. C., & Nonacs, R. M. (2008). Dissociative disorders. In T. A. Stern, J. F. Rosenbaum, M. Fava, J. Biederman, & S. L. Rauch (Eds.), *Massachusetts General Hospital comprehensive clinical psychiatry* (pp. 481–486). St. Louis: Mosby.

Smith, F. A. (2008). Factitious disorders and malingering. In T. A. Stern, J. F. Rosenbaum, M. Fava, J. Biederman, & S. L. Rauch (Eds.), *Massachusetts General Hospital comprehensive clinical psychiatry* (pp. 331–336), St. Louis: Mosby.

Stangier, U., Adam-Schwebe, S., Müller, T., & Wolter, M. (2008). Discrimination of facial appearance stimuli in body dysmorphic disorder. *Journal of Abnormal Psychology, 117*(2), 435–443.

Stickley, T., & Nickeas, R. (2006). Becoming one person: Living with dissociative identity disorder. *Journal of Psychiatric and Mental Health Nursing, 13,* 180–187.

Vennemann, B., Perdekamp, M., Weinmann, W., Faller-Marquardt, M., Pollak, S., & Brandis, M. (2007). A case of Munchausen syndrome by proxy with subsequent suicide of the mother. *Forensic Science International, 158*(2), 195–199.

Yates, W. R. (2008). *Somatoform disorders.* Retrieved September 6, 2008 from WebMD website: http://www.emedicine.com/med/topic3527.htm

Yutzy, S. H., & Parish, B. S. (2008). Somatoform disorders. In R. E. Hales, S. C. Yudofsky, & G. O. Babbard (Eds.), *Textbook of psychiatry* (5th ed., pp. 609–642). Washington, DC: Author.

A PATIENT SPEAKS

Hello, my name is Patty, and I am an alcoholic. When I was 16 years of age, my friends and I started skipping school on a regular basis to buy alcohol and drugs. At first it was just for kicks. Eventually I ended up drinking on almost a daily basis and stole from parents to buy drugs and alcohol. The more I drank, the worse things got at home. My whole existence revolved around drugs and alcohol. In the process I was losing everything. My poor parents had no idea what to do. I lied, stole, and hurt everyone who ever really cared for me.

Around this time I was diagnosed with bipolar disorder. Unfortunately, I was allergic to the only medication they had for bipolar disease at that time. I was left untreated for the next 16 years.

I married, but my drinking escalated, and my marriage deteriorated and ended. I was able to care for my son, Teddy, only with my parents' help. I started nursing school, and things were finally looking up. I graduated and became an LPN. For the first time ever I was proud of myself and had accomplished something great. It wasn't long before I fell off the wagon again. My parents took care of my son.

One day I went to New York City to get some dope and never came home. I was living on the street. All I cared about was the next high. I quickly became one of those homeless people you step over on the street… selling aluminum cans for a quarter just to buy one cigarette. All that mattered was staying high.

The day I went home, I was emaciated and was virtually on my death bed. My parents took me to a hospital, and I was in life-threatening withdrawal from drugs and alcohol. I almost died.

Later, looking at pictures of my son, I knew I had missed so many precious times with him that I will never get back. Hurting people you love is one of the things you can't take back or make up for. Now, even after 10 years of being clean and sober, I doubt my sister will ever forgive me. I love my sister. When I was pregnant with my first son, she helped me and stepped in for me when I was gone. I will never forget that. Thank you, Lisa.

I was unaware that addiction was a disease until I went to Alcoholics Anonymous (AA). I stopped feeling helpless, and I saw that other people who had similar problems were alive and well and able to stay sober. I owe my sobriety to the people in those rooms of AA over the years.

The important things to me now are family, religion, and my home. I have a terrific husband and another wonderful little boy, and my life is full. Staying sober is a daily struggle. Being bipolar and a recovering alcoholic and drug addict makes for a challenging existence. I have learned to stay around people that truly understand me and stay away from people who don't. If you don't, you set yourself up for a miserable life. I hope my story might help someone else struggling with this disease and help others know that when treated like a disease, alcoholism can be treated successfully.

CHAPTER **23**

Crisis and Disaster

Christine Heifner Graor and Carolyn M. Scott

Key Terms and Concepts

adventitious crisis, 532
crisis intervention, 529
critical incident stress debriefing (CISD), 539
maturational crisis, 530
phases of crisis, 532

primary care, 539
secondary care, 539
situational crisis, 531
tertiary care, 539

Objectives

1. Differentiate among the three types of crisis. Provide an example of each from the reader's own experience.
2. Delineate six aspects of crisis that have relevance for nurses involved in crisis intervention.
3. Develop a handout describing areas to assess during crisis. Include at least two sample questions for each area.
4. Discuss four common problems in the nurse-patient relationship that are frequently encountered by beginning nurses when starting crisis intervention. Discuss two interventions for each problem.

5. Compare and contrast the differences among primary, secondary, and tertiary intervention, including appropriate intervention strategies.
6. Explain to a classmate four potential crisis situations that patients may experience in hospital settings.
7. Provide concrete examples of interventions to minimize the situations.
8. List at least five resources in the community that could be used as referrals for a patient in crisis.

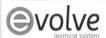 Visit the Evolve website for an **Audio Glossary & Flashcards, Concept Map Creator**, and additional resources related to the content in this chapter: **http://evolve.elsevier.com/Varcarolis/foundations**

The U.S. Department of Homeland Security raises the terror alert to "high" and warns citizens to be watchful for any suspicious behavior. A tornado touches down in a small Midwestern town, levels an entire neighborhood, and leaves 10 residents dead and many more homeless. Hurricane Katrina rips into the gulf coast, and the levees in New Orleans fail, leaving 80% of the city flooded and approximately 1836 people dead. A child is killed in a drive-by shooting by a bullet intended for a neighborhood drug dealer. A 35-year employee in a manufacturing company is laid off, and after months of desperately trying to pay the family's bills, he finds his family and himself homeless. A teenage boy armed with several guns enters his high school and randomly shoots everyone who crosses his path. A young nursing student discovers she is pregnant, and the father of the baby abandons

her. What do these situations have in common? Each of these situations could be the precipitant of a crisis—leaving individuals, families, and whole communities struggling to cope with the impact of the event.

Everyone experiences crises. The experience itself is not pathological but rather represents a struggle for equilibrium and adaptation. Roberts (2005, p. 778) defines a crisis as:

> ... an acute disruption of psychological homeostasis in which one's usual coping mechanisms fail and there exists evidence of distress and functional impairment. The subjective reaction to a stressful life experience that compromises the individual's stability and ability to cope or function. The main cause of a crisis is an intensely stressful, traumatic, or hazardous event, but two other conditions are also necessary: (1) the individual's perception of the event as

the cause of considerable upset and/or disruption and (2) the individual's inability to resolve the disruption by previously used coping mechanisms.

Crisis both threatens personality organization and presents an opportunity for personal growth and development. Successful crisis resolution results from the development of adaptive coping mechanisms, reflects ego development, and suggests the employment of physiological, psychological, and social resources. Therefore, crisis is an essential component of individual growth and development.

Crises are acute and time-limited, usually lasting 4 to 6 weeks. They are associated with events that are experienced with overwhelming emotions of increased tension, helplessness, and disorganization. A state of crisis is produced by three interconnected conditions: (a) a hazardous event that poses a threat, (b) an emotional need that represents earlier threats and increased vulnerability, and (c) an inability to respond adaptively (Parad & Caplan, 1965).

As shown in Figure 23-1 (Aguilera, 1998), the outcome of crisis depends on (a) the realistic perception of the event, (b) adequate situational supports, and (c) adequate coping mechanisms.

- People vary in the way they absorb, process, and use information from the environment (Aguilera, 1998).
- Situational supports include the nurses and other health professionals who use crisis intervention to assist those in crisis. **Crisis intervention** is "a short-term therapeutic process that focuses on the rapid resolution of an immediate crisis or emergency using available personnel, family, and/or environmental resources" (American Nurses Association et al., 2007, p. 65). In general, interventions are broad, creative, and flexible (Saunders, 2007).
- Coping skills are acquired through a variety of sources, such as cultural responses, the modeling behaviors of others, and life opportunities that broaden experience and promote the adaptive development of new coping responses (Aguilera, 1998). Many factors compromise a person's ability to cope with a crisis event (e.g., the number of other stressful life events with which the person is currently coping, the presence of other unresolved losses with which the person may be dealing, the presence of concurrent psychiatric disorders, the presence of concurrent medical problems, the presence of excessive fatigue or pain, the quality and quantity of a person's usual coping skills).

CRISIS THEORY

An early crisis theorist, **Erich Lindemann**, conducted a classic study in the 1940s on the grief reactions of close relatives of victims who died in the Coconut Grove nightclub fire in Boston. This study formed the foundation of crisis theory and clinical intervention. Lindemann was convinced that even though acute grief is a normal reaction to a distressing situation, preventive interventions could eliminate or decrease potential serious personality disorganization and the devastating psychological consequences of the sustained effects of severe anxiety. He believed that the same interventions that were helpful in bereavement would prove just as helpful in dealing with other types of stressful events. Therefore, he proposed a crisis intervention model as a major element of preventive psychiatry in the community.

In the early 1960s, **Gerald Caplan** (1964) advanced crisis theory and outlined crisis intervention strategies. Since that time, our understanding of crisis and effective intervention has continued to be refined and enhanced by numerous contemporary clinicians and theorists (Behrman & Reid, 2002; Roberts, 2005). The 1961 report of the Joint Commission on Mental Illness and Health addressed the need for community mental health centers throughout the country. This report stimulated the establishment of crisis services, which are now an

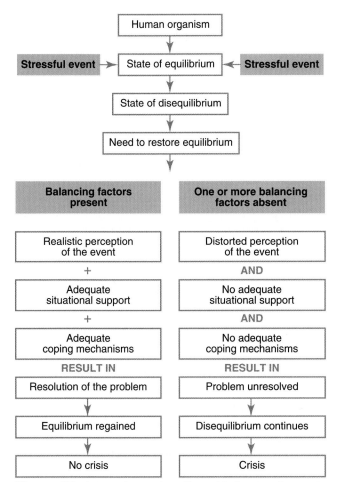

Figure 23-1 Paradigm: The effect of balancing factors in a stressful event. (From Aguilera, D.C. [1998]. *Crisis intervention: Theory and methodology* [8th ed.]. St. Louis: Mosby.)

important part of mental health programs in hospitals and communities.

Donna Aguilera and **Janice Mesnick** (1970) provided a framework for nurses for crisis assessment and intervention, which has grown in scope and practice. Aguilera's work (1998) continues to set a standard in the practice of crisis assessment and intervention.

Albert R. Roberts's seven-stage model of crisis interventions (Figure 23-2) (Roberts 2005; Roberts & Ottens, 2005) is a more contemporary model that is useful in helping individuals who have suffered from an acute situational crisis, as well as people who are diagnosed with acute stress disorder. In an effort to establish consensus on mass trauma intervention principles, Hobfoll and colleagues (2007) identified five essential, empirically supported elements of mass trauma interventions that promote: (1) a sense of safety, (2) calming, (3) a sense of self-efficacy and collective efficacy, (4) connectedness, and (5) hope.

The effects of disasters such as the 9/11 World Trade Center terrorist attack and Hurricane Katrina have emphasized the need for crisis assessment and intervention by community mental health providers. Regardless of the type of crisis and whether traumatized individuals are victims, families, rescue workers, or observers, those with access to crisis assessment and intervention are more likely to feel safe, supported, empowered, and able to make sense of their response to the disaster, compared to those without access (Hobfoll et al., 2007; Phoenix, 2007; Saunders, 2007).

Components of crisis assessment are derived from established crisis theory and constitute a sound knowledge base for the application of the nursing process to treatment of a patient in crisis. An understanding of three areas of crisis theory enables application of the nursing process; the areas are: (1) types of crisis, (2) phases of crisis, and (3) aspects of crisis that have relevance for nurses.

TYPES OF CRISES

There are three basic types of crisis situations: (1) developmental, or maturational, crises; (2) situational crises; and (3) disasters, or adventitious crises. Disadvantaged and stigmatized people, such as those with preexisting mental health problems, substance abuse, or limited external resources, are especially vulnerable during a stress event and prone to crises (Saunders, 2007).

Maturational Crisis

A process of maturation occurs across the life cycle. Erik Erikson (1902-1994) conceptualized the process by identifying eight stages of ego growth and development (see Table 2-2). Each stage represents a time where physical, cognitive, instinctual, and sexual changes prompt an internal conflict or crisis, which results in either psychosocial growth or regression. Therefore, each developmental stage represents a **maturational crisis** (that is, a critical period of increased vulnerability and heightened potential—a turning point).

When a person arrives at a new stage, formerly used coping styles are no longer effective, and new coping mechanisms have yet to be developed. Thus for a time the person is without effective defenses. This often leads to increased tension and anxiety, which may manifest as variations in the person's normal behavior. Examples of events that can precipitate a maturational crisis include leaving home during late adolescence, marriage, the birth of a child, retirement, and the death of a parent. Successful resolution of these maturational tasks leads to development of basic human qualities.

Erikson believed that the way these crises are resolved at one stage affects the ability to pass through subsequent stages, because each crisis provides the starting point for movement toward the next stage. If a person lacks support systems and adequate role models, successful resolution may be difficult or may not occur. Unresolved problems in the past and

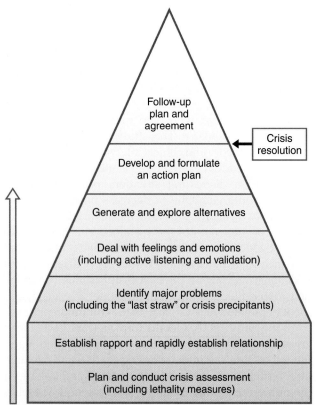

Figure 23-2 Roberts's seven-stage model of crisis intervention. (From Roberts, A. R., & Ottens, A. J. (2005). The seven-stage crisis intervention model: A road map to goal attainment, problem solving, and crisis resolution. *Brief Treatment and Crisis Intervention, 5,* 329–339.)

inadequate coping mechanisms then adversely affect what is learned in each developmental stage. When a person experiences severe difficulty during a maturational crisis, professional intervention may be indicated.

Factors may disrupt individuals' progression through the maturational stages. For example, alcohol and drug addiction disrupts progression through the maturational stages. Unfortunately, this interruption occurs too often among individuals during their adolescent years. When the addictive behavior is controlled (e.g., by the late teens or mid-20s), the young person's growth and development resume at the point of interruption. For example, a young person whose addiction is arrested at 22 years of age may have the psychosocial and problem-solving skills of a 14-year-old. Often these teenagers do not receive treatment, and their adult coping skills are diminished or absent.

Situational Crisis

A situational crisis arises from events that are extraordinary, external rather than internal, and often unanticipated (Roberts, 2005). Examples of events that can precipitate a situational crisis include the loss or change of a job, the death of a loved one, an abortion, a change in financial status, divorce, and severe physical or mental illness. Whether or not these events precipitate a crisis depends on factors such as the degree of support available from caring friends, family members, and others; general emotional and physical status; and the ability to understand and cope with the meaning of the stressful event. As in all crises or potential crisis situations, the stressful event involves loss or change that threatens a person's self-concept and self-esteem. To varying degrees, successful resolution of a crisis depends on resolution of the grief associated with the loss.

EVIDENCE-BASED PRACTICE

Posttraumatic Stress Disorder Following Disaster

Neria, Y., Nandi, A., & Galea. S. (2007). Post-traumatic stress disorder following disasters: A systematic review. *Psychological Medicine, 38*(4), 467–480.

Problem

"Disasters are traumatic events that may result in a wide range of mental and physical health consequences" (p. 467). Studies show that more than 15% of females and 19% of males are exposed to disasters during their lifetime. The most frequently occurring post-disaster psychopathology is post-traumatic stress disorder (PTSD), which is the most commonly studied post-disaster psychiatric disorder.

Purpose of Study

The purpose of this study was to systematically assess the evidence about PTSD following exposure to disasters.

Methods

The researchers performed a systematic search of peer-reviewed literature, using databases from Medline, PsycINFO, and PILOTS. Eligible studies for this review included reports based on the DSM criteria of PTSD symptoms from 1980 (when PTSD was first introduced in *DSM-III*) to February 2007.

Key Findings

- The researchers identified 284 reports of post-disaster PTSD (human-made disasters [90]; technological disasters [65]; natural disasters [116]; and multiple types of disasters, such as flooding and chemical contamination [13]). The body of research conducted after disasters in the past 3 decades suggests that the burden of PTSD among persons exposed to disasters is substantial.
- Regardless of the disaster type, the prevalence of PTSD in the first year after exposure ranges from 30% to 40% in those directly exposed to the disaster, 10% to 20% among first responders and rescue workers, and 5% to 10% in the general population.
- Post-disaster PTSD is associated with sociodemographic and background factors (e.g., low-income, recent immigration, specific ethnicities, mental illness), event exposure characteristics, social support factors, and personality traits.

Implications for Nursing Practice

During disasters and crises, nurses are challenged to address the immediate needs of individuals while considering the specific vulnerabilities of various groups. Since the most frequently occurring post-disaster psychopathology is PTSD, nurses should especially assess and plan intervention for PTSD in disaster victims, first responders and rescuers, and the general population (e.g., those experiencing loss of family members, friends, or colleagues or those suffering property loss, forced to relocate, or exposed to the event through the media). Nurses, as first responders, should be especially cognizant of their own vulnerability to PTSD.

Adventitious Crisis

An **adventitious crisis** is not a part of everyday life; it results from events that are unplanned and may be accidental, caused by nature, or human-made. This type of crisis results from (1) a natural disaster (e.g., flood, fire, earthquake), (2) a national disaster (e.g., acts of terrorism, war, riots, airplane crashes), or (3) a crime of violence (e.g., rape, assault or murder in the workplace or school, bombing in crowded areas, spousal or child abuse).

Commonly experienced, post-trauma phenomena include acute stress disorder, posttraumatic stress disorder, and depression. Therefore, the need for psychological first aid (crisis intervention) and debriefing after any crisis situation for all age groups cannot be overstressed.

Situational and adventitious crises can challenge the basic assumptions that underlie individuals' worldviews. Roberts (2005, p. 687) proposes that "a person's vulnerability to a stressful event depends to a certain extent on the newness, intensity, and duration of the stressful event." It is also possible to experience more than one type of crisis situation simultaneously, and as expected, the presence of more than one crisis further taxes individual coping skills. Consider a 51-year-old woman who may be going through a midlife crisis (maturational) when her husband dies suddenly of cancer (situational). Think about the victims of Hurricane Katrina, many of whom were members of vulnerable groups and experiencing maturational or situational crises prior to the hurricane. They were then confronted with the devastation of the hurricane and the simultaneous onset of multiple stress events (e.g., the deaths of family members and friends, the loss of homes and belongings, the loss of jobs, the loss of community supports, and even the loss of personal identification) (Saunders, 2007).

PHASES OF CRISIS

Caplan (1964) identified four distinct phases of crisis.

Phase 1

A person confronted by a conflict or problem that threatens the self-concept responds with increased feelings of anxiety. The increase in anxiety stimulates the use of problem-solving techniques and defense mechanisms in an effort to solve the problem and lower anxiety.

Phase 2

If the usual defensive response fails and the threat persists, anxiety continues to rise and produce feelings of extreme discomfort. Individual functioning becomes disorganized. Trial-and-error attempts at solving the problem and restoring a normal balance begin.

Phase 3

If the trial-and-error attempts fail, anxiety can escalate to severe and panic levels, and the person mobilizes automatic relief behaviors, such as withdrawal and flight. Some form of resolution (e.g., compromising needs or redefining the situation to reach an acceptable solution) may be made in this stage.

Phase 4

If the problem is not solved and new coping skills are ineffective, anxiety can overwhelm the person and lead to serious personality disorganization, depression, confusion, violence against others, or suicidal behavior.

APPLICATION OF THE NURSING PROCESS

Nurses, perhaps more than any other group of health professionals, deal with people who are experiencing disruption in their lives. Because people typically experience increased stress and anxiety in medical, surgical, and psychiatric hospital settings, as well as in community settings, nurses are often positioned and primed to initiate and participate in crisis intervention. Crisis theory defines aspects of crisis that are basic to crisis intervention and relevant for nurses (Box 23-1).

ASSESSMENT

General Assessment

As shown in Figure 23-1, a person's equilibrium may be adversely affected by one or more of the following: (1) an unrealistic perception of the precipitating event, (2) inadequate situational supports, and (3) inadequate coping mechanisms (Aguilera, 1998). It is crucial to assess these factors when a crisis situation is evaluated, because data gained from the assessment guide both the nurse and the patient in setting realistic and meaningful goals and in planning possible solutions to the problem situation.

The nurse's initial task is to promote a sense of safety by assessing the patient's potential for suicide or homicide. If the patient is suicidal, homicidal, or unable to

BOX 23-1 Foundation for Crisis Intervention

- A crisis is self-limiting and usually resolves within 4 to 6 weeks.
- At the resolution of a crisis, the patient will emerge at one of three different functional levels:
  - A higher level of functioning.
  - The same level of functioning.
  - A lower level of functioning.
- The goal of crisis intervention is to return the patient to at least the pre-crisis level of functioning.
- The form of crisis resolution depends on the patient's actions and others' interventions.
- During a crisis, people are often more receptive than usual to outside intervention. With intervention, the patient can learn different adaptive means of problem solving to correct inadequate solutions.
- The patient in a crisis situation is assumed to be mentally healthy, to have functioned well in the past, and to be presently in a state of disequilibrium.
- Crisis intervention deals only with the patient's present problem and resolution of the immediate crisis (e.g., the "here and now").
- The nurse must be willing to take an active, even directive, role in intervention, which is in direct contrast to conventional therapeutic intervention that stresses a more passive and nondirective role.
- Early intervention probably increases the chances for a good prognosis.
- The patient is encouraged to set realistic goals and plan a focused intervention with the nurse.

take care of personal needs, hospitalization should be considered (Aguilera, 1998). Sample questions to ask include:

- Do you feel you can keep yourself safe?
- Have you thought of killing yourself or someone else? If yes, have you thought of how you would do this?

After establishing that the patient poses no danger to self or others, the nurse assesses three main areas: (1) the patient's perception of the precipitating event, (2) the patient's situational supports, and (3) the patient's personal coping skills.

VIGNETTE

A 25-year-old woman named Madison is brought to the emergency department by police after being beaten by her husband. Madison is seen by the medical personnel and then interviewed by the psychiatric mental health nurse working in the emergency department. The nurse calmly introduces herself and tells Madison she would like to spend some time with her. The nurse says, "It looks as if things are pretty overwhelming.

Is that how you're feeling?" The nurse makes the observation that things must be very bad if Madison stays with an abusive husband. Madison sits slumped in a chair, her hands in her lap, head hanging down, and tears in her eyes. ■

Assessing Perception of Precipitating Event

The nurse's task is now to assess the individual or family and the problem. The more clearly the problem can be defined, the more likely effective solutions will be identified. Sample questions that may facilitate assessment include:

- Has anything particularly upsetting happened to you within the past few days or weeks?
- What was happening in your life before you started to feel this way?
- What leads you to seek help now?
- Describe how you are feeling right now.
- How does this situation affect your life?
- How do you see this event affecting your future?
- What would need to be done to resolve this situation?

VIGNETTE

Nurse: Madison, tell me what has happened.

Madison: I can't go home …. No one cares …. No one believes me …. I can't go through it again.

Nurse: Tell me what you can't go through again.

(Madison starts to cry, shaking with sobs. The nurse sits quietly for a while and then speaks.)

Nurse: Tell me what is so terrible. Let's look at it together.

After a while, Madison tells the nurse that her husband has been beating her regularly, although particularly after a night of drinking. The beatings have become much worse over time, and Madison states, "I'm afraid that eventually I'll end up dead." ■

Assessing Situational Supports

Next the nurse determines available resources by assessing the patient's support systems. Family and friends are often involved to aid the patient by offering material or emotional support. If these resources are unavailable, the nurse or counselor acts as a temporary support system while relationships with individuals or groups in the community are established. Sample questions are:

- Who do you live with?
- Who do you talk to when you feel overwhelmed?
- Who can you trust?
- Who is available to help you?
- Where do you go to worship (or talk to God)?
- Where do you go to school or to other community-based activities?

- During difficult times in the past, who did you want most to help you?
- Who is the most helpful?

VIGNETTE

Nurse: Madison, who can you go to? Do you have any other family?

Madison: No. My family is in another state. We stay pretty much alone.

Nurse: Do you have anyone you can talk to?

Madison: I really don't have any friends. My husband's jealousy makes it difficult for me to have friends. He doesn't like anyone that I would want as a friend.

Nurse: What about people at your place of worship or co-workers?

Madison: My co-workers are nice, but I can't tell them things like this. They wouldn't believe me anyway.

The nurse learns that Madison does well at her job. Madison explains that her job helps her forget her problems for a little while. Getting good job reviews also has another reward: it is the only time her husband says anything nice about her. ■

Assessing Personal Coping Skills

Finally, the nurse assesses the patient's personal coping skills by evaluating the patient's anxiety level and identifying the patient's established patterns of coping. Common coping mechanisms may be overeating, drinking, smoking, withdrawing, seeking out someone to talk to, yelling, fighting, or engaging in other physical activity (Behrman & Reid, 2002). Sample questions to ask include:

- What do you usually do to feel better?
- Did you try it this time? If so, what was different?
- What helped you through difficult times in the past?
- What do you think might happen now?

VIGNETTE

Nurse: What do you think would help your situation?

Madison: I don't want to be in an abusive marriage. I just don't know where to turn.

The nurse tells Madison that she wants to work with her to find a solution and that she is concerned for Madison's safety and well-being. ■

Self-Assessment

Nurses need to constantly monitor and acknowledge personal feelings and thoughts when dealing with a patient in crisis. It is important to recognize your own level of anxiety to prevent the patient from closing off his or her expression of painful feelings to you. Self-awareness of your negative feelings and reactions can prevent unconscious suppression of the patient's personal distress in an effort to manage your own discomfort. Closing off feelings in the patient renders the nurse ineffective. There may be times when, perhaps for personal reasons, you feel you cannot deal effectively with a patient's situation. If this happens, ask another colleague to work with the individual. Consulting a more experienced colleague or mentor or seeking supervision will help you separate the patient's needs from your own and identify how to work through uncomfortable or painful personal issues or bias to better care for those in crisis.

Beginning nurses in crisis intervention often face common problems that must be dealt with before they can become comfortable and competent in the role of a crisis counselor. Four of the more common problems are:

1. The nurse needs to be needed.
2. The nurse sets unrealistic goals for patients.
3. The nurse has difficulty dealing with the issue of suicide.
4. The nurse has difficulty terminating the nurse-patient relationship.

Table 23-1 gives examples, results, appropriate interventions, and desired outcomes of common problems in the nurse-patient relationship faced by beginning nurses. It is crucial that expert supervision be available as an integral part of the crisis-intervention training process.

Even experienced nurses working in disaster situations can become overwhelmed when witnessing catastrophic loss of human life (e.g., acts of terrorism, plane crashes, school shootings) and/or mass destruction of people's homes and belongings (e.g., floods, fires, tornadoes). In fact, researchers find that mental health care providers may experience psychological distress from working with traumatized populations, a phenomenon of secondary traumatic stress or "vicarious traumatization" (Dunkley & Whelan, 2006). As stressed before, nurses need to constantly monitor personal feelings and thoughts when dealing with patients in crisis (Phoenix, 2007), and disaster nurses need both supportive ties and access to debriefing.

Debriefing is an important step for staff in coming to terms with overwhelming violent or otherwise disastrous situations. Such intervention helps staff put the crisis in perspective and begin their own recovery. Debriefing is discussed in detail later in the chapter.

TABLE 23-1 Common Problems in the Nurse-Patient Relationship

Example	Result	Intervention	Outcome
Problem 1: Nurse needs to feel needed.			
Nurse: Allows excessive phone calls between sessions. Gives direct advice without sufficient knowledge of patient's situation. Attempts to influence patient's lifestyle on a judgmental basis.	Patient becomes dependent on nurse and relies less on own abilities. Nurse reacts to patient's not getting "cured" by projecting feelings of frustration and anger onto patient.	*Nurse:* Evaluates personal needs versus patient's needs with an experienced professional. Discourages patient's dependency. Encourages goal setting and problem solving by patient. Takes control only if patient is suicidal or homicidal.	Patient is free to grow and problem-solve own life crises. Nurse's skills and effectiveness grow as comfort with role increases and own goals are clarified.
Problem 2: Nurse sets unrealistic goals for patients.			
Nurse: Expects physically abused woman to leave battering partner. Expects man who abuses alcohol to stop drinking when loss of family or job is imminent.	Nurse feels anxious and responsible when expectations are not met; anxiety resulting from feelings of inadequacy are projected onto the patient in the form of frustration and anger.	*Nurse:* Examines realistic expectations of self and patient with an experienced professional. Reevaluates patient's level of functioning and works with patient on his level. Encourages setting of goals by patient.	Patient feels less alienated, and a working relationship can ensue. Nurse's ability to assess and problem-solve increases as anger and frustration decrease.
Problem 3: Nurse has difficulty dealing with a suicidal patient.			
Nurse selectively inattends by: Denying possible clues. Neglecting to follow up on verbal suicide clues. Changing topic to less threatening subject when self-destructive themes come up.	Patient is robbed of opportunity to share feelings and find alternatives to intolerable situation. Patient remains suicidal. Nurse's crisis intervention ceases to be effective.	*Nurse:* Assesses own feelings and anxieties with help of an experienced professional. Evaluates all clues or slight suspicions and acts on them (e.g., "Are you thinking of killing yourself?"—if yes, nurse assesses suicide potential and need for hospitalization).	Patient experiences relief in sharing feelings and evaluating alternatives. Suicide potential can be minimized. Nurse becomes more adept at picking up clues and minimizing suicide potential.
Problem 4: Nurse has difficulty terminating after crisis has resolved.			
Nurse is tempted to work on other problems in patient's life to prolong contact with patient.	Nurse steps into territory of traditional therapy without proper training or experience.	*Nurse works with an experienced professional to:* Explore own feelings about separations and termination. Reinforce crisis model; crisis intervention is a preventive tool, not psychotherapy. Nurse becomes better able to help patient with his/her feelings when nurse's own feelings are recognized.	Patient is free to go back to his or her life situation or request appropriate referral to work on other issues of importance to patient.

From Wallace, M. A., & Morley, W. E. (1970). Teaching crisis intervention. *American Journal of Nursing, 70*(7), 1484–1487.

Assessment Guidelines Crisis

1. Identify whether the patient's response to the crisis warrants psychiatric treatment or hospitalization to minimize decompensation (suicidal behavior, psychotic thinking, violent behavior).
2. Identify whether the patient is able to identify the *precipitating event.*
3. Assess the patient's understanding of his or her present *situational supports.*
4. Identify the patient's usual *coping styles,* and determine what coping mechanisms may help the present situation.
5. Determine whether there are certain religious or cultural beliefs that need to be considered in assessing and intervening in this patient's crisis.
6. Assess whether this situation is one in which the patient needs primary intervention (education, environmental manipulation, or new coping skills), secondary intervention (crisis intervention), or tertiary intervention (rehabilitation).

CONSIDERING CULTURE

Variations in Disaster Response

Researchers find varied post-disaster reactions *among* ethnic groups, as well as varied post-disaster reactions *within* ethnic groups. For example, Hispanics of Dominican or Puerto Rican origins were more likely to report symptoms consistent with probable post-traumatic stress disorder (PTSD) after the September 11 terrorist attacks than other Hispanics and non-Hispanics. The higher prevalence of probable PTSD in the Dominicans and Puerto Ricans is explained by their likelihood to have lower incomes, be younger, have less social support, have had greater exposure to the September 11 attacks, and to have experienced a peri-event panic attack upon hearing about the attacks.

Galea, S., Vlahov, D., Tracy, M., Hoover, D., Resnick, H., & Kilpatrick, D. (2004). Hispanic ethnicity and post-traumatic stress disorder after a disaster: Evidence from a general population survey after September 11, 2001. *Annals of Epidemiology, 14*(8), 520–531.

DIAGNOSIS

The North American Nursing Diagnosis Association International (NANDA-I) (2009) provides nursing diagnoses that can be considered for patients experiencing anxiety and anxiety disorders. When a person is in crisis, the nursing diagnosis of *Ineffective coping* is often useful. Because anxiety may escalate to moderate or severe levels, the ability to solve problems is usually impaired. Ineffective coping may be evidenced by inability to meet basic needs, inability to meet role

TABLE 23-2 Potential Nursing Diagnoses for Crisis Intervention

Signs and Symptoms	Nursing Diagnosis
Inability to meet basic needs, decreased use of social support, inadequate problem solving, inability to attend to information, isolation	*Ineffective coping* *Risk for compromised resilience*
Denial, exaggerated startle response, flashbacks, horror, hypervigilance, intrusive thoughts and dreams, panic attacks, feeling numb, substance abuse, confusion, incoherent	*Post-trauma syndrome* *Rape-trauma syndrome* *Anxiety (moderate, severe, panic)* *Acute confusion* *Sleep deprivation*
Minimizes symptoms, delays seeking care, displays inappropriate affect, makes dismissive comments when speaking of distressing events	*Ineffective denial*
Overwhelmed, depressed, states has nothing in life worthwhile, self-hatred, feelings of being ineffectual, sees limited alternatives, feels strange, perceives a lack of control	*Risk for suicide* *Chronic low self-esteem* *Disturbed personal identity* *Hopelessness* *Powerlessness*
Has difficulty with interpersonal relationships, isolated, has few or no social supports	*Social isolation* *Impaired social interaction*
Changes in family relationships and functioning, difficulty performing family caregiver role	*Interrupted family processes* *Caregiver role strain*

Data from North American Nursing Diagnosis Association International (NANDA-I). (2009). *NANDA-I nursing diagnoses: Definitions and classification 2009-2011.* Oxford, United Kingdom: Author.

expectations, alteration in social participation, use of inappropriate defense mechanisms, or impairment of usual patterns of communication. The "related-to" component will vary with the individual patient. Table 23-2 identifies potential nursing diagnoses for people in crisis and provides signs and symptoms that might be present to support the diagnosis.

In the preceding vignette, the assessment of Madison's (1) perception of the precipitating event, (2) situational supports, and (3) personal coping skills provides the nurse enough data to formulate two diagnoses and work with Madison in setting goals and planning interventions:

The nurse formulates the following nursing diagnoses:

Anxiety (moderate/severe) related to mental and physical abuse, as evidenced by ineffectual problem solving and feelings of impending doom

Compromised family coping related to the constant threat of violence ■

OUTCOMES IDENTIFICATION

Relevant outcomes of the *Nursing Outcomes Classification (NOC)* (Moorhead et al., 2008) for a person experiencing a crisis include *Coping, Decision Making, Role Performance,* and *Stress Level.* The planning of realistic outcomes is done with the patient and family, which results in outcomes congruent with the patient's cultural and personal values. Without the patient's involvement, the outcome criteria (goals at the end of 4 to 8 weeks) may be irrelevant or unacceptable solutions to that person's crisis. Table 23-3 lists selected *NOC* outcomes with supporting intermediate and short-term indicators for a patient in crisis.

The nurse consults a social worker about Madison, and the three meet together. All agree that Madison should not return to her home. Madison and the nurse then establish goals and plan interventions. The goals are as follows:

- Madison will return to her pre-crisis state within 2 weeks.
- With the support of the staff, Madison will find a safe environment.
- With the support of the staff, Madison will have at least two outside supports available within 24 hours.
- Madison will receive continued evaluation and support until the immediate crisis is over (6 to 8 weeks). ■

TABLE 23-3 *NOC* Outcomes for Patient in Crisis

Nursing Outcome and Definition	Intermediate Indicators	Short-Term Indicators
Coping: Personal actions to manage stressors that tax an individual's resources	Modifies lifestyle as needed Uses effective coping strategies Reports decrease in physical symptoms of stress Reports decrease in negative feelings	Identifies effective coping patterns Identifies ineffective coping patterns Reports decrease in stress Uses personal support system Verbalizes need for assistance
Decision-Making: Ability to make judgments and choose between two or more alternatives	Chooses among alternatives	Identifies relevant information Identifies alternatives Weighs alternatives
Role Performance: Congruence of an individual's role behavior with role expectations	Able to meet role expectations	Performs family role behaviors Describes role changes with illness or disability Describes role changes with elderly dependents/with new family member/when family member leaves home Performs family/parental/intimate/community/work/friendship role behaviors
Stress Level: Severity of manifested physical or mental tension resulting from factors that alter an existing equilibrium		Elevated blood pressure Increased radial pulse rate Upset stomach Restlessness Sleep disturbances Interruption of thought process Forgetfulness Frequent cognitive mistakes Inability to concentrate on tasks Emotional outbursts

Data from Moorhead, S., Johnson, M., Maas, M., & Swanson, E. (2008). *Nursing outcomes classification (NOC)* (4th ed.). St. Louis: Mosby.

PLANNING

Nurses are called upon to plan and intervene through a variety of crisis-intervention modalities, such as disaster nursing, mobile crisis units, group work, health education and crisis prevention, victim outreach programs, and telephone hotlines. Therefore, the nurse may be involved in planning and intervention for an individual (e.g., cases of physical abuse), for a group (e.g., students after a classmate's suicide event or shooting), or for a community (e.g., disaster nursing after tornadoes, shootings, and airplane crashes). Data from the answers to the following questions guide the nurse in determining immediate actions (Aguilera, 1998):

- How much has this crisis affected the patient's life? Can the patient still go to work? Attend school? Care for family members?
- How is the state of disequilibrium affecting significant people in the patient's life (wife, husband, children, other family members, boss, boyfriend, girlfriend)?

IMPLEMENTATION

Crisis intervention is a function of the basic-level nurse and has two initial goals:

1. **Patient safety.** External controls may be applied for protection of the patient in crisis if the patient is suicidal or homicidal.

2. **Anxiety reduction.** Anxiety-reduction techniques are used so inner resources can be mobilized.

During the initial interview, the patient in crisis first needs to gain a feeling of safety. Solutions to the crisis may be offered so the patient is aware of other options. Feelings of support and hope will temporarily diminish anxiety. The nurse needs to play an active role by indicating that help is available. The availability of help is conveyed by the competent use of crisis-intervention skills and genuine interest and support. It is not conveyed by the use of false reassurances and platitudes, such as "everything will be all right." Crisis intervention requires a creative and flexible approach through the use of traditional and nontraditional therapeutic methods. The nurse may act as educator, advisor, and role model, always keeping in mind that it is the patient who solves the problem, not the nurse. The following are important assumptions when working with a patient in crisis:

- The patient is in charge of his or her own life.
- The patient is able to make decisions.
- The crisis counseling relationship is one between partners.

The nurse helps the patient refocus to gain new perspectives on the situation. The nurse supports the patient during the process of finding constructive ways to solve or cope with the problem. It is important for the nurse to be mindful of how difficult it is for the patient to change behavior. Table 23-4 offers guidelines for nursing interventions and corresponding rationales.

TABLE 23-4 Guidelines for Crisis Intervention

Intervention	Rationale
Assess for suicidal or homicidal thoughts or plans.	Safety is always the first consideration.
Take initial steps to make patient feel safe and less anxious.	A person who feels safe and less anxious is able to more effectively problem-solve solutions with the nurse.
Listen carefully (e.g., make eye contact, give frequent feedback to verify and convey understanding, summarize what patient says).	A person who believes someone is really listening is more likely to believe that someone cares about his or her situation and help may be available. This offers hope.
Crisis intervention calls for directive and creative approaches. Initially the nurse may make phone calls to arrange babysitters, schedule a visiting nurse, find shelter, or contact a social worker.	A person who is confused, frightened, or overwhelmed may be temporarily unable to perform usual tasks.
Identify needed social supports (with patient's input) and mobilize the priority.	A person's need for shelter, help with care for children or elders, medical workup, emergency medical attention, hospitalization, food, safe housing, and self-help groups is determined.
Identify needed coping skills (problem solving, relaxation, assertiveness, job training, newborn care, self-esteem building.	Increasing coping skills and learning new ones can help with current crisis and help minimize future crises.
Involve patient in identifying realistic, acceptable interventions.	The person's involvement in planning increases his or her sense of control, self-esteem, and compliance with plan.
Plan regular follow-up (e.g., phone calls, clinic visits, home visits) to assess patient's progress.	Plan is evaluated to see what works and what does not.

After talking with the nurse and the social worker, Madison seems open to going to a safe house for battered women. She also agrees to talk to a counselor at a mental health facility. The nurse sets up an appointment at which she, Madison, and the counselor will meet. The nurse will continue to see Madison twice a week. ■

Counseling

Primary Care

Psychotherapeutic crisis interventions are directed toward three levels of care: (1) primary, (2) secondary, and (3) tertiary. Primary care promotes mental health and reduces mental illness to decrease the incidence of crisis. On this level the nurse can:

- Work with a patient to recognize potential problems by evaluating the patient's experience of stressful life events.
- Teach the patient specific coping skills, such as decision making, problem solving, assertiveness skills, meditation, and relaxation skills.
- Assist the patient in evaluating the timing or reduction of life changes to decrease the negative effects of stress as much as possible. This may involve working with a patient to plan environmental changes, make important interpersonal decisions, and rethink changes in occupational roles.

Secondary Care

Secondary care establishes intervention during an acute crisis to *prevent* prolonged anxiety from diminishing personal effectiveness and personality organization. The nurse's primary focus is to ensure the safety of the patient. After safety issues are dealt with, the nurse works with the patient to assess the patient's problem, support systems, and coping styles. Desired goals are explored and interventions planned. Secondary care lessens the time a patient is mentally disabled during a crisis. Secondary-level care occurs in hospital units, emergency departments, clinics, or mental health centers, usually during daytime hours.

Tertiary Care

Tertiary care provides support for those who have experienced a severe crisis and are now recovering from a disabling mental state. Social and community facilities that offer tertiary intervention include rehabilitation centers, sheltered workshops, day hospitals, and outpatient clinics. Primary goals are to facilitate optimal levels of functioning and prevent further emotional disruptions. People with severe and persistent mental problems are often extremely susceptible to crisis, and community facilities provide the structured environment that can help prevent problem situations. Box 23-2 lists *Nursing Interventions Classification (NIC)* interventions for responding to a crisis (Bulechek et al., 2008).

Critical Incident Stress Debriefing. Critical incident stress debriefing (CISD) is an example of a tertiary intervention directed toward a group that has experienced a crisis (Everly et al., 2000). CISD consists of a seven-phase group meeting that offers individuals the opportunity to share their thoughts and feelings in a safe and controlled environment. It is used to debrief staff on an inpatient unit following a patient suicide or an incident of violence, to debrief crisis hotline

---

BOX 23-2 Crisis Intervention

Definition: Use of short-term counseling to help the patient cope with a crisis and resume a state of functioning comparable to or better than the pre-crisis state
Activities:

- Provide an atmosphere of support.
- Avoid giving false reassurances.
- Provide a safe haven.
- Determine whether the patient presents a safety risk to self or others.
- Initiate necessary precautions to safeguard the patient or others at risk for physical harm.
- Encourage expression of feelings in a nondestructive manner.
- Assist in identification of the precipitants and dynamics of the crisis.
- Encourage patient to focus on one implication at a time.
- Assist in identification of personal strengths and abilities that can be used in resolving the crisis.
- Assist in identification of past/present coping skills and their effectiveness.
- Assist in development of new coping and problem-solving skills, as needed.
- Assist in identification of available support systems.
- Link the patient and family with community resources, as needed.
- Provide guidance about how to develop and maintain support system(s).
- Introduce the patient to persons (or groups) who have successfully undergone the same experience.
- Assist in identification of alternative courses of action to resolve the crisis.
- Assist in evaluation of the possible consequences of the various courses of action.
- Assist the patient to decide on a particular course of action.
- Assist in formulating a time frame for implementation of the chosen course of action.
- Evaluate with the patient whether the crisis has been resolved by the chosen course of action.
- Plan with the patient how adaptive coping skills can be used to deal with crises in the future.

From Bulechek, G. M., Butcher, H. K., & Dochterman, J. M. (2008). *Nursing interventions classification (NIC)* (5th ed.). St. Louis: Mosby.

volunteers, to debrief schoolchildren and school personnel after multiple school shootings, and to debrief rescue and health care workers who have responded to a natural disaster or a terrorist attack such as that on the World Trade Center (Hammond & Brooks, 2001).

The phases of CISD are:

- *Introductory phase*—Meeting purpose is explained; an overview of the debriefing process is provided; confidentiality is assured; guidelines are explained; team members are identified; and questions are answered.
- *Fact phase*—Participants discuss the facts of the incident; participants introduce themselves, tell their involvement in the incident, and describe the event from their perspective.
- *Thought phase*—Participants discuss their first thoughts of the incident.
- *Reaction phase*—Participants talk about the worst thing about the incident—what they would like to forget, what was most painful.
- *Symptom phase*—Participants describe their cognitive, physical, emotional, or behavioral experiences at the incident scene and describe any symptoms they felt following the initial experience.
- *Teaching phase*—The normality of the expressed symptoms is acknowledged and affirmed; anticipatory guidance is offered regarding future symptoms; group is involved in stress-management techniques.
- *Reentry phase*—Participants review material discussed, introduce new topics, ask questions, and discuss how they would like to bring closure to the debriefing. Debriefing team members answer questions, inform, and reassure; provide written material; provide information on referral sources; and summarize the debriefing with encouragement, support, and appreciation.

VIGNETTE

The nurse performs secondary crisis intervention and meets with Madison twice weekly for 4 weeks. Madison is motivated to work with the social worker and the nurse to find another place to live. The nurse suggests several times that Madison start to see a counselor in the outpatient clinic after the crisis is over so that she can talk about some of her pain. Madison is ambivalent and is already thinking she will return to her husband. ■

EVALUATION

NOC includes a built-in measurement for each outcome and for the indicators that support the outcome. Each indicator is measured on a five-point Likert scale, which helps the nurse evaluate the effectiveness of the crisis intervention. This evaluation is usually performed 4 to 8 weeks after the initial interview, although it can be done earlier (e.g., by the end of the visit, the anxiety level will decrease from 1 = severe to 3 = moderate). If the intervention has been successful, the patient's level of anxiety and ability to function should be at pre-crisis levels. Often a patient chooses to follow up on additional areas of concern and is referred to other agencies for more long-term work. Crisis intervention frequently serves to prepare a patient for further treatment.

VIGNETTE

Madison returned to her husband 3 weeks after the battering episode. She has convinced herself that he has changed his behavior, despite the fact that he has not sought any help to control his anger.

After 6 weeks, Madison and the nurse decide that the crisis is over. Madison is aloof and distant. The nurse evaluates Madison as being in a moderate amount of emotional pain, but Madison feels she is doing well. The nurse's assessment indicates that Madison has other serious issues (e.g., low self-esteem, childhood abuse), and the nurse strongly suggests that she could benefit from further counseling. The decision, however, is up to Madison, who says she is satisfied with the way things are and again states that if she has any future problems, she will return to the safe house counselor. ■

Case Study and Nursing Care Plan 23-1   Crisis

Ms. Greg, the psychiatric clinical nurse specialist, is called to the neurological unit. She is told that Mr. Raymond, a 43-year-old man with Guillain-Barré syndrome, is presenting a serious nursing problem, and the staff has requested a consult. The disease has caused severe muscle weakness to the point that Mr. Raymond is essentially paralyzed; however, he is able to breathe on his own.

The nurse manager says that Mr. Raymond is hostile and sexually abusive, and his abusive language, demeaning

attitude, and angry outbursts are having an adverse effect on the unit as a whole. The staff nurses state that they feel ineffective and angry and have tried to be patient and understanding; however, nothing seems to get through to him. The situation has affected the morale of the staff and, the nurses believe, the quality of their care.

Mr. Raymond, a Native American, was employed as a taxicab driver. Six months before his hospital admission, he had given up drinking after years of episodic alcohol abuse.

His fiancée visits him every day. He needs a great deal of assistance with every aspect of his activities of daily living. Because of his severe muscle weakness, he has to be turned and positioned every 2 hours and fed through a gastrostomy tube.

ASSESSMENT

Ms. Greg gathers data from Mr. Raymond, the nursing staff, and Mr. Raymond's fiancée.

Perception of the Precipitating Event

During the initial interview, Mr. Raymond speaks to Ms. Greg angrily, using profanity and making lewd sexual suggestions. He also expresses anger about needing a nurse to "scratch my head and help me blow my nose." He still cannot figure out how his illness suddenly developed. He says the doctors told him that it was too early to know for sure if he would recover completely, but that the prognosis was good.

Support System

Ms. Greg speaks with Mr. Raymond's fiancée. Mr. Raymond's relationships with his fiancée and with his American Indian cultural group are strong. With minimal ties outside their reservation, neither Mr. Raymond nor his fiancée have much knowledge of supportive agencies.

Personal Coping Skills

Mr. Raymond comes from a strongly male-dominated subculture where the man is expected to be a strong leader. His ability to be an independent person with the power to affect the direction of his life is central to his perception of being acceptable as a man.

Mr. Raymond feels powerless, out of control, and enraged. He is handling his anxiety by displacing these feelings onto the environment, namely, the staff and his fiancée. This redirection of anger temporarily lowers his anxiety and distracts him from painful feelings. When he intimidates others, he feels temporarily in control and experiences an illusion of power. He uses displacement to relieve his painful levels of anxiety when he feels threatened.

Mr. Raymond's unconscious use of displacement is maladaptive, because the issues causing his distress are not being resolved. His anxiety continues to escalate. Furthermore, his behavior leads others to minimize interactions with him, which further increases his sense of isolation and helplessness.

Self-Assessment

Ms. Greg meets with the staff twice. The staff discuss feelings of helplessness and lack of control stemming from their feelings of rejection by Mr. Raymond. They talk of their anger about Mr. Raymond's demeaning behavior and frustration about the situation. Ms. Greg points out to the staff that Mr. Raymond's feelings of helplessness, lack of control, and anger at his situation are the same feelings the staff are experiencing. Displacement of his feelings of helplessness and frustration by intimidating the staff gives Mr. Raymond a brief feeling of control. It also distracts him from his own feelings of helplessness.

The nurses become more understanding of the motivation for the behavior Mr. Raymond employs to cope with moderate to severe levels of anxiety. The staff begins to focus more on the patient, less on personal reactions, and decide on two approaches they can try as a group. First, they will not take Mr. Raymond's behavior personally. Second, Mr. Raymond's displaced feelings will be refocused back to him.

On the basis of her assessment, Ms. Greg identifies three main problem areas of importance and formulates the following nursing diagnoses:

DIAGNOSIS

1. *Ineffective coping* related to inadequate coping methods, as evidenced by inappropriate use of defense mechanisms (displacement)

Supporting Data

- Anger directed toward staff and fiancée
- Profanity and crude sexual remarks aimed at staff
- Isolation related to staff withdrawal
- Continued escalation of anxiety

2. *Powerlessness* related to lack of control over his health care environment, as evidenced by frustration over inability to perform previously uncomplicated tasks

Continued

Supporting Data

- Anger over nurses' having to "scratch my head and blow my nose"
- Minimal awareness of available supports in larger community

3. *Ineffective coping* related to exhaustion of staff's supportive capacity toward patient, as evidenced by staff withdrawal and limited personal communication with patient

Supporting Data

- Staff feels ineffective.
- Morale of staff is poor.
- Nurses believe that the quality of their care has been adversely affected.

OUTCOMES IDENTIFICATION

Ms. Greg speaks to Mr. Raymond and tells him she would like to spend time with him for 15 minutes every morning to talk about his concerns. She suggests that he might be able to handle his feelings in alternative ways and notes that they can also explore community resources. Mr. Raymond gruffly agrees, saying, "You can visit me if it will make you feel better." They make arrangements to meet each morning at 7:30 AM for 15 minutes.

For each nursing diagnosis, the following outcomes are set:

Nursing Diagnosis	Short-Term Goal
1. *Ineffective coping* related to inadequate coping methods, as evidenced by inappropriate use of defense mechanisms (displacement)	1. Mr. Raymond will be able to name and discuss at least two feelings about his illness and lack of mobility by the end of the week.
2. *Powerlessness* related to lack of control over health care environment, as evidenced by frustration over inability to perform previously uncomplicated tasks	2. Mr. Raymond will be able to name two community organizations that can offer him information and support by the end of 2 weeks.
3. *Ineffective coping* related to exhaustion of staff supportive capacity toward patient, as evidenced by staff withdrawal and limited personal communication with patient	3. Staff and nurse consultant will discuss reactions and alternative nursing responses to Mr. Raymond's behavior twice within the next 7 days.

PLANNING

Ms. Greg creates a nursing care plan and shares it with the staff.

Nursing diagnosis: *Ineffective coping* related to inadequate coping methods, as evidenced by inappropriate use of defense mechanisms (displacement)

Outcome criteria: By discharge, Mr. Raymond will state that he feels more comfortable discussing difficult feelings.

Short-Term Goal	Intervention	Rationale	Evaluation
1. By the end of the week, Mr. Raymond will be able to name and discuss at least two feelings about his illness and lack of mobility.	1a. Nurse will meet with patient daily for 15 minutes at 7:30 AM.	1a. Night is usually the most frightening for patient; in early morning, feelings are closer to surface.	**GOAL MET** Within 7 days, Mr. Raymond speaks to nurse more openly about feelings.
	1b. When patient lashes out, nurse will remain calm.	1b. Patient perceives that nurse is in control of her feelings. This can reassure patient and increase patient's sense of security.	
	1c. Nurse will consistently redirect and refocus anger from environment back to patient (e.g., "It must be difficult to be in this situation").	1c. Refocusing feelings offers patient opportunity to cope effectively with his anxiety and decreases need to act out.	
	1d. Nurse will come on time each day and stay for allotted time.	1d. Consistency sets stage for trust and reinforces that patient's anger will not drive nurse away.	

Nursing diagnosis: *Powerlessness* related to lack of control over health care environment, as evidenced by frustration over inability to perform previously uncomplicated tasks

Outcome criteria: By discharge, Mr. Raymond will contact at least one community support source.

Short-Term Goal	Intervention	Rationale	Evaluation
1. By the end of the 2 weeks, Mr. Raymond will name and discuss at least two community organizations that can offer information and support.	1a. Nurse will spend time with patient and fiancée. Role and use of specific agencies will be discussed. 1b. Nurse will introduce one agency at a time. 1c. Nurse will not push patient to contact any of the agencies.	1a. Both patient and fiancée will have opportunity to ask questions with nurse present. 1b. Gradual introduction allows time for information to sink in and minimizes feeling of being pressured or overwhelmed. 1c. Patient is able to make own decisions once he has appropriate information.	**GOAL MET** By the end of 10 days, Mr. Raymond and his fiancée can name two community resources they are interested in. At the end of 6 weeks, Mr. Raymond has contacted the Guillain-Barré Society.

IMPLEMENTATION

Ms. Greg goes into Mr. Raymond's room at 7:30 AM the following morning and sits by his bedside. At first, Mr. Raymond's comments are hostile.

Dialogue	Therapeutic Tool/Comment
Nurse: Mr. Raymond, I'm here as we discussed. I'll be spending 15 minutes with you every morning. We could use this time to talk about some of your concerns.	Nurse offers herself as a resource, gives information, and clarifies her role and patient expectations. Night is Mr. Raymond's most difficult time. In the early morning, he will be the most vulnerable and open for therapeutic intervention and support.
Mr. Raymond: Listen, sweetheart, my only concern is how to get a little sexual relief, get it?	
Nurse: Being hospitalized and partially paralyzed can be overwhelming for anyone. Perhaps you wish you could find some relief from your situation.	Nurse focuses on the process "need for relief," not the sexual content, and encourages discussion of feelings. Sexual issues often challenge new nurses, and discussing their feelings and appropriate interventions with an experienced professional is important for their growth and the quality of the care they give.
Mr. Raymond: What do you know, Ms. Know-it-all? I can't even scratch my nose without getting one of those fools to do it for me … and half the time those bitches aren't even around.	
Nurse: It must be difficult to have to ask people to do everything for you.	Nurse restates what the patient says in terms of his feelings and continues to refocus away from the environment back to the patient.
Mr. Raymond: Yeah …. The other night a fly kept landing on my face. I had to shout for 5 minutes before one of those bitches came in, just to take the fly out of the room.	
Nurse: Having to rely on others for everything can be a terrifying experience for anyone. It sounds extremely frustrating for you.	Nurse acknowledges that frustration and anger would be a natural response for anyone in this situation. This encourages the patient to talk about these feelings instead of acting them out.

Continued

Dialogue	Therapeutic Tool/Comment
Mr. Raymond: Yeah …. It's a bitch … like a living hell.	

Ms. Greg continues to spend time with Mr. Raymond. He gradually talks more about his feelings and acts with less hostility toward the staff. As he begins to feel more in control, he becomes less defensive about others' caring for him. After 2 weeks, Ms. Greg decreases her visits to twice a week. Mr. Raymond is beginning to experience gross motor movements but is not walking yet. He still displaces much of his frustration and lack of control onto the environment, but he is better able to acknowledge the reality of his situation. He can also identify and briefly talk about his feelings.

Dialogue	Therapeutic Tool/Comment
Nurse: What's happening? Your face looks tense this morning, Mr. Raymond.	Nurse observes the patient's clenched fists, rigid posture, and tense facial expression.
Mr. Raymond: I had to wait 10 minutes for a bedpan last night.	
Nurse: And you're angry about that.	Nurse verbalizes the implied.
Mr. Raymond: Well, there were only two nurses on duty for 30 people, and the aide was on her break…. You can't expect them to be everywhere … but still ….	
Nurse: It may be hard to accept that people can't be there all the time for you.	Nurse validates the difficulty of accepting situations one does not like when one is powerless to make changes.
Mr. Raymond: Well … that's the way it is in this place.	

EVALUATION

After 6 weeks, Mr. Raymond is able to get around with assistance, and his ability to perform his activities of daily living is increasing. Although Mr. Raymond still feels angry and overwhelmed at times, he is able to identify more of his feelings and acts them out less often. He is able to talk to his fiancée about his feelings, and he lashes out at her less. He is looking forward to going home, and his boss is holding his old job.

Mr. Raymond makes arrangements with the Guillain-Barré Society for a meeting, and he is thinking about Alcoholics Anonymous but believes he can handle this problem himself.

Staff feel more comfortable and competent in their relationships with Mr. Raymond. The goals have been met. Mr. Raymond and Ms. Greg agree that the crisis is over and terminate their visits. Mr. Raymond is given the number of the crisis unit and encouraged to call if he has questions or feels the need to talk.

KEY POINTS TO REMEMBER

- A crisis is not a pathological state but a struggle for emotional balance.
- Crises offer opportunities for emotional growth but can also lead to personality disorganization.
- There are three types of crisis: maturational, situational, and adventitious.
- Crises are usually resolved within 4 to 6 weeks.
- Crisis intervention therapy is short term, from 1 to 6 weeks, and focuses on the present problem only.
- Resolution of a crisis takes three forms: a patient emerges at a higher level, at the pre-crisis level, or at a lower level of functioning.
- Social support and intervention can promote successful resolution.
- Crisis therapists take an active and directive approach with the patient in crisis.
- The patient is an active participant in setting goals and planning possible solutions.
- Crisis intervention is usually aimed at the mentally healthy patient who generally is functioning well but is temporarily overwhelmed and unable to function.
- The crisis model can be adapted to meet the needs of patients in crisis who have long-term and persistent mental problems.
- The steps in crisis intervention are consistent with the steps of the nursing process.

- Specific qualities in the nurse that can facilitate effective intervention are a caring attitude, flexibility in planning care, an ability to listen, and an active approach.
- The basic goals of crisis intervention are to reduce the individual's anxiety level and to support the effort to return to the patient's pre-crisis level of functioning.
- Critical incident stress debriefing is a group approach that helps groups of people who have been exposed to a crisis situation.

CRITICAL THINKING

1. List the three important areas of the crisis assessment once safety concerns have been identified. Give examples of two questions in each area that need to be answered before planning can take place.
2. Samantha, a 21-year-old junior in nursing school, tells her nursing instructor that her father (age 45 years) has just lost his job. Her father has been drinking heavily for years, and Samantha is having difficulty coping. Because of her father's alcoholism and the increased stress in her family, Samantha wants to leave school. Her mother has multiple sclerosis and thinks Samantha should quit school to take care of her.
   A. How many different types of crisis are going on in this family? Discuss each crisis from the viewpoint of each individual family member.
   B. If you were providing crisis counseling for this family, what areas would you assess? What kinds of questions would you ask to evaluate each member's individual needs and the needs of the family as a unit (perception of events, social supports, coping styles)?
   C. Formulate some tentative goals you might set in conjunction with the family.
   D. Identify specific referral agencies in your area that would be helpful if members of this family were willing to expand their use of outside resources and stabilize the situation.
   E. How would you set up follow-up visits for this family? Would you see the family members together, alone, or in combination during the crisis period (4 to 6 weeks)? How would you decide whether follow-up counseling was indicated?

CHAPTER REVIEW

1. John had a psychotic episode when he was 15 years old. He did not respond well to treatments available at the time and continued to have a significant number of residual symptoms. At the age of 42, he began taking Clozaril (clozapine), which significantly reduced his remaining symptoms, allowing him to leave his group home and live independently for the first time. However, once he was doing better and living in his own apartment, he was unsure of what to do with his time, what he wanted to be, how to go about getting a job, and how to meet his needs

for romantic companionship appropriately. What type of crisis situation is represented by this case?
   1. Maturational crisis
   2. Situational crisis
   3. Adventitious crisis
   4. Phase 4 crisis

2. Mr. James witnessed a car suddenly careen out of control and onto the sidewalk where he and his best friend were walking. Mr. James's friend pushed him out of the way at the last second but was struck and killed instantly. Mr. James was treated for minor injuries and released but was referred for mental health evaluation because he was very distraught over the death of his friend. Which response should be used *first* during your assessment of Mr. James?
   1. "Tell me about what happened that day."
   2. "What would you like to accomplish during your treatment?"
   3. "Do you think you are coping well with this very tragic event?"
   4. "Tell me what has been going through your mind since the accident."

3. Mr. James confides that he feels so guilty that his friend died while pushing him to safety that he has found himself having impulses to kill himself by crashing his car. He says he almost did so yesterday when his guilt suddenly became overwhelming. Which intervention would be most therapeutic?
   1. Admit Mr. James to an inpatient mental health unit to assure his safety until his condition can improve.
   2. Work with Mr. James's family to ensure that he does not have access to a car, and set up emergency counseling sessions.
   3. Persuade Mr. James to agree to remain safe pending counseling, as admitting him would only further traumatize him.
   4. Consult with a prescribing physician or APRN so that Mr. James can be started immediately on antianxiety and antidepressant medications.

4. Sherie Johnson, a mother of two teenagers and veteran nurse with 15 years of experience in the crisis center, fails to show up for work several days in a row not long after providing crisis intervention to area high school students following a shooting at their school. Coworkers complain that she is not taking her share of crisis calls. As Sherie's manager, you attempt to address the issue, but she responds irritably and denies than anything is wrong. Sherie most likely:
   1. is becoming burned out on crisis work.
   2. is experiencing vicarious traumatization.
   3. has developed a hidden substance abuse problem.
   4. has lost her objectivity, owing to having children of her own.

5. A patient experiences a crisis after witnessing the brutal assault of her friend during a robbery on the way to their cars after work. Which outcome for the patient exposed to this highly traumatic event is the most appropriate?
    1. The patient reports greater satisfaction with her life within 2 months.
    2. The patient attends all treatment sessions specified in her treatment plan.
    3. Within 3 weeks, the patient reports that she no longer feels distressed.
    4. The patient returns to her pre-crisis level of functioning within 2 weeks.

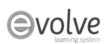

Visit the Evolve website for an **Audio Chapter Summary, Chapter Review Answers & Rationales, Critical Thinking Answer Guidelines**, and additional resources related to the content in this chapter: **http://evolve.elsevier.com/Varcarolis/foundations**

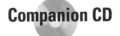

Companion CD Use the Companion CD to prepare for tests and the NCLEX® Examination with **Test-Taking Strategies** for psychiatric mental health nursing and hundreds of **Review Questions**.

References

Aguilera, D. C. (1998). *Crisis intervention: Theory and methodology* (8th ed.). St. Louis: Mosby.

Aguilera, D. C., & Mesnick, J. (1970). *Crisis intervention: Theory and methodology*. St. Louis: Mosby.

American Nurses Association, American Psychiatric Nurses Association, and International Society of Psychiatric-Mental Health Nurses. (2007). *Scope and standards of psychiatric-mental health nursing practice*. Washington, DC: American Nurses Publishing.

Behrman, G., & Reid, W. J. (2002). Post-trauma intervention: Basic tasks. *Brief Treatment and Crisis Intervention, 2,* 39–48.

Bulechek, G. M., Butcher, H. K., & Dochterman, J. M. (2008). *Nursing interventions classification (NIC)* (5th ed.). St. Louis: Mosby.

Caplan, G. (1964). *Symptoms of preventive psychiatry*. New York: Basic Books.

Dunkley, J., & Whelan, T. (2006). Vicarious traumatisation: Current status and future directions. *British Journal of Guidance and Counselling, 34*(1), 107–116.

Everly, G. S., Jr., Lating, J. M., & Mitchell, J. T. (2000). Innovations in group crisis intervention: Critical incident stress debriefing (CISD) and critical incident stress management (CISM). In A. R. Roberts (Ed.), *Crisis interventions handbook: Assessment, treatment, and research* (2nd ed., pp. 77–100). New York: Oxford University Press.

Hammond, J., & Brooks, J. (2001). The world trade center attack. Helping the helpers: The role of critical incident stress management. *Critical Care, 5,* 315–317.

Hobfoll, S., Watson, P., Bell, C., Bryant, R., Brymer, M., Friedman, M. J., et al. (2007). Five essential elements of immediate and mid-trauma mass trauma intervention: Empirical evidence. *Psychiatry, 70,* 283–315.

Moorhead, S., Johnson, M., Maas, M., & Swanson, E. (2008). *Nursing outcomes classification (NOC)* (4th ed.). St. Louis: Mosby.

North American Nursing Diagnosis Association International (NANDA-I). (2009). *NANDA-I nursing diagnoses: Definitions and classification 2009-2011*. Oxford, United Kingdom: Author.

Parad, H. J., & Caplan, G. (1965). Framework for studying families in crisis. In H. J. Parad (Ed.), *Crisis intervention: Selected readings* (pp. 53–72). New York: Family Service Association of America.

Phoenix, B. (2007). Psychoeducation for survivors of trauma. *Perspectives of Psychiatric Care, 43,* 123–131.

Roberts, A. R. (2005). *Crisis intervention handbook: Assessment, treatment, and research* (3rd ed.). New York: Oxford.

Roberts, A. R., & Ottens, A. J. (2005). The seven-stage crisis intervention model: A road map to goal attainment, problem solving, and crisis resolution. *Brief Treatment and Crisis Intervention, 5,* 329–339.

Saunders, J. M. (2007). Vulnerable populations in an American Red Cross shelter after Hurricane Katrina. *Perspectives in Psychiatric Care, 43*(1), 30–37.

Wallace, M. A., & Morley, W. E. (1970). Teaching crisis intervention. *American Journal of Nursing, 70,* 1484–1487.

CHAPTER **24**

Suicide

M. Selena Yearwood and Nancy Christine Shoemaker

Key Terms and Concepts

completed suicides, 548
copycat suicide, 551
lethality, 553
no-suicide contract, 558
parasuicide, 552
postvention, 556
primary intervention, 556

psychological autopsies, 549
SAD PERSONS scale, 553
secondary intervention, 556
suicidal ideation, 552
suicide, 548
suicide attempt, 552
tertiary intervention, 556

Objectives

1. Describe the profile of suicide in the United States, noting psychosocial and cultural factors that affect risk.
2. Identify three common precipitating events.
3. Describe risk factors for suicide, including coexisting psychiatric disorders.
4. Name the most frequent coexisting psychiatric disorders.
5. Use the SAD PERSONS scale to assess suicide risk.
6. Describe three expected reactions a nurse may have when beginning work with suicidal patients.
7. Give examples of primary, secondary, and tertiary (postvention) interventions.
8. Describe basic-level interventions that take place in the hospital or community.
9. Identify key elements of suicide precautions and environmental safety factors in the hospital.

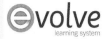 Visit the Evolve website for an **Audio Glossary & Flashcards, Concept Map Creator**, and additional resources related to the content in this chapter: **http://evolve.elsevier.com/Varcarolis/foundations**

Don't grieve for me, for now I'm free,
I'm following the path that God laid for me.
I took his hand when I heard him call,
I turned away, and left it all.

Tasks left undone must stay that way,
I've found true peace at the close of day.
If parting now has left a void,
then fill it with remembered joy.

Perhaps my time seemed all too brief,
don't lengthen it now with undue grief.
Lift up your hearts and remember me,
God wants me now, he set me free.

– From a suicide note

Sadly, it is the rare individual who has yet to encounter, directly or indirectly, the significant public health problem that is suicide. Approximately every 16 minutes, a human life ends as the result of suicide (McIntosh, 2006). Nursing students and practicing nurses at all levels encounter individuals suffering from the pain and hopelessness that all too frequently culminates in the act of parasuicide (nonfatal self-injury with a clear intent to cause bodily harm or death), suicide attempt, or completed suicide. These individuals can be identified in inpatient settings, outpatient treatment settings, and in the community. Studies show that one in five suicide victims had contact with mental health services during the month prior to their death, and 45% had contact with a primary care provider during this same period of time (Ortiz, 2006).

Nurses at the primary, secondary, and tertiary levels of intervention can play a crucial role in the care of these patients, their families, and the survivors of suicide (family and friends of a person who has committed suicide). Suicide is often a permanent solution to a temporary problem and is largely preventable; yet all too often, efforts are only directed towards individuals who are at immediate risk. It is critical for the health care community to become advocates for this problem and begin to mobilize the community in reducing and preventing factors that may contribute to suicide (Ortiz, 2006). This chapter reviews the facts about suicide and discusses approaches for assessment and care of suicidal patients and their loved ones.

EPIDEMIOLOGY

In the United States, suicide is the 11th leading cause of death—32,000 people kill themselves each year (Centers for Disease Control [CDC], 2008). Even when people survive suicide attempts, the results are often catastrophic and contribute to 395,000 annual visits to the emergency room. Consider the young man with schizophrenia who is so depressed and confused from his illness, he takes an overdose and kneels down in front of his couch to pray for forgiveness as he dies. His father finds him lifeless. The young man lives, but being in a kneeling position for so long cut off the circulation to his legs, necessitated their amputation, and led to lifelong disability.

It is important to consider that the number of suicides may actually be double or triple the reported statistics due to underreporting in general. Purposefully aiming the car at a bridge abutment and crashing may look like an accident. But in fact, many reported accidents, homicides, and deaths ruled as "undetermined" are actually suicides. In a study on war veterans, the rate of significant depressive symptoms was 31% higher than that of the general population. At highest risk for completed suicide was young veterans also diagnosed with post-traumatic stress disorder (PTSD) and substance abuse (Zivin et al., 2007). Box 24-1 provides some facts about suicide, including data for specific age groups.

Risk Factors

Suicide is not a psychiatric disorder per se; rather, it is the manifestation of inner pain, hopeless, and helplessness suffered by persons experiencing *Suicidal ideation*. Psychiatric disorders accompany 90% of completed suicides (Brendel et al., 2008). The percentage of completed suicides attributable to specific psychiatric disorders is listed in Table 24-1.

It is estimated that two thirds of people who commit suicide are experiencing depression at the time. About 15% of patients who have major depression or bipolar disorder (during the depressed phase) will commit suicide (Brendel et al., 2008). Loss of relationships, financial difficulty, and impulsivity are factors in this population.

Suicide risk is 50 times higher among patients with schizophrenia than the general population, especially during the first few years of the illness. It is the number-one leading cause of early death in this population. About 40% of all patients with schizophrenia attempt suicide at least once; males have a rate of 60%. Up to 10% of these patients die from suicide, usually related to depressive symptoms rather than to command hallucinations or delusions.

Patients with alcohol or substance use disorders also have a higher suicide risk. Years of abuse and comorbidity with depression or antisocial personality disorder are also factors associated with increased risk. Up to 15% of alcohol/substance abusers commit suicide (Sadock & Sadock, 2008).

Keep in mind that suicide is not necessarily synonymous with a mental disorder. The act of purposeful self-destruction represented by taking one's own life is usually accompanied by intensely conflicted feelings of pain, hopelessness, guilt, and self-loathing, coupled with the belief that there are no solutions, and things will not improve.

People who survive serious suicide attempts often report that it is these feelings that fuel the sense of isolation and despair. They describe an all-consuming psychic pain that shuts out thoughts of the loved ones and heartache they will leave behind. To understand this phenomenon, imagine the pain of your hand on a hot stove burner. At that moment, you are unlikely to think of anything but putting an immediate end to the pain. Emotional pain can render the individual void of thought and without even enough motivation to leave a suicide note; only about 30% of suicide victims leave a note (Koehler, 2007).

Besides psychiatric disorders, other risk factors for suicide include (Sadock & Sadock, 2008):

- *Male gender.* Men commit suicide four times more often than women.
- *Increasing age.* For men, suicide rates peak after the age of 45; for women, rates peak after 55.
- *Race.* White males commit two out of every three suicides in the United States.
- *Religion.* Religiosity is associated with decreased rates of suicide. Protestants and Jews have higher rates of suicide than Roman Catholics.
- *Marriage.* Being married, especially with children in the home, significantly reduces the risk of suicide. Divorced men are more likely than divorced women to kill themselves.
- *Profession.* Professionals are generally considered at higher risk for suicide, particularly if there is a fall in status. Law enforcement personnel, dentists, artists, mechanics, insurance agents, and lawyers are also at higher risk.

BOX 24-1 Suicide Facts

General

- Suicide is the 11th leading cause of death for all ages.
- Suicide accounts for 1.3% of all deaths in the United States.
- More than 32,000 suicides occur annually. This is the equivalent of 89 suicides per day; one suicide every 16 minutes, or 11.01 suicides per 100,000 population.
- The National Violent Death Reporting System examined toxicology tests of those who committed suicide in 13 states: 33.3% tested positive for alcohol; 16.4% for opiates; 9.4% for cocaine; 7.7% for marijuana; and 3.9% for amphetamines.

Gender Statistics

- Males take their own lives at nearly four times the rate of females and represent 79.4% of all U.S. suicides.
- During their lifetime, women attempt suicide about two to three times more often than men.
- Suicide is the 8th leading cause of death for males and the 17th leading cause for females.
- Among males, adults aged 75 years and older have the highest rate of suicide (nearly 38 per 100,000 population).
- Among females, those in their 40s and 50s have the highest rate of suicide (nearly 8 per 100,000 population).
- Firearms are the most commonly used method of suicide among males (approximately 58%).
- Poisoning is the most common method of suicide for females (39%).

Racial and Ethnic Statistics

- Among American Indians/Alaska Natives aged 15 to 34 years, suicide is the second leading cause of death.
- Suicide rates among American Indian/Alaskan Native adolescents and young adults aged 15 to 34 (21.7 per 100,000) are 2.2 times higher than the national average for that age group (10 per 100,000).
- Hispanic female high-school students in grades 9 to 12 reported a higher percentage of suicide attempts (14%) than their White, non-Hispanic (7.7%) or Black, non-Hispanic (9.9%) counterparts.

Age Statistics

- In 2007, 14.5% of U.S. high school students reported that they had seriously considered attempting suicide during the 12 months preceding the survey. More than 6.9% of students reported that they had actually attempted suicide one or more times during the same period.
- Suicide is the third leading cause of death among 15- to 24-year-olds (one suicide for every 100 to 200 attempts).
- Suicide is the second leading cause of death among 25- to 34-year-olds, accounting for 12.3% of all deaths in this age group annually.
- Among adults aged 65 years and older, there is one suicide for every four suicide attempts and a rate of 14.7 suicides per 100,000 people.

Attempted Suicide

- In 2005, 372,722 people were treated in emergency departments for self-inflicted injuries.
- In 2006, 162,359 people were hospitalized due to self-inflicted injury.
- There is one suicide for every 25 attempted suicides.

Data from Centers for Disease Control and Prevention. (2008, Summer). *Suicide facts at a glance.* Retrieved April 6, 2009 from http://www.cdc.gov/ncipc/dvp/Suicide/suicide_data_sheet.pdf

---

TABLE 24-1 Percentage of Suicides Attributable to Psychiatric Disorders

Disorders	Percentage
Affective illnesses (major depression and bipolar disorder)	50
Drug or alcohol abuse	25
Schizophrenia	10
Personality disorders	5

From Brendel, R. W., Lagomasino, I. T., Perlis, R. H., & Stern, T. A. (2008). The suicidal patient. In T. A. Stern, J. R. Rosenbaum, M. Fava, J. Biederman, & S. L. Rauch (Eds.), *Massachusetts General Hospital comprehensive clinical psychiatry* (pp. 733–745). St. Louis: Mosby.

- *Physical Health.* About half the people who commit suicide have physical illnesses. Loss of mobility, disfigurement, and chronic pain are especially associated with suicide.

Suicidal individuals are often ambivalent about death, and therein lies the key to helping them examine alternative actions to reduce their pain. Extensive data are available about risk factors for suicide, based on epidemiological studies and **psychological autopsies** (i.e., retrospective reviews of the deceased person's life within several months of death to establish likely diagnoses at the time of death). There is also evidence concerning protective factors (those that tend to reduce risk). Refer to Box 24-2 for a description of significant psychosocial risk and protective factors for suicide.

BOX 24-2 Suicide Risk Factors and Protective Factors

Risk Factors
- Suicidal ideation with intent
- Lethal suicide plan
- History of suicide attempt
- Co-occurring psychiatric illness
- Co-occurring medical illness
- History of childhood abuse
- Family history of suicide
- Recent lack of social support (isolation)
- Unemployment
- Recent stressful life event (e.g., death, other loss)
- Hopelessness
- Panic attacks
- Feeling of shame or humiliation
- Impulsivity
- Aggressiveness
- Loss of cognitive function (e.g., loss of impulse control)
- Access to firearms and other highly lethal means
- Substance abuse (without formal disorder)
- Impending incarceration
- Low frustration tolerance
- Sexual orientation issues

Protective Factors
- Sense of responsibility to family (spouse, children)
- Pregnancy
- Religious beliefs
- Satisfaction with life
- Positive social support
- Access to health care
- Effective coping skills
- Effective problem-solving skills
- Intact reality testing

Data from American Psychiatric Association. (2003). Practice guidelines for the assessment and treatment of patients with suicidal behaviors. *American Journal of Psychiatry, 160* (11 Suppl.), 12.

EVIDENCE-BASED PRACTICE

Suicide as Occupational Hazard: Nurses and Doctors at Risk

Agerbo, E., Gunnell, D., Bonde, J. P., Mortensen, P., & Nordentoft, M. (2007). Suicide and occupation: The impact of socioeconomic, demographic and psychiatric differences. *Psychological Medicine, 37*(8), 1131–1140.

Problem
Possessing suicide risk factors increases the possibility that a person will commit suicide. Certain occupations are associated with higher suicide rate; understanding the characteristics of people who may attempt suicide is important in planning preventive interventions.

Purpose of Study
Researchers wanted to know more about which occupations were associated with increased risk of suicide. This study examined the roles of work, social and economic considerations, and psychiatric conditions in the occurrence of suicide.

Methods
The researchers reviewed routine records from 3,195 people who committed suicide and 63,900 people who died from causes other than suicide. They compiled information related to cause of death, occupation, psychiatric admissions, marital status, and socioeconomic status.

Key Findings
- Suicide risk is high among physicians, architects, and engineers.
- Suicide risk is low in primary school teachers.
- Social and economic characteristics of people are the primary explanation for the increased risk.
- Physicians and nurses both have high rates of suicide; increased risk may be due to use of self-poisoning (overdose or lethal medication), a method they know how to use effectively.
- For people with a psychiatric illness, occupation has little to do with risk, except for physicians.

Implications for Nursing Practice
Assessing patients for suicide risk should be completed no matter the occupation or socioeconomic status. Knowing that professionals are at increased risk may counter stereotypes of suicide being committed by people who have little to lose. Especially important is considering that our peers—nurses and doctors—may be in need of closer scrutiny for suicide prevention than we may imagine. Asking the tough questions about suicidal ideation supersedes the boundaries of "professional courtesy."

ETIOLOGY

Biological Factors

Suicidal behavior tends to run in families (Sadock & Sadock, 2008). Margaux Hemingway's death in 1996 was the fifth suicide among four generations of writer Ernest Hemingway's (1899-1961) family. Yet it is difficult to distinguish biochemical or genetic predisposition to suicide from predisposition to depression or alcoholism. Twin and adoption studies suggest the presence of genetic factors in suicide. Suicide rates in twins are higher among monozygotic (identical) twins than among dizygotic (fraternal) twins. Studies found a significantly higher incidence of suicide among biological relatives of adoptees who committed suicide than among the biological relatives of control subjects.

Low serotonin levels are related to depressed mood. Studies have found low levels of serotonin or its metabolites in the cerebrospinal fluid of suicidal patients (Brendel et al., 2008). Postmortem exams of suicide victims also reveal a low level of serotonin in the brainstem or the frontal cortex.

Psychosocial Factors

Sigmund Freud originally theorized that suicide resulted from unacceptable aggression toward another person that is turned inward. Karl Menninger added to Freud's thought by describing three parts of suicidal hostility: the wish to kill, the wish to be killed, and the wish to die (Sadock & Sadock, 2008). Aaron Beck identified a central emotional factor underlying suicide intent: hopelessness. Certain cognitive styles that contribute to higher risk are rigid all-or-nothing thinking, inability to see different options, and perfectionism (APA, 2003).

Recent theories of suicide have focused on the lethal combination of suicidal fantasies accompanied by loss (love, self-esteem, job, and freedom due to imminent incarceration), rage or guilt, and identification with a suicide victim (copycat suicide). A *copycat suicide* follows a highly publicized suicide of a public figure, an idol, or a peer in the community. Adolescents are at especially high risk, owing to their immature prefrontal cortex, the portion of the brain that controls the executive functions involving judgment, frustration tolerance, and impulse control.

Cultural Factors

Cultural factors, including religious beliefs, family values, and attitude toward death, have an impact on suicide rates. In the United States, whites have the highest number of deaths by suicide. Groups with the highest rate of suicide are American Indians and Alaskan Natives, about 16 per 100,000; and white Americans, about 13 per 100,000 (Karch et al., 2008).

Among African Americans, men commit suicide more often than women, and the peak rate occurs in adolescence and young adulthood. Protective factors for this group as a whole include religion and the role of the extended family, both of which provide a strong social support system. Similarly, among Hispanic Americans, Roman Catholic religion (in which suicide is a sin) and the importance given to the extended family decrease the risk for suicide (Considering Culture box). There is also the philosophy of *fatalismo*, a belief that divine providence regulates the world—the individual is deemed unable to control adverse events and is more likely to accept misfortune instead of blaming the self.

CONSIDERING CULTURE

Cultural and Familial Factors: Suicidal Ideation among Latino Youths

Suicidal ideation, plans, and behaviors are higher for both sexes of Latino youth (Centers for Disease Control and Prevention, 2006). Psychological profiles of suicidal Latina adolescent females show that a unique situation involving cultural and familial factors is frequently associated with suicidal behaviors. In Hispanic cultures, *familismo* has been defined as the value that places the family as the primary unit, as opposed to the Western tradition that places the individual at the core. Adulthood is primarily defined as the socialization processes that prepare the adolescent for

parenthood, in contrast to the Western focus on occupational roles. Unique pressure is exerted on adolescent females to maintain the family unit, both nuclear and extended, and promote harmony in family relationships. Suicidal behaviors are often an impulsive and sudden means to escape stressful situations, usually related to arguments and conflicts with family members, most notably spouses and mothers. Cultural traditions that socialize women to maintain closeness and family obligations while limiting the expression of anger may result in increased suicidal behaviors.

Centers for Disease Control and Prevention. (2006). Youth risk behavior surveillance—United States, 2005. *Morbidity and Mortality Weekly Report, 55*, SS-5.

U.S. Department of Health & Human Services, Substance Abuse and Mental Health Services Administration. (2001). *Summary of findings from the 2000 National Household Survey of Drug Abuse.* Office of Applied Studies, NHSDA Series H-13, DHHS Publication No. (SMA) 01-3549. Rockville, MD: Author.

Zayas, L. H., & Pilat, A. M. (2008). Suicidal behavior in Latinas: Explanatory cultural factors and implications for intervention. *The American Association of Suicidology, 38*(3), 334–342.

Among Asian Americans, suicide rates are noted to increase with age. Beliefs that reduce suicide include adherence to religions that tend to emphasize interdependence between the individual and society (i.e., self-destruction is seen as disrespectful to the group or selfish). However, the high value given to the reputation of the family may lead at times to the conclusion that suicide is preferable if it prevents shame to the family. A belief in reincarnation may make death a potential honorable solution to life problems.

A different sort of suicide exists in some cultures. Suicide bombing has grown exponentially in recent years, most recently in the Middle East. While not condoned by Islam, suicide bombers may believe that it is an honor to die in defense of their faith, that real happiness exists beyond this life, and that for martyrs, dying is not real death but a ticket straight to heaven.

Societal Factors

No discussion about current societal attitudes and trends would be complete without an examination of the way in which suicide is viewed in a general context. In the United States, Oregon's Death with Dignity Act of 1994 legally allowed terminally ill patients a physician-assisted suicide. The patient must be thoroughly screened by a physician and deemed to be both terminally ill and psychiatrically sound. However, concern has been raised that as many as 25% of the patients in Oregon who have been assisted to die actually have clinical depression (Ganzini & Dobscha, 2008). The Netherlands allows for this practice in nonterminal cases of "lasting and unbearable" suffering (Appel, 2007). Belgium authorizes physician-assisted suicide for nonterminal cases when suffering is deemed to be "constant and cannot be alleviated." And no country has laws as liberal as Switzerland, in which assisted suicide has been legal since 1918 and allows nonresidents to terminate their lives without a physician involved in the process (Appel, 2007).

The ethical and moral dilemmas in this evolving trend are clear. There are now debates about whether chronic and serious mental illness is no different in the depth and breadth of suffering than chronic and serious physical illness (Appel, 2007). Until more effective treatment or a cure is found, some individuals who obtain little or no benefit from existing psychiatric treatments may choose to end suffering. At the core of the argument supporting assisted suicide are the twin goals of minimizing human suffering and maximizing individual autonomy.

APPLICATION OF THE NURSING PROCESS

The process of suicide risk assessment is comprehensive and based on identifying specific risk factors, taking a psychosocial and medical history, and interacting with the patient during the interview. The nurse usually completes this assessment in conjunction with other clinicians, since comparison of data from two interviewers is often a significant element of the evaluation.

Not all patients who show **suicidal ideation** or who make a **suicide attempt** truly want to die. **Parasuicide** is a self-injury that appears to have clear intent to cause bodily harm or death. Parasuicide is a risk factor for suicide—about half of all people who kill themselves have a history of parasuicide. Especially prevalent in the adolescent and young adult populations, self-injury (usually in the form of cutting) is most often done with the intent to either alleviate psychic pain or to pierce the psychic numbness these individuals describe (Cleaver, 2007). They do not engage in this type of behavior as a means of seeking attention and will often go to great lengths to conceal the evidence. Parasuicide often carries a lethal risk of death or permanent injury.

Nonacute suicidal or self-destructive thoughts and feelings can be treated in the outpatient setting. Alternate services available to suicidal patients include crisis intervention and assertive community treatment (ACT), addiction treatment, social services, and legal assistance. These types of interventions are evidence-based and cost effective, as well as individualized and realistic—all essential aspects of the person-centered recovery model (ANA [American Nurses Association] et al., 2007).

ASSESSMENT
Verbal and Nonverbal Clues

Almost all people considering suicide send out clues, especially to people they think of as supportive. Nurses often fit into this category. There may be overt or covert verbal clues and nonverbal signals. Examples include:
Overt statements
- "I can't take it anymore."
- "Life isn't worth living anymore."
- "I wish I were dead."
- "Everyone would be better off if I died."

Covert statements
- "It's okay now. Soon everything will be fine."
- "Things will never work out."
- "I won't be a problem much longer."

- "Nothing feels good to me anymore and probably never will."
- "How can I give my body to medical science?"

Most often it is a relief for people contemplating suicide to finally talk to someone about their despair and loneliness. Asking about suicidal thoughts does not "give a person ideas" and is, in fact, a professional responsibility similar to asking about chest pain in cardiac conditions. Talking openly leads to a decrease in isolation and can increase problem-solving alternatives for living. People who contemplate suicide, attempt suicide, and even those who regret the failure of their attempt, are often extremely receptive to talking about their suicide crisis. Specific questions to ask about suicidal ideation include the following (APA, 2003):

- Have you ever felt that life was not worth living?
- Have you been thinking about death recently?
- Did you ever think about suicide?
- Have you ever attempted suicide?
- Do you have a plan for committing suicide?
- If so, what is your plan for suicide?

The following dialogue illustrates how the nurse can make covert messages more open:

Nurse: You haven't eaten or slept well for the past few days, Mary.

Mary: No, I feel pretty low lately.

Nurse: How low are you feeling?

Mary: Oh, I don't know. Nothing seems to matter to me anymore. It's all so meaningless ….

Nurse: Tell me about it, Mary. I want to understand how you're feeling. What is meaningless?

Mary: Life … the whole thing … nothingness. Life is a bad joke.

Nurse: Are you saying you don't think life is worth living?

Mary: Well … yes. It's all so hopeless anyway.

Nurse: Are you thinking of killing yourself?

Mary: Oh, I don't know. Well, sometimes I think about it. I probably would never go through with it.

Nurse: Mary, let's talk more about what you're thinking and feeling. This is important. I'll need to share your thoughts with other members of the staff.

The nurse should be alert for nonverbal behavioral clues, including showing a sudden brightening of mood with more energy (especially after recently being prescribed an antidepressant medication), giving away possessions, or organizing financial affairs.

Evidence-based clinical practice guidelines emphasize the importance of establishing a therapeutic relationship with the patient and asking about possible suicidal feelings (APA, 2003). This is the single most important assessment (and intervention), yet health care professionals report a surprisingly small amount of probing. Possible reasons for this lack of probing include lack of personal comfort, lack of professional confidence, and time constraints (Harvard Mental Health Letter, 2006). Crisis intervention techniques involve listening for the emotional feeling message underlying the verbal message, especially when the patient presents as angry, hostile, and overwhelmed.

Lethality of Suicide Plan

The evaluation of a suicide plan is extremely important in determining the degree of suicidal risk. Three main elements must be considered when evaluating lethality (APA, 2003): (1) Is there a specific plan with details? (2) How lethal is the proposed method? (3) Is there access to the planned method? People who have definite plans for the time, place, and means are at high risk.

Based on the lethality of a method, which indicates how quickly a person would die by that mode, a method can be classified as higher or lower risk. Higher-risk methods, also referred to as *hard methods*, include:

- Using a gun
- Jumping off a high place
- Hanging
- Poisoning with carbon monoxide
- Staging a car crash

Examples of lower-risk methods, also referred to as *soft methods*, include:

- Slashing one's wrists
- Inhaling natural gas
- Ingesting pills

When the proposed method is available, the situation is more serious. A man who has access to a high building and states that he will jump from it or a woman who has a gun and says that she will shoot herself are at serious risk for suicide. When people are experiencing psychotic episodes, they are at high risk—regardless of the specificity of details—because impulse control and judgment are grossly impaired. A person suffering psychosis is particularly vulnerable when depressed or having command hallucinations.

Assessment Tools

Many tools have been developed to aid a health care worker in assessing suicidal potential. Patterson and co-workers (1983) devised an assessment aid with the acronym *SAD PERSONS* to evaluate 10 major risk factors for suicide (Table 24-2). The SAD PERSONS scale is a simple and practical guide for triaging potentially suicidal patients, particularly in an emergency department environment. Ten categories are described in the assessment tool, and the person being evaluated is assigned one point for each applicable characteristic. The total point score for the individual correlates with an action scale that assists health care workers determine whether hospital admission is advisable. If a patient scores in the 3- to 4-point ranges, it is then necessary for a psychiatric/mental health professional to conduct a full mental status examination and interview.

TABLE 24-2 SAD PERSONS Scale

S	Sex	1 if male
A	Age	1 if 25 to 44 years or 65+ years
D	Depression	1 if present
P	Previous attempt	1 if present
E	Ethanol use	1 if present
R	Rational thinking loss	1 if psychotic for any reason
S	Social supports lacking	1 if lacking, especially recent loss
O	Organized plan	1 if plan with lethal method
N	No spouse	1 if divorced, widowed, separated, or single male
S	Sickness	1 if severe or chronic

Guidelines for Action

Points	Clinical Action
0-2	Send home with follow-up
3-4	Closely follow up; consider hospitalization
5-6	Strongly consider hospitalization
7-10	Hospitalize or commit

From Patterson, W. M., Dohn, H. H., Bird, J., & Patterson, G. A. (1983). Evaluation of suicidal patients: The SAD PERSONS scale. *Psychosomatics, 24*(4), 343–345, 348–349.

The SAD PERSONS tool does not address whether or not the individual is taking either illicit or prescribed drugs that may have a significant impact on the patient. Other shortcomings are that the tool is dated (1983), and there is a need for a uniform and evidence-based screening tool that can be used in clinical environments (Price, 2007).

Prescription medications such as antidepressants should be evaluated for their contribution to suicide risk. The U.S. Federal Drug Administration (FDA) black box warning for selective serotonin reuptake inhibitor (SSRI) antidepressants includes children and young adults up to age 24. It states that careful monitoring should occur during the first few weeks of treatment, as well as when the dosage is changed (Harvard Mental Health Letter, 2007). Some patients develop extreme restlessness and agitation (akathisia) that can make life intolerable. The use of SSRIs in patients with depression related to undiagnosed bipolar disorder can result in mania, which carries an especially high risk for suicide. This type of mania can also be the result of steroid use. Prescribed medications should be carefully monitored and assessed during screening for suicide potential (Harvard Mental Health Letter, 2007).

Self-Assessment

All health care professionals who work with suicidal people need collaboration with other clinicians. Fear, grief, anger, puzzlement, and condemnation of suicidal feelings/intent are common feelings. If these intense emotional responses are not acknowledged, countertransference may limit effective intervention. Understanding the suicidal patient, as well as acknowledging, understanding, and accepting the emotions that arise from working with and caring for these patients, is essential.

Assessment Guidelines Suicide

1. Assess risk factors, including history of suicide (in family, friends), degree of hopelessness and helplessness, and lethality of plan.
2. If there is a history of suicide attempt, assess intent, lethality, and injury.
3. Determine whether the patient's age, medical condition, psychiatric diagnosis, or current medications put the patient at higher risk.
4. Further assessment is necessary if the patient suddenly goes from sad or depressed to happy and peaceful. Often a decision to commit suicide gives a feeling of relief and calm.
5. If the patient is to be managed on an outpatient basis, also assess social supports and helpfulness of significant others.

DIAGNOSIS

The nursing diagnosis with the highest priority is *Risk for suicide* related to various emotional states and situational circumstances. Feelings of hopelessness, anger, frustration, abandonment, and rejection are common among people who are suicidal. Table 24-3 identifies a number of nursing diagnoses that may apply. It is also important that related nursing diagnoses are prioritized. Diagnoses such as *Self-care deficit, Social isolation, Sleep pattern disturbance, Anxiety,* and *Altered nutrition* are very applicable to the immediate care of the patient.

OUTCOMES IDENTIFICATION

Relevant *Nursing Outcomes Classification (NOC)* outcomes include *Suicide Self-Restraint, Coping, Hope, Social Support, Spiritual Health,* and *Self-Esteem* (Moorhead et al., 2008). Refer to Table 24-4 for examples of short-term and intermediate indicators for suicidal patients.

PLANNING

The plan of care for the suicidal patient is based on risk factors. When a psychiatric disorder is present, the treatment plan includes appropriate nursing

TABLE 24-3 Potential Nursing Diagnoses for the Suicidal Patient

Signs and Symptoms	Potential Nursing Diagnoses
Gives overt or covert clues (e.g., "I can't stand the pain."), has a plan (gun), is in high-risk category on assessment (elderly or teenager, isolated, depressed, has had a recent loss), has a psychiatric diagnosis (substance abuse, depression, borderline personality disorder, psychosis)	*Risk for suicide* *Risk for injury* *Risk for self-directed/other-directed violence*
Overwhelmed with situational crises, relies heavily on drugs or alcohol, has few supportive systems, shows poor problem-solving skills, has "tunnel vision"; no family available or crisis in the family, poor family communication	*Ineffective coping* *Disabled family coping* *Impaired social interaction*
Lacks hope for the future; believes nothing can change intolerable situation; has intense feelings of isolation, deprivation, lack of love, having nowhere to turn; believes he or she has no control over the future	*Hopelessness* *Powerlessness* *Social isolation* *Spiritual distress* *Loneliness* *Chronic sorrow*
Believes that he or she is no good, worthless, ineffective, a burden to others, can't do anything right	*Situational low self-esteem* *Chronic low self-esteem*
Does not understand age-related crises; does not know of available resources	*Deficient knowledge*

Data from North American Nursing Diagnosis Association International (NANDA-I) (2009). *NANDA-I nursing diagnoses: Definitions and classification 2009-2011*. Oxford, United Kingdom: Author.

TABLE 24-4 *NOC* Outcomes for Suicidal Patients

Nursing Outcome and Definition	Intermediate Indicators	Short-Term Indicators
Suicide Self-Restraint: Personal actions to refrain from gestures and attempts at killing self	Maintains self-control without supervision	Discloses plan for suicide if present Refrains from attempting suicide
Coping: Personal actions to manage stressors that tax an individual's resources	Reports decrease in stress	Verbalizes need for assistance
Hope: Optimism that is personally satisfying and life-supporting	Sets goals	Expresses will to live
Self-Esteem: Personal judgment of self-worth	Verbalizations of self-acceptance	Feelings about self-worth
Social Support: Perceived availability and actual provision of reliable assistance from others	Emotional assistance provided by others	Willingness to call on others for help
Spiritual Health: Connectedness with self, others, higher power, all life, nature, and the universe that transcends and empowers the self	Connectedness with others	Interaction with others to share thoughts, feelings, and beliefs

From Moorhead, S., Johnson, M., Maas, M. L., & Swanson, E. (Eds.). (2008). *Nursing outcomes classification (NOC)* (4th ed.). St. Louis: Mosby.

approaches (e.g., care for patients with depression or schizophrenia). The patient's significant others need to be involved because the patient's perception of isolation is a significant cause of hopelessness. Case Study and Nursing Care Plan 24-1 on pages 560-562 presents the case of a suicidal young woman treated in the outpatient setting.

IMPLEMENTATION

Nursing interventions for suicide take place at three different levels: primary, secondary, and tertiary. Because improving *overall* community mental health can reduce the incidence of suicide more effectively than extensive efforts directed at identifying imminently suicidal individuals, more attention focused on **primary interventions** that involve community-wide participation can improve outcomes (Ortiz, 2006).

Primary Intervention

Primary intervention includes activities that provide support, information, and education to prevent suicide (Box 24-3). Primary intervention can be practiced in a wide variety of community settings such as schools, homes, churches, hospitals, and work settings. Elementary school children are screened using evidence-based tools that focus on both risk factors and warning signs (Joe & Bryant, 2007). Several high schools are adopting suicide prevention curricula that involve elements of education, peer support and referral, and discussions about risk factors and warning signs (Ciffone, 2007).

An evolving role for nurses that has significant influence on positive primary interventions community-wide is that of the parish nurse. Evidence suggests that enhanced education for nurses is needed to change attitudes and increase competence and compassion in caring for patients with suicidal behaviors (Patterson et al., 2007).

BOX 24-3 Goals of the National Strategy for Suicide Prevention

- Promote awareness that suicide is a preventable public health problem.
- Develop broad-based support for suicide prevention.
- Develop and implement strategies to reduce the stigma associated with being a consumer of mental health, substance abuse, and suicide-prevention services.
- Develop and implement suicide prevention programs.
- Promote efforts to reduce access to lethal means and methods of self-harm.
- Implement training for recognition of at-risk behavior and delivery of effective treatment.
- Develop and promote effective clinical and professional practices.
- Improve access to and community linkages with mental health and substance abuse services.
- Improve reporting and portrayals of suicidal behavior, mental illness, and substance abuse in the entertainment and news media.
- Promote and support research on suicide and suicide prevention.
- Improve and expand surveillance systems.

From U.S. Department of Health & Human Services, Public Health Service. (2001). *National strategy for suicide prevention: Goals and objectives for action.* Rockville, MD: Author; and U.S. Department of Health & Human Services, Office of the Surgeon General. (1999). *The Surgeon General's call to action to prevent suicide.* Washington, DC: Author.

Secondary Intervention

Secondary intervention is treatment of the actual suicidal crisis. It is practiced in clinics, hospitals, jails, and on telephone hotlines. Involving the entire community, especially in primary and secondary interventions, is essential to reducing suicides. Oftentimes, secondary interventions are the determinants of life or death, and nurses with good crisis intervention skills are in a position to use, role model, and teach these skills to others.

Tertiary Intervention

Tertiary intervention (or postvention) refers to interventions with the family and friends of a person who has committed suicide. This is done to both reduce the traumatic aftereffects and explore effective means of addressing survivor problems using primary and secondary interventions. Nurses understand grief/loss well and are in positions to refer, consult, and collaborate in the best interests of those left behind. This is vital, since the suicide rate increases for those left behind. (Vessier-Batcher & Douglas, 2006). Survivors of suicide are in immediate need of supportive avenues for coping with such complicated grief.

The *Nursing Interventions Classification (NIC)* offers the following topics pertinent to the care of the suicidal patient: *Suicide Prevention, Hope Instillation, Coping Enhancement, Self-esteem Enhancement, Family Mobilization, and Support System Enhancement* (Bulechek et al., 2008).

In the hospital or community setting, the basic level registered nurse (RN) utilizes counseling, health teaching, case management, and psychobiological interventions. During the acute suicidal crisis, suicide precautions are carried out as a specialized form of milieu therapy. It is important to understand that when a patient is admitted to an inpatient psychiatric unit, the nurse must carefully assess and then prioritize care. As previously noted, the vast majority (90%) of suicidal patients have a psychiatric illness underlying their suicide attempt. Oftentimes these patients have also been self-medicating their pain with alcohol and/or other drugs. Their lack of rational thought, low frustration tolerance, and impulsivity may require close monitoring for harm directed at self and also towards others.

Milieu Management

Suicide Precautions

In accordance with unit policies and procedures, the patient is observed continuously by nursing staff. Refer to Table 24-5 for a general description of suicide precautions. This intense attention from the nurse provides for safety and allows for constant reassessment of risk.

TABLE 24-5 Suicide Precautions with Constant One-to-One Observation

Staff Assessment	Possible Patient Symptoms	Nursing Responsibilities
Patient with suicidal ideation or delusions of self-mutilation who, according to assessment by unit staff, presents clinical symptoms that suggest a clear intent to follow through with the plan or delusion	• Patient is currently verbalizing a clear intent to harm self. • Patient is unwilling to make a no-suicide contract. • Patient shows no insight into existing problems. • Patient has poor impulse control. • Patient has already attempted suicide in the recent past by a particularly lethal method (e.g., hanging, gun, carbon monoxide poisoning).	1. Conduct one-to-one nursing observation and interaction 24 hours a day (never let patient out of staff's sight). 2. Maintain arm's length at all times. 3. Chart patient's whereabouts and record mood, verbatim statements, and behavior every 15 to 30 minutes per protocol. 4. Ensure that meal trays contain no glass or metal silverware. 5. During observation when patient is sleeping, **hands should always be in view**, not under the bedcovers. 6. Carefully observe patient swallow each dose of medication. 7. The nurse and physician should explain to the patient what they will be doing and why; both document this in the chart.

Monitoring flow sheets for suicide precautions are more clinically useful if they include a description of affect as well as behavior. For example, instead of noting "Patient watching television," the nurse can describe the patient's affect at each observation interval (hostile, fearful, calm, etc.). Flow sheets should also indicate clear accountability for staff starting and ending their periods of observation. In addition to observing the patient, the nurse is responsible for monitoring the environment for safety hazards. Review Box 24-4 for guidelines on how to minimize physical risks in the milieu.

Studies show that acute care of suicidal patients is usually effective. Suicide risk is highest in the first few days of admission and during times of staff rotation, particularly rotation of psychiatric residents. Assessment of suicidal risk must be an ongoing process; assessment should be performed particularly before a change in level of observation or upon sudden improvement or worsening of symptoms.

Counseling

Counseling skills, including interviewing, crisis care, and problem-solving techniques, are used in both the inpatient and outpatient settings. The key element is establishing a working alliance to encourage the patient to engage in more realistic problem solving. Helpful staff characteristics include warmth, sensitivity, interest, and consistency. After hospitalization, the nurse may see these patients in the clinic, in a

BOX 24-4 Environmental Guidelines for Minimizing Suicidal Behavior on the Psychiatric Unit

- Use plastic eating utensils.
- Do not assign patient to a private room, and ensure the door remains open at all times.
- Jump-proof and hang-proof the bathrooms by installing break-away shower rods and recessed shower nozzles.
- Keep electrical cords to a minimal length.
- Install unbreakable glass in windows. Install tamper-proof screens or partitions too small to pass through. Keep all windows locked.
- Lock all utility rooms, kitchens, adjacent stairwells, and offices. All nonclinical staff (e.g., housekeepers, maintenance workers) should receive instructions to keep doors locked.
- Take all potentially harmful gifts (e.g., flowers in glass vases) from visitors before allowing them to see patients.
- Go through personal belongings with patient present, and remove all potentially harmful objects (e.g., belts, shoelaces, metal nail files, tweezers, matches, razors, perfume, and shampoo).
- Ensure that visitors do not bring in or leave potentially harmful objects in patient's room (e.g., matches, nail files).
- Search patient for harmful objects (e.g., drugs, sharp objects, cords) on return from pass.

partial hospital program, or in home care. One particular aspect of counseling is the use of a **no-suicide contract** (also called a *no-harm contract*). This is a written contract in which the patient agrees not to harm himself or herself but to take an alternative action if feeling suicidal (e.g., talk with staff, call a crisis line). In reading about the current best evidence regarding the overall ineffectiveness of no-suicide contracts, nurses must also consider the realities of the current average 3- to 5-day hospital stay.

Health Teaching and Health Promotion

The nurse teaches the patient about psychiatric diagnoses, medications and complementary therapies, and age-related crises. Teaching is also important regarding community resources, coping skills, stress management, and communication skills. When possible, the family or significant others are included to strengthen the patient's support system.

A focus on personal strengths and positive thoughts and emotions (e.g., hope) is essential (Harvard Mental Health Letter, 2008). Talk therapy, in addition to medications, should be incorporated.

Case Management

Case management is an important aspect of nursing care for the suicidal patient. The patient's perception of being alone without supports often blinds the person to the real support figures who are present. Reconnecting the patient with family and friends is a major focus, whether in the hospital or the community. Aftercare referral, including information on the following resources may be given: substance treatment centers, crisis hotlines, support groups for patients or families, and recreational activities to enhance socialization and self-esteem. Encouraging the patient to get reacquainted with a previous spiritual support system can also be beneficial.

Pharmacological Interventions

A significant nursing intervention to assist the suicidal patient in regaining self-control is the careful administration of medication. All medications given to high-risk patients are monitored carefully, although lethal overdose is nearly impossible with SSRIs, unlike the risky tricyclic antidepressants and monoamine oxidase inhibitors. Mouth checks may be used to be sure patients are not saving (hoarding) medications in the hospital; in the community, provision of a limited-day supply or family supervision is required.

Treatment for suicidal patients is suggested by the APA (2003). Antidepressants should be ordered for patients who have depressive or anxiety disorders, with an emphasis on administering an adequate dosage and providing appropriate clinical evaluation during the

use of SSRIs. Close monitoring must occur, especially when medication is initiated and during times of dosage adjustment. Astute nursing care involves careful patient (and family, if appropriate) teaching about the identified benefits and risks of antidepressant therapy.

There is clear evidence that long-term lithium treatment for bipolar disorder and major depression significantly reduces suicide and suicide attempts. Because lithium does frequently cause side effects and necessitate periodic blood work to test for therapeutic levels, patient and family education is important to support adherence.

For patients experiencing psychotic or bipolar manic episodes, antipsychotic medication is usually ordered. Atypical antipsychotics are usually preferable to the traditional ones because they have fewer adverse effects. Some studies have shown a reduced suicide rate among patients with schizophrenia receiving clozapine. Its use must be monitored closely, however, because of the risk of severe medical side effects (e.g., agranulocytosis, myocarditis, and altered glucose metabolism).

Finally, antianxiety medication may help to treat panic and insomnia. Thus far, no clinical studies have examined the effect of antianxiety treatment on suicide risk. But short-term use of long-acting benzodiazepines may be helpful for management of panic symptoms. As previously mentioned, akathisia-like symptoms can sometimes occur with the use of SSRI medications. This side effect must be carefully assessed and appropriate treatment given as necessary.

An alternative somatic treatment for acute suicidal risk is electroconvulsive therapy (ECT). Evidence suggests that ECT decreases acute suicidal ideation. This treatment is useful for certain types of patients with depression or psychosis whose behavior is considered life threatening and for whom waiting for medication to take effect is not feasible. It is also safe and effective for pregnant patients, patients with certain medical conditions who cannot tolerate medication, and patients who do not respond to multiple trials of medication. Refer to Chapter 13 for further discussion of ECT.

Postvention for Survivors of Completed Suicide

A discussion of suicidal patients is incomplete without noting the issues surrounding a completed suicide. Surviving family and friends can experience overwhelming guilt and shame, compounded by the difficulty of discussing the frequently taboo subject of suicide. The usual social supports of neighbors and church are sometimes lacking for these mourners. Within 6 months of a suicide, 45% of bereaved adults report mental deterioration with symptoms of depression or PTSD. Adolescent siblings of youth suicide victims have a 7-times higher risk of developing major depressive disorder over the 6-month period.

Adolescent friends who suffer traumatic grief are more likely to report suicidal ideation within 6 years of the suicide (APA, 2003). Family members of a suicide victim develop a 4.5-times greater risk of suicide than those in families in which no suicide occurred. Despite their suffering, only approximately 25% of survivors seek treatment (APA, 2003).

One survivor wrote a personal account several years after the suicide of her daughter:

> If only I hadn't responded with anger and frustration during our last phone call…she was angry herself, and seemed to want to pick a fight with me—which was the pattern. If I could have looked past her angry words and instead tuned into the desperation behind them, maybe I could have gotten her to open up to me. Now I can only look back and consider the many, many times I should have picked up on the severity of her illness and how she struggled with it. Her experience has also caused me to look at my own depression and realize how especially vulnerable I am now. If I have any advice for others based on my experience, it is to get connected, listen, and be a real part of the lives of those you love. That's the only way you'll know when something is just not right, and how desperate someone really is. That also applies to friends and family of us survivors. Don't treat us like we're "contagious." And please do talk about our loss. The worst thing possible is to avoid mention of our lost loved one.

Survivors give the following suggestions to health care professionals:

- If being a survivor is the main reason treatment has been sought, remember that the survivor, not the deceased, is the patient. Focus on the patient's thoughts and feelings, and do a thorough assessment as you usually would.
- If you are a friend or relative of a suicide survivor, remember that the most difficult time for these survivors is not so much in the immediate aftermath of the suicide; rather, it is in the weeks, months, and *years* following it. Make frequent efforts to reach out to these individuals, especially on the most difficult anniversary dates. Do not be afraid of talking about the deceased person—in fact, speak of them often. While this may seem counterintuitive and uncomfortable for most, survivors of suicide universally want their loved one to be remembered in this way. Talking reduces the hurt, isolation, and stigma.
- If being a survivor comes out as an incidental finding during an assessment, ask open-ended questions and evaluate how much the loss has been resolved.
- Recommend community resources and survivor support groups, and show empathy about the loss of someone to suicide. Know about local Survivors of Suicide (SOS) support groups in your area, and refer the survivors and their families as soon as possible following the suicide.

Staff members who have cared for a suicide victim are similarly traumatized by suicide. Staff may also experience symptoms of PTSD, with guilt, shock, anger, shame, and decreased self-esteem (APA, 2003). Group support is essential as the treatment team conducts a thorough psychological postmortem assessment. The event is carefully reviewed to identify the potential overlooked clues, faulty judgments, or changes that are needed in agency protocols. Most facilities have a clear policy about communication with families after suicide. Although some lawyers advise having no contact except through them, others recommend designating a spokesperson who can address the feelings of the family without discussing the details of the patient's care. Referrals should be given to family members to try to assist them in dealing with their grief and to address any emotional problems that develop, especially in adolescents.

As for documentation, all staff need to ensure that the record is complete and that any late entries are identified. Courts require that the patient be periodically evaluated for suicidal risk, that the treatment plan provide for high-level security, and that staff members follow the individual treatment plan. Despite following institution protocols, treatment plans, and the appropriate standards of practice, suicides do occasionally still happen. This is especially the case for patients in the community. Human behavior is simply not predictable.

Advanced Practice Interventions

The psychiatric advanced practice RN (APRN) may treat suicidal patients directly with psychotherapy, psychobiological interventions, clinical supervision for direct care staff, or consultation in nonpsychiatric settings (e.g., medical unit, nursing home, or forensic site). Following hospitalization, the APRN provides aftercare for the patient with coexisting psychiatric disorders, including individual therapy and family therapy.

EVALUATION

Evaluation of a suicidal patient is ongoing. The nurse must be constantly alert to changes in the suicidal person's mood, thinking, and behavior. The nurse also looks for indications that the patient is communicating thoughts and feelings more readily and that the patient's social network is widening. For example, if the person is able to talk about his or her feelings and engage in problem solving with the nurse, this is a positive sign. Is the patient increasing his or her social activities and expanding his or her interests? The nurse must remember that *suicidal behavior is the result of interpersonal turmoil*. If an episode of major depression is the main admitting diagnosis and a serious suicidal gesture resulted from this depression, both problems are initially assessed and treated. When the patient is no longer an acute suicide risk, treating the depression becomes the main focus of care. Essentially, the nurse evaluates each short-term goal and establishes new ones as the patient progresses toward the long-term goal of resolving suicidal ideation.

Once stabilized, the patient may qualify for transfer to an intensive outpatient (IOP) treatment program, which involves continuing treatment after discharge, or a partial hospitalization program (PHP) that allows patients to go home in the evening to practice new coping skills. Community-based support groups are also available that are both effective and do not charge a fee. Nurses need to be knowledgeable about, and proactive in, referring patients to these support groups. Nurses should try to be knowledgeable about reimbursement systems and treatment options available for the increasing numbers of uninsured or underinsured patients.

Case Study and Nursing Care Plan 24-1   A Suicidal Patient in the Outpatient Setting

Kaitlyn is a 23-year-old single waitress who is brought to the emergency department by ambulance after a suicide attempt. Her live-in boyfriend had narrowly prevented her from shooting herself with a gun kept in their apartment. She has a minor scalp wound and remains under observation for a few hours after treatment. She is then interviewed by the psychiatric nurse and psychiatrist on call.

She states that she has been under increasing stress for the past 2 months since entering a management training program at work. Kaitlyn ultimately failed at this venture and lost her job. She expresses a great deal of desperation owing to the accumulation of several bills and the upcoming Christmas holidays. She admits to keeping these feelings to herself and self-medicating her growing fear and anxiety with drugs and alcohol. She states that she feels "like a total loser."

Because Kaitlyn continues to state that she wants to kill herself, because of her reluctance to open up and share her feelings with anyone, and because her score on the SAD PERSONS scale is 4, the decision is made to hospitalize her. After careful assessment, Kaitlyn is placed on antidepressant therapy and carefully monitored. Additionally, problems relating to her depressive state are assessed and monitored (poor appetite, insomnia, self-care deficit, and anxiety). After 3 days on suicide precautions, she is no longer acutely suicidal and agrees to continue treatment in the outpatient division of the hospital. In this system, outpatient nurses rotate through the emergency department. Kaitlyn requests assignment to the nurse who saw her initially.

ASSESSMENT

Self-Assessment

Mrs. Ruiz is a registered nurse with a bachelor's degree and 5 years' experience. She remembers Kaitlyn from the emergency evaluation and expresses reluctance to take the assignment. She seeks out the clinical supervisor to discuss the case. In talking about her feelings, she realizes that she wants to avoid this patient for two reasons. The first is that Kaitlyn's impatience, agitation, and anger make her feel anxious and inadequate. The second is that Mrs. Ruiz disapproves of Kaitlyn's attempt to end her life. "She is so young and has her whole life in front of her. How bad can her problems be? My Catholic faith makes suicide difficult to accept."

Mrs. Ruiz also notes the countertransference involved, in that Kaitlyn reminds her of her own daughter. Mrs. Ruiz recognizes her own feelings and can now better focus on Kaitlyn's issues: She feels angry and helpless after losing her job and facing financial concerns; and her isolation seems self-imposed because she pushes people away and keeps her feelings to herself, probably because of low self-esteem. After consultation, Mrs. Ruiz agrees with her supervisor that she can work with Kaitlyn.

Objective Data

Reported first suicide attempt in a 23-year-old female
Self-medicating with alcohol and substances (denies chronic use)
Isolated without social support systems
Recent failure at work and subsequent loss of job
Mounting debt at holiday season
No history of bipolar disorder or related behaviors

Subjective Data

"I love my boyfriend, but I don't like to talk about my problems."
"I have a lot of friends, but they don't really know me; I keep secrets from everyone."
"I just feel so down and depressed."
"I'm constantly getting in over my head and screwing up."
"I don't want my family to find out what a mess I've made of things ... again."

DIAGNOSIS

1. *Risk for suicide* related to feeling overwhelmed and depressed secondary to loss of job and mounting debt, as evidenced by suicide attempt

Supporting Data
- Suicide attempt with lethal intent
- "I don't want to live and have to face everyone with this mess I've made."
- Mounting debt at the holiday season
- Recent job loss

2. *Impaired social interaction* related to feelings of fear and shame, as evidenced by avoiding disclosure of issues and feelings with family and significant others.

Supporting Data
- "I'm too ashamed to face everyone now."
- "I feel like I'm all alone with my mess. I'm so disgusted and angry!"
- "My job was where my friends were."
- "I can't even tell my boyfriend."

OUTCOMES IDENTIFICATION

1. Patient will consistently use suicide prevention resources and social support groups within the community (long-term outcome).
2. Patient will develop insight and trust in order to establish supportive social contacts (long-term outcome).

PLANNING

The initial plan is to establish a working relationship with Kaitlyn, involving her in planning her own treatment and identifying alternative actions for suicidal ideation in the future.

IMPLEMENTATION

Kaitlyn's plan of care is personalized as follows:

Nursing diagnosis: *Risk for suicide* related to feeling overwhelmed and depressed secondary to loss of job and mounting debt

Outcome criteria: Patient will consistently use suicide prevention resources and social support groups within the community.

Short-Term Goal	Intervention	Rationale	Evaluation
1. Kaitlyn will immediately seek help when feeling self-destructive.	1a. Assess suicide status.	1a. Ongoing periodic check of suicidal status. Higher rate of suicide for those who have attempted suicide.	**GOAL MET** Kaitlyn agrees to talk to the nurse about suicidal feelings. If clinic is closed, she will call the crisis hotline (first session). Kaitlyn also agreed to a family session that included her boyfriend, and the gun was removed from her apartment.
	1b. Even if Kaitlyn denies suicidal ideas, make a future plan.	1b. Demonstrates concern and offers alternatives if suicidal thoughts return.	
	1c. Monitor efficacy of antidepressant therapy and assess for side effects.	1c. Ongoing periodic. Important to assess for increase in suicidal feelings, agitation, and monitor for lifting of depressive state.	1c. No adverse side effects noted. Noted increase in socialization, improved hygiene, reported improvement in sleep and appetite. Patient states her mood is improving, and she feels more hopeful.

Continued

Short-Term Goal	Intervention	Rationale	Evaluation
2. Kaitlyn will talk about painful feelings by the first week.	2a. Remain neutral in face of anger. 2b. Refocus attention back to Kaitlyn and the emotions underlying her anger. 2c. Give frequent opportunities for discussion of feelings through verbal invitation and stated concern.	2a. Diminishes power struggles and discourages continuing acting-out behaviors. 2b. Arguments and power struggles keep attention away from important issues. 2c. Aggressive, hostile communications are cover for painful feelings. When patient can express feelings in words, there is less need to act them out.	**GOAL MET** During the initial sessions, angry communication is constant. By the end of the first week, Kaitlyn states, "You really want to know." Kaitlyn talks of feeling like a failure as a daughter, girlfriend, and employee.
3. Kaitlyn will explore other employment opportunities by the end of the second week.	3. Alternative solutions can be problem-solved once feelings and problems are identified.	3. Acceptable alternatives increase a future orientation and decrease hopelessness. Patient can experience feelings of control over situation.	**GOAL MET** By the end of the second week, Kaitlyn talks about attending a regional job fair that will be held after the holidays. She has accepted a referral to social services for the purpose of registering for unemployment benefits and debt management.

Nursing diagnosis: *Impaired social interaction* related to feelings of fear and shame, as evidenced by avoiding disclosure of issues and feelings with family and significant others
Outcome criteria: Patient will develop insight and trust in order to establish supportive social contacts.

Short-Term Goal	Intervention	Rationale	Evaluation
1. Kaitlyn will discuss feelings of isolation and loneliness by the end of the third week.	1. Provide opportunities for Kaitlyn to honestly express feelings and thoughts regarding her self-imposed isolation.	1. Before change can take place, clarification of personal feelings and thoughts is necessary.	**GOAL MET** By the end of the third week, Kaitlyn speaks of feeling alone and demonstrates insight into the dynamics of keeping secrets, yet desperately wanting a real and honest connection to loved ones.
2. Kaitlyn will identify three positive aspects of self by the end of the third week.	2a. Validate Kaitlyn's strengths. 2b. Encourage self-evaluation of both positive and negative aspects of Kaitlyn's life.	2a. Both positive and negative feedback aid in more realistic perception of self. 2b. Patient can begin to see herself more clearly, with increase in self-esteem.	**GOAL MET** By the end of the third week, Kaitlyn states that she thinks she is a hard worker, good friend, and a caring daughter and girlfriend.
3. Kaitlyn will state that she enjoys one new, healthy activity with at least one other person by the end of the fourth week.	3a. Review previous activities that Kaitlyn enjoyed before she lost her job. 3b. Have Kaitlyn choose an activity she is willing to participate in.	3a. Change focus from negative present to positive aspects of patient's past. Can help increase hope and self-esteem. 3b. Participating in own problem solving and decision making offers patient a sense of control and an increase in self-esteem.	**GOAL MET** By the end of the fourth week, Kaitlyn states that she started skiing again and is surprised that she and her boyfriend had a good time.

EVALUATION

See individual outcomes and evaluation within the care plan.

KEY POINTS TO REMEMBER

- Suicide is a significant public health problem in the United States.
- Specific biological, psychosocial, and cultural factors are known to increase the risk of suicide.
- Most suicidal patients can be helped by treatment of a coexisting psychiatric disorder.
- Certain medical conditions and psychiatric diagnoses are associated with increased risk for suicide.
- Every suicide attempt must be taken seriously, even if the person has a history of multiple attempts.
- The nurse can have a real impact on suicide prevention through primary, secondary, and tertiary interventions.
- Nursing care of the suicidal patient is challenging but rewarding: patients' desperate feelings evoke intense reactions in staff, but most people with suicidal ideation respond to treatment and do not complete suicide.
- If a patient completes suicide, family, friends, and health care workers are traumatized and need support, possibly including referrals for psychiatric treatment.

CRITICAL THINKING

1. Locate and review the suicide protocol at your hospital unit or community center. Are there any steps you anticipate having difficulty carrying out? Discuss these difficulties with your peers or clinical group.
2. How would you respond to another staff member who expresses guilt over the completed suicide of a patient on your unit?
3. Identify three common and expected emotional reactions that a nurse might have when initially working with people who are suicidal.
   A. How do you think you might react?
   B. What actions could you take to deal with the event and obtain support?

CHAPTER REVIEW

1. Which assessment statement(s) would be appropriate for a patient who may be suicidal? *Select all that apply.*
   1. Do you ever think about suicide?
   2. Are you thinking of hurting yourself?
   3. Do you sometimes wish you were dead?
   4. Has it ever seemed like life is not worth living?
   5. If you were to kill yourself, how would you do it?
   6. Does it seem like others might be better off if you were dead?

2. Which person is at the highest risk for suicide?
   1. A 50-year-old married white male with depression who has a plan to overdose if circumstances at work do not improve.

2. A 45-year-old married white female who recently lost her parents, suffers from bipolar disorder, and attempted suicide once as a teenager.
3. A young, single white male who is alcohol dependent, hopeless, impulsive, has just been rejected by his girlfriend, and has ready access to a gun he has hidden.
4. An older Hispanic male who is Catholic, is living with a debilitating chronic illness, is recently widowed, and states: "I wish that God would take me too."

3. Which intervention(s) maximize the safety of an actively suicidal patient on an inpatient mental health unit? *Select all that apply.*
   1. Place the patient on every-15-minute checks.
   2. Place the patient in a room near the nurses' station.
   3. Assign the patient to a private room to facilitate monitoring.
   4. Install breakaway curtain rods, coat hooks, and shower rods.
   5. Search the patient, his room, and his belongings for dangerous items.
   6. Substitute blankets and thicker cloth items for sheets and thinner cloth items.
   7. Withhold visitation privileges to prevent the patient from obtaining dangerous items via visitors.

4. Which are accurate statements about no-suicide contracts? *Select all that apply.*
   1. Refusal to sign a no-suicide contract suggests higher risk.
   2. No-suicide contracts have been shown to reduce the risk of suicide.
   3. No-suicide contracts include alternate actions a patient should take if suicidal.
   4. Short lengths of stay tend to reduce the effectiveness of no-suicide contracts.
   5. Nurses should encourage ambivalent patients to sign a no-suicide contract.
   6. Such contracts may inhibit some suicidal behavior but cannot be relied upon for safety.

5. Which intervention(s) would be therapeutic for a patient experiencing suicidal ideation? *Select all that apply.*
   1. Focus primarily on developing solutions to the problems that are leading the patient to feel suicidal.
   2. Assess the patient thoroughly, and reassess the patient at regular intervals as levels of risk fluctuate.
   3. Meet regularly with the patient to provide opportunities for the patient to express and explore feelings.
   4. Administer antidepressant, mood-stabilizing, and anti-anxiety medications cautiously and conservatively because of their potential to increase suicide risk.
   5. Help the patient to identify positive self-attributes and question negative self-perceptions that are unrealistic.

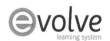

Visit the Evolve website for an **Audio Chapter Summary, Chapter Review Answers & Rationales, Critical Thinking Answer Guidelines**, and additional resources related to the content in this chapter: **http://evolve.elsevier.com/Varcarolis/foundations**

Companion CD Use the Companion CD to prepare for tests and the NCLEX® Examination with **Test-Taking Strategies** for psychiatric mental health nursing and hundreds of **Review Questions**.

References

American Nurses Association (ANA), American Psychiatric-Mental Health Nurses Association, & International Society of Psychiatric-Mental Health Nurses. (2007). *Psychiatric mental health nursing: Scope and standards of practice.* Silver Spring, MD: American Nurses Association.

American Psychiatric Association. (2003). Practice guideline for the assessment and treatment of patients with suicidal behaviors. *American Journal of Psychiatry, 160*(11 Suppl.), 1–60.

Appel, J. M. (2007). A suicide right for the mentally ill? A Swiss case opens a new debate. *Hastings Center Report, 37*(3), 21–23.

Brendel, R. W., Lagomasino, I. T., Perlis, R. H., & Stern, T. A. (2008). The suicidal patient. In T. A. Stern, J. R. Rosenbaum, M. Fava, J. Biederman, & S. L. Rauch (Eds.), *Massachusetts General Hospital comprehensive clinical psychiatry* (pp. 733–745). St Louis: Mosby.

Bulechek, G. M., Butcher, H. K., & Dochterman, J. M. (Eds.). (2008). *Nursing interventions classification (NIC)* (5th ed.). St. Louis: Mosby.

Centers for Disease Control and Prevention. (2006). Youth risk behavior surveillance—United States, 2005. *Morbidity and Mortality Weekly Report, 55*, SS–5.

Centers for Disease Control and Prevention. (2008, Summer). *Suicide facts at a glance.* Retrieved April 6, 2009 from http://www.cdc.gov/ncipc/dvp/Suicide/suicide_data_sheet.pdf

Ciffone, J. C. (2007). Suicide prevention: An analysis and replication of a curriculum-based high school program. *Social Work, 52*(1), 41–49.

Cleaver, K. (2007). Characteristics and trends of self-harming behaviour in young people. *British Journal of Nursing, 16*(3), 148–152.

Ganzini, L., & Dobscha, S. K. (2008). Prevalence of depression and anxiety in patients requesting physicians' aid in dying: A cross-sectional survey. *British Medical Journal* [online]. Retrieved December 16, 2008 from http://www.bmj.com/cgi/content/abstract/337/oct07_2/a1682

Harvard Medical School. (2006, September). Improving care for depression. *Harvard Mental Health Letter, 23*(3), 1–2.

Harvard Medical School. (2007, July). Antidepressants and suicide. *Harvard Mental Health Letter, 24*(1), 1–4.

Harvard Medical School. (2008, May). Positive psychology in practice. *Harvard Mental Health Letter, 24*(11), 1–3.

Joe, S., & Bryant, H. (2007). Evidence-based suicide prevention screening in schools. *Children & Schools, 29*(4), 219–227.

Karch, D. L., Lubell, K. M., Friday, J., Patel, N., & Williams, D. D. (2008). Surveillance for violent deaths—National Violent Death Reporting System, 16 States, 2005. *Morbidity and Mortality Weekly Report, 57*(SS03), 1–43, 45.

Koehler, S. A. (2007). The role of suicide notes in death investigation. *Journal of Forensic Nursing, 3*(2), 87–92.

McIntosh, J. L. (2006). *U.S.A. suicide: 2003 official final data.* Retrieved April 29, 2008, from http://www.suicidepreventioncenter.org/files/2003datapgb.pdf

Moorhead, S., Johnson, M., Maas, M., & Swanson, E. (2008). *Nursing outcomes classification (NOC)* (4th ed.). St. Louis: Mosby.

North American Nursing Diagnosis Association International (NANDA-I). (2009). *NANDA-I nursing diagnoses: Definitions and classification 2009–2011.* Oxford, United Kingdom: Author.

Ortiz, M. (2006). Staying alive! A suicide prevention overview. *Journal of Psychosocial Nursing and Mental Health Services, 44*(12), 43–49.

Patterson, P., Whittington, R., & Boggs, J. (2007). Testing the effectiveness of an educational intervention aimed at changing attitudes to self-harm. *Journal of Psychiatric and Mental Health Nursing, 14*, 100–105.

Patterson, W. M., Dohn, H. H., Bird, J., & Patterson, G. A. (1983). Evaluation of suicidal patients: The SAD PERSONS scale. *Psychosomatics, 24*, 343–345, 348–349.

Price, N. (2007). Improving emergency care for patients who self harm. *Emergency Nurse, 15*(8), 30–36.

Sadock, B. J., & Sadock, V. A. (2008). *Kaplan and Sadock's concise textbook of clinical psychiatry* (3rd ed.). Philadelphia: Lippincott Williams & Wilkins.

Vessier-Batcher, M., & Douglas, D. (2006). Coping with complicated grief in survivors of homicide and suicide decedents. *Journal of Forensic Nursing, 2*(1), 25–32.

Zayas, L. H., & Pilat, A. M. (2008). Suicidal behavior in Latinas: Explanatory cultural factors and implications for intervention. *The American Association of Suicidology, 38*, 334–342.

Zivin, K., Kim, M., McCarthy, J., Austin, K., Hoggatt, K., & Walters, H. (2007). Suicide mortality among individuals receiving treatment for depression in the veterans affairs health system: Associations with patient and treatment setting characteristics. *American Journal of Public Health, 97*, 2193–2197.

CHAPTER 25

Anger, Aggression, and Violence

Lorann Murphy and Verna Benner Carson

Key Terms and Concepts

aggression, 565
anger, 565
de-escalation techniques, 572
restraint, 574

seclusion, 574
trauma-informed care, 568
validation therapy, 580
violence, 566

Objectives

1. Compare and contrast three theories that explore the determinants for anger, aggression, and violence.
2. Compare and contrast interventions for a patient with healthy coping skills with those for a patient with marginal coping behaviors.
3. Apply at least four principles of de-escalation with a moderately angry patient.
4. Describe two criteria for the use of seclusion or restraint over verbal intervention.

5. Discuss two types of assessment and their value in the nursing process.
6. Role-play with classmates by using understandable but unhelpful responses to anger and aggression in patients; discuss how these responses can affect nursing interventions.

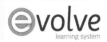 Visit the Evolve website for an **Audio Glossary & Flashcards, Concept Map Creator**, and additional resources related to the content in this chapter: **http://evolve.elsevier.com/Varcarolis/foundations**

Anger, aggression, and violence are the subject of daily news headlines. Evidence of the scope and prevalence of the problem can been seen in an expanding list of terminology used to describe specific types of aggression. *Road rage* is a dangerous habit rampant in high-stress industrialized societies and is accompanied by cursing, offensive gestures, and cutting others off while driving. *Air rage* is manifested as objectionable behavior, aggressive utterances, threats, and violence within the confines of an aircraft. *Desk rage* includes lashing out at work. Hospitals, as 24-hour-a-day, high-stress environments, have even earned a term for their own brand of confrontation: *ward rage.*

CLINICAL PICTURE

Anger is an emotional response to frustration of desires, a threat to one's needs (emotional or physical), or a challenge. It is a normal emotion that can even be viewed as positive when it is expressed in a healthy way. It can be used as a motivator or an aid in survival (Kassinove & Tafrate, 2006), but problems begin to occur when anger is expressed through aggression or violence.

Aggression is an action or behavior that results in a verbal or physical attack. Aggression tends to be used synonymously with violence; however, aggression is not always inappropriate and is sometimes necessary for self-protection. On the other hand, **violence** is always an objectionable act that involves intentional use of force that results in, or has the potential to result in, injury to another person.

Coping with a patient's anger is a challenge. Effective nursing intervention becomes more difficult when the anger is directed at the nurse. Nursing interventions for anger and aggression should begin when patients experience increased anxiety. Consult Chapter 11 for interventions that can be used when anxiety is escalating.

EPIDEMIOLOGY

As a nurse, you can be sure that you will deal with violent behavior. The Centers for Disease Control and Prevention (CDC) (2008) reported more than 50,000 deaths from suicide and homicide in 2005. The National Hospital Ambulatory Medical Care Survey reported that in 2005 there were 1.7 million emergency room visits for treatment of assault. The CDC (2008) suggests that the widespread incidence of aggression and violence indicates that these are common components of social interactions in many environments, including hospitals.

Violence can occur anywhere in the hospital, but it is most frequent in the following areas (Estryn-Chandler, 2008):

- Psychiatric units
- Emergency departments
- Geriatric units

Assault on inpatient psychiatric units is of worldwide concern. Although anyone working in a hospital may become a victim of violence, nurses and aides (who have the most contact with patients) are at higher risk. A nurse is estimated to have a 1 in 10 chance of injury as a result of an act of aggression from a patient (Foster et al., 2007).

Refer to Chapter 26 for statistics related to abuse of children, elders, and intimate partners; and Chapter 27 for statistics on sexual assault.

COMORBIDITY

Although anger is a universal emotion, not everyone responds to the anger with aggression and violence. A great deal of research has been done on aggression and violence in persons with post-traumatic stress disorders (PTSD) and substance abuse disorders (Sirotich, 2008). Anger also coexists with depression, anxiety, psychosis, and personality disorders (Kassinove & Tafrate, 2006).

Anger and hostility have effects on physical well-being; they are risk factors for hypertension and cardiovascular disease, including ischemic heart disease and cerebral vascular attacks (Kassinove & Tafrate, 2006). Suppression of anger has been shown to increase diastolic blood pressure and heart rate (Jorgensen & Kolodziej, 2007). Suppressed anger has also been shown to increase a person's perception of pain (Quartana & Burns, 2007).

ETIOLOGY

Biological Factors

Many neurological conditions are associated with anger and aggression. For example, certain brain tumors, Alzheimer's disease, temporal lobe epilepsy, and traumatic injury to certain parts of the brain result in changes to personality that include increased violence. Many patients with brain injury have severe behavior disorders that disrupt their lives, including aggressiveness.

One area of the brain known to be associated with aggression is the limbic system, which mediates primitive emotion and behaviors necessary for survival. The limbic system contains several structures that appear to have a role in the production of aggression. The area of the brain called the *amygdala* mediates anger experiences, judging events as either aversive or rewarding. In animal studies, stimulation of the amygdala produces rage responses, whereas lesions in the same structure produce docility. The temporal lobe of the brain shares some structures with the limbic system. Memory is thought to be integrated in the temporal lobe; memory of previous insult is important in the cognitive appraisal of threat in the face of new stimuli. This lobe is also the source of complex partial seizures, which may give rise to aggressive behavior (Ito et al., 2007).

The prefrontal cortex also has been identified as playing an important role in aggressive behavior. This was first noted in persons who had lesions or injury that caused aggressive behavior (Siever, 2008). Individuals with antisocial personality disorder have been shown to have less grey matter in their prefrontal cortexes (Narayan et al., 2009). In EEG analyses, a correlation has been found between left frontal activity and anger (Harmon-Jones, 2007).

Neurotransmitters play a vital role in anger and aggression. Serotonin, dopamine, norepinephrine, gamma-aminobutyric acid (GABA), glutamate, and acetylcholine all have an impact on anger and aggression (Siever, 2008). Studies have shown a relationship between impulsive aggression and low levels of serotonin (Gross & Sanders, 2008). Depressed patients with impulsivity and anger may have decreased dopamine receptors (Dougherty et al., 2006). Dopamine has also been linked to aggressive outbursts (de Almeida et al., 2005).

Some individuals are biologically more predisposed than others to respond to life events with irritability, easy frustration, and anger. This predisposition may be a function of genetics or of neurological development that occurs in the context of certain infant and childhood environments. These two risk factors appear to combine in an exponential way. Nevertheless, if all the dimensions of anger are centrally mediated, then successful interventions can be designed to target any of its manifestations. This is likely the reason biological, pharmacological, behavioral, and cognitive strategies are all useful in the management of anger and aggression.

Psychological Factors

Freud wrote in *Civilization and Its Discontents* that the conflict between sexual needs and societal norms was the source of mankind's dissatisfaction, aggression, hostility, and ultimately violence. More recently, Menninger (2007) asserted that the struggle for control over our lives is fundamental in every person. If that control is threatened, we experience trauma, and it is from that trauma that anger, aggression, and violence may originate. Interventions should be focused on realizing that the patient may be experiencing trauma and helping the patient feel as though he has some control in his or her life.

Early behaviorists held that emotions, including anger, were learned responses to environmental stimuli (Skinner, 1953). The stimulus is often a perceived threat, and this cognition leads to the emotional and physiological arousal necessary to take action. Although the threat is usually understood as an alert to physical danger, Beck (1976) noted that perceived assault on areas of personal domain, such as values, moral code, and protective rules, can also lead to anger. For example, clinic patients kept waiting for long periods of time without explanation may interpret this as neglect and a lack of respect. Anger may escalate when the initial appraisal is followed by cognitions such as "They have no right to treat me this way. I am a person too." These additional cognitions lead to escalating behavior that can erupt into violence unless the situation is defused through successful interventions.

In some individuals, the period of escalation can be rapid. In contrast, patients less predisposed to anger might interpret the wait as a sign that the clinic is busy. These patients might be frustrated by the situation, but in the absence of anger, they might access and utilize skills such as asking how much longer the wait is likely to be, finding distractions in the environment, or rescheduling the appointment.

Social learning theorists conducted research that showed children learn aggression by imitating others and that people repeat behavior that is rewarded (Bandura, 1973). Thus children who watch television violence or experience violence in the home learn violent ways of resolving problems. Not only is television violence portrayed as an option for resolving conflict, but most of those violent acts are presented as having no negative consequences. It has also been shown that a positive parental attitude toward fighting increases the likelihood for youth aggression, hostility, and suspension from school (Solomon et al., 2008) (Considering Culture box).

CONSIDERING CULTURE

The Culture of Bullying in Schools

School violence has been a concern throughout the world for almost 2 decades. Between 1992 and 1996, there were 116 school-related homicides in the United States. Bullying is another less extreme form of violence that is far more prevalent and has significant consequences.

Bullying is any negative activity intended to bother or harm someone else, including teasing, kicking, hitting, and spitting. It has been found that approximately 26% of school-age children are involved in bullying, either as victim or aggressor (Glew et al., 2008). It has been estimated that 160,000 school days are missed as a consequence of bullying (Randall, 2008). Victims are more likely to feel unsafe at school, have lower GPAs, and feel sad most days. But of most concern is that they have a higher likelihood of saying it was acceptable to bring a gun to school.

There has been a great call for action. Some schools have adopted zero tolerance policies to any form of violence. The role of the school nurse is an integral part of intervention. The nurse should be aware of some of the signs of victimhood, such as frequent injuries in one child, new depressive symptoms, frequent "illnesses," or coming to the office at the same time daily. The nurse must assess and intervene according to the assessment.

To decrease bullying, schools must adopt a team approach, implement programming, and change policies to prevent violence from occurring.

Centers for Disease Control and Prevention. (2008). School-associated homicides—United States, 1992-2006. *Morbidity and Mortality Weekly Report, 57*(2), 34–36.
Glew, G. M., Fan, M., Katon, W., & Rivara, F. P. (2008). Bullying and school safety. *Journal of Pediatrics, 152*(1), 123–128.
Hahn, R., Fuqua-Whitley, D., Wethington, H., Lowy, J., Crosby, A., Fullilove, M. et al. (2007). *American Journal of Preventive Medicine, 33*(2 Suppl), S114–S129.
Randall Consulting, Inc. (2008). *Stopping school violence.* <http://www.stoppingschoolviolence.com> Accessed 16.01.2009.

APPLICATION OF THE NURSING PROCESS

ASSESSMENT
General Assessment

When patients are experiencing anger, it may manifest as increased demands, irritability, frowning, redness of the face, pacing, twisting of the hands, or clenching and unclenching of the fists. Speech may either be increased in rate and volume or may be slowed, pointed, and quiet. Any change in behavior from what is typical for that patient must be addressed. Box 25-1 identifies signs and symptoms that indicate the risk of escalating anger leading to aggressive behavior.

It is also important to assess the patient's history of aggression or violence. Most of our reactions to stimuli come from our previous experiences; therefore, identifying patients' triggers is essential. Initial and ongoing assessment of the patient can reveal problems before they escalate to anger and aggression. Such assessment also leads directly to the appropriate nursing diagnosis and intervention.

Trauma-informed care is an older concept of providing care that has recently been reintroduced. It is based on the notion that disruptive psychiatric patients often have histories that include violence and victimization (Estryn-Chandler, 2008). These traumatic histories can impede patients' ability to self-soothe, result in negative coping responses, and create a vulnerability to coercive interventions (such as restraint) by staff. Trauma-informed care focuses on the patient's past experiences of violence or trauma and the role it currently plays in their lives.

Careful assessment can reduce the potential for violence. In a study conducted at New York State Psychiatric Institute, patients filled out a questionnaire that identified things that made them upset, how they responded to being upset, and how they wanted to be treated when they became upset. Examples of how they wanted to be treated included talking with them and allowing them time out alone. Making use of the patients' suggestions resulted in a decreased amount of time in restraints (Evidence-Based Practice box) and seclusion and a reduction in the number of fights and assaults on the unit (Hellerstein et al., 2007).

BOX 25-1 Predictors of Violence

1. Signs and symptoms that usually *(but not always)* precede violence:
   - Hyperactivity: most important predictor of imminent violence (e.g., pacing, restlessness)
   - Increasing anxiety and tension: clenched jaw or fist, rigid posture, fixed or tense facial expression, mumbling to self (patient may have shortness of breath, sweating, and rapid pulse)
   - Verbal abuse: profanity, argumentativeness
   - Loud voice, change of pitch; or very soft voice, forcing others to strain to hear
   - Intense eye contact or avoidance of eye contact
2. Recent acts of violence, including property violence
3. Stone silence
4. Alcohol or drug intoxication
5. Possession of a weapon or object that may be used as a weapon (e.g., fork, knife, rock)
6. Isolation that is new
7. Milieu characteristics conducive to violence:
   - Overcrowding
   - Staff inexperience
   - Provocative or controlling staff
   - Poor limit setting
   - Arbitrary revocation of privileges

EVIDENCE-BASED PRACTICE

Reducing the Use of Restraints

Sclafani, M. J., Humphrey, F. J., Repko, S., Ko, H. S., Wallen, M. C., & DiGiacomo, A. (2008). Reducing patient restraints: A pilot approach using clinical case review. *Perspectives in Psychiatric Care, 44*(1), 32–39.

Problem
The excessive reliance on the use of mechanical restraints to minimize disruptive patient behaviors is being met with increasing initiatives to reduce their use. National, state, and local initiatives, as well as federal regulations and accreditation standards, have resulted in strong advocacy for restraint elimination. There is also increasing awareness on the part of service providers and their unions regarding the damaging effects restraints have on patients, clinicians, and caretakers.

Purpose of Study

The purpose of this study was to implement alternatives to the use of mechanical restraints and evaluate the effectiveness of these approaches in contrast to approaches that had relied on the significant use of restraints.

Methods

A group of interdisciplinary consultants used a variety of approaches in working with both the unit staff and two selected patients at an acute psychiatric hospital. Both patients had a history of violent behaviors that resulted in the frequent use of mechanical restraints. This pilot study focused on enhancing clinical care provided to patients who are dually diagnosed with mental illness and developmental disabilities. Staff education and training, in conjunction with patient-centered approaches, significantly decreased the use of restraints.

Key Findings

- During the 16-month period of this pilot study, there was a steady decline in the use of restraints from 36 episodes per month to 0.

- The use of patient coaching (helping people discover and improve their coping skills) and group and individual problem-solving approaches significantly decrease the need to use mechanical restraints.
- Staff education and training that focus on person-centered approaches, positive reinforcements, and strength-based treatment assist in creating more humane living conditions and a therapeutic milieu for patients.

Implications for Nursing Practice

Nurses served as an integral part of both the consultation team and the unit staff in this pilot study. The study revealed the success of the interdisciplinary team working together to understand the needs of a particular population and intervene more effectively. Evidence-based strategies can significantly improve the care of vulnerable patients, as well as strengthen the cohesion and effectiveness of the staff.

Self-Assessment

Like patients, nurses have their own histories. The nurse's ability to intervene safely depends on self-awareness of strengths, needs, concerns, and vulnerabilities. Without this awareness, nursing interventions are marked by impulsive or emotion-based responses, which may be nontherapeutic. Self-awareness includes knowledge of personal responses to anger and aggression, including choice of words and tone of voice, as well as nonverbal communication via body posture and facial expressions. Awareness of the personal and cultural norms is also essential. In addition, staff must be aware of personal dynamics that may trigger emotions and reactions that are not therapeutic with specific patients. Finally, the nurse must assess situational factors (e.g., fatigue, insufficient staff) that may decrease normal competence in the management of complex patient problems.

Self-assessment promotes calm responses to patient anger and potential aggression. These responses are further supported by the:
- Creation of an environment that encourages staff to speak openly about their feelings
- Use of humor
- Development of a professional support system
- Variance of clinical work

Assessment Guidelines Anger and Aggression

1. A history of violence is the single best predictor of future violence.
2. Patients who are delusional, hyperactive, impulsive, or predisposed to irritability are at higher risk for violence.
3. Assess patient risk for violence:
   - Does the patient have a wish or intent to harm?
   - Does the patient have a plan?
   - Does the patient have means available to carry out the plan?
   - Does the patient have demographic risk factors: male gender, age 14 to 24 years, low socioeconomic status, inadequate support system, prison time?
4. Aggression by patients occurs most often in the context of limit setting by the nurse.
5. Patients with a history of limited coping skills, including lack of assertiveness or use of intimidation, are at higher risk of using violence.
6. Assess self for personal triggers and responses likely to escalate patient violence, including patient characteristics or situations that trigger impatience, irritation, or defensiveness.
7. Assess personal sense of competence when in any situation of potential conflict; consider asking for the assistance of another staff member.

DIAGNOSIS

Patients may have coping skills that are adequate for day-to-day events but may be overwhelmed by the stresses of illness or hospitalization. Other patients may have a pattern of maladaptive coping that is marginally effective and consists of a set of coping strategies that is unhealthy and may increase the possibility of anger and aggression. When the nursing assessment identifies potential for anger or aggression, *Ineffective coping* (overwhelmed or maladaptive), *Stress overload, Risk for self-directed violence,* and *Risk for other-directed violence* are important nursing diagnoses to consider (North American Nursing Diagnoses Association International, 2009).

OUTCOMES IDENTIFICATION

When interventions are planned for angry and aggressive patients, having clearly defined outcome criteria is important for identifying the behaviors that staff can encourage if their interventions have been successful. The *Nursing Outcomes Classification (NOC)* outlines specific outcome criteria for use with angry and aggressive patients (Moorhead et al., 2008). Table 25-1 describes selected potential outcomes for aggressive behaviors.

PLANNING

Planning interventions necessitates having a sound assessment, including past history (previous acts of violence, co-morbid disorders), present coping skills, and willingness and capacity of the patient to learn alternative and nonviolent ways of handling angry feelings.

Does the patient have:
• Good coping skills but is presently overwhelmed?

• Marginal coping skills and uses anger or violence as a way to cover other feelings and gain a sense of mastery or control?
• A personality disorder or chronic psychotic disorder and is prone to violence?
• Cognitive deficits that predispose to anger in the form of misinterpretation of environmental stimuli?

Does the situation call for:
• Psycho-educational approaches to teach the patient new skills for handling anger?
• Immediate intervention to prevent overt violence (de-escalation techniques, restraint/seclusion, and/or medications)?

Does the environment provide:
• Privacy for the patient?
• Enough space for patients or is there overcrowding?
• A healthy balance between structured time and quiet time?
• Adequate personnel available to safely and effectively deal with a potentially violent situation?

Do the skills of the staff call for:
• Additional education for staff in verbal de-escalation techniques?
• Counseling of staff regarding use of punitive and arbitrary approaches to patients?
• Additional training in restraint techniques?

IMPLEMENTATION

Ideally, intervention begins prior to any sign of escalation. It is important to develop a relationship of trust with the patient by having numerous brief, nonthreatening, nondirective interactions (e.g., talking about the weather, sports, or something of interest to the patient).

TABLE 25-1 *NOC* Outcome Indicators for Aggression Self-Control		
Nursing Outcome and Definition	**Intermediate Indicators**	**Short-Term Indicators**
Aggression Self-Control: Self-restraint of assaultive, combative, or destructive behaviors toward others	Maintains self-control without supervision Upholds contract to restrain aggressive behaviors	Identifies when angry/frustrated Vents negative feelings appropriately Expresses needs in a nondestructive manner Refrains from striking others Refrains from destroying property Uses specific techniques to control anger/frustration Identifies situations that precipitate hostility

Data from Moorhead, S., Johnson, M., Maas, M. L., & Swanson, E. (2008). *Nursing outcome classification (NOC)* (4th ed.). St. Louis: Mosby.

In settings in which staff can reasonably expect episodes of patient anger and aggression, regular teaching and practice of verbal and nonverbal interventions are essential. This fosters nurses' increased confidence in their own abilities and those of co-workers.

Psychosocial Interventions

As you try to determine what the patient is feeling, you have already begun to intervene. During this process, you are attempting to hear the patient's feelings and concerns. Frequently this can be accomplished by telling the patient that you are concerned and want to listen. The patient needs reassurance that people are interested and willing to help. It is essential to acknowledge the patient's needs, regardless of whether the expressed needs are rational or possible to meet. It is important to clearly and simply state your expectations for the patient's behavior: "I expect that you will stay in control."

However, patient behavior may escalate quickly, or the patient may mask early signs of distress. Nurses may be distracted and miss those early signs. Other patients may be acutely ill and not amenable to early nursing interventions. In these situations, the problem with anger may not be resolved before the risk for violence arises. When anger and aggression are the priority problems, de-escalation of anger is the primary nursing intervention. Seclusion, restraint, or pharmacological means of de-escalation may be necessary to ensure the safety of patients and staff.

When you approach the patient, convey that you are calm, controlled, open, nonthreatening, and caring. Maintain a relaxed posture. If you are experiencing fear, you may find that this is quite challenging. Maintaining a calm exterior while your interior is in an upheaval requires considerable self-discipline and will come with experience.

It is important to demonstrate respect for the patient's personal space. Your eyes should be on the same level as the patient's to decrease a sense of intimidation and communicate to the patient that you are speaking as equals. Allow the patient enough personal space so that you are not perceived as intrusive but not so much space that the patient cannot speak in a normal voice. Be sure you have left yourself an escape route if the patient becomes out of control. Always stay about 1 foot farther than the patient can reach with arms or legs.

Patients who are poised for violence need much more space than those who are not. While you are giving the patient space, the patient may be invading your space with verbal abuse and the use of profanity. This may be the only way feelings can be expressed. As uncomfortable as this may be, you cannot take the patient's words personally or respond in kind. It is also important not to end the conversation because of the patient's verbal abusiveness or to forbid the patient from communicating in this way.

When anger is escalating, a patient's ability to process decreases. It is important to speak to the patient slowly and in short sentences, using a low and calm voice. Never yell, but continue to model controlled behavior. Use open-ended statements and questions such as "You think people are always unkind to you?" rather than challenging statements such as "What is wrong with you?" Avoid ending statements with "okay?" because it may create ambivalence in the patient and give the erroneous impression that choices exist. It is also important to avoid punitive, threatening, accusatory, or challenging statements to the patient; rather, find out what is behind the angry feelings and behaviors. Honestly verbalize the patient's options, and encourage the individual to assume responsibility for choices made. You may want to give two options, such as "Do you want to go to your room or to the quiet room for a while?" This approach decreases the sense of powerlessness that often precipitates violence.

It is vital to pay attention to the environment. Choose a quiet place to talk to the patient but one that is visible to staff. This is most beneficial in helping a patient regain control. Staff should know who is working with the patient, keep an eye on the interaction, and be prepared to intervene if the situation escalates. At this point, other patients should be moved away, and the environment around the patient should be free from any object that could be used as a weapon.

Considerations for Staff Safety

There are six basic considerations for ensuring safety:

1. Avoid wearing dangling earrings or necklaces. The patient may become focused on these and grab at them, causing serious injury. Such jewelry should be removed before dealing with an agitated patient.
2. Ensure that there is enough staff for backup. Only one person should talk to the patient, but staff need to maintain an unobtrusive presence in case the situation escalates.
3. Always know the layout of the area. Correct placement of furniture and elimination of obstacles or hazards are important to prevent injury if the patient requires physical interventions.
4. Do not stand directly in front of the patient or in front of the doorway; this position could be interpreted as confrontational. It is better to stand off to the side and encourage the patient to have a seat.
5. If a patient's behavior begins to escalate, provide feedback. "You seem to be very upset." Such an observation allows exploration of the patient's feelings and may lead to de-escalation of the situation.

6. Avoid confrontation with the patient, either through verbal means or through a "show of force" with security guards. Verbal confrontation and discussion of the incident must occur when the patient is calm. A show of force by security guards may serve to escalate the patient's behavior; therefore, security personnel are better kept in the background until they are needed to assist.

Box 25-2 lists some principles underlying de-escalation techniques.

Pharmacological Interventions

When a patient is showing increased signs of symptoms of anxiety or agitation, it is perfectly appropriate to offer the patient a prn (as-needed) medication to alleviate symptoms. When used in conjunction with psychosocial interventions and de-escalation techniques, this can prevent an aggressive or violent incident. The nurse's ongoing assessment of behavior changes will give the patient the opportunity to obtain pharmacological relief from symptoms.

Antianxiety agents and antipsychotics are used in the treatment of acute symptoms of anger and aggression. These agents, their form of delivery, and considerations are listed in Table 25-2. During aggressive or violent incidents, haloperidol has historically been the most widely used antipsychotic, but with the intro-

duction of intramuscular (IM) atypical antipsychotics, the use of olanzapine and ziprasidone has become more widespread, in part because of the severe side effects of haloperidol. A combination of antipsychotic (haloperidol or perphenazine) and a benzodiazepine (lorazepam) can be given IM. Diphenhydramine or benztropine is added to the injection to reduce extrapyramidal side effects.

It is the nurse's role to assess for appropriateness of prn medications. It is important to remember that patients often feel traumatized by the use of IM injections, so oral medications should always be used if appropriate (Gilburt et al., 2008). The nurse also educates the patient about the medication, the reason it is being given, and the potential side effects of the medication, even if the patient is out of control.

The long-term treatment of anger, aggression, and violence is based on treating the underlying psychiatric disorder. SSRIs, lithium, anticonvulsants, benzodiazepines, atypical antipsychotics, and beta-blockers are all used successfully for specific patient populations. Anger and aggression related to attention deficit disorder/attention deficit hyperactivity disorder may be reduced through the use of psychostimulants. Table 25-3 gives an overview of the drugs used to treat chronic aggression.

Health Teaching and Health Promotion

One of the most important roles a nurse plays in a patient's recovery is that of role model and educator. You can model appropriate responses and ways to cope with anger, teach patients a variety of methods to appropriately express anger, and educate patients regarding coping mechanisms, de-escalation techniques, and self-soothing skills that can be used to manage behavior. It is also helpful to assist the patient in identifying triggers for angry or aggressive behavior. One method that can be used if the patient is not out of control is a "do over." The patient who responds inappropriately can try again to respond in a more appropriate way while being coached by the nurse.

Case Management

A multidisciplinary approach is important for all patients but especially a patient with behavioral issues. A plan of care must be implemented and carried out by all members of the health care team. A focus on intervention strategies should be discussed during treatment team meetings. The plan for discharge with appropriate follow-up, possibly with an anger-management course, must be put into place. The consistency of intervention among all team members is key to the patient's success.

BOX 25-2 De-escalation Techniques: Practice Principles

- Maintain the patient's self-esteem and dignity.
- Maintain calmness (your own and the patient's).
- Assess the patient and the situation.
- Identify stressors and stress indicators.
- Respond as early as possible.
- Use a calm, clear tone of voice.
- Invest time.
- Remain honest.
- Establish what the patient considers to be his or her need.
- Be goal oriented.
- Maintain a large personal space.
- Avoid verbal struggles.
- Give several options.
- Make clear the options.
- Utilize a nonaggressive posture.
- Use genuineness and empathy.
- Attempt to be confidently aware.
- Use verbal, nonverbal, and communication skills.
- Be assertive (not aggressive).
- Assess for personal safety.

From Mason, T., & Chandley, M. (1999). *Management of violence and aggression* (p. 73). Philadelphia: Churchill Livingstone.

TABLE 25-2 Drugs Used for Acute Management of Violent Behavior

Generic (Trade)	Forms	Considerations
ANTIANXIETY AGENTS (BENZODIAZEPINES)		
Lorazepam (Ativan)	PO, SL, IM, IV	Drug of choice in this class Use with caution with hepatic dysfunction
Alprazolam (Xanax)	PO	Paradoxical (opposite response) with personality disorders and older adults
Diazepam (Valium)	PO, IM, IV	Rapid onset of calming and sedating Long half-life; use with caution in older adults
CONVENTIONAL ANTIPSYCHOTICS		
Haloperidol (Haldol)	PO, IM, IV	Favorable side-effect profile. Due to risk of neuroleptic malignant syndrome, keep hydrated, check vital signs, and test for muscle rigidity
Chlorpromazine (Thorazine)	PO, PR, IM	Very sedating Injections can cause pain; watch for hypotension
ATYPICAL ANTIPSYCHOTICS		
Risperidone (Risperdal)	PO	Calms while treating underlying condition Watch for hypotension Increased risk of stroke in older adults
Olanzapine (Zyprexa)	PO, IM	Useful in patients unresponsive to haloperidol Calms while treating underlying condition Avoid when using lorazepam Increased risk of stroke in older adults
Ziprasidone (Geodon)	PO, IM	Use cautiously with QT prolongation Less sedating
COMBINATIONS		
Haloperidol (Haldol), lorazepam (Ativan), and diphenhydramine (Benadryl) or benztropine (Cogentin)	IM	Commonly used in the acute setting Men who are young and athletic are at increased risk of dystonia Consider akathisia if agitation increases
Perphenazine (Trilafon), lorazepam (Ativan), and diphenhydramine (Benadryl) or benztropine (Cogentin)	IM	Consider this combination if patient has difficulty taking haloperidol

Data from Gross, A. F., & Sanders, K. M. (2008). Aggression and violence. In T. S. Stern, J. F. Rosenbaum, M. Fava, J. Biederman, & S. L. Rauch (Eds.), *Massachusetts General Hospital comprehensive clinical psychiatry* (pp. 895–905). St. Louis: Mosby; and Martinez, M., Marangell, L. B., & Martinez, J. M. (2008). Psychopharmacology. In R. E. Hales, S. C. Yudofsky, & G. O. Gabbard (Eds.), *Textbook of psychiatry*. Arlington, VA: American Psychiatric Publishing.

Milieu Management

A thorough consideration of the environment is important when considering anger and aggression on the unit. It is important to be proactive not reactive. It is hard to imagine how the stimulation of a psychiatric unit might be experienced by someone whose anxiety is extremely high or who is delusional or confused.

If the patient has enough control, sometimes simply taking a timeout in his own room is sufficient. A multisensory room is another form of time out. It is also known as a *Snoezelen*, named partly from the Dutch word for "dozing." This quiet room is partially lit, has relaxing music available, and comfortable furniture and soft pillows. It promotes feelings of security and safety.

TABLE 25-3 Drugs Used for Long-Term Management of Chronic Aggression

Class	Population	Considerations
Selective serotonin reuptake inhibitors (SSRIs)	Antisocial personality, schizophrenia, dementia, brain injury	Reduces irritability, impulsivity, and aggression Stabilizes mood Use cautiously with bipolar disorder
Lithium	Antisocial personality, prison inmates, mental retardation, brain injury	TSH levels measured prior to treatment Due to anti-aggressive properties, blood levels can be lower than those necessary to treat mania
Anticonvulsants	Prison inmates, antisocial/borderline personality, substance use, attention-deficit disorders, brain injury, schizophrenia	Significantly reduces impulsive aggression Similar doses with bipolar disorder Multiple drug interactions Periodic blood levels Monitor CBC and LFTs
Gabapentin	Anxiety disorder, personality disorders	No interactions with other anticonvulsants
Benzodiazepines	Anxiety disorder	Potential for abuse, dependence, and withdrawal May cause paradoxical aggression
Atypical antipsychotics	Schizophrenia, psychosis, mania, borderline personality, mental retardation	Clozapine superior to other atypicals Fewer side effects and greater adherence than conventional antipsychotics Risperidone reduces irritability in autistic disorder
Beta-blockers	Schizophrenia, brain injury, dementia, mental retardation	Propranolol contraindicated with asthma, COPD, and IDDM Sedation side effects may explain anti-aggressive effects
Psychostimulants	ADD/ADHD in children and adults	Potential for addiction and abuse

ADD/ADHD, Attention deficit disorder/attention deficit hyperactivity disorder; *CBC*, complete blood count; *COPD*, chronic obstructive pulmonary disease; *IDDM*, insulin-dependent diabetes mellitus; *LFTs*, liver function tests; *TSH*, thyroid-stimulating hormone.
Data from Gross, A. F., & Sanders, K. M. (2008). Aggression and violence. In T. S. Stern, J. F. Rosenbaum, M. Fava, J. Biederman, & S. L. Rauch (Eds.), *Massachusetts General Hospital comprehensive clinical psychiatry* (pp. 895–905). St. Louis: Mosby; Scott, C. L., Quanbeck, C. D., & Resnick, P. J. (2008). Assessment of dangerousness. In R. E. Hales, S. C. Yudofsky, & G. O. Gabbard (Eds.), *Textbook of psychiatry* (pp. 1655–1672). Arlington, VA: American Psychiatric Publishing; and Stahl, S. M. (2008). *Stahl's essential psychopharmacology* (3rd ed.). New York: Cambridge University Press.

Realize that behavior rarely occurs in a vacuum. The nurse must examine the milieu as a whole and identify the stressors patients have to deal with, especially patients who have an antisocial personality disorder. These individuals have a tendency to create havoc and make it appear that another patient is at fault, either for their own pleasure or for their own purposes (e.g., escaping the unit or getting into the medication room). So even while dealing with an incident, staff must be aware of what could be happening in the surrounding environment.

Use of Restraints or Seclusion

Occasionally, despite numerous interventions, a patient will become violent and require restraint or seclusion. When this happens, it is essential to have an organized approach to the seclusion or restraint. According to the U.S. Department of Health & Human Services, Centers for Medicare and Medicaid Services (2008), **seclusion** refers to "the involuntary confinement of a patient alone in a room, or area from which the patient is physically prevented from leaving" (p. 96). The goal of seclusion is never punitive. Rather, *the goal is safety of the patient and others.*

Restraint is defined as "any manual method, physical or mechanical device, material or equipment that immobilizes or reduces the ability of a patient to move his or her arms, legs, body or head freely" (p. 90). Seclusion or physical restraint is used only after alternative interventions have been tried, including verbal intervention, behavioral care plan, medication, decrease in sensory stimulation, removal of a particular problematic stimulus, presence of a significant other, frequent observation, or use of a sitter who provides 24-hour, one-on-one observation of the patient. Seclusion or restraint is used only if the patient presents a clear and present danger to self or others.

Prior to an episode of seclusion, a patient must be assessed for contraindications for seclusion: pregnancy, COPD, head or spinal injury, seizure disorder, abuse, history of surgery or fracture, morbid obesity, and sleep apnea. A patient may not be held in seclusion or restraint without an order from a licensed practitioner. Once in restraint, a patient must be directly observed and formally assessed at frequent, regular intervals for level of awareness, level of activity, safety within the restraints, hydration, toileting needs, nutrition, and comfort. The frequency of observation is mandated by licensing and accreditation agencies.

Each team member is trained in the correct use of physical restraining maneuvers, as well as the use of physical restraints. The team is organized before approaching the patient so that each team member knows his or her individual responsibility regarding limb securing. Before approaching the patient, the team is prepared with the correct number and size of restraints and with medication, if ordered. The patient must be given every opportunity to regain control so that the least restrictive method can be used. If restraints are to be used, the patient is informed at this point of the team's intent and the reason for the actions. The team remains calm and acts as quickly as possible.

Once the patient is restrained, the nurse must get an order for the restraint episode from the appropriate health care provider. The nurse may also get an order for medication and administer it to the patient. The team leader continues to relate to the patient in a calm, steady voice, communicating decisiveness, consistency, and control. A restraint episode is typically not planned, so these may not be an accurate reflection of what happens. Guidelines for the use of mechanical restraints are given in Box 25-3.

BOX 25-3 Guidelines for Use of Mechanical Restraint

Indications for Use
- To protect the patient from self-harm
- To prevent the patient from assaulting others

Legal Requirements
- Multidisciplinary involvement
- Appropriate health care provider's signature according to state law
- Patient advocate or relative notification
- Restraint/seclusion discontinuation as soon as possible
- No use of weapons

Documentation
- Patient's behavior leading to restraint/seclusion
- Least-restrictive measures used prior to restraint
- Interventions used
- Patient response to interventions
- Plan of care for restraint/seclusion use implemented
- Ongoing evaluations by nursing staff and appropriate health care providers

Clinical Assessments
- Patient's mental state at time of restraint
- Physical exam for medical problems possibly causing behavior changes
- Need for restraints

Observation
- Have staff in constant attendance
- Complete written record every 15 minutes

- Range of movement
- Monitor vital signs
- Observe blood flow in hands/feet
- Observe that restraint is not rubbing
- Provide for nutrition, hydration, and elimination

Release Procedure
- Patient must be able to follow commands and stay in control.
- Termination of restraints
- Debrief with patient

Restraint Tips
- Patient must be able to follow commands and stay in control.
- Physical holding of a patient against their will is a restraint.
- Physical holding of a patient for medication administration is a restraint.
- Four side rails up is a restraint except in seizure precautions.
- Keeping a patient in his room by physical intervention is seclusion.
- Tucking sheets in so tightly patient cannot move is a restraint.
- Orders for seclusion/restraint cannot be prn ("as needed").

While the patient is restrained and in seclusion, close monitoring to determine the patient's ability to reintegrate into unit activities is mandatory. Reintegration should be gradual and geared to the patient's ability to handle increasing amounts of stimulation. If the reintegration proves to be too much for the patient and results in increased agitation, the individual is returned to the room or another quiet area. Patients must be able to follow commands and control behaviors before reintegration can occur.

Generally, a structured reintegration is the best approach. It can begin by reducing four-point restraints to three-point restraints. Once the patient no longer requires the locked seclusion room or restraints and is able to exercise self-control, he or she can return to the unit. After being returned to the unit the patient should be observed carefully to maintain safety. In some cases, the patient may require further seclusion or restraint and another order must be obtained.

Immediately after the seclusion or restraint episode, the staff must debrief with each other. Staff analysis of the episode of violence, referred to as *critical incident debriefing*, is crucial for a number of reasons. First, a review is necessary to ensure that quality care was provided to the patient. Staff members need to critically examine their response to the patient. Questions to be answered include:

- Could we have done anything that would have prevented the violence? If yes, then what could have been done, and why was it not done in this situation?
- Did the team respond as a team? Were team members acting according to the policies and procedures of the unit? If not, why not?
- How do staff members feel about this patient? About this situation? Feelings of fear and anger must be discussed and handled. Otherwise the patient may be dealt with in a punitive and nontherapeutic manner. Employee morale, productivity, use of sick leave time, transfer requests, and absenteeism are all affected by patient violence, especially if a staff member has been injured. Staff members must feel supported by their peers, as well as by the organizational policies and procedures established to maintain a safe environment.
- Is there a need for additional staff education regarding how to respond to violent patients?
- How did the actual restraining process go? What could be done differently? Do not focus only on whether they were acting like a team.
- If injury occurred, has it been reported and cared for? It has been shown that there is vast underreporting of violence against health care staff.

When the patient is reintegrated into the unit, discussion with the patient is an important part of the therapeutic process. Going over what has occurred allows the patient to learn from the situation, to identify the stressors that precipitated the out-of-control behavior, and to plan alternative ways of responding to these stressors in the future.

The nurse must provide documentation in situations in which violence was either averted or actually occurred, including:

- Assessment of behaviors that occurred as the patient was escalating
- Nursing interventions and the patient's responses
- Evaluation of the interventions used
- Detailed description of the patient's behaviors during the assaultive stage
- All nursing interventions used to defuse the crisis
- Patient's response to those interventions
- Observations of the patient and interventions performed while the patient was in restraints and/or seclusion
- The way the patient was reintegrated into the unit milieu
- Documentation required by CMS and The Joint Commission

Box 25-4 lists selected Nursing Interventions Classification *(NIC)* for *Anger Control Assistance* (Bulechek et al., 2008).

BOX 25-4 *NIC* Interventions for Anger-Control Assistance

Definition: Facilitation of the expression of anger in an adaptive, nonviolent manner
Activities*:

- Establish basic trust and rapport with patient.
- Use calm, reassuring approach.
- Determine appropriate behavioral expectations for expression of anger, given patient's level of cognitive and physical functioning.
- Limit access to frustrating situations until patient is able to express anger in an adaptive manner.
- Encourage patient to seek assistance from nursing staff or responsible others during periods of increasing tension.
- Monitor potential for inappropriate aggression, and intervene before its expression.
- Prevent physical harm if anger is directed at self or others (e.g., restrain and remove potential weapons).
- Provide reassurance to patient that nursing staff will intervene to prevent patient from losing control.
- Use external controls (e.g., physical or manual restraint, time-outs, and seclusion) as needed to calm patient who is expressing anger in a maladaptive manner.

---

*Partial list.
Data from Bulechek, G. M., Butcher, H. K., & Dochterman, J. M. (2008). *Nursing interventions classification (NIC)* (5th ed.). St. Louis: Mosby.

Let's take a closer look at intervening in different settings with patients who are exhibiting anger and have the potential for aggression and violence.

Caring for Patients in General Hospital Settings

Patients With Healthy Coping Who Are Overwhelmed

A patient loses autonomy and control when hospitalized, which can cause a great deal of related distress. When this stress is combined with the uncertainty of illness, a patient may respond in ways that are not usual for them. A careful nursing assessment, with history and information from family members, helps evaluate whether a patient's anger is a usual or an unusual way of managing stress. Interventions for patients whose usual coping strategies are healthy involve finding ways to reestablish or substitute similar means of dealing with the hospitalization. This problem solving occurs in collaboration with the patient in interactions that demonstrate the nurse acknowledges the patient's distress, validates it as understandable under the circumstances, and indicates a willingness to search for solutions. Validation includes making an apology to the patient when appropriate, such as when a promised intervention (e.g., changing a dressing by a certain time) has not been delivered or sympathizing with them about the "horrible food" and assisting them to make tastier choices on the menu.

Patients who have become angry may be unable to moderate this emotion enough to problem solve with their nurses; others may be unable to communicate the source of their anger. Often, the nurse—knowing the patient and the context of the anger—can make an accurate guess at what feeling is behind the anger. Naming this feeling can lead to a dissipation of the anger, help the patient to feel understood, and lead to a calmer discussion of the distress. Some of the feelings that can precipitate anger are listed in Box 25-5. The following vignette provides an example of nursing interventions that are helpful in dissipating anger in a hospital situation. In this situation, it is most important that the medical nurse takes time to sit down with the patient while listening.

VIGNETTE

Rachel, a 41-year-old woman with a history of peripheral vascular disease, surgeries for vascular grafts, and repair of graft occlusions, is admitted to the hospital with severe pain in her left foot. Tests reveal that vessels to the foot are occluded. Additional surgery is ruled out, and medication is prescribed. Unfortunately, the medication is ineffective, and the foot begins to necrotize. Physicians discuss amputation with the patient. Rachel refuses the surgery, demands a series of unproven alternative therapies, and is extremely angry with all members of the hospital staff. The treatment team becomes increasingly impatient to schedule surgery before the tissue death worsens and because the patient is beginning to exhibit signs of systemic infection. This impatience aggravates the patient's feelings of being out of control and erodes her belief that she is a competent partner in her treatment.

Intervention. The nurse is aware that before that Rachel became disabled by progressive vascular disease, she had been employed for many years as a buyer at a local department store. The nurse knows too that the patient's family lives some distance from the hospital and is unable to visit regularly. Nursing intervention is twofold. First, Rachel's anger and unwillingness to discuss her condition ends when the nurse empathizes with her feelings of fear and being out of control. Once the anger is reduced, the nurse is able to help Rachel negotiate more time for the final decision; this allows her to process anticipatory grieving (including stages of denial, anger, and bargaining). In this interval, the patient's wish to explore alternative therapies is addressed via second and third medical opinions. Rachel is also able to spend more time discussing her concerns with her family. ■

Patients With Marginal Coping Skills

Patients whose coping skills were marginal before hospitalization need a different set of interventions than those with basically healthy ways of coping. Patients with maladaptive coping are poorly

---

BOX 25-5 Feelings That May Precipitate Anger

- Discounted
- Embarrassed
- Frightened
- Found out
- Guilty
- Humiliated
- Hurt
- Ignored
- Inadequate
- Insecure
- Unheard
- Out of control of the situation
- Rejected
- Threatened
- Tired
- Vulnerable

equipped to use alternatives when their initial attempts to cope are unsuccessful or are found to be inappropriate. Such patients frequently manifest anger that moves quickly from anxiety to aggression. For some, anger and intimidation are primary strategies used to obtain their short-term goals of feelings of control or mastery. For others, the anger occurs when limited or primitive attempts at coping are unsuccessful and alternatives are unknown. For these patients, anger and violence are particular risks in inpatient settings.

This is especially true for hospitalized patients with chemical dependence who may be anxious about being cut off from their substance of choice. They may have well-founded concerns that any physical pain will be inadequately addressed. Many patients with marginal coping also have personality styles that externalize blame. That is, they see the source of their discomfort and anxiety as being outside themselves; relief must therefore also come from an outside source (e.g., the nurse, medication).

Interventions begin with attempts to understand and meet the patient's needs. For instance, baseline anxiety can be moderated by the provision of comfort items before they are requested (e.g., decaffeinated coffee, deck of cards). This can build rapport and acts symbolically to reassure. Anxiety can also be minimized by reducing ambiguity. This strategy includes clear and concrete communication. An interaction providing clarity about what the nurse can and cannot do is most usefully ended by offering something within the nurse's power to provide (e.g., leaving the patient with a "yes"). Most hospitals have some sort of withdrawal protocol assuring the patient that they will not go through withdrawal without medication. This can be very anxiety relieving if the patient has a chemical dependency problem.

Interventions for anxiety might also include the use of distractions such as magazines, action comics, and video games. Generally, distractions that are colorful and do not require sustained attention work best, although this varies according to the patient's interests and abilities. Finally, patients with a high level of baseline anxiety and limited coping skills are helped when their interactions with the treatment team are predictable. This may include speaking with the physician at a specific time each day and consistency in nursing assignments. Individuals from outside the unit such as a chaplain or a volunteer may help by giving the patient more attention.

Because these patients have limited coping skills, once anxiety is moderated, nursing interventions include teaching alternative behaviors and strategies. For patients who externalize blame, such teaching may best be preceded by a gentle challenge. The challenge serves to engage the patient's interest in teaching that might otherwise be seen as irrelevant. This intervention is also important in that the nurse has (1) avoided a punitive or demeaning response that might have fueled escalation of the patient's anger, (2) taught a number of strategies, and (3) provided the patient with choices and thus with more control.

Often anger may be communicated via long-term verbal abuse. If attempts to teach alternatives have not been successful, three interventions can be used:

1. The first is to leave the room as soon as the abuse begins; the patient can be informed that the nurse will return in a specific amount of time (e.g., 20 minutes) when the situation is calmer. A matter-of-fact, neutral manner is important because fear, indignation, and arguing are gratifying to many verbally abusive patients. Alternatively, if the nurse is in the midst of a procedure and cannot leave immediately, the nurse can break off conversation and eye contact, completing the procedure quickly and matter-of-factly before leaving the room. The nurse avoids chastising, threatening, or responding punitively to the patient.

2. Withdrawal of attention to the abuse is successful only if a second intervention is also used. This step requires attending positively to, and thus reinforcing, nonabusive communication by the patient. Interventions can include discussing non–illness related topics, responding to requests, and providing emotional support.

3. Patients who are verbally abusive may respond best to the predictability of routine, such as scheduled contacts with the nurse (e.g., every 30 or 60 minutes). Use of such contacts provides nursing attention that is not contingent on the patient's behavior and therefore does not reinforce the abuse. Of course, the patient's illness or injury may sometimes require nursing visits for assessment or intervention outside the scheduled contact times. These visits can be carried out in a calm, brief, matter-of-fact manner.

Implementing appropriate interventions can be difficult when the nurse is feeling threatened. Remaining matter-of-fact with patients who habitually use anger and intimidation can be difficult; these people are often skillful at making personal and pointed statements. It is important to remember that patients do not know their nurses personally and thus have no basis on which they can make judgments. Nurses can also vent their own responses elsewhere with other staff or family members (while maintaining confidentiality) or via critical incident debriefing.

A 21-year-old man who was in an automobile accident is bedridden with a pelvic fracture. During his first day of admission, he yells at each nurse who walks by his room, using expletives in his demands that the nurse enter the room.

Intervention. The nurse who is assigned to the patient for the evening stops in his doorway after he yells at her and asks in mild disbelief, "Is this working for you? Do nurses really come in here when you yell at them that way?" The patient responds sullenly, justifying his behavior by complaining about his care. However, the nurse's challenge has caught his attention, and she goes on to suggest (i.e., teach) alternative strategies for contacting her and other nurses. The strategies are immediately put into use by the patient. ▪

Caring for Patients in Inpatient Psychiatric Settings

It is important to know that not all psychiatric patients are violence-prone, and aggression appears to be correlated less with certain illnesses than with certain patient characteristics. The two most significant predictors of violence are a history of violence and a history of impulsivity.

Situational factors contribute to patient anger and aggression. For instance, feelings of vulnerability and powerlessness resulting from trying to come to grips with depersonalized hospital routines, intrusive procedures, and restrictions on freedom can lead to anger and possibly aggression. Additional causes of patients' anger include (1) unrealistic expectations that their nurses will be angels of mercy, (2) the feeling that their physical and psychological needs are being ignored, and (3) the feeling that health care providers fail to recognize the uniqueness and wholeness of the patient.

If staff can identify patients who have a potential for violence, early intervention becomes possible. Nurses can work with these patients to recognize early signs of anger and can teach them strategies to manage the anger and prevent aggression.

A 19-year-old man has a 2-year history of quadriplegia. He also has a history of drug abuse that began in grade school, an inability to set or work toward long-term goals, and a primary coping style of anger and intimidation. The patient is admitted to an inpatient psychiatric unit because of increasing suicidal ideation. He clearly communicates to staff that his preferred means of coping with anger is to "cuss people out" and run into them with his wheelchair. However, in the hospital, the consequence of wheelchair assaults is that the patient is secluded in his room, which he finds intolerable. The patient asks the staff to help him manage his anger.

Intervention. The nurse assigned to this young man sets aside time to interview him regarding the triggers for his anger. He identifies several issues that "make him angry." These typically relate to feeling unheard and controlled by the staff. Together the nurse and patient examine alternative ways for him to deal with these situations, such as telling the staff he doesn't feel they are listening to him and letting them know he needs to be involved in planning his care so he can have an increased sense of control. The patient and nurse role-play a situation in which the patient is told by a staff member that he must attend a group session. Such a situation would usually result in the patient's becoming angry and aggressive, but in the role play he is willing to "try out" alternative communication techniques to communicate his feelings to the staff member and thus to handle his anger. In addition, the patient is willing to enter into a behavioral contract with the nurse which states that he will not curse at staff nor assault anyone with his wheelchair. Instead, he will let the staff know when he is feeling angry and what the triggering issue is so that a nonaggressive resolution can be found.

Response. Because this patient is intelligent and motivated to gain increased personal control, he responds positively to these suggestions. In addition, once it becomes clear that issues of feeling unheard and out of control underlie most episodes of anger, the patient is able to target these issues for problem solving. He rapidly develops effective and appropriate ways to make himself heard and understood. He also becomes adept at communicating when he feels out of control and at finding ingenious ways of negotiating control on issues that are particularly important to him. The patient's suicidal impulses, which occur when he is frustrated, also diminish. ▪

Caring for Patients With Cognitive Deficits

Patients with cognitive deficits are particularly at risk for acting aggressively. Such deficits may result from delirium, dementias (e.g., Alzheimer's disease, multi-infarct dementia), or brain injury (see Chapter 17). Traditional approaches to disorientation and to the agitation it can cause have relied heavily on reality orientation and medication. Reality orientation consists of providing the correct information to the patient about place, date, and current life circumstances. For many patients, this is comforting because it reminds them of pertinent information and helps them feel grounded. For others, reality orientation does not work. Because of their cognitive disorder, they can no longer "enter into our reality"; they become frightened, more agitated, and may become aggressive. Orientation aids, such as a calendar and a clock, can provide easy reference and increased autonomy. Such aids must be prominent and easily read by patients with diminished eyesight. Sedating medication may calm agitation, but the risks often outweigh the benefits. Sedation only further clouds a patient's sensorium, which makes disorientation worse and increases the risk of falls and injuries. It is better to examine alternative interventions.

Typically a patient experiencing delirium will be in and out of reality. At times they will appear perfectly fine, and at others they will have a clouded sensorium. They will sometimes fall asleep as you are talking to them. Often patients with delirium will have visual hallucinations, commonly of children, animals, or bugs. Occasionally they will show periods of paranoia. The best intervention for delirium is to find and treat the medical cause. The next choice is to medicate the symptoms with a low-dose antipsychotic and discontinue it as the delirium clears.

Patients with any clouding of the sensorium have difficulty interpreting environmental stimuli. Another set of interventions involves making the environment as simple, predictable, and comfortable as possible. Simplicity includes decreasing sensory stimuli. In the hospital, this might include placing the patient's bed away from doorways that enter onto the hall and choosing not to turn on the television. Establishing a routine of activities for each day and displaying the day's schedule prominently in the patient's room can provide predictability. The comfort of the patient is enhanced by provision of familiar photographs and objects from home. The availability of a rocking chair can provide a rhythmic source of self-soothing.

Sometimes the patient with a cognitive disorder experiences such severe agitation and aggression that it is referred to as a *catastrophic reaction*. The patient may scream, strike out, or cry because of overwhelming fear. Adopting a calm and unhurried manner is the best approach to take with such a patient. To respond effectively to episodes of agitation, it is crucial to identify the antecedents (i.e., what preceded the episode) and the consequences of such episodes. Once antecedents are understood, interventions are often obvious.

VIGNETTE

An 81-year-old woman with Alzheimer's disease always becomes agitated during her morning care; this comes to be a time dreaded by her caregivers. Careful observation of antecedents to the episodes of agitation reveals a natural course to the morning problems. The patient is initially calm when care begins. However, one staff person gives morning care to the patient and her roommate at the same time, moving between the two. Observation of the process reveals that the patient becomes distracted by cues being given to her roommate and often startles when the caregiver returns to her. As this process continues over several minutes, the patient becomes increasingly distressed and then agitated. When a change is made so that the patient's care is provided by one person who remains with her throughout the process, the patient's morning agitation ends. ◼

Patients who misperceive their setting or life situation may be calmed by **validation therapy**. Some disoriented older patients believe that they are young and feel the need to return to important tasks that were a significant part of those earlier years. For example, a woman may insist that she must go home to take care of her babies. Telling the patient that her babies have grown up and there is no home to return to is not only cruel but nontherapeutic and will result in increased agitation. It is often more helpful to reflect back to the patient the feelings behind her demand and to show understanding and concern for her worry.

Rather than attempting to reorient the patient, the nurse should ask the patient to further describe the setting or situation that is reported to be a problem (e.g., the need to return home). During the conversation, the nurse can comment on what appears to be underlying the patient's distress, thus validating it. In the earlier example, the woman who believes that she needs to return home to care for her children is asked to tell the nurse more about her children. The nurse may note that the patient misses her children and that the current setting gets lonely at times:

Nurse: "Mrs. Green, you miss your children, and this can be a lonely place."

As the nurse shows interest in aspects of the patient's life, the nurse establishes himself or herself as a safe, understanding person. In turn, the patient often becomes calmer and more open to redirection. As patients reminisce in this fashion, they often bring themselves into the present:

Patient: "Of course, they're all grown and doing well on their own now."

Refer to Chapter 17 for a more detailed discussion of interventions for people with cognitive impairments. Refer to Chapter 29 for a more detailed discussion of the use of validation and reminiscent therapeutic modalities for older adults.

EVALUATION

Evaluation of the care plan is essential for patients who are potentially angry and aggressive. A well-considered plan has specific outcome criteria (see Table 25-1). Evaluation provides information about the extent to which the interventions have achieved the outcomes. Revision focuses on all aspects of the nursing process:

- Was the assessment accurate and thorough?
- Were the nursing diagnoses applicable to the assessment data? Did the nursing diagnoses accurately drive nursing interventions?
- Was the plan comprehensive and individualized?

The initial plan may have included assessment of the environmental stimuli that precede a patient's agitation. Once these are identified, the plan provides interventions that are specific to those stimuli. However, the plan can work only if staff members evaluate the effectiveness of the approach by noting the extent to which agitation is decreased. Evaluation may reveal that the patient's agitation has decreased except in specific situations. The plan is then revised to include these situations.

KEY POINTS TO REMEMBER

- Angry emotions and aggressive and violent actions are difficult targets for nursing intervention.
- Nurses benefit from an understanding of how the angry, aggressive, or violent patient should be handled.
- Understanding patient cues to escalating aggression, appropriate goals for intervention for individuals in a variety of situations, and helpful nursing interventions is important for nurses in any setting.
- The expression of anger can lead to increased anger and to negative physiological changes.
- Psychosocial, cognitive, and biological theories provide explanations for anger and aggression.
- It is helpful for providers of care to know what cues should be looked for and what should be assessed when a patient's anger is escalating (verbal cues; nonverbal cues that include facial expression, breathing, body language, and posture).
- A patient's past aggressive behavior is the most important indicator of future aggressive episodes.
- Working with angry and aggressive patients is a challenge for all nurses, and a careful understanding and recognition of one's personal responses to angry or threatening patients can be crucial.
- Many approaches are effective in helping patients deescalate and maintain control.
- Different interventions are used, depending on the patient's coping abilities, cognitive status, and potential for violence.
- Specific medications such as antipsychotics, mood stabilizers, and antianxiety medications may be useful.
- Restraints may be necessary to ensure the safety of both the patient and other patients and the staff.
- Each unit has a clear protocol for the safe use of restraints and for the humane management of care during the time the patient is restrained, as well as clear guidelines for understanding and protecting the patient's legal rights.

CRITICAL THINKING

1. Jennifer admits a 24-year-old man with mania to an inpatient unit. She notes that the patient is irritable, has trouble sitting during the interview, and has a history of assault.
   A. Identify appropriate responses the nurse can make to the patient.
   B. What interventions should be built into the care plan?
   C. Identify at least three long-term outcomes to consider when planning care.

2. What are the two indicators for the use of seclusion and restraint rather than verbal interventions? Give rationales for your answers.

3. Discuss the use of restraint and seclusion with your clinical group or in class. Choose a side and defend it (even if you do not necessarily believe it) regarding the following:
   A. There are always better alternatives to seclusion and restraint.
   B. Seclusion and restraint is underutilized—people who have tried to limit its use have gone too far.
   C. Using chemical restraint with medication is/is not preferable to seclusion and restraint.

CHAPTER REVIEW

1. Which statement about violence and nursing is accurate?
   1. Unless working in psychiatric mental health settings, nurses are unlikely to experience patient violence.
   2. About 1 in 10 nurses will face an injury due to patient violence during their careers.
   3. Emergency, psychiatric, and step-down units have the highest rates of violence towards staff.
   4. Violence primarily affects inexperienced or unskilled staff who cannot calm their patients.

2. A nurse working with a patient who describes himself as "always angry" should assess the patient for which problem(s)? *Select all that apply.*
   1. Pain
   2. Dementia
   3. Tachycardia
   4. Hypertension
   5. Traumatic brain injury

3. Which statement(s) by a patient indicate an increased likelihood of violent behavior? *Select all that apply.*
   1. "People push me, but they can only push me so far."
   2. "I have a right to feel angry, and right now I am angry."
   3. "You are really stupid. I'd get better nursing care from a monkey."
   4. "A man has to do what a man has to do when somebody crosses him."
   5. "This is frustrating; I wish people would leave me alone. That's what would help me."

4. A nurse, Sarah, responds to loud, angry voices coming from the day room, where she finds that Mr. Christopher is pacing and shouting that he "isn't going to take this (expletive) anymore." Which reaction by Sarah is likely to be helpful in deescalating Mr. Christopher?
   1. Act calm, quiet, and in control.
   2. State, "You are acting inappropriately and must calm yourself now."
   3. Match the patient's volume level so that he is able to hear over his own shouting.
   4. Stand close to the patient so you can intervene physically if needed to protect others.

5. Andrea is a patient anxiously waiting her turn to speak with staff. The nurse is very busy, however, and asks if Andrea can wait a few minutes so she can finish her task. The nurse is distracted and forgets her promise temporarily, and 45 minutes pass before the nurse remembers and approaches Andrea. On seeing the nurse, Andrea accuses the nurse of lying and refuses to speak with her. Which response by the nurse is most likely to be therapeutic at this time?

1. "You seem angry that I didn't speak with you when I promised I would."

2. "Look, I'm sorry for being late, but screaming at me is not the best way to handle it."

3. "You are too angry to talk right now. I'll come back in 20 minutes and we can try again."

4. "Why are you angry? I told you that I was busy and would get to you soon as I could."

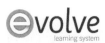

Visit the Evolve website for an **Audio Chapter Summary, Chapter Review Answers & Rationales, Critical Thinking Answers Guidelines,** and additional resources related to the content in this chapter: **http://evolve.elsevier.com/Varcarolis/foundations**

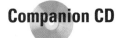 **Companion CD**   Use the Companion CD to prepare for tests and the NCLEX® Examination with **Test-Taking Strategies** for psychiatric mental health nursing and hundreds of **Review Questions.**

References

Bandura, A. (1973). *Aggression: A social learning analysis.* New York: Prentice Hall.

Beck, A. (1976). *Cognitive therapy and the emotional disorders.* New York: International Universities Press.

Bulechek, G. M., Butcher, H. K., & Dochterman, J. M. (2008). *Nursing interventions classification (NIC)* (5th ed.). St. Louis: Mosby.

Centers for Disease Control. (2008). Surveillance for Violent deaths—National violent death reporting system, 16 states, 2005. *Morbidity and Mortality Weekly Report, 57*(SS03), 1–43, 45. Retrieved from http://www.cdc.gov/mmwr/preview/mmwrhtml/ss5703a1.htm

de Almeida, R. M., Ferrari, P. F., Parmigiani, S., & Miczek, K. A. (2005). Escalated aggressive behavior: Dopamine, serotonin, and GABA. *European Journal of Pharmacology, 526*(1-3), 51–64.

Dougherty, D. D., Bonab, A. A., Ottowitz, W. E., Livni, E., Alpert, N. M., & Rauch, S. L. (2006). Decreased striatal D1 binding as measured using PET and [11C]SCH23,390 in patients with major depression with anger attacks. *Depression and Anxiety, 23*(3), 175–177.

Estryn-Chandler, G. (2008). From traditional inpatient to trauma-informed treatment: Transferring control from staff to patient. *Journal of the American Psychiatric Nurses Association, 14*(5), 363–371.

Foster, C., Bowers, L., & Nijman, H. (2007). Aggressive behaviour on acute psychiatric wards: Prevalence, severity and management. *Journal of Advanced Nursing, 58*(2), 140–149.

Gilburt, H., Rose, D., & Slade, M. (2008). The importance of relationships in mental health care study of service users' experiences of psychiatric hospital admission in the UK. *BioMed Central Health Services Research, 8*(92), 1–22.

Gross, A. F., & Sanders, K. M. (2008). Aggression and violence. In T. S. Stern, J. F. Rosenbaum, M. Fava, J. Biederman, & S. L. Rauch (Eds.), *Massachusetts General Hospital comprehensive clinical psychiatry* (pp. 895–905). St. Louis: Mosby.

Harmon-Jones, E. (2007). Trait anger predicts relative left frontal cortical activation to anger-inducing stimuli. *International Journal of Psychophysiology, 66*(2), 154–160.

Hellerstein, D. J., Staub, A. M., & Lequesne, E. (2007). Decreasing the use of restraint and seclusion among psychiatric inpatients. *Journal of Psychiatric Practice, 13*(5), 1–16.

Ito, M., Okazaki, M., Takahashi, S., Muramatsu, R., Kato, M., & Onuma, T. (2007). Subacute postictal aggression in patients with epilepsy. *Epilepsy Behavior, 10*(4), 611–614.

Jorgensen, R. S., & Kolodziej, M. E. (2007). Suppressed anger, evaluative threat, and cardiovascular reactivity: A tripartite profile approach. *International Journal of Psychophysiology, 66*(2), 102–108.

Kassinove, H., & Tafrate, R. F. (2006). Anger related disorders: Basic issues, models, and diagnostic considerations. In E. L. Feindler (Ed.), *Anger-related disorders: A practitioner's guide to comparative treatments* (pp. 1–27). New York: Springer.

Menninger, W. W. (2007). Uncontained rage: A psychoanalytic perspective on violence. *Bulletin of the Menninger Clinic, 71*(2), 115–131.

Moorhead, S., Johnson, M., Maas, M. L., & Swanson, E. (2008). *Nursing outcome classification (NOC)* (4th ed.). St. Louis: Mosby.

Narayan, V. M., Narr, K. L., Kumari, V., Woods, R. P., Thompson, P. M., Toga, A. W., & Sharma, T. (2007). Regional cortical thinning in subjects with violent antisocial personality disorder or schizophrenia. *American Journal of Psychiatry, 164,* 1418–1427.

North American Nursing Diagnosis Association International. (2009). *NANDA-I nursing diagnoses: Definitions and classification 2009-2011.* Philadelphia: Author.

Siever, L. J. (2008). Neurobiology of aggression and violence. *American Journal of Psychiatry, 165*(4), 429–442.

Sirotich, F. (2008). Correlates of crime and violence among persons with mental disorder: An evidence-based review. *Brief Treatment Crisis Interventions, 8*(2), 171–194.

Skinner, B. (1953). *Science and human behavior*. New York: Macmillan.

Solomon, B. S., Bradshaw, C. P., Wright, J., & Cheng, T. L. (2008). Youth and parental attitudes toward fighting. *Journal of Interpersonal Violence, 23*, 544–560.

United States Department of Health and Human Services, Centers for Medicare and Medicaid Services. (2008). *Revised interpretive guidelines for seclusion and restraint.* Retrieved April 7, 2009 from http://www.cms.hhs.gov/EOG/downloads/EO%200306.pdf

CHAPTER 26

Child, Older Adult, and Intimate Partner Abuse

Judi Sateren and Verna Benner Carson

Key Terms and Concepts

crisis situation, 589
economic abuse, 585
emotional abuse, 585
family violence, 585
health care record, 595
neglect, 585
perpetrators, 587
physical abuse, 584

primary prevention, 601
safety plan, 598
secondary prevention, 602
sexual abuse, 585
shelters or safe houses, 598
survivor, 589
tertiary prevention, 602
vulnerable person, 589

Objectives

1. Identify three indicators of (a) physical abuse, (b) sexual abuse, (c) neglect, and (d) emotional abuse.
2. Discuss the epidemiological theory of abuse in terms of stresses on the perpetrator, vulnerable person, and environment that could escalate anxiety to the point at which abuse becomes the relief behavior.
3. Compare and contrast three characteristics of perpetrators with three characteristics of a vulnerable person.
4. Describe four areas to assess when interviewing a person who has experienced abuse.
5. Identify two common emotional responses the nurse might experience when faced with a person subjected to abuse.

6. Formulate four nursing diagnoses for the survivor of abuse, and list supporting data from the assessment.
7. Write out a safety plan with the essential elements for a victim of intimate partner abuse.
8. Compare and contrast primary, secondary, and tertiary levels of intervention, giving two examples of intervention for each level.
9. Describe at least three possible referrals for an abusive family, including the telephone numbers of appropriate agencies in the community.
10. Discuss three psychotherapeutic modalities useful in working with abusive families.

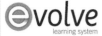 Visit the Evolve website for an **Audio Glossary & Flashcards, Concept Map Creator,** and additional resources related to the content in this chapter: **http://evolve.elsevier.com/Varcarolis/foundations**

Family abuse is any physical injury or mental anguish (e.g., putdowns, demeaning actions, controlling behavior) inflicted by one family member upon another or the deprivation of essential services by a caregiver. To be effective in working with victims, the nurse needs an understanding of the conditions for violence and the types of maltreatment. Fundamental to this entire discussion is self-understanding (see the Self-Assessment section later in the chapter).

CLINICAL PICTURE

Types of Abuse

Five specific types of abuse have been identified: (1) physical abuse, (2) sexual abuse, (3) emotional abuse, (4) neglect, and (5) economic abuse. **Physical abuse** is the infliction of physical pain or bodily harm (e.g., slapping, punching, hitting, choking, pushing, restraining, biting, throwing, burning). Sexual abuse is any form of sexual contact or exposure without consent, or in circumstances in which the victim is incapable of giving consent. Sexual abuse of adults is usually referred to as *sexual assault* or *rape* and is discussed in Chapter 27. Emotional abuse is the infliction of mental anguish (e.g., threatening, humiliating, intimidating, and isolating). It can take the form of any of the following:

- Terrorizing an individual through verbal threats
- Demeaning an individual's worth or putting the person down
- Directing blatant or subtle hostility and hatred toward an individual—or omitting positive behaviors
- Persistently ignoring an individual and her or his needs
- Consistently belittling and criticizing an individual
- Withholding warmth and affection from an individual
- Threatening an individual with abandonment or institutionalization (nursing home, psychiatric hospital)

Neglect can take several forms:

- Physical neglect is failure to provide for basic needs or to protect from harm.
- Emotional neglect is failure to attend to basic emotional needs and nurturing.
- Educational neglect is failure to provide a child with experiences, including formal education necessary for intellectual growth and development.
- Medical neglect is failure to provide basic medical, dental, or psychiatric care.

Economic abuse is the withholding of financial support or the illegal or improper exploitation of funds or other resources for one's personal gain.

Cycle of Violence

Walker (1979) describes a pattern of behavior that perpetrators of violence may use to control their partners. Periods of intense violence alternate with periods of safety, hope, and trust. The **tension-building stage** is characterized by relatively minor incidents, such as pushing, shoving, and verbal abuse. During this time, the victim often ignores or accepts the abuse for fear that more severe abuse will follow. Abusers then rationalize that their abusive behavior is acceptable. As the tension escalates, both participants may try to reduce it. The abuser may try to reduce the tension with the use of alcohol or drugs, and the victim may try to reduce the tension by minimizing the importance of the incidents ("I should have had the house neater … dinner ready").

During the **acute battering stage**, the abuser releases the built-up tension by brutal beatings. Severe injuries can and do result. The **honeymoon stage** may be characterized by kindness and loving behaviors. The abuser, at least initially, feels remorseful and apologetic and may bring presents, make promises, and tell the victim how much she or he is loved and needed. The victim usually believes the promises, feels needed and loved, and drops any legal proceedings or plans to leave that may have been initiated during the acute battering stage.

Unfortunately, without intervention, the cycle will repeat itself. Over time, the periods of calmness and safety become briefer, and the periods of anger and fear are more intense. There are intervals of stability, but the violence increases over time. With each repeat of the pattern, the victim's self-esteem becomes more and more eroded. The victim either believes the violence was deserved or accepts the blame for it. This can lead to feelings of depression, hopelessness, immobilization, and self-deprecation. Figure 26-1 illustrates the cycle of violence.

EPIDEMIOLOGY

Abuse within families is among the most important U.S. public health issues and is therefore a significant nursing concern. It is estimated that half of all people in the United States have experienced abuse in their families. The American Academy of Family Physicians defines family violence as the "intentional intimidation, abuse or neglect of children, adults or elders by a family member, intimate partner or caretaker in order to gain power and control over the victim" (2008, para. 1). While the true prevalence of child, elder, and intimate partner abuse is unknown (because of underreporting and variability in reporting methods, instruments, sites, and reporters), it is clear that abuse is a significant problem.

Child Abuse

In 2006 in the United States, there were 3.3 million referrals for child abuse, involving 6 million children; about 905,000 children were found to be victims (U.S. Department of Health & Human Services [USDHHS], 2008). The most common form of abuse was neglect (64%), followed by physical abuse (16%), sexual abuse (9%), and emotional abuse (7%). Table 26-1 gives statistics related to abuse rates and fatalities among different ethnicities.

Girls are slightly more likely to be abused and make up 51.5% of victims. In general, the younger the child—girl *or* boy—the more vulnerable she or he is to abuse. Infants under the age of 1 account for about 24% of abuse cases (USDHHS, 2008). More than 75% of children who die are younger than 4 years of age. Infants die more frequently from abuse or neglect—boys at a rate of 18.5 per 100,000 and girls at a rate of 14.7 per 100,000. Sexual abuse is uncommon in infants (0.4% of all abuse in infants) and increases with age, maintaining a steady rate of about 16% of all abuse beginning around puberty (age 12).

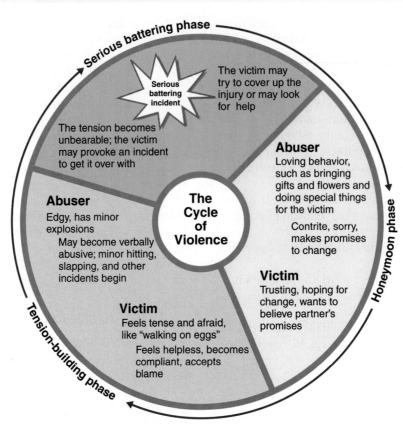

Figure 26-1 The cycle of violence. (Redrawn from YWCA of Annapolis and Anne Arundel County, 1517 Ritchie Highway, Arnold, MD 21012.)

TABLE 26-1	Rates of Abuse and Fatalities Among Different Ethnicities	
Race or Ethnicity	**Rates of Abuse per 1000 Children**	**% of Total Child Fatalities**
African American	19.8	29%
American Indian or Alaska Native	15.9	0.8%
Children of multiple races	15.4	1.3%
Hispanic	10.8	17%
White	10.7	43%
Asian	2.5	1.1%

Almost 80% of perpetrators are the victim's parents (USDHHS, 2008). About 40% of all abuse is from the mother acting alone, about 18% is from the father acting alone, about 18% is from both parents, and 7% is by one parent along with another person.

Intimate Partner Abuse

Spousal abuse is also referred to as *intimate partner violence* and *domestic violence*. The U.S. Bureau of Justice Statistics [BJS], (2007) provides some data regarding

this problem. Females are victimized about 6 times more often than males. In persons aged 12 and older, about 3 white females per 1000 persons report abuse, about 4.5 black females per 1000 persons report abuse, and white males report abuse at a rate of 0.7 per 1000 persons.

Not only are more women the victims of spousal abuse, but when severity of abuse is taken into account, they are clearly dominated. Women are 7 to 14 times more likely to be choked, beaten up, or threatened with a gun or drowning (Beck, 2008). Nearly half of married couples have instances of abuse, and homosexual couples seem to have nearly the same rates of abuse as heterosexual couples. One out of 10 homicides is due to spousal murder, and about a third of females who are killed are or were in an intimate relationship with their killer.

Socioeconomic status is related to abusive relationships; generally, the lower the income, the greater the amount of domestic violence (Table 26-2).

Older Adult Abuse

According to the American Psychological Association [APA] (2008), about 2 million older adults in the United States are reported to be physically abused, psychologically abused, or neglected. The APA suggests that the number may be far higher and that

TABLE 26-2 Average Annual Nonfatal Intimate Partner Abuse Rate*

Annual Household Income of Victim	Intimate Partner Victimization Rate	
	Females	**Males**
Less than $7500	12.7	1.5
$7500 to $24,999	6.2	1.5
$25,000 to $49,999	5.2	0.8
$50,000 or more	2.0	0.6

*Per 1000 persons age 12 or older by income and gender (2001-2005). Data from U.S. Bureau of Justice Statistics. (2007). *Intimate partner violence in the U.S.: Victim characteristics.* <http://www.ojp.usdoj.gov/bjs/intimate/table/incgen.htm> Accessed 11.12.2008.

for every case reported, five go unreported. Further complicating the picture is that the older adult himself or herself may actually be the caregiver which creates the potential for self-neglect (Milosavljevic & Brendel, 2008). Older adults can be used abused by family members in domestic settings or in institutions by paid caregivers.

VIGNETTE

Walter, a 53-year-old man, came to the ambulatory care clinic looking very fatigued and complaining of pain in his left shoulder "since last night." Holding his left arm close to his side, Walter averted his eyes from those of the receptionist, nurse, and doctor. When asked if anything had occurred that might have caused the pain, he answered, "I fell." Asked why he had not sought care the previous night, Walter stated, "I ... I ... thought it would go away overnight." Upon further examination and x-ray imaging, it was determined that the patient had sustained a fractured clavicle. Additional direct, supportive questioning elicited the information that the patient had been injured when pushed down the stairs by his 17-year-old stepson. ■

COMORBIDITY

The secondary effects of abuse (e.g., anxiety, depression, suicidal ideation) are health care issues that can last a lifetime. Depression and posttraumatic stress disorder (PTSD) are two of the most prevalent disorders resulting from childhood trauma. Family violence is common in the childhood histories of juvenile offenders, runaways, violent criminals, prostitutes, and those who in turn are violent toward others. Exposure to abuse can adversely affect a child's development, because the energy needed to successfully accomplish developmental tasks goes to coping with abuse (Bensley et al., 2003; Desai et al., 2002).

Abused adolescents report more psychopathological changes, poorer coping and social skills, a higher incidence of dissociative identity disorder, and poorer impulse control than do other adolescents. Women who are victims of prolonged childhood sexual abuse are more likely to develop major psychiatric distress. When health care providers do not routinely assess for history of sexual abuse, symptoms arising in times of crisis may be labeled as adult psychopathological disorders and not understood as possible post-trauma response (Stevens, 2003). Box 26-1 identifies some of the long-term effects of family violence.

The occurrence of one type of abuse is a fairly strong predictor of the occurrence of another type. This connection calls for more coordinated efforts at prevention and intervention. To this end, the President's Family Justice Center Initiative was passed in 2004 to provide for planning and development of a comprehensive domestic abuse victim service and support centers (U.S. Department of Justice, 2004).

ETIOLOGY
Environmental Factors

Abuse occurs across all segments of society in the United States. Social factors that reinforce violence include the wide acceptance of corporal punishment; increasingly violent movies, video games, websites, and comic books; violent themes in music; and the increase in the total volume of pornography (which is strongly associated with physical abuse of women).

The occurrence of abuse requires the following participants and conditions:

1. A perpetrator
2. Someone who by age or situation is vulnerable (e.g., children, women, older adults, and the mentally ill or physically challenged person)
3. A crisis situation

Perpetrator

The propensity for violence is rooted in childhood and manifested by a general lack of self-regard, dissatisfaction with life, and inability to assume adult roles. Often the abuser lacked good role models and was deprived of the opportunity to develop problem-solving skills. Witnessing or experiencing family violence, neglect, or abusive parenting (Box 26-2) are contributing factors. Perpetrators, those who initiate violence, often consider their own needs to be more important than anyone else's and look toward others to meet their needs.

The term *perpetrator* applies to any member of a household who is violent toward another member (e.g., siblings, same-sex partners, extended family members). Violence and abuse are found in all segments of society. Both male and female perpetrators perceive themselves as having poor social skills. They

BOX 26-1 Long-Term Effects of Family Violence

- People involved in family violence are found to have a higher incidence of:
  - Depression
  - Suicidal feelings
  - Self-contempt
  - Inability to trust
  - Inability to develop intimate relationships in later life
- Victims of severe violence are also at higher risk for experiencing recurring symptoms of posttraumatic stress disorder:
  - Flashbacks
  - Dissociation—out-of-body experiences
  - Poor self-esteem
  - Compulsive or impulsive behaviors (e.g., substance abuse, excessive spending, gambling, and promiscuity)
  - Multiple somatic complaints
- Children who witness violence in their homes:
  - After the age of 5 or 6 years show an indication of identifying with the aggressor and losing respect for the victim.

- Are at greater risk for developing behavioral and emotional problems throughout their lives.
- Some mental and behavioral disorders are associated with violence in childhood:
  - Depressive disorders
  - Posttraumatic stress disorder
  - Somatic complaints, technically not a "disorder"
  - Low self-esteem, same as above
  - Phobias (agoraphobia, social and specific phobias)
  - Antisocial behaviors
  - Child or spouse abuse
- Adolescents are more likely to have behavioral symptoms such as:
  - Failing grades
  - Difficulty forming relationships
  - Increased incidence of theft, police arrest, and violent behaviors
  - Seductive or promiscuous behaviors
  - Running away from home

BOX 26-2 Characteristics of Abusive Parents

- A history of abuse, neglect, or emotional deprivation as a child
- Family authoritarianism: raise children as they were raised by their own parents
- Low self-esteem, feelings of worthlessness, depression
- Poor coping skills
- Social isolation (may be suspicious of others): few or no friends, little or no involvement in social or community activities
- Involvement in a crisis situation: unemployment, divorce, financial difficulties
- Rigid, unrealistic expectations of child's behavior
- Frequent use of harsh punishment
- History of severe mental illness, such as schizophrenia
- Violent temper outbursts
- Looking to child for satisfaction of needs for love, support, and reassurance (often unmet because of parenting deficits in family of origin)
- Projection of blame onto the child for parents' "troubles" (e.g., stepparent may project hostility toward new mate onto a child)
- Lack of effective parenting skills
- Inability to seek help from others
- Perception of the child as bad or evil
- History of drug or alcohol abuse
- Feeling of little or no control over life
- Low tolerance for frustration
- Poor impulse control

describe their relationships with their partners as being the closest they have ever known, which is typical in enmeshed and codependent relationships. They lack supportive relationships outside the relationship.

Men who abuse believe in male supremacy, being in charge, and being dominant. "Acting out" physically makes them feel more in control, more masculine, and more powerful. Parent-child interactions, peer group experiences, observations of the partner dyad, and the influence of the media (television, comics, video games, movies) all support the same message: Males can expect to be in a position of power in relationships and may use physical aggression to maintain that position.

Extreme pathological jealousy is characteristic of an abuser. Many refuse to allow their partners to work outside the home; others demand that their partners work in the same place as they do so they can monitor activities and friendships. Many accompany their partners to and from all activities and forbid them to have personal friends or participate in recreational activities outside the home. When this is not possible, a perpetrator may restrict mobility by monitoring the odometer and keeping stopwatches. Even after imposing such restrictions, abusers often accuse their partners of infidelity. Many perpetrators maintain their possessiveness by controlling the family finances so tightly that there is barely enough money for daily living.

Minority groups, particularly those experiencing poverty and social marginalization, may have the label of perpetrator or abuser applied to them more often than those who are more socioeconomically advantaged (Malley-Morrison & Hines, 2003). It is important to recognize that a wide variety of cultural norms dictate relationships among intimate partners and child rearing practices. Learning about the cultural backgrounds of patients can prevent mistaking common cultural norms for abuse.

Individuals are more likely to engage in family violence when they use substances. Alcohol and other drugs (illicit or prescribed) tend to weaken inhibitions and lead to a disregard of social rules prohibiting violence. The consumption of alcohol and drugs is often used as a rationalization by the victim to excuse the behavior. ("He was drunk and didn't know what he was doing.") But when drug and alcohol use is reduced or eliminated, family violence still occurs.

Vulnerable Person

The **vulnerable person** is the family member upon whom abuse is perpetrated. This individual is variously referred to as the *victim*, *survivor*, or *victim/survivor*. Using the term **survivor** recognizes the recovery and healing process that follows victimization and does not have the connotation of passivity that *victim* has. In some situations, violence does not occur until after the legal marriage of couples who have lived together or dated for a long time.

Women. Pregnancy may trigger or increase violence. National estimates of assaults to pregnant women range from 1% to 20%, depending on the definition of assault and the population studied (Saltzman et al., 2003). The partner may resent the added responsibility a baby entails, or he may resent the relationship the baby will have with his mate. Violence also escalates when the wife makes a move toward independence, such as visiting friends without permission, getting a job, or going back to school. Victims are at greatest risk for violence when they attempt to leave the relationship.

Children. Children are most likely to be abused if they are younger than 3 years of age; are perceived as being different because of temperamental traits, congenital abnormalities, or chronic disease; remind the parents of someone they do not like (perhaps an ex-spouse); are different from the parents' fantasy of what the child should be like; or are a product of an unwanted pregnancy. Interference with emotional bonding between parents and child (e.g., because of a premature birth or prolonged illness requiring hospitalization) has also been found to increase the risk for future abuse. Adolescents are abused at least as frequently as younger children. However, such abuse is often overlooked, perhaps because adolescents tend to be viewed as capable of defending themselves.

Older Adults. Older adults may become vulnerable because they are in poor mental or physical health or are disruptive (e.g., a person with Alzheimer's disease). One to two million adults over the age of 65 are exploited, injured, or otherwise mistreated by their caregivers every year in the United States (National Research Council Panel to Review Risk and Prevalence of Elder Abuse and Neglect, 2003). The dependency needs of older adults are usually what put them at risk for abuse. The typical victim is female, over 75 years of age, Caucasian, living with a relative, and experiencing a physical and/or mental impairment. Dealing with the care of older adults can be stressful for caregivers in the best of cases, but in families in which violence is a coping strategy, the potential for abuse is great. Other scenarios include the older man cared for by a daughter he abused as a child and who now is abusive toward him, the older woman abused by her husband as part of a longstanding abusive relationship, or the caregiver who becomes angry because of the failing health of a loved one.

Crisis Situation

Anyone may be at risk for abuse in a **crisis situation**—a situation that puts stress on a family with a violent member. A person with effective impulse control, problem-solving skills, and a healthy support system is less likely to resort to violence. However, stressful life events tax coping skills, leaving the perpetrator incapable of dealing with the situation. Social isolation caused by frequent moves or an inability to make friends contributes to ineffective coping during crisis situations. Refer to Chapter 23 for more on crisis and crisis intervention.

APPLICATION OF THE NURSING PROCESS

ASSESSMENT
General Assessment

Victims of violence are encountered in every health care setting. Therefore, all patients should be screened for possible abuse. Because of the number of victims of violence seen in emergency departments, the Emergency Nurses Association (ENA) issued a position statement urging "emergency nurses to take an active role in the development, implementation, and ongoing maintenance of hospital and community protective service teams to ensure consistent and accurate assessments and protection of all individuals and/or families at risk for domestic violence, maltreatment and neglect" (ENA, 2003, p. 2). Complaints may be vague and can include chronic pain, insomnia, hyperventilation, or gynecological problems. Attention to the interview process and setting are important to facilitate accurate assessment of physical and behavioral indicators of family violence (Stevens, 2003). All assessments should include questions to elicit a history of sexual abuse, family violence, and drug use or abuse. It is helpful to have an institutional policy that facilitates screening in private; the assessment should be completed with the victim alone.

Interview Process and Setting

Important and relevant information about the family situation can be gathered by routine assessment conducted with tact, understanding, and a calm, relaxed attitude. Important interviewing guidelines are listed in Box 26-3. A person who feels judged or accused of wrongdoing is likely to become defensive, and any attempts at changing coping strategies in the family are thwarted. It is better to ask about ways of solving disagreements or methods of disciplining children rather than to use the words *abuse* or *violence.*

When interviewing, sit near the patient and spend some time establishing trust and rapport before focusing on the details of the violent experience. Establishing trust is crucial if the patient is to feel comfortable enough to self-disclose. The interview should be nonthreatening and supportive. The person who experienced the violence should be allowed to tell the story without

interruption. Reassure the patient that he or she did nothing wrong. Verbal approaches may include:

- Tell me about what happened to you.
- Who takes care of you? (for children and dependent older adults)
- What happens when you do something wrong? (for children) *or* How do you and your partner/caregiver resolve disagreements? (for women and dependent older adults)
- What do you do for fun?
- Who helps you with your child(ren)/parent?
- What time do you have for yourself?

Questions that are open-ended and require a descriptive response can be less threatening and elicit more relevant information than questions that are direct or can be answered with *yes* or *no* (see Chapter 10):

- What arrangements do you make when you have to leave your child alone?
- How do you discipline your child?
- When your infant cries for a long time, how do you get him/her to stop?
- What about your child's behavior bothers you the most?

When trust has been established, openness and directness about the situation can strengthen the relationship with those experiencing or perpetrating violence. The Nursing Research Consortium on Violence and Abuse (2001) developed a five-question assessment tool that has been used extensively to assist in the routine identification of intimate partner abuse (Figure 26-2).

Areas to include in an abuse assessment include: (a) violence indicators, (b) levels of anxiety and coping responses, (c) family coping patterns, (d) support systems, (e) suicide potential, (f) homicide potential, and (g) drug and alcohol use. The following vignette illustrates the key points in assessing a woman in crisis at the initial interview, as well as suggested follow-up.

BOX 26-3 Interview Guidelines

Do:

- Conduct the interview in private.
- Be direct, honest, and professional.
- Use language the patient understands.
- Ask the patient to clarify words not understood.
- Be understanding.
- Be attentive.
- Inform the patient if you must make a referral to Children's or Adult Protective Services, and explain the process.
- Assess safety, and help reduce danger (at discharge).

Do Not:

- Try to "prove" abuse by accusations or demands.
- Display horror, anger, shock, or disapproval of the perpetrator or situation.
- Place blame or make judgments.
- Allow the patient to feel "at fault" or "in trouble."
- Probe or press for answers the patient is not willing to give.
- Conduct the interview with a group of interviewers.
- Force a child or anyone else to remove clothing.

VIGNETTE

Darnell Peters is a 42-year-old married woman in a relationship she describes as "bad for a long time. We don't communicate." She is brought to the emergency department by ambulance with swollen eyes, lips, and nose and lacerations to her face. She tells the nurse that her husband had been in bed asleep for hours before she joined him. On getting into bed, she attempted to redistribute the blankets. Suddenly he leaped from the bed, started punching her in the face, and began to throw her against the wall. She called out to her 11-year-old son to call the police. The police arrived, called an ambulance, and took Mr. Peters to jail.

The nurse takes Mrs. Peters to an individual examination room (to emphasize confidentiality) for a full assessment. Mrs. Peters states that her relationship with her husband is always stormy. "He is always putting me down and yelling at me." He started hitting

---

ABUSE ASSESSMENT SCREEN

1. Within the last year, have you been hit, slapped, kicked, or otherwise physically hurt by someone?

☐ Yes ☐ No

If yes, by whom? _____

Total number of times: _____

2. Since you've been pregnant, have you been hit, slapped, kicked, or otherwise physically hurt by someone?

☐ Yes ☐ No

If yes, by whom? _____

Total number of times: _____

Mark the area of injury on the body map below.

3. Within the last year, has anyone forced you to have sexual activities?

☐ Yes ☐ No

If yes, who? _____

Total number of times: _____

4. Have you ever been emotionally or physically abused by your partner or someone important to you?

☐ Yes ☐ No

If yes, by whom? _____

Total number of times: _____

5. Are you afraid of your partner or anyone listed above?

☐ Yes ☐ No

Score each incident according to the following scale:

    1 = Threats of abuse including use of a weapon

    2 = Slapping, pushing; no injuries and/or continuing pain

    3 = Punching, kicking, bruises, cuts, and/or continuing pain

    4 = Beating up, severe contusions, burns, broken bones

    5 = Head injury, internal injury, permanent injury

    6 = Use of weapon, wound from weapon

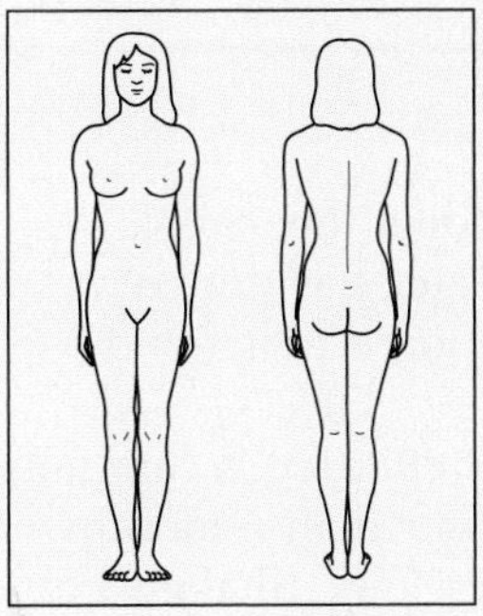

SCORE

_____

_____

_____

_____

_____

_____

Figure 26-2 Abuse assessment screen. (Developed by the Nursing Research Consortium on Violence and Abuse. [2001]) *Abuse assessment screen.* Retrieved April 7, 2009 from http://www.nnvawi.org/Abuse%20Assessment.pdf

her 5 years earlier when she became pregnant with her second and last child. The beatings have increased in intensity over the past year, and this emergency department visit is the fifth this year. Tonight is the first time she has ever called the police.

Mrs. Peters has visibly lost control. Periods of crying alternate with periods of silence. She appears apathetic and depressed. The nurse remains calm and objective. After Mrs. Peters has finished talking, the nurse explores alternatives designed to help her reduce the danger when she is discharged. "I'm concerned that you will be hurt again if you go home. What options do you have?" Acknowledging the escalating intensity of the violence, Mrs. Peters is able to make arrangements with a shelter to take in her and her two children until after she has secured a restraining order.

The nurse charts the abuse referrals. The keeping of careful and complete records helps ensure that Mrs. Peters will receive proper follow-up care and will assist Mrs. Peters when and if she pursues legal action. ◾

Types of Abuse

Physical Abuse

A series of minor complaints, such as headaches, back trouble, dizziness, and accidents—especially falls—may be covert indicators of violence. Overt signs of battering include bruises, scars, burns, and other wounds in various stages of healing, particularly around the head, face, chest, arms, abdomen, back, buttocks, and genitalia. Injuries that should arouse the nurse's suspicion are listed in Box 26-4.

If the explanation does not match the injury seen, or if the patient minimizes the seriousness of the injury, abuse may be suspected. Ask patients directly, but in a nonthreatening manner, if the injury has been caused by someone close to them. Observe the nonverbal response, such as hesitation or lack of eye contact, as well as the verbal response. Then ask specific questions such as: "When was the last time it happened? How often does it happen? In what ways are you hurt?" Inconsistent explanations serve as a warning that further investigation is necessary. Vague explanations should alert the nurse to possible abuse. ("She

---

BOX 26-4 Common Presenting Problems of Victims of Abuse

Emergency Department
- Bleeding injuries, especially to head and face
- Internal injuries, concussions, perforated eardrum, abdominal injuries, severe bruising, eye injuries, strangulation marks on neck
- Back injuries
- Broken or fractured jaw, arms, pelvis, ribs, clavicle, legs
- Burns from cigarettes, appliances, scalding liquids, acids
- Psychological trauma, anxiety, attacks of hyperventilation, heart palpitations, severe crying spells, suicidal tendencies
- Miscarriage

Ambulatory Care Settings
- Perforated eardrum, twisted or stiff neck and shoulder muscles, headache

- Depression, stress-related conditions (e.g., insomnia, violent nightmares, anxiety, extreme fatigue, eczema, loss of hair)
- Talk of having "problems" with husband or son, describing person as very jealous, impulsive, or an alcohol or drug abuser
- Repeated visits with new complaints
- Bruises of various ages and specific shapes (fingers, belt)

Any Setting
- Signs of stress due to family violence: emotional, behavioral, school, or sleep problems and increase in aggressive behavior
- Injuries in a pregnant woman
- Recurrent visits for injuries attributed to being "accident prone"

---

fell from a chair [from a lap, down the stairs]." "He was running away." "The hot water was turned on by mistake.") The key to identification is a high index of suspicion.

Nonspecific bruising in older children is common. Any bruises on an infant younger than 6 months of age should be considered suspicious. **Shaken baby syndrome**, one of the most serious types of child abuse, is the result of the brain moving in the opposite direction as the baby's head (Johnson, 2002). A baby who has been shaken may present with respiratory problems, bulging fontanelles, and central nervous system damage, resulting in seizures, vomiting, and coma.

Sexual Abuse

There are a variety of emotional and behavioral consequences of sexual abuse, including depression, anxiety, suicide, aggression, chronic low self-esteem, and PTSD. Childhood sexual abuse is likely to be a significant factor in the development of depression in many women (Bensley et al., 2003). Sexual abuse of boys appears to be common, underreported, underrecognized, and untreated (Desai et al., 2002).

VIGNETTE
Ms. Randall, 83 years old, is admitted from an adult foster home for evaluation of deterioration in her mental status. She is confused and disoriented as to time and place and is unable to give a coherent history. Blood and urine are collected for diagnostic evaluation. The laboratory report notes semen in the urine. Adult Protective Services is called to begin an investigation into the adult family home. ■

Emotional Abuse

Emotional abuse may exist on its own or as a result of co-occurring physical or sexual abuse. Although it is less obvious and more difficult to assess than physical violence, it can be identified through indicators such as low self-esteem, reported feelings of inadequacy, anxiety and withdrawal, learning difficulties, and poor impulse control. Many consider emotional abuse to have the most significant and negative effects on victims.

Neglect

Neglected children and older adults often appear undernourished, dirty, and poorly clothed. Neglect is also manifested by inadequate medical care, such as lack of immunizations or untreated medical conditions.

Economic Abuse

Failure to provide for the needs of the victim when adequate funds are available is a sign of economic maltreatment. Another sign is bills that are left unpaid by the person in charge of finances, which may result in disconnection of the heat or electricity (Stevens, 2003).

Level of Anxiety and Coping Responses

Nonverbal responses to the assessment interview can be indicative of the victim's anxiety level (see Chapter 12). Agitation and anxiety bordering on panic are often present in victims experiencing violence. Because they live in terror, abused individuals remain vigilant, unable to relax or sleep. Signs of the effects of living with chronic stress and severe levels of anxiety may be present (e.g., hypertension, irritability, gastrointestinal disturbances). Hesitation, lack of eye contact, and use of vague statements such as "It's been rough lately" indicate that the situation is difficult to talk about.

Coping mechanisms used by many victims to endure living in violent and terrifying situations often prevent the dissolution of the relationship. These coping mechanisms may take the form of flawed beliefs or myths (Table 26-3). Because of feelings of confusion, shame, despair, and powerlessness, victims may withdraw from interaction with others, increasing their isolation.

VIGNETTE

Bilateral corneal abrasions in a woman coming to the walk-in clinic raises the suspicion of an astute nurse, who notes the patient's vague responses to history questions and her unrelenting checking of the clock, followed by the urgent statement, "I've got to get home."

TABLE 26-3 Myth versus Fact: Family Abuse

Myth	Fact
Ninety-five percent of abuse victims are women.	Recent surveys report that from 30% to 40%, perhaps 50%, of abuse victims are men.
The victim's behavior often causes violence.	The victim's behavior is *not* the cause of the violence. Violence is the abuser's pattern of behavior, and the victim cannot learn how to control it.
Men have the right to keep their wives and/or children in line.	No person has the right to beat or hurt another person.
Intimate partner abuse is a minor problem.	There is a *real* danger that victims may be killed by abusive partners.
Battered women are masochistic and like to be beaten. (The abuse cannot be that bad or they would leave.)	Women do not like, ask, or deserve to be abused. Economic considerations are usually the only reason they stay.
Victims of intimate partner abuse could leave if they really wanted to.	There are numerous factors influencing a decision to leave, including fear of injury or death, financial dependence, welfare of children, etc.
Family abuse is most prevalent in poorly educated people from poor, working-class backgrounds.	Abuse occurs in families of all socioeconomic, religious, cultural, and educational backgrounds.
Family matters are private, and families should be allowed to take care of their own problems.	Intervention in family abuse is justified; abuse always escalates in frequency and intensity, can end in death, and is passed on to future generations.
Victims of abuse tacitly accept the abuse by trying to conceal it, by not reporting it, or by failing to seek help.	When attempting to disclose their situation, many victims are met with disbelief. This discourages them from persevering.
Myths victims commonly believe: "I can't live without him/her." "If I hadn't done _____, it wouldn't have happened." "He/She will change." "I stay for the sake of the children." "Jealousy and possessiveness prove his/her love."	These myths are coping mechanisms used to allay panic in a situation of random and brutal violence. They give the illusion of control and rationality.
Alcohol and stress are the major causes of physical and verbal abuse.	This myth offers an explanation of and tolerance for verbal abuse and battering. There are no excuses, and it is not acceptable behavior. Abuse is a learned behavior, not an uncontrollable reaction. People are abusive because they have acquired the belief that violence and aggression are acceptable and effective responses to real or imagined threats.
Violence occurs only between heterosexual partners.	Gay and lesbian partners experience violence for reasons similar to those in heterosexual relationships.
Pregnancy protects a woman from battering.	Battering frequently begins or escalates during pregnancy.

On further questioning, the woman reveals that she is often quite fatigued because of caring for her five children, all younger than 7 years of age. Yet her husband, who works until 2 AM, expects her to be awake when he comes home from work and have a warm meal ready in the oven. "He hits me if I'm asleep." She had taped her eyes open so that even if she were lying down when he came home she would look awake. "I didn't even think about taking my contacts out." ∎

Family Coping Patterns

To effectively assess abuse, the nurse must show a willingness to listen and avoid any judgmental tone. It is important to assess family strengths as well as stressors. Questioning about memories of early family relationships can provide additional information about attitudes in the home and the way they might influence coping. Asking parents about how they were disciplined as children may provide insight into their childrearing attitudes and practices. Living with and caring for children and older adults can cause frustration, stress, and anger. Unless there are appropriate outlets for stress, abuse can occur. Box 26-5 is a useful guide for assessing the risk of child and/or older adult abuse in the home.

Support Systems

The person experiencing abuse is usually in a dependent position, relying on the perpetrator for basic needs. This dependence, along with the isolation the perpetrator imposes on the person, limits the victim's access to support systems. Children's options are especially limited, as are those of the physically and mentally challenged. Assessing for support should focus on intrapersonal, interpersonal, and community resources (e.g., the school system for school-aged victims).

Suicide Potential

A person experiencing violence may feel desperate to leave yet be trapped in a detrimental relationship, and suicide may seem like the only option. The threat of suicide may also be used by an emotionally abusive person in an attempt to manipulate the victim into caving in to demands ("Don't leave me or I'll kill myself." "I took all my pills …. I said I would the next time you were late.")

A suicide attempt may be the presenting symptom in the emergency department. With sensitive questioning conducted in a caring manner, the nurse can elicit the history of violence. Often the means of attempted suicide is overdose with a combination of alcohol and other central nervous system depressants, or sleeping medications that have been prescribed in previous visits to physicians' offices, clinics, or emergency departments.

When the crisis of the immediate suicide attempt has been resolved, careful questioning to determine lethality is in order. For example, if the patient still feels that life is not worth living, has a suicide plan, and has the means to carry it out, admission to an inpatient psychiatric unit must be considered. On the other hand, if the patient is talking about future plans and about staying "for the sake of the children," outpatient referrals are appropriate.

BOX 26-5 Factors to Assess During a Home Visit

For a Child
- Responsiveness to infant's signals
- Caregiver's facial expressions in response to infant
- Playfulness of caregiver with infant
- Nature of physical contact during feeding and other caretaking activities
- Temperament of infant
- Caregiver's history of harsh discipline or abuse as a child
- Parental attitudes:
  - Feelings of inadequacy as a parent
  - Unrealistic expectations of child
  - Fear of "doing something wrong"
  - Attribution of negative qualities to newborn
  - Misdirected anger
  - Continued evidence of isolation, apathy, anger, frustration, projection
  - Adult conflict
- Environmental conditions:
  - Sleeping arrangements
  - Child management
  - Home management
  - Use of supports (formal and informal)
- Need for immediate services for situational (economics, child care), emotional, or educational information:
  - Information about hotlines, baby-sitters, homemakers, parent groups
  - Information about child development
  - Information about child care and home management services

For an Older Adult
- Absence of lack of access to basic necessities (food, water, medications)
- Unsafe housing
- Lack of or inadequate utilities, ventilation, space
- Poor physical hygiene
- Lack of assistive devices, such as hearing aids, eyeglasses, wheelchair
- Medication mismanagement (outdated prescriptions, unmarked bottles)

Homicide Potential

Ask whether the patient feels safe going home and if so, whether a safety plan is in place for when the violence recurs. The potential for lethality should be assessed (Campbell, 2004), recognizing that certain factors place a vulnerable person at greater risk for homicide, including the following:

- The presence of a gun in the home
- Alcohol and drug abuse
- History of violence on the part of the perpetrator in other situations
- Extreme jealousy and obsessiveness on the part of the perpetrator regarding the relationship with the victim and attempt to control all the victim's daily activities

Persons victimized by violence should be asked if they have ever felt like killing the perpetrator and if so, whether they have the current desire and means to do so. If the answer is yes, intervention is required.

Drug and Alcohol Use

A person experiencing violence may self-medicate with alcohol or other drugs as a way of escaping an intolerable situation. The drugs are usually central nervous system depressants (e.g., benzodiazepines) prescribed by physicians in response to the patient's presentation with vague complaints, which are often stress related (e.g., insomnia, gastrointestinal upsets, anxiety, difficulty concentrating).

The degree of intoxication can be determined by history, physical examination, and blood alcohol level. If an abused patient is intoxicated on presentation, allow the patient time to sober up before initiating referral. Referral information will not be understood or assimilated if the patient is intoxicated. The patient should not be discharged to the abuser. Assess for a chronic alcohol or drug problem (see Chapter 18) and provide appropriate treatment referrals. Treatment choices can include both inpatient and outpatient options.

Maintaining Accurate Records

Because of the possibility of future legal action, it is essential that the health care record contain an accurate and detailed description of the victim's medical history, the psychosocial history of the family, and observations of the family interactions during the interviews. Especially important in documentation of findings from the initial assessment are (1) verbatim statements of who caused the injury and when it occurred; (2) a body map to indicate size, color, shape, areas, and types of injuries, with explanations (see Figure 26-2); and (3) physical evidence of sexual abuse, when possible. Procedures for evidence collection must be followed carefully, or legal action can be thwarted. If the abuse has just occurred, ask the patient to return in a day or two for more photographs; bruises may be more evident at that time. The patient must be assured of the confidentiality of the record and of its power, should legal action be initiated. Even if intervention does not occur at this time, the record is begun; the next provider will be aware of the problem and will be in a better position to offer support.

Self-Assessment

In all areas of psychiatric mental health nursing and counseling, the nurse should be aware of personal emotions and thoughts. Acknowledging feelings that arise in response to those experiencing abuse stimulates an examination of personal views toward abuse and the status of children, women, and older adults. Strong negative feelings can cloud one's judgment and interfere with objective assessment and intervention, no matter how well we try to cover or deny personal bias. Intense and overwhelming feelings may be aroused by working with those experiencing violence. Common responses of health care professionals to violence are listed in Table 26-4.

The nurse who has a personal history of abuse may identify too closely with the victim, and personal issues connected with the abuse may surface, further clouding judgment (Thomas, 2003). Many nurses do not believe they are adequately prepared or have not had enough supervisory experience to intervene in cases of abuse. Supervision needs to be made available to nurses working with victims of abuse.

Multidisciplinary team conferences can be especially helpful in clarifying reactions and neutralizing intense emotions. Information from physicians, psychologists, nurses, and social workers can assist in refocusing efforts to work constructively with a family in crisis. Sharing perceptions and feelings with other professionals can help reduce feelings of isolation and discomfort.

Assessment Guidelines   Family Violence

During your assessment and counseling, maintain an interested and empathetic manner. Refrain from displaying horror, anger, shock, or disapproval of the perpetrator or the situation. Assess:

1. Presenting signs and symptoms of victims of abuse
2. Potential problems in vulnerable families; for example, some indicators of vulnerable parents who might benefit from education and instruction in effective coping techniques
3. Physical, sexual, and/or emotional abuse and neglect and economic maltreatment of older adults
4. Family coping patterns
5. Patient's support system
6. Drug or alcohol use
7. Suicidal or homicidal ideas
8. Post-trauma syndrome

If the patient is a child or older adult, identify the protective agency in your state that must be notified.

TABLE 26-4 Common Responses of Health Care Professionals to Violence

Response	Source
Anger	Anger may be felt toward the person responsible for the abuse, toward those who allowed it to happen, and toward society for condoning its occurrence through attitudes, traditions, and laws.
Embarrassment	The victim is a symbol of something close to home: the stress and strain of family life unleashed as uncontrollable anger.
Confusion	One's view of the family as a haven of safety and privacy is challenged.
Fear	A small percentage of perpetrators are dangerous to others.
Anguish	The nurse may have experienced abuse.
Helplessness	The nurse may want to do more, eliminate the problem, or cure the victim and/or perpetrator.
Discouragement	Discouragement may result if no long-term solution is achieved.
"Blame the victim" mentality	Health care workers can get caught up in "blaming the victim" for behaviors they see as provoking the abuse. There is never an excuse for abuse, and no one has the right to hurt another person. "Blaming the victim" can occur when health care professionals feel overwhelmed. Supervision is a must for therapeutic intervention.

DIAGNOSIS

Nursing diagnoses are focused on the underlying causes and symptoms of family violence. *Risk for injury, Risk for violence* (self-directed or other-directed), *Anxiety, Fear, Disabled family coping, Powerlessness,* and *Caregiver role strain* apply. Feelings of helplessness, hopelessness, and powerlessness contribute to the diagnoses of *Disturbed body image* and *Chronic low self-esteem.* The crisis of family abuse precipitates *Interrupted family process* or *Impaired parenting* as the family system becomes less able to meet the emotional, physical, and security needs of its members.

Pain related to physical injury or trauma would most certainly take high priority and need immediate attention. Table 26-5 lists potential nursing diagnoses for abuse.

The identification of desired outcomes and design of nursing interventions that facilitate achieving those outcomes should be developed as much as possible in collaboration with the survivor and primary support person. These outcomes should be continually reassessed and revised as new information about the survivor's needs emerges. A comprehensive plan can also be the coordinating framework for the work of an multidisciplinary team.

TABLE 26-5 Potential Nursing Diagnoses for Family Violence

Signs and Symptoms	Potential Nursing Diagnoses
Bruises, cuts, broken bones, lacerations, scars, burns, wounds in various phases of healing, particularly when explanations do not match injury or explanations are vague	*Risk for injury* *Pain* *Risk for infection* *Impaired skin integrity* *Risk for post-trauma syndrome*
Isolation, fear, feelings of shame and low self-esteem, feelings of worthlessness, depression, feelings of helplessness	*Powerlessness* *Ineffective coping* *Fear* *Risk for self-directed violence* *Chronic or situational low self-esteem* *Helplessness* *Spiritual distress*
Vaginal-anal bruises, sores, discharge, peritoneal pain, positive venereal disease test results	*Rape-trauma syndrome* *Risk for infection*

Data from North American Nursing Diagnosis Association International (NANDA-I) (2009). *NANDA-I nursing diagnoses: Definitions and classification 2009–2011.* Oxford, United Kingdom: Author.

OUTCOMES IDENTIFICATION

The *Nursing Outcomes Classification (NOC)* (Moorhead et al., 2008) identifies the following indicators for the outcome of *Abuse Cessation*, which is defined as "evidence that the victim is no longer hurt or exploited":

- Physical abuse has ceased.
- Emotional abuse has ceased.
- Sexual abuse has ceased.
- Financial exploitation has ceased.

NOC offers other abuse-specific outcomes, including *Abuse Protection, Abuse Recovery, Abuse Recovery: Emotional; Abuse Recovery: Financial; Abuse Recovery: Physical; and Abuse Recovery: Sexual*. In addition, it is appropriate to include outcomes focusing on improved coping, self-esteem, social support, and pain control, to name a few.

Table 26-6 can be used as a guideline for specific outcome criteria, along with short-term and intermediate indicators for victims of child, intimate partner, and elder abuse, as well as the abuser.

PLANNING

Nurses and other health care workers encounter abuse frequently, not only in health care settings but also in their communities and families. Unfortunately, abuse within families is seldom recognized by those outside the family, including nurses. The nurse is often the first point of contact for people experiencing abuse and thus is in an ideal position to contribute to prevention, detection, and effective intervention. The Joint Commission requires staff education in family violence and abuse, as well as the development of standards of care to guide clinical practice (Family Violence Prevention Fund, 2004a, 2004b).

The Nursing Network on Violence Against Women encourages the development of a nursing practice that focuses on health issues relating to the effects of abuse on women's lives. Altering the pattern of violence against women can also affect child abuse, because the main predictor of violence toward children is violence toward their mothers. Ultimately, the general tolerance of violence in the United States must be addressed if long-lasting changes are to be made.

Most hospitals and community centers provide protocols for dealing with child, intimate partner, or elder abuse that may or may not meet all the needs of a given patient. Unless it is a case of child abuse in which the child has been removed from the home, most interventions performed after necessary emergency care will take place within the community. Plans should center around the patient's safety first. Whenever it is possible or in the best interests of the patient, plans should be discussed with the patient. Planning should also take into consideration the needs of the abuser(s) (e.g., parents, caretakers, spouse or partner) if he or she is willing to learn alternatives to abuse and violence.

IMPLEMENTATION

Reporting Abuse

Nurses are legally mandated to report suspected or actual cases of child and vulnerable adult abuse. The appropriate agency may be the state or county child welfare agency, law enforcement agency, juvenile court, or county health department. Each state has specific guidelines for reporting, including whether the report can be oral, written, or both, and within what time period the suspected abuse or neglect must be reported (immediately, within 24 hours, or within 48 hours).

TABLE 26-6 *NOC* Outcomes for Family Abuse	
Nursing Outcome and Definition	**Short-Term and Intermediate Indicators**
Abuse Cessation: Evidence that the victim is no longer hurt or exploited	Evidence that physical abuse has ceased Evidence that emotional abuse has ceased Evidence that sexual abuse has ceased
Abuse Recovery: Physical: Extent of healing of physical injuries due to abuse	Timely treatment of injuries Healing of physical injuries Resolution of physical health problems
Abuse Recovery: Financial: Extent of control of monetary and legal matters following financial exploitation	Control of social security and pension income Protection in financial resources Control of withdrawal of money from account(s)
Abusive Behavior Self-Restraint: Self-restraint of abusive and neglectful behaviors toward others	Obtains needed treatment Controls impulses Discusses the abusive behavior

Data from Moorhead, S., Johnson, M., Maas, M., & Swanson, E. (2008). *Nursing outcomes classification (NOC)* (4th ed.). St. Louis: Mosby.

Every abused person is a crime victim, and assault with a weapon is reportable in most states. All 50 states have marital rape statutes. The following vignette gives an example of a child-abuse case to report.

VIGNETTE

Two nurses who work in a family practice clinic are suspicious of child abuse. A 12-year-old girl has recurrent urinary tract infections. She is always brought to clinic visits by her father, who accompanies her into the bathroom when she is providing urine samples. He answers all questions for the girl, even when they are directed to her. He has recently refused the next diagnostic test to attempt to ascertain the reason for the recurrent infections.

After pressure by the nurses, the physician agrees to ask the girl some questions in private. The nurses think the physician has discounted the problem, asked superficial questions, and dismissed their concerns. However, the nurses are not successful in their attempt to separate the girl from her father for a discussion. They decide to report their concerns to Children's Protective Services. They inform the father, who becomes outraged at their accusations and threatens to change doctors. Subsequent investigation confirms the likelihood of sexual abuse, and the child is placed in temporary foster care with follow-up counseling. The father refuses treatment and threatens to sue the nurses. Four months later, the father leaves the family. ▪

The case in the preceding vignette illustrates that a reasonable basis for suspecting abuse, not proof, is all that is required to report. Nurses must attempt to maintain both an appropriate level of suspicion and a neutral, objective attitude. One can be too concerned and jump to conclusions (which is what the physician in this case thought the nurses were doing) or not be concerned enough and rationalize an incomplete examination to avoid confrontation (which is what the nurses thought the physician was doing). Given these opposing stances, the case was reported, as required by law and ethical standards, and Children's Protective Services was given the opportunity to investigate.

Competency may be a consideration in a situation of elder abuse. Unless the older adult has been found legally incompetent, he or she has the right to self-determination. Many older abused women are battered women who have grown old. They are not incompetent simply by virtue of their age; therefore, they would not legally be considered vulnerable adults.

Some institutions and health care agencies have developed guidelines for dealing with actual or suspected situations of abuse. These protocols list possible behaviors or conditions of older adults and the most appropriate intervention. Establishing such protocols is highly recommended because it gives support to the nurse's actions.

Quality nursing care for those experiencing abuse must be culturally sensitive. This means the nurse must be aware of the cultural issues that may affect response to violence and to intervention. For example, Cambodian women control their responses to stress and violence through nonconfrontation and withdrawal, which are designed to restore equilibrium. Culture is important because it is central to how people organize their experience. Even the most acculturated people have a tendency to revert to their cultural past in organizing coping strategies after a stressful event. If there is a language barrier, the nurse should speak slowly and clearly in English, without using jargon, and allow time for the response. If the patient speaks no English, a trained medical interpreter should be provided. A family member should *not* be used as interpreter (to ensure confidentiality and protect the person from future retaliation).

Counseling

Counseling includes crisis intervention measures. It is important to emphasize that people have a right to live without fear of violence, physical harm, or assault. Telling an abused person that "no one deserves to be hit" can be a powerful statement in and of itself. The role of the nurse is to support the victim, counsel about safety, and facilitate access to other resources as appropriate. By listening, giving support, discussing options, and describing alternative ways of living, the nurse initiates an awareness of other possibilities.

All persons experiencing abuse should be counseled about developing a **safety plan**, a plan for a rapid escape when abuse recurs. Patients should be asked to identify the signs of escalation of violence and to pick a particular sign that will tell them in the future that "now is the time to leave." If children are present, they can all agree on a code word that, when spoken by the parent, means "It is time to go." If the individual plans ahead, it may be possible to leave before the violence occurs. It is important that the plan include a destination and transportation. The nurse should suggest packing the items listed in Box 26-6 ahead of time. The packed bag should be kept in a place where the perpetrator will not find it.

If the abused person chooses to leave, **shelters or safe houses** (for both sexes) are available in many communities. They are open 24 hours a day and can be reached through hotline information numbers, hospital emergency departments, YWCAs, or the local office of the National Organization for Women. The address of the house is usually kept secret to protect abused persons from attack by the perpetrator. Besides offering protection, many of these shelters and safe houses serve important education and consciousness-raising functions. Patients should be given the number of the

BOX 26-6 Personalized Safety Guide

Suggestions for Increasing Safety While in the Relationship

- I will have important phone numbers available to my children and myself.

- I can tell _____ and _____ about the violence and ask them to call the police if they hear suspicious noises coming from my home.

- If I leave my home, I can go to (list four places) _____, _____, _____, or _____.

- I can leave extra money, car keys, clothes, and copies of documents with _____.

- If I leave, I will bring _____ (see checklist below).

- To ensure safety and independence, I can keep change for phone calls with me at all times; open my own savings account; rehearse my escape route with a support person; and review safety plan on _____ (date).

Suggestions for Increasing Safety When the Relationship Is Over

- I can change the locks; install steel or metal doors, a security system, smoke detectors, and an outside lighting system.

- I will inform _____ and _____ that my partner no longer lives with me and ask them to call the police if he or she is observed near my home or my children.

- I will tell people who take care of my children the names of those who have permission to pick them up. The people who have permission are _____, _____, and _____.

- I can tell _____ at work about my situation and ask _____ to screen my calls.

- I can avoid stores, banks, and _____ that I used when living with my battering partner.

- I can obtain a protective order from _____. I can keep it on or near me at all times, as well as have a copy with _____.

- If I feel down and ready to return to a potentially abusive situation, I can call _____ for support or attend workshops and support groups to gain support and strengthen my relationships with other people.

Important Phone Numbers

- Police _____
- Hotline _____
- Friends _____
- Shelter _____

Checklist of Items to Take

- ☐ Identification
- ☐ Bwirth certificates for me and my children
- ☐ Social Security card
- ☐ School and medical records
- ☐ Money, bank books, credit cards
- ☐ Keys to house, car, office
- ☐ Driver's license and registration
- ☐ Medications
- ☐ Change of clothes
- ☐ Welfare identification
- ☐ Passport(s), green card, work permit
- ☐ Divorce papers
- ☐ Lease or rental agreement, house deed
- ☐ Mortgage payment book, current unpaid bills
- ☐ Insurance papers
- ☐ Address book
- ☐ Pictures, jewelry, items of sentimental value
- ☐ Children's favorite toys and/or blankets

nearest available shelter, even if they decide for the present to stay with their partners. Referral phone numbers may be kept for years before the decision to call is made. Having the number and a contact person all that time contributes to thinking about options.

Case Management

Community mental health centers are becoming increasingly involved in the delivery of services to victims and perpetrators of abuse. Nurses working in these settings have the opportunity to coordinate community, medical, criminal justice, and social services to provide comprehensive assistance to families in crisis. Strategies must encompass needs for housing, child care, economic stability, physical and emotional safety, counseling, legal protection, career development or job training, education, ongoing support groups, and health care.

The myriad of agencies and people that those seeking help must reach can be daunting and confusing. A nurse functioning in a case manager role can assist the patient in choosing the best options and coordinating the interventions of several agencies. Box 26-7 lists selected *NIC* interventions for *Abuse protection support* for children, intimate partners, and older adults (Bulechek et al., 2008).

BOX 26-7 Interventions for Abuse Protection Support for Children, Intimate Partners, and Older Adults

Abuse Protection Support: Children
Definition: Identification of high-risk, dependent child relationships and actions to prevent possible or further infliction of physical, sexual, or emotional harm or neglect of basic necessities of life
*Activities**

- Identify mothers who have a history of late (4 months or later) or no prenatal care.
- Identify parents who have had another child removed from the home or have placed previous children with relatives for extended periods.
- Identify parents with a history of domestic violence or a mother who has a history of numerous "accidental" injuries.
- Determine whether a child demonstrates signs of physical abuse, including numerous injuries in various stages of healing; unexplained bruises and welts; unexplained pattern, immersion, and friction burns; facial, spiral, shaft, or multiple fractures; unexplained facial lacerations and abrasions; human bite marks; intracranial, subdural, intraventricular, and intraocular hemorrhaging; whiplash shaken infant syndrome; and diseases that are resistant to treatment and/or have changing signs and symptoms.
- Encourage admission of child for further observation and investigation as appropriate.
- Monitor parent-child interactions and record observations.
- Report suspected abuse or neglect to proper authorities.

Abuse Protection Support: Intimate Partners
Definition: Identification of high-risk, dependent domestic relationships and action to prevent possible or further infliction of physical, sexual, or emotional harm or exploitation of a domestic partner
*Activities**:
- Screen for risk factors associated with domestic abuse (e.g., history of domestic violence, abuse, rejection, excessive

criticism, or feelings of being worthless and unloved; difficulty trusting others or feeling disliked by others; feeling that asking for help is an indication of personal incompetence; high physical care needs; intense family care responsibilities; substance abuse; depression; major psychiatric illness; social isolation; poor relationships between domestic partners; multiple marriages; pregnancy; poverty; unemployment; financial dependence; homelessness; infidelity; divorce; or death of a loved one).
- Document evidence of physical or sexual abuse using standardized assessment tools and photographs.
- Listen attentively to individual who begins to talk about own problems.
- Encourage admission to a hospital for further observation and investigation, as appropriate.
- Provide positive affirmation of worth.
- Report any situations in which abuse is suspected in compliance with mandatory reporting laws.

Abuse Protection Support: Older Adults
Definition: Identification of high-risk, dependent elder relationships and actions to prevent possible or further infliction of physical, sexual, or emotional harm; neglect of basic necessities of life; or exploitation
*Activities**:
- Identify older patients who perceive themselves to be dependent on caretakers due to impaired health status, functional impairment, limited economic resources, depression, substance abuse, or lack or knowledge of available resource and alternatives for care.
- Identify family caretakers who have a history of being abused or neglected in childhood.
- Monitor patient-caretaker interactions and record observations.
- Report suspected abuse or neglect to proper authorities.

---

*Partial list.
Data from Bulechek, G. M., Butcher, H. K., & Dochterman, J. M. (2008). *Nursing interventions classification (NIC)* (pp. 97–104). St. Louis: Mosby.

Milieu Management

Interventions are geared toward stabilizing the home situation and maintaining an abuse-free environment. Some mental health agencies have family-based units in which a caseworker or clinician visits the home instead of the family going to the agency. Providing and maintaining a therapeutic environment in the home ideally involves three levels of help for abusive families:

1. Provide the family with economic support, job opportunities, and social services.
2. Arrange social support in the form of a public health nurse, lay home visitor, daycare teacher, schoolteacher, social worker, respite worker, or any other potential contact person who has a good relationship with the family.
3. Encourage and provide family therapy.

Promotion of Self-Care Activities

The primary goal of intervention is empowerment. Supporting the patient to act on her or his own behalf can decrease feelings of helplessness and hopelessness. The initial phase of recovery begins when a patient first makes steps to leave the abusive relationship. Giving referral numbers and providing an opportunity for the patient to call from your office, or inquiring at the next visit whether the patient was successful in reaching the appropriate agency, demonstrates confidence in the patient's ability to take care of herself or himself.

Specific referrals regarding emergency financial assistance and legal counseling should be made available to each patient. Vocational counseling is another referral that may be appropriate. Patients should be given referrals to parenting resources that enable them to explore alternative approaches to discipline (e.g., no hitting, slapping, or other expressions of violence).

Health Teaching and Health Promotion

In families at risk for abuse, health teaching and promotion includes meeting with both the individual and the family and discussing associated risk factors. The patient, caregiver, and family need to learn to recognize behaviors and situations that might trigger violence.

Normal developmental and physiological changes should be explained to enable family members to gain a more positive view of the victim and the crisis situation. Gaining a more complete understanding can help family members broaden their insight and thus increase their compassion. They may then begin to anticipate new stress situations and be able to prepare for them before a crisis occurs.

Nurses who work on a maternity unit are often in a position to identify risk factors for abuse between new parents and initiate appropriate interventions, including education about effective parenting and coping techniques. Information about these interventions should be shared with the patient's health care team for appropriate monitoring and follow-up. Parents who are candidates for special attention include:

- New parents whose behavior toward the infant is rejecting, hostile, or indifferent.
- Teenage parents, who require special help in handling the baby and discussing their expectations of the baby and their support systems.
- Parents with cognitive deficits, for whom careful, explicit, and repeated instructions on caring for the child and recognizing the infant's needs are indicated.
- Parents who grew up watching their mothers being abused. This is a significant risk factor for perpetuation of family violence.

Nurses can also recognize when children are at risk and make referrals to community resources, including emergency child care facilities, emergency telephone numbers, numbers of 24-hour crisis centers or hotlines, and respite programs in which volunteers take the child for an occasional weekend so parents can get some relief. Community health nurses can make home visits to identify risk factors for abuse in the crucial first few months of life during which the style of parent-child interactions is established. See Box 26-5 for important factors for the community health nurse to assess during a home care visit. Such observations made by nurses in clinic and public health settings are fundamental in case finding and evaluation.

Prevention of Abuse

Primary Prevention

Primary prevention consists of measures taken to prevent the occurrence of abuse. Identifying individuals and families at high risk, providing health teaching, and coordinating supportive services to prevent crises are examples of primary prevention. Specific strategies include (1) reducing stress, (2) reducing the influence of risk factors, (3) increasing social support, (4) increasing coping skills, and (5) increasing self-esteem. Community health nurses are in a unique position to assess family functioning in the home during visits for other medical problems. In addition, the community health nurse and clinic nurse maintain contact with the family over time, which allows for assessment of changes. They are also in an excellent position to connect parents to appropriate resources in the community that can meet their needs. All nurses can work to reduce society's acceptance of violence by working toward social policy change.

Secondary Prevention

Secondary prevention involves early intervention in abusive situations to minimize their disabling or long-term effects. Nurses can establish screening programs for individuals at risk, participate in the medical treatment of injuries resulting from violent episodes, and coordinate community services to provide continuity of care. Stress and depression can be reduced by providing supportive psychotherapy, support groups, pharmacotherapy, and contact information for community resources. Social dysfunction or lack of information can be addressed by counseling and education. Caregiver burden can be reduced by arranging assistance in caregiving, nursing, or housekeeping or (in cases in which caregiving needs exceed even optimal caregiver capacity) by placing the patient in a more appropriate setting. The following vignette illustrates a successful secondary prevention effort.

VIGNETTE

Gavin, aged 4 years, is brought into the physician's office by 15-year-old Ashley, the child's babysitter, with second-degree burns on his right hand. Ashley frequently babysits for Gavin and his younger brother Tyler, aged 2, and older brother Logan, aged 6. Ashley appears apprehensive and says she is very concerned. Ashley tells the nurse that the children have told her in the past that their mother has threatened them with burning if they do not behave. Gavin told her that his mother once held his hands on a cold stove and told him that if he was bad, she would burn him. Ashley is shocked that Gavin's mother would do such a thing, but at the same time, she says she feels guilty for "telling on Ms. J."

Ashley also states that the older brother, Logan, told her what happened to Gavin but was afraid that if his mother found out, she would burn him also. Ashley says she is aware that the mother hits the children, but she did not believe that anyone would burn her own child. The nurse reports the incident to the physician, and the mother is called and asked to come to the office. Meanwhile, the nurse asks Ashley to come with Gavin while she examines him. Gavin appears frightened and in pain.

Nurse: Tell me about your hand, Gavin. *(Gavin looks down and starts to cry.)* It's OK if you don't want to talk about it, Gavin.

Gavin: *(Does not look at the nurse and speaks softly.)* My mommy burned my hand on the stove.

Nurse: Tell me what happened before that.

Gavin: Mommy was mad because I didn't put my toys away.

Nurse: What does your mommy usually do when she gets mad?

Gavin: She yells mostly. Sometimes she hits us. Mommy is going to be so mad at Logan for telling.

Nurse: Tell me about the hitting.

Gavin: Mommy hits us a lot since daddy left. *(Gavin starts to cry to himself.)*

On examination, the nurse notices a ringed pattern of burns resembling the burner on an electric stove across Gavin's right palm. There are blisters on the fingers. Gavin appears well nourished and properly dressed. He is at his approximate developmental age except for some language delay. Because of the physical evidence and history, there is strong suspicion of child abuse. Children's Protective Services is notified, and the family situation is evaluated for possible placement of Gavin in protective custody. The initial evaluation concludes that there is no indication of serious potential harm to the child and that Gavin should return home. The mother, who is initially defensive, starts to cry and states, "I can't cope with being alone, and I don't know where to turn."

Nursing interventions center on caring for Gavin's immediate health needs, finding supports for the mother to help her cope with crises, providing a counseling referral for the mother to learn alternative ways of expressing anger and frustration, informing the mother of parents' groups, providing referrals to play groups or daycare for the children to help increase their feelings of self-esteem and security, and providing a break and instruction in parenting for the mother. ■

Tertiary Prevention

Tertiary prevention, which often occurs in mental health settings, involves nurses facilitating the healing and rehabilitative process by counseling individuals and families, providing support for groups of survivors, and assisting survivors of violence to achieve their optimal level of safety, health, and well-being. Legal advocacy programs for survivors of intimate partner violence are an example of tertiary prevention (Chamberlain, 2008). Complementary therapies, such as mindfulness-based stress reduction, can also assist survivors in the healing process.

Advanced Practice Interventions

Psychotherapy is carried out by a nurse who is educated at the master's level in psychiatric nursing and is certified or eligible for certification. Therapy is most effective after crisis intervention, when the situation is less chaotic and tumultuous. A variety of therapeutic modalities are available for treatment of abusive families.

Individual Psychotherapy

The goals of individual therapy for a survivor are empowerment, the ability to recognize and choose productive life options, and the development of a solid sense of self. People who have experienced abuse as a child or have left a violent relationship may choose individual therapy to address symptoms of depression, anxiety, somatization, or PTSD.

Many of the psychological symptoms shown by women who have been abused can be understood as complex survival strategies and responses to violence. This constellation of symptoms has been referred to as the "battered woman syndrome," the PTSD category in the *Diagnostic and Statistical Manual of Mental Disorders,* fourth edition, text revision *(DSM-IV-TR)* (American Psychiatric Association [APA], 2000).

Nurses must address the guilt, shame, and stigmatization experienced by survivors of abuse (Campbell et al., 2003). It is helpful for nurses to understand that the patient's feelings and behaviors may be reflective of the grieving process, since he or she has experienced numerous losses as a result of the abusive relationship.

Individual psychotherapy is often indicated for the perpetrator, particularly when an individual psychopathological process is identified. Therapy for the perpetrator is most effective when it is court mandated, because the perpetrator is more likely to complete the course of treatment. Many perpetrators meet the *DSM-IV-TR* criteria for intermittent explosive disorder, which involves repeated episodes of assault or destruction of property out of proportion to precipitating stressors that cannot be accounted for by another mental disorder, the physiological effects of a substance, or a general medical condition. Nurses engaged in therapy with perpetrators have a duty to warn potential victims if they conclude that the perpetrator is a danger. Refer to Chapter 7 for a more detailed discussion of the duty to warn and duty to protect.

Family Psychotherapy

Because abuse is a symptom of a family in crisis, each part of the family system needs attention. Also, because change in one member of the family system affects the whole system, support and understanding are needed by all members. Interventions may maximize positive interactions among all family members. Family or marital therapy should take place *only* if the perpetrator has had individual therapy and has demonstrated change as a result and if both parties agree to participate.

Expected outcomes are that the perpetrator will recognize destructive patterns of behavior and learn alternative responses. Intermediate goals are that members of the family will openly communicate and learn to listen to each other. Refer to Chapter 35 for a more detailed discussion of family therapy.

Group Psychotherapy

Participation in therapy groups provides assurances that one is not alone and that positive change is possible. Because many survivors of abuse have been isolated over time, they have been deprived of validation and positive feedback from others. Working in a group can help diminish feelings of isolation, strengthen feelings of self-esteem and self-worth, and increase the potential for realistic problem solving in a supportive atmosphere.

The real problem in an abusive relationship is the perpetrator. Groups often use cognitive-behavioral techniques to help the abuser see abusive actions as behavioral patterns that can be changed. In therapy groups, perpetrators are taught to recognize the thoughts preceding an abusive incident, the responses to the thoughts, and how to interrupt negative feelings about their partners. Perpetrators who have never discussed problems with anyone before are encouraged to discuss their thoughts and feelings. Group therapy can help create a community of healing and restoration. Refer to Chapter 34 for a more detailed discussion of group therapy.

EVALUATION

Failures of interventions with abusive families often are due to problems within the social, economic, and political systems in which we live. A very real problem is that of social exclusion, by which disadvantaged individuals are prohibited from obtaining formal helping services (Hilbert & Krishnan, 2000). Nurses can direct their interventions to the social environment and can question, among other things, the acceptance of corporal punishment as a technique for guiding behavior in children, the unequal burden of caregiving responsibilities placed on women, the low priority given to education and preparation for parenthood, and the belief that older adults have little social value.

Evaluation of brief interventions can be based on whether the survivor acknowledges the violence, is willing to accept intervention, and is removed from the abusive situation. Evaluation of long-term interventions should be made on an ongoing basis. Because abuse is a symptom of a family in crisis, diagnosis, interventions, and evaluation should be carried out by a multidisciplinary team that includes a physician, a nurse, a social worker, an attorney, and perhaps a psychiatrist. Follow-up is crucial in helping decrease the frequency of family abuse.

Case Study and Nursing Care Plan 26-1   Family Violence

Mrs. Robb, a recently widowed 84-year-old woman, moved to her son's apartment 3 months ago. She had been living in her third-floor walk-up in the city. Because of her declining health, crime in the neighborhood, and the need to climb three flights of stairs, and with her son John's encouragement, she went to live with him. He and his wife Judy, who have been married for almost 20 years, have five children 6 to 18 years of age, all living in a rather cramped three-bedroom apartment.

Mrs. Robb is being cared for by a visiting nurse, who monitors her blood pressure and adjusts her medication. Over a series of visits, the nurse, Ms. Green, notices that Mrs. Robb is looking unkempt, pale, and withdrawn. While taking her blood pressure, Ms. Green observes bruises on Mrs. Robb's arms and neck. When questioned about the bruises, Mrs. Robb appears anxious and nervous. She says that she slipped in the bathroom. Mrs. Robb becomes increasingly apprehensive and stiffens up in her chair when her daughter-in-law Judy comes into the room, asking when the next visit is. The nurse notices that Judy avoids eye contact with Mrs. Robb.

When the injuries are brought to Judy's attention, she responds by becoming angry and agitated, blaming Mrs. Robb for causing so many problems. She will not explain the reason for the change in Mrs. Robb's behavior or the origin of the bruises to the nurse. She merely comments, "I have had to give up my job since my mother-in-law came here. It's been difficult and crowded ever since she moved in. The kids are complaining. We are having trouble making ends meet since I gave up my job. And my husband is no help at all."

ASSESSMENT

Self-Assessment

Ms. Green has worked in a number of situations with violent families, but this is the first time she has encountered elder maltreatment. She discusses her reactions with the other team members. She is especially angry at Judy, although she is able to understand the daughter-in-law's frustration. The team concurs with Ms. Green that there seems to be potential for positive change in this family. If abuse does not abate, more drastic measures will need to be taken and legal services contacted.

Objective Data

Physical symptoms of violence (bruises, unkempt appearance, withdrawn attitude)

Stressful, crowded living conditions

No eye contact between Mrs. Robb and her daughter-in-law

Economic hardships leading to stress

No support for the daughter-in-law from the rest of the family for care of Mrs. Robb

Subjective Data

Mrs. Robb states she slipped in the bathroom, but physical findings do not support this explanation.

Judy states, "It's been difficult and crowded ever since she moved in."

Mrs. Robb exhibits withdrawn and apprehensive behavior.

DIAGNOSIS

On the basis of the data, the nurse formulates the following nursing diagnoses:

1. *Risk for injury* related to increase in family stress, as evidenced by signs of violence

Supporting Data

- Mrs. Robb states she slipped in the bathroom, but physical findings do not support this explanation.
- Physical symptoms of violence (bruises, unkempt appearance, withdrawn attitude)
- Stressful, crowded living conditions

2. *Ineffective coping* related to helplessness, as evidenced by inability to meet role expectations

Supporting Data

- Mrs. Robb appears unkempt, anxious, depressed.
- Mrs. Robb exhibits withdrawn and apprehensive behavior.

3. *Risk for other-directed violence* related to increased stressors within a short period, as evidenced by probable elder abuse and feelings of helplessness verbalized by the primary caregiver

Supporting Data

- Judy states, "It's been difficult and crowded ever since she moved in."
- No eye contact between Judy and Mrs. Robb
- Signs and symptoms of physical abuse on Mrs. Robb
- Judy says, "My husband is no help at all."

4. *Caregiver role strain* related to extreme feelings of being overwhelmed and of helplessness

Supporting Data

- Family not helping with care of mother-in-law; burden of care on Judy
- Economic hardships leading to stress when Judy gave up her job to care for Mrs. Robb

OUTCOMES IDENTIFICATION

Overall outcome: Abuse cessation: Evidence that the victim is no longer hurt or exploited
Short-term indicators:

- Evidence that physical abuse has ceased
- Evidence that emotional abuse has ceased

PLANNING

Ms. Green discusses several possible outcomes with members of her team, giving attention to the priority of outcomes and to whether they are realistic in this situation. She also plans to report the elder abuse to Adult Protective Services and to work with Mrs. Robb, Judy, and the rest of the family to improve this situation for everyone.

IMPLEMENTATION

Mrs. Robb's plan of care is personalized as follows:
Nursing diagnosis: *Risk for injury* related to increase in family stress, as evidenced by signs of violence
Outcome criteria: Abuse cessation

Short-Term Goal	Interventions	Rationale	Evaluation
1. On each visit made by the nurse, the patient will state that abuse has decreased, using a scale from 1 to 5 (1 being the least abuse).	1a. Follow state laws and guidelines for reporting elder abuse. 1b. Assess severity of signs and symptoms of abuse. 1c. Do a careful home assessment to identify other areas of abuse and neglect. 1d. Discuss with patient factors leading to abuse and concern for safety.	1a. Provides maximum protection under the law. Provides data for future use. 1b. Accurate charting (body map, pictures with permission, verbatim statements) helps follow progress and provides legal data. 1c. Check for inadequacy of food, presence of vermin, blocked stairways, medication safety issues, etc. All indicate abuse and neglect. Determine the kinds of problems in the home, and plan intervention. Identify community resources that could help the elder and caregivers. 1d. Allows family stressors and potential areas for intervention to be identified. Validates that situation is serious and increases patient's knowledge base.	**GOAL MET** Patient states that after family talked to the nurse and planned strategies, physical abuse no longer occurs.

Continued

Short-Term Goal	Interventions	Rationale	Evaluation
2. Within 2 weeks, patient will be able to identify at least two supportive services to deal with emergency situations.	2. Discuss with patient supportive services such as hotlines and crisis units to call in case of emergency situations.	2. Maximizes patient's safety through use of support systems.	**GOAL MET** Patient has been talking to two old friends she had stopped talking to because of shame and depression. She has called the hotline once to get information on transportation to the senior center in town.
3. Within 3 weeks, family members will be able to identify difficult issues that increase their stress levels.	3. Discuss with family members their feelings, and identify at least four areas that are most difficult for the various family members.	3. Listening to each family member and identifying unmet needs helps both family and nurse identify areas that require changing and appropriate interventions.	**GOAL MET** Family members identify areas such as overwork, lack of free time, lack of privacy, and financial difficulties, all of which increase their stress levels.
4. Within 3 weeks, family will seek out community resources to help with anger management, need for homemaker support, and other needs.	4. Identify potential community supports, skills training, respite places, homemakers, financial aids, etc., that might help meet family's unmet needs.	4. When stressed, individuals solve problems poorly and do not know about or cannot manage to organize outside help. Finances are often a problem.	**GOAL MET** The daughter-in-law is glad to get out of the house for anger management classes, and the son states he will try to take on more responsibility, but he often feels guilty and angry too. Reluctantly, he and his wife agree to try a support group with other caregivers in similar situations.

EVALUATION

Eight weeks after Ms. Green's initial visit, Mrs. Robb appears well groomed, friendly, and more spontaneous in her conversation. She comments, "Things are better with my daughter-in-law." No bruises or other signs of physical violence are noticeable. She is considerably more outgoing and has even taken the initiative to contact an old friend. Mrs. Robb has talked openly to her son and daughter-in-law about stress in the family. Mrs. Robb says that she went for a walk when her daughter-in-law Judy appeared tense and returned to find that the tension had lessened. Neither Mrs. Robb nor her family has initiated plans for alternative housing.

KEY POINTS TO REMEMBER

- Abuse can occur in any family and can be predicted with some accuracy by examining the characteristics of perpetrators, vulnerable people, and crisis situations in which violence is likely.
- Abuse can be physical, sexual, emotional, or economic or caused by neglect.
- Assessment includes identifying indicators of abuse, levels of anxiety, coping mechanisms, support systems, suicide and homicide potential, and alcohol and drug abuse.

CRITICAL THINKING

1. A colleague who has witnessed a child being abused states "I don't think it's any of our business what people do in the privacy of their own homes."

   A. What would you be legally required to do?
   B. What are your ethical responsibilities?

2. Congratulations! You successfully convinced your colleagues to assess routinely for abuse. Now they want to know how to do it. How would you go about teaching them to assess for child abuse? Intimate partner abuse? Elder abuse?

3. Your health maintenance organization's routine health screening form for adolescents, adults, and older adults has just been changed to include questions about family abuse. How would you respond to patients who indicate on this form that abuse occurs in their home?

4. Write out a safety plan that could be adopted by individuals who are being abused.

A. Identify at least four referrals in your community for an abused person.

B. Identify two referrals in your community for a violent person, partner, or parent.

CHAPTER REVIEW

1. A man becomes frustrated when his children cry repeatedly and shoves his wife into the refrigerator. His wife explains to the neighbor who witnessed this that, "I should have made the children go to bed earlier so they wouldn't be so cranky." This is an example of:
   1. masochism.
   2. emotional abuse.
   3. tension reduction.
   4. secondary prevention.

2. Which statement(s) about perpetrators and victims of abuse is accurate? *Select all that apply.*
   1. Thirty or more percent of victims of intimate partner and family abuse are male.
   2. Abusive behavior is usually the result of intoxication or stress.
   3. Perpetrators tend to respond best to treatment if it is court ordered.
   4. Victims do not report abuse, because they tacitly are accepting of it.
   5. Victims of abuse stay in the relationship because they really do not want to leave.
   6. Disruptive behavior may make older adults with dementia vulnerable to abuse.

3. A staff nurse, Chandra, is assisting a 30-year-old victim of domestic violence in the emergency department. The patient suffered numerous bruises and abrasions, is reluctant to be examined, seems very ashamed, and is very fearful that Children's Services will take custody of her young daughter, who has not been assaulted and is safe, if the police become involved. Which intervention is indicated?
   1. Report the assault to the police, since reporting of domestic violence is mandatory.

2. Probe the patient for information to use as evidence in prosecuting the perpetrator.
3. Press the patient to disrobe so that she can be examined for signs of hidden injuries.
4. Guide and assist the patient to develop a safety plan for rapid escape should abuse recur.

4. Ms. Patel, a student nurse, is assigned to a patient recovering from injuries received during an episode of domestic violence, the third such assault for which she has received treatment. Ms. Patel left home at age 17 to escape an abusive father. Which statements about this situation are accurate? *Select all that apply.*
   1. Ms. Patel may be prone to blame the patient for her injuries and abuse.
   2. Ms. Patel's personal experiences give her special insight into the needs of this patient.
   3. Ms. Patel's experiences are likely to make her more empathetic towards victims.
   4. Caring for victims of abuse will help Ms. Patel cope with her own abuse experiences.
   5. Ms. Patel may experience overwhelming anguish as a result of caring for abuse victims.
   6. Ms. Patel would likely benefit from clinical supervision related to caring for abuse victims.

5. Perpetrators of domestic violence tend to:
   1. belong to lower socioeconomic groups and be poorly educated.
   2. have relatively poor social skills and to have grown up with poor role models.
   3. believe they, if male, should be dominant and in charge in relationships.
   4. force their mates to work and expect them to support the family.
   5. be controlling and willing to use force to maintain their power in relationships.
   6. prevent their mates from having relationships and activities outside the family.

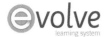 Visit the Evolve website for an **Audio Chapter Summary, Chapter Review Answers & Rationales, Critical Thinking Answer Guidelines,** and additional resources related to the content in this chapter: **http://evolve.elsevier.com/Varcarolis/foundations**

Companion CD Use the Companion CD to prepare for tests and the NCLEX® Examination with **Test-Taking Strategies** for psychiatric mental health nursing and hundreds of **Review Questions**.

References

American Academy of Family Physicians. (2008). *Family and intimate partner violence and abuse.* Retrieved December 10, 2008 from http://www.aafp.org/online/en/home/policy/policies/f/familyandintimatepartner-violenceand-abuse.html

American Psychiatric Association. (2000). *Diagnostic and statistical manual of mental disorders* (4th ed., text rev.) *(DSM-IV-TR).* Washington, DC: Author.

American Psychological Association. (2008). *Elder abuse and neglect: In search of solutions.* Retrieved April 7, 2009 from http://www.apa.org/pi/aging/eldabuse.html

Beck, B. J. (2008). Domestic violence. In T. A. Stern, J. F. Rosenbaum, M. Fava, J. Biederman, & S. L. Rauch (Eds.), *Massachusetts General Hospital comprehensive clinical psychiatry* (pp. 1125–1132). St. Louis: Mosby.

Bensley, L., Van Eenwyk, J., & Wynkoop Simmons, K. (2003). Childhood family violence history and women's risk for intimate partner violence and poor health. *American Journal of Preventive Medicine, 25*(1), 38–44.

Bulechek, G. M., Butcher, H. K., & Dochterman, J. M. (2008). *Nursing interventions classification (NIC)* (5th ed.). St. Louis: Mosby.

Campbell, J. C. (2004). Helping women understand their risk in situations of intimate partner violence. *Journal of Interpersonal Violence, 19*(12), 1464–1477.

Campbell, J. C., Torres, S., McKenna, L. S., Sheridan, D. J., & Landenburger, K. (2003). Nursing care of survivors of intimate partner violence. In J. C. Campbell & J. C. Humphreys (Eds.), *Family violence and nursing practice* (pp. 307–360). Philadelphia: Lippincott Williams & Wilkins.

Chamberlain, L. (2008). A prevention primer for domestic violence: Terminology, tools, and the public health approach. In: P. A. Harrisburg (Ed.), *VAWnet, a project of the National Resource Center on Domestic Violence/Pennsylvania Coalition Against Domestic Violence.* Retrieved 8/6/08, from http://www.vawnet.org

Desai, S., Arias, I., Thompson, M. P., & Basile, K. C. (2002). Childhood victimization and subsequent adult revictimization assessed in a nationally representative sample of women and men. *Violence and Victims, 17*(6), 639–653.

Emergency Nurses Association. (2003). *Emergency Nurses Association position statements: Domestic violence, maltreatment, and neglect.* Retrieved February 18, 2005, http://www.ena.org/about/position/domesticviolence.asp

Family Violence Prevention Fund. (2004a). *Comply with JCAHO Standard PC.3.10 on victims of abuse.* Retrieved February 18, 2005, from http://endabuse.org/programs/display.php3?DocID=266

Family Violence Prevention Fund. (2004b). *Staff education for elder abuse, neglect and exploitation.* Retrieved February 18, 2005, from http://endabuse.org/programs/display.php3?DocID=268

Hilbert, J. C., & Krishnan, S. P. (2000). Addressing barriers to community care of battered women in rural environments: Creating a policy of social inclusion. *Journal of Health and Social Policy, 12*(1), 41–52.

Johnson, C. F. (2002). Physical abuse: Accidental versus intentional trauma in children. In J. E. B. Meyers, L. Berliner, J. N. Briere, C. T. Hendrix, T. A. Reid, & C. A. Jenny (Eds.), *The APSAC handbook on child maltreatment* (pp. 249–268). Thousand Oaks, CA: Sage Publications.

Malley-Morrison, K. & Hines, D. (2003). *Family violence in a cultural perspective: Defining, understanding and combating abuse.* Thousand Oaks, CA: Sage Publications.

Milosavljevic, N., & Brendel, R. W. (2008). Abuse and neglect. In T. A. Stern, J. F. Rosenbaum, M. Fava, J. Biederman, & S. L. Rauch (Eds.), *Massachusetts General Hospital comprehensive clinical psychiatry* (pp. 1133–1142). St. Louis: Mosby.

Moorhead, S., Johnson, M., Maas, M., & Swanson, E. (2008). *Nursing outcomes classification (NOC)* (4th ed.). St. Louis: Mosby.

National Research Council Panel to Review Risk and Prevalence of Elder Abuse and Neglect. (2003). *Elder maltreatment: Abuse, neglect and exploitation in an aging America.* Washington, DC: Author.

Nursing Research Consortium on Violence and Abuse. (2001). *Abuse assessment screen.* Retrieved April 7, 2009 from http://www.nnvawi.org/Abuse%20Assessment.pdf

Stevens, L. (2003). *Clinical update: Improving screening of women for violence—basic guidelines for physicians.* Retrieved February 17, 2004, from http://www.medscape.com/viewprogram/2777

Thomas, S. P. (2003). Anger: The mismanaged emotion. *Dermatology Nursing, 15*(4), 351–357.

U.S. Bureau of Justice Statistics. (2007). *Intimate partner violence in the U.S.: Victim characteristics.* Retrieved December 11, 2008 from http://www.ojp.usdoj.gov/bjs/intimate/table/incgen.htm

U.S. Department of Health & Human Services. (2008). *Child maltreatment 2006.* Washington, DC: U.S. Government Printing Office.

U.S. Department of Justice, Office on Violence against Women. (2004). *President's Family Justice Center initiative.* Retrieved February 22, 2004, from http://www.ojp.usdoj.gov/vawo/pfjci.htm

Walker, L. E. (1979). *The battered woman* (2nd ed.). New York: Springer.

CHAPTER **27**

Sexual Assault

Margaret Jordan Halter and Verna Benner Carson

Key Terms and Concepts

acquaintance (or date) rape, 611
acute phase, 612
attempted rape, 610
blame, 618
controlled style of coping, 615
expressed style of coping, 614

long-term reorganization phase, 613
rape, 610
rape-trauma syndrome, 612
sexual assault, 609
spousal (or marital) rape, 611

Objectives

1. Define sexual assault, attempted rape, and rape.
2. Discuss the underreporting of sexual assault.
3. Describe the profile of the victim and the perpetrator of sexual assault.
4. Distinguish between the acute and long-term phases of the rape-trauma syndrome, and identify some common reactions during each phase.
5. Identify and give examples of five areas to assess when working with a person who has been sexually assaulted.
6. Formulate two long-term outcomes and two short-term goals for the nursing diagnosis *rape-trauma syndrome*.

7. Analyze one's own thoughts and feelings regarding the myths about rape and its impact on survivors.
8. Identify six overall guidelines for nursing interventions related to sexual assault.
9. Describe the role of the sexual assault nurse examiner to a colleague.
10. Discuss the long-term psychological effects of sexual assault that might lead to a survivor's seeking psychotherapy.
11. Identify three outcome criteria that would signify successful interventions for a person who has suffered a sexual assault.

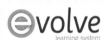 Visit the Evolve website for an **Audio Glossary & Flashcards, Concept Map Creator**, and additional resources related to the content in this chapter: **http://evolve.elsevier.com/Varcarolis/foundations**

In 2008, a 42-year-old Austrian woman, Elisabeth Fritzl, reported to police that she had been imprisoned in the soundproofed, windowless cellar of her family home since the age of 18. Her own father, Josef Fritzl, lured her there, locked her in, and repeatedly raped her for the next 24 years. This abuse resulted in seven children, one of whom died shortly after birth. Three of the surviving children were taken upstairs to be raised by Fritzl and his wife. He explained to his wife that the children had been left on the doorstep by their daughter, Elisabeth, who had run away to join a cult. The other three children remained in the cellar with their mother, never seeing the light of day, and were forced to be present for the continual rape of their

mother by their father/grandfather. When the moldy, dark conditions caused the eldest daughter, Kersten, 19, to become mortally ill, Elisabeth begged Fritzl to get her treatment. Fritzl relented and took her to a hospital, where Elisabeth would later be taken to visit. It was there that Elisabeth revealed the nature of her daughter's illness and her own abuse, on the condition that she would never have to see her father again.

This story is horrific and demonstrates some of the most contemptible violations that can be perpetrated by one human being on another. In this chapter, we will further explore one of these violations, namely sexual assault. Sexual assault is any type of sexual activity to which the victim does not consent,

609

and it ranges from inappropriate touching to penetration (i.e., intercourse). Sexual assault also can occur verbally over the telephone or online. Being forced into activities such as prostitution, posing for pornographic photographs, and appearing in pornographic videos are all examples of sexual assault. Children, older adults, women, and men can all be victims of sexual assault.

Rape is one type of sexual assault. Rape is nonconsensual vaginal, anal, or oral penetration, obtained by force or by threat of bodily harm or when a person is incapable of giving consent. It is usually men who rape, and most victims are women. The term attempted rape includes physical attempts and verbal threats of rape.

The Federal Bureau of Investigation (FBI) (2008) considers rape to be the second most violent crime in a group of crimes that includes murder, robbery, and aggravated assault. Victims are traumatized, both physically and emotionally, and are often seen in health care settings. Nurses are instrumental in not only providing holistic care for those who have been sexually assaulted through rape, but also in helping to preserve evidence that could lead to prosecution of the perpetrator(s). Therefore, it is essential that nurses be adequately informed about their roles and responsibilities with regard to these patients.

For the remainder of this chapter, victims of sexual assault will be referred to using the female pronoun in recognition of the fact that women are more frequently raped. However, the principles discussed apply to anyone who is raped.

EPIDEMIOLOGY

In the United States, the FBI Uniform Crime Reporting (UCR) Program calculates rates of rape to include one count for each forcible rape, attempted forcible rape, or assault with intent to rape for each female victim of any age. Incestuous sexual assault (occurring among family members) is included in the statistics. According to the FBI (2008), the most commonly reported sexual assault is rape of force (92%). Assault with attempt to rape is reported less frequently (8%). In 2007, the number of forcible rapes was estimated at 90,427—a 2.5% decrease from 92,757 in 2006. The forcible rape rate was estimated at about 59 offenses per 100,000 females, a decrease from an estimated rate of 61 in 2006.

This reduction of sexual assault is part of an overall trend and may be due to several factors, including policies that support longer sentences for perpetrators, "three-strikes" laws, and mandatory minimum sentences. Another factor may be increased assertiveness of females in younger generations who have grown up knowing that "no means no." Women today are also more willing to report sexual abuse, which may be a deterring factor.

As with other violent crimes, people of lower socioeconomic classes are more often victims (U.S. Department of Justice, 2008). Although about 80% of victims are white, proportionately African Americans are more likely to be sexually assaulted. One third of all sexual assaults occur inside the home, and most of the time (72%), no weapon is involved. Young females between the ages of 12 and 19 are at particular risk for sexual assault. During the college and university years, 20% to 25% of all females are victims of attempted or completed rape. Among high school students, 8% of females and 4% of males reportedly have been forced to have sex (Centers for Disease Control and Prevention [CDC], 2007).

The percentage of males who are sexually assaulted is commonly cited as 9% to 10% of all rapes, but it is likely that male victimizations are vastly underreported. This may be due to shame at being dominated by a stronger male. Also, since perpetrators are nearly always men, this brings the stigma of homosexuality into the picture, which for many victims makes reporting nearly worse than the crime.

Also, the statistics for men and women often do not accurately reflect the crime. The FBI (2008) categorizes sexual attacks on males not as sexual assault but as aggravated assaults or sex offenses, depending on the extent of injury that is sustained. When men are assaulted, the perpetrator is more likely to be intoxicated, know his victim, and live with him (Carlson, 2007). A male who is raped is more likely to experience physical trauma and to have been victimized by several assailants. Reports of male-to-male rape occur primarily in locked institutions, such as prisons and maximum-security hospitals. Males experience the same devastation, physical injury, and emotional consequences as females. Although they may cover their responses, they too benefit from care and treatment.

Profile of Sexual Perpetrators

According to the U.S. Department of Justice (2008), perpetrators are almost always men (95%). Perpetrators of sexual assault tend to be young—30% are under the age of 21, and another 23% are under the age of 30. About 43% of abusers are under the influence of alcohol or drugs at the time of the offense. While we often think of the stranger lurking in the shadows in parking lots as the typical perpetrator, this is not true. For all types of sexual assault, the victim is acquainted with the perpetrator 61% of the time. Looking at the statistics for rape alone, the percentage increases to 72%. When race is known, white victims are more commonly identified in assaults by white perpetrators (46%) than by African American perpetrators (32%). African American victims are more commonly assaulted by African American perpetrators (67%).

CLINICAL PICTURE

Relationships Between Victims and Perpetrators

The terms spousal (or marital) rape and acquaintance (or date) rape describe the nature of the relationship between victim and rapist. In recent years, the courts have recognized spousal (or marital) rape, in which the perpetrator (nearly always the male) is married to the person raped. In acquaintance (or date) rape, the perpetrator is known to, and presumably trusted by, the person raped. The psychological and emotional outcomes of rape seem to vary depending on the level of intimacy between the victim and the perpetrator. Sexual distress is more common among women who have been sexually assaulted by intimates, fear and anxiety are more common in those assaulted by strangers, and depression occurs in both groups.

Acquaintance (or date) rape has increased in incidence in the United States in recent years, with drugs, often combined with alcohol, being used to commit sexual assault. Most cases of acquaintance rape involve the use of alcohol on the part of the perpetrator, the victim, or both (American Prosecutors Research Institute, 2007). Other so-called "date-rape drugs" may render a woman incapable of resisting the attack and are purported to facilitate acquaintance rape. Often these drugs are given to the unknowing victim. Once the drugs are ingested, victims lose their ability to ward off attackers, develop amnesia, and become unreliable witnesses. Because the symptoms mimic those of alcohol, victims are not always screened for these drugs. The increase in prevalence and incidence of drug-assisted rape led to the passage of the Drug-Induced Rape Prevention and Punishment Act in 1996. This law allows up to 20 years' imprisonment and fines for anyone who intends to commit a violent crime by administering a controlled substance to an unknowing individual (U.S. Department of Justice, 1997). Table 27-1 provides information about date-rape drugs.

Psychological Effects of Sexual Assault

Most people who are raped suffer severe and long-lasting emotional trauma. Long-term psychological effects of sexual assault may include depression, suicide, anxiety, and fear; difficulties with daily functioning; low self-esteem; sexual dysfunction; and somatic complaints. Victims of incest may experience a negative self-image, depression, eating disorders, personality disorders, self-destructive behavior, and substance abuse. A history of sexual abuse in psychiatric patients is associated with a characteristic pattern of symptoms that may include depression, anxiety disorders, chemical dependency, suicide attempts, self-mutilation, compulsive sexual behavior, and psychosis-like symptoms (Read et al., 2007). Timely intervention can reduce the devastating aftermath of rape.

TABLE 27-1 **Drugs Associated With Date Rape**			
Drug, Alternate Names, and Status in the United States	**Form, Mechanism of Action, and Onset**	**Effect on Victim**	**Overdose Symptoms and Treatment**
GHB (gamma-hydroxybutyrate) Also known as *G, Georgia home boy, liquid ecstasy, salty water, and scoop* Legal in the United States for narcolepsy Often made in home labs	Liquid, white powder, or pill with a salty taste Schedule III central nervous system depressant A metabolite of gamma-aminobutyric acid Onset within 5-20 minutes; duration is dose related and from 1-12 hours	Produces relaxation, euphoria, and disinhibition Incoordination, confusion, deep sedation, and amnesia Tolerance and dependence exhibited by agitation, tachycardia, insomnia, anxiety, tremors, and sweating	Respiratory depression, seizures, nausea, vomiting, bradycardia, hypothermia, agitation, delirium, unconsciousness, and coma Intubation for severe respiratory distress; atropine for bradycardia, and benzodiazepines for seizure activity Vomiting should be induced when possible
Rohypnol (flunitrazepam)* Also known as *forget-me pill, roofies, club drug, roachies, R2, and rophies* Not legal in the United States	Pill that dissolves in liquids Schedule IV potent benzodiazepine; 10 times stronger than diazepam Impact is within 10-30 minutes and lasts 2-12 hours	More potent when combined with alcohol; causes sedation, psychomotor slowing, muscle relaxation, and amnesia Dependence and tolerance may develop	Overdose unlikely Airway protection and gastrointestinal decontamination

Continued

TABLE 27-1 Drugs Associated With Date Rape—cont'd

Drug, Alternate Names, and Status in the United States	Form, Mechanism of Action, and Onset	Effect on Victim	Overdose Symptoms and Treatment
Ketamine Also known as *black hole, bump, K, kit kat, purple,* and *Special K* Legal in the United States for anesthesia	Comes as a liquid or a white powder An anesthetic frequently used in veterinary practice; also a hallucinogenic substance related to PCP (phencyclidine) Onset within 30 seconds intravenously and 20 minutes orally; duration only 30-60 minutes; amnesia effects may last longer	Causes dissociative reaction, with a dreamlike state leading to deep amnesia and analgesia and complete compliance of the victim May become confused, paranoid, delirious, combative, with drooling and hallucinations	Airway maintenance and use of anticholinergics such as atropine and benzodiazepines

*Two other benzodiazepines, clonazepam (Klonopin) and alprazolam (Xanax), are also used.
Data from Lehne, R. A. (2010). *Pharmacology for nursing care* (7th ed.). Philadelphia: Saunders; and U.S. Department of Health and Human Services. (2008). *Date rape drugs.* <http://www.womenshealth.gov/faq/date-rape-drugs.cfm> Accessed 10.12.08.

Rape-Trauma Syndrome

The **rape-trauma syndrome** is a variant of posttraumatic stress disorder (PTSD) and consists of an acute phase and a long-term reorganization process that occurs after an actual or attempted sexual assault. Each phase has separate symptoms. See Chapter 12 for a more detailed discussion of PTSD.

Acute Phase

The **acute phase** of the rape-trauma syndrome occurs immediately after the assault and may last for 2 to 3 weeks. This is the stage at which patients usually are seen by emergency department personnel, and nurses are most involved in dealing with initial reactions. During this phase, there is a great deal of disorganization in the person's lifestyle, and somatic symptoms are common. This disorganization can be described in terms of impact, somatic, and emotional reactions (Box 27-1).

The most common initial reactions are shock, numbness, and disbelief. Outwardly, the person may appear self-contained and calm and may make remarks such as "It doesn't seem real," or "I don't believe this really happened to me." Sometimes, cognitive functions may be impaired, and the traumatized person may appear extremely confused and have difficulty concentrating and making decisions. Alternatively, the person may become hysterical or restless or may cry or even smile. These reactions to crisis are typical and reflect cognitive, affective, and behavioral disruptions.

BOX 27-1 Acute Phase of Rape-Trauma Syndrome

Impact Reaction
Expressed Style
Overt behaviors:
- Crying, sobbing
- Smiling, laughing, joking
- Restlessness, agitation, hysteria
- Volatility, anger
- Confusion, incoherence, disorientation
- Tenseness

Controlled Style
Ambiguous reactions:
- Confusion, incoherence, disorientation
- Masked facies
- Calm, subdued appearance
- Shock, numbness, confusion, disbelieving appearance
- Distractibility, difficulty making decisions

Somatic Reaction
Evidenced within first several weeks after a rape:

Physical Trauma
- Bruises (breasts, throat, or back)
- Soreness

Skeletal Muscle Tension
- Headaches
- Sleep disturbances
- Grimaces, twitches

BOX 27-1 Acute Phase of Rape-Trauma Syndrome—cont'd

Gastrointestinal Symptoms
- Stomach pains
- Nausea
- Poor appetite
- Diarrhea

Genitourinary Symptoms
- Vaginal itching
- Vaginal discharge
- Pain or discomfort

Emotional Reaction
- Fear of physical violence and death
- Denial
- Anxiety
- Shock
- Humiliation
- Fatigue
- Embarrassment
- Desire for revenge
- Self-blame
- Lowered self-esteem
- Shame
- Guilt
- Anger

Data from Burgess A. W. (1995). Rape trauma syndrome: A nursing diagnosis. *Occupational Health Nursing, 33*(8), 405; and Burgess, A. W., & Holstrom, L. L. (1974). The rape victim in the ER. *American Journal of Nursing, 73*(10), 1740.

People who have experienced an emotionally overwhelming event may find it too painful to discuss. Examples of this response are found in statements such as "I don't want to talk about it," or "I just want to forget what happened." Behaviors that minimize the magnitude of the event include reluctance to seek medical attention and failure to follow up with legal counsel.

Long-Term Reorganization Phase

The **long-term reorganization phase** of rape-trauma syndrome occurs 2 or more weeks after the rape. Nurses who initially care for survivors can help them anticipate and prepare for the reactions they are likely to experience, which include:
- **Intrusive thoughts** of the rape that break into the survivor's conscious mind during the day and during sleep. These thoughts commonly include anger and violence toward the assailant, flashbacks (reexperiencing of the traumatic event), dreams with violent content, and insomnia.

- **Increased activity**, such as moving, taking trips, changing telephone numbers, and making frequent visits to old friends. This activity stems from the fear that the assailant will return.
- **Increased emotional lability**, including intense anxiety, mood swings, crying spells, and depression.

Fears and phobias develop as a defensive reaction to the rape. Typical phobias include:
- Fear of the indoors, if the rape occurred indoors
- Fear of the outdoors, if the rape occurred outdoors
- Fear of being alone; common for most women after an assault
- Fear of crowds. Women may believe any person in the crowd might be a rapist.
- Fear of sexual encounters and activities. Many women experience acute disruption of their sex lives with their partners. Rape is especially disruptive for those with no previous sexual experience.

As mentioned, the consequences of sexual assault may be severe, debilitating, and long term. Intervention and support for the survivor can help prevent some of the complications of anxiety, depression, suicide, difficulties with daily functioning and interpersonal relationships, sexual dysfunction, and somatic complaints.

APPLICATION OF THE NURSING PROCESS

ASSESSMENT

According to the U.S. Department of Justice, 32% of sexual assault victims seek help in a hospital emergency department. The attention the victim receives depends on the protocol of the particular hospital. The Emergency Nurses Association position statement on care of sexual assault victims (2007) suggests the following interventions:
- Use a nonjudgmental and empathetic approach.
- Provide rapid assessment of the needs and support required to prevent further trauma.
- Treat and document injuries.
- Provide a private environment, and limit personnel to examining health care professionals, a translator if needed, and (with the consent of the patient) a specially trained advocate, if indicated.
- Assist with or conduct a physical examination.
- Obtain pertinent laboratory tests (e.g., human immunodeficiency virus [HIV] testing, hepatitis profiles).

- Assist with or perform collection of evidence, with appropriate documentation and preservation of evidence.
- Evaluate for and treat sexually transmitted diseases.
- Conduct pregnancy risk evaluation and prevention.
- Provide crisis intervention and arrange follow-up counseling.

Unfortunately, the care sexual assault victims receive varies from facility to facility. In one recent study in the Midwest, researchers found that virtually all emergency departments provided acute medical care (Patel et al., 2008); however, only two thirds of these agencies offered rape counseling and sexually transmitted infection management. Counseling and emergency contraceptives were provided by 40% of facilities; only about 30% provided HIV management. Just 10% of the facilities provided all of these services to victims of sexual assault.

General Assessment

The nurse should talk with the survivor, the family or friends who accompany the survivor, and the police to gather as much data as possible for assessing the crisis. The nurse then assesses the survivor's (1) level of anxiety, (2) coping mechanisms, (3) available support systems, (4) signs and symptoms of emotional trauma, and (5) signs and symptoms of physical trauma. Information obtained from the assessment is then analyzed, and nursing diagnoses are formulated.

Level of Anxiety

A patient experiencing severe to panic levels of anxiety will not be able to problem solve or process information. Approaches such as support, reassurance, and appropriate therapeutic techniques can lower the patient's anxiety and facilitate mutual goal setting and the assimilation of information. Refer to Chapters 12 and 13 for more detailed discussions of the levels of anxiety and therapeutic interventions.

Coping Mechanisms

The same coping skills that have helped the survivor through other difficult problems in her lifetime will be used in adjusting to the rape. In addition, new ways of getting through the difficult times may be developed for both the short- and long-term adjustment. Behavioral responses include crying, withdrawing, smoking, abusing alcohol and drugs, talking about the event, becoming extremely agitated, confused, disoriented, incoherent, and even laughing or joking. These behaviors are examples of an **expressed style of coping** (see Box 27-1).

Cognitive coping mechanisms are the thoughts people have that help them deal with high anxiety levels. A positive cognitive response might be, "At least I am alive and will get to see my children again." Not-so-positive responses may become generalized as a way to sum up the situation: "It's my fault this happened; my mother warned me about working in such a trashy place" may develop into an ego-damaging refrain. If such thoughts are verbalized, the nurse will know what the survivor is thinking. If not, the nurse can ask questions such as, "What are you thinking and feeling?" or "What can I do to help you in this difficult situation?" or "What has helped in the past?"

Available Support Systems

The availability, size, and usefulness of a survivor's social support system must be assessed. Often partners or family members do not understand the survivor's feelings about the sexual assault, and they may not be the best supports available. Pay careful attention to verbal and nonverbal cues of the survivor that may communicate the strength of the social network.

VIGNETTE

Ms. Ruiz, age 18, is brought to the emergency department by a concerned neighbor. She was found wandering aimlessly outside her house, sobbing and muttering, "He had no right to do that to me." Because of Ms. Ruiz's distraught appearance and her statement, the triage nurse suspects sexual assault and brings Ms. Ruiz to the office of the psychiatric nurse, Carol Davies. Ms. Davies introduces herself, explains her role, and states that she is there to help. Ms. Davies then asks Ms. Ruiz what happened. After careful, sensitive, nonthreatening questioning, Ms. Ruiz divulges that she had been out with her boyfriend, who took her to a "rave" party and then raped her. She got a ride back home, but no one else was at home. She was so upset and afraid, she did not go inside, and her neighbor had seen her.

After the entire history and examination are completed, plans for discharge are discussed. Ms. Ruiz states that no one will be home until Sunday night, 2 days away, and that she does not feel comfortable calling any friends, because she does not want them to know what happened. The neighbor, Ms. Green, told the nurse earlier that Ms. Ruiz can stay with her family.

Nurse: Earlier, your neighbor, Ms. Green, told me that you are welcome to spend the weekend with her family.

Ms. Ruiz: (Loudly, sharply, with eyes wide) Oh no, I couldn't do that.

Nurse: You don't like that idea?

Ms. Ruiz: Oh, I just wouldn't want to bother them.

Nurse: Ms. Green seems quite concerned about your welfare.

Ms. Ruiz: Oh, yes, she's very nice. (Pause)

Nurse: But not someone you would want to spend the weekend with?

Ms. Ruiz: Her children are too noisy. I've got homework to do.

Nurse: You might not get the quiet you need to study. (Pause) Yet you also do not want to be alone?

Ms. Ruiz: (Wringing a tissue in her hands, head hanging, voice soft) I can't go in her house anymore.

Nurse: Something about being in that house disturbs you?

Ms. Ruiz: Mr. Green (deep sigh, pause) used to … uh … take advantage of me when I would baby-sit his children.

Nurse: Take advantage?

Ms. Ruiz: Yes…(sobbing) he used to try to get me to have sex with him. He said he'd blame it on me if I told anyone.

Nurse: What a frightening experience that must have been for you.

Ms. Ruiz: Yes.

Nurse: I can see why you would not want to spend the night there. Let's continue to explore other options.

A suitable place to stay is finally arranged. Ms. Ruiz is given counseling referrals that will help her deal with the process of reorganization after this current rape experience. Her counselor will explore her feelings about past sexual abuse she has suffered at the hands of her neighbor when she is ready. ▪

Signs and Symptoms of Emotional Trauma

Nurses work with sexual assault survivors most frequently in the emergency department soon after the rape has occurred. Rape is a psychological emergency and should receive immediate attention. Some emergency departments provide the services of sexual assault nurse examiners (SANEs) or clinicians specially trained to meet the needs of sexual assault survivors. They are trained to assess the extent of psychological and emotional trauma that may not be readily apparent, especially if the person uses the **controlled style of coping** during the acute phase of the rape trauma (see Box 27-1).

A nursing history should be obtained and carefully recorded. When taking a history, the nurse determines only the details of the assault that will be helpful in addressing the immediate physical and psychological needs of the survivor. The nurse allows the survivor to talk at a comfortable pace; poses questions in nonjudgmental, descriptive terms; and refrains from asking "why" questions. The survivor frequently finds that relating the events of the rape is traumatic and embarrassing.

If suicidal thoughts are expressed, the nurse assesses what precautions are needed by asking direct questions, such as "Are you thinking of harming yourself?" and "Have you ever tried to kill yourself before or after this attack occurred?" If the answer is yes, the nurse conducts a thorough suicide assessment (plan, means to carry it out), as described in Chapter 24.

Signs and Symptoms of Physical Trauma

It is essential that nurses provide psychological support while collecting and preserving legal evidence such as hair, skin, and semen samples that may be crucial for conviction of the perpetrator. The most characteristic physical signs of sexual assault are injuries to the face, head, neck, and extremities. Any physical injuries should be carefully documented, both in narrative and pictorial form using preprinted body maps, hand-drawn copies, or photographs.

The nurse takes a brief gynecological history, including the date of the last menstrual period and the likelihood of current pregnancy, and assesses for a history of sexually transmitted disease. If the survivor has never undergone a pelvic examination, the steps of the examination will need to be explained. The nurse plays a crucial role in giving support and minimizing the trauma of the examination, because the survivor may experience it as another violation of her body. Recognizing this, the nurse can explain the examination procedure in a way that will be reassuring and supportive. Allowing the survivor to participate in all decisions affecting care helps her regain a sense of control over her life.

The survivor has the right to refuse either a legal or a medical examination. Consent forms must be signed before photographs are taken, a pelvic examination occurs, and any other procedures that might be needed to collect evidence and provide treatment are carried out. The correct preservation of body fluids and swabs is essential, because DNA samples may identify the rapist. A shower and fresh clothing should be made available to the survivor as soon after the examination and collection of specimens as possible.

Providing prophylactic treatment for syphilis, chlamydiosis, and gonorrhea—according to guidelines of the Centers for Disease Control and Prevention—is common practice. HIV exposure is often a concern of sexual assault survivors. This concern should always be addressed and the rape survivor given the information needed to evaluate the likelihood of risk. With this information, the person and her sexual partner(s) can make educated choices about HIV testing and safer sex practices until testing can be done.

About 5% of women who are raped become pregnant as a result (Rape, Abuse & Incest National Network, 2008). Pregnancy prophylaxis can be offered in the emergency department or at follow-up, after the results of the pregnancy test are available.

All data are carefully documented, including verbatim statements by the survivor, detailed observations of emotional and physical status, and all results of the physical examination. All laboratory tests performed are noted and findings recorded as soon as they are available. One of the greatest concerns is that crucial evidence may be lost or overlooked. The Emergency Nurses Association position statement on forensic evidence collection (2003) underscores the role of the nurse in collecting and securing medical and legal evidence.

Self-Assessment

Nurses' attitudes influence the physical and psychological care received by rape survivors. Knowing the myths and facts surrounding sexual assault can increase your awareness of your personal beliefs and feelings regarding rape. If you examine personal feelings and reactions *before* encountering a rape survivor, you will be better prepared to give empathetic and effective care. Examining your feelings about abortion is also important, because a patient might choose an abortion if a pregnancy results from rape. Table 27-2 compares rape myths and facts.

Assessment Guidelines Sexual Assault

1. Assess psychological trauma, and document the patient's verbatim statements.
2. Assess level of anxiety. If in a severe to panic level of anxiety, the patient will not be able to problem solve or process information.
3. Assess physical trauma. Use a preprinted body map, and ask permission to take photographs.
4. Assess available support system. Often partners or family members do not understand the trauma of rape, and they may not be the best supports to draw on at this time.
5. Identify community supports (e.g., attorneys, support groups, therapists) that work in the area of sexual assault.
6. Encourage the patient to talk about the experience, but do not press the patient to tell.

DIAGNOSIS

The nursing diagnosis *Rape-trauma syndrome* applies to the physical and psychological effects of a sexual assault. According to North American Nursing Diagnosis

TABLE 27-2 Myth versus Fact: Rape

Myth	Fact
Many women really want to be raped.	Women do not ask to be raped—no matter how they are dressed, what their behavior is, or where they are at any given time. Studies show that violence toward women in the media leads to attitudes that foster tolerance of rape.
Most rapists are oversexed.	Sex is used as an instrument of violence in rape. Rape is an act of aggression, anger, or power.
Most women are raped by strangers.	The majority (69%) of rape victims are raped by someone they knew.
No healthy adult female who resists vigorously can be raped by an unarmed man.	Most men can overpower most women because of differences in body build. Also, the victim may panic, which makes her actions less effective than usual.
Most charges of rape are unfounded.	There is no evidence to show that there are more false reports for rape than for other crimes. Most rape victims do not even report the rape.
Rapes usually occur in dark alleys.	Over 50% of all rapes occur in the home.
Rape is usually an impulsive act.	Most rapes are planned; over 50% involve a weapon.
Nice girls don't get raped.	Any woman is a potential rape victim. Victims range in age from 6 months to 90 years.
There was not enough time for a rape to occur.	There is no minimal time limit that characterizes rape. It can happen very quickly.
Do not fight or try to get away, because you will just get hurt.	There are no verifiable data to substantiate the theory that a victim will be injured if he or she tries to get away.
Only females are raped.	There are a growing number of male rape victims.
Rape is a sexual act.	Rape is a violent expression of aggression, anger, and need for power.

Association International (2009), rape-trauma syndrome is defined as a "sustained maladaptive response to a forced, violent sexual penetration against the victim's will and consent" (p. 239). It includes an acute phase of disorganization of the survivor's lifestyle and a long-term phase of reorganization.

OUTCOMES IDENTIFICATION

The long-term outcome includes the absence of any residual symptoms after the trauma. The *Nursing Outcomes Classification (NOC)* identifies additional outcomes appropriate for the rape survivor: *Abuse Protection, Abuse Recovery: Emotional, Abuse Recovery: Sexual, Coping, Personal Resiliency, Sexual Functioning,* and *Stress Level* (Moorhead et al., 2008). Some of the suggested indicators for these outcomes include:

- Patient will demonstrate positive interpersonal relationships.
- Patient will demonstrate adequate social interactions.
- Patient will demonstrate healing of physical injuries.
- Patient will demonstrate evidence of appropriate opposite-/same-sex relationships.
- Patient will verbalize accurate information about sexual functioning.
- Patient will express comfort with body.
- Patient will express sexual interest.
- Patient will report increased psychological comfort.

- Patient will report a decrease in physical symptoms of stress.

PLANNING

Unless the survivor has sustained serious physical injury, treatment is offered, and the patient is released. However, because the ramifications of rape are experienced for an extended time after the acute phase, the plan of care includes information for follow-up care. The survivor needs information about available community supports and how to access them. Nurses may also encounter rape survivors in other settings when they are no longer in acute distress but still dealing with the aftermath of rape. Such settings include inpatient facilities, the community, and the home. A comprehensive plan of care addresses the continuing needs of the rape survivor in any setting.

IMPLEMENTATION

The occurrence of rape can be the most devastating experience in a person's life and constitutes an acute adventitious (unexpected) crisis. Typical crisis reactions reflect cognitive, affective, and behavioral disruptions. For survivors to return to their previous level of functioning, it is necessary for them to fully mourn their losses, experience anger, and work through their fears. Box 27-2 provides *Nursing Interventions Classification (NIC)* interventions for rape-trauma syndrome (Bulechek et al., 2008).

BOX 27-2 Interventions for Rape-Trauma Syndrome

Definition: Provision of emotional and physical support immediately following a reported rape
Activities:
- Provide support person to stay with patient.
- Explain legal proceedings available to patient.
- Explain rape protocol, and obtain consent to proceed through protocol.
- Document whether patient has showered, douched, or bathed since incident.
- Document mental state, physical state (clothing, dirt, and debris), history of incident, evidence of violence, and prior gynecological history.
- Determine presence of cuts, bruises, bleeding, lacerations, or other signs of physical injury.
- Implement rape protocol (e.g., label and save soiled clothing, vaginal secretions, and vaginal hair combings).
- Secure samples for legal evidence.
- Implement crisis intervention counseling.
- Offer medication to prevent pregnancy, as appropriate.
- Offer prophylactic antibiotic medication against sexually transmitted disease.
- Inform patient of availability of human immunodeficiency virus testing, as appropriate.
- Give clear, written instructions about medication use, crisis support services, and legal support.
- Refer patient to rape advocacy program.
- Document according to agency policy.

From Bulechek, G. M., Butcher, H. K., & Dochterman, J. M. (Eds.). (2008). *Nursing interventions classification (NIC)* (5th ed.). St. Louis: Mosby.

Counseling

The rape survivor may be too traumatized, ashamed, or afraid to go to the hospital. Cultural definitions of what constitutes rape may also affect the decision to seek treatment. For these reasons, 24-hour telephone and online hotlines—such as the Rape, Abuse, and Incest National Network (RAINN)—are initiated through instant messaging and provide direct communication with volunteers trained in rape crisis support. These types of support focus on helping the person through the period of acute distress by assessing what has happened and determining what kind of assistance is needed. Counselors provide empathetic listening, the survivor is encouraged to go to the emergency department, and the main focus is on the immediate steps the survivor may take.

The most effective approach for counseling in the emergency department or crisis center is to provide nonjudgmental care and optimal emotional support. Confidentiality is crucial. The most helpful things the nurse can do are to listen and to let the survivor talk. A victim who feels understood is no longer alone and feels more in control of the situation.

It is especially important to help the survivor and significant others to separate issues of vulnerability from blame. Although the person may have made choices that made her more vulnerable, she is not to blame for the rape. She may, however, decide to avoid some of those choices in the future (e.g., walking alone late at night or excessive use of alcohol). Focusing on one's behavior (which is controllable) allows the survivor to believe that similar experiences can be avoided in the future.

VIGNETTE

Mary comes to see that it was not her fault that she was raped. However, she is now adamant about not walking from the bus stop alone late at night, and from now on will take a cab, get a lift from a friend, or take a safer alternative route when she goes home. ■

If the survivor consents, involve her support system (e.g., family or friends) and discuss with them the nature and trauma of sexual assault and possible delayed reactions that may occur. One survivor expressed the aftermath of her assault as follows:

> It takes a few days to hit you. It was bad. It was really rough for my husband. I needed to be reassured. I needed to be told that there was nothing I could do to prevent it. Understanding helps. (Anonymous)

Social support effectively moderates somatic symptoms and subjective health ratings. The survivor who is able to confide comfortably in one or two friends or family members, especially immediately after the assault, is likely to experience fewer somatic manifestations of stress. In many cases, family and friends need support and reassurance as much as the survivor

does. This is especially true for those from traditional cultures, particularly those cultures who believe that sexual assault brings shame to the entire family. The longstanding cultural myth that women are the property of men still prevents some people from empathizing with the woman's severe psychic injury and from being supportive. Instead, in these cases, the woman is devalued.

Promotion of Self-Care Activities

When preparing the survivor for discharge, the nurse provides all referral information and printed follow-up instructions, detailing potential physical concerns and emotional reactions, legal matters, victim compensation (state financial assistance paid through perpetrators' fines and fees), and ways that family and friends can help. This is important because the amount of verbal information the patient can retain likely will be limited due to high levels of anxiety. Written material can be referred to repeatedly over time. Legal referrals (e.g., names of attorneys who specialize in rape cases and options for low-cost legal assistance) can also be given.

Case Management

The emotional state and other psychological needs of the survivor should be reassessed by telephone or personal contact within 24 to 48 hours of discharge from the hospital. Repeat referrals should be made for resources or support services. Effective crisis intervention and continuity of care require outreach activities and services beyond the emergency medical setting.

Survivors may avoid seeking treatment from psychiatric mental health care providers because medical treatment is more socially sanctioned, and they are likely to be experiencing physical symptoms of stress. Thus the outpatient nurse can make a more focused assessment of stress-related symptoms and/or depression and ascertain the need for mental health referral. Reporting symptoms and seeking medical treatment are adaptive coping behaviors and can be reinforced as such.

Follow-up visits should occur at least 2, 4, and 6 weeks after the initial evaluation. At each visit, the survivor should be assessed for psychological progress, the presence of a sexually transmitted disease, and pregnancy. Case Study and Nursing Care Plan 27-1 on pages 619-621 describes the care of a patient who has been raped.

Advanced Practice Interventions

Psychotherapy

The advanced practice nurse may offer individual or group psychotherapy for either the rape survivor or the perpetrator.

Survivors. Most of those who have been raped are eventually able to resume their previous lifestyle and level of functioning after supportive services and crisis counseling. However, many continue to experience emotional trauma, including flashbacks, nightmares, fear, phobias, and other symptoms associated with PTSD (see Chapter 12). Some people who survive rape may be susceptible to a psychotic episode or an emotional disturbance so severe that hospitalization is required. Others whose emotional lives may be overburdened with multiple internal and external pressures may require individual psychotherapy.

Depression and suicidal ideation too frequently follow rape. Depression is more common in those who do not disclose the assault to significant others because they have concerns about being stigmatized, have children living at home, or have a pending civil lawsuit. Any exposure to stimuli related to the traumatic event may activate a reliving of the traumatic state.

People who have been raped are likely to benefit from group therapy or support groups. These modalities may be particularly beneficial for survivors from cultures that are group oriented rather than individualistic and for women who derive much of their self-definition from cultural norms. Group therapy can make the difference between a person's coming out of the crisis at a lower level of functioning or gradually adapting to the experience with an increase in coping skills.

Perpetrators. Psychotherapy is essential for perpetrators of sexual assault if behavioral change is to occur.

Unfortunately, most perpetrators do not acknowledge the need for behavioral change, and no single method or program of treatment has been found to be totally effective. The nurse's awareness of his or her own feelings and reactions will be crucial to avoid interference with the therapeutic process.

EVALUATION

Rape survivors are considered to be recovered if they are relatively free of any signs or symptoms of PTSD; that is, if they are:

- Sleeping well with very few instances of episodic nightmares or broken sleep
- Eating as they were before the rape (Patients may respond to the crisis of rape by undereating or overeating.)
- Calm and relaxed or only mildly suspicious, fearful, or restless
- Getting support from family and friends (Some strain might still be present in relationships, but it should be minimal.)
- Generally positive about themselves (On occasion, doubts about self-worth may occur.)
- Free from somatic reactions (If mild symptoms persist and minor discomfort is reported, the survivor should be able to talk about it and feel in control of the symptoms.)
- Showing a return to pre-rape sexual functioning and interest

In general, the closer the survivor's lifestyle is to the pattern that was present before the rape, the more complete the recovery has been.

Case Study and Nursing Care Plan 27-1 Rape

Latisha Smith, a 36-year-old single mother of two, goes out one evening with some friends. Her children are at a slumber party, and she "needs to get away and have a little rest and relaxation." She and her friends go bowling. Later in the evening, Latisha is tired and ready to go home. A man who has joined the group offers to take her home. She has seen the man at the bowling alley before but does not know much about him. Not in the habit of going home alone with men she does not know, she hesitates. A friend whom she trusts encourages her to go with James because he is a "nice man."

James drives Latisha home. He then asks if he can come into her house to use the bathroom before driving the long distance to his house. She reluctantly agrees and sits on the living room couch. After using the bathroom, James sits next to Latisha and begins to kiss her

and fondle her breasts. As she protests, James becomes more forceful in his advances. Latisha is confused and frightened. She manages to get away from him briefly, but he begins grabbing, squeezing, and biting her. He tells her gruffly, "If you don't do what I say, I'll break your neck." She screams, but he proceeds to rape her. James becomes nervous that the noise will alert the neighbors and races out of the house. A neighbor does in fact arrive just after James flees. The neighbor calls the police and then brings Latisha to the local hospital emergency department for a physical examination, crisis intervention, and support.

In the emergency department, Latisha is visibly shaken. She keeps saying, over and over, "I shouldn't have let him take me home. I should have fought harder, I shouldn't have let him do this."

Continued

The nurse takes Latisha to a quiet cubicle. She does not want Latisha to stay alone and asks the neighbor to stay with her. The nurse then notifies the doctor and the rape-victim advocate. When the nurse comes back, she tells Latisha that she would like to talk to her before the doctor comes. Latisha looks at her neighbor and then down. The nurse asks the neighbor to wait outside for a while and says she will call her later.

Latisha: *It was horrible. I feel so dirty.*

Nurse: *You have had a traumatic experience. Do you want to talk about it?*

Latisha: *I feel so ashamed. I never should have let that man take me home.*

Nurse: *You think that if you hadn't gone home with a stranger this wouldn't have happened?*

Latisha: *Yes …. I shouldn't have let him do it to me anyway, I shouldn't have let him rape me.*

Nurse: *You mentioned that he said he would break your neck if you didn't do as he said.*

Latisha: *Yes, he said that … he was going to kill me, it was awful.*

Nurse: *It seems you did the right thing in order to stay alive.*

As the nurse continues to talk with Latisha, Latisha's anxiety level seems to lessen. The nurse talks to Latisha about the kinds of experiences rape victims often have after the rape and explains that the reactions she might have 2 or 3 weeks from now are normal in these circumstances. The nurse continues to collect the necessary information. She says that the doctor will want to examine Latisha and explains the procedure to her. She then asks Latisha to sign a consent form. While preparing Latisha for examination, the nurse notices bite marks and bruises on both breasts. She also notes Latisha's lower lip, which is cut and bleeding. The nurse keeps detailed notes on her observations and draws a body map of the injuries. After the examination, Latisha is given clean clothes and a place to shower.

ASSESSMENT

Self-Assessment

The nurse has worked with rape survivors before and has helped develop the hospital protocol. It took a while for her to be able to remain both neutral and responsive, because her own anger at rapists had initially interfered. She also remembers a time when a woman came in stating that she was raped but was so calm, smiling, and polite that the nurse initially did not believe her story. She had not at that point examined her own feelings or dealt with the popular societal myths regarding rape. It was only later, when she had talked to more experienced health care personnel, that she learned that crisis reactions can seem bizarre, confusing, and contradictory.

The nurse learned that staying with the survivor, encouraging her to express her reactions and feelings, and listening are effective methods of reducing feelings of anxiety. Once the nurse learned through supervision and peer discussion to let go of her personal anger at the attacker and her ambivalence toward the survivor, her care and effectiveness improved greatly. All of this growth took time and support from more experienced nurses and other members of the health care team.

Objective Data

Crying and sobbing
Bruises and bite marks on each breast
Lip cut and bleeding
Rape reported to the police

Subjective Data

"He was going to kill me."
"It was horrible. I feel so dirty."
"I shouldn't have let him rape me."

DIAGNOSIS

The nurse formulates the following diagnosis:
Rape-trauma syndrome

Supporting Data

- "I shouldn't have let him rape me."
- "He was going to kill me."
- Crying and sobbing
- Bruises and bite marks on both breasts
- Rape reported to the police
- "It was horrible. I feel so dirty."

OUTCOMES IDENTIFICATION

Overall outcome: Abuse Recovery: Emotional
Short-term indicator: Latisha will demonstrate appropriate affect for the situation.

Intermediate indicator: Latisha will demonstrate confidence.

Short-term and intermediate outcome indicators are measured on a five-point Likert scale from 1 (none) to 5 (extensive).

PLANNING

The nurse plans to provide emotional and physical support to Latisha while she receives care in the emergency setting and to make sure that Latisha is aware of the importance of follow-up care.

IMPLEMENTATION

Latisha's plan of care is personalized as follows.

Short-Term Goal	Intervention	Rationale
1. Latisha will demonstrate appropriate affect by discharge from the emergency department.	1a. Remain neutral and nonjudgmental, and assure survivor of confidentiality.	1a. Lessens feelings of shame and guilt and encourages sharing of painful feelings.
	1b. Do not leave survivor alone.	1b. Deters feelings of isolation and escalation of anxiety.
	1c. Allow patient negative expressions and behavioral self-blame while using reflective techniques.	1c. Fosters feelings of control.
	1d. Assure survivor she did the right thing to save her life.	1d. Decreases burden of guilt and shame.
	1e. When anxiety level is down to moderate, encourage problem solving.	1e. Increases survivor's feeling of control in her own life. (When in severe anxiety, a person cannot problem-solve.)
	1f. Tell survivor of common reactions experienced by people in long-term reorganization phase (e.g., phobias, flashbacks, insomnia, increased motor activity).	1f. Helps survivor anticipate reactions and understand them as part of recovery process.
	1g. Explain emergency department procedure to survivor.	1g. Lowers anticipatory anxiety.
	1h. Explain physical examination.	1h. Allows for questions and concerns; victim may be too traumatized and may refuse.
	1i. Nurse/female rape advocate should stay with survivor during physical examination.	1i. Physical examination may be experienced as a second assault. Nurse provides comfort and support.

EVALUATION

Latisha is able to express her feelings in the emergency department, as well as talk about the possible reactions she might experience as she moves through the reorganization phase. The indicator is achieved at a level of 3 (moderate).

KEY POINTS TO REMEMBER

- Sexual assault is a common and often underreported crime of violence in the United States.
- Females are far more likely to victims of sexual assault and tend to know their perpetrators. Sexual assault of males tends to be underreported, owing to the humiliation and stigma attached to such victimization.
- Psychoactive substances play a major role in sexual assault, and alcohol is the most commonly used date-rape drug. Other disinhibiting and amnestic substances play a role in forcible sex acts.
- A rape survivor experiences a wide range of feelings, which may or may not be exhibited to others.
- Feelings of fear, degradation, anger and rage, helplessness, and nervousness; sleep disturbances; disturbed

relationships; flashbacks; depression; and somatic complaints are all common following sexual assault.

- The circumstances of the initial medical evaluation may be frightening and stressful. Police interrogation, repeated questioning by health professionals, and the physical examination itself all have the potential to add to the trauma of the sexual assault.
- Nurses, in their role as case managers, can serve to minimize repetition of questions and support the survivor as she goes through the entire ordeal.
- Survivors require long-term health care that can include counseling to minimize long-term effects of the rape and assist in early return to a normal living pattern.
- Telephone and online resources are available to assist rape survivors.

CRITICAL THINKING

1. Isaac, 18 years of age, is brutally beaten and sexually assaulted by an unidentified male as he makes his way home from a party in an unfamiliar part of town. He is found semiconscious by a passerby and taken to the emergency department. Isaac has extensive bruises around his head, chest, and buttocks and has sustained a cracked rib and anal tears. Ms. Santinez, a nurse and rape counselor in the emergency department, works with Isaac using the hospital's rape protocol. Isaac appears stunned and confused and has difficulty focusing on what the nurse says. He states repeatedly, "This is crazy, this can't be happening …. I can't believe this has happened to me …. Oh, my God, I can't believe this."

   A. What areas of Isaac's assessment should be given highest priority by Ms. Santinez and her staff while he is in the emergency department?

   B. Chart the signs and symptoms of Isaac's physical and emotional trauma and verbatim statements in as much detail as you can.

   C. What are some of the pivotal issues that need to be addressed in terms of assessing Isaac's signs and symptoms of physical trauma? Although the risk of pregnancy is not present, what other real physical risks need to be assessed?

   D. What are some of the signs and symptoms of rape-trauma syndrome? Of rape-trauma silent reaction?

   E. Identify the short-term outcome criteria for Isaac that ideally would be met before he leaves the emergency department.

   F. What information does Isaac need to have regarding potential signs and symptoms that may occur in the near future? Why is this important for him to understand at present?

   G. Identify specific indicators that will be met if Isaac recovers with minimal trauma from the event. How would you evaluate these criteria?

CHAPTER REVIEW

1. The nurse is caring for a patient in the emergency department who has been raped just hours earlier. Which behaviors should the nurse expect if the patient were exhibiting controlled-style reactions?
   1. Shock, numbness
   2. Volatility, anger
   3. Crying, sobbing
   4. Smiling, laughing

2. The nurse is caring for a patient who has just been raped. Which is the appropriate *initial* nursing response?
   1. "I will get you the number for the crisis intervention specialist."
   2. "May I get your consent to test you for pregnancy and HIV?"
   3. "You are safe here."
   4. "I need to look at your bruises and cuts."

3. A patient who has been raped has chosen to accept pregnancy prophylaxis medication. If the nurse does not believe in abortion, what is the appropriate nursing action?
   1. Examine own feelings about abortion before entering the patient's room.
   2. Encourage patient to take more time to consider her options.
   3. Provide the patient with the number to Planned Parenthood.
   4. Administer the pregnancy prophylaxis medication as ordered.

4. The nurse is working at a telephone hotline center when a rape victim calls. If the rape victim states she is fearful of going to the hospital, what is the appropriate nursing response?
   1. "You don't need to go to the hospital if you don't want to."
   2. "I'm here to listen to you, and we can talk about your feelings."
   3. "Did you do something to make the other person attack you?"
   4. "Why are you afraid to seek medical attention?"

5. The nurse is caring for a patient who is in the long-term reorganization phase of rape-trauma syndrome. Which symptom(s) should the nurse anticipate? *Select all that apply.*
   1. Development of fear of locations that resemble the rape location
   2. Emergence of acceptance of the rape
   3. Dreams with violent content
   4. A shift from anxiety to calm
   5. Onset of phobia of being alone

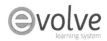

Visit the Evolve website for an **Audio Chapter Summary, Chapter Review Answers & Rationales, Critical Thinking Answer Guidelines,** and additional resources related to the content in this chapter: **http://evolve.elsevier.com/Varcarolis/foundations**

Companion CD   Use the Companion CD to prepare for tests and the NCLEX® Examination with **Test-Taking Strategies** for psychiatric mental health nursing and hundreds of **Review Questions.**

References

American Prosecutors Research Institute. (2007). *Prosecuting alcohol-facilitated sexual assault.* Retrieved December 10, 2008 from http://www.ndaa.org/pdf/pub_prosecuting_alcohol_facilitated_sexual_assault.pdf

Bulechek, G. M., Butcher, H. K., & Dochterman, J. M. (Eds.). (2008). *Nursing interventions classification (NIC)* (5th ed.). St. Louis: Mosby.

Carlson, M. (2007). Male rape rates in the National Violence Against Women Survey. Paper presented at the annual meeting of the American Society of Criminology, Atlanta Marriott Marquis, Atlanta, Georgia, Nov 14, 2007. Retrieved December 10, 2008 from http://www.allacademic.com/meta/p200729_index.html

Centers for Disease Control and Prevention. (2007). *Understanding sexual violence fact sheet.* Retrieved December 10, 2008 from http://www.cdc.gov/ncipc/pub-res/images/SV%20Factsheet.pdf

Drug-Induced Rape Prevention and Punishment Act, 21 U.S.C. § 841(b)(7) (1996).

Emergency Nurses Association. (2003). *Emergency Nurses Association position statements: Forensic evidence collection.* Retrieved February 20, 2005, from http://www.ena.org/about/position/forensicevidence.asp

Emergency Nurses Association. (2007). *Emergency Nurses Association position statements: Care of sexual assault victims.* Retrieved December 10, 2008 from http://www.ena.org/about/position/PDFs/D7BB8F1B2D0B4FC296F6E12926FFDB4F.pdf

Federal Bureau of Investigation. (2008). *Forcible rape: Crime in the United States.* Retrieved December 10, 2008 from http://www.fbi.gov/ucr/cius2007/offenses/violent_crime/forcible_rape.html

Moorhead, S., Johnson, M., Maas, M. L., & Swanson, E. (Eds.). (2008). *Nursing outcome classification (NOC)* (4th ed.). St. Louis: Mosby.

North American Nursing Diagnosis Association International (NANDA-I). (2009). *NANDA-I nursing diagnoses: Definitions and classification 2009-2011.* Oxford, United Kingdom: Author.

Patel, A., Patel, D., Piotrowski, Z.H., & Panchal, H. (2008). Comprehensive medical care for victims of sexual assault: A survey of Illinois hospital emergency departments. *Contraception, 77,* 426-430.

Rape, Abuse and Incest National Network. (2008). *Who are the victims?* Retrieved December 10, 2008 from http://www.rainn.org/get-information/statistics/sexual-assault-victims

Read, J., Hammersley, P., & Rudegeair, T. (2007). Why, when and how to ask about childhood abuse. *Advances in Psychiatric Treatment, 13,* 101–110.

U.S. Department of Justice, Office of the Attorney General. (1997, September 23). *Memorandum for all United States attorneys.* Retrieved February 21, 2005, from http://www.usdoj.gov/ag/readingroom/drugcrime.htm

U.S. Department of Justice. (2008). *Criminal victimization in the United States, 2006 statistical tables.* Publication NCJ 223436. Retrieved December 10, 2008 from http://www.ojp.usdoj.gov/bjs/pub/pdf/cvus0602.pdf

Interventions for Special Populations

A PATIENT SPEAKS

I am a 35-year-old female, and I was born in Tennessee. I grew up with my parents and my two younger sisters. My mother said that I was a jolly, friendly baby and that everyone was always holding and playing with me. Growing up, I was very quiet and shy and I did not make friends easily. I was an average student and I graduated from high school. I started working as a secretary and I also took some college courses. I have never married, although I have had a few male acquaintances.

When I was 26, I began to hear voices. I remember thinking that I was hearing people talking outside. And I was thinking, "Am I crazy? It sounds like they are talking about me." Except that the talking never stopped. No matter where I went, I kept hearing people talking. I had what I considered to be a weird life, so I just brushed it off as something else weird. Then one day it dawned on me that something was not right, and I sat down in a stupor and realized that I was hearing things. I was really scared. There were four different voices: a loud, shrill female voice that kept telling me to kill myself; another female voice that sounded like a nerd; a male voice that was kind of deep but sweet; and another male voice that had an "I don't care" attitude. They told me all sorts of things, like they did not know who they were, or I was going to die before the next day. They even told me a story about my childhood best friend and her family going to hell. They had a lot of personality and they often said things that sounded comical. They talked nonstop unless I fell asleep for a little while. My mother noticed me sitting around staring, and took me to a hospital.

I was diagnosed with schizophrenia and started on medication, which made me so tired that I thought that I was dying. I stayed in the hospital for 2 weeks and then I started seeing a community psychiatrist. I have taken several different medications, and the psychological change that took place is that the four voices decreased to two constant voices (although, under stress, I still hear four). I never used alcohol or illegal drugs to cope with my illness.

With regard to the stigma of mental illness, I really do not talk much about my illness to anyone unless it is necessary. The times that I do talk, people may act a little hesitant. Currently, my social support system includes my family and several other groups. My relationship with my mother is good and we talk often. I have just completed an online nursing assistant course, although I am not sure if I want to go into that work right now. I enjoy working on the computer, exercising, and listening to music or news programs. I really like my living situation—I have my own apartment in a group of apartments supervised by a mental health case manager. I have not had an actual friend since high school because I feel tense around people. I am not working right now, but I hope to become self-supporting some day, by which I mean not having to depend on Social Security. For now, I am continuing to learn how to be happy and strong.

CHAPTER **28**

Disorders of Children and Adolescents

Elizabeth Hite Erwin and Cherrill W. Colson

Key Terms and Concepts

Objectives

1. Explore factors and influences contributing to child and adolescent mental disorders, and develop intervention strategies for these young patients.
2. Explain how characteristics associated with resiliency can mitigate ecological influences.
3. Identify characteristics of mental health and positive youth development in children and adolescents.
4. Discuss holistic assessment of a child or adolescent.

5. Explore areas in the assessment of suicide that may be unique to children or adolescents.
6. Compare and contrast at least six treatment modalities for children and adolescents.
7. Describe clinical features and behaviors of at least three child and adolescent psychiatric disorders.
8. Formulate three nursing diagnoses, stating patient outcomes and interventions for each.

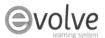 Visit the Evolve website for an **Audio Glossary & Flashcards, Concept Map Creator,** and additional resources related to the content in this chapter: **http://evolve.elsevier.com/Varcarolis/foundations**

L
ike any other illness in children, a psychiatric disorder can disrupt the normal pattern of childhood development and may carry devastating consequences in terms of hopes, dreams, and aspirations. Stigma and misconceptions can cause patients and families to attempt to conceal the conditions or even limit help seeking and professional care. Fortunately, this often silent public health epidemic is being addressed by increasingly sophisticated screening and treatment methods that show promise in reducing the impact of

mental illness in children and on into adolescence and adulthood.

Younger children are more difficult to diagnose than older children because of limited language skills and cognitive and emotional development. Additionally, children undergo more rapid psychological, neurological, and physiological changes over a briefer period than adults. The rapidity and complexity of this development must be taken into consideration during assessment for psychiatric disorders. Clinicians and parents often wait to see whether symptoms are the result of a developmental lag or trauma response that will eventually correct itself; therefore, intervention may be delayed—for instance, until the child reaches school age. Usually a number of factors influence a child's or adolescent's mental health, so a variety of interventions are needed to improve psychological, social, physical, educational, and spiritual well-being.

Important psychiatric disorders that can occur in children and adolescents—mood disorders, anxiety disorders, schizophrenia, and substance abuse—are described elsewhere in this text. These are conditions that may be present during childhood or adolescence but are most often diagnosed when a child reaches maturity. Anxiety and depression are discussed here as they relate specifically to the child and adolescent.

Meeting the mental health needs of youth and their families is a challenge for the nurse, because need steadily increases while funding and access to care steadily decrease, and existing services remain fragmented in many communities. Considering all the developmental changes and associated vulnerabilities and resiliencies that occur during adolescence, it is clear that this is an optimal time to target intervention. This chapter describes the nurse's role in assessment and interventions for selected mental disorders, as well as broad treatment modalities that are implemented through the nursing process with children and adolescents and their families.

EPIDEMIOLOGY

One in five children and adolescents in the United States suffers from a major mental illness that causes significant impairments at home, at school, with peers, and in the community. The prevalence rate for depression in adolescence is about 15%, with up to 30% of adolescents reporting clinically significant levels of depressive symptoms at some point (Evans & Seligman, 2005). Suicide ranks as the third leading cause of death for youth aged 15 to 24 years and sixth for those aged 5 to 15 years (National Mental Health Association [NMHA], 2004). It is estimated that two thirds of young people with mental health problems are not receiving needed services.

Mental illness can continue into adulthood; 74% of 21-year-olds with mental disorders experienced problems in childhood. Unfortunately, lack of services and premature termination of treatment are two main problems, especially for vulnerable populations (poor children with single mothers, minority children, and those with serious presenting problems at intake) (Hoagwood et al., 2001). The suffering experienced by children and adolescents with mental disorders is significant, and the cost to society is high.

It is especially important to understand that the prevalence of some of the disorders of childhood and adolescence have been rising over successive generations. Certain changes in the nature of adolescence and in the environment are considered to be responsible in part for these increases. For example, adolescence is more extended—in many cases until the child completes an education and obtains employment—and puberty is occurring earlier, particularly in developed countries such as the United States. In addition, access to firearms and potentially harmful substances has increased at the same time as there is less supervision from parents or other adults and more time with peers (Evans & Seligman, 2005).

The U.S. government's recognition of childhood and adolescent mental health problems and efforts toward identifying effective treatments were identified in *Mental Health: A Report of the Surgeon General*

(U.S. Department of Health & Human Services [USDHHS], 1999). However, barriers to assessment and treatment remain, including: (1) lack of clarity about conditions for screening children; (2) lack of coordination among multiple systems; (3) lack of resources and long waiting lists for services; (4) lack of mental health providers; and (5) cost and inadequate reimbursement (Children's Defense Fund, 2004). More research is needed to understand the reasons for underutilization and early termination of services, and funding is needed to improve coordination among existing resources to provide programs for young people at varying degrees of need for mental health services (U.S. Public Health Service, 2000).

COMORBIDITY

Children and adolescents with mental health disorders often meet the criteria for more than one diagnostic category. **Attention deficit hyperactivity disorder (ADHD)**, a prominent comorbid condition, occurs in 90% of individuals with juvenile-onset bipolar disorder, 90% of children with oppositional defiant disorder, and 50% of those with conduct disorder. Childhood depression has a high incidence of comorbidity: 20% to 80% of children with depression have conduct or oppositional disorders, 30% to 75% have anxiety disorders, and 5% to 60% display symptoms of ADHD (Inder, 2000). Multiple services are often needed by those with coexisting diagnoses, such as special education evaluation and services, after-school services, family counseling, and behavior management.

RISK FACTORS

Mental illness can become serious or severe and persistent if early detection and effective intervention are not implemented. A child with a parent who has depression has risks of developing an anxiety disorder, conduct disorder, and alcohol dependence. The parent's inability to model effective coping strategies can lead to learned helplessness, creating anxiety or apathy and an inability to master the environment. A child with a conduct disorder may develop an antisocial personality and enter the criminal justice system. In fact, two thirds of youth in the juvenile justice system have one or more diagnosable mental disorders (Children's Defense Fund, 2004).

Children who have been abused and neglected are at great risk for developing emotional, intellectual, and social handicaps as a result of their traumatic experiences (USDHHS, 1999). Neglect is the most prevalent form of child abuse in the United States. According to the National Child Abuse and Neglect Data System (2008), 899,000 children were victims of abuse and neglect in 2005. Of those who died, 42.2% of their deaths occurred from neglect, 24.1% from physical abuse and neglect, and 27.3% as a result of multiple abuse types. In addition, an estimated 9.3% of cases involved sexual abuse.

Other studies suggest even more children suffer abuse and neglect than is reported to child protective services agencies, with girls more frequently victims of sexual abuse. However, boys are also sexually abused, but the numbers are suspected to be underreported due to shame and stigma. The nurse must understand that sexual abuse varies from fondling to forcing a child to observe lewd acts to sexual intercourse. All instances of sexual abuse are devastating to a child who lacks the mental capacity or emotional maturation to consent to this type of a relationship. All instances of suspected abuse of a minor child are required to be reported to the local child protective services.

Witnessing violence is traumatizing and a well-documented risk factor for many mental health problems, including depression, anxiety, PTSD, aggressive and delinquent behavior, drug use, academic failure, and low self-esteem (Farrell et al., 2007). Children who have been abused also are at risk for identifying with the aggressor, and they may act out, bully others, become abusers in adulthood, or otherwise develop dysfunctional patterns in close interpersonal relationships.

Children may bully and act violently toward each other, and gang involvement is a growing problem among adolescents. It is estimated there are 27,000 gangs and 788,000 members across the United States (U.S. Department of Justice, 2009). Youth ages 11 to 13, a time of particular vulnerability, are primarily solicited to become gang members because decision-making capacities are limited, and they may look up to older peers for status and belonging. Certain risk factors seem to predispose a person to gang membership, including past trauma, learning disability, poor school performance, poverty, and family disorganization (Wood et al., 2002). Gang members often inflict violence on others, including vandalism, theft, and aggression. Many end up in the juvenile court system, where they exhibit comorbid mental health problems that may remain untreated.

It is important for nurses working in juvenile detention, school, and community settings to assess for PTSD and safety of environment for young people who have been traumatized or experienced abuse and a history of violence. Interventions should focus on teaching coping skills to deal with trauma, supporting efforts to achieve socially appropriate goals, and facilitating integration into healthy social support systems.

ETIOLOGY

Mental illness in children and adolescents, as in adults, is caused by multiple factors, and distinguishing among the genetic, psychosocial, and environmental factors makes diagnosis challenging. Increasing numbers of children are born with or develop disordered brain function related to malnutrition, human immunodeficiency virus (HIV) infection, fetal alcohol syndrome, drug addiction, and brain injury. In addition, they are exposed to environmental stressors in the family, school, peer group, and community that have an impact on their social, emotional, cognitive, psychological, and spiritual development (Bronfenbrenner, 2006).

The degree of a child's vulnerability to mental illness changes over time. The resiliency of the child and the presence of positive environmental factors (e.g., parental role models, a healthy school environment) enable a child to learn and adapt. This can decrease vulnerability to mental disorders or improve functioning to the fullest possible level if a disorder exists.

Biological Factors

Genetic

Hereditary factors are implicated in a number of mental disorders, including autism, bipolar disorders, schizophrenia, attention-deficit problems, and mental retardation. Because not all genetically vulnerable children develop mental disorders, it is assumed that resilience and a supportive environment are key factors in avoiding the development of mental disorders. According to the *Diagnostic and Statistical Manual of Mental Disorders,* 4th edition, text revision *(DSM-IV-TR)* (American Psychiatric Association [APA], 2000), some disorders have a direct genetic link, such as mental retardation associated with Tay-Sachs disease, phenylketonuria, and fragile X syndrome.

Brain Development and Biochemicals

Dramatic changes occur in the brain during childhood and adolescence, including a declining number of synapses (they peak at age 5), myelination of brain fibers, changes in the relative volume and activity level in different brain regions, and interactions of hormones. Myelination increases the speed of information processing, improves the conduction speed of nerve impulses, and enables faster reactions to occur. Myelination of fibers in the cortex of the brain occurs most rapidly during childhood but continues until well after puberty (Luna & Sweeney, 2004). The teen years are also marked by changes in the frontal and prefrontal cortex regions, leading to improvements in executive functions, organization and planning skills, and inhibiting responses (Evans & Seligman, 2005). These changes, including cerebellum maturation and hormonal changes, reflect the emotional and behavioral fluctuations characteristic of adolescence. Early adolescence is typically characterized by low emotional regulation and intolerance for frustration; emotional and

EVIDENCE-BASED PRACTICE:

Prevention of Violence Among African American Adolescents

Farrell, A. F., Erwin, E. H., Bettencourt, A., Mays, S., Vulin-Reynolds, M., Sullivan, T. et al. (2008). Individual factors influencing effective nonviolent behavior and fighting in peer situations: A qualitative study with urban African American adolescents. *Journal of Clinical Child and Adolescent Psychology, 37*(2), 397–411.

Problem

Efforts to promote positive adolescent development and prevent youth violence require a clear understanding of the factors that influence effective nonviolent response and adaptation, particularly in challenging environments. Aggression is a common problem among adolescents, both those with mental disorders and other school-age youth, especially those living in urban areas with high rates of crime and violence.

Purpose of Study

The purpose of this study was to use qualitative methods to explore how middle-school African American adolescents reason about solving peer problems in a peaceful, nonviolent manner. The researchers want to use this information to develop better interventions that are more realistic and more grounded in the lived experience of inner-city, African American youth.

Methods

Interviewers conducted 109 semi-structured interviews with male and female African American (95%) youth (aged 11 to 15). Students were given three different written descriptions of problem situations and responses (e.g., "Situation: You told a friend something private, and they told it to other people." Response: "I'd talk to my friend and ask why they broke their promise not to tell."). Interviewers asked the participant to imagine the problem was happening to them and how easy it would be to make the response, how likely they would be to make the response, and why they would or would not make the response.

Key Findings

The following themes emerged as barriers or supports for nonviolent, peaceful responses and for fighting in response to teen peer problems:
- Personal resources
  - Problem-solving skills (good, bad, deficient in some way, such as generating alternatives)
  - Self-efficacy for either responding nonviolently or for fighting
  - Emotion-regulation skills ("handling it when someone pushes your buttons")
- Beliefs and values
  - Prosocial values and goals ("I'm going to stay out of trouble," "I value her friendship.")
  - Beliefs about the world (based on past experiences), supporting or against fighting
- Consequences
  - Perceived the response wouldn't work in their world ("I'd get beat up if I tried it.")
  - Absence or lack of fear of consequences (denial or really sees no consequences)
  - Feared fighting (might get hurt) or not fighting (seen as weak, a future victim)
- Appraisal of the situation
  - Attributes of the other person (e.g., likeability, size, how the other person acts)
  - Perceived closeness, connection, or history with the person (in my group or not)

Implications for Nursing Practice

Nurses who work with adolescents and provide cognitive-behavioral interventions can use these findings in their work. We can explore the belief systems of adolescents to challenge ideas supporting aggression (e.g., "He deserved it.") and discuss and support prosocial goals that are compromised if aggression is used to solve problems. The ability to regulate emotions is key for these youth, and teaching them to manage their feelings in highly charged situations such as problems with friends is critical to their success in using nonviolent strategies at school and in the community.

behavioral control usually increase over the course of adolescence.

Alterations in neurotransmitters have also been implicated as playing a role in causing child and adolescent disorders. Decreased norepinephrine and serotonin levels are related to depression and suicide, and elevated levels are related to mania and pathological fear. Abnormalities in dopamine receptors and dopamine transporters are implicated in ADHD, certain addictions, and schizophrenia (Sadock & Sadock, 2008).

Temperament

Temperament, according to Thomas and Chess (1977), is the style of behavior a child habitually uses to cope with the demands and expectations of the environment. This style is present in the infant, is modified by maturation, and develops in the context of the social environment (Gemelli, 2008). All people have temperaments, and the fit between the child and parent's temperament is critical to the child's development. The caregiver's role in shaping that relationship is of primary importance, and the nurse can intervene to teach parents ways to modify their behaviors to improve the interaction. If there is incongruence between parent and child temperament, and the caregiver is unable to respond positively to the child, there is a risk of insecure attachment, developmental problems, and future mental disorders.

By the time children enter grade school, they show temperament and behavior traits that are powerful indicators of an inclination to use and abuse drugs in later life, including shyness, aggressiveness, and rebelliousness. External risk factors include substance use among peers, parental drug use, and involvement in legal problems such as truancy or vandalism. Researchers have also identified childhood protective factors that shield some children from drug use, including self-control, parental monitoring, academic achievement, anti-drug use policies, and strong neighborhood attachment (National Institute on Drug Abuse, 2008).

Resilience

Most children with risk factors for the development of mental illness develop normally. The term resilience has been used to denote the relationship between a child's constitutional endowment and success negotiating stressful environmental factors. Studies have shown that a *resilient child* has the following characteristics: (1) adaptability to changes in the environment, (2) ability to form nurturing relationships with other adults when the parent is not available, (3) ability to distance self from emotional chaos, (4) good social intelligence, and (5) good problem-solving skills (Gallagher & Chase, 2002; Hall & Pearson, 2003). Other studies have identified the cushioning effects of family stability in the face of poverty and adversity. The nurse's role is to identify and foster these qualities to keep at-risk children from developing emotional and mental problems.

Environmental Factors

To a greater degree than adults, children are dependent on others. During childhood, the main context is the family. Parents model behavior and provide the child with a view of the world. If parents are abusive, rejecting, or overly controlling, the child may suffer detrimental effects at the developmental point(s) at which the trauma occurs. There is strong evidence that a number of familial risk factors correlate with child psychiatric disorders, including (1) severe marital discord, (2) low socioeconomic status, (3) large families and overcrowding, (4) parental criminality, (5) maternal psychiatric disorders, and (6) foster-care placement.

External factors in the environment can either support or put stress on children and adolescents and shape their development. Young people are vulnerable in an environment in which systems (e.g., schools, court systems) and people (e.g., parents, counselors) have power and control.

Cultural Considerations

Children in minority groups may be at risk for a variety of problems. Yeh and colleagues (2004) found a disproportionate number of children in minority groups are labeled with mental and learning disorders and suffer from this stigma throughout life. In addition, because of the lack of same-culture role models, these children experience increased risk. Differences in cultural expectations, presence of stresses, and lack of support by the dominant culture may have profound effects on children not of the dominant culture and increase the risk of mental, emotional, and academic problems. Working with children and adolescents from diverse backgrounds requires an increased awareness of one's own biases, as well as the patient's needs. The social and cultural context of the patient, including factors as such as age, ethnicity, gender, sexual orientation, worldview, religiosity, and socioeconomic status should be taken into consideration when assessing and planning care (APA, 2005).

CHILD AND ADOLESCENT PSYCHIATRIC MENTAL HEALTH NURSING

In 2007, the American Nurses Association (ANA), together with the American Psychiatric Nurses Association (APNA) and International Society of Psychiatric-Mental Health Nurses (ISPN), defined the basic-level functions in the combined child and adult *Psychiatric-Mental Health Nursing: Scope and Standards of Practice.* Child psychiatric mental health nurses utilize evidence-based psychiatric practices to provide care that is responsive to the patient and family's specific problems, strengths, personality, sociocultural context, and preferences, which is evident in practice guidelines such as the New Practice Parameters for Child/Adolescent Psychiatric Inpatient Treatment (ISPN, 2007).

Although the number of young people with acute mental illness in our society is increasing, inpatient and residential treatment time has steadily decreased. Treatment for children often consists of brief hospitalization followed by interventions conducted in a wide

CONSIDERING CULTURE

Hostility Toward Gay, Lesbian, and Bisexual Adolescents

On February 12, 2008, E.O. Green Junior High School student Brandon McInerney shot and killed fellow student Larry King, who was openly gay. This is a story of the tragic murder of a young boy who was discovering his sexuality in a school environment that struggled with protecting his rights to personal expression while setting limits on inappropriate, sometimes dangerous behavior. School officials reported King was a "troubled child" who flaunted his sexuality and was provocative with other students, especially the boys. The story describes the difficulties schools and communities may have in coping with the needs of youth with emotional and behavioral difficulties and can open dialogue for nurses in how to increase community readiness to work with gay, lesbian, and bisexual youth.

Statistics on hate crimes since 1992 indicate approximately 17,000 crimes have been related to sexual orientation. Teenagers and children as young as 10 may experience feelings of identification with the same gender or sexual attraction. Young people often disclose these feelings to friends, and they may be met with social rejection, anger, ridicule, bullying, and violence. Studies have shown that gay, lesbian, and bisexual youth (GLB) are at risk for a variety of negative outcomes, including dramatically increased suicidality, mental health problems, high-risk sexual behaviors, poorer school outcomes, homelessness, and substance abuse. Externally, GLB youth are subjected to higher rates of violence and victimization than heterosexual youth.

Readiness for enhanced community is a nursing diagnosis related to adapting and problem solving to meet the demands and needs of the community (in this case, it includes the school) and accessing social supports. In addition to providing counseling for GLB youth, nurses could play a key role in (1) educating schools and parents about the needs of GLB to change attitudes, (2) helping the community apply for and obtain funds for additional programs, (3) encouraging communication and collaboration among community members on these issues, and (4) serving as advocates for GLB youth.

< http://www.venturacountystar.com/news/2008/feb/12/no-headline---nxxwcshooting13/> Accessed 14.05.2009.
Abrams, J. House passes extended hate crimes bill, *Guardian Unlimited*, 05-03-2007. Accessed 05.03.2007.

spectrum of community support settings, including day treatment programs, partial hospitalization programs, clinics, schools, and psychiatric home care. To be considered eligible for inpatient hospitalization, the child or adolescent typically must be an eminent danger to self or others. In short-term inpatient facilities, the nurse has less time to form a therapeutic relationship with the child and family, making it more difficult to facilitate lasting behavioral changes. Residential and group home facilities for long-term placement are more difficult to secure because facilities may not be available, the cost is high, and consistent evidence of their effectiveness in reducing symptoms and improving long-term functioning is lacking (Evans & Seligman, 2005).

As psychiatric care moved from inpatient facilities to the community, child and adolescent psychiatric mental health nurses have responded, becoming an integral part of these programs. Advanced practice registered nurses, including clinical nurse specialists and nurse practitioners, have established outpatient practices, school-based primary prevention, and other innovative treatment programs for young people. Research on interventions for young people at risk for developing mental illness is also being carried out in nontraditional settings such as homeless shelters, online, and in mentoring programs.

Assessing Development and Functioning

A child or adolescent with mental illness is one whose progressive personality development and functioning is hindered or arrested due to biological, psychosocial, and spiritual factors, resulting in functional impairments. In comparison, a child or adolescent who does not have a mental illness matures with only minor regressions, coping with the stressors and developmental tasks of life. Learning and adapting to the environment and bonding with others in a mutually satisfying way are signs of mental health (Box 28-1). The degree of mental health and illness can be viewed on a continuum, with one's level on the continuum changing over time. Many mental illnesses are chronic but can be managed effectively with evidenced-based treatments.

Assessment Data

The type of data collected to assess mental health depends on the setting, the severity of the presenting problem, and the availability of resources. Box 28-2 identifies essential assessment data, including history of the present illness; medical, developmental, and family history; mental status, and neurological developmental characteristics. Agency policies determine which data are collected, but a nurse should be

BOX 28-1 Characteristics of a Mentally Healthy Child or Adolescent

- Trusts others and sees his or her world as being safe and supportive
- Correctly interprets reality, makes accurate perceptions of the environment and one's ability to influence it through actions (e.g., self-determination)
- Behaves in a way that is developmentally appropriate and does not violate social norms
- Has a positive, realistic self-concept and developing identity
- Adapts to and copes with anxiety and stress using age-appropriate behavior
- Can learn and master developmental tasks and new situations
- Expresses self in spontaneous and creative ways
- Develops and maintains satisfying relationships

prepared to make an independent judgment about what to assess and how to assess it. In all cases, a physical examination is part of a complete assessment for serious mental problems.

Data Collection

Methods of collecting data include interviewing, screening, testing (neurological, psychological, intelligence), observing, and interacting with the child or adolescent. Histories are taken from multiple sources, including parents, other caregivers, the child or adolescent and other adults, such as teachers, when possible. Structured questionnaires and behavior checklists can be completed by parents and teachers. A genogram can document family composition, history, and relationships (see Chapter 35). Numerous assessment tools are available, and with training, nurses can use them to effectively monitor symptoms and behavioral change.

BOX 28-2 Types of Assessment Data

History of Present Illness
- Chief complaint
- Development and duration of problems
- Help sought and results
- Effect of problem on child's life at home and school
- Effect of problem on family and siblings' lives

Developmental History
- Pregnancy, birth, neonatal data
- Developmental milestones
- Description of eating, sleeping, and elimination habits and routines
- Attachment behaviors
- Types of play
- Social skills and friendships
- Sexual activity

Developmental Assessment
- Psychomotor skills
- Language skills
- Cognitive skills
- Interpersonal and social skills
- Academic achievement
- Behavior (response to stress, to changes in environment)
- Problem-solving and coping skills (impulse control, delay of gratification)
- Energy level and motivation

Neurological Assessment
- Cerebral functions
- Cerebellar functions

- Sensory functions
- Reflexes
  NOTE: Functions can be observed during developmental assessment and while playing games involving a specific ability (e.g., "Simon says touch your nose.")

Medical History
- Review of body systems
- Traumas, hospitalizations, operations, and child's response
- Illnesses or injuries affecting central nervous system
- Medications (past and current)
- Allergies

Family History
- Illnesses in related family members (e.g., seizures, mental disorders, mental retardation, hyperactivity, drug and alcohol abuse, diabetes, cancer)
- Background of family members (occupation, education, social activities, religion)
- Family relationship (separation, divorce, deaths, contact with extended family, support system)

Mental Status Assessment
- General appearance
- Activity level
- Coordination and motor function
- Affect
- Speech
- Manner of relating
- Intellectual functions
- Thought processes and content
- Characteristics of play

The observation-interaction part of a mental health assessment begins with a semi-structured interview in which the nurse asks the young person about the home environment, parents, and siblings and the school environment, teachers, and peers. In this format, the child is free to describe current problems and give information about his or her developmental history. Play activities, such as games, drawings, and puppets are used for younger children who cannot respond to a direct approach. The initial interview is key to observing interactions among the child, caregiver, and siblings (if available) and building trust and rapport.

Mental Status Examination

Assessment of mental status of children is similar to that of adults. It provides information about the mental state at the time of the examination and identifies problems with thinking, feeling, and behaving. Broad categories to assess include safety, general appearance, socialization, activity level, speech, coordination and motor function, affect, manner of relating, intellectual function, thought processes and content, and characteristics of play.

Developmental Assessment

The developmental assessment provides information about the child or adolescent's maturational level. These data are then reviewed in relation to the child's chronological age to identify developmental strengths or deficits. The Denver II Developmental Screening Test for infants and children up to 6 years of age is a popular assessment tool. For adolescents, tools may be tailored to specific areas of assessment, such as neuropsychological, physical, hormonal, and biochemical. One tool to assess risk is the Youth Risk Behavior Survey for children and adolescents.

Abnormal findings in the developmental and mental status assessments may be related to stress and adjustment problems or to more serious disorders. Children may outgrow a difficulty, but nurses need to evaluate behaviors indicative of stress or minor regressions, as well as those indicative of more serious psychopathology, and identify the need for further evaluation or referral. Stress-related behaviors or minor regressions may be handled by working with parents. However, as young people develop maladaptive coping behaviors and use these behaviors over time, they are at risk of developing mental disorders. Serious psychopathology requires evaluation by an advanced practice nurse in collaboration with clinicians from other child and adolescent mental health and pediatric disciplines.

Suicide Risk

Suicide is the second leading cause of death in adolescence (Sadock & Sadock, 2008); therefore, assessment of suicidality is an essential nursing skill. Some children make idle threats about killing themselves, but to determine the cause of the distress and the risk of violence, the nurse must listen carefully to any young person expressing the wish to hurt self or others. The number one predictor of suicidal risk is a past suicide attempt. Areas to explore when assessing suicidal risk include:

- Past suicidal thoughts, threats, or attempts
- Existence of a plan, lethality of the plan, and accessibility of the methods for carrying out the plan
- Feelings of hopelessness, changes in level of energy
- Circumstances, state of mind, and motivation
- Viewpoints about suicide and death (e.g., Has a family member or friend attempted suicide?)
- Depression and other moods or feelings (e.g., anger, guilt, rejection)
- History of impulsivity, poor judgment, or decreased decision making
- Drug or alcohol use
- Prescribed medications and any recent adherence issues

Additional questions may be asked about these areas for teens, including acting-out behaviors, artwork with a violent theme, listening to music or reading books with morbid themes, and recent changes in behavior or social life (eating, sleeping, isolating, loss of a relationship).

Assessing lethality in a young child's suicide plan is complicated by the distorted concept of death, immature ego functions, and an immature understanding of lethality. For instance, a child who is highly suicidal may believe a few aspirin will cause death. The incorrect judgment about the lethality does not diminish the seriousness of the intent. Another child simply seeking attention may threaten to jump off a bridge believing this would not be fatal. Some teens may make a pact to kill themselves or become upset after a friend has committed suicide or died accidentally. Early intervention is essential, and parents need to understand that suicidal thoughts or self-threatening behavior (e.g., cutting, reckless driving, binge drinking) must be taken seriously and evaluated by mental health professionals as an emergency.

Cultural Influences

Psychiatric professionals recognize the importance of culture in evaluating psychiatric disorders, especially when working with families. The *DSM-IV-TR* identifies culture-bound syndromes of mental illness that are not diagnostic categories in Western medicine (see Chapter 6). Sensitivity to cultural influences in mental illness is a necessity to show respect for cultural preferences in providing individualized care and avoid behavior stereotyping and incorrect assessment.

The use of "nonstandard" English dialects can make speech difficult to assess and contribute to stereotyping. To facilitate accuracy in assessment, a child should be interviewed in his or her native language to fully understand any problems (Ackley & Ladwig, 2008).

General Interventions

The interventions described in this section can be used in a variety of settings: inpatient, residential, outpatient, day treatment, outreach programs in schools, and home visits. Many of the modalities can encompass activities of daily living, learning activities, multiple forms of play and recreational activities, and interactions with adults and peers.

Family Therapy

The family is seen as critical to improving the function of a young person with a psychiatric illness; family counseling is often a key component of treatment. In family therapy, specific goals are defined and outlined for each member, identifying ways to improve and work to achieve the goals for the family or subunits within the family (e.g., parental, sibling). Homework assignments are often used for family members to practice newly learned skills outside the therapeutic environment. In addition to therapy involving a single family, multiple-family therapy useful for interaction to (1) learn how other families solve problems and build on strengths, (2) develop insight and improve judgment about their own family, (3) learn and practice new information, and (4) develop lasting and satisfying relationships with other families.

Group Therapy

Group therapy for younger children takes the form of play to introduce ideas and work through issues. For grade-school children, it combines play, learning skills, and talk about the activity. The child learns social skills by taking turns and sharing with peers. For adolescents, group therapy involves learning skills and talking, focusing largely on peer relationships and working through specific problems. Adolescent group therapy might use a popular media event or personality as the basis for a group discussion. Groups have been used effectively to deal with specific issues in a child's life (e.g., bereavement, physical abuse, substance use, dating, or chronic illnesses like juvenile diabetes).

Milieu Management

Milieu management is the mechanism for structuring inpatient, residential, and day treatment programs. According to the *Psychiatric-Mental Health Nursing: Scope and Standards of Practice* (ANA, 2007), the nurse collaborates with other health care providers in structuring and maintaining the therapeutic environment to:

- Provide physical and psychological security
- Promote growth and mastery of developmental tasks
- Ameliorate psychiatric disorders and promote well being

The physical milieu for inpatient or residential care is designed to provide a safe, comfortable place to live, play, and learn, with areas for both private time and group activity. There may be a gym, outdoor playground, swimming pool, recreational facilities, and even pets. A daily schedule sets the structure for what activities will occur (e.g., school, therapy sessions, outings, family or home visits). The multidisciplinary team shares and articulates a philosophy regarding how to provide physical and psychological security, promote personal growth, and work with problematic behaviors. This philosophy is reflected in the rules of the facility and is typically written in a handbook given to patients and families upon admission. The child or adolescent's behavior, emotions, and cognitive processes are the focus of the therapeutic interventions in the milieu. The therapeutic factors operating in the milieu's structure, activities, and interactions with staff are listed in Box 28-3.

Behavioral Therapy

Behavioral therapy involves rewarding desired behavior to reduce maladaptive behaviors. In a healthy relationship, a child's developmentally appropriate behaviors are validated by a significant adult (**operant conditioning**). Behavior management in psychiatry is classified according to the level of restrictiveness and

---

BOX 28-3 Therapeutic Factors in the Milieu

- Safe, therapeutic environment with roles, boundaries, and limits
- Reduction of stressors
- Structure for coping with stress
- Ability to express feelings without fear of rejection or retaliation
- Availability of emotional support and comfort
- Assistance with reality testing and support for weak or missing ego functions
- Interventions for impulsive, aggressive, or inappropriate behaviors
- Opportunities for learning and testing new adaptive behaviors and mastering developmental tasks
- Consistent, constructive feedback from trained and supportive adult staff
- Reinforcement of positive behaviors and development of self-esteem
- Corrective emotional experiences
- Availability of role models for making healthy identifications and positive attachments
- Opportunities to develop peer relationships and practice handling peer pressure
- Opportunities to be spontaneous and creative
- Opportunities to explore issues related to self-esteem and identity formation

intrusiveness. To ensure that the civil and legal rights of individuals are not violated, and effective treatment is provided, techniques are selected according to the **principle of least restrictive intervention**. This principle requires that more-restrictive interventions should be used *only* after less-restrictive interventions have been attempted to manage the behavior. Intrusive techniques (such as physical restraints) are implemented to manage behavior and maintain safety only when very severe or dangerous behaviors (i.e., those that may result in injury to the patient or others) are exhibited.

Most child and adolescent treatment settings use a behavior modification program to motivate and reward age-appropriate behaviors. One popular method is the **point and level system**, in which points are awarded for desired behaviors, and increasing levels of privileges can be earned. The value for specific behaviors and privileges for each level are spelled out, and points earned each day are recorded. Older youth can be made responsible for keeping their own point sheet and for requesting points for their behaviors. Children who work on individual behavioral goals (e.g., seeking help in problem solving) can earn additional points. Points are used to obtain a specific reward, which can be part of the system or be negotiated on an individual or group basis.

Seclusion and Restraint

Hospitalized patients are often a high risk to themselves, and effective use of prevention strategies for dangerous behavior begins at intake. Promoting a therapeutic environment for all patients involves (1) actively engaging the patient and family in treatment planning to avoid the use of seclusion or restraint, (2) maintaining adequate staffing patterns with motivated staff experienced in working with patients who have been violent and abused, (3) accurate assessment of the acuity of the individuals and group makeup of the unit, and (4) the use of positive and less restrictive alternatives (e.g., de-escalation strategies, time-space interviews) (Masters & Belonci, 2002).

Controversy continues over the use of locked seclusion and physical restraint in managing dangerous behavior, and evidence suggests both are psychologically harmful and can be physically harmful. Deaths have resulted, primarily by asphyxiation due to physical holds during restraints (Masters & Belonci, 2002). However, at times a child's behavior is so destructive or dangerous that physical restraint or seclusion is needed. All nurses who might be involved in therapeutic holding or physical restraint of children and adolescents must receive training to decrease the risk of injury to themselves and the child. This intervention requires prompt, firm, nonretaliatory protective restraint that is gentle and safe and reduces the risk of injury to self or others. Children are released as soon as they are no longer dangerous, usually a few minutes, and most facilities strive to avoid all intensive interventions that restrict movement, such as holds and restraints.

The decision to restrain or seclude a child is made by the registered nurse who is working with the patient. A physician, nurse practitioner, or other advanced level practitioner must authorize this action, either at the same time or after the fact. All patients in seclusion or restraints must be monitored constantly. Vital signs, including pulse and blood pressure, and range of motion in extremities must be monitored every 15 minutes. Hydration, elimination, comfort, and other psychological and physical needs should be monitored. The patient's family should be informed of any incident of seclusion or restraint, and they should be encouraged to discuss the event with their child and reinforce the treatment plan to reduce the likelihood of future incidents (Masters, 2009).

Once the child is calm, the staff should discuss what happened with the patient. This helps to strengthen the nurse-patient relationship, which may have been disrupted, and also enables staff to learn from the event to prevent it from happening in the future. Debriefings with staff are important to determine if injury has occurred and identify how the situation could have been avoided by using less restrictive alternatives.

Quiet Room

A unit may have an unlocked **quiet room** for a child who needs an area with decreased stimulation for regaining and maintaining self-control. Variations on the quiet room include the **feelings room**, which is carpeted and supplied with soft objects that can be punched and thrown, and the **freedom room**, which contains items for relaxation and meditation, like music and yoga mats. The child is encouraged to express freely and work through feelings of anger or sadness in privacy and with staff support. When a child has difficulty being in touch with or expressing feelings, staff provide practice sessions and act as role models.

Time-Out

Asking, negotiating, or directing a child or adolescent to take a **time-out** from an activity is another method for intervening to halt disruptive behaviors or encourage self-control. Taking a time-out may require going to a designated room or sitting on the periphery of an activity until self-control is regained and the episode is reviewed with a staff member. The child's individual behavioral goals are considered in setting limits on behavior and using time-out periods. If they are overused or used as an automatic response to a behavioral infraction, time-outs lose their effectiveness.

Cognitive-Behavioral Therapy

As discussed in Chapter 2, cognitive-behavioral therapy (CBT) is an evidence-based treatment approach. Simply put, it is based on the premise that negative and self-defeating thoughts lead to psychiatric pathology and that learning to replace these thoughts with more realistic and accurate appraisals results in improved functioning. Researchers and clinicians have discovered that CBT is also useful in children (Abernethy & Schlozman, 2008). Disorders such as obsessive-compulsive disorder, aversion to school, and depression are all responsive to CBT.

Play Therapy

Play is often described as the work of childhood through which the child learns to master impulses and adapt to the environment. Play is a medium of communication that can be used to assess developmental and emotional status, determine diagnosis, and institute therapeutic interventions. Melanie Klein (1955) and Anna Freud (1965) were the first to use play as a therapeutic tool in their psychoanalysis of children in the 1920s and 1930s. Axline (1969) identified the guiding principles of play therapy, which are still used by mental health professionals:

- Accept the child as he or she is and follow the child's lead.
- Establish a warm, friendly relationship that helps the child express feelings completely.
- Recognize the child's feelings and reflect them back so the child can gain insight into the behavior.
- Accept the child's ability to solve personal problems.
- Set limits only to provide reality and security.

There are many forms of play therapy that can be used individually or in groups. The term *play therapy* usually refers to a one-to-one session the therapist has with a child in a playroom. Most playrooms are equipped with a range of developmentally appropriate toys for both genders, including art supplies, clay or play dough, dolls and dollhouses, hand puppets, toys, building blocks, and trucks and cars. The dolls, puppets, and dollhouse provide the child with opportunities to act out conflicts and situations involving the family, work through feelings, and develop more adaptive ways of coping. The following vignette shows how play therapy can help a child cope with a significant loss.

VIGNETTE

Hannah, a 6-year-old, begins having nightmares and refusing to go to school after her grandmother, who was also her babysitter, dies. Her parents do not let her attend the funeral, thinking it will upset her. Hannah becomes fearful and preoccupied with the death. In play sessions, she repeatedly uses dolls to act out her grandmother's hospitalization, death, and funeral. She then pretends to bury her grandmother in a small, coffin-like box. Her parents have told Hannah that "Grandma has gone to heaven." Hannah demonstrates the concept by removing "Grandma" from the box and placing her high up on a bookshelf in the playroom, looking down on the rest of the doll family. ■

Mutual Storytelling

Mutual storytelling is a psychodramatic technique developed by Gardner (1971) to help young children express themselves verbally. The child is asked to make up a story with a beginning, middle, and ending. At the end of the story, the child is asked to state the lesson or moral of the story. The nurse determines the psychodynamic meaning of the story and selects one or two of its important themes. Using the same characters and a similar setting, the nurse retells the story, providing a healthier resolution. The lesson of the story is also reformulated to help the child become consciously aware of the better resolution. If the child has trouble starting a story, the nurse can assist by beginning the story with "Once upon a time in a faraway land there lived a …" and then asking the child to continue. After the child has identified the main characters, the nurse may need to keep prompting with comments, such as "and then…" until the story is completed. The story can be recorded as audio or video, which allows for a review to reinforce the learning.

Therapeutic Games

The use of therapeutic games is ideal for children who have difficulty talking about their feelings and problems. Playing a game with a child facilitates the development of a therapeutic alliance and provides an opportunity for conversation. The game might be as simple as checkers, but specific therapeutic games are more effective in eliciting children's fears and fantasies. Gardner (1979) developed a series of therapeutic games for children, one of which, Board of Objects, can be used with children 4 to 8 years of age. The game pieces are small items (people, animals, various objects) that are placed on a checkerboard. The players roll dice. One side of each is colored red. If a red side lands face up, the player selects an object. To get a reward chip, the player must say something about the object; if the player tells a story about the object, he or she gets two reward chips. The child's statement or story can be used in a therapeutic interchange (e.g., to communicate empathy or make a statement suggesting a more adaptive way to cope with a difficult situation). In the end, the player with the most chips (usually the child) wins.

A board game appropriate for latency-age children (6 to 12 years) is Gardner's Talking, Feeling, and Doing Game (1986). The player throws dice to advance his or her playing piece along a pathway of different-colored squares. Depending on the color landed upon, the player draws a talking, feeling, or doing card, which gives instructions or asks a question. A reward chip is given when the player responds appropriately. For example, a feeling card might read, "All the girls in the class were invited to a birthday party except one. How did she feel?" If this game is played with more than one child, the nurse can elicit additional responses and engage the whole group in the therapeutic interchange. The nurse may stack the deck to make sure that cards relating to the child's problems will be selected.

Bibliotherapy

Bibliotherapy involves using child and adolescent literature to help the child express feelings in a supportive environment, gain insight into feelings and behavior, and learn new ways to cope with difficult situations. When children listen to or read a story, they unconsciously identify with the characters and experience a catharsis of feelings. The books selected by the nurse should reflect the situations or feelings the child is experiencing. It is important to assess not only the needs of the child but also the child's readiness for the particular topic and the child's level of understanding. A children's librarian has access to a large collection of stories and knows which books are written specifically to help children deal with particular subjects; however, the nurse should read the book first to be sure the content is age appropriate and fits with the treatment plan and be prepared to discuss it with the patient. Whenever possible, the nurse consults with the family to make sure the books do not violate the family's belief systems. A choice of several books is offered, and a book is never forced on the child.

Therapeutic Drawing

Many children and adolescents love to draw and paint and will spontaneously express themselves in artwork. Their drawings capture the thoughts, feelings, and tensions they may not be able to express verbally, are unaware of, or are denying. For some, however, this modality may be too threatening or not engaging. Children and adolescents can be encouraged to draw themes, such as people, families, or themselves or more abstract themes, such as feelings. To use this modality, the nurse needs to be familiar with the drawing capabilities expected of children at particular developmental levels, and additional training is recommended. In the following vignette, the art therapist and the nurse use a family art session to identify family dynamics and begin interventions.

VIGNETTE

Andrew, an intelligent 15-year-old with obsessive-compulsive behaviors and severe insecurity, lives with his parents and younger sister. In an art session, all family members are given paper on an easel and asked to draw themselves and the other members of the family. Andrew draws his parents and sister as being the same size and standing together shoulder to shoulder. He draws himself as a tiny figure in a box that appears to be suspended in space. When questioned, he reports feeling as though he were trapped in a falling elevator and disconnected from the family.

The family is surprised that he feels isolated (he is a normal size in their drawings). After completing a series of drawings and discussing them, the family is asked to draw a joint picture that requires them to work together. The picture they draw shows a smiling family standing by a house near a tree and a fence. The picture suggests that the family does view Andrew as separate and different, for although he is standing beside the family, he is placed behind the fence. This observation is discussed, and as an intervention, the family is given the task of finding ways to make Andrew feel included. ■

Psychopharmacology

Medicating children typically works best when combined with another treatment such as cognitive-behavioral therapy (Sadock & Sadock, 2008). Medications that target specific symptoms can make a real difference in a family's ability to cope and quality of life, and they can enhance the child or adolescent's potential for growth. Table 28-1 lists some child and adolescent disorders and identifies some of the medications used in the treatment of these disorders.

Pervasive Developmental Disorders

A **pervasive developmental disorder (PDD)** is characterized by severe and pervasive impairment in reciprocal social interaction and communication skills, usually accompanied by stereotypical behavior, interests, and activities (APA, 2000). Some degree of mental retardation is often evident in these disorders, and they are typically diagnosed in early childhood. The *DSM-IV-TR* classifies these disorders as developmental disorders (as opposed to clinical disorders) on Axis II. Three common subtypes of PDD are autistic disorder, Asperger's disorder, and Rett's disorder. Each may vary in terms of level of severity.

CLINICAL PICTURE

Autistic Disorder

Autistic disorder is a complex neurobiological and developmental disability that typically appears during a child's first 3 years of life. However, half of all autism cases are not *diagnosed* until a child is school age. Autism affects the normal development of the

TABLE 28-1 Drug Treatment of Child and Adolescent Disorders and Symptoms

Disorder or Symptom	Type of Drug	Examples and Comments
Pervasive developmental disorders	Antipsychotics	Risperidone (Risperdal) reduces hyperactivity, fidgetiness, and labile affect. Olanzapine (Zyprexa) reduces hyperactivity, social withdrawal, use of language, and depression.
Autistic disorder	Antipsychotics Propranolol (Inderal) Selective serotonin reuptake inhibitors (SSRI)	Haloperidol (Haldol) can reduce irritability and labile affect. Propranolol reduces rage outbursts, aggression, and severe anxiety. Clomipramine (Anafranil) may help treat anger and compulsive behavior.
Attention deficit hyperactivity disorder (ADHD)	Stimulants Antidepressants α-adrenergic agonists	Methylphenidate (Ritalin) Mixture of salts and L-amphetamine (Adderall) Dexmethylphenidate (Focalin) Pemoline (Cylert) All improve symptoms of ADHD. Nortriptyline (Aventyl) Bupropion (Wellbutrin) Fluoxetine (Prozac) All produce improvements in hyperactivity, attention, and global functioning. Clonidine (Catapres) can be used for aggressiveness, impulsivity, and hyperactivity in patients with ADHD.
Conduct disorders	Antipsychotics Stimulants Antidepressants Mood stabilizers Alpha-adrenergic agonists	Risperidone decreases aggression. Methylphenidate decreases antisocial behaviors. Bupropion improves symptoms of conduct disorder. Carbamazepine (Tegretol) and lithium both have demonstrated efficacy in decreasing aggression. Clonidine may help with impulsive and disordered behaviors.
ANXIETY DISORDERS		
Panic and school phobia	SSRIs Tricyclic antidepressants (TCAs)	Citalopram (Celexa), fluoxetine, and paroxetine (Paxil) Imipramine (Tofranil) is commonly used.
Obsessive-compulsive disorder (OCD)	SSRIs TCAs Atypical anxiolytics	Fluoxetine and paroxetine Clomipramine Buspirone (BuSpar) is used as adjunct treatment for refractory OCD.
Separation anxiety disorder	TCAs SSRIs	Imipramine Fluoxetine
Social phobia	TCAs Anxiolytics	Imipramine Buspirone
Posttraumatic stress disorder (PTSD)	Atypical antipsychotics	Risperidone is used to control the flashbacks and aggression in PTSD.
ANXIETY SYMPTOMS		
Insomnia	Antihistamines	Diphenhydramine (Benadryl)
DEPRESSIVE SYMPTOMS		
Major depression and dysthymia	SSRIs TCAs Atypical antidepressants	Fluoxetine is effective in decreasing depressive symptoms. No significant differences have been found between responses to TCAs and to placebo. Venlafaxine (Effexor): one small study reported no difference between venlafaxine and placebo. Nefazodone (Serzone) effective in treating depressive symptoms.
Psychotic symptoms	Antipsychotics	Quetiapine (Seroquel) Risperidone

Data from Wagner, K. D. (2004). Treatment of childhood and adolescent disorders. In Schatzberg, A. F., & Nemeroff, C. B. (2004). *Textbook of psychopharmacology* (3rd ed., pp. 949–1007). Washington, DC: American Psychiatric Publishing.

brain in social interaction and communication skills. People with autism typically have difficulties in verbal and nonverbal communication, social interactions, and leisure or play activities.

There is a genetic component to autism. The concordance rate for identical twins is 70% to 90% (Smoller et al., 2008). Autism is four times more common in boys than girls (Sadock & Sadock, 2008). It has no racial, ethnic, or social boundaries and is not influenced by family income, educational levels, or lifestyles.

Early intervention for children with autism can greatly enhance their potential for a full, productive life. Unfortunately, many families with an autistic child may not know it. Problems with left hemispheric functions (e.g., language, logic, reasoning) are evident, yet music and visual-spatial activities may, in rare cases, be enhanced, such as in savant syndrome (Ursano, et al., 2008). The prognosis is related to the child's overall intellectual level and the development of social and language skills (APA, 2000). Often, symptoms are first noticed when the infant fails to be interested in others or to be socially responsive through eye contact and facial expressions. Some children show improvement during development, but puberty can be a turning point toward either improvement or deterioration. Without intensive intervention, individuals with severe autism may not be able to live and work independently, and only about one third achieve partial independence with restricted interests and activities.

Three presenting symptoms of autism, as adapted from the *DSM-IV-TR*, include:

1. Impairment in communication and imaginative activity
   - Language delay or absence of language
   - Stereotypical or repetitive use of language
   - Lack of spontaneous make-believe play or imaginative play
   - Failure to imitate other's activities or words
2. Impairment in social interactions
   - Lack of responsiveness to or interest in social activities
   - Limited eye-to-eye contact and facial responses
   - Indifference or aversion to affection and physical contact
   - Not able to share enjoyment, interest, or achievement with others
   - Failure to develop friendships or cooperative or imaginative play with peers
3. Markedly restricted, stereotypical patterns of behavior, interest, and activities
   - Rigid adherence to routines and rituals with catastrophic reactions to changes in the environment (e.g., moving furniture)
   - Stereotypical and repetitive motor mannerisms (hand or finger flapping, spinning, head banging, or hand biting)
   - Preoccupation with repetitive activities (pouring water, twirling string)
   - Other abnormalities in behavior

Asperger's Disorder

Asperger's disorder differs from autistic disorder, appearing to have a later onset and no significant delay in cognitive and language development (APA, 2000). The etiology is unknown, although there appears to be a familial pattern. Restricted and repetitive patterns of behavior and idiosyncratic interests (e.g., fascination with remembering train schedules or dates) may develop. Problems with social relationships become more noticeable upon entering school and may continue into adulthood.

Rhett's Disorder

Rhett's disorder differs from autistic disorder and Asperger's disorder in that it is observed only in females, with onset before 4 years of age (APA, 2000). The exact cause is unknown, but it is associated with electroencephalographic abnormalities, seizure disorder, abnormal gait, impaired head growth, and severe or profound mental retardation. These girls experience severely impaired language development, and many have social interaction problems.

APPLICATION OF THE NURSING PROCESS

ASSESSMENT

Assessment Guidelines Pervasive Developmental Disorders

1. Assess for developmental delays, uneven development, or loss of acquired abilities. Use baby books and diaries, photographs, films, or videotapes.
2. Assess the quality of the parent-child relationship for evidence of bonding, anxiety, tension, and quality of caregiver-child temperaments.
3. Be aware that children with behavioral and developmental problems are at risk for abuse, and be knowledgeable about community programs providing support services for parents and children, including parent education, counseling, and after-school programs.

DIAGNOSIS

The child with PDD has severe impairments in social interactions and communication skills, often accompanied by stereotypical behavior, interests, and activities.

The stress on the family can be severe, owing to the chronic nature of the disease. The severity of the impairment is evident in the degree of responsiveness to or interest in others, the presence of associated behavioral problems (e.g., head banging), and the ability to bond with peers. Table 28-2 lists potential nursing diagnoses.

OUTCOMES IDENTIFICATION

Nursing Outcomes Classification (NOC) (Moorhead et al., 2008) identifies a number of outcomes appropriate for the child with PDD. Table 28-3 includes examples of *NOC* outcomes and supporting indicators that target developmental competencies and coping skills.

IMPLEMENTATION

Children with PDD are treated in therapeutic nursery schools, specialized private autism schools, day treatment programs, and special education classes in public or private schools, and their education and treatment are mandated under the Children with Disabilities Act.

TABLE 28-2 Potential Nursing Diagnoses for Disorders of Childhood and Adolescence

Signs and Symptoms	Nursing Diagnosis
Lack of responsiveness or interest in others, empathy, or sharing	*Impaired social interaction* *Risk for impaired attachment*
Severe behavior problems creating stress on family members	*Caregiver role strain* *Interrupted family processes* *Chronic sorrow* *Spiritual distress*
Lack of cooperation or imaginative play with peers Disruptive, hostile behavior leading to difficulty in making or keeping friends	*Activity intolerance* *Situational low self-esteem*
Language delay or absence, stereotyped or repetitive use of language	*Impaired verbal communication*
Inability to feed, bathe, dress, or toilet self at age-appropriate level	*Delayed growth and development*
Head banging, face slapping, hand biting	*Risk for trauma*
Catastrophic reactions (e.g., severe temper tantrums, rage reactions)	*Risk for other-directed violence*
Impulsiveness, anger, and aggression	*Risk for self-mutilation*
Thoughts or verbalizations regarding self-harm	*Risk for self-directed violence*
Frequent disregard for bodily needs	*Self-care deficit* *Risk for situational low self-esteem*
Conflict with authority, refusal to comply with requests	*Powerlessness* *Readiness for enhanced power*
Failure to follow age-appropriate social norms	*Ineffective coping*
Blaming of others for problems or for causing his or her actions	*Defensive coping* *Impaired individual resilience*
Fear of being separated from parent (e.g., going to school or a party)	*Anxiety* *Relocation stress syndrome*
Depression	*Stress overload* *Spiritual distress*
Refusal to attend school	*Ineffective coping* *Readiness for enhanced parenting*
Inability to concentrate, withdrawal, difficulty in functioning, feeling down, change in vegetative symptoms	*Risk for suicide*
Re-experiences of past trauma (dreams, illusions, flashbacks)	*Post-trauma syndrome* *Rape-trauma syndrome*
Fear of objects, people, or situations	*Anxiety*

North American Nursing Diagnosis Association International (NANDA-I). (2009). *NANDA-I nursing diagnoses: Definitions and classification 2009-2011*. Oxford, United Kingdom: Author.

TABLE 28-3 *NOC* Outcomes for Pervasive Developmental Disorders		
Nursing Outcome and Definition	**Intermediate Indicators**	**Short-Term Indicators**
Child Development: 3 Years: Milestones of physical, cognitive, and psychosocial progression by 3 years of age	Speech understood by strangers	Gives own first name
Child Development: 4 Years: Milestones of physical, cognitive, and psychosocial progression by 4 years of age	Engages in creative play	Draws person with three parts
Child Development: 5 Years: Milestones of physical, cognitive, and psychosocial progression by 5 years of age	Follows simple rules of interactive games with peers	Recognizes most letters of the alphabet
Communication: Expressive: Expression of meaningful verbal and/or nonverbal messages	Directs messages appropriately	Uses spoken language: Vocal
Play Participation: Use of activities by a child from 1 year through 11 years of age to promote enjoyment, entertainment, and development	Expresses emotions during play activities	Expresses satisfaction with play activities

From Moorhead, S., Johnson, M., Maas, M., & Swanson, E. (2008). *Nursing outcomes classification (NOC)* (4th ed.). St. Louis: Mosby.

Treatment plans include behavior management plans with a reward system and teaching parents to provide structure, rewards, consistency in rules, and expectations at home in order to shape and modify behavior and foster the development of socially appropriate skills. It is important that the nurse recognize and capitalize on the individual's and family's strengths and incorporate them into the plan of care. Pharmacological agents such as risperidone, clomipramine, and desipramine are used with some success in conjunction with ongoing psychiatric medication management.

Attention Deficit Hyperactivity Disorder and Disruptive Behavior Disorders

CLINICAL PICTURE

Attention Deficit Hyperactivity Disorder

Children with attention deficit hyperactivity disorder (ADHD) show an inappropriate degree of inattention, impulsiveness, and hyperactivity. Some children can have attention deficit disorder without hyperactivity (ADD). In order to diagnose a child with ADHD/ADD, symptoms must be present before age 7 and be present in at least two settings (e.g., at home and school).

Preschoolers with ADHD exhibit excessive gross motor activity that becomes less pronounced as the child matures. The disorder is most often detected when the child has difficulty adjusting to elementary school. Attention problems and hyperactivity contribute to low frustration tolerance, temper outbursts, labile moods, poor school performance, peer rejection, and low self-esteem (Sadock & Sadock, 2008).

Children with ADHD are often concurrently diagnosed as having oppositional defiant disorder or conduct disorder. Presenting symptoms of ADHD include:

- Inattention
  - Has difficulty paying attention during tasks (especially those requiring sustained attention) or play, even if they are enjoyable activities
  - Has difficulty listening, even with prompts and redirection
  - Is easily distracted, loses things, and is forgetful in daily activities
- Hyperactivity
- Fidgets, climbs, unable to sit still or play quietly
- Does not pay attention to social cues
- Acts as if "driven by a motor" and constantly "on the go"
- Talks excessively
- Impulsivity
- Blurts out answers before the question has been completed
- Has difficulty waiting for own turn or being patient
- Interrupts, intrudes in others' conversations and games

Oppositional Defiant Disorder

Oppositional defiant disorder is a recurrent pattern of negativistic, disobedient, hostile, defiant behavior toward authority figures without going so far as to seriously violate the basic rights of others (APA, 2000). Such children exhibit persistent stubbornness and argumentativeness, limit testing, unwillingness to give in or negotiate, touchiness and quick annoyance, and refusal to accept blame for misdeeds. The behaviors lead to significant impairment in home, social relationships, school, or occupational functioning. Children and adolescents with oppositional defiant disorder justify their behavior as a response to unreasonable demands or situations. This disorder is usually evident before 8 years of age and is more common in males until puberty; after that point, the rate is equal between males and females.

Conduct Disorder

Conduct disorder is characterized by a persistent pattern of behavior in which the rights of others are violated and age-appropriate societal norms or rules are disregarded (APA, 2000). It is one of the most frequently diagnosed disorders of childhood and adolescence. Complications associated with conduct disorder are academic failure, school suspensions and dropouts, juvenile delinquency, drug and alcohol abuse and dependency, and juvenile court involvement. Psychiatric disorders that frequently coexist with conduct disorder are anxiety, depression, ADHD, learning disabilities, and substance dependency. There are four types of conduct disorder: (1) aggression toward people and animals, (2) property destruction, (3) theft, and (4) serious violations of rules.

There are two subtypes of conduct disorder—child onset and adolescent onset—both of which can occur in mild, moderate, or severe forms. Predisposing factors are ADHD, oppositional child behaviors, parental rejection, inconsistent parenting with harsh discipline, early institutional living, chaotic home life, large family size, absent or alcoholic father, antisocial and drug-dependent family members, and association with delinquent peers.

Childhood-onset conduct disorder occurs prior to age 10 years and is found mainly in males who are physically aggressive, have poor peer relationships, show little concern for others, and lack feelings of guilt or remorse. These children frequently misperceive others' intentions as hostile and believe their aggressive responses are justified. Violent children also often display antisocial reasoning, such as "he deserved it," when rationalizing aggressive behaviors (Farrell et al., 2008). Children with childhood-onset conduct disorder attempt to project a strong image, but they actually have a low self-esteem. They also display limited frustration tolerance, irritability, and temper outbursts. Individuals with childhood-onset conduct disorder are more likely to have problems that persist through adolescence and without intensive treatment, later develop antisocial personality disorder as adults.

In **adolescent-onset conduct disorder**, youths tend to act out misconduct with their peer group (e.g., early onset of sexual behavior, substance abuse, risk-taking behaviors). Males are apt to fight, steal, vandalize, and have school discipline problems, whereas girls tend to lie, are truant, run away, abuse substances, and engage in prostitution. The male-to-female ratio is not as high as for the childhood-onset type, indicating more girls become aggressive during this period of development.

APPLICATION OF THE NURSING PROCESS

ASSESSMENT

Assessment Guidelines   Attention Deficit Hyperactivity Disorder and Disruptive Behavior Disorders

1. Assess the quality of the relationship between the child or adolescent and parents or caregivers for evidence of bonding, anxiety, tension, and quality of fit between temperaments, which can contribute to the development of disruptive behaviors.
2. Assess parents' or caregivers' understanding of growth and development, effective parenting skills, and handling of problematic behaviors; a lack of knowledge and poor parenting contributes to the development of these problems.
3. Assess cognitive, psychosocial, and moral development for lags or deficits, because immaturity in developmental competencies results in disruptive behaviors. Assess for legal involvement.
4. Assess parenting practices for rules, roles, and responsibilities in the family, relationships with siblings and extended family, history of conflict, and presence of support system (e.g., extended family members, clergy, after school program).
5. Assess the school history for problems and strengths in school, grades, occupational goals, disciplinary problems, and placements.

Attention Deficit Hyperactivity Disorder
1. Observe for level of physical activity, attention span, talkativeness, frustration tolerance, impulse control, and the ability to follow directions.
2. Assess social skills, friendship history, problem solving skills, and school performance. Academic failure and poor peer relationships lead to low self-esteem, depression, and further acting out.
3. Assess for associated comorbidities such as depression.

Oppositional Defiant Disorder

1. Identify issues that result in power struggles and triggers for outbursts—when they begin and how they are handled.
2. Assess the child's or adolescent's view of his/her behavior and its impact on others (e.g., at home, school, and with peers). Explore feelings of empathy and remorse.
3. Explore how the child or adolescent can exercise control and take responsibility, problem solve for situations that occur, and plan to handle things differently in the future. Assess barriers and motivation to change and potential rewards to engage patient.

Conduct Disorder

1. Assess the seriousness, types, and initiation of disruptive behavior and how it has been managed.
2. Assess anxiety, aggression and anger levels, motivation, and the ability to control impulses.
3. Assess moral development, problem solving, belief system, and spirituality for the ability to understand the impact of hurtful behavior on others, to empathize with others, and to feel remorse.
4. Assess the ability to form a therapeutic relationship and engage in honest and committed therapeutic work leading to observable behavioral change (e.g., signing a behavioral contract, drug testing, and living according to "home rules").
5. Assess for substance use (past and present).

DIAGNOSIS

Children and adolescents with ADHD, oppositional defiant disorder, and conduct disorder display disruptive behaviors that are impulsive, angry/aggressive, and often dangerous. They are often in conflict with others, are noncompliant, do not follow age-appropriate social norms, and have inappropriate ways of meeting their needs. Refer to Table 28-2 for potential nursing diagnoses.

OUTCOMES IDENTIFICATION

NOC identifies a number of outcomes appropriate for the child with ADHD, oppositional defiant disorder, or conduct disorder. Table 28-4 lists a sampling of *NOC* outcomes and supporting indicators that target hyperactivity, impulse self-control, the development of self-identity and self-esteem, positive coping skills, and family functioning.

IMPLEMENTATION

The interventions for ADHD include administration of pharmacological agents for the inattention and hyperactive-impulsive behaviors, behavior modification, family counseling, special education programs for the academic difficulties, and cognitive-behavioral therapy and play therapy for the younger child. Children and teens in specialized programs (e.g., day treatment programs) may receive additional services, such as recreational or art therapy.

TABLE 28-4 *NOC* Outcomes for Attention Deficit Hyperactivity Disorder and Disruptive Behavior Disorders

Nursing Outcome and Definition	Intermediate Indicators	Short-Term Indicators
Hyperactivity Level: Severity of patterns of inattention of impulsivity in a child from 1 year through 17 years of age	Inappropriate aggressive behavior decreases	Lack of active listening
Impulse Self-Control: Self-restraint of compulsive or impulsive behaviors	Maintains self-control without supervision	Identifies harmful impulsive behaviors
Self-Esteem: Personal judgment of self-worth	Feelings about self-worth are expressed	Acceptance of self-limitations
Coping: Personal actions to manage stressors that tax an individual's resources	Reports increase in psychological comfort	Identifies effective coping patterns
Family Normalization: Capacity of the family system to maintain routines and develop strategies for optimal functioning when a member has a chronic illness or disability	Maintains usual parenting expectations for affected child, seeks help from a health care professional as appropriate	Acknowledges existence of impairment and its potential to alter family routines

Data from Moorhead, S., Johnson, M., Maas, M., & Swanson, E. (2008). *Nursing outcomes classification (NOC)* (4th ed.). St. Louis: Mosby; and Ackley, B., & Ladwig, G. (2008). *Nursing diagnosis handbook: An evidence-based guide to planning care.* St. Louis: Mosby.

Paradoxically, the mainstay of treatment for ADHD is the use of psychostimulant drugs. Responses to these drugs can be dramatic and can quickly increase attention and task-directed behavior while reducing impulsivity, restlessness, and distractibility (Lehne, 2010). Methylphenidate (Ritalin) is the most widely used psychostimulant because of its safety and simplicity of use. However, there is a risk of abuse and misuse, such as selling the medication on the street or use by people for whom the medication was not intended.

Insomnia is a common side effect while taking the stimulant ADHD medications (Lehne, 2010). Treating with the minimum effective dose is essential, as is administering the medication no later than 4:00 in the afternoon. Other side effects include headache, abdominal pain, and lethargy. Growth retardation secondary to appetite suppression has been associated with the use of stimulants, although studies have provided contradictory findings.

A nonstimulant selective norepinephrine reuptake inhibitor, atomoxetine (Strattera), is approved for childhood and adult ADHD. Although the stimulants result in greater symptom improvement, this drug eliminates the risk of abuse. Therapeutic responses develop slowly, and it may take up to 3 weeks for full improvement (Lehne, 2010). The most common side effects are gastrointestinal disturbances, reduced appetite, weight loss, dizziness, fatigue, and insomnia. It may also cause a small increase in blood pressure and heart rate. Rarely, serious allergic reactions occur.

The dosing schedule of these medications is important. Drug preparations vary in their onset of action and duration of action. This may result in dosing once a day (in the morning) or up to three times a day. Once-a-day dosing is easier and avoids the uncertainty and potential stigma of taking medications at school, so long-acting medications tend to be more attractive. See Table 28-5 for a summary of the FDA-approved medications used to treat ADHD.

TABLE 28-5 Drug Treatment of Patients with ADHD

Classification	Trade Name	Indications	Duration	Schedule
Methylphenidate	Ritalin	Ages 6-12	3-5 hours	2 or 3 times a day
Immediate release	Methylin	Ages 6 and older	3-5 hours	
Extended or sustained release	Ritalin SR	Ages 6-12	6-8 hours	1 or 2 times a day
	Metadate ER	Ages 6-15	6-8 hours	1 or 2 times a day
	Metadate CD	Ages 6-15	6-8 hours	Once a day
	Ritalin LA	Ages 6-12	7-9 hours	Once a day
	Concerta	Ages 6-65	Up to 14 hours	Once a day
Transdermal patch	Daytrana	Ages 6-12	10-12 hours (up to 3 hours after removal)	Once a day
Dexmethylphenidate SR	Focalin	Ages 6 and older	4-5 hours	2 times a day
Extended release	Focalin XR	Ages 6 and older	6-8 hours	Once a day
Dextroamphetamine *Short acting*	Dexedrine	Ages 3-16	4-6 hours	2 or 3 times a day
Intermediate acting	Dexedrine Spansules	Ages 6-16	6-10 hours	1 or 2 times a day
Lisdexamfetamine dimesylate	Vyvanse	Ages 6-12	10-12 hours	Once a day
Amphetamine mixture *Intermediate acting*	Adderall	Ages 6 and older	4-6 hours	2 times a day
Extended release	Adderall–XR	Ages 6 and older	10-12 hours	1 or 2 times a day
Atomoxetine *Extended release*	Strattera	Ages 6-65	24 hours	Once a day

Data from Lehne, R. A. (2010). *Pharmacology for nursing care* (7th ed.). Philadelphia: Saunders; and Huffman, J. C., & Stern, T. A. (2008). Side effects of psychotropic medications. In T. S. Stern, J. F. Rosenbaum, M. Fava, J. Biederman, & S. L. Rauch (Eds.), *Massachusetts General Hospital comprehensive clinical psychiatry* (pp. 705–720). St. Louis: Mosby.

Interventions for severe oppositional defiant and conduct disorders focus on correcting the faulty personality (ego and superego) development, which include firmly entrenched patterns, such as blaming others and denial of responsibility for their actions. Children and adolescents with these disorders also must generate more mature and adaptive coping mechanisms and prosocial goals, a process that is gradual and cannot be accomplished during short-term treatment. With conduct disorder, inpatient hospitalization for crisis intervention, evaluation, and treatment planning, as well as transfer to therapeutic foster care, group homes or long-term residential treatment, is often needed. Oppositional youth are generally treated on an outpatient basis, using individual, group, and family therapy, with much of the focus on parenting issues.

Unfortunately, studies indicate that many children who are simply placed in group homes and in some residential programs do not maintain improvements following discharge. However, intensive programs such as multisystemic therapy, therapeutic foster care, and use of interdisciplinary, community-based treatment teams for children with serious emotional and behavioral disturbances have been found to improve outcome and reduce offenses over the long term (Hoagwood et al., 2001). These types of programs are more promising in improving positive adjustment, decreasing negative behaviors, and improving family stability.

To control the **aggressive behaviors**, a wide variety of pharmacological agents have been tried, including antipsychotics, lithium, anticonvulsants, and antidepressants, with limited effect (USDHHS, 1999). Cognitive-behavioral therapy is used to change the pattern of misconduct by fostering the development of internal controls and working with the family to improve coping and support. Development of problem solving, conflict resolution, empathy, and social skills is an important component of the treatment program.

Families are actively engaged in therapy and given support in using parenting skills to provide nurturance and set consistent limits. They are taught techniques for behavior modification, monitoring medication for effects, collaborating with teachers to foster academic success, and setting up a home environment that is consistent, structured, and nurturing and promotes achievement of normal developmental milestones. If families are abusive, drug dependent, or highly disorganized, the child may require out-of-home placement. The following nursing interventions are helpful when working with parents and caregivers:

- Explore the impact of the child's behaviors on family life, and of the other members' behavior on the child.
- Assist the immediate and extended family to access available and supportive individuals and systems.
- Discuss how to make home a safe environment, especially in regard to weapons and drugs; attempt to talk separately to members whenever possible.
- Discuss realistic behavioral goals and how to set them; problem solve potential problems.
- Teach behavior modification techniques. Practice the techniques through role play with the parents in different problem situations that might arise with their child.
- Give support and encouragement as parents learn to apply new techniques.
- Provide education about medications.
- Refer parents or caregivers to a local self-help group.
- Advocate with the educational system if special-education services are needed.

Techniques for managing disruptive behaviors are listed in Box 28-4.

BOX 28-4 Techniques for Managing Disruptive Behaviors

Behavioral contract: A verbal or written agreement between the patient and nurse or other parties (e.g., family, treatment team, teacher) about behaviors, expectations, and needs. The contract is periodically evaluated and reviewed and typically coupled with rewards and other contingencies, positive and negative.

Counseling: Verbal interactions, role playing, and modeling to teach, coach, or maintain adaptive behavior and provide positive reinforcement. It is most effective for motivated youth and those with well-developed communication and self-reflective skills.

Modeling: A method of learning behaviors or skills by observation and imitation that can be used in a wide variety of situations. It is enhanced when the modeler is perceived to be similar (e.g., age, interests) and attending to the task is required.

Role playing: A counseling technique in which the nurse, the patient, or a group of youngsters act out a specified script or role to enhance their understanding of that role, learn and practice new behaviors or skills, and practice specific situations. It requires well-developed expressive and receptive language skills.

Planned ignoring: When behaviors are determined by staff not to be dangerous and attention seeking, they may be ignored. Additional interventions may be used in conjunction (e.g., positive reinforcement for on-task actions).

Use of signals or gestures: Use a word, a gesture, or eye contact to remind the child to use self-control. To help

Continued

BOX 28-4 Techniques for Managing Disruptive Behaviors—cont'd

promote behavioral change, this may be used in conjunction with a behavioral contract and a reward system. An example is placing your finger to your lips and making eye contact with a child who is talking during a quiet drawing activity.

Physical distance and touch control: Moving closer to the child for a calming effect, perhaps putting an arm around the child (with permission). Evaluate the effect of this, because some children may find this more agitating and may need more space and less physical closeness. It also may involve putting the nurse or a staff member between certain children who have a history of conflict.

Redirection: A technique used following an undesirable or inappropriate behavior to engage or re-engage an individual in an appropriate activity. It may involve the use of verbal directives (e.g., setting firm limits), gestures, or physical prompts.

Additional affection: Involves giving a child planned emotional support for a specific problem or engaging in an enjoyable activity. It can be used to redirect a child away from an undesirable activity as well. This might be involvement in an activity, such as a game of basketball or working on a puzzle. This shows acceptance of the child while ignoring the behavior and can increase rapport in the nurse-patient relationship.

Use of humor: Use well-timed, appropriate kidding about some external, nonpersonal (to the child) event as a diversion to help the child save face and relieve feelings of guilt or fear.

Clarification as intervention: Breaking down a problem situation that a child experiences can help the child understand the situation, other people's roles, and his or her own motivation for the behavior. This can be done verbally and using worksheets, depending on the age and functional level of the child.

Restructuring: Changing an activity in a way that will decrease the stimulation or frustration (e.g., shorten a story or change to a physical activity). This requires flexibility and planning in advance to have an alternative in mind in case the activity is not going well.

Limit setting: Involves giving direction, stating an expectation, or telling a child what to do or where to go. This should be done firmly, calmly, without judgment or anger, preferably in advance of any problem behavior occurring, and consistently when in a treatment setting among multiple staff. An example would be, "I would like for you to stop turning the light on and off."

Simple restitution: Refers to a procedure in which an individual is required or expected to correct the adverse environmental or relational effects of his or her misbehavior by restoring the environment to its prior state, making a plan to correct his or her actions with the nurse, and implementing the plan (e.g., apologizing to the persons harmed, fix the chairs that are upturned). Simple restitution is not punitive in nature, and there are typically additional activities involved (e.g., counseling).

Physical restraint: Use therapeutic holding to control and protect the child from own impulses to act out and hurt self or others.

Anxiety Disorders

The combined prevalence of anxiety disorders is higher than virtually all other mental disorders of childhood and adolescence (NMHA, 2004). The 1-year prevalence in children ages 9 to 17 is 13%. Not all anxiety is abnormal in childhood or adolescence, and a number of fears are a part of normal development. Young people may worry about grades, peer problems, or family issues. Anxiety becomes problematic when the child or adolescent fails to move beyond the fears associated with a particular problem or when the anxiety interferes with functioning over an extended period of time.

There is evidence of genetic contributions to anxiety disorders (Hollander & Simeon, 2008). However, genetic predisposition does not mean a disorder will develop. From a prevention standpoint, early intervention and support can be effective. Cognitive theorists propose that anxiety is the result of dysfunctional efforts to make sense of life events.

The physiological, behavioral, and cognitive characteristics of anxiety in youth are clinically similar to those in adults. Evans and Seligman (2005) noted that SSRIs such as fluvoxamine (Luvox) have been found to be first-line treatment for childhood separation anxiety disorder. They are well tolerated and have a favorable side-effect profile; however, further study is needed in their use in adolescence. Separation anxiety disorder and posttraumatic stress disorder in children and adolescents are discussed in the following sections.

CLINICAL PICTURE
Separation Anxiety Disorder

Children and adolescents with **separation anxiety disorder** become excessively anxious when separated from or anticipating separation from their home or parental figures (APA, 2000). Separation anxiety disorder may develop after a significant stress, such as the death of a relative or pet, an illness, a move or change in schools, or a physical or sexual assault. The prevalence in children is estimated to be 4%, with a higher incidence in females. It is common in first-degree biological relatives of an affected individual, and the incidence may be higher in children whose mothers have a panic disorder. Although remission rates are high, the disorder can persist and lead to panic disorder with agoraphobia. A **depressed mood** often accompanies the anxiety.

DSM-IV-TR characteristics of separation anxiety disorder are:

- Excessive distress when separated or anticipating separation from home or parental figures
- Excessive worries one will be lost or kidnapped, that parents will be harmed, or that the home will be violated or damaged
- Fear of being home alone or in situations without significant adults
- Refusal to sleep unless near a parental figure, refusal to sleep away from home
- Refusal to attend school or other activities without parents
- Physical symptoms of anxiety

Posttraumatic Stress Disorder

Children exposed to traumatic events such as acute injuries from accidents or witnessing significant harm to others may develop an acute stress disorder (Bostic & Prince, 2008). This is manifested in anxiety, dissociative symptoms, emotionally re-experiencing the trauma, and avoidance. Children whose symptoms last longer than one month will be diagnosed with **posttraumatic stress disorder (PTSD)**. This disorder can occur at any age, including childhood. Younger children with PTSD tend to exhibit behaviors indicative of internalized anxiety. In older children and adolescents, the anxiety is more often externalized. There may be comorbid disorders such as depression, and other behaviors such as self-mutilation, depending on the severity and longevity of the trauma that precipitated the PTSD.

APPLICATION OF THE NURSING PROCESS

ASSESSMENT

Assessment Guidelines   Anxiety Disorders

1. Assess the quality of the parent-child relationship for evidence of anxiety, conflicts, or quality of fit between their temperaments.
2. Assess relationships among other family members.
3. Observe parent-child interactions to determine patterns.
4. Assess for recent stressors and their severity, duration, and proximity to the child.
5. Assess parent or caregiver understanding of developmental norms, parenting skills, and handling of problematic behaviors
6. Assess the developmental level, and determine whether regression has occurred.
7. Assess for symptoms of anxiety and coping style.

Separation Anxiety Disorder

Assess the child's previous and current ability to separate from parents or caregivers. (The separation or individuation process may not be completed, or the child may have regressed.)

Posttraumatic Stress Disorder

Assess for personal exposure to an extreme traumatic stressor and evidence of internalized or externalized anxiety symptoms. Explore understanding of the meaning of the event, feelings of safety and security.

DIAGNOSIS

The chief characteristic of the anxiety disorders is disabling anxiety. Refer to Table 28-2 for potential nursing diagnoses.

OUTCOMES IDENTIFICATION

NOC identifies a number of outcomes appropriate for children with an anxiety disorder. The two most relevant outcomes focus on decreasing the anxiety level of the child or adolescent and increasing the ability to control anxiety (Table 28-6).

IMPLEMENTATION

The nursing interventions for an anxious child or adolescent include the following:

- Help prevent the child or adolescent from experiencing panic levels of anxiety by acting as a parental surrogate, providing a safe environment, and providing for biological and psychosocial needs.
- Accept regression, but give emotional support and praise to enable progression, healing, and reintegration into activities of daily living.
- Increase self-esteem and feelings of competence in the ability to perform, achieve, and influence the present and future.
- Help the child or adolescent accept and work through traumatic events without the use of cognitive distortions or unrealistic fears.
- Teach and practice positive self-talk and reframing to reduce cognitive distortions.

TABLE 28-6 *NOC* Outcomes for Anxiety Disorders

Nursing Outcome and Definition	Intermediate Indicator	Short-Term Indicator
Anxiety Level: Severity of manifested apprehension, tension, or uneasiness arising from an unidentifiable source	Decreased school achievement and performance in activities of daily living	Problem behaviors escalate
Anxiety Self-Control: Personal actions to eliminate or reduce feelings of apprehension, tension, or uneasiness from an unidentifiable source	Controls anxiety response and demonstrates return of basic problem-solving skills	Monitors intensity of anxiety

Data from Moorhead, S., Johnson, M., Maas, M., & Swanson, E. (2008). *Nursing outcomes classification (NOC)* (4th ed.). St. Louis: Mosby; and Ackley, B.,& Ladwig, G. (2008). *Nursing diagnosis handbook: An evidence-based guide to planning care.* St. Louis: Mosby.

- Teach coping skills (e.g., deep breathing, counting to 10, exercise, guided imagery, listening to music, distraction) to manage feelings.

Children and adolescents with anxiety disorders are most often treated on an outpatient basis, using cognitive-behavioral techniques in individual, group, or family therapy. Medications such as antidepressants, antianxiety agents, and beta blockers are also used. Cognitive therapy focuses on the underlying fears and concerns, and behavior modification is used to shape behavior and reinforce self-control behaviors. Children who refuse to start school are introduced gradually into the school environment, with a supportive adult present for part of the day. When adolescents develop school phobia, the goal is to return them to the classroom at the earliest possible date and give parents support in setting limits on truancy.

Refer to Table 28-1 for a summary of medications used in the treatment of childhood and adolescent clinical and developmental disorders.

Other Disorders of Children and Adolescents

MOOD DISORDERS

The most frequently diagnosed mood disorders in children and adolescents are **major depressive disorder, dysthymic disorder**, and **bipolar disorder**. Symptoms of mood disorders in young people may be similar to the symptoms in adults (see Chapters 13 and 14), with feelings of sadness, pessimism, hopelessness, and anhedonia (inability to experience happiness); social withdrawal; and suicidal ideation. Children may have somatic complaints, be critical of themselves and others, and feel unloved. Adolescents may have psychomotor retardation and hypersomnia (APA, 2000). Both children and adolescents often manifest irritability leading to aggressiveness. They are less likely than adults to have psychotic symptoms.

Factors associated with child and adolescent depression are physical and sexual abuse or neglect; homelessness; parental problems, including marital discord, death, divorce or separation, or separation from parents; learning disabilities; chronic illness; and conflicts with others such as peers. The complications of depression are school failure and dropout, substance abuse, sexual acting out, pregnancy, running away, illegal behavior, and suicide.

INTEGRATIVE THERAPY

Yoga for Adolescents

Low self-esteem contributes to feelings of depression, suicide, teen pregnancy, and other health-related problems of adolescence. To live a healthy and safe life, teens need to feel good about themselves and be confident. This study demonstrated that a 16-week yoga course, occurring as part of a physical education program for eighth-grade students, enhanced their self-esteem. The psychological benefits of yoga in general include an increase in somatic and kinesthetic awareness, positive mood, well-being, self-acceptance, and decreases in negative feelings. It also has physical benefits in improving strength and flexibility.

Before teaching yoga, the nurse must assess for any physical limitation to yoga, obtain parental consent, and encourage children to progress safely, listening to their bodies and not forcing movements that might be painful.

Bridges, K., & Madlem, M. (2007). Yoga, physical education, and self-esteem: Off the court and onto the mat for mental health. *Californian Journal of Health Promotion. 5*(2), 13-17.

TOURETTE'S DISORDER

Tourette's disorder is characterized by motor and verbal tics that cause marked distress and significant impairment in social and occupational functioning (APA, 2000). Tics typically appear between 2 and 7 years of age. Motor tics usually involve the head but can involve the torso or limbs, and they change in location, frequency, and severity over time. Other motor tics are tongue protrusion, touching, squatting, hopping, skipping, retracing steps, and twirling when walking. Vocal tics include spontaneous production of words and sounds. Coprolalia (uttering of obscenities) occurs in fewer than 10% of cases. The disorder is usually permanent, but periods of remission may occur, and symptoms often diminish during adolescence and sometimes disappear by early adulthood. A familial pattern exists in about 90% of cases. Tourette's disorder often coexists with depression, OCD, and ADHD (Flaherty, 2008).

Symptoms associated with Tourette's disorder are obsessions, compulsions, hyperactivity, distractibility, and impulsivity. In addition, a child or adolescent with tics may have low self-esteem as a result of feeling ashamed, self-conscious, and rejected by peers and may severely limit behavior in public situations for fear of displaying tics. Central nervous system stimulants increase severity of tics, so medications must be carefully monitored in children with coexisting ADHD.

ADJUSTMENT DISORDER

Adjustment disorder is a psychological response to identifiable stressor(s), with symptoms developing within 3 months of the stressor(s) (APA, 2000). Symptoms are typically not severe enough to require hospitalization, but reactions are severe enough to cause impairments in areas such as school and social relationships. The subtypes of adjustment disorder are classified according to the presenting symptoms: adjustment disorder (1) with anxiety, (2) with mixed anxiety and depressed mood, (3) with disturbance of conduct, (4) with mixed disturbance of emotions and conduct, and (5) unspecified.

FEEDING AND EATING DISORDERS

Three feeding and eating disorders are pica, rumination disorder, and feeding and eating disorder of infancy or early childhood (APA, 2000). Anorexia and bulimia nervosa, which also can occur in childhood and adolescence, are described in detail in Chapter 16. **Pica** is the persistent eating of nonnutritive substances without an aversion to eating food. Infants and toddlers may eat paint, plaster, string, or cloth.

This behavior is frequently associated with mental retardation. **Rumination disorder** is the repeated regurgitation and rechewing of food without apparent nausea, retching, or gastrointestinal problems. In a **feeding and eating disorder**, the child fails to eat adequate amounts of food, despite availability, and there is no medical condition or mental retardation. However, because the child fails to gain weight or has a significant weight loss, he or she can then develop nutritional problems that lead to developmental delays.

Interventions for these disorders include working with the family to provide a safe and well-monitored environment that prohibits placing unsafe items in the child's mouth, removal of unsafe items, working with associated care providers (e.g., pediatricians and nutritionists), and provision of praise and support for parents and caregivers to manage the child's behavior.

KEY POINTS TO REMEMBER

- One in five children and adolescents in the United States suffers from a major mental illness that causes significant impairments at home, at school, with peers, and in the community.
- An estimated two thirds of all young people with mental health problems are not receiving proper treatment.
- Factors known to affect the development of mental and emotional problems in children and adolescents include genetic influences, biochemical (prenatal and postnatal) factors, temperament, psychosocial developmental factors, social and environmental factors, and cultural influences.
- The characteristics of a resilient child include an adaptable temperament, the ability to form nurturing relationships with surrogate parental figures, the ability to distance the self from emotional chaos in parents and family, and good social intelligence and problem-solving skills.
- Seclusion and restraint should be used as last resorts after less restrictive interventions have failed and only in the case of dangerous behavior toward self or others. Seclusion and restraint require continuous monitoring by trained staff and must be nonpunitive. Parents should be notified if such measures are used.
- The most commonly diagnosed child psychiatric disorders are anxiety disorders, conduct and oppositional defiant disorder, ADHD, adjustment reactions, and depression. The PDDs are rare.
- Treatment of childhood and adolescent disorders requires a multimodal approach in almost all instances, and family involvement is seen as critical to improvement in outcomes.
- Nurses can be important advocates for children with severe emotional and behavioral disorders.

- Cognitive-behavioral therapies, social skills groups, family therapy, parent training in behavioral techniques, and individual therapy focused on self-esteem issues have been found useful.
- Skills training may focus on a variety of areas, depending on the child's or adolescent's presenting symptoms, and require an individualized assessment to determine each child's need.

CRITICAL THINKING

1. Owen, a 4-year-old boy, has been diagnosed with a PPD—autism.
   A. Describe the specific behavioral data you would find on assessment in terms of (1) communication, (2) social interactions, (3) behaviors and activities.
   B. Name at least three realistic outcomes for a child with PPD.
   C. Which interventions do you think are the most important for a child with PPD? Identify at least six.
   D. What kinds of support should the family receive?

2. Natasha is a 7-year-old girl in the second grade who has been diagnosed with ADHD.
   A. What clinical behaviors might she be exhibiting at home and in the classroom? Give behavioral examples for her (1) inattention, (2) hyperactivity, and (3) impulsivity.
   B. Identify at least six intervention strategies one might use for her, including medication management.
   C. Describe the concept of time-out.

3. Connor is an 8-year-old boy who has been diagnosed with conduct disorder.
   A. Explain to one of your classmates his probable behaviors in terms of (1) aggression toward others, (2) destruction of property, (3) deceitfulness, and (4) violation of rules.
   B. What are three outcomes for this child? What is the overall prognosis for children with this disorder?
   C. What are four ways you could support Connor's parents? Where could you refer this family within your own community?

CHAPTER REVIEW

1. The nurse is assessing a teenage patient for suicidal risk. Which patient statement would require immediate further nursing assessment?
   1. "The idea of death really scares me."
   2. "I only smoked one time in my life."
   3. "My mom keeps a bunch of pills in her nightstand."
   4. "I've never tried to kill myself before."

2. The nurse is preparing to assess a child who primarily speaks Spanish but is fluent in English. Which is the appropriate method for gathering information?
   1. Begin the assessment in English.
   2. Utilize a Spanish dictionary to ask questions of the child.
   3. Ask the child if he understands English.
   4. Obtain an interpreter who is fluent in Spanish.

3. The nurse is caring for a 9-year-old patient who will be entering a freedom room. Which activity should the nurse anticipate the child would engage in?
   1. Listening to a CD
   2. Throwing pillows
   3. Sitting in the periphery of the room
   4. Punching soft objects

4. A 7-year-old male who has met earlier normal expectations in cognitive and language development develops a fascination with the bus schedule in his neighborhood and has difficulty establishing friendships with other school children. Which condition should the nurse anticipate?
   1. Mild autism
   2. Severe autism
   3. Rhett's disorder
   4. Asperger's disorder

5. The nurse is caring for a patient with attention deficit hyperactivity disorder (ADHD). Which medication order should the nurse question?
   1. Strattera (atomoxetine)
   2. Lithobid (lithium)
   3. Wellbutrin (bupropion)
   4. Concerta (methylphenidate)

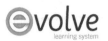 Visit the Evolve website for an **Audio Chapter Summary, Chapter Review Answers & Rationales, Critical Thinking Answer Guidelines,** and additional resources related to the content in this chapter: **http://evolve.elsevier.com/Varcarolis/foundations**

Companion CD Use the Companion CD to prepare for tests and the NCLEX® Examination with **Test-Taking Strategies** for psychiatric mental health nursing and hundreds of **Review Questions**.

References

Abernethy, R. S., & Schlozman, S. C. (2008). An overview of the psychotherapies. In T. S. Stern, J. F. Rosenbaum, M. Fava, J. Biederman, & S. L. Rauch (Eds.), *Massachusetts General Hospital comprehensive clinical psychiatry* (pp. 129–140). St. Louis: Mosby.

Ackley, B. J., & Ladwig, G. B. (2008). *Nursing diagnosis handbook: An evidence-based guide to planning care.* St. Louis: Mosby.

American Nurses Association (ANA), American Psychiatric-Mental Health Nurses Association, & International Society of Psychiatric-Mental Health Nurses. (2007). *Psychiatric mental health nursing: Scope and standards of practice.* Silver Spring, MD: American Nurses Association.

American Psychiatric Association. (2000). *Diagnostic and statistical manual of mental disorders* (4th ed., text rev.) *(DSM-IV-TR).* Washington, DC: Author.

American Psychological Association. (2005). Criteria for evaluating treatment guidelines. *American Psychologist, 57,* 1052–1059.

Axline, V. (1969). *Play therapy.* New York: Ballantine Books.

Bostic, J. Q., & Prince, J. B. (2008). Child and adolescent psychiatric disorders. In T. A. Stern, J. F. Rosenbaum, M. Fava, J. Biederman, & S. L. Rauch (Eds.), *Massachusetts General Hospital comprehensive clinical psychiatry* (pp. 937–959). St. Louis: Mosby.

Bronfenbrenner, U. (2006). *Ecology of human development: Experimentation by nature and design.* Cambridge, MA: Harvard University Press.

Children's Defense, Fund. (2004). *The state of America's children 2004.* Washington, DC: Author.

Evans, D., & Seligman, M. E. P. (2005). Introduction. In D. Evans, E. Foa, R. Gur, H. Hendin, C. O'Brien, M. Seligman, & B. T. Walsh (Eds.), *Treating and preventing adolescent mental health disorders.* New York: Oxford University Press.

Farrell, A., Erwin, E., Allison, K., Meyer, A., Sullivan, T., Camou, S., et al. (2007). Problematic situations in the lives of urban African American middle school students: A qualitative study. *Journal of Research on Adolescence, 17*(2), 413–454.

Farrell, A., Erwin, E., Bettencourt, A., Mays, S., Vulin-Reynolds, M., Sullivan, T., et al. (2008). Individual factors influencing effective nonviolent behavior and fighting in peer situations: A qualitative study with urban African American Adolescents. *Journal of Clinical Child and Adolescent Psychology, 37*(2), 397–411.

Flaherty, A. W. (2008). Movement disorders. In T. A. Stern, J. F. Rosenbaum, M. Fava, J. Biederman, & S. L. Rauch (Eds.), *Comprehensive clinical psychiatry* (pp. 1091–1105). Philadelphia: Elsevier.

Freud, A. (1965). *Normality and pathology in childhood: Assessments of development.* New York: International Universities Press.

Gallagher, R., & Chase, A. (2002). *Building resilience in children in the face of fear and tragedy.* Retrieved September 16, 2004, from http://AboutOurKids.org./aboutour/articles/crisis_resilience.html

Gardner, R. A. (1971). *Therapeutic communication with children: The mutual story-telling technique.* New York: Jason Aronson.

Gardner, R. A. (1979). Helping children cooperate in therapy. In J. D. Noshpitz & S. I. Harrison (Eds.), *Basic handbook of child psychiatry: Therapeutic interventions* (pp. 414–432). New York: Basic Books.

Gardner, R. A. (1986). The talking, feeling and doing game. In C. E. Schaefer & S. E. Reid (Eds.), *Game play: Therapeutic use of childhood games* (pp. 41–72). New York: Wiley.

Gemelli, R. J. (2008). Normal child and adolescent development. In R. E. Hales, S. C. Yudofsky, and G. O. Gabbard (Eds.), *Textbook of psychiatry* (5th ed., pp. 245–300). .Washington, DC: American Psychiatric Publishing.

Hall, D. K., & Pearson, J. (2003). *Resilience—Giving the skills to bounce back.* Retrieved September 16, 2004, from http://www.voicesforchildren.ca/report-Nov2003-1.htm

Hoagwood, K., Burns, B., Kiser, L., Ringeisen, H., & Schoenwald, S. (2001). Evidence-based practice in child and adolescent mental health services. *Psychiatric Services, 52,* 1179–1189.

Hollander, E., & Simeon, D. (2008). Anxiety disorders. In R. E. Hales, S. C. Yudofsky, & G. O. Gabbard (Eds.), *Textbook of psychiatry* (5th ed., pp. 505–607). Arlington, VA: American Psychiatric Publishing.

Inder, T. (2000). *Advances and application of psychopharmacology in pediatrics.* Paper presented at Advancing Children's Health 2000: Pediatric Academic Societies and American Academy of Pediatrics Year 2000 Joint Meeting. Retrieved April 2, 2005, from http://trainland.tripod.com/advancing.pdf

International Society of Psychiatric Nurses. (2007). *Practice parameters: Child and adolescent inpatient psychiatric treatment.* Retrieved January 30, 2009 from http://www.ispn-psych.org/docs/PracticeParameters.pdf

Klein, M. (1955). The psychoanalytic play technique. *American Journal of Orthopsychiatry, 25,* 223–237.

Lehne, R. A. (2010). *Pharmacology for nursing care* (7th ed.). Philadelphia: Saunders.

Luna, B., & Sweeney, J. A. (2004). The emergence of collaborative brain function: FMRI studies of the development of response inhibition. *Annals of the New York Academy of Sciences, Jun,* (1021), 296–309.

Masters, K. (2009). Risk management: Part 1 seclusion and restraint. *Audio Digest Psychiatry, 38*(6), Retrieved May 5, 2009, from http://www.cme-ce-summaries.com/psychiatry/ps3806.html

Masters, K., & Belonci, C. (2002). Practice parameter for the prevention and management of aggressive behavior in child and adolescent psychiatric institutions, with special reference to seclusion and restraint. *Journal of the American Academy of Child and Adolescent Psychiatry, 41,* (2 Suppl.), 4–25.

Moorhead, S., Johnson, M., Maas, M., & Swanson, E. (2008). *Nursing outcomes classification (NOC)* (4th ed.). St. Louis: Mosby.

National Child Abuse and Neglect Data System. (2008). Retrieved August 20, 2008: http://www.childwelfare.gov/pubs/factsheets/fatality.cfm

National Institute on Drug Abuse. (2008). Preventing drug abuse among children and adolescents. Retrieved May 4, 2009 from http://www.nida.nih.gov/Prevention/risk.html

National Mental Health Association. (2004). *Children's mental health statistics.* Retrieved September 15, 2004, from http://www.nmha.org/children/prevent/stats.cfm

Sadock, B. J., & Sadock, A. (2008). *Kaplan & Sadock's concise textbook of clinical psychiatry.* (3rd ed.). Philadelphia: Lippincott Williams & Wilkins.

Smoller, J. W., Sheidley, B. R., & Tsuang, M. T. (2008). *Psychiatric genetics: Applications in clinical practice.* Arlington, VA: American Psychiatric Publishing.

Thomas, A., & Chess, S. (1977). *Temperament and development.* New York: Brunner/Mazel.

U.S. Department of Health & Human Services. (1999). *Mental health: A report of the Surgeon General.* Rockville, MD: U.S.

Department of Health & Human Services, Center for Mental Health Services, National Institutes of Health. Retrieved March 9, 2004, from http://www.surgeongeneral.gov/library/mentalhealth/ toc.html#chapter3

U.S. Public Health Service. (2000). Report of the surgeon general's conference on children's mental health: A national action agenda. Washington, DC: Department of Health and Human Services.

U.S. Department of Justice. (2009). *Highlights of the 2007 national youth gang survey*. Retrieved May 4, 2009 from http://www.ncjrs.gov/pdffiles1/ojjdp/225185.pdf

Ursano, A. M., Kartheiser, P. H., & Barnhill, L. J. (2008). Disorders usually first diagnosed in infancy, child-hood, or adolescence. In R. E. Hales, S. C. Yudofsky, & G. O. Gabbard (Eds.), *Textbook of psychiatry* (5th ed., pp. 861–920). Washington, DC: American Psychiatric Publishing.

Wood, J., Foy, D. W., Goguen, C. A., Pynoos, R., & James, C. B. (2002). Violence exposure and PTSD among delinquent girls. *Journal of Aggression, Maltreatment, & Trauma, 6*(1), 109–126.

Yeh, M., Hough, R. L., McCabe, K., Lau, A., & Garland, A. (2004). Parental beliefs about the causes of child problems: Exploring racial/ethnic patterns. *Journal of the American Academy of Child and Adolescent Psychiatry, 43*(5), 605–612.

CHAPTER **29**

Psychosocial Needs of the Older Adult

Leslie A. Briscoe and Evelyn Yap

Key Terms and Concepts

adult day care, 673
advance directives, 663
ageism, 662

late-life mental illness, 654
Patient Self-Determination Act (PSDA), 663

Objectives

1. Discuss facts and myths about aging.
2. Describe mental health disorders that may occur in older adults.
3. Analyze how ageism may affect attitudes and willingness to care for older adults.
4. Explain the importance of a comprehensive geriatric assessment.
5. Describe the role of the nurse in different settings of care.

6. Identify the requirements for the use of physical and chemical restraints.
7. Discuss the importance of pain assessment, and identify three tools used to assess pain in older adults.
8. Identify legislation and legal documents that protect the rights of older patients, and describe their impact on nursing care.
9. Recognize the significance of health care costs for older adults.

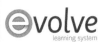 Visit the Evolve website for an **Audio Glossary & Flashcards, Concept Map Creator,** and additional resources related to the content in this chapter: **http://evolve.elsevier.com/Varcarolis/foundations**

The aging of the population is a global phenomenon occurring at a record-breaking rate, especially in developing countries around the world. The U.S. economy, as well as health and social services, are affected by this marked increase in the proportion of the older adults in the population. By the year 2030, 23% of the population in the United States will consist of individuals older than 65 years of age. Among older adults, the fastest-growing subgroups are the minorities, the poor, and those aged 85 years and older. In 2005, the percentage of adults older than 65 was 12%; by 2050 this will rise to 19% (Passel & Cohn, 2008).

As people live longer, they are more likely to deal with chronic illness and disability. At least 80% of individuals older than age 65 have one chronic condition; many older people have more than one. The likelihood of developing one or more chronic illnesses increases notably with age: individuals 75 years of age and older are the most prone to chronic illnesses and functional

disabilities. After age 85, there is a one-in-three chance of developing dementia, immobility, incontinence, or another age-related disability.

Statistics indicate that women generally outlive men. This has significant ramifications for society at large and for the health care system in particular. Not only do women constitute the largest proportion of older adults, they also use health care services more frequently than men and seek services earlier, even for minor conditions. The Institute of Medicine (2008) recognizes an impending crisis as health care costs soar, resources dwindle, and the Baby Boomers age.

Chronological age is considered an arbitrary indicator of function because there are significant variables that contribute to the capabilities of older adults. Surveys focusing on how older adults see themselves reveal that nearly half of people 65 years and older consider themselves to be middle-aged or young.

Only 15% of people aged 75 years and older consider themselves "very old" (Ebersole et al., 2004). A common classification for people 65 and older is:

- **Young old**—65 to 75 years
- **Middle old**—75 to 85 years
- **Old old**—85 to 100 years
- **Elite old (centenarians)**—100+ years of age

Aging is accompanied by increased medical and psychiatric illness. This increase is brought about in part by increasingly stressful life events (e.g., the loss of a spouse, family members, and independence) and co-morbid illness (Cremens, 2008). Polypharmacy also contributes to health problems, especially since there is a gradual reduction in renal, hepatic, and gastric function—all of which are needed to metabolize and degrade medications.

MENTAL HEALTH ISSUES RELATED TO AGING

Late-Life Mental Illness

Older adults who develop late-life mental illness are less likely than young adults to be accurately diagnosed and receive mental health treatment. Psychiatric issues such as depression, memory loss, and prolonged grieving are not a normal part of aging and should be diagnosed and treated. Treating psychiatric disorders prolongs the individual's ability to remain independent and increases the ability to take the lead in personal decision making.

Depression

Depression is not a normal part of aging and is often underidentified because of comorbid medical conditions. Depression is often confused with dementia, and delirium is often misdiagnosed as dementia. A careful, systematic assessment is necessary to properly distinguish among the three. The cardinal differences in depression, dementia, and delirium are:

1. Onset of mental-status change and course of illness
2. Level of consciousness
3. Attention span

All three illnesses are treatable if properly identified.

Depression and Suicide Risk

The demographic group with the highest rate of suicide is white males over the age of 75 years: 37.9 per 100,000 (Centers for Disease Control, 2005). One explanation for the high rate may lie in changes of occupational status and measures of success in men at the time of retirement and thereafter. With retirement, a man may lose status, influence, and contact with fellow workers in the community, which may precede clinical depression.

Depression that is accompanied by psychosis carries a higher risk of suicide (Cremens, 2008). Depression accounts for up to 70% of late-life suicides. Research has shown that older adults who commit suicide suffer from the most treatable kind of depression but do not receive needed mental health services (National Institute of Mental Health [NIMH], 2004). Early identification of and treatment for depression, therefore, are key measures for suicide prevention. Other factors that can lead to suicide are feelings of hopelessness, uselessness, and despair. For older adults, suicide may be seen as a final gesture of control at a stage when independence is at risk or activities are limited. Severe medical illness,

CONSIDERING CULTURE

Older African Americans' View of Depression

Older African Americans are underrepresented in treatment settings. Understanding their beliefs and perceptions would assist mental health care providers to overcome barriers and better identify depression. In a recent qualitative study, 51 older African Americans responded to questions about depression, and four major themes were identified:

- "Keeping the Bully Out"—The belief that depression is something bad and can be kept out or avoided.
- "God Will Provide"—The role of God, faith, and prayer is vital to preventing depression.
- "Losing Control"—The experience of depression is a physical manifestation, which takes control.

- "That's Not Me"—Participants were very clear that being depressed did not pertain to them.

These responses indicate that stigma remains associated with depression in this population. There is a clear belief that people who have depression are weak, choose to be depressed, or perhaps do not have enough faith. In this population, physical manifestations of depression may also be more prominent and a more acceptable way of expressing symptoms. This may lead to misdiagnosis and lack of treatment. Health care providers need to be keenly aware of the mind-body-spirit connection when assessing and treating older African American patients.

Shellman, J., Mokel, M., & Wright, B. (2007). "Keeping the Bully Out": Understanding older African Americans' beliefs and attitudes toward depression. *Journal of the American Psychiatric Nurses Association, 13*(4), 230–236.

functional disability, alcohol abuse, history of suicide attempts, comorbid anxiety, and psychotic depression are added risk factors for suicide (Dharmarajan & Norman, 2003). Unlike younger persons, whose suicidal gestures may be a cry for help, older adults more frequently have a real desire to die.

Even though the suicide rate among older adults is high (Figure 29-1), suicide in this group is probably underreported. Suicide is often not listed on the death certificate, even if it is suspected. The numbers also do not reflect those who passively or indirectly commit suicide by abusing alcohol, starving themselves, overdosing or mixing medications, stopping life-sustaining drugs, or simply losing the will to live. Unfortunately, primary care providers continue to under-recognize and undertreat; many are slow to refer older adults to mental health care providers, despite the evidence that treatment of depression is cost-effective and decreases the amount of health care expenditures utilized (NIMH, 2004). Review Chapter 24 for an in-depth discussion of suicide.

Selective serotonin reuptake inhibitors (SSRIs) are the first-line treatment for depression; this category is often helpful if anxiety, worry, or rumination is problematic. If pain or diabetic neuropathy is a comorbid condition, serotonin norepinephrine reuptake inhibitors (SNRIs) are often prescribed. Tricyclic antidepressants (TCAs) are utilized for those with chronic pain. Treatment-resistant depression can be treated with psychostimulants such as methylphenidate; MAOIs are older treatments but remain effective. A new MAOI patch was recently approved by the U.S. Food and Drug Administration (FDA) for the treatment of depression.

Anxiety Disorders

Cassidy and Rector (2008) identify anxiety disorders in late life as "The Silent Geriatric Giant." Older adults often have multiple physical complaints, medication problems, pain, sleep disturbances, as well as psychiatric illness. Anxiety is twice as prevalent as dementia, and four to eight times as common as major depressive disorders. Again, accurate diagnosis of the anxiety disorder is difficult. The most common sources of anxiety are phobias and generalized anxiety disorder (Cremens, 2008). Comorbid conditions, including depression, bipolar disorder, dementia, and alcoholism may contribute to anxiety.

Anxiety disorders may have been present earlier in life but did not significantly impair functioning. Once the stress of aging, retirement, loss, or physical frailty occurs, the previous coping strategies may no longer be effective. Older adults with anxiety often have physical complaints or describe fears of illness. Treatment for anxiety disorders typically includes an SSRI. Antianxiety agents are also used, but they should be used cautiously, since they may result in confusion, oversedation, and paradoxical agitation. Anxiety disorders are discussed in greater detail in Chapter 12.

Delirium

Delirium occurs secondary to a general medical condition. It causes fluctuations in consciousness and changes in cognition which develop over a short period of time (hours to days). There is usually evidence from history, examination, or diagnostic testing that the disturbance is caused by physiological changes due to underlying pathology (Caplan et al., 2008). Patients may be disoriented and often appear demented; therefore, it is crucial to obtain data from family or caregivers about a baseline level of functioning. A patient who is newly confused, falling, disrobing, and fighting with staff should be assessed for delirium.

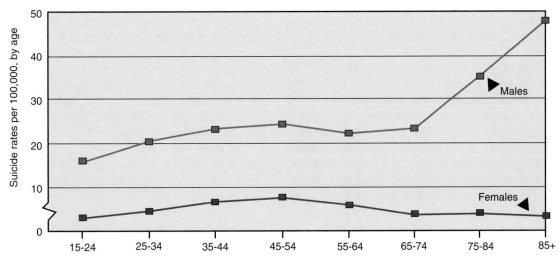

Figure 29-1 Suicide rates in the United States by age and gender. (From National Center for Health Statistics (NCHS), Health, United States, 2005.)

Nursing staff often have more contact with family and the opportunity to collect vital data about the patient's baseline level of functioning. Asking questions such as "Has your mother been shopping and cooking for herself?" or "Does she pay her own bills?" or "Does she ever get lost when driving?" may give subtle clues about whether the changes are acute or have been coming on slowly. Other questions that can be revealing include "Has your father been started on any new medication?" or "Has your father fallen or hit his head recently?"

Treatment of delirium begins with identifying the cause. Adverse drug reactions, infections, electrolyte imbalances, anemia, thyroid dysfunction, vitamin deficiencies, and other problems must be ruled out. A multidisciplinary approach is often helpful to identify causation: doctors of clinical pharmacology are very helpful in identifying possible drug-related effects; geriatricians provide a comprehensive approach to physical assessment; and psychiatry consultation can provide mental status evaluation, medication review, and recommendations for treatment of behaviors. If agitation or combative behaviors are present, it is not uncommon to provide short-term use of antipsychotic medications. Benzodiazepines are often avoided owing to side effects and possible worsening of delirium.

Dementia

Dementia is usually of the Alzheimer's or vascular type. Both are characterized by aphasia (difficulty finding words), apraxia (difficulty carrying out motor functions despite intact functioning), agnosia (failure to recognize objects), and disturbances in executive functioning (organizing, planning, abstracting, insight, judgment) (Wright et al., 2008). Changes in executive functioning may include forgetting how to make old family recipes, inability to manage bill paying, and limited insight and judgment, leading to increased vulnerability to exploitation.

Another symptom that often is not discussed is sexual disinhibition. Older patients may be overly flirtatious, grope caregivers or family during care, make sexually inappropriate comments, expose genitalia, or masturbate openly. These types of behaviors can cause staff and family to be very uncomfortable and confused about how to respond. It is important for the nurse to be open and understanding about such behaviors and to recognize them as symptoms of a brain dysfunction (frontal lobe). Chapter 17 presents a more complete description of delirium and dementia.

Alcohol Abuse

Although heavy drinking tends to decline with age, it continues to be a serious problem that can create particular problems for older adults. The risk factors for heavy drinking in older adults are being male and single, having less than a high-school education, low income, and smoking (Karlamangla et al., 2006). Identifying alcohol and substance abuse is often difficult because personality and behavioral changes frequently go unrecognized in older adults.

The stressful or reactive factors that precipitate late-onset alcohol abuse are often related to environmental conditions and may include retirement, widowhood, and loneliness. These stressors in the older adult, who may have retired, may not drive, and may be isolated from family and friends, are often greater than the problems faced by the middle-aged adult, who has to manage a job or career and care for a family and household. Work and family responsibilities may help keep a potential alcoholic from drinking too much. Once these demands are gone, and the structure of daily life is disrupted, there is little impetus to remain sober.

Caution is required when medicating the older adult who abuses alcohol. Central nervous system toxicity from psychoactive drugs increases with aging. Ingestion of antidepressants or tranquilizers can be particularly harmful because their effect is further potentiated by alcohol. The toxicity of other drugs (e.g., acetaminophen) is enhanced by alcohol and by the age-related decrease in clearance (Luggen, 2004). Whenever there is a suspicion or indication that an older adult is abusing alcohol, the health care provider should conduct a screening test. The CAGE-AID screening tool (Wagenaar et al., 2001) (Box 29-1) and the MAST-G (Box 29-2) are instruments commonly used to assess older adults.

Signs of alcohol abuse in younger individuals (e.g., alcohol-induced pancreatitis or liver disease, blackouts, major trauma) occur infrequently in older adults. Instead, the older alcoholic displays vague geriatric syndromes of contusions, malnutrition, self-neglect, depression, and falls (Wagenaar et al., 2001). Diarrhea, urinary incontinence, decreased functional status, failure to thrive, and apparent dementia may also be present. Although confusion and disorientation in an older patient are often associated with dementia or Alzheimer's disease, they could be caused by other factors, including alcohol abuse. Assessment of these conditions is necessary to differentiate the normal physiological changes of aging from those due to excessive drinking.

Treatment plans should emphasize social therapies. Older adults who abuse alcohol tend to be more passive than younger adults who abuse alcohol and may

EVIDENCE-BASED PRACTICE

Aging, Loss, and Loneliness

Rosedale, M. (2007). Loneliness: An exploration of meaning. *Journal of the American Psychiatric Nurses Association, 13*(4), 201–209.

Problem

Older adults have a unique experience as they age filled with loss: career, productivity, health, spouse, family, friends, independence, and finally loss of life. The hope of aging well does not eliminate the inevitable loss and grieving that comes with old age. It is important as caregivers to appreciate the emotional conflicts and stressors that may go unspoken. For example, how does one recover after the loss of a spouse of 40+ years? Can a widow express the thought, "Who will love me and say I'm beautiful now?" after a lifetime with one man. This is a common experience.

Purpose of Study

Rosedale (2007) has explored and worked to clarify the concept of loneliness. Her research came from investigating loneliness in breast cancer survivors. She identified the importance of psychiatric nurses asking questions to gain understanding about their patients. Words like "Tell me about your experience of loneliness" give permission to share this very intimate part of the human experience.

Methods

A comprehensive search of the literature was conducted. In this overview of loneliness, 190 relevant articles and books were reviewed.

Key Findings

- The concept of loneliness was studied from several views, including philosophical, psychological, integrative, and nursing.
- Most aspects identified a sense of separation, isolation, or lack of support as key. The feeling of loneliness was also associated with invalidation of meaning, dissatisfaction, and transition.
- Also notable was that most views supported a potential for new possibilities.

Implications for Nursing Practice

As caregivers, nurses need to be keenly sensitive and help patients share their experience with loneliness and loss, yet see the potential for new possibilities.

BOX 29-1   CAGE-AID Screening Tool

C—Have you ever felt you ought to **C**ut down on your drinking (drug use)?

A—Have people **A**nnoyed you by criticizing your drinking (drug use)?

G—Have you ever felt bad or **G**uilty about your drinking (drug use)?

E—Have you ever had a drink (used drugs) first thing in the morning (**E**ye-opener) to steady your nerves or get rid of a hangover?

AID—**A**dapt to **I**nclude **D**rugs. One positive answer indicates a possible problem; two positive answers indicate a probable problem.

From Ewing, J. A. (1984). Detecting alcoholism: The CAGE questionnaire. *Journal of the American Medical Association, 252*, 1905–1907.

---

benefit from interpersonal involvement with professional health care personnel. Older people respond easily to emotional and social support, and family therapy should be encouraged. Group therapy with other middle-aged and older adults with alcoholism, as well as self-help groups like Alcoholics Anonymous, can also be effective.

According to the Center for Substance Abuse Treatment (CSAT)–Treatment Improvement Protocol for Older Adults (TIP) Consensus Panel, there are six recommendations:

1. Age-specific group treatment that is supportive and nonconfrontational and aims to build or rebuild the patient's self-esteem
2. A focus on coping with depression, loneliness, and loss (e.g., death of spouse, retirement)
3. A focus on rebuilding the patient's social-support network
4. A pace and content of treatment appropriate for the older person
5. Staff members who are interested and experienced in working with older adults
6. Linkages with medical services, services for the aging, and institutional settings for referral into and out of treatment, as well as case management

Although the older adult with alcohol/substance abuse is difficult to treat, the prognosis for a person

---

BOX 29-2 Michigan Alcoholism Screening Test—Geriatric Version (MAST-G)

Please answer "Yes" or "No" to each question by marking the line next to the question. When you finish answering the questions, please add up how many "Yes" responses you checked, and put that number in the space provided at the end.

1. After drinking, have you ever noticed an increase in your heart rate or beating in your chest?	___ Yes	___ No
2. When talking to others, do you ever underestimate how much you actually drank?	___ Yes	___ No
3. Does alcohol make you sleepy so that you often fall asleep in your chair?	___ Yes	___ No
4. After a few drinks, have you sometimes not eaten or been able to skip a meal because you didn't feel hungry?	___ Yes	___ No
5. Does having a few drinks help you decrease your shakiness or tremors?	___ Yes	___ No
6. Does alcohol sometimes make it hard for you to remember parts of the day or night?	___ Yes	___ No
7. Do you have rules for yourself that you won't drink before a certain time of the day?	___ Yes	___ No
8. Have you lost interest in hobbies or activities you used to enjoy?	___ Yes	___ No
9. When you wake up in the morning, do you ever have trouble remembering part of the night before?	___ Yes	___ No
10. Does having a drink help you sleep?	___ Yes	___ No
11. Do you hide your alcohol bottles from family members?	___ Yes	___ No
12. After a social gathering, have you ever felt embarrassed because you drank too much?	___ Yes	___ No
13. Have you ever been concerned that drinking might be harmful to your health?	___ Yes	___ No
14. Do you like to end an evening with a nightcap?	___ Yes	___ No
15. Did you find your drinking increased after someone close to you died?	___ Yes	___ No
16. In general, would you prefer to have a few drinks at home rather than go out to social events?	___ Yes	___ No
17. Are you drinking more now than in the past?	___ Yes	___ No
18. Do you usually take a drink to relax or calm your nerves?	___ Yes	___ No
19. Do you drink to take your mind off your problems?	___ Yes	___ No
20. Have you ever increased your drinking after experiencing a loss in your life?	___ Yes	___ No
21. Do you sometimes drive when you have had too much to drink?	___ Yes	___ No
22. Has a doctor or nurse ever said they were worried or concerned about your drinking?	___ Yes	___ No
23. Have you ever made rules to manage your drinking?	___ Yes	___ No
24. When you feel lonely, does having a drink help?	___ Yes	___ No
TOTALS:	**___ Yes**	**___ No**

Scoring: A score of 3 points or less is considered to indicate no alcoholism; a score of 4 points is suggestive of alcoholism; a score of 5 points or more indicates alcoholism.

From Menninger, J. (2004). Assessment and treatment of alcoholism and substance-related disorders in the elderly. *Bulletin of the Menninger Clinic, 66*(2), 166–183.

---

who has lived to this point without recourse to substances—and their use is precipitated by losses and stressors—is excellent. This individual often responds very positively to a recovery program, especially if it is accompanied by environmental interventions (Salisbury, 1999). It is important that health care providers recognize this recovery potential. Proper education and awareness of a positive outcome for the geriatric problem drinker can increase the availability of resources; if the prognosis is good, providers and agencies should be more willing to spend resources on

treatment. Nurses can be pioneers in the developing need for substance abuse rehabilitation focused on older adults.

Pain

Pain is common among older adults and affects their sense of well-being and quality of life. Up to 85% of the older population is thought to have conditions that predispose them to pain, such as arthritis, peripheral vascular disease, and diabetic neuropathy

(Luggen, 2000). Pain is often associated with depression. Jann and Slade (2007) describe three categories of depressive symptoms: emotional (mood, motivation, apathy, anxiety), cognitive (concentration, memory), and physical (insomnia, fatigue, headache, and stomach, back, and neck pain).

The older adult's functioning and ability to perform activities of daily living such as walking, toileting, and bathing can be affected by pain, especially pain from musculoskeletal disease. Pain can lead to increased stress, delayed healing, decreased mobility, disturbances in sleep, decreased appetite, and agitation with accompanying aggressive behaviors. Chronic pain can cause depression, low self-esteem, social isolation, and feelings of hopelessness (Wynne et al., 2000).

Barriers to Accurate Pain Assessment

Binaso (2002) identifies beliefs and misconceptions held by older adults about pain that may interfere with appropriate assessment and treatment. Older adults may believe that pain is a punishment for past behaviors, an inevitable part of aging, indicative of pending death, related to serious illness, expensive to test and diagnose, or a sign of weakness. External obstacles include inadequate assessment by health professionals, complicated clinical presentation, assumptions by health care professionals that pain is part of aging, and communication deficits due to cognitive impairment.

Changes in behavior may indicate pain and should be assessed, especially in patients who have difficulty communicating their needs (e.g., those with dementia). Unlike younger adults, older adults may understate their pain using words such as *discomfort*, *hurting*, or *aching*. Multiple painful problems may occur together, making differentiation of new pain from preexisting pain difficult. Sensory impairments, memory loss, dementia, and depression can add to the difficulty of obtaining an accurate pain assessment. An interview with family members, caregivers, or friends is vital.

Assessment Tools

When pain is suspected, the nurse begins with a physical assessment for medical origins of the pain and assesses the pain itself. To aid older adults who may have sensory deficits or cognitive impairments, simply worded questions and simple drawings may be necessary. The **Wong-Baker FACES Pain Rating Scale** (Hockenberry & Wilson, 2008) (Figure 29-2) is an active assessment instrument. The FACES scale shows facial expressions on a scale from 0 (a smile) to 5 (crying grimace). Respondents are asked to choose the face that depicts the pain they feel. Studies have shown that 86% of nursing-home residents can successfully use the FACES scale (Flaherty, 2000).

The present pain intensity (PPI) rating from the **McGill Pain Questionnaire (MPQ)** (Davis & Srivastana, 2003) is another tool accepted for use with older patients. Patients are asked to respond by selecting the description (from "no pain" [0] to "excruciating pain" [5]) that they believe identifies the pain they feel. Wynne (2000) found that the PPI rating of the MPQ was the most useful instrument for pain assessment in nursing-home residents, including both the cognitively intact and the impaired.

The **Pain Assessment in Advanced Dementia (PAINAD) scale** is used to evaluate the presence and severity of pain in patients with advanced dementia who no longer have the ability to communicate verbally (Figure 29-3). The scale evaluates five domains: breathing, negative vocalization, facial expression, body language, and consolability (Box 29-3). The score guides the caregiver in the appropriate pain intervention (Lane et al., 2003; Warden et al., 2003).

Pain Management

Pharmacological Pain Treatments. The cause of the pain should be addressed along with treatment of the pain itself. Pain should be managed with pharmacological and/or alternative measures. Pharmacological pain management relies on the use of prescriptive and non-prescriptive medications, frequently based on the recommendation of the health care provider. These include analgesics, opioid analgesics, and adjuvant medications. Consultation with a pain-management specialist is often helpful with chronic pain syndromes. Some considerations in pharmacological pain management in older adults are listed in Box 29-4.

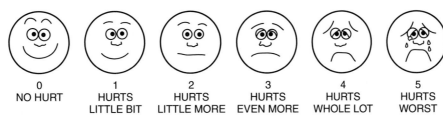

0	1	2	3	4	5
NO HURT	HURTS LITTLE BIT	HURTS LITTLE MORE	HURTS EVEN MORE	HURTS WHOLE LOT	HURTS WORST

Figure 29-2 Wong-Baker FACES Pain Rating Scale. (From Hockenberry, M., & Wilson, D. [2008]. Wong's essentials of pediatric nursing [8th ed., p. 1301]. St. Louis: Mosby.)

	0	1	2	Score
Breathing Independent of vocalization	Normal	Occasional labored breathing; short period of hyperventilation	Noisy, labored breathing; long period of hyperventilation; Cheyne-Stokes respirations	
Negative Vocalization	None	Occasional moan or groan; low-level speech with a negative or disapproving quality	Repeated troubled calling out; loud moaning or groaning; crying	
Facial Expression	Smiling or inexpressive	Sad; frightened; frown	Facial grimacing	
Body Language	Relaxed	Tense; distressed pacing; fidgeting	Rigid; fists clenched; knees pulled up; pulling or pushing away; striking out	
Consolability	No need to console	Distracted or reassured by voice or touch	Unable to console, distract, or reassure	
			TOTAL	

Figure 29-3 Pain Assessment in Advanced Dementia (PAINAD) scale. (From Warden, V., Hurley, A. C., & Volicer, L. [2003]. Development and psychometric evaluation of the Pain Assessment in Advanced Dementia [PAINAD] scale. *Journal of the American Medical Directors Association, 4*(1), 9–15.)

BOX 29-3 The Five Elements of the Pain Assessment in Advanced Dementia (PAINAD) Scale

1. Breathing

Normal breathing is effortless breathing characterized by quiet, rhythmic respirations.

Occasional labored breathing is characterized by episodic bursts of harsh, difficult, or wearing respirations.

Short period of hyperventilation is characterized by intervals of rapid, deep breaths lasting a short period of time.

Long period of hyperventilation is characterized by excessive rate and depth of respirations lasting a considerable time.

Cheyne-Stokes respirations are characterized by rhythmic waxing and waning of breathing from very deep to shallow respirations with periods of apnea.

2. Negative Vocalization

None is characterized by speech or vocalization that has a neutral or pleasant quality.

Occasional moan or groan: Occasional moaning is characterized by mournful or murmuring sounds, wails, or laments. *Occasional groaning* is characterized by louder than usual inarticulate involuntary sounds, often abruptly beginning and ending.

Low-level speech with negative or disapproving quality is characterized by muttering, mumbling, whining, grumbling, or swearing in a low volume with a complaining, sarcastic, or caustic tone.

Repeated, troubled calling out is characterized by phrases or words being used over and over in a tone that suggests anxiety, uneasiness, or distress.

Loud moaning or groaning: Loud moaning is characterized by mournful or murmuring sounds, wails, or laments in a much louder than usual volume. *Loud groaning* is characterized by louder than usual inarticulate involuntary sounds, often abruptly beginning and ending.

Crying is characterized by an utterance of emotion accompanied by tears. There may be sobbing or quiet weeping.

3. Facial Expression

Smiling or inexpressiveness: Smiling is characterized by upturned corners of the mouth, brightening of the eyes, and a look of pleasure or contentment. *Inexpressive* refers to a neutral, at ease, relaxed, or blank look.

Sad is characterized by an unhappy, lonesome, sorrowful, or dejected look. Eyes may be teary.

Frightened is characterized by a look of fear, alarm, or heightened anxiety. Eyes may appear wide open.

Frown is characterized by a downward turn of the corners of the mouth. Increased facial wrinkling in the forehead and around the corners of the mouth may appear.

Facial grimacing is characterized by a distorted, distressed look. The brow is more wrinkled, as is the area around the mouth. Eyes may be squeezed shut.

BOX 29-3 The Five Elements of the Pain Assessment in Advanced Dementia (PAINAD) Scale—Cont'd

4. Body Language

Relaxed is characterized by a calm, restful, mellow appearance. The person seems to be taking it easy.

Tense is characterized by a strained, apprehensive, or worried appearance. The jaw may be clenched.

Distressed pacing is characterized by activity that seems unsettled. There may be a fearful, worried, or disturbed element present. The rate may be faster or slower.

Fidgeting is characterized by restless movement. Squirming about or wiggling in the chair may occur. The person might be hitching a chair across the room. Repetitive touching, tugging, or rubbing body parts can also be observed.

Rigid is characterized by stiffening of the body. The arms and/or legs are tight and inflexible. The trunk may appear straight and unyielding (exclude contractures).

Fists clenched are characterized by tightly closed hands. They may be opened and closed repeatedly or held tightly shut.

Knees pulled up is characterized by flexing the legs and drawing the knees upward toward the chest (exclude contractures).

Pulling or pushing away is characterized by resistiveness upon approach or to care. The person is trying to escape by yanking or wrenching himself or herself free or by shoving you away.

Striking out is characterized by hitting, kicking, grabbing, punching, biting, or other forms of personal assault.

5. Consolability

No need to console is characterized by a sense of well-being. The person appears content.

Distracted or reassured by voice or touch is characterized by a disruption in the behavior when the person is spoken to or touched. The behavior stops during the period of interaction, with no indication that the person is at all distressed.

Unable to console, distract, or reassure is characterized by the inability to soothe the person or stop a behavior with words or actions. No amount of verbal or physical comforting will alleviate the behavior.

Scoring: (See Figure 29-5 for point allocation.)

0-1 = No significant pain

2-3 = Mild to moderate pain

4-6 = Moderate to severe pain

7-10 = Severe to very severe pain

From Lane, P., Kuntupis, M., MacDonald, S., McCarthy, P., Panke, J., Warden, V., & Volicer, L. (2003). A pain assessment tool for people with advanced Alzheimer's and other progressive dementias. *Home Healthcare Nurse, 21*(1), 36.

BOX 29-4 Tips for Pharmacological Pain Management in Older Adults

- Remember that older adults often receive pain medication less often than younger adults, which results in inadequate pain relief. Compensate for this.
- Safe administration of analgesics is complicated because of possible interactions with drugs used to treat multiple chronic disorders, nutritional alterations, and altered pharmacokinetics in older adults.
- Analgesics reach a higher peak and have a longer duration of action in older adults than in younger individuals. Start with one fourth to one half the adult dose, and titrate up carefully.
- Give oral analgesics around the clock at the beginning. Administer on an as-needed basis later on, as indicated by the patient's pain status.
- If acute confusion occurs, assess for other contributing factors before changing the medication or stopping analgesic use. Confusion in postoperative patients has been found to be associated with unrelieved pain rather than with opiate use.

- **Acetaminophen** is an effective analgesic in older adults. Although there is an increased risk of end-stage renal disease with long-term use, it does not produce the gastrointestinal bleeding seen with **nonsteroidal anti-inflammatory drugs (NSAIDs).**
- Analgesics and adjuvants, such as **anticholinergics** and **pentazocine**, may produce increased confusion in older adults. **NSAIDs** can have the same effect during their initial period of administration.
- **Opiates** have a greater analgesic effect and longer duration of action than nonopioid analgesics. Avoid the use of **meperidine**, whose active metabolite may stimulate the central nervous system and lead to confusion, seizures, and mood alterations. If this drug is selected, do not use it for more than 48 hours. Avoid intramuscular administration because of tissue irritation and poor absorption. **Morphine** is a safer choice than meperidine because its duration of action is longer, so a smaller overall dose is required.
- Assess bowel function daily, because constipation can be a frequent side effect of opiates.

Data from Davis, M., & Srivastava, M. (2003). Demographics, assessment and management of pain in the elderly. *Drugs and Aging, 20*(1), 23–35.

As an individual ages, the body's ability to eliminate drugs via the kidney decreases. Nurses must be aware of this change, which can result in overdosing. Fear of narcotic overmedication, which can cause respiratory depression and falls, may lead the nurse to give less pain medication to older adults than is needed for effective treatment (Celia, 2000). It is critical for nurses to evaluate the effectiveness of pain interventions at regular intervals and to be attentive to behavioral changes or verbal responses that indicate that the patient is experiencing pain. It is a common misconception to assume that the ability to perceive pain decreases with aging. No physiological changes in pain perception in older adults have been demonstrated. In fact, older adults may feel pain even more keenly than younger persons do. Careful and continuing assessments and an understanding of pain physiology are necessary for effective pain management of older adults.

Nonpharmacological Pain Treatments. Nonpharmacological treatments for pain include vagal nerve stimulation, exercise, hydrotherapy, heat and cold packs, chiropractics, and transcutaneous electrical nerve stimulation (TENS). Yoga, biofeedback, hypnosis, acupuncture, massage, shiatsu, Reiki, guided imagery, reflexology, and therapeutic touch are integrative therapies for managing pain. Herbal remedies include cayenne, capsaicin, ginger extract, echinacea, kava kava, and willow bark. It is important to ask older adults if they are utilizing any alternative treatments for pain relief. Pain-management education is important for both the patient and caregivers. The key to successful pain management lies in the application of a variety of techniques that the patient must learn and practice. See Chapter 36 for a full discussion of integrative therapies.

HEALTH CARE CONCERNS OF OLDER ADULTS

Financial Burden

Health care expenses for older adults are nearly four times higher than the expenses for the rest of the population, and with the predicted growth in this population, health prevention and maintenance of functional ability must be a priority in nursing care. Patients will be looking to nurses for help navigating the health care system, locating affordable care, and finding the means to follow important medical recommendations.

Caregiver Burden

Another phenomenon with the aging population is the increase in caregiver burden. A common scenario would be the two-income family in the middle of raising children and planning for their future retirement, who are now faced with aging parents in need of help. Dwindling health care benefits, shorter lengths of stay for hospitalization, limited home-care options, and complicated procedures to access care have increased the need for adult children to advocate for and provide care to aging parents. Unfortunately, this scenario is not common for older adults who have lived with a chronic mental illness. Schizophrenia and bipolar disorders take a toll on family members and intimate relationships, and it is not uncommon for those with severe mental illness to have no family available for support as they age. Grown children may be estranged because of a parent's frequent hospitalization, poor parenting ability, or paranoid symptoms. The support system of those aging with chronic mental illness often becomes case managers, community nurses, and mental health providers.

Access to Care

The disparity of mental health coverage in the United States has developed into a fragmented system of care so complicated that some patients become resigned to go without care. Nurses may feel powerless to change shortfalls in the health care system; however, they can take advantage of their numbers and the respect given to the profession to be strong advocates for improving health care.

Ageism

In Western cultures, growing older is not viewed as a privilege, and old age does not tend to confer a revered social status upon those who have attained it. Ageism has been defined as a bias against older people because of their age. It is based on erroneous beliefs that older adults are unattractive, unintelligent, asexual, unemployable, and senile. Ageism is not limited to the way the young may view the old, though; it can also be exhibited by older adults themselves. Indeed, the attitudes of older adults toward their contemporaries, particularly those with mental disabilities, are often negative—perhaps because the threat of contagion by association with the frail and infirm may raise feelings of vulnerability. Ageism differs from other forms of discrimination in that it cuts across gender, race, religion, and socioeconomic status to reach the majority of those over age 65.

Ageism and Public Policy

The results of ageism can be observed in every level of society. Financial and political support for programs for older adults is difficult to obtain. Their needs often are addressed only after those of younger, albeit smaller, population groups. However, the Grey Panthers and the American Association of Retired Persons (AARP) are powerful lobbying groups that are fighting to change this trend.

Ageism and Drug Testing

Only since 1999 has the United States Federal Drug Administration (FDA) required research specific to those over the age of 65. Barriers to inclusion in clinical trials are linked to older adults being on multiple medications or already having an existing chronic illness. Information about medications for the general population has to be generalized for older adults, and appropriate (generally lower) doses may not have been tested or be available (Rochon, 2008).

HEALTH CARE DECISION MAKING

Advance Directives

Since the 1960s, the public's desire to participate in decision making about health care has increased. This interest in patient advocacy was recognized when Congress passed the Patient Self-Determination Act (PSDA) in 1990, requiring that health care facilities provide clear written information for every patient regarding his or her legal rights to make health care decisions, including the right to accept or refuse treatment. It also establishes the right of a person to provide directions (advance directives) for clinicians to follow in the event of a serious illness. Such a directive indicates preferences for the types of medical care or amount of treatment desired. The directive comes into effect should physical or mental incapacitation prevent the patient from making health care decisions. These wishes can be communicated through one or more of the following instruments: (1) a living will, (2) a directive to physician, and (3) a durable power of attorney for health care. These documents must be in writing, and the patient's signature must be witnessed; depending on state and institutional provisions, notarization of the documents may be required.

Health care institutions that receive federal funds are required to (1) provide to each patient at the time of admission written information regarding his or her right to execute advance health care directives and (2) inquire if the patient has made such directives. The patient's admission records should state whether such directives exist. The American Nurses Association (1992) recommends that specific questions about advance directives be part of every nurse's admission assessment. Box 29-5 reproduces these questions and describes the responsibilities of health care workers under the Patient Self-Determination Act.

In 21 states, by signing a **psychiatric advance directive**, those with serious mental illness can designate a health care agent to make treatment decisions during an illness relapse (Elbogen et al., 2006). The National

---

BOX 29-5 Nurses' Responsibilities and the Patient Self-Determination Act of 1990

Part of Nursing Admission Assessment

- Nurses should know the laws of the state in which [they] practice . . . and should be familiar with the strengths and limitations of the various forms of advance directive.
- The ANA recommends that the following questions be part of the nursing admission assessment:
  1. Do you have basic information about advance care directives, including living wills and durable power of attorney?
  2. Do you wish to initiate an advance care directive?
  3. If you have already prepared an advance care directive, can you provide it now?
  4. Have you discussed your end-of-life choices with your family or designated surrogate and health care workers?

Responsibilities of Health Care Workers Under the Patient Self-Determination Act of 1990

- Hospitals, skilled nursing facilities, home health agencies, hospice organizations, and health maintenance

organizations serving Medicare and Medicaid patients must:

1. Maintain written policies and procedures for providing information to their patients for whom they provide care.
2. Give written material to patients concerning their rights under state law to make decisions about medical care, including the right to accept or refuse surgical or medical care and to formulate advance directives and provide written policies and procedures for the realization of these rights.
3. Document in patients' records whether they have advance directives.
4. Not discriminate in care or in other ways against patients who have or have not prepared advance directives.
5. Make sure that policies are in place to ensure compliance with state laws governing advance directives.

Data from Schlossberg, C., & Hart, M. A. (1992). Legal perspectives. In M. Burke & M. Walsh (Eds.), *Gerontologic nursing care of the frail elderly* (p. 469). St. Louis: Mosby; and American Nurses Association. (1992). *Position statement on nursing and the patient self-determination act.* Washington, DC: Author.

Resource Center on Psychiatric Advance Directives provides information about this method of treatment planning for those with serious mental illnesses like schizophrenia and bipolar disorder. Both disorders characteristically have patterns of relapse, often combined with poor insight for needed intervention.

Living Will

A **living will** is a personal statement of how and where one wishes to die (Ebersole et al., 2004). It is activated only when the person is terminally ill and incapacitated, and a competent patient may alter a living will at any time. The question of whether an incompetent person can change a living will is addressed on a state-by-state basis. Executing a living will does not always guarantee its application.

Directive to Physician

In a **directive to physician**, a physician is appointed by the individual to serve as proxy. Many of the features of a directive to physician parallel those of a living will, such as activation only when a terminal illness is present, need for verification of the terminal illness by the physician, and requirement of patient competency at the time of signing. The directive to physician designating the physician as surrogate can be particularly useful in cases of terminal illness when an individual has no family. The physician must agree in writing to be the patient's agent and must also be one of the two physicians who made the original determination that the patient is terminally ill. Unlike the living will, the directive to physician can be revoked orally at any time without regard to patient competency.

Durable Power of Attorney for Health Care

The **durable power of attorney for health care** differs from living wills and directives to physicians in that a person other than a physician is appointed to act as the patient's agent. The patient must be competent and of age when making the appointment and must also be competent in order to revoke the power. Individuals do not have to be terminally ill or incompetent to allow the empowered individual to act on their behalf. No physician's certification is required.

Guardianship

A **guardianship** is an involuntary trust relationship in which one party, the guardian, acts on behalf of an individual, the ward. The law regards the ward as incapable of managing his or her own person and/or affairs. Through investigation and an evaluation process, probate court determines if guardianship is warranted. A physician's expert opinion indicating incompetence is required to initiate the proceeding. Many people with mental illness, mental retardation, traumatic brain injuries, and organic brain disorders such as dementia have guardians. It is important that health care workers identify patients who have guardians and communicate with the guardians when health care decisions are being made.

The Nurse's Role in Decision Making

The nurse is often responsible for explaining the legal policies of the institution to both the patient and family and can help them understand advance directives. There are usually three common approaches to care:

1. Full code: All life saving measures are initiated.
2. Do not resuscitate–comfort care arrest (DNR–CCA): All life saving measures are initiated, except in the case of a full cardiac arrest and intubation.
3. Do not resuscitate–comfort care only (DNR–CCO): Medical care is focused on providing pain-free quality of life and comfort free of invasive procedures and intubation.

Ethical dilemmas can occur when a patient has a feeding tube and a DNR–CCO status is initiated later. The nurse serves as an advocate and knowledgeable resource for the patient and family. The patient is encouraged to verbalize thoughts and feelings during this sensitive time of decision making.

Nurses are responsible for being knowledgeable about both the state regulations on advance directives and the potential obstacles in completing the directives for the state in which they practice. Maintaining an open and continuing dialogue among patient, family, nurse, and physician is of principal importance. The nurse supports any surrogates appointed to act on the patient's behalf and seeks consultation for ethical issues the nurse feels unprepared to handle.

Every health care facility receiving federal funds is required to have written policies, procedures, and protocols in compliance with the Patient Self-Determination Act. Nurses must prepare themselves to deal with the legal, ethical, and moral issues involved when counseling about advance directives. The law does not specify who should talk with patients about treatment decisions, but in many facilities nurses are being asked to discuss this issue with the patient. If the advance directive of a patient is not being followed, the nurse intervenes on the patient's behalf. If the problem cannot be resolved with the physician, the facility's protocol providing for notification of the appropriate supervisor is followed.

Although nurses may discuss options with their patients, they may not assist patients in writing advance directives, because this is considered a conflict of interest. The existence of an advance directive serves as a guide to health care providers in advocating for the older patient's rightful wishes in this process.

NURSING CARE OF OLDER ADULTS

Nurses encounter older adults in a variety of settings, and in each of these settings, the nurse is responsible for application of the nursing process to the individual patient's situation.

Studies suggest that because nursing students are not given enough information about older adults and often are not exposed to older patients, they may hold ageist views when they begin their nursing careers, which has significant implications for practice, education, and research (Lueckenotte, 2000). Morris and Mentes (2006) discuss the challenges of geropsychiatric nursing education, citing the lack of standardized curriculum and credentialing. It is important for all nurses to gain a better understanding of the aging process. Adequate theory and principles of practice are needed to provide safe and excellent care for older adults.

An outline of some major developmental theories of aging is provided in Box 29-6. Although these theories provide the framework for formulating appropriate nursing interventions in caring for older adults, there is no specific theory that encompasses all the developmental stages.

Positive attitudes toward older adults and their care need to be instilled during basic nursing education. Education programs must include:
- Information about the aging process
- Discussion of attitudes relating to the care of older adults
- Sensitization of participants to their patients' needs
- Exploration of the dynamics of nurse-patient and staff-patient interactions
- Providing respect to the older patient and appreciating their wisdom and life experience

Box 29-7 provides some facts and myths about aging that influence how society perceives the older adult.

Assessment Strategies

Nurses who work with older adults benefit from specific knowledge about normal aging, drug interactions, and chronic disease. Those who work with older patients who have mental health problems need to have specific skills in interviewing and assessing and special knowledge of effective treatment modalities. The National Institutes of Health recommend a

---

BOX 29-6   Major Theories of Aging

Biological
Aging is influenced by molecular, cellular, or physiological systems and processes.
- **Gene theory:** Harmful genes become active in later life.
- **Error theory:** Error in protein synthesis results in impaired cellular function.
- **Free radical theory:** Reactive molecules damage DNA.
- **Wear-and-tear theory:** Internal and external stressors harm cells.
- **Programmed aging theory:** Biological or genetic clock plays out on genes.
- **Neuroendocrine theory:** There is neurohormonal regulation of life until death.
- **Immunological theory:** Immune system diversifies with age.

Psychological
- **Kohlberg's theory:** Crises and turning points in adult life are moral dilemmas.
- **Piaget's theory:** Cognitive operations in youth influence aging.
- **Erikson's theory:** Integrity is built on morality and ethics.

- **Bandura's theory:** Self-efficacy is essential for longevity.
- **Sullivan's theory:** Interpersonal responses influence behavior.
- **Freud's theory:** Focuses on control of instinctual responses.
- **Psychobiological theory:** Neurotransmitters modulate behaviors, emotions, and thoughts.
- **Dialectical theory:** Crises and transitions release positive and negative forces that lead to developmental progress.
- **Behavioral theory:** Learning determines the organization of behavior.

Psychosocial
- **Maslow's theory:** Self-actualization and the evolution of developmental needs occur as the individual ages.
- **Disengagement theory:** Mutual withdrawal occurs between the aging person and others.
- **Activity theory:** Actions, roles, and social pursuits are important for satisfactory aging.
- **Continuity theory:** Life satisfaction and activity are expressions of enduring personality traits.

Adapted from Hess, P. (2004). Theories of aging. In Ebersole, P., Hess, P., & Luggen, A. S. (Eds.), *Toward healthy aging: Human needs and nursing response* (6th ed.). St. Louis: Mosby.

BOX 29-7 Facts and Myths About Aging

Facts

- The senses of vision, hearing, touch, taste, and smell decline with age.
- Muscular strength decreases with age. Muscle fibers atrophy and decrease in number.
- Regular sexual expressions are important to maintain sexual capacity and effective sexual performance.
- At least 50% of restorative sleep is lost as a result of the aging process.
- Older adults are major consumers of prescription drugs because of the high incidence of chronic diseases in this population.
- Older adults have a high incidence of depression.
- Many individuals experience difficulty when they retire.

- Older adults are prone to become victims of crime.
- Older widows appear to adjust better than younger ones.

Myths

- Most adults past the age of 65 are demented.
- Sexual interest declines with age.
- Older adults are unable to learn new tasks.
- As individuals age, they become more rigid in their thinking and set in their ways.
- The aged are well off and no longer impoverished.
- Most older adults are infirm and require help with daily activities.
- Most older adults are socially isolated and lonely.

---

comprehensive geriatric assessment, which includes a focus on physical and mental health; functional, economic, and social status; and environmental factors that might impinge on the person's well-being (Dharmarajan & Norman, 2003). Figure 29-4 provides an example of a comprehensive geriatric assessment.

A thorough assessment, including a physical assessment and diagnostic testing, must precede any treatment and/or diagnosis of a mental illness in older adults. Common tests include thyroid, kidney, and liver function; complete blood count; comprehensive metabolic panel; vitamin B_{12}, folic acid, and therapeutic drug levels; urinalysis; serology (RPR); β-type natriuretic peptide (BNP); and computed tomography (CT) of the head. A review of current medications and possible adverse reactions or drug-drug interactions must also occur (Rochon, 2008). Confusion can be caused by anticholinergics, antihistamine, and benzodiazepines. Psychosis has been linked to steroids and even cholesterol-lowering medications, and depression has been linked with beta-blockers, alpha adrenergics, and opiates. Serious medical conditions such as cancer, anemia, diabetes, infections, electrolyte imbalance, malnutrition, dehydration, and cardiac disease can manifest in symptoms such as fatigue or anorexia before more specific physical manifestations occur. Nurses are in a unique position to advocate for and coordinate appropriate medical evaluation for older adults.

An examination and interview of an older adult conducted in unfamiliar surroundings can produce anxiety. Unlike younger patients, who may be comfortable discussing personal issues—family conflicts, feelings of sadness, sexual practices, finances, and bodily functions—older adults may view these topics as private or taboo. As a result, they may be uncomfortable discussing them. It is important to respect these feelings while reviewing essential history by:

- Conducting the interview in a private area
- Introducing oneself and asking the patient what he or she would like to be called (use of the first name is rarely appropriate unless one is invited to do so)
- Establishing rapport and putting the patient at ease by sitting or standing at the same level as the patient
- Ensuring that lighting is adequate and noise level is low in recognition of the fact that hearing and vision may be impaired
- Using touch (with permission) to convey warmth, while at the same time respecting the patient's comfort level with personal touch
- Summarizing the interaction, inviting feedback and questions, and thanking them for giving their time and information

Assessment of the cognitive, behavioral, and emotional status of the older adult is very important in managing the nursing care of the patient. This is particularly vital for detecting dementia, delirium, and depression, because their prevalence increases with age (Dharmarajan & Norman, 2003). The periodic repetition of these assessment tools serves to evaluate the effectiveness of intervention. The Geriatric Depression Scale (Short Form) (Box 29-8) is a subjective questionnaire (Sheikh & Yesavage, 1986), and the Cornell Scale for Depression in Dementia is an objective screening tool for caregivers to help identify the presence of depressive symptoms (Alexopoulos, 1988).

It is also essential to assess for suicidal thoughts and suicidal intent by asking specific questions such as:

- Have you ever thought about killing yourself?
- Have you ever felt that life is not worth living?
- Have you ever tried to hurt yourself in the past?

Thoughts of harming others also must be assessed. Interventions for the prevention of suicide in older adults are discussed in greater depth later in this chapter. Also see Chapter 24 for a more detailed discussion of suicide assessment and intervention.

COMPREHENSIVE GERIATRIC ASSESSMENT						
Name:		Date of birth:			Gender:	

Physical Health

Chronic disorder

Vision	Adequate	Inadequate	Eyeglasses:	Y	N	Needs evaluation

Hearing	Adequate	Inadequate	Hearing aids:	Y	N	

Mobility	Ambulatory:	Y	N	Assistive device:		
	Falls:	Y	N			Needs evaluation

Nutrition	Albumin:		TLC:		HCT:	
	Weight:		Weight loss or gain: Y	N		Needs evaluation

Incontinence	Y	N	Treatment:	Y	N	Needs evaluation

Medications	Total number:	Reviewed & revised:	Y	N	
	Adverse effects/allergy:				

Screening	Cholesterol:	TSH:	B12:	Folate:
	Colonoscopy: Date:		N/A	
	Mammogram: Date:		N/A	
	Osteoporosis: Date:		N/A	
	Pap smear: Date:		N/A	
	PSA: Date:		N/A	

Immunization	Influenza:	Date:	
	Pneumonia:	Date:	
	Tetanus:	Date:	Booster:

Counseling	Diet	Exercise	Calcium	Vitamin D
	Smoking	Alcohol	Driving	Injury prevention

Mental Health

Dementia	Y	N	MMSE score:	Date:	Cause (if known):	
Depression	Y	N	GDS score:	Date:	Treatment:	Y	N

Functional Status

ADL	Bathing:	I	D	Dressing:	I	D	Toileting:	I	D
	Transferring: I	D		Feeding:	I	D	Continence: Y	N	

Figure 29-4 Comprehensive geriatric assessment. *ADL*, Activities of daily living; *B₁₂*, vitamin B12; *D*, dependent; *GDS*, Geriatric Depression Scale; *HCT*, hematocrit; *I*, independent; *MMSE*, Mini-Mental State Examination; *N*, no; *PSA*, prostate-specific antigen; *TLC*, total lymphocyte count; *TSH*, thyroid-stimulating hormone; *Y*, yes.

Older adult abuse is another area to explore during a nursing assessment and is discussed in depth in Chapter 26. Questions about being hit, pushed, kicked, and slapped are important, but it is also imperative to inquire about care being withheld. Not being fed, cleaned,

helped, or cared for are critical issues. Asking initially, "How are you being treated at home?" or "Are you afraid of anyone?" may encourage further exploration. Financial exploitation is another issue that is difficult to uncover. Older adults may feel ashamed or embarrassed to admit

BOX 29-8 Geriatric Depression Scale (Short Form)

1. Are you basically satisfied with your life?   Yes/No

2. Have you dropped many of your activities and interests?   Yes/No

3. Do you feel that your life is empty?   Yes/No

4. Do you often get bored?   Yes/No

5. Are you in good spirits most of the time?   Yes/No

6. Are you afraid that something bad is going to happen to you?   Yes/No

7. Do you feel happy most of the time?   Yes/No

8. Do you often feel helpless?   Yes/No

9. Do you prefer to stay at home rather than going out and doing new things?   Yes/No

10. Do you feel you have more problems with memory than most?   Yes/No

11. Do you think it is wonderful to be alive now?   Yes/No

12. Do you feel pretty worthless the way you are now?   Yes/No

13. Do you feel full of energy?   Yes/No

14. Do you feel that your situation is hopeless?   Yes/No

15. Do you think that most people are better off than you are?   Yes/No

From Sheikh, J. I., & Yesavage, J. A. (1986). Geriatric Depression Scale (GDS): Recent evidence and development of a shorter version. In T. L. Brink (Ed.), *Clinical gerontology: A guide to assessment and intervention* (pp. 165–173). New York: Hawthorn Press.

they have been taken advantage of by family, friends, or strangers (Spangler & Brandl, 2007). Box 29-9 provides helpful interview techniques to use with older adults.

Intervention Strategies

Certain psychotherapeutic methods are especially useful for older adults:

- Applying crisis intervention techniques (see Chapter 23)
- Providing empathetic understanding and active listening
- Encouraging ventilation of feelings and normalizing emotional responses
- Reestablishing emotional equilibrium when anxiety is moderate to severe
- Providing health education and explaining alternative solutions
- Assisting in the use of problem-solving approaches
- Allowing adequate time to process information
- Ensuring hearing aids are working or using an amplifier to facilitate good communication

An older adult may require acute inpatient mental health care for signs and symptoms of severe psychiatric conditions, such as non-dementia psychiatric illnesses, major depression with suicidal thoughts, bipolar disorder, and schizophrenia (Hoover et al., 2008). The number of patients with non-dementia psychiatric illnesses treated on an inpatient basis is declining, owing to Medicare's attempt to contain costs by seeking the least-restrictive setting and improved outpatient care. Inpatient treatment is still recommended when the patient is at high risk of self-harm (whether intentional or unintentional) or poses a risk of harm to other people.

BOX 29-9 Helpful Techniques for Interviewing Older Adults

- Gather preliminary data before the session, and keep questionnaires relatively short.
- Ask about often-overlooked problems, such as difficulty sleeping, incontinence, falling, depression, dizziness, or loss of energy.
- Pace the interview to allow the patient to formulate answers; resist the tendency to interrupt prematurely.
- Use yes-or-no or simple-choice questions if the older patient has trouble coping with open-ended questions.
- Begin with general questions such as "How can I help you most at this visit?" or "What's been happening?"
- Be alert for information on the patient's relationships with others, thoughts about families or co-workers, typical responses to stress, and attitudes toward aging, illness, occupation, and death.
- Assess mental status for deficits in recent or remote memory, and determine if confusion exists.
- Be aware of all medications the patient is taking, and assess for side effects, efficacy, and possible drug interactions.
- Determine how fast the condition of the patient has been changing to assess the extent of the patient's concerns.
- Include the family or significant other in the interview process for added input, clarification, support, and reinforcement.

From National Institute on Aging. (2008, October). *Talking with your older patient: A clinician's handbook.* Retrieved May 5, 2009, from http://www.nia.nih.gov/NR/rdonlyres/99DFC896-8E13-4BC7-9F85-EED95AA6A293/0/clinicianhandbk11708FINALPDF.pdf

Specialized geropsychiatric units provide a comprehensive and specialized approach to care. These units utilize a multidisciplinary approach to assessment, treatment planning, implementation, and evaluation of care. Ideally, the team consists of a geriatric psychiatrist, geriatrician, social worker, nurses, a pharmacist, psychologist, dietician, occupational therapist, physical therapist, and other specialists as indicated. Nurses play the major role in providing continuous care from admission to discharge.

Psychosocial Interventions

The basic-level nurse uses counseling skills to assist the patient in talking about present problems, examining his or her present situation, looking at alternatives, and planning for the future. Sometimes counseling is provided through group therapy, because this helps to decrease the sense of disorientation and isolation. Remotivation therapy (Box 29-10) and reminiscence therapy are also appropriate interventions for the basic-level nurse.

The advanced practice nurse may provide individual and/or group psychotherapy to older adults with depression. Groups are useful because they can diminish social isolation and loneliness and help the members understand that they are not alone in their situation. Group members can learn creative ways to raise their mood and increase quality of life (Yalom, 2005). Table 29-1 outlines the purpose, format, and desired outcomes for each by type of psychotherapeutic group. Individual therapies, specifically cognitive-behavioral, interpersonal, and psychodynamic therapy, are also

---

BOX 29-10   Example of Remotivation Session (Bodies of Water)

Step 1: Climate of Acceptance

The leaders personally welcomed each participant as he or she arrived at the group session. After the leaders introduced themselves, each group member made a self-introduction. The leader used a calendar to orient the members to the date and time of the current remotivation session. The theme for session four was introduced by the leader as "Bodies of Water—Rivers, Lakes, and Oceans." All group members had some familiarity with bodies of water because of their residence in Seattle.

Step 2: Creating a Bridge to Reality

The world globe was used as a visual aid to stimulate discussion on bodies of water. The leader asked questions such as "How are bodies of water formed from glaciers?" Pictures of glaciers, rivers, and lakes were shown.

The leader read poems about tide pools, seashells, and fishing written by anonymous grade-school children. Discussion was stimulated by the leader's asking, "What can we do at the ocean?" Visual aids and props were provided for direct sensory stimulation. Some examples of these aids and props were (1) different types of seashells, (2) fishing tackle and bait, (3) suntan lotion, (4) sun hat, and (5) sunglasses.

An anonymous author's poem about fishing was read to the group. This was followed by recorded music with lyrics about fishing experiences.

Step 3: Sharing the World We Live In

Group discussion focused on jobs related to bodies of water. Topics the participants discussed in regard to self or others included crabbing, clamming, shrimping, and fishing. Visual aids were provided to stimulate further discussions of past related experiences involving bodies of water. Pictures of river rafting, canoeing, scuba diving, and sailing were shared.

Step 4: An Appreciation of the World of Work

This time was used for the members to think about work in relation to others. More experiences in past related work roles, as well as hobbies and pastimes, were discussed. The group then participated in singing a familiar old song, "Love Letters in the Sand," written in 1931 by J. Fred Coots and revived in 1957 when sung by Pat Boone.

Step 5: Climate of Appreciation

The group members were thanked individually by the leaders for coming to the group and sharing their experiences. The next remotivation session theme and meeting date were announced prior to terminating the session.

Group Response to Session Four

Most members of the group appeared to enjoy discussing their experiences in relation to bodies of water. Many members recalled fishing and boating experiences. Other members expressed interest in this topic by their nonverbal participation in touching and smelling some physical props and observation of visual aids. All but two participants touched the seashells and smelled the fish eggs. One lady in the group stood up and modeled the sun hat and glasses, while a man demonstrated how to reel in the line on a fishing pole. Several participants remarked on how beautiful the pictures of the glaciers were. All but a couple of group members sang to the recorded lyrics on fishing. One member stood up and danced to the music while many others clapped to her movements.

From Janssen, J. A., & Giberson, D. L. (1988). Remotivation therapy. *Journal of Gerontological Nursing, 14*(6), 31–34.

TABLE 29-1 Useful Group Therapy Modalities for Older Adults

Remotivation Therapy	Reminiscence Therapy (Life Review)	Psychotherapy
PURPOSE OF GROUP		
Resocialize regressed and apathetic patients Reawaken interest in the environment	Share memories of the past Increase self-esteem Increase socialization Increase awareness of the uniqueness of each participant	Alleviate psychiatric symptoms Increase ability to interact with others in a group Increase self-esteem Increase ability to make decisions and function more independently
FORMAT		
Groups are made up of 10 to 15 people. Meetings are held once or twice a week. Meetings are highly structured in a classroom-like setting. Group uses props. Each session discusses a particular topic. See Box 29-10 for the five basic steps used in each session.	Groups are made up of 6 to 8 people. Meetings are held once or twice weekly for 1 hour. Topics include holidays, major life events, birthdays, travel, and food.	Group size is 6 to 12 members. Group members should share similar: • problems • mental status • needs • sexual integration Group meets at regularly scheduled times (certain number of times a week, specific duration of session) and place.
DESIRED OUTCOMES		
Increases participants' sense of reality Offers practice of health roles Realizes more objective self-image	Alleviates depression in institutionalized older adults Through the process of reorganization and reintegration, provides avenue by which members: • achieve a new sense of identity • achieve a positive self-concept	Decreases sense of isolation Facilitates development of new roles and reestablishes former roles Provides information for other group Provides group support for effecting changes and increasing self-esteem

From Matteson, M. A., & McConnell, E. S. (Eds.). (1988). *Gerontological nursing: Concepts and practice* (p. 80). Philadelphia: Saunders.

useful. The best outcomes result from combining some kind of therapy with medication. Primary care providers therefore must acquire the skills to enable sensitive assessment for depression and suicide risk and must be knowledgeable about methods of intervention. Collaboration with mental health providers is best practice.

Pharmacological Interventions

Evidence about the biology of mental illness and the discovery of new psychotropic medications has expanded the role of the geropsychiatric nurse. Nurses play a vital role in monitoring, reporting, and managing medication side effects such as acute dystonia, akathisia, pseudo-parkinsonism, neuroleptic malignant syndrome (NMS), serotonin syndrome, and anticholinergic effects. Physical assessment of response to medication is also important; this includes monitoring vital signs, pain, lab work, elimination (bowel and bladder), changes in gait,

prevention of falls, and neurological checks when appropriate. The nurse assesses for underlying medical problems. Often patients with chronic persistent mental illnesses, such as schizophrenia, do not report or misinterpret visceral cues, pain, and vital symptoms of illness (Reeves & Torres, 2003).

Health Teaching and Health Promotion

The nurse provides health teaching to both patient and caregiver on a variety of issues, including the nature of the patient's illness, symptom management, maintenance of safety, self-care strategies, management of medications (Box 29-11), coping skills, steps necessary for recovery, and resources that will support recovery. When providing written information, large print is often helpful.

Promotion of Self-Care Activities

Hospitalization may result in regression that ranges from needing assistance to requiring total care in

---

BOX 29-11 Patient and Family Teaching: Drug Safety

- Learn about your medicines:
  - Read medicine labels and package inserts, and follow the directions.
  - If you have questions, ask your doctor or other health care professionals.
- Talk to your team of health care professionals about your medical conditions, health concerns, and all the medicines you take (prescription and over-the-counter medicines), as well as dietary supplements, vitamins, and herbal supplements.
  - The more they know, the more they can help.
  - Do not be afraid to ask questions.
- Keep track of side effects or possible drug interactions, and let your doctor know right away about any unexpected symptoms or changes in the way you feel.
- Make sure to go to all doctor appointments and to any appointments for monitoring tests done by your doctor or at a laboratory.

- Use a calendar, pill box, or something to help you remember what medications you need to take and when.
- Write down information your doctor gives you about your medicines or your health condition.
- Take a friend or relative to your doctor's appointments if you think you need help to understand or remember what the doctor tells you.
- Have a "medicine check-up" at least once a year.
  - Go through your medicine cabinet to get rid of old or expired medicines.
  - Ask your doctor or pharmacist to go over all the medicines you now take. Remember to tell them about all the over-the-counter medicines, vitamins, dietary supplements, and herbal supplements you take.
- Keep all medicines out of the sight and reach of children.

---

accomplishing the activities of daily living. A goal for nurses is to encourage the patient to regain independence in the realm of personal care. Hospitalization may be an opportunity for the patient to receive much-needed assessment of the skin, feet, hair, mouth, and perineal areas. These assessments can often uncover hidden infections, unhealed wounds, and growths that may otherwise have been missed and lead to needed medical attention.

Milieu Management

The major roles of the nurse in terms of milieu management are to assist the patient in adjusting to the environment, keep the patient safe at all times (e.g., make sure roommates are compatible, call lights are within reach, patients at risk for falling are placed close to the nurses' station), minimize the adverse effects of hospitalization on functional capacity (e.g., encourage patients to walk and to do so as

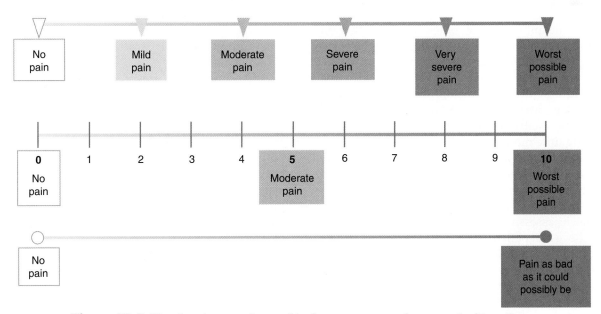

Figure 29-5 Visual analogue scales used in the management of cancer pain. (From Jacox A., et al. [1994, March]. *Management of cancer pain* [Clinical Practice Guideline No. 9, AHCPR Publication No. 94-0952]. Rockville, MD: U.S. Department of Health needs Human Services, Public Health Service, Agency for Health Care Policy and Research.)

independently as possible), provide reality orientation, and engage in therapeutic communication with the patient. It helps to know that reorienting a patient is not always therapeutic, especially if the patient has dementia and reorientation causes agitation. Using distraction techniques is often the intervention of choice.

Another vital aspect of milieu management is the prevention and reduction of agitation by maintaining a visible presence on the unit and anticipating the patient's needs (Johnson & Delaney, 2007). Crisis intervention techniques may be utilized if an agitated patient does not respond to redirection or verbal attempts to deescalate agitation. As a crisis situation unfolds, staff response will largely determine the outcome, and a well-trained crisis team improves these outcomes. The crisis team leader is usually a nurse for several reasons:

1. Nurses provide professional care 24 hours a day, 7 days a week and have detailed knowledge of patients.
2. The nurse is aware of the patient's medical condition.
3. The nurse is able to guide the team and help prevent injury of a patient who needs physical restraint but has osteoporosis.

After the crisis has been deescalated, the team leader, the team, and other patients (as indicated) help restore a sense of safety and calm. As the agitated patient gains control, it is important to help the individual ease back into the milieu with dignity.

Care Settings

Skilled Nursing Facilities

As acute hospital care of older adults with non-dementia psychiatric illnesses is decreasing, the use of long-term skilled nursing facilities is increasing (Hoover et al., 2008). The use of these facilities to treat older adults with severe mental illness is controversial, and opponents fear that "nursing homes" will become the mental institutions of the 21st century, providing little more than custodial care.

Whereas some long-term care settings provide specialized psychiatric mental health care, most do not. There may be little consistency in the education of nurses and nursing assistants in appropriate psychiatric assessment and intervention. Clinicians may believe that patients who refuse personal hygiene, medication, or wound care are exercising their rights to refuse care, rather than recognizing the negative symptoms of schizophrenia. Nurses who accept these refusals may inadvertently contribute to a patient's deterioration.

The skilled nursing facility setting can be a stabilizing environment for a person with severe mental illness who thrives within the structure of a therapeutic environment. Providing a documented plan of care and intervening when behavioral symptoms increase is as important as monitoring and intervening when a resident has signs of infection.

Legislation has had a significant impact on the treatment of older adults in extended-care facilities. The **Patient Self-Determination Act** of 1990 declared that nursing-home residents have the right to be free from unnecessary drugs and physical restraints. There now is much greater awareness and focus on the use of nonpharmacological interventions for the treatment of agitation, wandering, confusion, yelling, and aggression. Drugs deemed "unnecessary" are generally antipsychotics, antianxiety agents, and sedatives. Federal regulations also mandate gradual dosage reduction of these medications for patients who are taking them unnecessarily. Patients with a history of depression, schizophrenia, obsessive-compulsive disorder, generalized anxiety disorder, or bipolar disorder need ongoing treatment to prevent relapse and re-emergence of symptoms. Nurses can play an important role in advocating for psychiatric evaluation and intervention to assist with (1) medication management, (2) monitoring and documenting behavioral changes, (3) notifying the physician of behavioral changes, and (4) planning care for the needs of those residents with mental illness.

Because of inappropriate use of restraints, which resulted in many injuries and deaths, legislation regarding their safe use was put into place. The requirements governing the use of restraints include:

1. Consultation with a physical and/or occupational therapist must be carried out.
2. The least restrictive measures must be considered, and this must be documented.
3. A physician's order is required.
4. Consent of the resident or family must be obtained.
5. Documentation must be provided that the restraint enables the resident to maintain maximum functional and psychological well-being.

Residential Care Settings

Nurses who work with older adults should be knowledgeable about residential care settings. This is especially important for older adults with chronic and persistent mental illness (e.g., schizophrenia), since placement becomes increasingly difficult. As discussed in Chapters 4 and 5, the mental health system has increasingly become focused on the goal of community living rather than institutional living, but resources necessary to meet this goal have been chronically underfunded. Patients who would benefit from residential care are often moved from the most structured environment (inpatient care) to unstructured and unsupervised living situations in the community.

Partial Hospitalization

Partial hospitalization, or acute psychiatric day hospital programs, are sometimes recommended for ambulatory patients who do not need 24-hour nursing care but require and would benefit from intensive, structured psychiatric treatment. A review of acute psychiatric day hospitals in the United Kingdom found that patients who received care in partial hospitalization programs showed a more rapid improvement in mental status than patients randomly assigned to inpatient care; this type of care also led to cost reductions ranging from 20.9% to 36.9%, compared with inpatient care (Marshall, 2003). Health education includes symptom monitoring and management, medication education and management, relapse and stress prevention, and problem solving of health maintenance issues to enable the patient to adapt to active functioning in the community. The nurse also reviews with the team, in collaboration with the patient and family or caregiver, additional referrals for needed services (e.g., Meals on Wheels, transportation services, church activities, and home-care services).

Day Treatment Programs

Multipurpose senior centers provide a broad range of services, including: (1) health promotion and wellness programs; (2) health screening; (3) social, educational, and recreational activities; (4) meals; and (5) information and referral services. For those in need of nursing care and custodial care services, adult day care is an appropriate choice. There are three types of day care programs: (1) social day care, (2) adult day health or medical treatment programs, and (3) maintenance day care. In each type, older adults are cared for during the day and stay in a home environment at night. The boundaries of these programs blend and overlap. All three models are meant to provide a safe, supportive, and nonthreatening environment and fulfill a vital function for older adults and their families. The programs allow older adults to continue their present living arrangements and maintain their social ties to the community; they also relieve families of the burden of 24-hour-a-day care for older adult dependents. If institutionalization becomes necessary, adult day care staff can work with patients and their families to assess the situation and make recommendations for placement.

Behavioral Health Home Care

Older adults typically prefer the continuum of services to be delivered in the least-restrictive setting, and that is usually in their homes. Home-based behavioral health care is particularly recommended to assist the homebound older adult adjust to and manage illness and disability either before or after hospitalization. It is often the role of the behavioral health home-care nurse to help a person affected by a cognitive brain disorder or a severe and persistent mental illness remain in the home or to facilitate a transfer to a temporary or permanent facility, if necessary. The National Association of Area Agencies on Aging assist with providing local home care services, such as housekeeping, meal preparation, and assistance with activities of daily living, to increase the older adult's ability to live independently.

The target population for behavioral health home care includes older adults who need help with activities of daily living, have behavioral issues related to their physical illness, or have an enduring mental illness. Nursing services are usually provided by a basic-level practitioner or a certified generalist nurse in community health or home health care, or by an advanced practice registered nurse certified in adult psychiatric mental health nursing. Chapter 5 discusses home psychiatric mental health care in greater detail.

Community-Based Programs

The hazards of institutionalization are numerous: increased mortality may be caused by the increased risk for nosocomial infections; injuries may occur due to initial disorientation to a new setting; and patients may develop learned helplessness, losing interest in self-care activities. There also may be a decrease in opportunities for socialization. In contrast, community-based programs are an alternative, the purpose of which is to promote the older adult's independent functioning and reduce the stress on the family system.

Community-based programs that provide specialized case management services assist older adults with coordination of care and assistance with entitlements (such as Meals on Wheels and transportation). Federal funding has increased the accessibility to home-care options with the creation of the Administration on Aging, a part of the U.S. Department of Health and Human Services. Constant assessment of the changing needs of older adults requires frequent contact and rapid intervention when they become sick or need additional services. Hospitalization can be averted if aggressive and skilled case management is in place, and nurses are uniquely qualified to fulfill the role of case manager.

Older adults living in the community may still be driving, which can become a safety concern for caregivers, family, and the public. If there is evidence that the older adult can no longer safely drive a vehicle (e.g., failing visual acuity, hearing loss, memory deficits, impaired mobility, movement disorders such as Parkinson's disease), or there have been occurrences of frequent small collisions, it is appropriate to notify the state bureau or department of motor vehicles for a driving evaluation to determine the capacity for safe operation of a vehicle.

KEY POINTS TO REMEMBER

- The older adult population continues to increase exponentially.
- The increase in the number of older adults poses a challenge not only to nurses but to the entire health care system to be prepared to respond to the special needs of this population.
- Attitudes toward older adults are often negative, reflecting ageism—a bias against older adults based solely on age.
- Ageism is found at all levels of society and even among health care providers, which affects the way we render care to our older patients.
- Nurses who care for older adults in various settings may function at different levels. All should be knowledgeable about the process of aging and be cognizant of the differences between normal and abnormal aging changes.
- Older adults face increasing problems of substance abuse and suicide.
- OBRA established guidelines and a philosophy of care that call for patients to be free from unnecessary use of drugs and physical restraints.
- Adequate pain assessment is important, and the nurse must bear in mind that older adults tend to understate their pain. Sufficient pain medication should be administered and the drugs carefully titrated.
- Nurses working with the mentally ill patient must know psychotherapeutic approaches relevant for the older adult. Advanced practice nurses may offer psychotherapy groups geared toward the special needs of this population.
- When it comes to dying and death, older adults' wishes and those of their families are frequently ignored. The implementation of the Patient Self-Determination Act, passed in 1990, can afford some patients autonomy and dignity in death.

CRITICAL THINKING

1. Mr. Jackson is a 70-year-old African American who has been admitted to the intensive care unit with a diagnosis of alcohol withdrawal delirium. He is confused and combative and threatens to strike the nurse unless he is allowed to leave. After getting an order from the primary care provider, the nurse applies wrist restraints to keep Mr. Lopez from striking her and leaving the room.
   A. What are the mandates of OBRA (1990) regarding the use of restraints?
   B. Is the nurse working in accordance with the mandates of OBRA (1990) regarding the use of restraints? Explain your rationale.

2. Mr. Lopez has received treatment for alcohol withdrawal. He is very quiet, refuses to eat, does not sleep at night, admits to thoughts of desperation, and wishes he could die. He also confides that he attempted suicide when his wife died five years earlier and that is when he started drinking heavily.

A. Culturally, what may be helpful to know about older African Americans' response to depression:
B. Which depression assessment tool is appropriate to use in assessing the severity of Mr. Lopez's condition? Explain your answer.

3. Mrs. Duff is 75 years old and lives with her daughter's family. She has moderate-advanced Alzheimer's disease. Although Mrs. Duff's family wants to keep her at home for as long as possible, they are overwhelmed by her needs and being unable to leave her alone. What community placements might be best for Mrs. Duff? Explain your answer.

CHAPTER REVIEW

1. The nurse is caring for an older adult patient. Which symptom should the nurse recognize as a normal part of aging?
   1. Depression
   2. Memory loss
   3. Situational grieving
   4. Delirium

2. The nurse is caring for a patient experiencing delirium. Which nursing response is appropriate when the patient's daughter asks, "Will he ever stop acting like this?"
   1. "I'm sorry, your father will likely be in this state from now on."
   2. "Once we know the cause of the delirium, we can begin treatment to attempt to reverse the process."
   3. "Delirium is caused by infections and electrolyte imbalances, and the damage is permanent."
   4. "A benzodiazepine will help alleviate the delirium."

3. A patient with dementia exhibits difficulty feeding himself despite the fact that there is nothing wrong with his motor functions. Which term should the nurse use to document this finding?
   1. Aphasia
   2. Apraxia
   3. Agnosia
   4. Disinhibition

4. An older adult patient experiencing pain states that she is going to use kava kava, which she has heard provides pain relief. Which nursing response is appropriate?
   1. "Kava kava is an appropriate herb to use for pain relief."
   2. "Older adults should not use herbal preparations."
   3. "Willow bark would be a better herbal supplement to use."
   4. "Are you using any other treatments for pain relief?"

5. The nurse is caring for a patient who is a "DNR-CCO." Which nursing action would be appropriate if the patient were to go into cardiac arrest?
   1. Immediately call for the code team
   2. Prepare for intubation by physician
   3. Administer morphine for pain control
   4. Initiate cardiopulmonary resuscitation

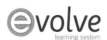

Visit the Evolve website for an **Audio Chapter Summary, Chapter Review Answers & Rationales, Critical Thinking Answer Guidelines**, and additional resources related to the content in this chapter: **http://evolve.elsevier.com/Varcarolis/foundations**

Companion CD Use the Companion CD to prepare for tests and the NCLEX® Examination with **Test-Taking Strategies** for psychiatric mental health nursing and hundreds of **Review Questions**.

References

Alexopoulos, G. S. (1988). Cornell scale for depression in dementia. *Biological Psychiatry, 23*(3), 271–284.

American Nurses Association. (1992). *Position statement on nursing and the patient self-determination act.* Washington, DC: Author.

Binaso, K. (2002). *Pain management for the geriatric patient.* Presented at the 37th Annual American Society of Health System Pharmacists Midyear Clinical Meeting, December 11, 2002, Atlanta, GA.

Caplan, J. P., Cassem, N. H., George, B. M., Park, J. M., & Stern, T. A. (2008). Delirium. In T. A. Stern, J. F. Rosenbaum, M. Fava, J. Biederman, & S. L. Rauch (Eds.), *Massachusetts General Hospital comprehensive clinical psychiatry* (pp. 217–229). St. Louis: Mosby.

Cassidy, K., & Rector, N. (2008). The silent geriatric giant: Anxiety disorders in late life. *Geriatrics and Aging, 11*(3), 150–156.

Celia, B. (2000). Age and gender differences in pain management following coronary artery bypass surgery. *Journal of Gerontological Nursing, 26*(5), 7–13.

Centers for Disease Control. (2005). *Suicide: Facts at a glance.* Retrieved May 5, 2009, from http://www.cdc.gov/ViolencePrevention/pdf/Suicide-DataSheet-a.pdf

Cremens, M. C. (2008). Geriatric psychiatry. In T. A. Stern, J. F. Rosenbaum, M. Fava, J. Biederman, & S. L. Rauch (Eds.), *Massachusetts General Hospital comprehensive clinical psychiatry* (pp. 963–971). St. Louis: Mosby.

Davis, M., & Srivastana, M. (2003). Demographics, assessment and management of pain in the elderly. *Drugs and Aging, 20*(1), 23–35.

Dharmarajan, T., & Norman, R. (Eds.). (2003). *Clinical geriatrics.* New York: Parthenon.

Ebersole, P., Hess, P., & Luggen, A. (2004). *Toward healthy aging: Human needs and nursing response* (6th ed.). St. Louis: Mosby.

Elbogen, E. B., Swartz, M. S., VanDorn, R., Swanson, M. K., & Scheyett, A. (2006). Clinical decision making and views about psychiatric advance directives. *Psychiatric Services, 57,* 350–355.

Flaherty, E. (2000). Assessing pain in older adults. *Journal of Gerontological Nursing, 26*(3), 5–6.

Hess, P. (2004). Intimacy, sexuality, and aging. In P. Ebersole, P. Hess, & A. S. Luggen (Eds.), *Toward healthy aging: Human needs and nursing response.* St. Louis: Mosby.

Hockenberry, M., & Wilson, D. (2008). *Wong's essentials of pediatric nursing* (8th ed). St. Louis: Mosby.

Hoover, D. R., Akincigil, A., Prince, J. D., Kalay, E., Lucas, J. A., Walkup, J. T., et al. (2008). Medicare inpatient treatment of elderly non-dementia psychiatric illnesses 1992–2002: Length of stay and expenditures by facility type. *Administration and Policy in Mental Health, 35,* 231–240.

Institute of Medicine. (2008). Retooling for an aging America: Building the healthcare workforce. Retrieved June 30, 2009, from http://books.nap.edu/catalog.ph?record id=12089

Jacox, A., Carr, D., Payne, R., Berde, C., & colleagues. (1994, March). *Management of cancer pain (Clinical Practice Guideline No. 9, AHCPR Publication No. 94–0952).* Rockville, MD: U.S. Department of Health and Human Services, Public Health Service, Agency for Health Care Policy and Research.

Jann, M. W., & Slade, J. H. (2007). Antidepressant agents for the treatment of chronic pain and depression. *Pharmacotherapy, 27,* 1571–1587.

Johnson, M. E., & Delaney, K. R. (2007). Keeping the unit safe: The anatomy of escalation. *Journal of the American Psychiatric Nurses Association, 13*(1), 42–52.

Karlamangla, A., Zhou, K., Reuben, D., Greendale, G., & Moore, A. (2006). Longitudinal trajectories of heavy drinking in adults in the United States of America. *Addiction (Abingdon, England), 101*(1), 91–99.

Kolanowski, A., & Piven, M. (2006). Geropsychiatric nursing: The state of the science. *Journal of the American Psychiatric Nurses Association, 12*(2), 75–99.

Lane, P., Kuntupis, M., MacDonald, S., McCarthy, P., Panke, J., Warden, V., et al. (2003). Assessment tool for patients with advanced Alzheimer's and other progressive dementias. *Home Healthcare Nurse, 21*(1), 30–37.

Lueckenotte, A. (2000). Gerontologic assessment. In A. Lueckenotte (Ed.), *Gerontologic nursing* St. Louis: Mosby.

Luggen, A. (2000). Pain. In A. Lueckenotte (Ed.), *Gerontologic nursing.* St. Louis: Mosby.

Luggen, A. (2004). Mental wellness and disturbances. In P. Ebersole, P. Hess, & A. S. Luggen (Eds.), *Toward healthy aging: Human needs and nursing response.* St. Louis: Mosby.

Marshall, M. (2003). Adult psychiatric day hospital. *British Medical Journal, 327*(7407), 116–117.

Menninger, J. (2004). Assessment and treatment of alcoholism and substance-related disorders in the elderly. *Bulletin of the Menninger Clinic, 66*(2), 166–183.

Morris, D., & Mentes, J. (2006). Geropsychiatric nursing education: Challenge and opportunity. *Journal of the American Psychiatric Nurses Association, 12*(2), 105–115.

Nadler-Moodie, M., & Gold, J. (2005). A geropsychiatric unit without walls. *Issues in Mental Health Nursing, 26,* 101–114.

National Institute of Mental Health. (2004). *Older adults: Depression and suicide facts.* Washington, DC: Author: Retrieved March 21, 2005, from http://www.nimh.nih.gov/publicat/elderlydepsuicide.cfm

Passel, J. S., & Cohn, D. (2008). U.S. population projections: 2005–2050. Pew Research Center. Retrieved January 21, 2009, from http://pewresearch.org/pubs/729/united-states-population-projections

Patient Self-Determination Act of 1990, 42 U.S.C. 1395.

Reeves, R. R., & Torres, R. A. (2003). Exacerbation of psychosis by misinterpretation of physical symptoms. *Southern Medical Journal, 96*(7), Retrieved May 5, 2009, from http://www.medscape.com/viewarticle/459197_print

Rochon, P. A. (2008). *Drug prescribing for older adults.* Retrieved May5,2009,fromhttp://www.uptodate.com/patients/content/topic.do;jsessionid = 54BA18D5CBC3B6473E881E83C1 ABE22B.0504?topicKey = ~hFWFDt6C2406eq&selectedTitle = 46~86&source = search_result

Salisbury, S. (1999). Alcoholism. In J. Stone (Ed.), *Clinical gerontological nursing* (p. 537). Philadelphia: Saunders.

Sheikh, J. I., & Yesavage, J. A. (1986). Geriatric Depression Scale (GDS): Recent evidence and development of a shorter version. In T. L. Brink (Ed.), *Clinical gerontology: A guide to assessment and intervention* (pp. 165–173). New York: Haworth Press.

Spangler, D., & Brandl, B. (2007). Abuse in later life: Power and control dynamics and a victim-centered response. *Journal of the American Psychiatric Nurses Association, 12,* 322–331.

Wagenaar, D., Mickus, M., & Wilson, J. (2001). Alcoholism in late life: Challenges and complexities. *Psychiatric Annals, 31*(11), 665–672.

Warden, V., Hurley, A. C., & Volicer, L. (2003). Development and psychometric evaluation of the Pain Assessment in Advanced Dementia (PAINAD) scale. *Journal of the American Medical Directors Association, 4*(1), 9–15.

Wright, C. I., Trinh, N., Blacker, D., & Falk, W. E. (2008). Dementia. In T. A. Stern, J. F. Rosenbaum, M. Fava, J. Biederman, & S. L. Rauch (Eds.), *Massachusetts General Hospital comprehensive clinical psychiatry* (pp. 231–246). St. Louis: Mosby.

Wynne, C., Ling, S. M., & Remsburg, R. (2000). Comparison of pain assessment instruments. *Geriatric Nursing, 21*(1), 20–23.

Yalom, I. D. (2005). *The theory and practice of group psychotherapy* (5th ed.). Cambridge, MA: Basic Books.

CHAPTER **30**

Serious Mental Illness

Edward A. Herzog and Nancy Christine Shoemaker

Key Terms and Concepts

anosognosia, 678
assertive community treatment (ACT), 684
deinstitutionalization, 678
institutionalized, 678
National Alliance on Mental Illness (NAMI), 679
outpatient commitment, 689
parity, 681
psychoeducation, 683
recovery model, 679

rehabilitation, 679
serious mental illness (SMI), 678
social skills training, 685
stigma, 680
supported employment, 686
supportive psychotherapy, 685
transinstitutionalization, 690
vocational rehabilitation, 686

Objectives

1. Discuss the effects of serious mental illness on daily functioning, interpersonal relationships, and quality of life.
2. Describe three common problems associated with serious mental illness.
3. Discuss five evidence-based practices for the care of the person with serious mental illness.
4. Explain the role of the nurse in the care of the person with serious mental illness.
5. Develop a nursing care plan for a person with serious mental illness.
6. Discuss the causes of treatment nonadherence, and plan interventions to promote treatment adherence.

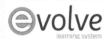 Visit the Evolve website for an **Audio Glossary & Flashcards, Concept Map Creator** and additional resources related to the content in this chapter: **http://evolve.elsevier.com/Varcarolis/foundations**

Categorizing mental illness according to levels of severity has tremendous implications for setting mental health policy, establishing insurance reimbursement standards, and facilitating access to appropriate care. In the United States, each state determines how to classify mental illness for the purpose of insurance coverage. The definitions used by the states generally fall into one of three categories. "Broad-based mental illness" refers to any diagnosis found within the *Diagnostic and Statistical Manual of Mental Disorders*, 4th edition, text revision *(DSM-IV-TR)*, whereas "serious mental illness" and "biologically-based mental illness" refer only to a limited number of *DSM-IV-TR* diagnoses.

The federal government's classifications of "severe and persistent mental illness (SPMI)" and "serious mental illness (SMI)" apply to those who are most deeply affected by psychiatric disorders. Disorders that fall into this category include severe forms of depression, panic disorder, and obsessive compulsive disorder, as well as schizophrenia and bipolar disorder. SPMI affects about 2.6% of all adults and results in significant impairment of global functioning, which may be continuous or episodic, and results in disability in 30% to 50% of cases (Substance Abuse and Mental Health Services Administration [SAMHSA], 2002).

In this chapter, we will focus on the broader classification of serious mental illness (SMI), which includes disorders in the SPMI group and affects about 5.4% of the U.S. population (SAMHSA, 2002). Individuals with SMI usually have difficulties in multiple areas, including activities of daily living (cooking, hygiene), relationships, social interaction, task completion, communication, leisure activities, safe movement about the community, finances and budgeting, health maintenance, vocational and academic activities, and coping with stressors. Associated issues for those with SPMI include poverty, stigma, unemployment, and inadequate housing.

SMIs are chronic or recurrent. Some patients experience remissions interrupted by exacerbations of varying lengths; the remissions may be essentially symptom-free but in most cases involve some degree of residual symptoms. For other patients, the illness follows a chronic and sometimes deteriorating course during which symptoms wax and wane but never remit.

People with serious mental illness are at risk for multiple physical, emotional, and social problems: they are more likely to be victims of crime, be medically ill, have undertreated or untreated physical illnesses, die prematurely, be homeless, be incarcerated, be unemployed or underemployed, engage in binge substance abuse, live in poverty, and report lower quality of life than persons without such illnesses (Glied, 2007; Aquila & Emanuel, 2003).

SMI carries with it varying degrees of disability, with skill deficits ranging from an inability to prepare meals to an inability to cope with everyday stressors. The impairments associated with SMI, along with related factors such as poverty, stigma, unemployment, and inadequate housing, can significantly impact the quality of life and can cause persons with SMI to live in a "parallel universe" separate from "normals" (the name some use to describe people who do not have mental illnesses) (Fitch, 2007). Symptoms or socially inappropriate behavior caused by SMIs can cause others to reject the patient and refuse friendship, housing, or employment.

SERIOUS MENTAL ILLNESS ACROSS THE LIFESPAN

SMI occurs in persons of any gender, age, culture, or geographical location. However, the population of people currently living with SMIs can be separated into two groups who have had different experiences with the mental health system: (1) those old enough to have experienced long-term institutionalization (common before approximately 1975), and (2) those young enough to have been hospitalized only for acute care during exacerbations of their disorders.

Older Adults

Before deinstitutionalization, the mass shift of patients with SMIs out of state hospitals and into the community that began in the 1960s and continued through the 1970s, psychiatric hospitals were the long-term residences for many people (see Chapter 4). Medical paternalism, in which the health care provider made all decisions for patients with SMIs, was a pervasive philosophical stance at that time. Thus, patients became institutionalized, (i.e., they became dependent on the services and structure of institutions and unable to function independently outside such institutions). It was difficult to distinguish whether behaviors were the result of the disease process or the altered responses that resulted from institutionalization.

VIGNETTE

During her adolescence and young adulthood, Marian was a resident at a facility that cared for people with SMI. On discharge, she moves to a community home, where she spends long periods sitting in front of the living room window. Marian does not ask to go out into the garden she watches for so many hours. Indeed, she rarely asks for anything, including snacks or recreational activities. The caregivers work with Marian for several months to help her to recognize her needs of the moment and then to articulate or act on them. There is a major celebration the day she walks into the kitchen and makes a peanut butter sandwich of her own volition. Some of the dependency caused by the institutionalization is being positively altered. ■

Younger Adults

People young enough never to have been institutionalized usually do not have problems of passivity and dependency. However, treatment via a series of short-term hospitalizations has given them limited experience with formal treatment and has contributed to some patients not truly believing a problem exists. This increases denial, which when coupled with anosognosia—inability to realize that one has an illness, owing to impairments caused by the illness itself—puts young adults with SMI at particular risk for additional problems, including legal difficulties, substance abuse, and unemployment.

VIGNETTE

After graduating from high school, Christopher enlists in the army and serves for 5 years. He settles on the West Coast and takes a job in the post office. In his first psychotic break, Christopher becomes paranoid and threatening at work and is hospitalized briefly. Upon discharge, Christopher refuses aftercare and will not take medication. He quits his job and moves to another city. For the next 15 years, Christopher works intermittently, is homeless off and on, and drinks heavily whenever he has money. He is only hospitalized when his behavior is threatening to others. He consistently resists aftercare recommendations, showing no insight into his illness. One day Christopher simply disappears. ■

DEVELOPMENT OF SERIOUS MENTAL ILLNESS

SMI has much in common with chronic physical illness: the original problem increasingly overwhelms and erodes basic coping mechanisms and increases the use of compensatory processes. As the disorder extends beyond the acute stage, more and more of the neighboring systems are involved. For example, in chronic congestive heart failure, the lungs and kidneys begin to deteriorate due to cardiac insufficiency. A person with schizophrenia may experience disturbed thought processes and social skills, which cause interactions with others to become increasingly awkward and anxiety provoking for both the patient and others. This in turn results in people becoming increasingly hesitant to interact with the affected person and the person's self-esteem weakens.

REHABILITATION VERSUS RECOVERY: TWO MODELS OF CARE

For many years, the concept of **rehabilitation**, which focused on managing patients' deficits and helping them learn to live with their illnesses, dominated psychiatric care. Staff directed the treatment and focused on helping patients function in their daily roles. Advocates and patients with SMI (many of whom prefer to call themselves "consumers" to emphasize the choices they have, or seek to have, over their treatment) have increasingly sought a different treatment approach. This **consumer movement** has criticized the rehabilitation model as being paternalistic and focused on living with disability rather than on quality of life and eventual cure.

The **recovery model** developed out of the consumer movement. It is supported by the **National Alliance on Mental Illness (NAMI)**, perhaps the leading mental health consumer-advocacy organization; the President's New Freedom Commission on Mental Health (2003) has based its recommendations for the future of mental health care on it (Mulligan, 2005). The recovery model is patient/consumer-centered and involves active partnership with care providers (Fisher & Ahern, 2002). It is a hopeful, empowering, strengths-focused model wherein staff assist the consumer in using strengths to achieve the highest quality of life possible (Mulligan, 2005). It encourages a high degree of patient independence and self-determination and focuses on achieving goals of the patient's choosing and leading increasingly productive and meaningful lives (Resnick & Rosenheck, 2006). The emphasis is on the person and the future rather than on the illness and the present. A patient in recovery stated, "Slowly I accepted my illness but wanted to live a full life in spite of it. I was desperate to succeed in the real world, and I entered college. There I expanded my social ties so I wouldn't have to be forced into the identity of schizophrenia. My teachers gave me courage and respect" (Group for the Advancement of Psychiatry [GAP], 2000, p. 22).

ISSUES CONFRONTING THOSE WITH SERIOUS MENTAL ILLNESS

Establishing a Meaningful Life

Finding meaning in life and establishing goals can be difficult for persons living with SMI, particularly if they also experience poor self-esteem or apathy. Patients may struggle with the possibility that they may never be the person they once expected to be. Finding a way to "reset" one's goals so that meaning can be found in new ways (e.g., helping others, volunteering, or simply surmounting a significant illness) is important to achieving a satisfactory quality of life and avoiding despair.

If a person cannot work or attend school, there is a significant amount of free time to be filled. If this same person does not own a car or live on a bus line, have money for movies or other pastimes, have access to parks or libraries, is afraid to go outside, or does not have enough confidence to join peers, options can be very limited. Unstructured free time and resulting boredom can be a significant problem, reducing access to potential support resources and sometimes leading to maladaptive coping via substance abuse or petty theft.

Comorbid Conditions

Physical Disorders

As noted in Chapter 15, persons with SMI are at greater risk from co-occurring physical illnesses, particularly hypertension, obesity, cardiovascular disease, and diabetes. The risk of premature death is 1.6 to 2.8 times greater than the general population, and on average, patients with SMI die 28 years prematurely (Miller et al., 2007). Contributing factors include failing to provide for their own health needs, inability to access or pay for care, and other obstacles, such as stigma or stereotyping. For example, expressing health care needs in an eccentric or unclear manner can influence the quality of care received. One patient with schizophrenia experienced a priapism—a medically dangerous extended period of penile erection—as a side effect of his medications. Due to his psychosis, he described the resulting paresthesias to emergency department staff as "demons sticking needles in my [penis]." Despite the obviousness of his erection, the priapism was not detected during a physical exam by the ED resident, suggesting that the patient's presentation, perhaps along with staff bias or inadequate understanding of mental illness, had resulted in a less thorough evaluation.

Depression and Suicide

Persons with SMIs may experience a profound sense of loss of their pre-illness life and potential. Consider a successful premed student who develops SMI, then 3 years later finds herself unemployed and living in a group home. There is a significant disconnect between her former life trajectory and her current living situation. This loss can lead to acute or chronic grief which, along with the chronicity of the illness and its demands and impact on daily life, can contribute to despair, depression, and risk of suicide, which occurs in 5% to 10% of persons with SMI (Pompili et al., 2007).

Substance Abuse

Comorbid substance abuse occurs in 50% of those with SMI (NAMI, 2007a). It may be a form of self-medication, countering the dysphoria or other symptoms caused by illness or its treatment (e.g., the sedation caused by one's medications). Nicotine use has always been higher in the population of those with SMI and is not declining as it has been in the general population. Substance abuse contributes to comorbid physical health problems, reduced quality of life, incarceration, relapse, and reduced effectiveness of medications (McCloughen, 2003).

Social Problems

Stigma

Stigma has been described as negative attitudes or behaviors toward a person or group based on a belief that they possess negative traits (Gonzalez et al., 2007). It is one of three primary obstacles identified as preventing access to quality health care and related services (President's New Freedom Commission on Mental Health, 2003). Stigma stems from a lack of understanding of mental illness and causes others to make assumptions about persons with SMI. It can result in discrimination and cause shame, anger, and further isolation (Stuart, 2006).

According to the Substance Abuse and Mental Health Services Administration (SAMHSA) (2008), only 25% of young adults believe that one can recover from mental illness. This stigma is perpetuated by stereotypical images in U.S. culture and limited corrective contact with persons with SMIs. Initiatives such as SAMHSA's "What a Difference a Friend Makes" program (2008) and NAMI's "Stigmabusters" campaign (2008) seek to improve understanding and acceptance through education and reduction of stigma. As one

patient explained, "We need to grieve the loss of normal lives, normal families, and normal places in society. For me this is a continuous process that never ends. We are placed at the very lowest rung on the ladder of society. We are believed by many to be ax-murdering fiends—all of us, even though statistics do not bear this notion out" (GAP, 2000, p. 9).

Isolation and Loneliness

Social isolation and loneliness are concerns of many people with chronic illnesses, not just those with SMIs. Stigma reduces social contact with "out" groups, such as persons with SMI, and individual factors such as poor self-image, poverty (which interferes with social/ recreational social activities), passivity, impaired hygiene, and similar factors also reduce interaction and interfere with relationships. Romantic relationships and opportunities for sexual expression, usually desired among persons with SMI illness just as in any population, are also affected by isolation (and by sexual dysfunction from medications). One response has been the creation of dating services specifically for persons with disabilities or mental illness.

Victimization

Stereotypes would have us believe that people with SMI are more likely to be violent than people who do not have mental illness. But the reverse is actually true: mentally ill people are more likely to be *victims* of violence than *perpetrators* (White et al., 2006; Schanda, 2005). Sexual assault or coerced sexual activity also occur in this vulnerable population. Impaired judgment, impaired interpersonal skills (e.g., unknowingly acting in ways that might provoke others, such as standing too close or not leaving when told to), passivity, poor self-esteem, dependency, living in high-crime neighborhoods, and seeming more vulnerable to criminals may contribute to this significant problem. Drug abuse and transient living conditions have been shown to be strong predictors of victimization among the population (White et al., 2006).

Economic Challenges

Unemployment and Poverty

Most persons derive at least part of their identity and sense of value from the work they do. Many persons with SMI would like to work, but symptoms such as cognitive slowing or disorganization interfere with obtaining or succeeding at work. Eighty-five percent of persons with SMI are unemployed, and disability entitlements received by 50% of those with SMIs do not provide much income. It can be difficult to find an employer open to hiring a person with SMI, and laws to prevent discrimination do not guarantee a job. Also, becoming employed and having an income may cause the person with SMI to become ineligible for public health care coverage. In the absence of employer-based coverage, he or she may be forced to pay for treatment out-of-pocket, creating an obstacle to treatment adherence and to health care in general (Rosenheck et al., 2006).

Atypical antipsychotic medications can be extremely expensive. Co-pays or Medicaid "spend-downs" (the monthly need to exhaust one's funds to re-establish Medicaid eligibility) are obstacles to treatment. Persons with insurance may find that their share of costs is prohibitively high, or their insurance provider limits the amount of care that will be covered or does not cover it at all. Providing mental health care coverage that is equal to that for physical health care, or parity, has been legislated in many states (and somewhat at the national level) but remains affected by "loopholes" that reduce mental health care coverage for many.

Housing Instability

Many persons with SMIs have limited funds, which equates to limited options for housing. Obtaining an affordable apartment may require one to live far from needed resources (e.g., stores, health care centers, support persons) or in unsafe neighborhoods. Living with family can produce interpersonal strains and conflict about patient behavior (e.g., nonadherence, impaired self-care) that often lead to estrangement and loss of housing with family.

An episode of inappropriate behavior could lead to eviction and a negative reputation among landlords, closing doors to future housing. Symptoms can cause behavior that leads to police arrest. One person asked a store clerk if he could pay him later for soda and, thinking concretely, mistook the clerk's sarcastic "Oh, sure" as genuine approval, only to leave with the soda and find himself charged with theft an hour later. A single bad decision caused an arrest that could leave him ineligible for housing subsidies or public housing. Even with a subsidy, waiting lists might be 2 years long. Finding and keeping good housing can be very challenging.

Caregiver Burden

Caregivers, particularly family members, have limits in terms of coping with the persistent and challenging needs of persons with SMI and may find themselves unable to shoulder the burden. They also age, become ill, and may require care themselves. For both the parent and child, living apart after 30 or 40 years can be a very difficult adjustment and lead to crises such as homelessness, conflict between caregiver and patient, and even relapse (e.g., when a caregiver is hospitalized, leaving the patient alone for the first time in his life). Making the transition from home to alternate living arrangements before a crisis occurs and making arrangements for financial support (such as living trusts) when finances allow can preserve stability and avert relapse.

Treatment Issues

Nonadherence

At any point in time, nearly half of all persons with mental illness are not receiving treatment or are nonadherent to treatment; this can double the likelihood of relapse (Amador, 2007). Most health care providers address this problem with medication education, but patients faced with repetitive medication groups and exhortations to take medications often become more resistant rather than insightful. Other obstacles, such as side effects, drug costs, interruptions in treatment, and rotating treatment providers increase the risk of nonadherence and threaten stability and prognosis. Box 30-1 describes nursing interventions that promote adherence.

BOX 30-1 Interventions to Improve Adherence to Treatment

- Select treatments and dosages that are most likely to be effective and well tolerated by each patient.
- Actively manage side effects to avert/minimize patient distress, which could result in nonadherence.
- Simplify treatment regimens to make them more acceptable and understandable to the patient (e.g., once-a-day dosing instead of twice daily).
- Tie treatment adherence to achieving the *patient's* goals (not staff's or society's) to increase motivation. Point out and reinforce improvements, connecting them to treatment adherence.
- Avert potential reasons for reducing or opting out of treatment by providing assistance with treatment costs and access.

- To improve patient insight and motivation, provide psychoeducation about SMI and the role of treatment in recovery. Take care not to assume that nonadherence means the patient does not understand. There are many reasons for nonadherence; applying psychoeducation when the problem is something *other* than a lack of knowledge is unlikely to succeed.
- Assign consistent, committed caregivers who have (or are skilled at building) positive therapeutic bonds with the patient and who will be able to work with the patient for extended periods of time.
- Involve the patient in support groups with members who have greater insight and first-hand experience with

Continued

BOX 30-1 Interventions to Improve Adherence to Treatment—cont'd

illness and treatment—people whose viewpoints the patient may be more likely to accept.

- Provide culturally-sensitive care. Cultural beliefs and practices (e.g., suspicious attitudes towards health care and authority figures or valuing self-sufficiency or privacy above health care) can undermine therapeutic relationships and result in rejection of treatment (Lutz & Warren, 2001).
- Carefully monitor medication decreases or changes to control side effects and/or improve the therapeutic effect (Wieden, 2007).
- When other interventions have not been successful, use medication monitoring, long-acting forms of medication

(depot injections or sustained release formats), and other techniques as indicated to increase the likelihood that needed medication will be in the patient's system.

- Never reject, blame, or shame the patient when nonadherence occurs. Instead, label it as simply an issue for continuing focus, often requiring numerous tries. **Never give up on a patient.** Instead, remind yourself that nonadherence is common, due to the brain disease (and not a reflection of inadequate nursing skill or apathy or denial on the patient's part), and almost always takes significant amounts of time (and tries) to establish and maintain.

Anosognosia

Many people assume that persons with mental illness who do not understand that they are mentally ill must be in denial (i.e., they know they are ill but cannot accept it). Although denial is a possibility, another is *anosognosia* (ă-nō'sog-nō'sē-ă), the inability to recognize one's deficits due to one's illness. In SMI, the brain—the organ one needs in order to have insight and make good decisions—is the organ that is diseased. A person whose illness results in the inability to recognize that he *has* an illness understandably may be resistant to taking drugs for the illness. This creates a serious roadblock and is a common impediment for treatment adherence (Amador, 2007). It can take months or years for a person with SMI to acknowledge having a mental illness.

Medication Side Effects

Psychotropic medications, especially antipsychotic agents, can produce a range of distressing side effects, from involuntary movements to increased risk of diabetes. Some side effects (e.g., dystonias) are treatable; others may diminish over time or can be compensated for via behavioral changes (e.g., changing position slowly to reduce dizziness from hypotension). Addressing side effects is essential to preventing nonadherence and maximizing quality of life. See Chapter 3 for a detailed discussion of antipsychotic drugs used in the treatment of SMI.

Treatment Inadequacy

NAMI estimates that up to half of all mentally ill persons are receiving treatment that does not match treatment guidelines, is not supported by research, or is outdated (NAMI, 2000). Some effective medications or other treatments supported by research are not covered by third-party payers. Consumers must be informed and diligent in ensuring that they are receiving the most effective treatment, and agencies and staff must be diligent in updating their programs and practice.

Residual Symptoms

Residual symptoms are those that do not improve completely or consistently with treatment. This can be very frustrating, and patients may feel that these symptoms mean they will not get better or that treatments are not working (promoting helplessness and hopelessness). The patient may then discontinue treatment, worsening the illness. Residual symptoms can also cause or worsen associated issues (e.g., inappropriate social behavior and impulsiveness that can add to stigmatization and isolation).

Relapse, Chronicity, and Loss

The majority of patients with a SMI face the possibility of relapse even when adhering to treatment, which may contribute to hopelessness and helplessness. Living with SMI paradoxically requires *more* effort and emotional resources from people *less* able to cope with such demands. Each relapse can cause loss of relationships, employment, and housing, adding that much more loss to the patient's life and making discharge planning significantly more complicated.

RESOURCES FOR PERSONS WITH SERIOUS MENTAL ILLNESS

Comprehensive Community Treatment

Ideally, the community-based mental health care system provides comprehensive, coordinated, and cost-effective care for the consumer with mental illness. However, in 2003, the President's New Freedom Commission on Mental Health concluded that services—particularly for those with serious mental illness—were fragmented and inefficient, with blurring of responsibility among agencies, programs, and levels of government. Many consumers were noted to "fall through the cracks," and those who received treatment had difficulty achieving financial independence because of limited job opportunities and the fear of losing health insurance in the workplace (President's New Freedom Commission on Mental Health, 2003).

The overall goal of community psychiatric treatment is to improve the consumer's ability to function independently in the community. State hospitals and psychiatric units in general hospitals provide inpatient care; outpatient care is provided by community mental health centers (CMHCs), private providers (psychiatrists, psychologists, counselors, social workers, and advance practice registered nurses [APRNs]), and private, public, and governmental agencies. Community services vary with local needs and resources; rural communities or those with limited finances may provide only mandated services (and limited access to them), whereas other communities may have a broad array of accessible services. Consumers sometimes find that needed services are not available or have long wait lists, and they may have difficulty identifying the best programs for their needs amidst the maze of agencies and services.

Community Services and Programs

Psychiatric or **medical-somatic services** center on prescribing medications and related biological aspects of treatment (e.g., monitoring physical health status). Services are provided by psychiatrists, advanced practice registered nurses, and sometimes physician assistants, with support from basic level nurses, who are also usually part of this team.

Case management is usually provided by paraprofessional staff (people trained to assist professionals) who help patients with day-to-day needs, treatment coordination, and access to services. They work in their patient's home, school, and vocational setting and provide comprehensive services coordinating the patient's overall care, brokering and facilitating access to services, and providing psychosocial education, guidance, and support (Aquila & Emanuel, 2003). Case managers may also provide **medication monitoring**, wherein they observe and facilitate the patient's use of medications to promote adherence. One evidence-based model of case management for patients with SMIs is **assertive community treatment (ACT)**, discussed later in this chapter.

Day programs provide structure and offer therapeutic activities to patients who come to the program 1 or more days per week. Social skills training, discussed later in this chapter, focuses on socialization, activities of daily living (ADLs), and prevocational training (the fundamentals needed before one can be successfully employed). Interviewing, dressing for work, and interacting professionally with co-workers are stressed. Day programs also provide social contact and peer support and allow staff to monitor the patient's status so that concerns can be detected and addressed quickly. A variety of staff, and sometimes consumers themselves, provide day program services.

Crisis intervention services focus on helping patients regain their ability to cope when facing overwhelming situations, such as psychological trauma or relapse. People with SMI frequently experience crises because of their vulnerability to stress and impaired cognition and problem solving. Stressors, such as changes in routines at home or work, physical or financial problems, or anniversaries of traumatic events may overwhelm coping mechanisms and result in crises. A person with SMI and limited coping abilities may respond to a small stressor first by seeking hospitalization; crisis intervention seeks to help that person manage the stressor and avert a crisis and inpatient care.

Crisis intervention includes four steps: (1) clarify the reality of the situation; (2) build on the patient's strengths and support system; (3) identify realistic, step-by-step goals; and (4) play an active role in the problem-solving process. Direct interventions, such as calling on existing resources for additional support or finding new resources for the patient, are emphasized. Services range from staff on-call, to respond 24 hours a day to their patients by phone or in person, to support lines ("warm" lines) or hotlines providing phone-based screening, support, crisis intervention, and referral services. Crisis residential or stabilization programs in some communities help persons who are in crisis and/or facing impending relapse, typically providing a stay of several days to 2 weeks during which acuity is too great to remain in a community residence but not high enough to require hospitalization.

Emergency psychiatric services involve emergency assessments, emergency inpatient psychiatric care, and sometimes emergency medication administration. Persons with SMI may be unable to recognize that their illness is worsening or that they are becoming unsafe; therefore, virtually all communities provide a 24-hour emergency psychiatric evaluation program that can initiate emergency inpatient admissions on an involuntary basis using a **mobile crisis team**, which consists of mental health professionals who can respond to patient residences, jails, or even street corners, and/or specially-trained personnel in a crisis center or emergency department setting. In some communities, law-enforcement officers are responsible for initiating involuntary psychiatric evaluations. Local probate courts can also order such evaluations upon petition by family members or other interested parties.

Group and individual psychotherapy includes counseling and related interventions based on a variety of models, usually provided by independently licensed mental health professionals (e.g., licensed independent social workers or APRNs). Approaches appropriate for those with SMI include (1) family therapy (focusing on helping family members function more effectively and providing skills and knowledge necessary to support loved ones with mental illnesses), (2) psychoeducation groups (focusing on education about mental health topics [e.g., psychotropic drugs] and building patient skills [e.g., conflict resolution]), and (3) support groups (providing support related to daily challenges of living with chronic illness). Three other approaches—cognitive therapy, cognitive-behavioral therapy (CBT), and supportive psychotherapy—are discussed later in this chapter.

Housing services include halfway houses, supervised or unsupervised group homes, "board-and-care" homes (wherein room, board, and limited supervision are provided by lay persons in their homes), independent community housing (apartments, houses), and programming for specialized populations, such as forensic patients (e.g., criminal offenders found "Not Guilty by Reason of Insanity," who no longer require inpatient care but require special or intensive monitoring and programming in the community). Housing services are designed to help the patient progress towards independent living, maintain stability, and avoid homelessness.

Partial hospital programs (PHPs) provide services similar to those received during inpatient psychiatric care on an outpatient basis and typically include most of the services available to inpatients. They are usually affiliated with inpatient psychiatric programs, and often their patients have been "stepped down" to the PHP program from the inpatient unit to further stabilize acute psychiatric conditions before fully releasing patients to community-based services. **Intensive outpatient programs (IOPs)** are similar but typically community based and focused on services for high-need persons.

Guardianship involves the appointment of a person (the guardian) to make decisions for the consumer during times when judgment is impaired. Guardians may be family members or attorneys and typically are appointed during a court process addressing the issue of whether or not a patient is competent to provide for his own needs. For consumers judged incompetent, the court may appoint a guardian or direct an involuntary, or probate, inpatient psychiatric admission. Consumers may also voluntarily agree to guardianship. Those with a guardian typically may not enter into contracts, consent to sexual activity, or authorize their own treatment. In some cases, the guardian's authority may be limited to the person's finances, as when a consumer is unable to manage money and meet basic needs for food and shelter; the guardian is responsible for using the consumer's funds to meet such needs. A **payee** is a person, often a volunteer or staff member, the consumer agrees to allow to manage his finances, usually via a contract.

Community outreach programs, often focused on homeless persons, send professional and nonprofessional teams into the community to engage patients with mental illness in needed services, foster self-care, and provide patient advocacy. **Multiservice centers** collaborate with outreach programs to supply hot meals, laundry and shower facilities, clothing, social activities, transportation to and from shelters, and provide access to a telephone and a mailing address for persons who are homeless or living in drop-in shelters.

VIGNETTE

After 3 years, Christopher returns home to his parents. He is soon arrested for threatening a policeman with a steel pipe, is found "Guilty but Insane," and is released on the condition that he receive psychiatric treatment. Because of his history of nonadherence, he goes to a clinic and receives intramuscular depot medication. He is also enrolled in a day program and is assigned a case manager, who helps him apply for Social Security Income and refers him to a group home when his aging parents state that he can no longer live with them. Because he wants to work, he is referred to Goodwill Industries. He gets a job unloading delivery trucks and stays on that job for the next 5 years. When the requirements of his conditional release are completed, he continues in treatment and continues working nearly full time. Because he is stable, his medication is changed to an oral atypical antipsychotic, and he continues to receive supervision in his group home. ∎

Substance Abuse Treatment

A variety of services exist for those who have a dual diagnosis of SMI and alcohol- or drug-related problems (sometimes referred to as *substance abuse/mentally ill* [SAMI] patients). Chemical dependency clinics provide therapeutic and rehabilitative services, including medical and psychosocial assessment, detoxification, crisis intervention, and medication such as methadone. Help for families is also available. Most clinicians endorse SAMI treatment that is integrated (i.e., delivered by a single provider rather than split between a mental health agency and a drug/alcohol agency), using personnel with dual areas of expertise, but this standard has not yet been met in some settings (NAMI, 2007a; Ziedonis et al., 2005). See Chapter 18 for a detailed discussion of treatment settings for patients with substance abuse issues.

EVIDENCE-BASED TREATMENT APPROACHES

Assertive Community Treatment

Assertive community treatment (ACT) has been shown to improve symptoms of SMI and reduce inpatient admissions, incarceration, and homelessness among persons with mental illness (Coldwell & Bender, 2007; Yang et al., 2005; Lamberti et al., 2004).

In the ACT model, rather than go to multiple departments or agencies to receive the range of services needed, the patient works with a team of professionals who provide a comprehensive array of services; the consumer is a patient of the team as a whole. At least one member of the team is available 24 hours a day for crisis needs, and the emphasis is on treating the patient within his own environment. Although ACT programs cost more to operate, proponents believe those costs are offset by reduced care costs elsewhere.

VIGNETTE

After 10 years of treatment adherence, Christopher, now age 50, announces that he wants to move out on his own and maybe get married. Despite respectful disagreement from his nurse therapist, he finds himself a room to rent. Over the next 2 months, his mental status remains stable: he is polite, quiet, and guarded as usual. However, his psychiatrist, who weighs him monthly, notices that he has lost 20 pounds. Christopher cannot identify any change in his eating habits, and he is referred to his primary care provider for an evaluation. He doesn't follow up with the primary care provider, and over the next 4 weeks, he loses another 10 pounds. His nurse therapist calls his work supervisor, who reports that Christopher is behaving differently: he is talking out loud to himself, becoming more isolated, and one morning he smelled of alcohol. She is supportive of Christopher and hopes he'll get treatment. At his next clinic appointment, the psychiatrist and therapist discuss these changes and recommend that Christopher go into the partial hospital program for medication reevaluation. He reluctantly agrees, denying that he has any problem. ■

Cognitive and Behavioral Therapy

Cognitive and behavioral therapy (CBT) has been shown to be effective in helping persons with SMI reduce and cope with symptoms such as auditory hallucinations (England, 2007). The cognitive component of CBT focuses on patterns of thinking and "self-talk" (i.e., what one says to oneself internally). It identifies cognitive distortions and negative self-talk and guides patients to substitute more effective forms of thinking. The behavioral component of CBT uses natural consequences and positive reinforcers (rewards) to shape the person's behavior in a more positive or adaptive manner.

Cognitive Enhancement Therapy

Cognitive Enhancement Therapy (CET) is based on the principle that the brain is able to change, and compromised neurological functions can be assumed by healthier areas of the brain. CET involves many hours (e.g., 60 or more) of computer-based drills and exercises that incrementally challenge functions, such as focusing attention, processing and recalling information, and interpreting social and emotional information (e.g., inferring a person's mood from his expression or tone of voice). Research has shown that CET leads to sustained improvement in these functional areas and improves social and vocational functioning (Eack et al., 2006; Hogarty et al., 2004).

Family Support and Partnerships

Families and significant others can face significant stresses related to the mental illness of a loved one, and both may suffer from insufficiencies in empathy and understanding (Brady & McCain, 2004). Having sound **family support and partnerships** is one of the strongest predictors of recovery; treatment is enhanced, and conflict is reduced when treatment providers work as empathic partners with patients and significant others. NAMI's Family-to-Family program, for example, focuses on the skills families need to cope with the illness and to promote recovery (NAMI, 2007c). NAMI meetings and support groups specific to various SMIs (e.g., the Depression and Bipolar Support Alliance) serve as an excellent source of support and practical guidance for patients and their significant others.

Social Skills Training

Social skills training focuses on teaching persons with SMI a wide variety of social and ADL skills. Persons with SMI often have social deficits that cause functional impairment; for example, persons unable to respond assertively may respond aggressively instead. Complex interpersonal skills, such as negotiating or resolving a conflict, are broken down into subcomponents which are then taught in a step-by-step fashion.

Supportive Psychotherapy

Supportive psychotherapy focuses on supporting the patient at the current stage of illness rather than confronting possible problems and pushing the patient towards change. It stresses empathic understanding, improved coping, and anxiety reduction; is informal in style; can be used by any member of the treatment team and in combination with other modalities; and has been shown to enhance the therapeutic alliance and improve long-term recovery prospects in patients with SMI (Hellerstein et al., 1998).

VIGNETTE

Christopher attends the partial hospital program for 4 weeks. In the first week, the nurse calls the therapist to report that he is severely paranoid: he will not eat or drink out of any open containers and is observed spitting out his pills. His medication is changed to a quickly disintegrating tablet form. He attends groups that focus on education about medication, chronic illness, substance use, and healthy habits. He begins to eat normally, gaining 5 pounds in 2 weeks. Finally, he admits that he has not taken any medication since he moved out of his group home. The discharge plan is referral to the psychosocial program again for structure and case management to assist with finding a new home, medical care, and eventual return to work, with a biweekly medication injection and supportive group therapy. Over the next 3 months, Christopher gradually returns to his baseline level of functioning. His case manager finds him another group home with his previous caregiver. He returns to work 2 days per week and still attends the day program for 3 days. Christopher never is able to identify the trigger for his relapse, but his nurse therapist now observes his physical status more closely and inquires specifically about his work and social activities at each session. ■

Vocational Rehabilitation and Related Services

Vocational rehabilitation and related services can vary widely but can include vocational training, financial support for attaining employment, or supported-employment services. Consumers with SMI are interested in competitive employment (Drake et al.,

2003). Benefits of employment (or volunteer work) are enhanced self-esteem, improved organizational abilities, and increased socialization and income. In the past, consumers were referred to state vocational rehabilitation agencies which emphasized extensive prevocational training and employment in sheltered workshops before placement in competitive jobs; success of this type of program (i.e., maintaining employment) was low. Outcomes improved when the consumer was placed in the job first and then given individualized training.

Programs using a **clubhouse model** (in which consumers run their own business, such as a coffee shop or housekeeping service) teach all members to perform a job in order to run the business. Such programs have led to the supported employment model, which has been shown to be more effective in helping persons with SMI achieve employment. There are four elements in this approach (Mueser et al., 2005; Cook et al., 2005):

1. Rapid placement in a competitive job preferred by the patient
2. Continuing support on the job (e.g., a coach at the worker's side, providing training and communicating with supervisors)
3. Close integration between the job coach and the mental health team
4. Perspective that job endings are a learning experience instead of a failure

EVIDENCE-BASED PRACTICE

Supported Employment

Becker, D., Whitley, R., Bailey, E. L., & Drake, R. E. (2007). Long-term employment trajectories among participants with severe mental illness in supported employment. *Psychiatric Services, 58*(7), 922–928.

Problem
Research on supported employment affirms its efficacy, but the long-term outcomes for this modality related to finding and maintaining work are less studied.

Purpose of Study
This study sought to determine the employment circumstances and history of patients 8 to 12 years after they had enrolled in supported-employment programs.

Methods
Thirty-eight volunteer patients were interviewed 8 to 12 years after they had initiated involvement in supported-employment programs. Patients were asked a variety of questions regarding their employment experiences and perceived barriers to employment, and data was analyzed using quantitative and qualitative methods.

Key Findings
- Psychiatric illness was a significant barrier to finding employment.
- Availability of long-term supports and working part-time were major facilitators of continued employment.
- Patients perceived individual placement and supported-employment interventions as important to their vocational success, aiding them in finding and negotiating their positions and in negotiating conditions of employment.

Implications for Nursing Practice
The study supports the long-term efficacy of supported employment. Nurses can contribute to vocational success by (1) reinforcing prevocational and vocational skills addressed in supported employment and (2) connecting unemployed or underemployed patients to supported-employment services.

OTHER POTENTIALLY BENEFICIAL SERVICES OR TREATMENT APPROACHES

While not yet evidence-based practices, research to date supports use of the following services and treatment approaches.

Advance Directives

Advance directives are legal documents that allow the consumer to direct how future relapses and treatment needs should be managed. For example, a consumer can give consent to hospitalization or forced antipsychotic medications and specify when these responses may be used, minimizing the consumer's loss of control over his treatment and avoiding the need for involuntary admission and court involvement.

Consumer-Run Programs

NAMI and other programs offer training that enables consumers to assist peers effectively in the recovery process. **Consumer-run programs** range from informal "clubhouses," which offer socialization, recreation, and sometimes other services to competitive businesses, such as snack bars or janitorial services, which provide needed services and consumer employment while encouraging independence and building vocational skills.

Wellness and Recovery Action Plans

Wellness and recovery action plans (WRAPs) (Copeland, 2007) and similar programs are psycho-educational programs that empower and train consumers in skills that promote recovery and prepare them to deal with stressors and crises. Training focuses on daily maintenance plans (things that must be done and resources needed to maintain wellness), identifying and managing triggers that could provoke a relapse, early identification of impending relapse, and crisis plans (for managing crises or impending relapse). Typically, a wide variety of useful tools, templates, and techniques are provided, and the programs lead to developing practical and concrete action plans for promoting recovery.

Technology

Technology holds the potential to reduce costs and improve treatment access and outcomes. Electronic records available wirelessly in multiple locations can assist in assessments or service delivery anywhere in the community. Personnel in remote locations are using distance therapy, speaking with patients by telephone or the internet through text-based chats or web-cameras when patients cannot otherwise access distant services or specialists. Although this method is not appropriate for everyone, distance therapy can assist staff in providing additional support and screening for problems.

Exercise

Exercise holds many benefits for persons with SMI, including improved activity tolerance and ability to cope with symptoms, reduced anxiety and depression, enhanced self-esteem, weight control or loss (important for patients with weight-related co-morbidities, such as diabetes and hypertension), and cost effectiveness (Beebe et al., 2005).

NURSING CARE OF PATIENTS WITH SERIOUS MENTAL ILLNESS

Nurses encounter patients with SMI in a variety of inpatient and community settings. All roles and techniques used by psychiatric mental health nurses in inpatient psychiatric settings also apply in the community and other settings.

Assessment Strategies

Important assessments include the following:
- Signs of risk to self or others (suicidality or homicidality)
- Depression or hopelessness
- Signs of relapse (especially increased impulsivity or paranoia, diminished reality testing, increased delusional thinking or command hallucinations)
- Inadequate attention to proper nutrition, adequate clothing or medical care, and carelessness while driving, smoking, or cooking (e.g., leaving pots on the stove and becoming distracted or falling asleep)
- Signs of treatment nonadherence and/or impending relapse (early detection and correction of relapse reduces its intensity and duration and prevents hospitalization, loss of housing, arrest, and loss of entitlements)
- Physical health problems, such as brain tumors or drug toxicity, which can cause psychiatric symptoms and be mistaken for mental illness or relapse
- Comorbid illnesses (ensuring that the patient provides appropriate self-care and receives adequate health care)

Table 30-1 lists potential nursing diagnoses that apply to the patient with SMI. Table 30-2 lists examples of specific nursing outcomes from *Nursing Outcomes Classification (NOC)* (Moorhead et al., 2008).

TABLE 30-1 Potential Nursing Diagnoses for the Patient with Serious Mental Illness

Signs and Symptoms	Nursing Diagnoses
Speaking too softly to be heard	*Impaired verbal communication*
Verbalization incongruent with the setting	*Impaired social interaction*
Silence in groups or withdrawal when approached	*Social isolation*
Failure to keep appointments Admitted missing of medication or observed return of symptoms	*Nonadherence*
Self-negating verbalization	*Chronic low self-esteem*
Fear of trying new things or situations Nonassertiveness or passivity	*Powerlessness*
Distortion of patient's health problem, often denial Neglect of other members of family Excessive concern for and supervision of patient	*Disabled family coping Caregiver role strain*

Data from North American Nursing Diagnosis Association International (NANDA-I). (2009). *NANDA-I nursing diagnoses: Definitions and classification 2009–2011.* Oxford, United Kingdom: Author.

BOX 30-2 *NIC* Interventions for Serious Mental Illness

Self-Care Assistance: IADL
Definition: Assisting and instructing a person to perform instrumental activities of daily living (IADL) needed to function in the home or community
Activities*:
- Instruct individual on appropriate and safe storage of medications.
- Instruct individual on alternative methods of transportation (e.g., buses and bus schedules, taxis, city or county transportation for disabled people).
- Assist individual in establishing methods and routines for cooking, cleaning, and shopping.

Family Support
Definition: Promotion of family values, interests, and goals
Activities*:
- Listen to family concerns, feelings, and questions.
- Accept the family's values in a nonjudgmental manner.
- Identify congruence between patient, family, and health professional expectations.

*Partial list.
Data from Bulecheck, G. M., Butcher, H. K. & Dochterman, J. M. (2008). *Nursing interventions classification (NIC)* (5th ed.). St. Louis: Mosby.

Intervention Strategies

Box 30-2 outlines two relevant *Nursing Interventions Classification (NIC)* interventions for the management of serious mental illness (Bulechek et al., 2008). Basic nursing interventions for patients with serious mental illness are:

- Empowering the patient is a focus of intervention strategies. Involving the patient in goal-setting and treatment selection increases the likelihood of treatment adherence and success.
- Rather than simply focusing on symptoms, emphasizing quality-of-life issues conveys an

TABLE 30-2 *NOC* Outcomes Related to Serious Mental Illness

Nursing Outcome and Definition	Intermediate Indicators	Short-Term Indicators
Self-Care: Instrumental Activities of Daily Living (IADL): Ability to perform activities needed to function independently in the home or community, with or without assistive device	Manages medications Manages money	Shops for groceries Prepares meals Uses phone Travels on public transportation
Family Coping: Family actions to manage stressors that tax family resources	Uses available social support Cares for needs of all members	Involves family members in decision making Establishes family priorities Plans for emergencies

Data from Moorhead, S., Johnson, M., Maas, M. & Swanson, E. (2008). *Nursing outcomes classification (NOC)* (4th ed.). St. Louis: Mosby.

interest in the person (rather than the illness) and reflects the patient's best interests (rather than the staff's preferences).

- Developing and maintaining relationships are keys to overcoming anosognosia and achieving treatment adherence. Persons with SMI often require extended periods of working with staff to form these connections.

- Supportive psychotherapy, focusing on the here and now, aids in maintaining therapeutic rapport and helps the patient maintain positive self-esteem and cope effectively rather than maladaptively.

- Impaired reality testing is the hallmark of SMI and contributes to hallucinations and delusional thinking. Training and encouraging the patient to seek independent information on whether experiences are real or not can help the patient identify these experiences as part of the illness and respond accordingly.

- SMIs predispose persons to isolation due to stigma, impaired social skills, and social discomfort. Isolation contributes to loneliness and reduces access to support. Activities which increase skill and comfort with interaction, provide opportunities for socialization (especially with supportive persons and positive role models, such as other patients who are further along in recovery), or which reduce aloneness, contribute to improved functioning and a higher quality of life.

- Support groups such as NAMI expose the patient to members who "have been there." In addition to providing support and socialization opportunities, such groups often have practical suggestions for issues and problems facing patients and significant others. Involvement in support groups is often empowering for the patient.

- Education and reinforcement is essential, since SMI may result in impaired judgment, desperation for connectedness, or other vulnerabilities which increase the risk for victimization, STDs, and undesired pregnancies.

- Care for the whole person is especially important with SMI patients who have higher burdens of physical illness, poorer hygiene and health practices, less access to effective medical treatment, and more premature mortality than the general population. Averting or reducing obesity through good nutritional and health practices can reduce the risk of co-morbidities such as metabolic syndrome; sound physical health conserves energy and resources for use in coping with SMI (Thomas, 2007).

- Involve persons with co-occurring substance abuse in AA/NA and dual-diagnosis service. Substance abuse rates are high in SMI populations, increase relapse, and interfere with recovery; achieving sobriety is most associated with AA and integrated treatment programs.

Evaluation

Identified outcomes serve as the basis for evaluation. Each *NOC* outcome has a built-in rating scale that helps the nurse to measure improvement.

CURRENT ISSUES

Involuntary Treatment

Involuntary treatment involves treatment mandated by a court and delivered without the patient's consent. Traditionally this has referred to involuntary inpatient admissions, but beginning in the 1980s, jurisdictions began to experiment with outpatient commitment, which provides mandatory treatment in a less restrictive setting. Typically ordered when a patient leaves the hospital or prison, it is intended for persons who would otherwise be likely to discontinue treatment and then come to represent a danger to society. Some consider outpatient commitment a form of assisted treatment in that it helps persons who do not realize they are mentally ill to maintain the best possible mental health status (Torrey & Zdanowicz, 2001). Research on the effectiveness of outpatient commitment has been mixed to date. One difficulty is determining how to respond if the person does not follow the ordered outpatient treatment: rehospitalization or reincarceration are expensive options, and neither may be sufficient to cause the patient to relent and cooperate with treatment (Allen & Smith 2001; Segal & Burgess, 2006).

Criminal Offenses and Incarceration

People with SMIs may commit crimes out of desperation, impaired judgment, or impulsivity; most often they are nonviolent crimes, such as petty theft or disorderly conduct. Police may also become involved with patients who seem unable to care for themselves, have become a public nuisance, or cannot be persuaded to accept treatment but do not meet criteria for involuntary treatment (usually imminent danger to self or others). Consider a patient with impaired judgment who does not dress adequately for cold weather and spends time in laundromats and libraries for warmth, causing disruption. When expelled, the individual is at risk of hypothermia. In such cases, the risk to self may not be "imminent," and hospitalization may not be possible. Loved ones or police may then seek the person's arrest simply to get him or her off the street for the patient's own safety.

Many advocates for the mentally ill feel that incarceration, even if it is viewed as "for the patient's good," is harmful. Imprisonment can lead to victimization, increased hopelessness, relapse due to increased stress and isolation or overstimulation, and cessation of entitlements such as SSI or Medicaid. Also, most mental health care in correctional settings is both expensive and inadequate, and a criminal record can reduce future access to housing or employment. Advocates instead seek diversion from jail to clinical care. Two interventions to achieve this end include (1) **educating police** so they can identify mental illness, distinguish it from criminal intent, and connect persons with SMI to help instead of jailing them, and (2) establishing **mental health courts**, which are designed to intercept persons whose crimes are secondary to mental illness. Such courts feature specially trained officials with authority to order treatment instead of imprisonment.

Transinstitutionalization

Transinstitutionalization is the shifting of a person or population from one form of institution to another, such as from state hospitals to jails, prisons, nursing homes, or shelters (Torrey, 1997). The percentage of people with SMI who are incarcerated or homeless has gone from 2% of the population in 1970 to 7% in 2000 (Glied, 2007). More than 10% of the prison population has SMI (NAMI, 2000). Although deinstitutionalization has given the appearance of providing care in less restrictive settings and provided for financial savings in certain constituencies, in some cases, the new setting is in fact another kind of institution, and the costs have been transferred to another payer (such as departments of corrections). Nursing homes may provide less care or less effective mental health care (or even no mental health treatment at all) and are sometimes less humane than yesterday's asylums (Torrey, 1997).

KEY POINTS TO REMEMBER

- Patients with SMI suffer from multiple impairments in thinking, feeling, and interacting with others.
- The course of SMI involves exacerbations and remissions, as do many chronic medical illnesses.
- Coordinated, comprehensive community services help the SMI patient to function at his or her optimal level.
- Persons with SMI often suffer complications due to insufficient housing, nonadherence to treatment, comorbid medical or substance use problems, and the stigma of mental illness.
- The family and support systems play a major part in the care of many persons with SMI and should be included as much as possible in planning, education, and treatment activities.
- The recovery model stresses hope, strengths, quality of life, patient involvement as an active partner in treatment, and eventual recovery.

CRITICAL THINKING

1. John Yang, 42, dually diagnosed with schizophrenia and alcohol/marijuana abuse, is brought to the clinic by his mother, Mrs. Yang. During this initial assessment, Mrs. Yang reports that she has been caring for her son at home since he was 15; however, since recently moving to town, she is at a loss about what is available in the community. John has been prescribed haloperidol (Haldol), but Mrs. Yang says he rarely takes it because of muscle rigidity and sexual side effects. They have tried many of the traditional antipsychotic drugs without success.
   A. Given your understanding of the problems faced by a person with a severe mental illness, what are some areas of John's life you might want to explore in your assessment? Consider relationships, employment history, cognitive abilities, social skills, and behavior. How would knowledge in these areas help your long-term planning?
   B. After you assess John's medication history, how can you be an advocate in terms of his nonadherence to traditional antipsychotics? What are some of the obstacles to adherence for a dually-diagnosed patient? What approach or change in treatment would offer the best chance of success?
   C. Of the resources mentioned in this chapter, what are some that might be appropriate for John?
   D. Identify three basic aims of psychoeducation for John and his mother.

2. You are doing your psychiatric rotation in a state hospital where many of the patients are diagnosed with schizophrenia. Although you had been apprehensive about this rotation, you are surprised to realize that patients respond well to you, that you are fascinated by this specialty area, and may consider it as a career. A fellow student remarks, "You must be crazy to want to work with these people."
   A. What social problem is represented by this student's remark?
   B. Identify other social prejudices that have been significant problems in the United States. What responses were effective in reducing and eliminating their impact?

CHAPTER REVIEW

1. A patient with schizophrenia does not feel that he needs medication because "there is nothing wrong with me." This is most likely an example of:
   1. denial.
   2. projection.
   3. anosognosia.
   4. paranoid ideation.

2. Sarah, a young woman with schizophrenia who has struggled with hygiene and other activities of daily living, has been on a 4-hour pass. She is tearful and reports that

when she sat down on the bus to return to the hospital, the woman she sat next to immediately moved to another seat. Which response(s) would most likely be therapeutic? *Select all that apply.*

1. Acknowledge Sarah's distress, and remind her that dinner will be ready in 30 minutes so she has time to settle in before eating.
2. State, "You sound discouraged. Sometimes people who do not understand mental illness can be hurtful," and offer to sit with her.
3. Advise Sarah that the woman's behavior was simply rude and can be ignored because it is something people with mental illness have to get used to.
4. Suggest to Sarah that perhaps her hygiene would benefit from improvement, and offer to help her improve her hygiene so that others will be less likely to reject her.

3. Christopher is a 25-year-old male who has been hospitalized three times for exacerbations of schizophrenia. Each time he was discharged, he became homeless and relapsed. Typically he is very disorganized, does not spend his money responsibly, loses his housing when he does not pay the rent, and in turn cannot be located by his case manager, leading to treatment nonadherence and relapse. Which response would be most therapeutic in this situation?

1. Advise Christopher that if he does not pay his rent, he will be placed in a group home instead of independent housing.
2. Discuss with Christopher the option of having a guardian who will assure that the rent is paid, and assure that his money is managed to meet his basic needs.
3. Suggest to Christopher's prescribing clinician that he be placed on a long-acting injectable form of antipsychotic medication to address the issue of treatment nonadherence.
4. Encourage Christopher's case manager to hold him responsible for the outcomes of his poor decisions by allowing such periods of homelessness to serve as a natural consequence.

4. Peggy has experienced repeated episodes of severe depression and mania. These episodes and related

hospitalizations have disrupted her full-time employment and created discord within her marriage. She argues with the outpatient staff about medications, does not believe she has a mental illness, and—although she takes her medications while hospitalized—she stops taking them after discharge. She will be discharged in 2 weeks. Which intervention is most likely to increase her adherence to medications?

1. Advise Peggy that she will be assigned to new outpatient staff to reduce the conflicts she is experiencing with her current providers.
2. Explain to Peggy that the medications will help her and that all medications have side effects she can learn to live with in time.
3. Involve her in a medication education group that will help her learn the types and names of psychotropic medications, their purpose, and possible side effects.
4. Explore with Peggy her perceptions of the medications and her experiences with them, and guide her to connect use of the medications with achieving her goals.

5. Which intervention(s) would be appropriate to promote recovery for persons with serious mental illness who live in the community? *Select all that apply.*

1. Meet regularly with the patients, and encourage them to make steady progress towards complete independence.
2. Introduce patients to others with similar illnesses, and encourage participation in social activities with peers.
3. Support the development of advance directives and involvement in social and employment activities run by other consumers.
4. Use public transportation to take patients to a museum, and share a nutritious dinner with them at an inexpensive restaurant.
5. Guide them to develop written plans that identify resources to maintain stability and steps to take when faced with unusual stressors.
6. Over time, guide the patients to identify and switch to sources of support outside the family to reduce dependence on their loved ones as their primary support resource.

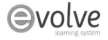 **learning system**

Visit the Evolve website for an **Audio Chapter Summary, Chapter Review Answers & Rationales, Critical Thinking Answer Guidelines,** and additional resources related to the content in this chapter: **http://evolve.elsevier.com/Varcarolis/foundations**

Companion CD Use the Companion CD to prepare for tests and the NCLEX® Examination with **Test-Taking Strategies** for psychiatric mental health nursing and hundreds of **Review Questions**.

References

Allen, M., & Smith, V. F. (2001). Opening Pandora's box: The practical and legal dangers of involuntary outpatient commitment. *Psychiatric Services, 52*, 342–346.

Amador, X. (2007). *I am not sick, I don't need help!* Peconic, NY: Vida Press LLC.

Aquila, R., & Emanuel, M. (2003, September 25). *Managing the long-term outlook of schizophrenia.* Retrieved February 28, 2005, from http://www.medscape.com/viewprogram/2680_pnt.

Beebe, L. H., Tian, L., Morris, N., Goodwin, A., Allen, S., & Kuldau, J. (2005). Effects of exercise on mental and physical health parameters of persons with schizophrenia. *Issues in Mental Health Nursing, 26*(6), 661–676.

Brady, N., & McCain, G. C. (2004). Living with schizophrenia: A family perspective. *Online Journal of Issues in Nursing, 10*(1). Retrieved June 27, 2007, from http://nursingworld.org/ojin/hirsch/topin4/tpc4_2htm.

Bulecheck, G. M., Butcher, H. K., & Dochterman, J. M. (2008). *Nursing interventions classification (NIC)* (5th ed.). St. Louis: Mosby.

Coldwell, C. M., & Bender, W. S. (2007). The effectiveness of assertive community treatment for homeless populations with severe mental illness: A meta-analysis. *American Journal of Psychiatry, 164*(3), 393–399.

Cook, J. A., Leff, H., Blyler, C., Gold, P., Goldberg, R., Mueser, K., et al. (2005). Results of a multisite randomized trial of supported employment interventions for individuals with severe mental illness. *Archives of General Psychiatry, 62*, 505–512.

Copeland, M. E. (2007). *About mental health recovery and WRAP.* Retrieved May 6, 2009, from http://mentalhealthrecovery.com/aboutus.php

Drake, R. E., Becker, D. R., & Bond, G. R. (2003). Recent research on vocational rehabilitation for persons with severe mental illness. *Current Opinions in Psychiatry, 16*, 451–455.

Eack, S. M., Hogarty, G., Greenwald, D., Hogarty, S., & Keshavan, M. (2006). Cognitive enhancement therapy improves emotional intelligence in early course schizophrenia: Preliminary effects. *Schizophrenia Research, 89*(2007), 308–311.

England, M. (2007). Efficacy of cognitive nursing interventions for voice hearing. *Perspectives in Psychiatric Care, 43*(2), 69–76.

Fisher, D. B., & Ahern, L. (2002). Evidence-based practices and recovery. *Psychiatric Services, 53*, 632–633.

Fitch, B. (2007, Mar 17). Growing through psychosis: The patient's journey toward mental health. Presentation at the Eighth Annual All-Ohio Institute on Community Psychiatry, Beachwood, OH.

Glied, S. (2007, Mar 16). Better, but not well: Mental health policy in the United States. *Presentation at the Eighth Annual All-Ohio Institute on Community Psychiatry*, Beachwood, OH.

Gonzalez, J. M., Perlick, D., Miklowitz, D., Kaczynski, R., Hernandez, M., Rosenheck, R., et al. (2007). STEP-BD family experience study group.. Factors associated with stigma among caregivers of patients with bipolar disorder in the STEP-BD study. *Psychiatric Services, 58*(1), 41–48.

Group for the Advancement of Psychiatry. (2000). *Now that we are listening.* Dallas, TX: Committee on Psychiatry and the Community Group for the Advancement of Psychiatry.

Hellerstein, D. J., Rosenthal, R. D., Pinsker, H., Samstag, L. W., Murau, J. C., & Winston, A. (1998). A randomized prospective study comparing supportive and dynamic therapies: Outcome and Alliance. *Journal of Psychotherapy Practice and Research, 7*(4), 261–271.

Hogarty, G. E., Flesher, S., Ulrich, R., Carter, M., Greenwald, D., Pogue-Giele, M., et al. (2004). Cognitive enhancement therapy for schizophrenia: Effects of a 2-year randomized trial on cognition and behavior. *Archives of General Psychiatry, 61*(9), 866–876.

Lamberti, J. S., Weisman, R., & Faden, D. I. (2004). Forensic assertive community treatment: Preventing incarceration of adults with severe mental illness. *Psychiatric Services, 55*, 1285–1293.

Lefley, H. P., & Hatfield, A. B. (1999). Helping parental caregivers and mental health consumers cope with parental aging and loss. *Psychiatric Services, 50*, 369–375.

Lutz, W. J., & Warren, B. J. (2001). Symptomatology and medication monitoring for public mental health consumers: A cultural perspective. *Journal of the American Psychiatric Nurses Association, 7*(4), 115–124.

McCloughen, A. (2003). The association between schizophrenia and cigarette smoking: A review of the literature and implications for mental health nursing practice. *International Journal of Mental Health Nursing, 12*, 119–129.

McCombs, J. S., Nichol, M., Johnstone, B., Stimmel, G., Shi, J., & Smith, R. (2000). Antipsychotic drug use patterns and the cost of treating schizophrenia. *Psychiatric Services, 51*(4), 525–527.

Miller, B. J., Paschall, C. B., & Svendsen, D. P. (2007, Mar 16). Mortality and medical co-morbidity in patients with serious mental illness. *Poster presentation at the Eighth Annual All-Ohio Institute on Community Psychiatry*, Beachwood, OH.

Moorhead, S., Johnson, M., Maas, M., & Swanson, E. (2008). *Nursing outcomes classification (NOC)* (4th ed.). St. Louis: Mosby.

Mueser, K. T., Bond, G. R., & Drake, R. E. (2001). Community-based treatment of schizophrenia and other severe mental disorders: Treatment outcomes? *Medscape Mental Health, 6*(1), 1–31.

Mueser, K. T., Corrigan, P., Hilton, D., Tanzman, B., Schaub, A., Gingerich, S., et al. (2002). Illness management and recovery: A review of the research. *Psychiatric Services, 53*, 1272–1284.

Mueser, K. T., Aalto, S., Becker, D., Ogden, J., Wolfe, R., Shiavo, D., et al. (2005). The effectiveness of skills training for improving outcomes in supported employment. *Psychiatric Services, 56*, 1254–1260.

Mulligan, K. (2005). Recovery model seeks more than symptom relief. *Psychiatric News, 40*(18), 6.

National Alliance for the Mentally Ill. (2000). *Omnibus mental illness recovery act.* Retrieved May 6, 2009, from http://www.nami.org/Template.cfm?Section = press_release_archive&template=/contentmanagement/contentdisplay.cfm&ContentID = 5734&title = NAMI%20Challenges%20Decision%20Makers%20To%20Make%20Mental%20Illness%20Recovery%20A%20Priority

National Alliance on Mental Illness. (2007a). *Dual diagnosis and integrated treatment of mental illness and substance abuse disorder.* Retrieved July 1, 2007, from http://www.nami.org/Content/ContentGroups/Helpline1/Dual_Diagnosis_and_Integrated_Treatment_of_Mental_Illness_and_Substance_Abuse_Disorder.htm

National Alliance on Mental Illness. (2007b). *PACT: Program of Assertive Community Treatment.* Retrieved July 2, 2007, from http://www.nami.org/Content/ContentGroups/Programs/PACT1/What_is_the_Program_of_Assertive_Community_Treatment_(PACT)_.htm

National Alliance on Mental Illness. (2007c). *About NAMI's education, training, & peer support programs.* Retrieved July 2, 2007, from http://www.nami.org/Content/NavigationMenu/Find_Support/Education_and_Training/Education_Training_and_Peer_Support_Center/Education,_Training_and_Peer_Support_Center.htm

National Alliance on Mental Illness. (2008). *Stigma busters: Fight stigma*. Retrieved December 30, 2008, from http://www.nami.org/template.cfm?section = about_stigmabusters

Pompili, M., Amador, X., Girardo, P., Harkavy-Friedman, J., Harrow, M., Kaplan, K., et al. (2007). Suicide risk in schizophrenia: Learning from the past to change the future. *Annals of General Psychiatry, 6*, 10. Retrieved July 2, 2007, from http://www.annals-general-psychaitr.com/content/6/1/10

President's New Freedom Commission on Mental Health. (2003). *Report of the President's New Freedom Commission on Mental Health*. Retrieved July 12, 2008, from http://www.mentalhealthcommission.gov/reports/FinalReport/downloads/FinalReport.pdf

Resnick, S. G., & Rosenheck, R. A. (2006). Recovery and positive psychology: Parallel themes and potential synergies. *Psychiatric Services, 57*, 120–122.

Rosenheck, R., Leslie, D., Keefe, R., McEvoy, J., Swartz, M., & Perkins, D. (2006). Barriers to employment for people with schizophrenia. *American Journal of Psychiatry, 163*, 411–417.

Schanda, H. (2005). Psychiatry reforms and illegal behaviour of the severely mentally ill. *Lancet, 365*, 367–369.

Segal, S. P., & Burgess, P. M. (2006). Conditional release: A less restrictive alternative to hospitalization? *Psychiatric Services, 57*, 1600–1606.

Stuart, H. (2006). Mental illness and employment discrimination. *Current Opinion in Psychiatry, 19*, 522–526.

Substance Abuse and Mental Health Services Administration. (2002). *Number of persons with serious mental illness by state, 2002*. Retrieved January 20, 2009, from http://mentalhealth.samhsa.gov/databases/databases_exe.asp?D1 = AK&Type = ASMI&Myassign = list

Substance Abuse and Mental Health Services Administration. (2008). *Campaign for mental health recovery*. Retrieved January 2, 2009, from www.whatadifference.org/docs/NASC_FactSheet.pdf

Thomas, P. (2007). The stable patient with schizophrenia—From antipsychotic effectiveness to adherence. *European Neuropsychopharmacology, 17*, S115–S122.

Torrey, E. F. (1997). *A well-intentioned disaster: The fallout from releasing the mentally ill from institutions*. Retrieved January 2, 2009, from http://chronicle.com/che-data/articles.dir/art-43.dir/issue-40.dir/40b00401.htm

Torrey, E. F., & Zdanowicz, M. (2001). Outpatient commitment: What, why, and for whom. *Psychiatric Services, 52*, 337–341.

U.S. Census Bureau. (2008). *The numbers count: Mental health disorders in America*. Retrieved January 2, 2009, from http://www.nimh.nih.gov/health/publications/the-numbers-count-mental-disorders-in-america.shtml

Wieden, P. J. (2007). Discontinuing and switching antipsychotic medications: understanding the CATIE schizophrenia trial. *Journal of Clinical Psychiatry, 68*(Suppl. 1), 12–19.

Wiederhold, B. K., & Wiederhold, M. D. (2003). An annual conference to advance the use of virtual reality in the treatment of mental disorders. *Psychiatric Services, 54*, 1209–1210.

White, M. C., Chafetz, L., Collins-Bride, G., & Nickens, J. (2006). History of arrest, incarceration, and victimization in community-based severely mentally ill. *Journal of Community Health, 31*(2), 123–135.

Yang, J., Law, S., Chow, W., Andermann, L., Steinberg, R., & Sadavoy, J. (2005). Assertive community treatment for persons with severe and persistent mental illness in ethnic minority groups. *Psychiatric Services, 56*, 1053–1056.

Ziedonis, D. M., Smelson, D., Rosenthal, R., Batki, S., Green, A., & Henry, R. (2005). Improving the care of individuals with schizophrenia and substance use disorders: Consensus recommendations. *Journal of Psychiatric Practice, 11*(5), 315–339.

CHAPTER 31

Psychological Needs of Patients With Medical Conditions

Roberta Waite and Elizabeth M. Varcarolis

Key Terms and Concepts

coping skills, 702
holistic approach, 694
human rights abuses, 702

psychiatric liaison nursing, 703
quality of life, 700
stigmatized persons with medical conditions, 702

Objectives

1. Describe the influence of stress on general medical conditions.
2. Construct a nursing diagnosis for an individual who has HIV and depression.
3. Explain the importance of nurses teaching relaxation techniques and coping skills to patients with medical illness.

4. Perform a comprehensive nursing assessment for a patient with a medical illness.
5. Assess the patient's coping skills by identifying (a) areas for psychoeducation teaching and (b) areas of strength.
6. Identify two instances in which a consultation with a psychiatric liaison nurse might have been useful for one of your medical-surgical patients.

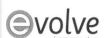 Visit the Evolve website for an **Audio Glossary & Flashcards**, **Concept Map Creator**, and additional resources related to the content in this chapter: **http://evolve.elsevier.com/Varcarolis/foundations**

The relationship between physical conditions and psychological factors are addressed by two separate though related classifications in the *Diagnostic and Statistical Manual of Mental Disorders*, fourth edition, text revision *(DSM-IV-TR)* (American Psychiatric Association [APA], 2000). Somatoform disorders, psychological problems that manifest themselves in physical symptoms such as chronic pain or preoccupation with illnesses, were discussed in Chapter 22. Now we turn our attention to people who have diagnosed or diagnosable general medical conditions that are influenced by psychological factors and psychiatric disorders.

Psychological factors have been found to influence a variety of physical illnesses. Stressful life events may result in further health risk and increase disability through stress-related physiological responses (Fava & Wise, 2007). When psychiatric disorders are present along with general medical conditions, they may increase the likelihood of adverse events, length of stay, and cost; they also may negatively impact on outcomes and increase morbidity and mortality (Levenson, 2008).

This chapter helps to prepare nurses to utilize a holistic approach in nursing care so that we may address both psychological and physiological needs. This is important for psychiatric mental health nurses who are caring for patients with physical illnesses. It is also essential that nurses who work outside of psychiatric settings be aware of the influence of psychological factors and psychiatric disorders on the course of general medical conditions and plan for care accordingly.

PSYCHOLOGICAL FACTORS AFFECTING MEDICAL CONDITIONS

Both the medical and mental health communities recognize the interrelationships between psychiatric and medical comorbidities. Psychological factors may present a risk for medical disease, or they may magnify and/or adversely affect a medical condition. The expanded diagnostic category **psychological factors affecting medical condition** in the *DSM-IV-TR*

(APA, 2000) includes the identification of psychological factors that interfere with medical treatment, pose health risks, or cause stress-related pathophysiological changes. This diagnosis includes both the psychological factor and the general medical condition. The multiaxial system of the *DSM-IV-TR* provides a framework for making such a diagnosis. As you may recall, the five categories are:

- Axis I: Clinical Disorders
- Axis II: Personality disorders and mental retardation
- Axis III: General medical conditions
- Axis IV: Psychosocial and environmental problems
- Axis V: Global Assessment of Functioning (GAF)

Axis I identifies the symptoms of the psychiatric disorder (e.g., depression, anxiety, substance abuse), whereas axis II codes the personality trait (e.g., type A). Axis III identifies the medical condition or maladaptive health behavior (human immunodeficiency virus [HIV], unsafe sex practices). For example, the diagnosis might read "a major depressive disorder affecting the immune system." Figure 31-1 lists the *DSM-IV-TR* criteria for psychological factors affecting medical condition.

The interaction of the axes has gained increasing attention for at least two reasons. First, researchers have gained an increased understanding of the basic physiological responses to stress (see Chapter 11); and second, there is deep interest in improving both the outcomes and the efficiency of health care delivery. Collaboration among providers of primary health care and mental health care can lead to more accurate diagnoses. Furthermore, treatment adherence for psychiatric disorders can be improved by addressing both psychiatric and physical problems, thereby reducing the stigma for seeking mental health care and making care more convenient. Obtaining remission, improving care of the family, and decreasing suicide behavior are major points of focus (Culpepper, 2003) (Box 31-1).

Stress is certainly a psychological factor. Axis IV (psychosocial and environmental problems) identifies stressors in an individual's life that might become a primary focus of treatment. Hans Selye (1956) was the first to introduce the concept of stress into the fields of medicine and physiology. Stress can lead to changes in physical and mental health in many ways (see Chapter 11). Cannon's identification of the fight-or-flight response (1914) and Selye's description of the general adaptation syndrome provided insight into the biological and molecular reactions to stressors in the sympathetic nervous system, the pituitary-adrenocortical axis, and the immune system. Extensive studies have left little doubt that psychosocial stress can affect the course and severity of illness.

DSM-IV-TR Criteria for Psychological Factors Affecting Medical Condition

A. A general medical condition (coded on axis III) is present.

B. Psychological factors adversely affect the general medical condition in one of the following ways:
(1) The factors have influenced the course of the general medical condition as shown by a close temporal association between the psychological factors and the development or exacerbation of, or delayed recovery from, the general medical condition.
(2) The factors interfere with the treatment of the general medical condition.
(3) The factors constitute additional health risks for the individual.
(4) Stress-related physiological responses precipitate or exacerbate symptoms of the general medical condition.

Choose name based on the nature of the psychological factors (if more than one factor is present, indicate the most prominent):

Mental disorder affecting... [indicate the general medical condition] (e.g., an axis I disorder such as major depressive disorder delaying recovery from a myocardial infarction)

Psychological symptoms affecting... [indicate the general medical condition] (e.g., depressive symptoms delaying recovery from surgery, anxiety exacerbating asthma)

Personality traits or coping style affecting... [indicate the general medical condition] (e.g., pathological denial of the need for surgery in a patient with cancer; hostile, pressured behavior contributing to cardiovascular disease)

Maladaptive health behaviors affecting... [indicate the general medical condition] (e.g., overeating, lack of exercise, unsafe sex)

Stress-related physiological response affecting... [indicate the general medical condition] (e.g., stress-related exacerbations of ulcer, hypertension, arrhythmia, or tension headache)

Other unspecified psychological factors affecting... [indicate the general medical condition] (e.g., interpersonal, cultural, or religious factors)

Figure 31-1 Diagnostic criteria for psychological factors affecting medical conditions. (From American Psychiatric Association. [2000]. *Diagnostic and statistical manual of mental disorders* [4th ed., text rev.]. Washington, DC: Author.)

Chronic stressors cause components of the immune system to be affected in detrimental ways. Research in the field of psychoneuroimmunology has provided insights into the relationship between psychological and physiological health in human immunodeficiency virus (HIV) and other diseases (Temoshok et al., 2008). This research explains the negative impact of perceived stress on HIV disease progression, primarily as a function of immunosuppression mediated by elevated

---

BOX 31-1 Patient-Specific Outcomes of Primary Care–Psychiatry Collaboration

- Accuracy of diagnosis
- Retention in care
- Adherence with the treatment plan
- Decreased medication problems
  - Adverse/toxic effects
  - Drug-drug interactions
- Stabilization on long-term care plan
- Attainment of remission
  - Symptom control
  - Functional improvement
- Improved medical outcomes
  - Preventive measures
  - Chronic disease management
- Improved care of family
- Decreased suicidal behaviors

From Culpepper, L. (2003, May 18). The successful intervention: Management of the patient with medical comorbidities. In *Psychiatry and medicine: Common patients, different perspectives.* Symposium conducted at the 156th Annual Meeting of the American Psychiatric Association, San Francisco, CA.

---

cortisol. A meta-analysis of more than 300 empirical articles suggests that psychological stressors may be associated with suppression of both cellular and humoral measures (Segerstrom & Miller, 2004). Being able to attenuate the stress response within this patient population is important because we can potentially positively affect not only the quality of life, but also the illness trajectory of persons living with HIV.

A variety of other medical disorders have been studied with regard to the effects of stress on the course of the illness. Table 31-1 identifies some common medical conditions that are negatively affected by stress and would benefit from stress reduction and support. In fact, anyone experiencing a serious medical condition needs a variety of supports and may benefit from learning new coping skills.

PSYCHOLOGICAL RESPONSES TO SERIOUS MEDICAL CONDITIONS

The diagnosis of a medical problem or condition is stressful for nearly everyone. However, the degree of stress is dependent upon the person's perception of the illness. People's questions can be many and varied when they find themselves faced with a serious medical problem:

- Will I be disfigured?
- Will I have a long-term disability?
- Will I be able to function as a wife or husband, parent, and member of society?

- Will I be able to continue to work?
- Will I suffer pain?
- Will I be stigmatized?

People who face the crisis of a serious medical diagnosis need the kind of emotional support that allows them to face their burdens without censure or fear of judgment (Jenkins, 2006). When strong emotional supports and social ties are not available, other questions may arise:

- How will I cope?
- How will this affect my life?
- Will I retain a reasonable quality of life?

The psychological impact of medical illness can be severe and can account for a higher rate of disruption in functional ability than just the medical illness alone would indicate. Among the most common psychological responses to physical illness are depression, anxiety, substance use, denial, hopelessness, and anger (Dunn, 2005). A psychological condition, however, may supersede or be comorbid with a medical condition. In general, individuals with medical disorders and psychological symptoms have poorer outcomes than those with the same medical disorders but without psychological problems (Levenson, 2008).

Depression

The risk of a major depressive disorder is high among individuals with a serious medical illness and is thought to be as high as 20% to 50% (Jiang, 2008). Often, depression is masked by the medical condition itself and goes unrecognized and thus untreated. Just a few of the medical illnesses that typically are associated with depression are cancer (depression rate as high as 50%), HIV (depression rate of 41%), diabetes (depression rate of 9% to 27%), and stroke (depression rate of 20% to 30%) (Gaynes et al., 2008; Herrmann, 2006; Pirl, 2004). Depression can amplify the pathophysiology of endocrine and cardiac disease and diminish functional ability (Jiang, 2008).

Depression is also a risk factor for nonadherence to medication and treatment regimen. Patients with depression have been found to be three times more likely to be nonadherent to medical treatment than are patients without depression (Culpepper, 2003). If not recognized and treated, depression can affect the severity of the medical disorder, increase personal distress, impair functioning, and interfere with adherence to a prescribed medical regimen. However, people with medical conditions who get treatment for co-occurring depression often experience improvement in their overall medical condition, show better adherence to recommendations for general medical care, and experience a better quality of life (Simon et al., 2005).

TABLE 31-1 Common Medical Conditions Negatively Affected by Stress

Medical Condition	Incidence	Genetic and Biological Correlates	Common Precipitating Factors	Holistic Therapies in Addition to Medical Management
Cardiovascular disease (e.g., coronary heart disease)	Rates higher in males until age 60 years Rates higher in white population than in African American population	Family history of cardiac disease a risk factor Other risk factors include hypertension, increased serum lipid levels, obesity, sedentary lifestyle, and cigarette smoking Psychosocial risk factors (stress, depression, loneliness) High anxiety risk in patient with prior cardiac events	Often, myocardial infarction occurs after sudden stress preceded by a period of losses, frustration, and disappointments	Relaxation training, stress management, group social support, and psychosocial intervention Support groups for type A personalities and type A modification helpful Anxiolytics (benzodiazepines) and antidepressants when indicated
Peptic ulcer (caused by *Helicobacter pylori* infection)	Occurs in 12% of men, 6% of women (more prevalent in industrialized societies)	Infection with *H. pylori* is associated with 95% to 99% of peptic ulcers Both peptic and duodenal ulcers cluster in families, but separately from each other	Periods of social tension and increased life stress After losses; often after menopause	Biofeedback can alter gastric acidity; cognitive-behavioral approaches are used to reduce stress (stress management)
Cancer	Men: most common in lung, prostate, colon, and rectum Women: most common in breast, uterus, colon, and rectum Death rate higher in men (especially African American men) than in women	Genetic evidence suggests dysfunction of cellular proliferation Familial patterns for breast cancer, colorectal cancer, stomach cancer, melanoma	Prolonged and intensive stress Stressful life events (e.g., separation from or loss of significant other 2 years before diagnosis) Feelings of hopelessness, helplessness, and despair (depression) may precede the diagnosis of cancer	Relaxation (e.g., meditation, autogenic training, self-hypnosis) Visualization Psychological counseling Support groups Massage therapy Stress management
Tension headache	Occurs in 80% of population when under stress Begins at end of workday or early evening		Associated with anxiety and depression	Psychotherapy usually prescribed for chronic tension headaches Learning to cope or avoiding tension-creating situations or people Relaxation techniques, stress management techniques, cognitive restructuring techniques
Essential hypertension	Rates higher in males until age 60 years	Family history of cardiac disease and hypertension a risk factor	Life changes and traumatic life events Stressful job (e.g., air traffic controller) Hypothesized to be found more in areas of social stress and conflict	Behavioral feedback, stress reduction techniques, meditation, yoga, hypnosis NOTE: pharmacological treatment considered primary for treatment of hypertension

Candace is a 61-year-old, single, head administrative para-legal who was recently hospitalized for congestive heart failure. She is referred by her physician because of excessive crying, insomnia, and irritability. Candace complains of waking up at night obsessing about small details and having chest pain. She states, "I feel very scared and alone, and I worry about my health and having to retire. I don't know where I would get the money to live or to pay for medical insurance if I get sick again. I am too old, and it is just too difficult to go on." These observations were reported to the nurse practitioner. After a thorough assessment and medical work-up it is determined that Candace is experiencing depression and severe anxiety which precipitated physiological symptoms from extreme distress. ■

Anxiety

Anxiety disorders are among the most common mental health problems seen in primary health care settings, with as many as one third of patients displaying significant symptoms (Weisberg et al., 2007). Anxiety disorders and medical illnesses are commonly comorbid, especially when pain, disability, hospitalization, economic loss, or fear of death is present (Katon et al., 2007). Psychological and social factors and the severity and presence of comorbid medical conditions play an important role in the level of anxiety experienced (Cohen et al., 2007).

Acute anxiety can influence a person's coping capacity, defensive structure, adaptive capacity, and resilience. Anxiety may also lead to heightened awareness of physical symptoms, as well as physiologically causing medical symptoms based on increased muscle tension and autonomic nervous system and hypothalamic-pituitary-axis dysregulation. The burden of physical symptoms and resulting functional impairment caused by complications of medical illness are likely to worsen episodes of anxiety (Katon & Roy-Byrne, 2007). Recognizing treatable anxiety disorders that are highly concurrent with medical comorbid conditions is important in alleviating distress and improving the course of the illness.

Verbalization can be an effective outlet for anxiety. However, the ability to effectively communicate one's feelings may be compromised by cultural expectations, disability, or lack of a listener. A sense of helplessness often accompanies anxiety in the person who feels a loss of control over events, such as when awaiting surgery or undergoing invasive treatments. In this case, defense mechanisms (e.g., denial or regression) may be used with greater frequency, or compulsive behaviors may surface. Unreasonable requests of caregivers may be a cover for feelings of inadequacy.

At 27 years of age, Todd tests positive for human immuno-deficiency virus (HIV) infection. During the posttest counseling session, the public health nurse at the health department gives him referrals and information regarding the virus. The nurse notes that Todd is having difficulty focusing on details and needs to have information repeated several times. The nurse gives him the opportunity to explore his feelings, but Todd has difficulty in this area because he was raised to believe that it is a strength to deal with crisis alone. Todd is also experiencing a great deal of denial in this initial period of loss. For these reasons, the nurse anticipates the most common and immediate concerns that might be facing a person who has just discovered that he is HIV positive and gently leads Todd into discussion of these concerns over a period of several weeks, with the use of reflective statements and silence. This approach gives Todd the opportunity to verbalize his feelings and begin to unburden himself in a safe environment. ■

Substance Abuse

Long-term abuse of various substances can lead to a variety of medical complications; for example, alcohol use is associated with hepatic conditions, marijuana use with lung disease, cocaine use with cardiac toxicity, and use of ecstasy (3,4-methylenedioxy-methamphetamine or MDMA) with neurotoxicity (problems with memory, reasoning, and impulse control). However, patients who are diagnosed with serious medical conditions often turn to alcohol and/or other substances of abuse to cope with overwhelming feelings of hopelessness, fear, anxiety, depression, or pain.

Linking medical and mental health services with substance abuse services is important because substance abuse is a concurrent diagnosis in large numbers of medical and mental health patients (Weisner & Matzger, 2003). Untreated substance abuse can increase the number of hospitalizations and the severity of the disorder (medical and/or mental health) in patients with a dual diagnosis (Rosack, 2003). Thus relevant research indicates that health care workers need to be diligent in their initial assessments and identify any coexisting or resulting psychological response or disorder. In most cases of physical illness, the focus is on the complaints of physical symptoms, and minimal attention is given to the psychological responses of the patient.

Grief and Loss

Serious medical illnesses are nearly always accompanied by grief and loss. Any type of treatment or procedure intended to treat a physical illness that creates a major permanent change is accompanied by feelings of loss. The dynamics involved in coping with these feelings are similar to those in a person who is dealing with his or her own impending death or the death of a loved one. The person must grieve for this loss, just as the dying person must work through the confusion and darkness until a degree of acceptance and relative peace is achieved. Negotiating the loss of physical well-being involves movement through feelings of frustration, vulnerability, and sadness to become a whole person once again. This journey encompasses both spiritual and emotional changes and for this reason requires spiritual assessment of the patient, as well as a focus on psychosocial issues.

VIGNETTE

Lillian is a 47-year-old woman being treated with hemodialysis. She has been complaining of frequent tension headaches and occasional stomach upsets before her treatment appointments. The hemodialysis nurse has always been impressed by Lillian's patience and compliant attitude in spite of her debilitating illness, which has robbed her of a normal family life. For this reason, the nurse suspects that Lillian's physical complaints could be a way of dealing with emotions, so the nurse makes a point of spending more time with Lillian to allow her to talk about her frustrations. Lillian expresses anger and some feelings of hopelessness. She resents others who are healthy, including the people who care for her. Frequent opportunities to verbalize these feelings gradually result in the lessening of her somatic complaints and a decrease in her sense of powerlessness and isolation. ▪

Denial

Denial is often a response to physical illness as an unconscious defense mechanism. Common responses to the initial symptoms of illness, receiving a diagnosis, and functional limitations and impairments evoke the complicated process of denial, acceptance, and adaptation (although not necessarily in that order). Denial may be evident when the diagnosed person and the family seem to have little knowledge or interest in learning about the condition or define the illness as acute rather than chronic. Nurses and other health care providers may actually foster such beliefs by withholding information about the meaning and likely consequences of a particular problem. Initial illness crises support explanations of the illness as acute and can be so overwhelming for patients and families as to prevent consideration of long-term course.

As symptoms and acute crises repeat over time, individuals begin to accept the chronicity of their illnesses and the effects of the illness on their daily lives. People begin to experience their bodies as altered and come to think of illness as real in ways that allow them to relate symptoms and the changes in their lives. They compare their present condition with that of the past, weighing the risks of continuing their regular activities and activity levels and then adapting those activity levels. The patient may feel estranged from the person they have become, betrayed by their own bodies, or guilty for not meeting standards of activity levels,

functioning, and appearance. Patients can also distance themselves from their illness, diagnosis, and bodies, objectifying their symptoms as a way of coping. Bodily changes affect individuals' identities in important ways, and some chronically ill patients work very hard at maintaining their pre-illness identity, sometimes to the detriment of their health (Green, 2004).

VIGNETTE

After a car accident, Carol is being assessed by the triage nurse in the emergency department for possible injuries. She complains of a slight headache and dizziness but denies having any other pain or symptoms. Carol is preoccupied with seeing that her 2-year-old son, who was also in the car, is being examined, so she denies her own need for medical attention. Carol's blood pressure is 86/50 mm Hg and her body posture indicates that she is guarding her abdomen. These observations are reported to the examining physician immediately because they indicate possible internal bleeding and danger of shock. Carol is eventually taken to the operating room so the bleeding may be stopped. ▪

Fear of Dependency

Responses to being dependent might be exhibited as the inability to accept warmth, nurturing, or tenderness from caregivers or as refusal to accept treatment or medical advice. This reaction is strongest in those who have unmet dependencies and those who have had negative experiences when help was sought in the past. Anger may mask acute embarrassment over being in a dependent position or may be used by the patient who feels the need to project an independent image. Others are fearful of not having their dependency needs met and do not express any negative feelings to caregivers. These people strive to be "good" patients out of fear that they will be abandoned if they are perceived to be difficult. Anxiety or anger they may suppress could be exhibited through increased somatic complaints.

VIGNETTE

Rebecca, a 50-year-old woman with HIV, worked as a home attendant until she fractured her leg and sustained a severe elbow injury when a patient she was assisting fell on her. The resultant disabilities prevented her from resuming her job as a home attendant. Prior to this incident, she was independent, hard working, self-supporting, and was able to manage a mild anxiety disorder through cognitive reframing and controlled breathing. She was forced to apply for financial support and rely on her son for assistance with transportation and taking care of her apartment. She began to experience shortness of breath, palpitations, and impaired concentration. ▪

NURSING CARE OF PATIENTS WITH MEDICAL CONDITIONS

Psychosocial Assessment

Psychosocial factors are relevant to the course of an illness, and the way a person thinks and feels can have a profound effect on how the disease progresses. Struggling with illness evokes a range of difficult emotions such as fear, anger, sadness, confusion, and guilt. Patients may feel overwhelmed and alone, while family members may feel helpless and at a loss emotionally (Meyerstein, 2005). How can a health care worker know what a patient thinks or feels unless the patient's psychosocial situation is assessed?

The elements of a thorough psychosocial assessment are described in detail in Chapter 8. The following are some highlights that can help the nurse plan necessary interventions. When working with someone who is medically ill, it is important to know if the person has:

- Someone who can share his or her concerns and who cares for him or her
- Friends and supports in the community

- Any coexisting conditions that could negatively affect adjustment to the illness, the course of the illness, adaptation to the illness, or ability to heal (e.g., depression; personality disorder; substance abuse; compulsive behaviors such as gambling, eating, or cybersex)
- Risky health behaviors (e.g., sedentary lifestyle, smoking, engaging in unsafe sex practices, and/or abusing alcohol or drugs)
- A cultural view of health and illness that helps or impedes the process of seeking adequate care

Table 31-2 provides an outline for a psychosocial assessment of a patient with a medical condition. A psychosocial assessment is performed in tandem with a thorough physical workup and mental status examination (see Chapter 8).

Quality of Life

For interventions to be most effective, the nurse must understand how a person's medical condition affects quality of life. For example, how is the medical illness affecting the ability to function in the home, at work, or in school? How are the patient's feelings about the illness (depression, anxiety, hopelessness) affecting

TABLE 31-2 Psychosocial Assessment of Patients With Medical Conditions	
Areas to Assess	**Specific Questions to Ask**
SOCIAL SUPPORTS AND CULTURAL ISSUES	
Family	What were the effects of the patient's illness, treatments, and recovery on the family in the past?
Friends	Who can the patient share painful feelings with?
	Does the patient have friends to joke and laugh with?
	Are there people the patient believes would stand by him or her?
Religious or spiritual beliefs	Does the patient find comfort and support in spiritual practices?
	Is the patient a member of a spiritual or religious group in the community (church, temple, other place of worship)?
	Does the patient find inner peace and strength in religious or spiritual practices?
	The following statements may be used in performing a spiritual assessment of a patient:
	• I [often/sometimes/seldom] believe that life has value, meaning, and direction.
	• I [often/sometimes/seldom] feel a connection with the universe.
	• I [often/sometimes/seldom] believe in a power greater than myself.
	• I [often/sometimes/seldom] believe that my actions make a difference.
	• I [often/sometimes/seldom] believe that my actions express my true self.
Cultural beliefs	Does the patient use specific culture-oriented treatments or remedies for his or her condition?
	Do the patient's cultural beliefs allow for adequate treatment by Western medical standards?
Work	Are there colleagues at work the patient can count on for support?
CONCURRENT PHYSICAL CONDITIONS AFFECTING PSYCHOSOCIAL WELL-BEING	
Physical pain	Is the patient in pain? If yes:
	• How does the patient cope with it?
	• Is the pain disabling?
	• Are there pain-reducing techniques that might help?

TABLE 31-2 Psychosocial Assessment Patients With Medical Conditions—cont'd

Areas to Assess	Specific Questions to Ask
Major illness	Does the patient have a co-occurring major illness that will negatively affect his or her current condition? Is the patient undergoing treatments that are affecting daily life more than expected? Are there interventions that would help the patient better cope with the sequelae of the illness and treatments? Has the patient been hospitalized in the past? If yes: • How many times? • For what? • How did the patient cope?
Addictions and mental health	Does the patient have a co-occurring mental health problem (depression, anxiety, compulsions)? Has the patient suffered a mental disease in the past? Does the patient participate in any compulsive behavior (e.g., smoking, overworking, excessive spending, gambling, cybersex)? Does the patient abuse substances (alcohol, drugs [illicit, over the counter, prescription])?

his or her relationships and ability to function? The World Health Organization's Quality of Life-BREF (WHOQOL-BREF) (2004) tool can be used to examine an individual's perceptions about quality of life in the context of culture, value systems, and personal goals, standards, and concerns. This tool was developed based on the statements made by patients with a range of diseases from a variety of cultures.

Coping Skills

Assessing how a patient has dealt with adversity in the past provides information about coping skills available for use now and in the future. Health care workers can also support the patient in gaining additional coping skills that may help an individual better manage a serious medical or surgical situation.

A person who has a life-threatening disease or chronic illness often deals with distressing physical side effects and changes in body image. For example, a patient who is given a colostomy to avoid death from cancer or ulcerative colitis is left with complex emotional as well as physical issues. This is especially true for women. The patient must learn techniques for dealing with not only the stoma but also the lifelong consequences and their effects on body image, appearance, and relationships. Concerns such as the following may arise (Manderson, 2005):

- Will my partner still be attracted to me?
- Will I continue to be interested in sexual relationships?
- Will I be embarrassed by my friends' reactions to my situation?
- Will people still think of me and relate to me the way they did before this illness?

For example, breast cancer survivors have been helped by the camaraderie with other survivors who openly share their techniques for dealing with appliances or prostheses. Other survivors can also show patients how to respond to well-intended but probing or embarrassing questions. Women who have previously traveled the same path are the best resources for helping others establish how to manage inevitable questions about their illness.

Table 31-3 highlights some of the characteristics that allow people to cope well and some of the

TABLE 31-3 Assessment of Coping Skills

Effective Coping Skills	Ineffective Coping Behaviors
Has optimistic attitude (sees glass as half full)	Has pessimistic attitude (sees glass as half empty)
Confronts the issues; acts accordingly	Minimizes critical health status or signals
Seeks information; gets guidance	Shows tendency to find escape or withdraw
Shares concerns; finds consolation	Blames someone or something else
Has capacity for healthy denial	Denies as much as possible; shows prolonged denial
Redefines the situation, reviews alternatives, examines consequences	Feels things are hopeless, were meant to be; has attitude of "What's the use?"
Constructively uses distractions: keeping busy; maintaining positive emotional ties with family, friends, community	Withdraws; broods; is overwhelmed with self-pity, anger, envy, guilt about having caused the illness

characteristics that may be changed or improved through psychosocial interventions or cognitive-behavioral approaches.

Spirituality and Religion

Nurses and other health care workers are becoming increasingly aware of the role spirituality or religion plays in many patients' lives and its importance as a source of peace. Support from a priest, pastor, rabbi, or other religious leader may be indicated, especially in a case of spiritual distress. Beliefs and practices are forces that promote resilience; practicing healthy coping depends upon the capacity to create meaning from experiences (Meyerstein, 2005).

Social Support

Medical conditions initially may elicit strong support from friends and family, but as time wears on, this support may begin to wane. Knowing who is there for the patient will be helpful in planning for later interventions. Does the patient have sufficient social supports (family, friends, and religious/spiritual help) to enable him or her to share thoughts and feelings? Would the patient benefit from a medical support group?

General Interventions

In an ideal situation, a multidisciplinary team of caretakers, including a psychiatric liaison nurse, an advanced practice nurse who provides consultation to nurses outside of psychiatry, would be involved in the treatment of patients with serious medical illness. Using the data from the holistic assessment, nurse clinicians, along with a physician, are in a position to provide useful and effective interventions.

People who have a medical condition are vulnerable to a variety of psychosocial stresses. How they cope with these stresses may make the difference between living with an acceptable quality of life or giving in to despair, withdrawal, helplessness, or hopelessness. Nurses are in a position to assess and understand patients' psychosocial stressors, identify needed coping skills, and teach stress-management techniques. Nurses can play an important role not only in providing and managing patients' immediate medical care but also in helping patients to improve their ability to cope and increase the quality of life during the course of a chronic medical illness.

Effective **coping skills** that can be taught are many and varied (e.g., assertiveness training, cognitive reframing, problem-solving skills, and social supports). A nurse is in a key position to assess, educate, or provide referrals to a patient to enable healthier ways of looking at and dealing with illness. Consider referring the patient for instruction in a variety of relaxation techniques, such as meditation, guided imagery, breathing exercises, and others, or teach the patient

such techniques yourself. Behavioral techniques are useful, and nurses with special training can offer their patients progressive muscle relaxation or biofeedback. Relaxation techniques, stress management, and supportive education should be part of the care of the patient with a medical condition, regardless of the medical diagnosis.

Although medical procedures may extend or promote life, they often take a toll on the patient's physical state because of the high degree of anxiety they evoke. The following have all been shown to affect a patient's recovery positively:

- Educating the patient regarding the specific medical treatment
- Referring the patient to community support groups (or systems)
- Teaching patients more effective coping skills that take into consideration patients' values, preferences, and lifestyle
- Focusing on a patient's strengths and reinforcing coping skills that work (e.g., prayerfulness, participation in hobbies, relaxation techniques)

There is growing evidence that psychotherapy can help people endure medical illness (Turvey & Klein, 2008). Beneficial psychotherapy approaches include:

- Cognitive-behavioral psychotherapy
- Guided imagery, biofeedback, acupressure, and hypnosis
- Psychodynamic psychotherapy

Box 31-2 provides guidelines for teaching patients and their families how to adapt to a major medical illness.

HUMAN RIGHTS ABUSES OF STIGMATIZED PERSONS WITH MEDICAL CONDITIONS

Some consumers of health care and some health care providers have voiced the need for examination of **human rights abuses** of people who are stigmatized by health care providers. These **stigmatized persons with medical conditions** include those who have mental illnesses, those who are HIV positive, and those who have undergone transgender surgeries or treatments. These are abuses that can result in inadequate care and lead to undue stress, worsening of physical illness, and even death. By assuming that persons with certain illnesses are bad, disgusting, or even just unusual, health care workers fail to acknowledge and understand that the psychosocial issues are similar to those of others and that the same nursing interventions for anger, anxiety, or grief are applicable. Examples of human rights abuse include:

- Failure to fully investigate somatic complaints made by emergency department patients with a history of psychiatric illness

---

BOX 31-2 Patient and Family Teaching: Coping With a Major Medical Illness

Learn all you can about your illness—Knowledge can help reduce anxiety. Keeping your anxiety at manageable levels helps you understand your options and helps you make decisions you believe are right for you.

Practice healthy behaviors—Good sleep hygiene, diet, and exercise are good policies. Even if you are physically limited, exercise promotes a positive state of well-being. Lack of sleep can increase pain, irritability, and fatigue. Proper nutrition in the face of a medical illness can preserve or promote a healthy immune system.

Take advantage of support groups that help manage your medical condition—Support groups that focus on your medical issue can provide you information, help you learn how to handle difficult situations related to your illness, reduce isolation, and offer a safe place to share difficult thoughts and feelings.

Consider entering psychotherapy—There is growing evidence that psychotherapy helps people endure medical illness. Benefits include less pain, better coping skills, and even longer survival, in some situations.

Find a way to express your feelings—Studies have examined the profound healing power of putting upsetting experiences into words (e.g., writing them down, keeping a journal). Acknowledging thoughts and feelings can help your nervous system relax.

Seek additional help if you become depressed, demoralized, anxious, or panicky or have unremitting pain—Your clinician might not be aware of these changes, and there are approaches (i.e., acupuncture, acupressure, biofeedback) that can give people control over their physiological responses and reduce the need for high doses of medication.

Find a creative outlet—Writing poetry or prose, painting or making collages, playing an instrument or singing (anything creative) are powerful tools in working with the feelings of fear, anger, and loss that are stirred by illness.

If you are a caregiver, do not neglect your own self-care—Take time for rest and restoration, time to renew yourself in important life interests and activities. If you become depleted, you cannot give to another what is depleted and you no longer possess.

Data from Zerbe, K. J. (1999). *Women's mental health in primary care.* Philadelphia: Saunders.

- Avoidance of contact with, or refusal to care for, persons who are stigmatized, which results in worsening illness or death
- Hasty labeling with a psychiatric diagnosis and prescription of antipsychotic drugs for persons who are experiencing normal emotional responses (e.g., sadness, anger) to chronic physical illness
- Inappropriate psychiatric admission of persons who are on medical units or in nursing homes, based on the financial needs of the institution or on the staff's inability to manage emotional responses to physical illness or the aging process

These situations may occur more frequently for individuals who lack family support or the personal resources to advocate for themselves (e.g., those from the lower socioeconomic classes, newly arrived immigrants, those living socially "unacceptable" lifestyles). The key to increasing awareness of human rights issues in psychiatric mental health care may be the integration of these concepts into nursing curricula. Humanitarian values are at the very heart of our profession and practice. Nurses are in a unique position to advocate for equal patient treatment, but many hesitate to confront employers about violations of basic patient rights, fearing reprisal. A committee composed of nurses and other hospital employees could be formed to review such cases and make recommendations to the hospital administration. In this age of managed care and cuts in hospital budgets, upholding human rights is one of nursing's greatest challenges.

PSYCHIATRIC LIAISON NURSE

Psychiatric liaison nursing is a subspecialty of psychiatric mental health nursing initiated in the early 1960s. Usually the psychiatric liaison nurse has a master's degree and a background in psychiatric and medical-surgical nursing. The psychiatric liaison nurse functions as a consultant to other nurses in managing psychological concerns and symptoms of psychiatric disorders and as a clinician who works directly to help the patient deal more effectively with physical and emotional problems. The psychiatric liaison nurse is a resource for members of a nursing staff who feel unable to intervene therapeutically with a patient who presents a management problem or has problems that impede care. The psychiatric liaison nurse first meets with the nurse who initiated the consultation and then reviews the medical records, talks with the physicians, and interviews the patient. After the patient interview, the liaison nurse discusses the assessment and suggestions with the referring nurse. If a psychiatric consultation is warranted, the psychiatric liaison nurse initiates the consultation by contacting the patient's physician. A case conference is sometimes needed to enhance communication and consistency in the care of a particular patient.

KEY POINTS TO REMEMBER

- There is irrefutable evidence that psychiatric disorders and psychological responses influence general medical conditions.
- A bidirectional effect exists between physical and emotional states of health. Physical illnesses are often accompanied by a spectrum of emotional responses, particularly anxiety and depression. Likewise, adverse emotional states often increase the severity of physical symptoms.
- The holistic philosophy of nursing dictates that all nurses, regardless of their roles or specialties, assess patients' psychosocial needs as well as their strengths.
- Health care personnel in the medical and mental health communities recognize the need to target both the psychological and medical problems of a patient to increase adherence to the care regimen, maximize quality of life, and promote healing.
- Understanding a patient's psychosocial needs and knowing when to intervene and where to refer the patient is essential for the nurse who truly practices holistic care and more effectively promotes health.
- Identifying the existence of depression, anxiety, and substance abuse and getting the patient treatment can help promote a positive outcome of the medical disorder and improve the patient's quality of life.
- A holistic approach to patient care includes assessment of physical, psychosocial, social, and spiritual needs.
- A growing concern about patients is the state of their spiritual lives. Including this dimension in the holistic nursing assessment allows nurses to see inner strengths in their patients that might be overlooked by a more traditional approach.
- The psychiatric liaison nurse is a nurse clinician who is in the key position of being able to help other health care personnel look at their patients in a holistic manner and to help those who care for these patients understand nonmedical issues that are impeding medical progress.

CRITICAL THINKING

1. Maria Valdez is a 45-year-old woman who has had a partial hysterectomy. Although she is asymptomatic and has a normal physical examination, her lab results indicate that she is HIV positive. Maria was unaware that her boyfriend of two years was engaging in unprotected sex with men.

   She and her ex-husband have been divorced for five years but maintain a good relationship and share custody of their three teenage children. Maria has a supportive extended family, several close friends, and she belongs to a church.

   After her diagnosis, Maria is encouraged to talk about her feelings and see a therapist. Maria states, "I will be able to do everything I did before. I feel healthy." The nurse has several concerns, including Maria's focus on self-care, acceptance, and understanding of her HIV-positive status, and willingness to disclose her status to sexual/intimate partners.
   A. How would you evaluate Maria's social support system?
   B. What other information about her situation would be helpful in your assessment (e.g., cultural beliefs about illness)?
   C. What recommendations or referrals could you make to Maria, and how would you approach her with these recommendations? Would you include contact data for any medically related/HIV-related support groups in the information you would give her?

2. Discuss how you would approach the physician regarding Maria's need to be evaluated for depression. What are some of the compelling reasons depression (and any coexisting mental condition) should be treated in any and all seriously ill medically patients?

3. What cognitive-behavioral coping skills have been proven useful for a patient who is HIV-positive?

CHAPTER REVIEW

1. Which statement about the psychological impact of medical illnesses is accurate?
   1. An experience of grief and loss is not typical of most serious medical illnesses.
   2. Depression is a significant issue in over 60% of persons with cancer or heart disease.
   3. Psychological responses to medical illnesses can delay recovery but do not worsen the outcome.
   4. Patients often have significant concerns regarding the impact a medical illness can have on their ability to function.

2. While taking the vital signs of a patient about to undergo surgery, you notice she is tearful. When asked, she tells you that her mother had the same surgery and later died of a postoperative infection. Which response is most likely to be therapeutic?
   1. Ask the patient if she would like to speak with the chaplain before surgery.
   2. Reassure the patient that she has an excellent surgeon and that complications for her surgery are rare.
   3. State, "Surgery can be very frightening ...", and sit down next to the patient to convey your availability to talk.
   4. State, "Many people become anxious before surgery, but this is a normal reaction. You will be fine."

3. An older adult male with heart disease feels both angry and guilty about his illness, blaming himself for becoming obese and inactive and feeling anger towards tobacco and fast-food companies. He presented in the emergency department today four hours after the onset of

unrelenting chest pain, reporting that it "didn't hurt that much" and that, given his prior experiences with chest pain, he "did not think it would matter much" whether he came in quickly or tried to "wait it out." Now awaiting the results of his ECG, he is reading magazines and talking about the likelihood that a new stent will again give him a new lease on life. Based on this information, how well would you expect this patient to be able to cope with his illness?
1. Poorly
2. Inadequately
3. Adequately
4. Exceptionally

4. A nurse on a medical-surgical unit is admitting a patient with a history of bipolar disorder and alcohol abuse. Which action would be most appropriate for assuring that this patient receives the best possible nursing care?
1. Consult with the psychiatric liaison nurse regarding assessment skills and interventions likely to benefit this patient.
2. Review Internet, textbook, or journal resources pertaining to the patient's mental health and substance abuse disorders.

3. Consult more experienced colleagues and the head nurse for tips on assessing and caring for persons with comorbid psychiatric disorders.
4. Focus primarily on the patient's physical health needs, and refer the patient for outpatient psychiatric care at discharge if the patient requests it.

5. Which statements about persons with mental illness who present with serious medical conditions are most accurate? *Select all that apply.*
1. Such patients are at higher risk of receiving inadequate care, owing to failure to fully assess somatic complaints.
2. Patients who have a medical *and* a mental illness tend to receive more care and more costly care because of their dual diagnoses.
3. Staff are more likely to minimize the amount of time spent with such patients compared to medically ill patients without mental illness.
4. Such patients risk being admitted to psychiatric settings instead of needed medical-surgical units, owing to staff's anxiety about caring for them.
5. Emotional responses to medical conditions may be mistakenly attributed to psychiatric illness rather than being addressed as normal responses to medical conditions.

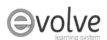

Visit the Evolve website for an **Audio Chapter Summary, Chapter Review Answers & Rationales, Critical Thinking Answer Guidelines,** and additional resources related to the content in this chapter: **http://evolve.elsevier.com/Varcarolis/foundations**

Companion CD   Use the Companion CD to prepare for tests and the NCLEX® Examination with **Test-Taking Strategies** for psychiatric mental health nursing and hundreds of **Review Questions.**

References

American Psychiatric Association. (2000). *Diagnostic and statistical manual of mental disorders (DSM-IV-TR)* (4th ed., text rev.). Washington, DC: Author.

Cohen, M., Batista, S., & Gorman, J. (2007). *Comprehensive textbook of AIDS psychiatry* (M. Cohen & J. Gorman, Eds.). Oxford University Press.

Culpepper, L. (2003, May 18). The successful intervention: Management of the patient with medical comorbidities. In *Psychiatry and medicine: Common patients, different perspectives.* Symposium conducted at the 156th Annual Meeting of the American Psychiatric Association, San Francisco, CA.

Dunn, S. (2005). Hopelessness as a response to physical illness. *Journal of Nursing Scholarship, 37*(2), 148–155.

Fava, G. A., & Wise, T. N. (2007). Issues for *DSM-V*: Psychological factors affecting either identified or feared medical conditions: A solution for somatoform disorders. *American Journal of Psychiatry, 164*, 1002.

Gaynes, B., Pence, B., Eron, J., & Miller, W. (2008). Prevalence and comorbidity of psychiatric diagnoses based on reference standard in an HIV+ patient population. *Psychosomatic Medicine, 70*(4), 505–511.

Green, C. (2004). Fostering recovery from life-transforming mental health disorders: a synthesis and model. *Social and Health Theory, 2*(4), 293.

Herrmann, N. (2006). Post-stroke depression. *Brain and Cognition, 63*(2), 195.

Jenkins, A. (2006). Face the feelings: patients may need emotional support to cope with life-threatening illness. *Nursing Standard, 20*(24), 31.

Jiang, W. (2008). Impacts of depression and emotional distress on cardiac disease. *Cleveland Clinic Journal of Medicine, 75*(2), S20-S25.

Katon, W., Lin, E., & Kroenke, K. (2007). The association of depression and anxiety with medical symptom burden in patients with chronic medical illness. *General Hospital Psychiatry, 29*, 147–155.

Katon, W., & Roy-Byrne, P. (2007). Anxiety disorders: Efficient screening is the first step in improving outcomes. *Annals of Internal Medicine, 146*(5), 390–392.

Levenson, J. L. (2008). Psychological factors affecting medical conditions. In R. E. Hales, S. C. Yudofsky, & G. O. Gabbard (Eds.), *Textbook of psychiatry* (5th ed., pp. 999–1024). Washington, DC: American Psychiatric Publishing.

Manderson, L. (2005). Boundary breaches: The body, sex and sexuality after stoma surgery. *Social Science & Medicine, 61*(2), 405–415.

Meyerstein, I. (2005). Sustaining our spirits: Spiritual study/discussion groups for coping with medical illness. *Journal of Religion and Health, 44*(2), 207–225.

Pirl, W. F. (2004). Evidence report on the occurrence, assessment, and treatment of depression in cancer patients. *Journal of National Cancer Institute Monographs, 32,* 32–39.

Rosack, J. (2003). Comorbidity common in addicts, but integrated treatment rare. *Psychiatric News, 38*(2), 30.

Selye, H. (1956). *The stress of life.* New York: McGraw-Hill.

Segerstrom, S. C., & Miller, G. E. (2004). Psychological stress and the human immune system: A meta-analytic study of 30 years of inquiry. *Psychological Bulletin, 130*(4), 601–630.

Simon, G., Von Korff, M., & Lin, E. (2005). Clinical and functional outcomes of depression treatment in patients with and without chronic medical illness. *Psychological Medicine, 35,* 271–279.

Temoshok, L. R., Wald, R. L., Synowski, S., & Garzino-Demo, A. (2008). Coping as a multisystem construct associated with pathways mediating HIV-relevant immune function and disease progression. *Psychosomatic Medicine, 70,* 555–561.

Turvey, C., & Klein, D. (2008). Remission from depression comorbid with chronic illness and physical impairment. *The American Journal of Psychiatry, 165*(5), 569–575.

Weisberg, R. B., Dyck, R., Culpepper, L., & Keller, M. (2007). Psychiatric treatment in primary care patients with anxiety disorders: A comparison of care received from primary care providers and psychiatrists. *The American Journal of Psychiatry, 164*(2), 276–283.

Weisner, C., & Matzger, H. (2003). Missed opportunities in addressing drinking behavior in medical and mental health services. *Alcoholism: Clinical & Experimental Research, 27*(7), 1132–1141.

World Health Organization. (2004). *World Health Organization Quality of Life – BREF.* http://www.who.int/substance_abuse/research_tools/en/english_whoqol.pdf Accessed 20.02.2009.

Zerbe, K. J. (1999). *Women's mental health in primary care.* Philadelphia: Saunders.

CHAPTER 32

Care for the Dying and for Those Who Grieve

Kathy Kramer-Howe and Elizabeth M. Varcarolis

Key Terms and Concepts

anticipatory grief, 711
bereavement, 715
caring presence, 709
disenfranchised grief, 718
Four Gifts of Resolving Relationships, 712

grief, 715
hospice, 708
mourning, 715
palliative care, 708

Objectives

1. Compare and contrast the specific goals of end-of-life care inherent in the hospice model with those of the medical model.
2. Analyze the effects of specific interventions nurses can implement when working with a dying person and his or her family and loved ones.
3. Analyze how the Four Gifts of Resolving Relationships (forgiveness, love, gratitude, and farewell) can be used to help people respond to a dying loved one.
4. Identify the relationship between the way a person responds to life and how the same person responds to death.

5. Explain how the distinction between the terms *grief* and *mourning* as presented in this chapter can help enhance the effectiveness of a holistic approach.
6. Differentiate among some of the characteristics of normal bereavement and dysfunctional grieving.
7. Explain how the various models of understanding grieving (dual process, four tasks of mourning) can enhance your care of those who grieve.
8. Discuss at least five guidelines for dealing with catastrophic loss and identify appropriate support for someone in acute grief.

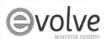 Visit the Evolve website for an **Audio Glossary & Flashcards**, **Concept Map Creator**, and additional resources related to the content in this chapter: **http://evolve.elsevier.com/Varcarolis/foundations**

Caring for patients with terminal illnesses or who are near death due to other conditions challenges and rewards nurses in deep and personal ways. In caring for the dying, nurses may grow personally by both accepting their patients' deaths and by developing a richer understanding of their own mortality. Nurses also have the opportunity to bring dignity to dying and help shape an enduring positive memory for family members and caregivers.

Nurses provide this care for dying patients primary in medical institutions. In a study by Teno and colleagues (2004), family members whose relatives had died were participants. Respondents identified that over 67% of deaths occur in such institutions, with the majority of the remaining deaths occurring at home.

For those who die at home, less than half of individuals received home hospice services. Some key findings from this study were that one in four people who died did not receive adequate pain medication; one in two received inadequate emotional support; and between 20% and 33% of those surveyed expressed dissatisfaction with physician communication and treatment decisions, emotional support to families, and provision of consistently respectful treatment to the dying person. Families receiving home hospice care were the most satisfied on all these measures, with over 70% rating hospice care as excellent (Teno et al., 2004).

Medical professionals in both institutional and home settings can be advocates for the terminally ill and their often overburdened caregivers. The hospice and palliative care treatment model asserts that dying persons and their families have the right to receive honest answers for difficult questions, have control over as much of their medical care and living situation as possible, have advance directives completed and followed, including instructions to suspend or withhold curative efforts, receive excellent palliative care and be comfortable, and be perceived as fully deserving of dignity and human worth.

HOSPICE AND PALLIATIVE CARE

Before the hospice movement began in England in the 1960s, dying people were routinely shunted into hospital rooms with phrases like "We're sorry, there's nothing more we can do for you," and with doctor's orders for prn pain medication. Despite the care of health professionals and visits from helpless relatives, dying people were often neglected, isolated, and left to die in pain.

In 1967, Dame Cicely Saunders established St. Christopher's Hospice in London to remedy this state of neglect (Stolberg, 1999). At St. Christopher's, patients' physical comfort was aggressively pursued with around-the-clock pain medication that allowed them to enjoy optimal quality of life. Effective pain management restored meaningful quality of life to many, enabling them to take care of legal and financial matters, engage in normal activities such as shopping, saying their goodbyes, restoring damaged relationships, and aligning themselves spiritually.

During the same time period in the United States, Dr. Elisabeth Kübler-Ross began actively listening to the terminally ill, and out of her groundbreaking work came a construct of the human response to death and loss that has entered the mainstream. Kübler-Ross (1969) identified distinctive phases, or cycles, in people's responses to terminal illness: **denial, anger, bargaining, depression, and acceptance.** She also realized that personal growth did not necessarily cease in the last stages of life; on the contrary, it often accelerated. Encouraged by her findings, hospices staffed by volunteers began to appear in the 1970s. St. Christopher's comprehensive model was adapted, and the multidisciplinary care team evolved to include a physician, nurse, social worker, pastor or chaplain, and an aide.

In 1983, Medicare instituted a hospice reimbursement, and most commercial insurers followed suit. Nonprofit and for-profit hospice organizations proliferated.

The National Hospice and Palliative Care Organization (NHPCO, 2008) reports that there are over 4,500 operating or planned hospices in the United States. These hospices served approximately 1.3 million people in 2006, with about 75% dying in a private residence, nursing home, or other residential facility.

Palliative care is a medical specialty that has grown out of the hospice movement and an increasing international awareness of the need for better care for the dying. The NHPCO (n.d.) describes hospice and palliative care as follows:

> Considered to be the model for quality, compassionate care for people facing a life-limiting illness or injury, hospice or palliative care involves a team-oriented approach to expert medical care, pain management, and emotional and spiritual support expressly tailored to the patient's needs and wishes. Support is provided to the patient's loved ones as well. At the center of hospice and palliative care is the belief that each of us has the right to die pain-free and with dignity.

VIGNETTE

Mr. Spence contracted amyotrophic lateral sclerosis at the age of 52. He lived at home until his care overwhelmed his family, and he has now been in a care center for 9 months. He is almost completely paralyzed but can still use a letter board with a head-mounted laser pointer. He has a warm smile and a pleasant gaze. He is experiencing shooting pains in his legs and has increasing difficulty with swallowing and breathing. Despite the fact that he can barely eat, he has refused a feeding tube. The staff feels helpless. How can they just stand by while he starves to death? Will he starve to death? One of the aides has decided to quit working with him because it has become so painful.

A hospice referral was made. A hospice nurse and social worker visited the care facility and offered practical help and guidance for staff, patient, and family in treating Mr. Spence. They talked with him about the future as his condition declined. Comfort-oriented medication and nonpharmacological care were reviewed, offering him as many choices as possible. Emotional, spiritual, and educational support were offered to the family and staff concerning the course of the illness, anticipatory grieving, and ways of using the remaining time to meet goals and nurture relationships. Mr. Spence, assisted by his family and a hospice volunteer, chose to work on a memoir about his illness and its impact on his growth as a person. ■

Hospice care is available to everyone, regardless of age, diagnosis, or the ability to pay. As a general rule, hospice care requires certification by the physician and hospice medical director that the patient is terminally ill with a life expectancy of 6 months or less if the disease runs its normal course. In addition, the patient elects hospice care rather than curative treatments. The Medicare Hospice Benefit currently stipulates two initial 90-day benefit periods followed by an unlimited number of 60-day periods, each requiring physician recertification. Four levels of care are mandated: routine home care, continuous home care (with short-term, around-the-clock nursing care at home), inpatient respite care, and general inpatient care for acute symptom management.

Hospice care includes physician services, nursing and nurse's aide visits, medical equipment, medications and some supplies related to the terminal illness, social work and counseling services, spiritual care, volunteer services, and bereavement services. Limited physical, dietary, speech, and occupational therapies are also available. The Medicare Hospice Benefit (under Medicare Part A) is the dominant source of payment for hospice services (83.7%), with the rest of patients being served by private insurance, Medicaid, self-pay, or charity care. Patients with cancer account for 44.1% of hospice admissions, with the remainder made up of chronic conditions such as cardiac disease, renal disease, neurological illnesses, amyotrophic lateral sclerosis, AIDS, Alzheimer's disease, cirrhosis, leukemia, and others. According to the NHPCO, the median length of stay in hospice care in 2007 was 20 days, and the mean was 67 days (NHPCO, 2008).

Hospice programs accept dying as a natural and inevitable part of life. A personalized plan of care is developed with the patient, reflected in the care, and regularly reviewed and updated by the multidisciplinary team.

NURSING CARE AT THE END OF LIFE

Providing nursing care for the terminally ill and supporting their families in any setting calls for a holistic approach. This holistic approach is a powerful tool in assisting people as they progress through the final stage of life.

Practice the Art of Presence

Caring for patients who are terminally ill requires some shifts in professional expectations. "Whole-person care" involves seeing the patient first and foremost as a human being and being attentive to all aspects of suffering. As front-line medical caregivers, nurses are trained to help patients get better, stronger, and more independent, but patients who are terminally ill are going to grow weaker, sicker, and ultimately die. Thus the nurse's sense of competency and professionalism based on positive results through action must yield to a willingness to embrace the mysteries of the dying process. Paradoxically, the **caring presence** of a health care professional who also feels helpless may bring solace and support to the dying person and the family.

To use the art of presence, two essential skills you can practice are listening and observing. Reflect back to the speaker what you heard by restating or summarizing the message. Observe the patient's nonverbal communications. Do you sense well-being? Sorrow? Suffering? Ask the patient and family open-ended questions like:

- Would you tell me what this is like for you?
- How do you see your condition right now?
- Where do you see things going?
- Are you worried about anything?
- What are you hoping for?

Practice staying silent and giving the patient or family member all the time needed to respond. Offer a reassuring touch. The presence of a caring nurse can invite and permit the patient to discover new dimensions of his or her own experiences, bringing greater wholeness.

Assess for Spiritual Issues

Spirituality, the dimension of human experience that can provide meaning for life, is integral to end-of-life care. To understand how a patient's spirituality may enhance comfort, conducting a comprehensive spiritual assessment is especially important. Patients report that they feel cared about when medical personnel are interested in their spirituality. However, they seem to prefer that such discussions occur in the context of ordinary conversation and human sharing (Hart et al., 2003). Spiritual themes, such as what patients value as meaningful, how they experience intimate connections, and when they have an intensely spiritual moment are often imbedded in ordinary conversations (Stephenson et al., 2003). These themes can provide clues to how an individual defines hope and healing, addressing such questions as: What energizes our lives? What will survive our personal death, if anything? How do we explain to ourselves the things that happen in life? When do we feel most peaceful? How have we surmounted life's hardest challenges? Caregivers can become skilled at listening for the patient's intrinsic spirituality, in addition to thoroughly assessing connections to a specific religion. For many patients, religion provides context, community, and comfort when facing end-of-life challenges. It is interesting to note that intrinsic spirituality—the ability to apply faith beliefs during difficult times—may be a more important indicator of positive bereavement outcomes than religious affiliation alone (Gamino & Sewell, 2004). Box 32-1 provides a spirituality assessment tool developed by a hospice nurse and social worker.

To assess spirituality in health care, the following guidelines (Kramer-Howe & Huls, 2004) may be helpful:

- **Start the conversation.** Allow yourself to be genuinely interested without feeling you have to be an expert or have all the answers. Just listen; ask questions in a spirit of seeking to understand, not to "fix" the patient.

BOX 32-1 Spiritual Assessment Tool: S.H.A.R.E.

Spirituality

What does spirituality mean to you? How would you describe your belief or faith system?

Secular/Spiritual

What is the meaning of what is happening to you in your life?
How do you need to respond?

Religious/Spiritual

What is God's place in what is happening to you?
How do you need to respond?

How Important?

What role does your faith/spirituality have in your life?

Secular/Spiritual

What is most important in your life?
How would your life change if this were taken away?

Religious/Spiritual

What has been most meaningful to you in your faith community?
What is meaningful right now?

Activity

What actions connect you to your beliefs?

Secular/Spiritual

What calms your anxieties?
What puts you in touch with a sense of strength, peace, or hope?

Religious/Spiritual

What faith practices (prayer, music, movement, meditation, etc.) do you use to calm or center yourself?

Relationship

How do your beliefs and values relate to your present circumstances (diagnosis, prognosis, comfort, hope, etc.)?

Secular/Spiritual

Do you think there is a reason why this is happening to you?
Do you feel incomplete about aspects of your life?

Religious/Spiritual

Has this illness changed your relationship with God?
Do you feel incomplete in your relation to your church or faith?
Do you have any unmet needs?

Empower

How can we be most effective in supporting your faith/belief?
If we could do just one thing to help you with this part of your life, what would it be?

Do not seek to fix or answer everything that comes up.

From Kramer-Howe, K., & Huls, P. T. (2004). *A spiritual assessment tool.* Phoenix, AZ: Hospice of the Valley.

- **Remember that this is the patient's story.** Avoid using the lens of your own belief system. This is the patient's and family's framework of values. You are there to learn and support, not to change their spirituality or faith (or lack thereof).
- **Refer to a counselor with spiritual expertise.** There will be times when a patient or family wishes to share with a counselor, or the multidisciplinary team thinks it would be helpful. As a nondenominational pastoral counselor with health care training and end-of-life experience, a hospice or hospital chaplain may be able to bring a perspective that complements formal religion. In other cases, only a representative of the patient's religion can bring the solace that is needed.
- **Hear unspoken questions.** Existential issues may be difficult to communicate in words. These include unspoken questions such as: "Do you know what I am hoping for today?" "Can you tell if I am feeling despair?" "Do you know what brings me courage and peace?" "Can you help calm my fears?" Answers to these questions may be encoded in repeated life stories, dreams, or the patient's reactions to news events, movies, or the behavior of others.
- **Be empowered by the process.** Assessment of patients' spirituality may help nurses explore their own, and they can grow more comfortable hearing and expressing spiritual concepts in everyday language. The care nurses provide will be enhanced by their sensitivity to the patient's unique spiritual story.

Provide Palliative Symptom Management

Excellent symptom management is a hallmark of palliative nursing. The goals of care are determined by the patient and/or the patient's advance directives and medical proxy. Palliative care offers a wide spectrum of interventions to alleviate symptoms, guided by patients' own reports and careful assessment. The most commonly reported end-of-life symptoms are pain, constipation, dyspnea, fatigue, depression, and delirium (Lee & Washington, 2008). It is gratifying to relieve pain or nausea or to give patients control over bowel medications and breathing treatments. For symptoms such as worry, fear, sadness, and low energy, however, better approaches might include education, normalization, counseling, integrative therapies (massage, music), and stress-reduction practices.

Each symptom should be assessed individually. Treatable, reversible, and temporary conditions can be mistakenly attributed to the terminal diagnosis. For example, if a patient reports feeling depressed, it is important to not assume that it is due to the dying process. If the patient becomes confused or lethargic, it is essential to rule out such things as medication effects, dehydration, delirium, urinary tract infections, or constipation before attributing it to terminal decline.

Become an Effective Communicator

The end-of-life care provider has an essential educational role with the family, especially those providing direct care at home. In a 2003 national poll conducted by the Hospice of the Florida Suncoast, 3000 caregivers with a dying or recently deceased family member were asked which kinds of support and information they considered most helpful. Over 900 responses indicated that caregivers value practical information about the illness, how to give medications, what to expect at the time of death, and how to make end-of-life decisions (Florida Policy Exchange Center on Aging & The Hospice Institute of the Florida Suncoast, 2003).

Having information about the patient's condition in preparation for the death has been shown to improve both bereavement outcomes and family satisfaction with hospice care (Rhodes, 2008). During stressful periods, two factors seem to make things more bearable: (1) the ability to have—or believe one can have—some control over the situation and (2) the ability to predict changes. Information and education from the hospice nurse can improve a family's sense of control by enabling them to make the most of the time they have with the patient. Information should be conveyed slowly, given repeatedly, written down, and reviewed often. Communication experts estimate that *people need at least six reiterations of new information when they are under stress.*

Families providing end-of-life care must live with the dual realities of impending death and continued life. The patient or family may ask the nurse questions such as "How long will this go on?" The impossibility of predicting death can create a sense of interminable waiting for patient or family. When the family seeks answers, a two-pronged approach can be helpful:

- Focus the family on the here and now, opportunities to find respite and comfort, and living one day at a time.

- Offer clinical data based on physical examination, and point out any changes from which family and patient can draw some conclusions.

The following vignette illustrates the confusion and misery that can result from lack of information, the desire to take control of one's life situation, and the inadequacy of the term *dying* to describe living with a terminal disease.

VIGNETTE

Susan, a 74-year-old divorced woman living alone, is told by her doctor that she is dying of liver cancer. Upon hearing that she cannot be cured, she assumes she will die in a few days or weeks. She goes home, settles all her affairs, calls everyone she cares about and says goodbye, accepts hospice care, and sits down to await death. As weeks and then months go by, Susan feels betrayed by her doctor, embarrassed to be alive, unsure how to behave, and uncomfortable with her friends and relatives. She has time to begin worrying about how her death will be, how much control she will lose, and how she can afford care at the end. She is confused and even disoriented by the unexpected apparent improvement in her symptoms.

Susan shares her feelings with the hospice nurse. The hospice nurse educates Susan about her cancer and how to interpret her symptoms. The hospice team addresses her emotions and needs in many ways. They encourage her to take a trip she had postponed and to begin seeing friends again. They educate her on the concept of "living with terminal illness" rather than dying from it. Susan needs to learn new approaches to living meaningfully with an uncertain future. When Susan finally enters the end stage of her disease, she is comfortable and cared for by her relatives at home. ■

Counsel About Anticipatory Grieving

Once a life-threatening diagnosis has been received or curative efforts are stopped, many people begin a time of grieving called **anticipatory grief** or *anticipatory mourning* (Rando, 1986). This type of grief is anticipatory in the sense that a future loss is being mourned in advance as people acknowledge the importance of the dying person, adjust their lives to accommodate the intervening time, and foresee how their futures will be altered by the loss.

The experience of anticipatory grief varies by individual, family, and culture. In a recent study of bereaved individuals, anticipatory grieving was described as adjusting one's own life to meet caregiving demands, gathering information and becoming informed, "doing it all" and being overwhelmed at times, and finalizing the connection with the dying person (Clukey, 2007). Aspects of finalizing the connection included spending time together, talking, making memories, life review, saying goodbye (often indirectly or metaphorically), touch, communication, taking care of business, and detaching from one another. A common emotional experience was anger (at the disease, the medical community, others, life), in addition to sadness, hurt, fear, anxiety, and hidden grief. Many people reflected that they did not experience their full grief until the patient died, thereby extinguishing all hope.

Indeed, "anticipatory grief is not simply grief begun in advance, it is different from post-mortem grief both in duration and form" (Fulton, 2003, p. 348). Although the nature and function of this particular type of mourning are still being examined, nurses can reassure families that grieving is normal, even before death, and that many of their distressing feelings can be attributed to grief processes. The following interventions can help the family and patient during this challenging period (Doka, 2001):

- **Validate expressions of anticipatory grief.** Listening, understanding, accepting, and explaining the grieving process can be freeing for the griever. Be open to whatever they are experiencing at that moment, and help them to feel comfortable with healthy expressions of anticipatory grieving.
- **Inform patients and families about the disease and its symptoms.** Assist the family to interpret and accept limitations as inevitable during end-of-life caregiving. This is a difficult time for everyone involved and requires new approaches and understanding. Common patient behaviors such as social withdrawal, mood swings, fatigue, and vacillation between acceptance and denial must be understood by family members as normal and even functional. Similarly, caregiver burden, resentment, and confusion are normal expressions of grief.
- **Invite patients and families to deal with emotional issues.** Encourage appropriate expressions of feelings within the family. Notice and appreciate peoples' expressions of grief, even if they do not match your preconceptions. Feelings can be elicited with phrases such as "Other people in your situation have often told me they felt [sad, guilty, angry, hopeless]. Have you experienced that?"
- **Acknowledge the losses and changes in their lives.** Many losses accumulate gradually and almost imperceptibly. Simply asking, "In what ways has your own life changed since [the diagnosis, the treatments, the ending of treatments, the hospitalization]?" can permit people to identify and begin to cope with these losses and to see how far they have already come.
- **Explore ways of coping.** Examining both productive and unproductive ways of adjusting to change can be helpful. Strategies for using available help, taking time off from caregiving duties, and distracting from grief can increase opportunities for respite and relief for both patient and caregivers.

Anticipatory grieving is a gift of time that "does not decrease or increase the amount of emotion generated by [the death], yet it can help work through feelings in advance and resolve unfinished business before the separation actually occurs" (Shearer & Davidhizar, 1994, p. 62). Box 32-2 lists some signs of anticipatory grief.

Explain the Four Gifts of Resolving Relationships

An important role of the nurse during end-of-life care is to invite families to accept the dying of their loved one and say goodbye. Sometimes this is called "giving permission" for the patient to die, which wrongly implies that family members and loved ones have control over the situation. Perhaps a more accurate description is that they "consent" to the inevitability of death.

Taking the opportunity to say goodbye has been correlated to more positive bereavement outcomes (Gamino & Sewell, 2004). The Four Gifts of Resolving Relationships is one means of opening conversations about the coming separation. The concept of the Four Gifts was interpreted from the writings of Elisabeth Kübler-Ross and used with her permission by Beverly Ryan, LCSW, of the Hospice of the Twin Cities in Minnesota. Dr. Kübler-Ross witnessed many couples and families in her workshops for the terminally ill shift from being distant, cold, or angry to becoming warm, loving, and close. She observed that this change resulted from a predictable sequence of communications, which were later formulated into the Four Gifts. People often intuitively recognize the gifts as processes they have already been experiencing. Perhaps these processes are innate within human relationships, but anxiety, sorrow, and denial can obstruct their expression.

The nurse can describe the gifts in simple terms and encourage families and patients to express them in their own ways. The gifts—forgiveness, love, gratitude, and farewell—can work for both the giver and the receiver. When given with sincerity and simplicity, they can precipitate a healing shift in relationships.

BOX 32-2 Signs of Anticipatory Grief

- Feelings of emptiness or of being lost
- A sense of being numb and fatigued
- A feeling of unreality and disbelief
- Periods of weeping or raging
- A desire to run away from the situation
- A need to protect the patient from suffering or death by overseeing every detail of care
- Worry about the future and the unknown
- Anger at the patient, medical professionals, or both
- Pronounced clinging to or dependency on the patient or other family members
- Fear of going crazy

Forgiveness. The first step is to admit to the wrongs and hurts experienced in the relationship. The intention here is to forgive, seek forgiveness, and release the hurt so healing can occur. Bear in mind two important caveats. One is that sometimes a face-to-face encounter is not possible (the patient is sedated, comatose, or experiencing dementia), and sometimes it is not advisable (it would cause more distress than it would relieve). Reconciliation requires two people who wish to heal a broken relationship. Forgiveness is a one-sided act which can be done unilaterally. The other caveat is that granting forgiveness does not mean condoning or accepting a truly injurious or abusive action. It does not make a wrong right. What it does is signal a desire to let go of blame and anger, to release one's own heart from the chains of resentment. As such, it is a gift to the one who offers forgiveness, whether reconciliation is possible or not.

Love. The second gift is to express love to each other. Many adult children wish to hear their parent say, "I love you, and I am proud of you." In some long-term marriages, these words have faded away to be replaced by daily togetherness and the practical caring of a shared life. It is not uncommon in bereavement for survivors to regret that they did not hear or say the words, "I love you" and long for that final recognition of the relationship's value. Ultimately, the message we need to hear at the end of life is that we are loved for being who we are not for what we have done or achieved.

Gratitude. Expressions of love naturally flow into gratitude for what each has been in the other's life. People look back over life together and remember the good times and the tough times. They can take out photograph albums, show videotapes, reminisce, and listen again to favorite stories. It is especially gratifying to acknowledge the things that were taken for granted. Fathers and husbands may never have been thanked for going to work every day for 30 or 40 years. Wives and mothers might not expect thanks for all the laundry, mending, and help with school projects. Many exhausted caregivers weep when they are told they really are doing a good job and are appreciated.

Farewell. Many people say they hate goodbyes because they bring up feelings of grief at the finality of parting. Also, it is awkward to say goodbye before someone is actually leaving. It may appear to be rushing the person or even causing the departure. Yet when the final separation of death awaits us, the act of saying goodbye is deeply appropriate and meaningful. In cases when there was no chance to say goodbye, or when the opportunity to say goodbye was not taken, survivors may express long-term regret. The words or gestures used do not matter as long as the meaning was adequately expressed.

VIGNETTE

Tom is a 28-year-old man with developmental disabilities and bipolar disorder. He arrives at his dying father's home to see him for the last time. Tom lives in a group home and has not seen his family for many months. The last time he visited, he had not taken his medication, and his behavior caused his family to avoid him. The hospice nurse tells Tom his father is dying and explains the Four Gifts. The young man sadly enters his father's bedroom and sits on the bed. He says, "Dad, I know you are going to die, and I want you to know that I am so sorry for the ways I have acted and the trouble I have caused. Please forgive me, Dad. You have always looked out for me, and I shouldn't have gone off my meds. I love you, Dad. You've never given up on me. Thank you for finding me the place where I live and people to love me and look after me. Thanks for being my Dad. I know I have to say goodbye. I promise I will keep taking my meds so I will behave right. I promise I'll listen to my counselors and have a good life. I love you so much, Dad. Goodbye." He weeps with his father, who holds him for a little while. Then he comes out of the room with a tear-streaked face, knowing he will never see his father alive again. He feels complete, however. He has said the important things with courage and taken proper leave of his father. ■

In the preceding vignette, Tom did not rehearse, resist, or complicate the Four Gifts but used the sequence to express the full range of his feelings. His story illustrates how simple and natural this process can be. Many families need no encouragement to forgive, cherish, thank, and release a loved one. The Four Gifts can be a helpful contribution, however, to families whose members are overwhelmed, cling to false hope, or are emotionally reticent.

Practice Good Self-Care

Finally, the demands inherent in end-of-life nursing lead to increased vulnerability to emotional attachments and compassion fatigue. This, along with daily exposure to grief and dying, calls nurses to practice conscious self-care in both their professional and private lives. Health care personnel naturally grow attached to some patients and may experience both anticipatory grieving and bereavement. To maintain emotional balance and health, it is essential to rely on the support of others and practice good self-care. This is a journey that promotes greater self-understanding, wisdom, and compassion. The multidisciplinary team approach is helpful in this process.

Caring for patients who are dying and those who grieve can bring up personal reactions, which may be triggered by a patient who is younger than the caregiver, resembles a significant person in the nurse's own life, is experiencing symptoms reminiscent of other difficult deaths, or offends the nurse's sense of fairness or acceptability. Workplace conditions such as inappropriate caseloads, rapid turnover in office staff, several losses in a short period of time, or too many demands for on-call time or overtime can intensify a nurse's vulnerability to feeling overwhelmed. Box 32-3 provides guidelines to help the health care professional maintain emotional health when working with death and the dying.

STYLES OF CONFRONTING THE PROSPECT OF DYING: SEVEN MOTIFS

People respond to the prospect of their own death in various ways. Researchers conducted in-depth interviews with individuals who knew they were dying and then searched for patterns of meaning among them. The researchers found seven distinct motifs, that is, "seven cohesive patterns characterizing the ways in which participants viewed the prospect of their own

---

BOX 32-3 Guidelines for Self-Care When Caring for the Dying

1. Remind yourself that what is happening to your patients and their families is not happening to you. This is their life drama right now but not your own.
2. When you notice that you are having a particularly strong emotional reaction, either positive or negative (countertransference), take it as a signal to explore your deeper issues or needs by talking with a trusted friend, counselor, or colleague.
3. Protect your private life by practicing time management, avoiding working outside of normal hours, protecting your pager or home telephone number, and taking regular days off and vacations.
4. Clearly state what you can and cannot do for your patients so your human and professional limitations are known up front.
5. Practice humility. There is much you can do, but there is also much that is unknown and unknowable.
6. Do your own mourning when your heart is touched and you need to acknowledge the importance of others in your life. Even after a person has died, you can honor the relationship you had in your memory. Attend funerals or create grieving rituals when this happens.
7. Create a healthy, balanced private life by releasing stress. Working with patients who are dying creates stresses at many levels. The challenge is to work them into your busy schedule and stay on course. Foremost among these methods are regular exercise, a balanced diet, adequate rest, vacations, fun and laughter, loving and accepting relationships, and a connection to higher meaning in life.

---

death" (Yedidia & MacGregor, 2001, p. 811). These motifs are intriguing and show that people tend to respond to their own deaths in a pattern similar to the way they responded to life.

Dying is not necessarily or solely a crisis of meaning requiring reassessments of the past, new coping skills, or new visions of the future. Rather, it occurs in the context of a lifetime of experience, perception, and ways of assigning meaning. Providing the best care for patients who are dying requires getting to know them in a broader context than simply that of the last stage of life. Judgments about the quality of their deaths should take into account their life motifs rather than anyone else's standards. A "good death" is one that is congruent with a person's personality, whether death is struggled against or met with inner strength and calmness.

The seven motifs and how they might influence a patient's end-of-life reactions are described here briefly, along with nursing interventions that may be helpful for each.

1. **Struggle: Living and dying are a struggle.** For these people, life has been hard and required tremendous effort. They may have dealt with abuse, mental illness, or addiction. Dying is a further manifestation of the struggle. In hospice care, psychotherapeutic efforts to reassess lifelong conflicts would not be successful, but basic safety, caring, affirmation, and comfort can provide a haven of rest.
2. **Dissonance: Dying is not living.** These people reflect positively on their past lives but do not think dying offers anything but the end of their story. They do not seek meaning in dying or wish to adapt to it. It represents an unacceptable quality of life that they hope will be over soon. Because physical symptoms are so unwelcome and burdensome, aggressive pain and symptom management is advised. Life-prolonging care would be unwelcome.
3. **Endurance: Triumph of inner strength.** These people are determined to continue with life on their own terms as they are dying. They take control of their emotions, sustain an upbeat outlook, and wish to be strong in the face of adversity. Introspection or reflection does not interest them. Their strength is more an intrinsic character trait than linked to a belief system. Treatment plans should capitalize on their inner strength, setting outcomes and rewarding challenges met. Their confidence should not be mistaken for denial but should be seen as an affirmation of their identity.
4. **Incorporation: Belief system accommodates death.** These people have a belief system, whether religious or secular, that encompasses both life and death. Although they may regret the timing of their death, they accept it as in accordance with a larger purpose or higher power. It is important

to acknowledge and respect the belief systems of these people and to harmonize it with the plan of care as much as possible.

5. **Coping: Working to find a new balance.** These people work hard to adjust to change; they want to cope and find a new equilibrium in their lives. They do not use a core of inner strength or rely on an overarching belief system. Seeking meaning or resolving old issues does not appeal to them. They try to be realistic and practical. An appropriate intervention would be to acknowledge and support the strength in their coping mechanisms.

6. **Quest: Seeking meaning in dying.** The opportunity to grow and to learn has been paramount throughout these people's lives. Dying presents a final opportunity to derive meaning and growth. They are reflective and exploratory. They value the opportunity to speak about their experiences and to know they are perceived as unique, whole individuals, apart from their age, symptoms, and disabilities.

7. **Volatile: Unresolved and unresigned.** These people have a history of confused, chaotic, and unresolved issues. They lack clarity of direction and express a lack of understanding or control over major forces in their lives. Psychosocial interventions may be welcomed in an effort to understand past conflicts and find relief, but these individuals may not be able to incorporate much purposeful change, and their deaths may engulf them, as have their lives. Acceptance and affirmation of their survival in life and their worthiness in dying can be helpful.

VIGNETTE

Arthur is a 62-year-old married man dying of liver failure brought on by an early life of heavy drug and alcohol use. He vehemently denies any belief in God or anything remotely "spiritual." When asked during a spiritual assessment what has brought him the most joy and sense of freedom in his life, he replies, "Oh, that's easy. Riding my Harley!" Conversely, his greatest loss during these days is not being able to ride his bike. Arthur has had a long illness with plenty of time to prepare himself and his family for a future without him, but when the hospice team visits, he typically leaves the room when death or dying is discussed and will not talk about it with his teenage children. Just before the onset of several days of acute delirium and agitation preceding his death, Arthur shares a dream with his wife that he has had on three consecutive nights. He has experienced himself riding his bike from city to city where he used to live, happily visiting friends and family. His wife uses this powerful image of freedom, joy, and connection to comfort herself and the children while Arthur lies dying and in the months of mourning that follow. ■

Based on the previous vignette, what would you identify as Arthur's dominant life motif? How might that information influence the plan of care, your own feelings as a nurse, and the efforts of the multidisciplinary team?

Using these seven motifs to understand a person's response to dying is just a starting place. Any one individual will use a combination of motifs and be part of a larger social or familial system that will influence responses. These descriptors, however, provide us with a framework within which to consider dying the continuation of an already complex and individualized life. It moves us from the ideal to the real and reminds us that dying is a deeply personal event deserving of dignity, care, and respect.

NURSING CARE FOR THOSE WHO GRIEVE

Loss is part of the human experience, and grieving is the response that enables people to accept and reconcile with the loss and adapt to change. We grieve the commonplace losses in our lives, be they loss of a relationship (divorce, separation, death, abortion), health (a body function or part, mental or physical capacity), a friendship, status or prestige, security (occupational, financial, social, cultural), or a dream. Other normal losses include changes in circumstances, such as retirement, promotion, marriage, and aging. These losses can promote growth through adaptation or may result in apathy, anger, and resentment.

Losing a significant person through death is a major life crisis. Long-term relationships deeply bond us to each other, shaping our world and our identity in it. Their loss can diminish aspects of our own self-concept and tear apart our assumptive world. Grief is experienced holistically, affecting us emotionally, cognitively, spiritually, and physically. Those who grieve sometimes describe the death of a loved one as an amputation. Writer Simone Weil (1998) called it an "almost biological disorder caused by the brutal unloosing of an energy hitherto absorbed by an attachment and now left undirected" (p. 42).

GRIEF REACTIONS, BEREAVEMENT, AND MOURNING

Grief encompasses all of an individual's reactions to loss. Normal grief reactions include depressed mood, insomnia, anxiety, poor appetite, loss of interest, guilt, dreams about the deceased, and poor concentration. Psychological states include shock, denial, and yearning or searching for the deceased. **Bereavement**, derived from the Old English word *berafian*, meaning "to rob," is the period of grieving following a death. **Mourning** refers to things people do to cope with their grief, including shared, social expressions of grief, such as funerals and bereavement groups. Everyone grieves, but not everyone engages in the work of mourning. The length of time, degree, and ritual for mourning are often typically determined by cultural, religious, and familial factors.

The study of human grief and bereavement has evolved over the past 40 years. Research examines questions such as: What constitutes normal, healthy grieving? What are predictors of complicated grief? What interventions, if any, benefit different populations of grieving people? When is medication useful for the bereaved? What is the impact of losses on family systems? What are cultural mediators of delivering grief support? How does complicated or unresolved grief affect public and private health care usage? What are best practices to intervene in special types of loss, such as traumatic loss, genocidal loss, societal loss, and wartime losses?

Models for understanding grief are being clinically tested and refined so health care systems can understand grieving, best utilize limited health care resources, and relieve suffering whenever possible.

Theory

The psychoanalytic model of grieving posits a distinct psychological process that involves disengaging strong emotional ties from a significant relationship and reinvesting those ties in a new and productive direction. This requires engaging in "grief work" that is thought to progress through predictable stages and phases. Since Kübler-Ross's groundbreaking work with the dying in the 1960s, her phases of denial, anger, bargaining, depression, and acceptance (Kübler-Ross 1969) have been identified by many with the stages of grieving. Some other models of grieving emphasize coping skills and adaptive tasks (Worden, 2009), dual processes of coping with bereavement stressors (Stroebe & Schut, 1999), and the potential for personal growth (Gamino & Sewell, 2004).

Therapeutic approaches to grief have drawn from the fields of traumatology (Shear et al., 2005), cognitive stress theory (Stroebe & Schut, 1999) and meaning reconstruction (Neimeyer, 2000). Therapeutic protocols for treating complicated grieving are being field tested (Shear et al., 2005), and other clinical studies are seeking predictors of bereavement adjustment (Gamino & Sewell, 2004). Complicated grief is being evaluated for its relevance to become a distinct diagnostic category (Parkes, 2007).

The goals of mourning have evolved from "doing the grief work, getting over it, and moving on with life." Many now regard mourning as a complex, individual, culturally embedded process of accepting the death, confronting the painful experience of grief, constructing an identity and a life in a transformed environment, and finding an enduring relationship with the deceased, based not on physical presence but on accurate memory. Depending on many factors, this process can take many months to a number of years. Our losses transform our lives, and we are never quite the same person again. Over time, people move from pain defining who they are and constant preoccupation with their loss to living with the residual pain and forever carrying the memory of the loved one.

Dual Process Model of Coping with Bereavement

Bereavement is an enormously challenging life stressor (Table 32-1). Healthy adaptation is crucial for long-term health and reengagement in life. Stroebe and Schut's dual process model (1999) identifies adaptive versus maladaptive coping activities in two interrelated spheres: loss orientation and restoration orientation. Their model attempts to address inadequacies in the "grief work" concept, such as a lack of specificity about grief stressors, cultural bias, favoring intuitive/female expressions of grief over instrumental styles (Martin & Doka, 2000), and discounting the value of denial and distraction in grieving.

In their dynamic model, *loss-oriented stressors* include concentrating on the loss experience, feeling the pain of grief, remembering, and longing. *Restoration-oriented stressors* reengage the mourner with the outer world, as in overcoming loneliness (seeking social support), mastering skills and roles once performed by the deceased person, finding a new identity, and facing many practical details of life. By identifying specific coping activities on both sides of the model, the nurse can strengthen a griever's skills and reinforce positive meanings.

Both orientations assert that denial, avoidance, and distraction from grief are beneficial, as long as they are not excessive. The process of alternating between the two spheres of coping is called *oscillation*. Oscillation is a dynamic process of confronting and avoiding various stressors of bereavement and is postulated to be an indication of healthy adaptation. However, a prolonged moving back and forth between these poles can be seen as an indication of complicated grieving.

Four Tasks of Mourning

Many theorists who have studied the grief process, including George Engel, Colin Parkes, Erich Lindemann, John Bowlby, and J. William Worden, have identified similar, commonly experienced psychological and behavioral phenomena, including:
- Shock and disbelief
- Sensation of somatic distress
- Preoccupation with the image of the deceased
- Guilt
- Anger
- Change in behavior (e.g., depression, disorganization, or restlessness)
- Reorganization of behavior directed toward a new object or activity

TABLE 32-1 Phenomena Experienced During Bereavement

Symptoms	Examples
SENSATIONS OF SOMATIC DISTRESS	
The bereaved may experience tightness in the throat, shortness of breath, sighing, mental pain, or exhaustion; food tastes like sand; things feel unreal. Pain or discomfort may be identical to the symptoms experienced by the dead person. Normally, symptoms are brief.	A woman whose husband died of a stroke complains of weakness and numbness on her left side.
PREOCCUPATION WITH THE IMAGE OF THE DECEASED	
The bereaved brings up and thinks and talks about numerous memories of the deceased. The memories are positive. This process goes on with great sadness. The idealization of the deceased lets the bereaved relive the gratifications associated with the deceased and helps resolve any guilt the bereaved feels concerning the deceased. The bereaved may also take on many of the mannerisms of the deceased through identification. Identification serves the purpose of holding on to the deceased. Preoccupation with the dead person can continue for many months before it lessens.	A man whose wife has recently died states, "I just can't stop thinking about my wife. Everything I see reminds me of her. We picked up this seashell on our honeymoon. I remember every wonderful moment we had together. The pain is so great, but the memories just keep coming." His friends notice that when he talks, his hand gestures and expressions are like those of his recently deceased wife.
GUILT	
The bereaved reproaches himself or herself for real or fancied acts of negligence or omissions in the relationship with the deceased.	"I should have made him go to the doctor sooner." "I should have paid more attention to her, been more thoughtful."
ANGER	
The anger the bereaved experiences may not be toward the object that gives rise to it. Often the anger is displaced onto the medical or nursing staff. Often it is directed toward the deceased. The anger is at its height during the first month but is often intermittent throughout the first year. The overflow of hostility disturbs the bereaved, resulting in the feeling that he or she is "going insane."	"The doctor didn't operate in time. If he had, Mary would be alive today." "How could he leave me like this … how could he?"
CHANGE IN BEHAVIOR: DEPRESSION, DISORGANIZATION, RESTLESSNESS	
A person may exhibit marked restlessness and an inability to organize his or her behavior. A depressive mood during routine activities is common, decreasing as the year passes and the intensity of the grief declines. Absence of depression is more abnormal than its presence. Loneliness and aimlessness are most pronounced 6 to 9 months after the death.	Six months after her husband died, Mrs. Faye states, "I just can't seem to function. I have a hard time doing the simplest tasks. I can't be bothered with socializing. I feel so down … so, so empty."
REORGANIZATION OF BEHAVIOR DIRECTED TOWARD A NEW OBJECT OR ACTIVITY	
Gradually, the person renews his or her interest in people and activities. The grieving thus releases the bereaved from one interpersonal relationship, and new ones are free to take its place.	Twenty months after her husband's death, Mrs. Faye tells a friend, "I'll be away this weekend. I am going fishing with my brother and his friend. This is the first time I've felt like doing anything since Harry died."

Worden organizes aspects of mourning into four tasks: (1) accept the reality of the loss, (2) experience the pain of grief, (3) adjust to an environment without the loved one (externally, internally, and spiritually), and (4) relocate and memorialize the loved one. He emphasizes that every loss must be assessed according to mediating factors such as the nature of the person who died, the nature of the attachment, the circumstances of the death, personality factors, family history, social circumstances, and concurrent changes resulting from the death (Worden, 2009). His model can be readily understood by the mourner as empowering and hopeful and serves as a specific guide for the nurse providing counseling or therapy.

Maladaptive Grieving

Worden also describes the ways in which some people fail to grieve adaptively (chronic grief, delayed grief, exaggerated grief, and masked grief reactions) and outlines therapeutic approaches for each. There are some similarities and important differences between complicated grief and major depression and posttraumatic stress disorder (PTSD). These differences suggest that complicated grief might one day constitute its own diagnostic category in the 5th edition of the *Diagnostic and Statistical Manual of Mental Disorders.* Bereavement exacerbates preexisting medical or psychiatric problems, and treatment needs to be both specific and multidimensional. Proposed diagnostic criteria for complicated grief are: (1) persistent pining for a lost person, (2) grief that lasts a period of 6 months or more after the death, and (3) bereavement that seriously impairs the mourner's ability to function in domestic and occupational roles (Parkes, 2007).

VIGNETTE

On a large, extended-family picnic, Mr. and Mrs. Lopez's youngest child was accidently crushed by the tires of a relative's truck as it backed up. The 3-year-old died in her parents' arms on the way to the hospital. Many family members, including the older siblings of the toddler, witnessed the event. After 6 months, the Lopez family was still in chaos and shock. Mrs. Lopez, especially, was unable to resume normal responsibilities. Her husband had returned to work and did his best to support her. The surviving children were exhibiting behavioral problems. The Lopezes sought out a grief counselor and attended support groups. The mixture of horror, shock, anger, disbelief, grief, and senselessness that engulfed them made their mourning complicated. Gradually some of the feelings softened, and the family began to regain some stable routines. After 2 years, Mrs. Lopez had progressed to the point of organizing support networks in her daughter's name for parents whose children had suffered similar deaths. ▪

Indications that a person may have the potential for dysfunctional grieving may be determined by careful assessment. Factors that can complicate bereavement are:

- Heavy emotional dependence on the deceased
- Unresolved conflicts between the bereaved and the deceased
- Young age of the deceased (often the most profound loss) or of the bereaved

- Lack of a meaningful relationship or support system
- A history of previous losses
- A lack of sound coping skills
- A death that was associated with a cultural stigma (e.g., acquired immunodeficiency syndrome, suicide)
- A death that was unexpected or associated with violence (e.g., murder, suicide)
- A history of depression, drug or alcohol abuse, or other psychiatric illness

Complicated grieving essentially means that the grief work is unresolved. Prolonged depression is the most common response to unresolved grief. Disturbances in mood are associated with biological changes in the body during stress-related depressive illness. Some examples include electrolyte disturbance, nervous system alterations, and faulty regulation of the autonomic nervous system. Always assess the potential for suicide. Box 32-4 offers guidelines that can help people and their families cope with bereavement. Table 32-2 identifies common grief experiences and describes the pathological intensification of these phenomena that indicates the need for psychotherapy.

Sometimes an individual experiences an intense loss that is not congruent with a socially recognized and sanctioned relationship—for example, the role of lover, caregiver, roommate, coworker, counselor, or health care worker. Typically these mourners do not have the opportunity to publicly grieve the loss. Doka (1989) refers to these experiences as **disenfranchised grief**—"the grief a person experiences when they incur a loss that is not and cannot be openly acknowledged, publicly mourned, or socially supported." This might include the grief felt by health care workers over the loss of a patient, as well as grief over deaths by abortion or miscarriage, suicide and substance abuse, deaths of friends, divorced partners, and even animal companions. To acknowledge and recognize such losses can help the griever begin the work of mourning.

Grief Engendered by Public Tragedy

Another kind of loss can be caused by public tragedies. Public tragedies involve a loss whose impact is felt broadly across a community or the general public. Because of the scale of the loss, many are affected, and the events often involve strong elements of surprise and shock (Corr, 2003). Common public tragedies include, among others:

- Terrorist attacks
- Assassinations
- Tornados, earthquakes, or flooding
- Large-scale wildfires
- School or work shootings

BOX 32-4 Guidelines for Dealing With Bereavement

Take the time you need to grieve. The hard work of grief uses psychological energy. Resolution of the numb state that occurs after loss requires a few weeks at least. A minimum of 1 year, to cover all the birthdays, anniversaries, and other important dates without your loved one, is normal before you can learn to live with your loss.

Express your feelings. Remember that anger, anxiety, loneliness, and even guilt are common grief reactions and that everyone needs a safe place to express them. Tell your personal story of loss as many times as you need to—this repetition is a helpful and necessary part of the grieving process. Trusted friends, bereavement groups, and counselors will continue to listen.

Establish a structure for each day and stick to it. Although it is hard to do, keeping to some semblance of structure makes the first few weeks after a loss easier. Getting through each day helps restore the confidence you need to accept the reality of loss.

Don't feel that you have to answer all the questions asked you. Although most people try to be kind, they may be unaware of their insensitivity. Down the road, you may want to read books about how others have dealt with similar circumstances. They often have helpful suggestions for a person in your situation.

As hard as it is, try to take good care of yourself. Eat well, talk with friends, get plenty of rest. Be sure to let your primary care clinician know if you are having trouble eating or sleeping. Make use of exercise. It can help you let out pent-up frustrations. If you are losing weight, sleeping excessively or intermittently, or still experiencing deep depression after 3 months, be sure to seek professional assistance.

Expect grief triggers and setbacks. You may begin to feel a bit better, only to have a brief emotional collapse. These are expectable reactions. Moreover, you may find that you dream about, visualize, think about, or search for your loved one. This too is a part of the grieving process.

Give yourself time. Don't feel that you have to resume all of life's duties right away.

Make use of rituals. Those who take the time to say goodbye at a funeral or a viewing tend to find that it helps the bereavement process. Continuing to remember and commune with your loved one's picture or memory during certain times of the day or week can be a comfort.

If you do not begin to feel better within a few weeks, at least for a few hours every day, be sure to tell your doctor. If you have had an emotional problem in the past (e.g., depression, substance abuse), be sure to get the additional support you need. Losing a loved one puts you at higher risk for a relapse of these disorders.

From Zerbe, K. J. (1999). *Women's mental health in primary care* (pp. 207-208). Philadelphia: Saunders.

TABLE 32-2 Common Experiences During Grief and Their Pathological Intensification

Phenomenon	Typical Response	Pathological Intensification
Dying	Emotional expression and immediate coping with the dying process	Avoidance; feeling of being overwhelmed, dazed, confused; self-punitive feelings; inappropriately hostile feelings
Death and outcry	Outcry of emotions with news of the death and turning for help to others or isolating self with self-soothing	Panic; dissociative reactions, reactive psychoses
Warding off (denial)	Avoidance of reminders and social withdrawal, focusing elsewhere, emotional numbing, not thinking of implications to self or of certain themes	Maladaptive avoidance of confronting the implications of death; drug or alcohol abuse, promiscuity, fugue states, phobic avoidance, feeling of being dead or unreal
Reexperience (intrusion)	Intrusive experiences, including recollections of negative experiences during relationship with the deceased, bad dreams, reduced concentration, compulsive reenactments	Flooding with negative images and emotions; uncontrolled ideation, self-impairing compulsive reenactments, night terrors, recurrent nightmares, distraught feelings resulting from the intrusion of anger, anxiety, despair, shame, or guilt; physiological exhaustion resulting from hyperarousal

Continued

TABLE 32-2 Common Experiences During Grief and Their Pathological Intensification—cont'd

Phenomenon	Typical Response	Pathological Intensification
Working through	Recollection of the deceased and a contemplation of self with reduced intrusiveness of memories and fantasies and with increased rational acceptance, reduced numbness and avoidance, more "dosing" of recollections, and a sense of working it through	Feeling of inability to integrate the death with a sense of self and continued life; persistent warding-off themes that may manifest as anxious, depressed, enraged, shame-filled, or guilty moods and psychophysiological syndromes
Completion	Reduction in emotional swings and a sense of self-coherence and readiness for new relationships; ability to experience positive states of mind	Failure to complete mourning, which may be associated with inability to work or create or to feel emotion or positive states of mind

From Horowitz, M. J. (1990). A model of mourning: Change in schemas of self and others. *Journal of the American Psychoanalytic Association, 38* (2), 297–324.

In any grief and loss assessment, it is important to explore the impact of public tragedies. As with other losses, acknowledging and validating the personal impact of the loss can be therapeutic.

Helping People Cope with Loss

The majority of people who suffer bereavement are resilient and recover from the experience. After decades of pathologizing grief, researchers are now examining healthy grief to find out what characterizes people who recover well in bereavement and even show positive personal growth. In an ongoing grief study at Texas A&M Health Science Center College of Medicine, information from mourners is being analyzed both quantitatively and qualitatively. Four constructs (Gamino & Sewell, 2004) that support personal growth are:

1. Seeing some good resulting from the death
2. Continuing the connection with the deceased
3. Invoking intrinsic spirituality to understand the death and aftermath
4. Going forward with life

For some resilient grievers, limited counseling support seems to be helpful (Grimby & Johansson, 2008), focusing on grief education, normalizing of experiences, and skilled supportive presence. Helpful interventions include writing letters (both to and from the deceased), performing simple rituals and ceremonies, "dosing" times of grieving throughout the day or week, working on projects to memorialize the deceased (planting a tree or creating a website), and planning ahead for holidays and anniversary dates.

Telling the story repeatedly is therapeutic for the bereaved. Active listening can assist in healing. Tschudin (1997) states that "listening and not talking, not interrupting, being comfortable with silence when indicated, and using prompts like 'go on,' etc.,

to encourage the person to continue talking" (p. 105) are the most helpful behaviors. It is important to avoid clichés, advice giving, comparisons to other losses, or statements that minimize the loss (see Chapter 10 for detailed discussion of communication techniques). Table 32-3 provides guidelines for helping people grieve, and Table 32-4 offers guidelines for communicating with a person suffering a profound loss.

Palliative Care for Patients with Dementia

Dementia is a leading cause of death among older adults in the United States; therefore, all caregivers should receive education on the unique elements of palliative dementia care in order to increase comfort and enhance quality of life. Persons with advanced dementia experience significant impairments in insight, language, and judgment, limiting their ability to communicate unmet needs and desires. Imagine not being able to convey that you were uncomfortable, had to urinate, or wanted to be some place quiet rather than a crowded day hall. Difficult behaviors such as irritability or refusal to cooperate with care are often a form of communication indicating discomfort in body, mind, or spirit. When caregivers use an *anticipatory* approach to care, they can frequently prevent or reduce behaviors that result when a person with dementia is unable to communicate important unmet needs.

Caregivers must remember to focus on the person, rather than the disease, and recognize the numerous opportunities that arise with every interaction to affirm the meaning of the individual's life, uphold dignity, and provide pleasurable sensory and spiritual experiences. The goal is to create meaningful connections for these patients. One effective method for customizing care that honors the unique preferences and

TABLE 32-3 Guidelines for Helping People in Acute Grief

Intervention	Rationale
Give your full presence: Use appropriate eye contact, attentive listening, and appropriate touch.	Talking is one of the most important ways of dealing with acute grief. Listening patiently helps the bereaved express all feelings, even ones he or she feels are "negative." Appropriate eye contact helps to convey the awareness that you are there and are sharing the person's sadness. Suitable human touch can express warmth and nurture healing. Inappropriate touch can leave a person confused and uncomfortable.
Be patient with the bereaved in times of silence. Do not fill silence with empty chatter.	Sharing painful feelings during periods of silence is healing and conveys your concern.
Know about and share with the bereaved information about the phenomena that occur during the normal mourning process, because they may concern some people (intense anger at the deceased, guilt, symptoms the deceased had before death, unbidden floods of memories). Give the bereaved support during the occurrence of these phenomena and a written handout to refer to.	Although the knowledge will not eliminate the emotions, it can greatly relieve a person who is thinking there is something wrong with having these feelings.
Encourage the support of family and friends. If no supports are available, refer the patient to a community bereavement group. (Bereavement groups are helpful even when a person has many friends or much family support.)	Friends can help with routine matters—for example: • Getting food into the house • Making phone calls • Driving to the mortuary • Taking care of the kids or other family members
Offer spiritual support and referrals when needed.	Dealing with an illness or catastrophic loss can cause the most profound spiritual anguish.
When intense emotions are in evidence, show understanding and support (see Table 32-4).	Empathetic words that reflect acceptance of a bereaved individual's feelings are healing.

lifelong interests of the patient is to use some form of life story or About Me form (Dougherty et al., 2007). This abbreviated biography guides and informs care to enhance the patient's enjoyment of life's simple pleasures.

It is also important to address health care decisions for advanced dementia such as resuscitation, hospitalizations, antibiotics, and nutrition/hydration. Health care providers should (1) identify the patient's goals for care and consider educating the family to minimize aggressive medical interventions, (2) eliminate medications that may detract from safety or quality of life, and (3) proactively manage issues such as pain and depression.

Families and friends spend a significant amount of time, finances, and emotions caring for a loved one with dementia. It is important to recognize and support the role of family caregivers as they navigate the day-to-day challenges and cope with many losses. The Marwit-Meuser Caregiver Grief Inventory (Marwit & Meuser, 2002) is a tool developed to identify the unique forms of grief experienced by caregivers of those with dementia.

IMPLICATIONS FOR FURTHER STUDY

We are emerging from a time when many grievers have been pathologized and treated with psychotropic drugs for depression, anxiety, and sleep disorders. A recent study found that compassionate primary caregivers, seeing symptoms of acute grief such as crying and sleep disturbances in their older adult patients, spontaneously prescribed benzodiazepines, contrary to all major guidelines on the subject (Cook et al., 2007). On the other end of the spectrum, grief has been overlooked by many health care providers as a possible underlying contributor to their patients' presenting problems. Internationally, grief recovery models are being adapted to diverse cultures to assist traumatized people, especially children and youth, begin to heal and reengage with life, hope, and the future. There is a growing urgency for practitioners to become knowledgeable and skilled at supporting human mourning in all health care settings. The realization of full human health and happiness may depend on it.

TABLE 32-4 Guidelines for Communication with a Bereaved Person

Situation	Sample Response
When you sense an over-whelming *sorrow*	"This must hurt terribly."
When you hear *anger* in the bereaved's voice	"I hear anger in your voice. Most people go through periods of anger when their loved one dies. Are you feeling angry now?"
If you discern *guilt*	"Are you feeling guilty? This is a common reaction many people have. What are some of your thoughts about this?"
If you sense a *fear* of the future	"It must be scary to go through this."
When the bereaved seems *confused*	"This can be a bewildering time."
In almost *any painful situation*	"This must be very difficult for you."

Adapted from Robinson, D. (1997). *Good intentions: The nine unconscious mistakes of nice people* (p. 249). New York: Warner Books.

KEY POINTS TO REMEMBER

- The hospice movement offers compassionate care for those who are dying. Hospice and palliative care focus on patients' physical and emotional comfort and offer holistic support for dying persons and their families.
- More hospitals are offering palliative expertise for end-of-life care, but in many hospitals, conflict continues to exist between the wishes of dying persons and their families and the medical model of treatment that focuses on the prolongation of life.
- In work with the terminally ill, nursing goals include providing physical and emotional comfort, helping with adjustments in lifestyle and relationships, and offering spiritual support. Health care workers need to shift their thinking so as to see the value of providing a caring human presence even in the face of helplessness.
- When providing end-of-life care to persons with dementia, challenging behaviors may communicate discomfort in mind, body, or spirit. Care should focus on providing meaningful connections with patients and between family members and their loved one.
- People who work with the dying need to maintain their own emotional health. End-of-life care is usually delivered by multidisciplinary teams so that no one discipline bears too much responsibility. Nurses need to learn to draw on team support, protect their private lives by setting clear personal boundaries, and recognize their human and professional limitations.
- Providing timely and ongoing information about the disease and its effects and about physical and psychological signs of death can help the family deal with anticipatory mourning.
- Health care workers involved in care of the dying can teach families communication skills, such as the Four Gifts of Resolving Relationships, that will help them to express love, share memories, say goodbye, and provide a sense of peace.
- Family members may experience anticipatory grief, and it is helpful for them to understand that it is normal, although difficult. It can be helpful to understand that the way an individual confronts dying usually harmonizes with the ways he or she has faced other important aspects of life.
- So that plans of treatment and approaches can be truly individualized, seven motifs have been proposed to sensitize health care workers to the different ways individuals deal with their impending death.
- Grief and mourning are distinct holistic processes and normal reactions to a loss, real or perceived, including the loss of a person, loss of security, loss of self-confidence, and loss of a dream. Essentially, a loss results in a change in self-concept.
- Common phenomena are evident during the experience of grief, and mourning is greatly influenced by cultural norms. However, everyone's experience of grieving is shaped by many mediating factors, such as the relationship to the person who died and the capacities of the mourner.
- Indicators of the potential for complicated or unresolved grief include social isolation, extensive dependency on the deceased person, unresolved interpersonal conflicts, loss of a child, violent and senseless death, and/or a catastrophic loss.
- Grief work is successful when the relationship to the deceased person has been restructured, energy is available for new relationships and life pursuits, and the mourner can remember realistically both the pleasures and the disappointments of the lost relationship. Outcomes for successful grief work have been identified.

CRITICAL THINKING

1. George is dying of pancreatic cancer. His wife and adult children are asking about using hospice. Help George's family to make an informed decision by comparing and contrasting the hospice model of care with the medical model of care for dying persons.

2. How can you use the Four Gifts in working with the families of dying people in your practice of nursing? Do you think you would find this a useful tool for a personal family member in the future?

3. What are some concrete ways in which you can help another to cope with a loss? Identify specific components in the following areas:
   A. How can you let the person tell his or her story, and what is the potential therapeutic value of doing so?
   B. Avoiding banal (overused or trite) advice, what are some things you might say that could offer comfort? Use the guidelines in Table 32-3 and Table 32-4 to describe how you would help a person who is suffering a profound loss.

CHAPTER REVIEW

1. The nurse is caring for a patient who is grieving. The patient has stated she is angry that she has been diagnosed with terminal cancer. Which behavior should the nurse anticipate next as the patient reconciles her anger?
   1. Denial that she has cancer
   2. Depression over the diagnosis of cancer
   3. Acceptance that her cancer is a reality
   4. Begging God to remove the cancer from her body

2. The nurse is planning hospice care for a dying patient. Which outcome is most appropriate?
   1. Patient will regain health
   2. Patient will remain pain-free
   3. Patient will not fear death
   4. Patient will decline all medications

3. Which patient statement regarding spirituality would require further nursing teaching?
   1. "I am not religious, so therefore I am not spiritual."
   2. "Death scares me."
   3. "My family is what gives my life meaning."
   4. "I believe in a higher power."

4. The nurse identifies that a patient is experiencing dysfunctional grieving related to the loss of her spouse. Which evaluation finding would indicate that a treatment plan is appropriate? The patient:
   1. no longer thinks of her spouse.
   2. copes without the need for a support system.
   3. states she should have taken her spouse to the doctor more often.
   4. laughs occasionally with her grandchildren.

5. The nurse is caring for a patient whose partner—with whom she was having an affair—died suddenly after a myocardial infarction. The patient had told no one about the affair, so no friends or family were aware that she experienced a loss. How should the nurse document the patient's grieving?
   1. Disenfranchised grief
   2. Dysfunctional grief
   3. Maladaptive grief
   4. Normal bereavement

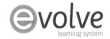

Visit the Evolve website for an **Audio Chapter Summary, Chapter Review Answers & Rationales, Critical Thinking Answer Guidelines,** and additional resources related to the content in this chapter: **http://evolve.elsevier.com/Varcarolis/foundations**

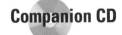 **Companion CD**   Use the Companion CD to prepare for tests and the NCLEX® Examination with **Test-Taking Strategies** for psychiatric mental health nursing and hundreds of **Review Questions.**

REFERENCES

Clukey, L. (2007). Just be there: hospice caregivers' anticipatory mourning experience. *Journal of Hospice and Palliative Nursing, 9*(3), 150–158.

Cook, J. M., Marshall, R., Masci, C., & Coyne, J. C. (2007). Physicians' perspectives on prescribing benzodiazepines for older adults: A qualitative study. *Journal of General Internal Medicine, 22*(3), 303–307.

Corr, C. A. (2003). Loss, grief, and trauma in public tragedy. In M. Lattanzi-Light & K. J. Doka (Eds.), *Living with grief: Coping with public tragedy* (pp. 63–76). Washington, DC: Hospice Foundation of America.

Doka, K. (1989). *Disenfranchised grief—Recognizing hidden sorrows.* New York: Lexington.

Doka, K. (2001). Grief, loss, and caregiving. In K. Doka & J. Davidson (Eds.), *Caregiving and loss.* Washington, DC: Hospice Foundation of America.

Dougherty, J., Gallagher, M., Cabral, D., Long, C. O., & McLean, A. (2007). About me: Knowing the person with advanced dementia. *Alzheimer's Care Quarterly, 8*(1), 12–16.

Florida Policy Exchange Center on Aging and The Hospice Institute of the Florida Suncoast. (2003, June). *Caregiving at life's end: The national needs assessment and implications for hospice practice.* Tampa and Largo, FL: Authors.

Fulton, R. (2003). Anticipatory mourning: A critique of the concept. *Mortality, 8,* 342–351.

Gamino, L. A., & Sewell, K. W. (2004). Meaning constructs as predictors of bereavement adjustment: A report from the Scott and White Grief Study. *Death Studies, 28,* 397–421.

Grimby, A., & Johansson, A. K. (2008). Does early bereavement counseling prevent ill health and untimely death? *American Journal of Hospice and Palliative Medicine, 24,* 475–478.

Hart, A., Kohlwes, R. J., Deyo, R., Rhodes, L. A., & Bowen, D. J. (2003). Hospice clients' attitudes regarding spiritual discussions with their doctors. *American Journal of Hospice and Palliative Care, 20*(2), 135–139.

Kramer-Howe, K., & Huls, P. T. (2004). *A spiritual assessment tool.* Phoenix, AZ: Hospice of the Valley.

Kübler-Ross, E. (1969). *On death and dying.* New York: Macmillan.

Lee, N. P., & Washington, G. (2008). Management of common symptoms at end of life in acute care settings. *Journal of Nurse Practitioners, 4,* 610–615.

Martin, T. L., & Doka, K. J. (2000). *Men don't cry...women do: Transcending gender stereotypes of grief.* Philadelphia: George A. Buchanan.

Marwit, S. J., & Meuser, T. M. (2002). Development and initial validation of an inventory to assess grief in caregivers of persons with Alzheimer's Disease. *The Gerontologist, 42,* 751–765.

National Hospice and Palliative Care Organization. (2008). *Hospice fact sheet.* Alexandria, VA: Author. Retrieved May 6, 2009, from http://www.nhpco.org/files/public/Statistics_Research/NHPCO_facts-and-figures_2008.pdf

National Hospice and Palliative Care Organization. (n.d.). What is hospice and palliative care. Retrieved May 5, 2009, from http://www.nhpco.org/i4a/pages/index.cfm?pageid=4648&openpage=4648

Neimeyer, R. A. (2000). The language of loss: Grief therapy as a process of meaning reconstruction. In R.A. Neimeyer (Ed.), *Meaning reconstruction and the experience of loss* (pp. 261–292). Washington DC: American Psychological Association.

Parkes, C. M. (2007). Complicated grief: The debate over a new *DSM-V* diagnostic category. In K. Doka (Ed.), *Living with grief: Before and after the death.* Washington, DC: Hospice Foundation of America.

Rando, T. A. (Ed.). (1986). *Loss and anticipatory grief.* Lexington, MA: Lexington Books.

Rhodes, R. L., Mitchell, S. L., Miller, S. C., Connor, S. R., & Teno, J. M. (2008). Bereaved family members' evaluation of hospice care: What factors influence overall satisfaction with services? *Journal of Pain and Symptom Management, 35*(4), 365–371.

Shear, K., Frank, E., Houck, P. R., & Reynolds, C. F. (2005). Treatment of complicated grief: A randomized study. *Journal of the American Medical Association, 293,* 2601–2608.

Shearer, R., & Davidhizar, R. (1994). It can never be the way it was. *Home Health Care Nurse, 12*(4), 60–65.

Stephenson, P., Draucker, C., & Martsolf, D. (2003). The experience of spirituality in the lives of hospice clients. *Journal of Hospice and Palliative Nursing, 5*(1), 51–58.

Stolberg, S. G. (1999, May 11). A conversation with Dame Cicely Saunders: Reflecting on a life of treating the dying. *New York Times,* Health and Fitness Section.

Stroebe, M., & Schut, H. (1999). The dual-process model of coping with bereavement: Rationale and description. *Death Studies, 23*(3), 197–224.

Teno, J. M., Clarridge, B.R., Casey, V., Welch, L. C., Wetle, T., Shield, R., et al. (2004). Family perspectives on end-of-life care at the last place of care. *Journal of the American Medical Association, 291*(1), 88–93.

Tschudin, V. (1997). *Counseling for loss and bereavement.* London: Baillière Tindall.

Weil, S. (1998). *Simone Weil: Writings selected with an introduction by Eric Springsted.* New York: Orbis Books.

Worden, J. W. (2009). *Grief counseling and grief therapy* (4th ed.). New York: Springer.

Yedidia, M., & MacGregor, B. (2001). Confronting the prospect of dying: Reports of terminally ill clients. *Journal of Pain and Symptom Management, 22,* 807–819.

CHAPTER 33

Forensic Psychiatric Nursing

L. Kathleen Sekula, Alison M. Colbert, and Judith W. Coram

Key Terms and Concepts

advanced practice forensic nurse, 726
competency evaluator, 729
consultant, 730
correctional nursing, 731
criminal profiler, 730
expert witness, 729
fact witness, 729
forensic nurse examiner, 728

forensic nurse generalist, 726
forensic nursing, 725
forensic psychiatric nurse, 727
hostage negotiator, 730
legal sanity, 729
nurse coroner/death investigator, 727
sexual assault nurse examiner (SANE), 727

Objectives

1. Define forensic nursing, forensic psychiatric nursing, and correctional nursing.
2. Describe the educational preparation required for the forensic nurse generalist and the advanced practice forensic nurse.
3. Identify the functions of forensic nurses.
4. Discuss the specialized roles in forensic nursing.
5. Identify three roles of psychiatric nurses in the specialty of forensic nursing.
6. Discuss the differences between a fact witness and an expert witness.
7. Compare and contrast the roles of forensic nurses and correctional nurses.

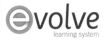 Visit the Evolve website for an **Audio Glossary & Flashcards, Concept Map Creator**, and additional resources related to the content in this chapter: **http://evolve.elsevier.com/Varcarolis/foundations**

According to the *World Report on Violence and Health* (World Health Organization [WHO], 2002), over 1.6 million people worldwide lose their lives annually to self-directed (suicide), interpersonal, or collective (societal) violence. In the United States, crime accounts for more deaths, injuries, and loss of property than all natural disasters combined (Disaster Center, 2007). Approximately 13 million people (5% of the U.S. population) are victims of crime on a yearly basis, and of those crimes, 1½ million are violent. Box 33-1 lists *Healthy People 2010* goals for preventing injury and violence in the United States (U.S. Department of Health & Human Services [USDHHS], 2000).

Forensics (an abbreviation derived from *forensic science*) is an umbrella term that refers to legal issues or working with the courts. In recent years, nurses formalized a broad category called *forensic nursing*, which brings together components of traditional nursing care and legal issues to serve victims and perpetrators of violence. In this chapter, we will explore a variety of roles that registered nurses assume within the legal system.

FORENSIC NURSING

The International Association of Forensic Nurses (IAFN) (2006b) defines **forensic nursing** as:
- The application of nursing science to public or legal proceedings
- The application of the forensic aspects of health care combined with the bio-psycho-social education of the registered nurse in the scientific investigation and treatment of trauma and/or death of victims and perpetrators of abuse, violence, criminal activity, and traumatic accidents.

BOX 33-1 *Healthy People 2010* **Goals: Injury and Violence Prevention**

- Reduce homicides.
- Reduce maltreatment and maltreatment fatalities of children.
- Reduce the rate of physical assault by current or former intimate partners.
- Reduce the annual rate of rape or attempted rape.
- Reduce sexual assault other than rape.
- Reduce physical assaults.
- Reduce physical fighting among adolescents.
- Reduce weapon carrying by adolescents on school property.

U.S. Department of Health and Human Services. (2000). *Injury and violence prevention.* <http://www.healthypeople.gov/Data/midcourse/html/focusareas/FA15Introduction.htm> Accessed 26.02.2009.

Forensic nurses provide direct services to crime victims and perpetrators of crime and consultation services to colleagues in nursing-, medical-, and law-related agencies. Other services provided by forensic nurses include expert court testimony in cases of trauma and/or questioned death, adequacy of service delivery, and specialized diagnoses of specific conditions as related to nursing.

The IAFN was formed in 1992 when 74 nurses—most of whom were sexual assault nurse examiners (SANEs)—came together to create an organization to represent nurses whose practice overlapped with key areas of forensic science and law (IAFN, 2006a). The group currently represents nurses who are forensic nurse generalists, SANEs, forensic psychiatric nurses, death investigators, coroners, correctional nurse specialists, and those in other forensic nursing specialties that continue to evolve. A year after its creation, the organization had more than tripled in size, and by 2008, the IAFN's membership had grown to more than 3000 nurses (IAFN, 2006a). The ANA officially recognized forensic nursing as a specialty practice area in 1995 and combined efforts with the IAFN to develop the *Scope and Standards of Forensic Nursing* in 1997.

The goals of the IAFN (2006a) are:
- To incorporate primary prevention strategies into our work at every level in an attempt to create a world without violence.
- To establish and improve standards of evidence-based forensic nursing practice.
- To promote and encourage the exchange of ideas and transmission of developing knowledge among its members and related disciplines.
- To establish standards of ethical conduct for forensic nurses.
- To create and facilitate educational opportunities for forensic nurses and related disciplines.

In the United States, there is no standard method of uniformly credentialing forensic nurses, so a variety of designations are used to describe their educational preparation and roles.

Education

Educational programs have been developed to prepare nurses for a career in forensic nursing. The IAFN calls for the incorporation of forensic content at all levels of nursing education. As students become more knowledgeable about forensic issues in the care of all patients, more graduate programs are offered that focus the nurse on forensic practice as a specialty area. The methods for acquiring forensic nurse training occur at all academic levels.

Forensic Nurse Generalist

To be called a **forensic nurse generalist**, the nurse with a baccalaureate or associate degree or diploma may acquire additional knowledge and skills by completing a certificate program that comprises continuing education in the area of forensic nursing. Nurses can also gain expertise by taking secondary education electives and/or pursuing a minor in legal topics.

The role of the forensic nurse generalist may vary according to clinical setting, but consistent within this role is the need to be proficient in assessment and treatment of victims of violence, evidence collection and preservation, proper documentation, the legal system, and setting standards of care for victims and perpetrators (Evans & Stagner, 2003). A forensic nurse generalist may work in a specialty area, such as on a trauma team or in an emergency department, critical care, or outpatient women's health clinic, or may serve as a general resource person for colleagues in the clinical setting. The forensic nurse generalist may also serve as a resource for the care provider who is working with a patient who has been a victim or perpetrator of violence. In addition to addressing patients' physical and psychological needs, forensic nurse generalists must be prepared to identify and care for victims of violence and know when evidence should be collected and preserved (Wick, 2000).

Advanced Practice Forensic Nurse

An **advanced practice forensic nurse** has completed graduate education with a broad focus in forensic nursing and obtained credentials as a clinical nurse specialist, certified nurse-midwife, or nurse practitioner. The education provides clinicians with nursing, medical, and legal content and focuses on the collaboration among disciplines in the care of victims and perpetrators. The advance practice registered nurse in forensics also has an educational background in psychiatric assessment and intervention skills, death investigation, forensic wound identification, evidence collection, family violence, sexual assault of all types and in varied populations, introductory law, and principles of criminal justice and forensic science.

Other advanced training takes place after the completion of a master's degree. Individuals who are prepared with a doctor of nursing practice (DNP) may evaluate and apply evidence-based forensic practice for the improvement of education, clinical practice, systems management, and nursing leadership. A doctor of philosophy (PhD) prepares nurses to initiate and conduct research in the area of forensics to ultimately enhance the practice of forensic nursing. Most forensic nursing researchers have completed a doctoral degree or have another advanced degree.

Postdoctoral education or fellowships are also available as additional coursework in the specialty of forensics and clinical experiences to enhance terminal nursing degrees. This type of education may result in a diploma.

Roles and Functions

Regardless of the preparation level of the nurse, the goal of forensic education is to provide nurses who are knowledgeable in the care of all victims and perpetrators of violence.

In forensic nursing, the nurse-patient relationship occurs based on the possibility that a crime has been committed, but it is not the role of the forensic nurse to make a decision as to guilt or innocence or whether a victim is being candid in reporting what happened. The roles of the forensic nurse center on the identification of victims, creation of appropriate treatment plans, and collection, documentation, and preservation of potential evidence. The forensic nurse possesses expertise in assessment and treatment roles related to competency, risk, and danger. Forensic nurses are educated in theories of violence and victimology, legal issues, and nursing science that enable them to objectively assess the circumstances of the case.

An understanding of both the victim and the perpetrator enhances evidence collection. Forensic nurses may apply medical-surgical knowledge to the care of victims and perpetrators or may function in the legal role primarily as they collect evidence, testify in court, or collaborate with law practitioners with relationship to a victim or perpetrator.

Sexual Assault Nurse Examiner

The **sexual assault nurse examiner (SANE)** was the first specialized forensic role for nurses, and it represents the largest subspecialty in forensic nursing. SANEs are forensic nurse generalists who seek training in the care of adult and pediatric victims of sexual assault (SANE-A and SANE-P respectively). The IAFN has established clear guidelines for the preparation of SANEs and provides certification for nurses, although not all nurses who work in this capacity have

certification. The training is relatively brief, and the course is typically 5 days and 40 contact hours and is available online or in the classroom setting.

Nurses recognize the need to provide consistent care for all victims; therefore, nurses and leaders in many communities in the United States have set standards for educating the public on sexual assault prevention techniques and establishing comprehensive care to victims through sexual assault response teams (SARTs), which utilize a multidisciplinary model in providing care. SANEs are involved in the formation of SARTs in many communities throughout the United States. Along with SANEs, members of a SART may include representatives from the health department, law enforcement agency, advocacy groups, the local department of children and family services, district attorneys' offices, local hospitals, victim-assistant programs, and other service areas, as pertinent (Sekula, 2006). The multidisciplinary approach provides a standard of care that includes expert care in the acute setting, advocacy for the acute and long-term needs of the victim, and referral for counseling for the survivors in an effort to decrease long-term effects resulting from the assault.

Nurse Coroner/Death Investigator

The **nurse coroner/death investigator** for nurses was first recognized in the mid 1990s. Traditionally, the coroner is a public official primarily charged with the duty of determining how and why people die. Increasingly, nurses are prepared as death investigators or deputy coroners. Nurses can practice as death investigators in medical examiners' or coroners' offices or independently in private offices. This expanding nursing role involves assessing the deceased through understanding, discovery, preservation, and use of evidence.

Nurses who work as nurse coroners/death investigators possess medical knowledge that allow them to make expert judgments of the circumstances of death based on observations of history, symptomatology, autopsy results, toxicology, other diagnostic studies, and evidence revealed in other areas of the case. The value of nurses serving in this capacity is bolstered by their knowledge of anatomy and physiology, pathophysiology, pharmacology, grief and grieving, growth and development, interviewing, outcomes measurement, and many other areas of nursing practice (Wooten, 2003). Nurses are able to expand the role of the coroner and improve services provided to families, health care agencies, and communities by employing the basic principles of holistic nursing care.

FORENSIC PSYCHIATRIC NURSING

A **forensic psychiatric nurse** is one who is prepared as a generalist or at the advanced practice level. In the generalist role, nurses are prepared at the entry level as a college/university-degree, associate-degree, or diploma graduate, which prepares them to function as direct care providers and patient advocates. At the advanced practice level, graduate education is required, which prepares nurses to function as psychiatric clinical nurse specialists or psychiatric nurse practitioners. Additional graduate work in forensics at the master's and post-master's level provides the knowledge needed to practice with forensic populations. This specialty requires skills in psychiatric mental health nursing assessment, evaluation, and treatment of victims or perpetrators.

Evidence collection is central to the role of the forensic psychiatric nurse. For example, evidence is collected by a careful evaluation of intent or diminished capacity in the perpetrator's thinking at the time of the crime. This evaluation aids in determining the degree of crime and may later influence the sentence. Forensic psychiatric nurses who work as competency evaluators collect evidence by spending many hours with a defendant and carefully documenting the dialogue. In this capacity, the role of the forensic psychiatric nurse is not to determine guilt or innocence but to provide assessment data that can help make a final diagnosis within the multidisciplinary forensic team (Sekula & Burgess, 2006).

Roles and Functions

The forensic psychiatric nurse may function as a psychotherapist, forensic nurse examiner, competency evaluator, fact or expert witness, consultant to law enforcement agencies or the criminal justice system, hostage negotiator, or criminal profiler. These roles may involve providing therapy, witness testimony, services to a prosecutor or defense attorney, and criminal profile reports. Roles of the forensic psychiatric nurse may be examined in relationship to the outcomes for which the nurse is contracted to accomplish. The nurse may be contracted by the legal system to interface with the perpetrator for a variety of services. They may also be contracted by the correctional system or a private entity to offer direct services to the perpetrator. The nurse may provide services to the victim in a variety of settings. A list of role functions of forensic psychiatric nurses is presented in Box 33-2.

Nurse Psychotherapist

In addition to the competencies possessed by the generalist, the forensic APRN in psychiatric mental health (APRN-PMH) may function as a psychotherapist, providing individual, family, and group therapy. Depending on educational preparation and individual state statutes, an APRN-PMH may have prescriptive privileges and initiate psychopharmacology treatment along with psychotherapy.

BOX 33-2 Forensic Psychiatric Nursing Functions

- Assesses:
  - Perpetrator's ability to formulate intent
  - Risk for violence and for committing additional crimes
  - Factors such as race and culture that influenced crime
  - Legal sanity
  - Competence to proceed to trial
  - Sexual predator behaviors
- Investigates criminal history and reviews police reports
- Provides competency therapy
- Writes and submits formal reports to court
- Serves as an expert witness
- Participates in police training
- Assists in jury selection
- Consults with attorneys, as well as law enforcement personnel at crime scene
- Offers opinions regarding parole and probation

Forensic Nurse Examiner

Important activities of the forensic nurse examiner are to conduct court-ordered evaluations regarding legal sanity or competency to proceed, to respond to specific medicolegal questions as requested by the court, and to render an expert opinion in a written report or courtroom testimony. An evaluation may be requested by the prosecution, the defense, or the judge. Evaluations are usually based on the defendant's history, along with behavior at the scene of the crime, in jail, or in the courtroom. A comprehensive report is based on clinical data, observations of the defendant's behavior, any forensic evidence contained in crime-scene reports or laboratory reports, summary of any psychological testing, and a thorough psychosocial history. The forensic nurse examiner interviews the defendant and notes behavior, past diagnoses, personality traits, emotions, cognitive abilities, any symptoms of mental disorder, and the psychodynamics of interpersonal relationships (Emiley, 2002).

The forensic nurse examiner must be able to separate personal opinion from professional opinion. Personal opinion is based on one's background, upbringing, education, and value system. Professional opinion is based on scientific principle, advanced education in a specific field of endeavor, and the unbiased standards set by research in that area. Although other members of the treatment staff on a forensic unit strive to be supportive, accepting, and empathetic, the forensic nurse examiner strives to remain neutral, objective, and detached.

Legal sanity is defined as the individual's ability to distinguish right from wrong with reference to the act charged, capacity to understand the nature and quality of the act charged, and capacity to form the intent to commit the crime. Legal sanity is determined for the specific time of the act. The forensic nurse examiner must reconstruct the defendant's mental state by reviewing evidence left at the scene, any witness statements, the self-report of the defendant's symptoms, and the defendant's disclosed motivation. Some of the issues addressed in the forensic nurse examiner's determination are (1) whether or not the defendant was using drugs, (2) whether the defendant's reasoning ability was affected by any medical condition, and (3) what the social context of the crime was.

In most states, the presence of a major mental disorder (usually referring to those that cause psychoses—delusions, hallucinations, and disorganized thought—such as schizophrenia) is a prerequisite for a finding of *legal insanity*; however, a defendant who has a mental illness does not have to use this defense. It is the defendant's choice. The forensic nurse specialist must have a clear knowledge of which legal standard is being used and must be able to articulate it to the court and jury. Legal tests of sanity may include the McNaughton rules, irresistible impulse, and guilty but mentally ill.

The *McNaughton Rules* derive from a trial in 1843 in which Daniel McNaughton was tried for the murder of a public official. McNaughton believed there was a conspiracy among the Tories of England to destroy him. In an attempt to assassinate the Prime Minister, who was the Tory leader, McNaughton mistakenly shot and killed the Prime Minister's secretary. McNaughton was judged to be criminally insane and acquitted of the murder (but institutionalized for the remainder of his life). There was a public outcry over the leniency of this verdict. The House of Lords convened a special session of the judges to give an advisory opinion regarding the law of England governing the insanity defense. The judges advised that to be considered legally insane, the accused person with a mental disorder either must not know the nature and quality of the act or must not know whether the act is right or wrong. Whether or not the individual is responsible for his or her action is the underlying issue in the McNaughton rules. *Irresistible impulse* was added to the McNaughton rules in 1929. This addition stipulates that even if the defendant knew the criminal act was wrong but could not control his or her behavior because of a psychiatric illness or a mental defect, the defendant is not guilty.

Guilty but mentally ill is another insanity defense. Those who plead guilty but mentally ill are remanded to the correctional system, where they receive treatment for their mental disorder. They are subject to the correctional system's parole decisions.

Whereas legal insanity is determined by defendant's thinking in the past at the time of the offense, *competence to proceed* is determined by the defendant's present thinking at the time of the trial. It is defined as the capacity to assist one's attorney and understand the legal proceedings. As many as 60,000 defendants are evaluated for competence to proceed annually in the United States (Poythress, 2001). Because competence to proceed is a determination of mental capacity in the present, the defendant's competency must be determined each time he or she goes to court. A prior finding of incompetence, even if due to a developmental disability or mental illness, does not preclude a subsequent finding of competency in a later, unrelated case.

Competency Evaluator

Under United States federal law, no person may be tried if deemed legally incompetent, and the defendant must be sent to a suitable facility (usually a locked unit in a psychiatric facility) for a specified time period for treatment to regain competency. Forensic psychiatric nurses working as competency evaluators have greatly enhanced the treatment of defendants deemed legally incompetent, which in the past usually meant only the prescribing of antipsychotic medications.

Roles of the competency evaluator include assessing mental health or illness, conducting a forensic interview, providing documentation, completing a formal report to the court, and testifying as an expert witness. Competency therapists work with the defendant in one-to-one and group activities, which should not be confused with psychotherapy. For competency therapists, the patient is the court, not the defendant, and the products of their work are a competent defendant and a completed report. Becoming an advocate for the defendant, rather than for the process, is a breach of professional boundaries (Jacobson, 2002).

Fact and Expert Witnesses

Three types of witnesses can be used in the courtroom trial: (1) the principals (plaintiffs and defendants), (2) fact witnesses, and (3) expert witnesses. Each witness has a specific role in the presentation of the case and establishing the required burden of proof (Matthews, 2001). The fact witness is now used routinely in medical malpractice cases as an individual considered by the court to be capable and qualified to summarize and explain complex and voluminous medical records and medical terminology to the jury (Matthews, 2001).

Any nurse can be subpoenaed by the court to testify as a fact witness. A fact witness testifies regarding what was *personally* seen or heard, performed, or documented regarding a patient's care and testifies first-hand experience only (Sekula & Burgess, 2006). An expert witness is recognized by the court as having a certain level of skill or expertise in a designated area and possesses superior knowledge because of education or specialized experience. A nurse may testify as a fact witness and an expert witness. For example, a SANE may testify the facts of a case in which she examined the victim and collected evidence and may also testify in the case because of her expertise as a certified SANE-A.

Forensic nurses with advanced degrees are more likely to be called upon as expert witnesses. To establish credibility as an expert witness and to have one's opinion given equal weight to that of other professionals in court, the forensic nurse specialist must have current and updated clinical expertise, trustworthiness, and a professional presentation style (Box 33-3). Clinical expertise is established by professional credentials, and trustworthiness by the degree of honesty in demeanor and opinion evidenced on the witness stand, as perceived by the judge or jury. The expert witness may be deemed an authority in a specialty area and trustworthy, but unless he or she has a professional presentation style (i.e., the ability to communicate in a concise and convincing fashion), the testimony given is of limited value.

Consultant

Over the last decades, deinstitutionalization (see Chapter 5) has precipitated a need for interagency cooperation between mental health and law enforcement agencies. Although controversial, individuals who previously would have been institutionalized are now commonly homeless and often (intentionally or unintentionally) the focus of law enforcement. The forensic psychiatric nurse can provide consultation to mental health agencies regarding care of the patient with legal issues and to law enforcement agencies regarding the status and suggested treatment of mentally ill patients in the legal system. In this role, the nurse may also act as an advocate for families and patients. The bottom line for the nurse who serves in this capacity is

the perpetrator's well-being, even if that results in civil detention and admission to a hospital.

A forensic psychiatric nurse may be used as a resource for education and information about mental illness by either side in a court case. In this consultant role, the nurse may be asked to listen to witness testimony for the purpose of guiding further cross-examination or to assist in the preparation for trial by giving information about mental illness, including personality disorders and paraphilias. The nurse may be asked to testify about mental health treatment options, medications, and community resources.

Hostage Negotiator

In the late 1970s, the Federal Bureau of Investigation (FBI) began expanding hostage-negotiation team structure by recommending the use of consultants who could address the mental state of the perpetrator and recommend appropriate negotiation strategies. In the 1980s, local police agencies began to develop specialized teams that included consultants. When the forensic psychiatric mental nurse functions as a hostage negotiator, the role may include:

- Being on call around the clock to assist law enforcement officers on the scene
- Providing suggestions regarding negotiation techniques
- Assessing the mental status of the perpetrator
- Providing a link to mental health agencies
- Participating in a critique of the hostage incident
- Assessing released hostages
- Assessing the stress level of the hostage negotiator
- Providing training in communication skills to law enforcement officers

The successful hostage negotiator thinks clearly under stress, is able to communicate with persons from all socioeconomic classes, demonstrates common sense and "street smarts," is able to cope with uncertainty, can accept responsibility with no authority, and is able to express commitment to the negotiation process.

Criminal Profiler

A criminal profiler attempts to provide law enforcement officials with specific information about the type of individual who may have committed a certain crime. This service is usually requested when the crime scene indicates psychopathology or when serial crime is suspected. Historically, criminal profilers came from a variety of backgrounds, including law enforcement, psychology, psychiatry, and criminal justice. The criminal profiler collects all the available data, attempts to reconstruct the crime, formulates a hypothesis, develops a profile, and tests it against the known data.

This is familiar territory for the forensic psychiatric nurse, who is comfortable with the nursing processes

---

BOX 33-3 Expert Witness: Credentials for Credibility

Establishment of Expertise
- Academic preparation
- Professional training
- Occupational and life experiences
- Involvement in professional organizations

Establishment of Trustworthiness and Objectivity
- Dress, manner, and performance that communicate professionalism
- Successful communication to jury

of assessment, diagnosis (analysis), planning, implementation, and evaluation. Ann Burgess, one of the founders of the IAFN, was the first identified nurse criminal profiler with the FBI (Burgess et al., 2000). Skilled profilers have the ability to isolate their own emotions and reconstruct the crime using the criminal's reasoning process (Fintzy, 2000). Although this requires time and thoughtful consideration, the insights gained are usually critical for diagnosis and treatment. Psychiatric mental health nurses can serve as profilers of specific perpetrators because of their knowledge of psychiatry and human behavior.

The forensic psychiatric nurse must be highly skilled in interpersonal communications and able to develop collegial relationships with those in other disciplines. Nurses should not practice in this area if they hold narrow views of the issues facing these patients or if they are motivated by the desire to punish (Evans, 2000). A prerequisite is the ability to listen and accept others' values and motivations in a nonjudgmental fashion. Forensic psychiatric nursing appeals to a particular type of nurse who thrives in a stimulating intellectual environment, seeks out opportunities to apply clinical skills to complex legal problems, and enjoys pushing the limits of traditional boundaries. Because of the value placed on tradition by the nursing profession, the forensic psychiatric nurse is sometimes viewed with skepticism in nursing and with caution in the legal system. These responses must be met with professionalism in practice, research, and education of future forensic psychiatric nurses.

CORRECTIONAL NURSING

Nursing care of patients who are incarcerated presents challenges to the way nurses think about the patient. There is debate as to the terminology used when referring to both correctional nurses and psychiatric mental health nurses within correctional settings. Education is key in determining the level of expertise and whether one merits the title *forensic nurse* (either psychiatric mental health or correctional). Working in a correctional setting does not qualify one as a forensic nurse; rather, it is the advanced education and clinical practice that qualifies one as a forensic nurse (Sekula et al., 2001).

The number of incarcerated individuals in the United States has increased significantly for both men and women over the last 2 decades. Incarcerated men and women have higher rates of serious and chronic physical and mental illnesses than the general population, requiring enormous health care efforts (Maeve & Vaughn, 2001).

Prisoners are the only U.S. population group with a constitutional right to heath care. Because most of their civil liberties are taken away from them when they are incarcerated, and their movements are (necessarily)

severely restricted, prisoners are unable to seek and secure health care services on their own. Therefore, correctional facilities are required to provide "adequate" health services to inmates, either directly or through community health services organizations. **Correctional nursing** is defined by the location of the work or the legal status of the patient, rather than by the role functions being performed. Today's inmates suffer from a disproportionately greater number of chronic illnesses and infectious diseases than the general population.

Treatment and services for inmates with chronic mental health diagnoses are a significant part of the job for correctional staff. According to the U.S. Department of Justice (2006), more than 1 in 3 state prisoners, 1 in 4 federal prisoners, and 1 in 6 jail inmates with a mental health problem received treatment during their incarceration, which amounts to hundreds of thousands of incarcerated adults. In addition to those receiving care are the thousands of incarcerated adults known to have a mental health problem who are not receiving treatment. In 2005, rates of inmates with a mental health problem were estimated at 56% of state prisoners (705,600), 45% of federal prisoners (78,800), and 64% of jail inmates (479,900). When compared to the rates in the general population (11% of whom have a mental health problem, with approximately 55,000 individuals hospitalized at an inpatient psychiatric hospital on any given day), it is clear that correctional facilities carry a disproportionate share of the burden for the provision of mental health services. General medical care becomes an extension of this issue because inmates with mental health problems are more likely to be charged with violating rules of the correctional facility and over twice as likely to be injured in a fight.

Correctional nurses provide care for many patients with serious mental illness who are caught in a cycle of homelessness, psychiatric hospitals, and jail. Frequently these individuals become incarcerated as a result of psychiatric emergencies that generally include threats made to others. Because psychiatric facilities for the management of such emergencies are scarce, often these patients end up in jail instead of in a hospital. Once they are in jail, their psychiatric condition often worsens without adequate psychiatric intervention. The fortunate patients end up in a secure treatment unit within the jail, where they receive proper medication and psychiatric mental health nursing care.

Because of the long-term effects on recidivism (repeat offenders) and resource allocation, policy makers and legislators are beginning to recognize the importance of providing treatment for patients who are incarcerated. In a U.S. Department of Justice survey (2006), the most common mental health symptoms were insomnia and hypersomnia. Many of the commonly reported symptoms were related to major depression. Delusions and hallucinations were the most commonly identified psychotic symptoms, with 25% of state inmates,

TABLE 33-1 Comorbid Substance Abuse Among Arrestee

	Men (Median)	Women (Median)
Heavy drug use*	37.0	36.2
Risk for drug dependence	39.1	40.5
Tested positive for alcohol	9.5	86.4
Risk for alcohol dependence	28.6	23.8

*Defined as 13 or more days of self-reported consumption of a drug in a 30-day period in the year before the interview.
Adapted from Zhang, Z. (2004). *Drug and alcohol use and related matters among arrestees 2003*. Washington, DC: U.S. Department of Justice.

15% of federal inmates, and 10% of jail inmates reporting at least one of the two symptoms. Especially critical within this population is treatment of those with a history of trauma or posttraumatic stress disorder (PTSD), owing to their long-term debilitating effects. The correctional setting, however, is not conducive to the intensive therapy required to adequately treat these issues; therefore, the needs of the vast majority of people with PTSD and/or trauma history in the correctional system are not appropriately addressed.

Another issue that must be considered in the treatment of those who are incarcerated is substance use and abuse. Table 33-1 illustrates the connection between drugs, alcohol, and arrests in the United States, providing details about substance use of all arrestees in 2003 by gender. Drug courts, mandatory drug treatment, and drug/alcohol treatment within correctional facilities have all been shown to decrease the likelihood of recidivism and increase the likelihood of abstinence from drugs and/or alcohol after release.

Correctional nurses working in facilities with comprehensive psychiatric services perform psychiatric mental health nursing role functions, rather than forensic nursing role functions, including completing comprehensive mental status examinations and implementing psychiatric care plans. The following vignette illustrates a challenging situation facing a correctional psychiatric nurse.

VIGNETTE
Suzanne is a 45-year-old woman incarcerated at a state facility in general population. She was convicted of assault with a deadly weapon, following a confrontation with a "friend." Her psychiatric diagnoses include major depression and PTSD (resulting from severe abuse in her childhood and from an intimate partner during her early 20s). Although she is not in a locked forensic unit, she is being treated with medication and seen by the facility's psychiatric mental health nurse practitioner (NP) for medication management. While watching television in the common area one morning, Suzanne attacked a fellow inmate for no apparent reason, screaming and clawing at anyone who approached her. Staff was unable to control her physically. She was placed in solitary confinement with mechanical restraints; these actions did nothing to control her screaming. She was seen by the NP on call, who reported that Suzanne was having a flashback related to her PTSD. The solitary confinement and mechanical restraints were only worsening her flashbacks. The staff and the NP were facing a common dilemma in correctional health care: custody versus caring. While the NP was focusing on the needs of the individual inmate, the correctional staff were focused on the goals of the correctional facility related to custody of violent offenders and protecting the environment. The successful correctional treatment team seeks to balance the two sides of this debate: creating an environment where possible rehabilitation of offenders is possible, without compromising the compulsory "punitive" aspects of incarceration. ■

KEY POINTS TO REMEMBER

- Forensic nursing is an emerging specialty area of practice that combines elements of traditional nursing, forensic science, and criminal justice.
- The IAFN was established in 1992 as the professional association representing this specialty.
- Forensic psychiatric nurses fulfill a variety of roles, including that of psychotherapist, forensic nurse examiner, competency therapist, fact witness, expert witness, consultant, hostage negotiator, criminal profiler, and correctional nurse.

CRITICAL THINKING

1. Compare and contrast the roles of forensic nurse and correctional nurse. How would you describe the nurse-patient relationship in forensic nursing? In what ways does this differ from the nurse-patient relationship in correctional nursing?

2. Imagine you are working on a psychiatric inpatient unit as a new graduate. A patient on the unit commits suicide, and you are called to testify as a fact witness. A nurse who is nationally recognized for her research on suicidal behavior is called as an expert witness.
   A. Describe what your role would be as a fact witness?
   B. How would the other nurse's role differ from yours?

CHAPTER REVIEW

1. Which statement regarding forensic nursing is accurate?
   1. Forensic nurses must all be prepared at the doctoral level.
   2. Forensic nurses only perform sexual assault examinations.
   3. Forensic nurse examiners conduct court-ordered evaluations regarding sanity or competency.
   4. Forensic psychiatric mental health nurses are not permitted to act as hostage negotiators.

2. Which type of patients would a correctional nurse typically see?
   1. Students
   2. Police officers
   3. Teachers
   4. Prisoners

3. The nurse is caring for an incarcerated patient. Which most frequently seen psychotic symptom in prisoners should the nurse anticipate?
   1. Delusions and hallucinations
   2. Posttraumatic stress disorder
   3. Depression
   4. Anxiety

4. The nurse is caring for a female patient who has been arrested. Which most common form of comorbid substance abuse for women should the nurse anticipate?
   1. Heavy drug use
   2. Risk for drug dependence
   3. Testing positive for alcohol
   4. Risk for alcohol dependence

5. The nurse is caring for a male patient who has been arrested. Which most common form of comorbid substance abuse for men should the nurse anticipate?
   1. Heavy drug use
   2. Risk for drug dependence
   3. Testing positive for alcohol
   4. Risk for alcohol dependence

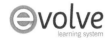

Visit the Evolve website for an **Audio Chapter Summary, Chapter Review Answers & Rationales, Critical Thinking Answer Guidelines,** and additional resources related to the content in this chapter: **http://evolve.elsevier.com/Varcarolis/foundations**

Companion CD Use the Companion CD to prepare for tests and the NCLEX® Examination with **Test-Taking Strategies** for psychiatric mental health nursing and hundreds of **Review Questions.**

References

Burgess, A. W., Dowdell, E. B., & Brown, K. (2000). The elderly rape victim: Stereotypes, perpetrators, and implications for practice. *Journal of Emergency Nursing, 26,* 516–518.

Disaster Center. (2007). *United States: Uniform crime report: State statistics from 1960–2007.* Retrieved February 26, 2009 from http://www.disastercenter.com/crime/

Emiley, S. F. (2002). Forensic psychological evaluations: Back to basics. *Forensic Examiner, 11*(1-2), 31–35.

Evans, M. (2000). Re-visioning the nurses' punitive attitudes within forensic psychiatric and correctional nursing: The significance of ethical sophistication. *Journal of Psychosocial Nursing, 38*(4), 8–13.

Evans, M. M., & Stagner, P. (2003). Maintaining the chain of custody: Evidence handling in forensic cases. *AORN Online, 78,* 563–569.

Fintzy, R. T. (2000). Criminal profiling: An introduction to behavioral evidence analysis. *American Journal of Psychiatry, 157,* 1532–1555.

International Association of Forensic Nurses. (2006a). *About IAFN.* Retrieved February 2, 2009, from http://www.iafn.org/displaycommon.cfm?an=3

International Association of Forensic Nurses. (2006b). *What is Forensic Nursing.* Retrieved February 2, 2009, from http://www.iafn.org/displaycommon.cfm?an=1&subarticlenbr=137

International Association of Forensic Nurses and American Nurses Association. (1997). *Scope and standards of forensic nursing practice.* Washington, DC: American Nurses Publishing.

Jacobson, G. (2002). Maintaining professional boundaries: Preparing nursing students for the challenge. *Journal of Nursing Education, 41,* 279–281.

Maeve, M. K., & Vaughn, M. S. (2001). Nursing with prisoners: The practice of caring, forensic nursing or penal harm nursing? *Advances in Nursing Science, 24*(2), 47–64.

Matthews, M. D. (Ed.). (2001). *The nurse and the legal system.* Philadelphia: Davis.

Poythress, N. (2001). The MacArthur adjudicative competence study: Executive summary. *Behavioral Sciences and the Law, 15,* 329–345.

Sekula, L. K. (Ed.). (2006). Forensic nursing in the 21st century (5, supplemental issue ed.). In C. H. Wecht (Ed.), *Forensic Sciences* (5th ed.).

Sekula, L. K., & Burgess, A. W. (Eds.). (2006). *Forensic and legal nursing* (Vol. 1). Boca Raton: CRC Press.

Sekula, L. K., Holmes, D., Zoucha, R., DeSantis, J., & Olshansky, E. (2001). Forensic psychiatric nursing. Discursive practices and the emergence of a specialty. *Journal of Psychosocial Nursing & Mental Health Services, 39*(9), 51–57.

U.S. Department of Health & Human Services. (2000). *Healthy People 2010* (2nd ed., Vol. 2). Washington, DC: U.S. Government Printing Office.

U.S. Department of Justice. (2006). *Mental health problems of prison and jail inmates*. Retrieved February 25, 2009 from http://www.ojp.usdoj.gov/bjs/pub/pdf/mhppji.pdf

U.S. Department of Justice-Federal Bureau of Investigation. (2006). United States Uniform Crime Report. Washington, DC: Author.

Wick, J. M. (2000). Don't destroy the evidence. *AORN Journal*, 75(5), 805–836.

Wooten, R. (2003). Applying the nursing process to death investigation. *Forensic Nurse, 8*, Available at <http://www.forensicnursemag.com/articles/3b1lifedeath.html>

World Health Organization. (2002). *World report on violence and health: Summary*. Geneva: World Health Organization.

Zhang, Z. (2004). *Drug and alcohol use and related matters among arrestees, 2003*. Washington, DC: U.S. Department of Justice.

Other Intervention Modalities

A NURSE SPEAKS

Working with patients who are actively hearing voices during group therapy is a rewarding, yet daunting, experience. Much of my current practice with one long-term group of six participants is counter to my early education over 40 years ago. Each member complied with the medication regimen, had extensive community support, and was diagnosed with some variant along the schizophrenic continuum. Of course, names and specifics have been altered. The frameworks used were a combination of Peplau's methods, Ericksonian hypnotherapy, and cognitive-behavioral therapy. These interventions were used with patients hearing nonthreatening, basically benign, yet critical voices, not with those hearing voices of lethal intent or command hallucinations.

The group members found the acceptance to talk about their voices and to talk with others who also experienced voices very helpful and healing. The participants informally started observing in themselves the intensity, duration, timing, numbers, and intent of the voices, and their relationship to them. They spontaneously started telling the group members ways they have coexisted and coped with the barrage of voices.

As leader, I normalized their experiences by reframing their negative voices as "inner critics" or "self-talk" that most people experience. We identified similarities to other peoples' self-talk in that the inner critic may continually comment on everything the person is doing, may play nonstop rap songs with sardonic overtones, or may yell lists of things not done well and all the mistakes the individual has made.

When one patient, Harold, described his need to put all his CDs in the attic of his halfway house to try to decrease the incessant stream of negativity, I matched his metaphor by suggesting that in his head he slowly turn the volume down on a make-believe CD player with each exhalation. Although he found this very helpful, he still kept his CDs in the attic. Kevin liked the suggestion that he develop a dialogue with his voices by saying things like: "Yep, that's a possibility. Thanks for the input." "I never thought of that. I'll give it a try." After reporting his ability to do this as his homework assignment, he then learned to pair his response with a physical activity, such as walking to the grocery store or around the block, to help divert his attention away from the voices.

Other suggestions for dealing with negative and disturbing voices were the following: (1) Consider that the voice may be targeting an area of greatest insecurities and make a plan to improve that area. (2) Compare your list of all your positive traits, compiled by self-identification and group input, with the list of faults given by the voices and recognize that your voices are not always correct. (3) Put things in perspective. Will it matter tomorrow, next week, next year? Most of the time, the answer is no. (4) Compare yourself with your own yardstick of traits and accomplishments, not with your perceptions of someone else who appears to be perfect on the outside, when that may not necessarily be an accurate estimation of what is going on inside of that person.

Some of the voices were positive and offered alternatives. Jane described voices that sometimes encouraged her. We labeled these as her "guardians" or "angels." One member actually brought in a book about angels, and everyone actively participated in a discussion of his or her opinion and described how we can tap their resources.

Sharon Shisler

CHAPTER **34**

Therapeutic Groups

Karyn I. Morgan and Nancy Christine Shoemaker

Key Terms and Concepts

conflict, 737
feedback, 737
group, 736
group content, 737
group norms, 737
group process, 737
group psychotherapy, 743

group themes, 737
group work, 736
psychoeducational groups, 742
self-help groups, 743
support groups, 743
therapeutic factors, 737

Objectives

1. Identify basic concepts related to group work.
2. Describe the phases of group development.
3. Define task and maintenance roles of group members.
4. Discuss the therapeutic factors that operate in all groups.

5. Discuss four types of groups commonly led by basic level registered nurses.
6. Describe a group intervention for (1) a member who is silent or (2) a member who is monopolizing the group.

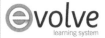 Visit the Evolve website for an **Audio Glossary & Flashcards**, **Concept Map Creator**, and additional resources related to the content in this chapter: **http://evolve.elsevier.com/Varcarolis/foundations**

We all live and interact among groups throughout our lives. We are born into a family group and grow up with various peer groups, such as those at school, work, and church and within the community. As adults, we establish our own family group. A **group** consists of two or more people who come together for the purpose of pursuing common goals and/or interests. Each group has characteristics that influence its progress and outcomes, including:

- Size
- Defined purpose
- Degree of similarity among members
- Rules
- Boundaries
- Content (what is said in the group)
- Process (underlying dynamics among group members)

Box 34-1 defines terms related to types of groups and group work. **Group work** is a method whereby individuals with a common purpose come together and benefit by both giving and receiving feedback within the dynamic and unique context of group life.

There are advantages and disadvantages of the group approach for psychiatric patients. Advantages include:

- Engaging multiple patients in treatment at the same time, thereby saving costs
- Participants benefit not only from the feedback of the nurse leader but also that of peers who may possess a unique understanding of the issues
- Providing a relatively safe setting to try out new ways of relating to other people and practicing new communication skills
- Promoting a feeling of belonging

BOX 34-1 Terms Central to Therapeutic Groups

Terms Describing Group Work

Group content—all that is said in the group

Group process—the dynamics of interaction among the members (e.g., who talks to whom, facial expressions, and body language)

Group norms—expectations for behavior in the group that develop over time and provide structure for members (e.g., starting on time, not interrupting)

Group themes—members' expressed ideas or feelings that recur and have a common thread (The leader can clarify a theme to help members recognize it more fully.)

Feedback—letting group members know how they affect each other

Conflict—open disagreement among members (Positive conflict resolution within a group is key to successful outcomes.)

Terms Describing Types of Groups

Heterogeneous group—a group in which a range of differences exists among members

Homogeneous group—a group in which all members share central traits (e.g., men's group, group of patients with bipolar disorder)

Closed group—a group in which membership is restricted; no new members are added when others leave

Open group—a group in which new members are added as others leave

Subgroup—an individual or a small group that is isolated within a larger group and functions separately (Members of a subgroup may have greater loyalty, more similar goals, or more perceived similarities to one another than they do to the larger group.)

BOX 34-2 Therapeutic Factors in Groups

Instillation of hope—The leader shares optimism about group treatment, and members share their improvements.

Universality—Members realize that they are not alone with their problems, feelings, or thoughts.

Imparting of information—Participants receive formal teaching by the leader or advice from peers.

Altruism—Members feel a reward from giving support to others.

Corrective recapitulation of the primary family group—Members repeat patterns of behavior in the group that they learned in their families; with feedback from the leader and peers, they learn about their own behavior.

Development of socializing techniques—Members learn new social skills based on feedback from others.

Imitative behavior—Members may copy behavior from the leader or peers and can adopt healthier habits.

Interpersonal learning—Members gain insight into themselves based on the feedback from others. This is a complex process that occurs later in the group after trust is established.

Group cohesiveness—This powerful factor arises in a mature group when each member feels connected to the other members, the leader, and the group as a whole; members can accept positive feedback and constructive criticism.

Catharsis—Intense feelings, as judged by the member, are shared.

Existential resolution—Members learn to accept painful aspects of life (e.g., loneliness, death) that affect everyone.

Data from Yalom, I. D. (2005). *The theory and practice of group psychotherapy* (5th ed.). New York: Basic Books.

Disadvantages include:

- Time constraints in which an individual member may feel cheated for floor time, particularly in large groups
- Concerns that private issues may be shared outside the group
- Dealing with disruptive member behavior during an emotionally vulnerable point

Not all patients benefit from group treatment. Persons who are acutely psychotic, acutely manic, or intoxicated have difficulty interacting effectively in groups and may interfere with other members' ability to remain focused on group goals and progress.

THERAPEUTIC FACTORS COMMON TO ALL GROUPS

Irvin D. Yalom (2005), one of the most noted researchers on group psychotherapy, is credited with identifying the factors that make groups therapeutic (Box 34-2). **Therapeutic factors** are aspects of the group experience that leaders and members have identified as facilitating therapeutic change. For example, as group members begin to share life experiences, feelings, and concerns, they may recognize for the first time that they are not "alone in the world," which allows them to connect with others. Yalom calls this factor *universality*—the patient's recognition that other people feel the same way or have had the same experiences. Recognizing universality can provide a profound sense of relief. Different factors operate at different phases of a group, and the leader may role-model several behaviors during the initial phase, such as instilling hope and imparting information. Just as with other types of treatment, each person's response to a group is highly individualized based on past experiences and level of participation.

PLANNING A GROUP

To develop a successful group, planning should include a description of specific characteristics, including:

- Name and objectives of the group
- Types of patients or diagnoses of members
- Group schedule (frequency, times of meetings, etc.)
- Description of leader and member responsibilities
- Methods or means of evaluating outcomes of the group

Planning and structure is especially important when group leaders are likely to change (in inpatient settings where staffing patterns change) or when several groups are running at the same time with a common goal (in a research study).

PHASES OF GROUP DEVELOPMENT

All groups go through developmental phases similar to those identified for individual therapeutic relationships (see Chapter 9). In each phase, the group leader has specific roles and challenges to address in support of positive interaction, growth, and change.

In the **orientation phase**, the group leader's role is to structure an atmosphere of respect, confidentiality, and trust. The purpose of the group is stated, and members are encouraged to get to know one another. Initially, members may be overly silent or overbearing because they have not yet established trust with one another. Therapeutic interaction is supported when the group leader points out similarities between members, encourages them to talk directly to each other rather than to the leader, and reminds members about ground rules for respectful interaction.

In the **working phase**, the group leader's role is to encourage focus on problem solving consistent with the purpose of the group. As group members begin to feel safe within the group, conflicts may be expressed, which should be viewed by the group leader as a positive opportunity for group growth. It is important for the leader to guide and support conflict resolution. Through successful resolution of conflicts, group members are empowered to develop confidence in their problem-solving abilities and better support one another in their individual efforts to grow and change.

In the **termination phase**, the group leader's role is to encourage members to reflect on progress they have made and identify post-termination goals. Members may experience feelings of loss or anger about the group ending; at times, these feelings can be directed toward other group members or the leader. It is important to openly address such feelings as part of the group's work toward successful termination.

GROUP MEMBER ROLES

We each have a unique style of interacting with others, and we gravitate toward specific comfort zones within groups. Consider your own behaviors within groups. You may tend to sit back and mainly observe, giving your opinion only after careful consideration. Or perhaps you feel it is important to keep everyone moving in a common direction or help maintain order and actively urge people to continue working. The way we behave in groups is a function of our innate personalities (e.g., shy or outgoing), socialization (e.g., birth order or exposure to groups), and the specific context of the group (e.g., a familiar and interesting topic or one outside your comfort zone).

Studies of group dynamics have identified informal roles that group members often assume, which may or may not be helpful in the group's development. The classic descriptive categories for these roles are task, maintenance, and individual roles (Benne & Sheats, 1948). *Task roles* serve to keep the group focused on its main purpose and get the work done. *Maintenance roles* function to keep the group together, help each person feel worthwhile, and create a sense of group cohesion. There are also *individual roles* that have nothing to do with helping the group but instead relate to specific personalities, personal agendas, and a desire to have needs met by shifting the group's focus to them. Awareness of roles that individual members assume can assist the group leader to identify behaviors that need to be confronted or reinforced. Table 34-1 describes the informal roles of group members.

GROUP LEADERSHIP
Responsibilities

The group leader has multiple responsibilities in initiating, maintaining, and terminating a group. The leader is often most directive in the orientation phase. During this phase, the structure, size, composition, purpose, and timing of the group are defined. Task and maintenance functions may be discussed and demonstrated. During the working phase, the leader facilitates communication and ensures that meetings begin and end on time. In the termination phase, the leader ensures that each member summarizes individual accomplishments and gives positive and negative feedback regarding the group experience.

Sensitivity to cultural diversity and cultural needs of individual members is a key responsibility of the group leader. The leader initially sets a foundation for open communication by defining the importance of mutual respect and rules for group conduct. As group members begin to engage with one another, the leader's sensitivity to issues that may have a cultural basis can be pivotal in facilitating efforts to maintain open communication and mutual respect.

TABLE 34-1 Informal Roles of Group Members

	Role	Function
Task Roles	Coordinator	Tries to connect various ideas and suggestions
	Elaborator	Gives examples and follows up meaning of ideas
	Energizer	Encourages the group to make decisions or take action
	Evaluator	Measures the group's work against a standard
	Information giver	Shares facts or own experience as an authority figure
	Information seeker	Tries to clarify the group's values
	Initiator-contributor	Offers new ideas or a new outlook on an issue
	Opinion giver	Shares opinions, especially to influence group values
	Orienter	Notes the progress of the group toward goals
	Procedural technician	Supports group activity by distributing papers, arranging seating, etc.
	Recorder	Keeps notes and acts as the group memory
Maintenance Roles	Compromiser	In a conflict, yields to preserve group harmony
	Encourager	Praises and seeks input from others
	Follower	Agrees with the flow of the group
	Gatekeeper	Monitors the participation of all members to keep communication open
	Group observer	Keeps records of different aspects of group process and reports to the group
	Harmonizer	Tries to mediate conflicts between members
	Standard setter	Verbalizes standards for the group
Individual Roles	Aggressor	Criticizes and attacks others' ideas and feelings
	Blocker	Disagrees with group issues; oppositional
	Dominator	Tries to control other members of the group with flattery or interruptions
	Help seeker	Asks for sympathy of group excessively
	Playboy	Acts disinterested in group process
	Recognition seeker	Seeks attention by boasting and discussing achievements
	Self-confessor	Verbalizes feelings or observations unrelated to group
	Special-interest pleader	Advocates for a special group, usually with own prejudice or bias

Data from Benne, K., & Sheats, P. (1948). Functional roles of group members. *Journal of Social Issues, 4*(2), 41.

Diversity may exist in many forms, including racial, ethnic, economic, and sexual orientation. Encouraging members to share and explore their cultural foundations and beliefs promotes genuine communication and provides the group with the opportunity to share similarities and differences in an environment of mutual respect.

Consider the example of a woman who came to group after a significant suicide attempt. She remained silent and withdrawn until the leader encouraged her to explore her feelings about the group. The patient revealed that she "wasn't smart like everyone else" and that she was "basically just trailer trash." Other group members began to share their similarities and differences in backgrounds, with a focus on their common needs, fears, and insecurities. When this woman finished the group, she acknowledged having learned an important lesson: she could give and get help from people she saw as different from her, and not everyone would treat her like she was "less than."

Styles of Leadership

There are three main styles of group leadership, and a leader selects the style that is best suited to the therapeutic needs of a particular group. The **autocratic leader** exerts control over the group and does not encourage much interaction among members. For example, staff leading a community meeting with a fixed, time-limited agenda may tend to be more autocratic. In contrast, the **democratic leader** supports extensive group interaction in the process of problem solving. Psychotherapy groups most often employ this leadership style. A **laissez-faire leader** allows the group members to behave in any way they choose and does not attempt to control the direction of the group. In a creative group, such as an art or horticulture group, the leader may choose a laissez-faire style, giving minimal direction to allow for a variety of responses.

In any group, the leader must be thoughtful about communication techniques, since these can have a tremendous impact on group content and process. Table 34-2 describes communication techniques frequently used by group leaders. It is also important to note that inpatient groups have significant differences from outpatient groups (Table 34-3), and consequently the role of the leader must be adapted accordingly.

Clinical Supervision

Clinical supervision is important for group leaders; it provides feedback about their performance and enhances

TABLE 34-2 Group Leader Communication Techniques

Technique	Example
Giving Information—provides resources and information that supports treatment goals	"Antidepressants may take as long as 4 weeks or more to show real therapeutic effects."
Clarification—asks the group member to expand and clarify what they mean	"What do you mean when you say 'I can't go back to work?'"
Confrontation—encourages the group member to explore inconsistencies in their communication or behavior	"Jane, you're saying 'nothing's wrong,' but you're crying."
Reflection—encourages the group member to explore and expand on feelings (rather than thoughts or events)	"I noticed you're clenching your fists. What are you feeling right now?" "It sounds like that really upset you."
Summarization—closes a discussion or group session by pointing out key issues and insights	"We've talked about different types of cognitive distortions, and everyone identified at least one irrational thought that has influenced their behavior in a negative way. In the next group, we'll explore some strategies for correcting negative thinking."
Support—gives positive feedback and acknowledgement	"It took a lot of courage to explore those painful feelings. You're really working hard on resolving this problem."

TABLE 34-3 Comparison of Outpatient and Inpatient Groups

Outpatient Groups	Inpatient Groups
The group has a stable composition.	The group is rarely the same for more than one or two meetings.
Patients are carefully selected and prepared.	Patients are admitted to the group with little prior selection or preparation.
The group is homogeneous with regard to ego function.	The group has a heterogeneous level of ego function.
Motivated, self-referred patients make up the group; therapy is growth oriented.	Patients are ambivalent, often therapy is compulsory; therapy is relief oriented.
Treatment proceeds as long as required: may continue for 1 to 2 years.	Treatment is limited to the hospital period, with rapid patient turnover.
The boundary of the group is well maintained, with few external influences.	Whatever happens on the unit affects the group.
Group cohesion develops normally, given sufficient time in treatment.	There is no time for cohesion to develop spontaneously; group development is limited to the initial phase.
The leader allows the process to unfold; there is ample time to set up group norms.	The group leader structures time and is not passive.
Members are encouraged to avoid extra group contact.	Patients eat, sleep, and live together outside of the group; extra group contact is endorsed.

Data from Mackenzie, K. R. (1997). *Time-managed group psychotherapy: Effective clinical applications.* Washington, DC: American Psychiatric Press.

their professional growth. Transference and counter-transference issues occur in groups just as in individual treatment (see Chapter 9), and a more objective input supports a focus on therapeutic goals. Co-leadership of groups is a common practice and has several benefits which include (1) providing training for less experienced staff, (2) allowing for immediate feedback between leaders after each session, and (3) offering two role models for teaching communication skills to members.

NURSE AS GROUP LEADER

Psychiatric mental health nurses are involved in a variety of therapeutic groups in acute care and long-term treatment settings. Registered nurses with basic preparations may lead activity, educational, task, and support groups. More complex skills are necessary for leading psychotherapy, and only advanced practice registered nurses are qualified for this type of group. For all group leaders, a clear theoretical framework is necessary to provide a foundation for analyzing the group interaction. Table 34-4 describes several theoretical frameworks commonly used in group work.

Registered nurses who are trained at the basic level (diploma, associate degree, baccalaureate degree) have holistic training and an educational background that enables them to provide strong leadership skills in a variety of groups. These include psychoeducational and support groups. Advanced practice registered

TABLE 34-4 Theoretical Foundations for Group Therapy		
Theory	**Concepts**	**Role of Therapist**
Psychodynamic/ psychoanalytic	Applies Freud's concepts of psychoanalysis to individual members and to the group itself; focus is on unconscious conflicts and transference; goal is insight	Helps members to recognize unconscious conflicts and encourages peer feedback
Interpersonal	Applies Sullivan's theories about interpersonal learning; focus is on understanding how current relationships repeat early significant relationships; goal is to rebuild individual's personality	Helps to reduce anxiety and encourages members to validate feelings and thoughts with each other
Communication	Applies a systems model, holding that the whole (group) is greater than the sum of its parts (members); focus is on subgroups and communication, both verbal and nonverbal; goal is to learn clear, congruent communication skills	Helps point out confusing or contradictory messages; acts as a role model for clear communication
Group process	Analyzes the group with a focus on individual roles and group patterns of behavior (phases, norms, etc.); goal is to resolve authority and intimacy issues	Helps develop a mature group in which members trust each other and give supportive feedback
Existential/Gestalt	Applies theories of Maslow and Rogers to encourage individuals to develop to full potential; focus is on the here and now to increase members' awareness of feelings; goal is self-actualization in which individual takes full responsibility for choices	Helps focus members on here-and-now experiences to promote self-learning; promotes emphasis on "what" of behaviors, not "why"
Cognitive-behavioral	Applies concepts of learning theory and Ellis's cognitive therapy; focus is on behavior and thinking patterns, with the group used to reinforce adaptive behavior and extinguish maladaptive patterns; usually time limited; goal is to change behavior or thinking patterns	Helps develop a trusting group in which members give supportive feedback to reinforce healthier behavior; may provide formal teaching, along with homework assignments

Data from Dies, R. (1992). Models of group psychotherapy: Sifting through confusion. *International Journal of Group Psychotherapy, 42,* 1–16; and Scheidlinger, S. (1997). Group dynamics and group psychotherapy revisited: Four decades later. *International Journal of Group Psychotherapy, 47*(2), 141–159.

nurses may lead these groups as well but are also qualified to facilitate other specialized group treatments.

Basic Level Registered Nurse

Psychoeducational Groups

Psychoeducational groups are groups set up to increase knowledge or skills about a specific somatic or psychological subject and allow members to communicate emotional concerns. These groups may be time limited or may be supportive for long-term treatment. Generally, written handouts or audiovisual aids are used to focus on specific teaching points. Psychiatric mental health nurses, who are holistically trained, are well prepared to teach a variety of health subjects.

Medication Education. The psychoeducational group for which the nurse most commonly assumes responsibility is the medication education group. Medication education groups are designed to teach patients about their medications, answer their questions, and prepare them for self-management. The group setting facilitates discussion. When patients have concerns about taking medications, it is often the group members themselves who are in the position to respond to these questions. "Yes, I got a dry mouth when I first started taking that, but it got better. Hang in there." Box 34-3 outlines an example of a medication education group protocol, and Figure 34-1 shows a tool used to evaluate a medication group.

Health Education. Nurses also frequently lead health education groups, including groups on sex education. Patients who have used poor judgment in sexual behavior because of mental illness are at high risk for human immunodeficiency virus (HIV) infection/acquired immunodeficiency syndrome (AIDS) and other sexually transmitted diseases. Topics for discussion may include:

- HIV/AIDS
- Modes of transmission and treatment of sexually transmitted diseases
- Education on condom use and other forms of safer sex practices
- The effect of illness and medication on sexuality

Dual-Diagnosis. Dual-diagnosis groups are designed to incorporate learning about co-existing mental illnesses and substance abuse. Since treatment issues for patients with a dual diagnosis can be complex, group leaders must have demonstrated competency in both mental health and chemical dependence treatment. The goal is to engage patients in treatment and decrease their use of substances in a step-by-step process. Research has shown that combined treatment for patients with serious mental illness produces improved outcomes (Drake et al., 2001).

BOX 34-3 Example of Medication Education Group Protocol

Description of Group

A group for all patients, regardless of level of concentration, that prepares patients for self-management of medication on discharge.

Criteria for Patient Selection

Open to all patients except those who are displaying suicidal or homicidal behaviors or the potential for assault

Visual Aids

Overhead transparencies, films, patient medication education sheets

Purpose

1. To educate patients on the primary function of their medications
2. To provide information on side effects (that benefits can outweigh risks)
3. To describe a mechanism to negotiate relationships with health care workers
4. To enhance a sense of self-control over treatment

Procedure

1. Orientation and introduction to the group
2. Brief description of major symptoms in a diagnosis
3. Overview of antipsychotics or antidepressants
4. Use of Albany Medical Center patient medication education sheets
5. Specific open question period

Behavioral Objectives

At the end of the 45-minute session, patients will be able to:

1. State one symptom they have that is treated by their medication.
2. Be able to ask at least one question about their medicine.
3. Identify one mechanism that helps in adhering to the medication regimen.

Theoretical Justification

Even people who think they are adherent only take 80% of doses. Counseling and therapy are always adjuncts to drug therapy.

Adapted from Ott, C. A. (2000). *Pediatric psychopharmacology.* South Easton, MD: American Healthcare Institute, a division of SC Publishing.

Symptom Management. For patients with a common symptom resulting from a disorder such as anger or anxiety, symptom management groups are ideal. The focus is on sharing positive and negative experiences so that members learn coping skills from

Criteria	Strongly Agree	Somewhat Agree	Agree	Disagree	Strongly Disagree
1. I know the name(s) of the medication(s) I am taking.					
2. I know what symptoms the medication(s) can help me with.					
3. I know the common side effects of my medication(s).					
4. I feel comfortable talking to my prescriber if I am having problems with my medication(s).					
5. It is important to take my medication(s) at the same time every day.					

Figure 34-1 Medication group evaluation tool.

each other. A primary goal is to increase self-control or prevent relapse by helping patients develop a plan for action at the first appearance of symptoms.

Stress Management. Often time limited, stress management groups teach members about various relaxation techniques, including deep breathing, exercise, music, and spirituality. One such technique that is increasingly demonstrating efficacy in stress management as well as other symptoms is mindfulness (Chadwick et al., 2005). Mindfulness groups focus on developing awareness of the present moment with the intent to induce relaxation and promote insight into thoughts, emotions, and physical responses. Although much of the research has focused on the use of this technique in outpatient settings, one recent study by Winship (2007) reports the benefits of this technique for acutely ill patients on an inpatient unit.

Support and Self-Help Groups

Support groups and self-help groups are structured for the purpose of providing patients with the opportunity to maintain or enhance personal and social functioning through cooperation and shared understanding of life's challenges (Hayes et al., 2006; Yalom, 2005). Examples include support groups for survivors of cancer, bereavement support, or support groups for families who have lost a loved one to suicide. Hayes and colleagues (2006) present evidence of the benefits of supportive group therapy for severe mental illness as well. Their findings also indicated that adding structured cognitive exercises enhanced the overall improvement in this population over supportive group therapy alone.

The nurse may serve as a resource for patients and must be aware of the wide array of self-help groups available. One of the most important functions of such groups is to demonstrate to individuals that they are not alone in having a particular problem. Thus these groups provide members with support, and their

members help each other by telling their stories and providing alternative ways to view and to resolve problems. Box 34-4 describes characteristics of support and self-help groups.

Advanced Practice Nurse

Group Psychotherapy

Group psychotherapy is a specialized treatment intervention in which a trained leader (or co-leaders) establishes a group for the purpose of treating patients with psychiatric disorders. *Psychiatric-Mental Health Nursing: Scope and Standards of Practice* (American Nurses Association [ANA], 2007) defines group psychotherapy as a role of the advanced practice registered nurse in psychiatric mental health (APRN-PMH). Expertise is necessary, since the group is used as a tool to bring about personality change (Sadock & Sadock, 2008). Often group psychotherapy is done in conjunction with individual psychotherapy as part of an ongoing plan of feedback in which intense one-to-one work is interspersed with an opportunity to relive and work through early life experiences.

Psychodrama Groups. Psychodrama groups are specialized groups in which members are encouraged to act out life experiences or situations for the purpose of learning and insight. Leaders should have training specific to this approach and graduate-level education.

Dialectical Behavior Treatment. Dialectical behavior treatment (DBT) groups are a type of group psychotherapy where patients are seen each week with the goal of improving interpersonal, behavioral, cognitive, and emotional skills and reducing self-destructive behaviors (Sadock & Sadock, 2008). DBT was originally developed for the treatment of patients with borderline personality disorders, but it has been extended to other illnesses. Unlike in other types of group therapy, DBT group members are discouraged from making observations

---

BOX 34-4 Support and Self-Help Groups

Target Population
- People who have shared the experience of a common problem, illness, crisis, or tragedy

Group Leader Activities
- May or may not be defined, may rotate among members
- Role is often more task oriented

Examples of Support Groups
- Bereavement groups for those who have experienced the loss of a loved one
- Suicide survivor groups for those who have lost a loved one to suicide
- NAMI (National Alliance for the Mentally Ill) groups for patient/family support, education, and advocacy
- Cancer support groups for families and patients coping with the ramifications of this illness
- Internet support groups for a growing number of people, providing online, real-time interaction and support

Examples of Self-Help Groups and Resources
- Twelve-step groups that use a common model for recovery:
  - Alcoholics Anonymous (AA)—the prototype for other 12-step groups
  - Gamblers Anonymous (GA)
  - Overeaters Anonymous (OA)

- Narcotics Anonymous (NA)
- Co-Dependents Anonymous
- Adult Children of Alcoholics (ACOA)
- Recovery International for people who have had a mental illness; groups use prescribed model for managing illness and recovery
- National Mental Health Consumers Self-Help Clearinghouse, an information clearinghouse to guide consumers to the nearly 500 diverse types of self-help groups in operation (Yalom, 2005)

Goals
- To provide health education and networking for resources
- To reduce anxiety and decrease feelings of isolation
- To provide support and encouragement of positive coping behaviors:
  - Decrease feelings of isolation
  - Provide mutual support
  - Provide psychoeducation and health education
  - Reduce stress
  - Help people cease self-destructive behaviors or come to terms with an overwhelming event or situation

Frequency and Duration
- Meets one or more times per week for an indefinite period of time
- Ongoing and open membership

---

about others in the group. This treatment also requires specialized training and advanced education.

Dealing With Challenging Member Behaviors

Research into group dynamics has identified certain behaviors of individual members that are challenging to manage within a group. Many defensive behaviors used by patients interfere with their ability to function or achieve satisfaction in their lives. Group therapy is about working through problem behaviors, but some can be especially disruptive to the group process and difficult for the leader to manage. The patient who monopolizes the group, the patient who complains but continues to reject help, the demoralizing patient, and the silent patient are examples (Yalom, 2005).

In dealing with any problematic behaviors in groups, members may appreciate help disclosing their own feelings and responses. The leader encourages the use of statements such as, "When you speak this way, I feel ...." The leader helps by noting that feelings are not right or wrong but simply exist. People tend to feel

less defensive when *I feel* statements rather than *you are* statements are used. This approach helps members feel like part of the group, not alienated from it.

Monopolizing Member

The compulsive speech of a person who monopolizes the group may be an attempt to deal with anxiety. As group tension grows, the patient's level of anxiety rises, and the patient's tendency to speak increases even more. Some people are just extremely talkative or may be hypertalkative due to hypomania or mania. In any case, no one else gets a chance to be heard, and other group members eventually lose interest and begin to withdraw.

VIGNETTE
Holly is the most talkative member of the group until the nurse intervenes. Initially, Holly talks at length about her early experiences related to losing both of her parents and having to live with her grandparents. The other members of the group become bored with the same old story, and they drift off. They have heard these stories many times, not only in group therapy but also during other activities. ■

There are several useful strategies for dealing with an overly talkative group member. One subtle method is to address the entire group with a reminder that in group work everyone should have an equal chance to contribute and that members should consider whether or not they are dominating the group's time. Another strategy is to request a response from group members who have not had a chance to talk about the day's topic. If the behavior continues, it may be necessary to speak directly to the monopolizing group member, either privately or in the group setting. In private, you can share your observations and suggest that perhaps nervousness may be a factor causing the talkativeness. Asking for clarification of your observations may lead to a greater understanding of what the group member is experiencing. You may then ask him or her to limit contributions to a specific number of times (e.g., two or three). In the group setting, the leader may ask the group if they would like to share observations or feedback about other members, thereby offering a chance for growth. This strategy is probably the most challenging but potentially the most rewarding in that members feel empowered, and the real therapeutic forces of groups are realized.

Complaining Member Who Rejects Help

The patient who complains but continues to reject help continually brings environmental or somatic problems to the group and often describes them in a manner that makes the problems seem insurmountable. In fact, the patient appears to take pride in the insolubility of his or her problems. The patient comes across as entirely self-centered, and the group's attempts to help are continually rejected.

The person who uses these tactics generally has highly conflicting feelings about his or her own dependency; any notice from the leader temporarily increases the patient's self-esteem. On the other hand, the patient has a pervasive mistrust of all authority figures. Most patients who complain but continue to reject help have been subjected to severe deprivation early in their lives and may have experienced emotional and/or physical abuse.

VIGNETTE

Michelle is always complaining about how horrible her relationship with her boyfriend is, and she manages to get the entire group worked up over the situation. Members tell her to leave him, not to spend all her time with him, and not to spend all her money on him, but each week she reports a new incident or crisis. In every session, the group members become concerned and offer encouragement, advice, and solutions. Each time, the group becomes angry at her lack of change, and she is frustrated by her own inability to change. She asserts that the group is not helpful. ■

The leader should acknowledge the patient's pessimism but maintain a neutral affect. If the patient stays in the group long enough, and the group develops a sense of cohesion, this individual can be helped to recognize relationship patterns. The leader should encourage the patient to look at the habitual "yes … but" behavior objectively.

Demoralizing Member

Some people whose behavior is self-centered, angry, or depressed may lack empathy or concern for other members of the group. They refuse to take any personal responsibility and can challenge the group leader and negatively affect the group process.

VIGNETTE

Becky comes to the support group on the inpatient psychiatric unit. She is very angry, stating, "I don't know why I come to these groups anyway! They don't help." Becky is to be discharged the next day to a 28-day alcohol rehabilitation program. She has a previously scheduled dental appointment before the rehabilitation intake interview, and she is being strongly encouraged by her therapist to reschedule the appointment. The therapist fears Becky is at high risk for drinking again, because she states that she constantly has the urge to drink. When a group member who is an addictions therapist confronts Becky about not being flexible and prioritizing her need for alcohol treatment, she explodes. "I thought this group was for support. This is outrageous!" Group members are obviously uncomfortable with her anger. ■

In this case, the group leader should listen to the comments objectively. Again, the leader may choose to speak to the group member in private and ask what is causing the anger. Sometimes this simple exchange can make the patient feel greater connection with the nurse and more important as a member of the group, which likely will decrease hostile behavior and increase the group's benefit. In the group setting, the leader can focus on positive group members whose comments may reduce the hostility of the negative group member.

Remember that angry patients may be extremely vulnerable, and devaluing or demoralizing keeps others at a distance and maintains the patient's own precarious sense of safety. Leaders must empathize with the patient in a matter-of-fact manner, such as, "You seem angry that the group wants to support you in putting sobriety ahead of your dental needs."

Silent Member

Patients who are silent in the group may be observing intently until they decide the group is safe for them, or they may believe they are not as competent as other, more assertive group members. Silence does not mean that the member is not engaged or involved, but it should be addressed for several reasons. The person who does not speak cannot benefit from others' feedback, and other group members are deprived of this group member's valuable insights. Furthermore, a silent group member may make others uncomfortable and create a sense of mistrust.

VIGNETTE

Anne has attended three group sessions for survivors of childhood sexual abuse. While she appears to be listening, she rarely makes eye contact with the leader or other group members. She will respond to yes or no questions, but when it comes to the open-ended type, such as "What do you think, Anne?" she tends to shrug her shoulders and respond with "I don't know." Other group members have tried to draw Anne out, as has the leader. Kathy, another group member, is beginning to exhibit frustration with Anne. "Look, I have shared some of the most private and painful memories of my childhood. I feel like you think you're too good to share what happened to you." ■

Anyone who has led a group can attest to the challenges of a silent member. There are several techniques that may help, including allowing the person to have extra time to formulate his or her thoughts before responding. Saying, "I'll give you a moment to think about that," and waiting or coming back to the group member later is often helpful. Another tactic is to make an assignment that every person in the group respond to a certain topic or question. For example, "Let's all think of a positive and assertive response to something that you generally feel helpless about. I'll give you a minute or so to think this over, and then I'm going to ask each of you to share."

Sometimes partnering with another group member will give the silent member the courage they need to participate. You may break the group into pairs who are asked to discuss a certain topic and then each report back to the group what they heard the other one say.

EXPECTED OUTCOMES

Expected outcomes of group participation will vary, depending on the type and purpose of the group. For education groups, such as a medication education group, the expected outcome would be demonstration of knowledge such as:

- Patient identifies three significant side effects of their prescribed medication
- Patient recognizes dangerous drug-drug and drug-food interactions for their prescribed medication
- Patient correctly identifies time of day and dose for each prescribed medication

For therapy groups, the expected outcomes will focus more on insights, behavior changes, and reduction in symptoms. For example, in an alcohol treatment group, an expected outcome might be that the patient develops insight into the connection between drinking and negative consequences. An expected behavioral outcome would be abstinence from alcohol use. In groups that focus primarily on emotional issues such as depression or anxiety, standardized tests can be used to measure symptom reduction as an outcome of group participation.

KEY POINTS TO REMEMBER

- When a new group is formed, similarities and differences in many dimensions, including diagnosis, age, gender, and culture, must be considered.
- A group format has advantages over individual therapy, including cost savings, increased feedback, an opportunity to practice new skills in a relatively safe environment, and instilling a sense of belonging.
- Research has identified 11 therapeutic factors that operate in groups and lead to therapeutic change for members. Yalom's Therapeutic Factors identify specific positive aspects of groups, such as universality of experience and the instillation of hope.
- Groups develop through predictable phases over time.
- For a group to continue and be productive, members must fulfill specific functions known as *task* or *maintenance roles*. Individual roles are not productive and are based on individual personalities and needs.
- Clinical supervision is important so that group leaders can objectively analyze group interactions and leadership techniques.
- Nurses have many opportunities to lead or co-lead therapeutic groups, both in the hospital and community setting.
- Psychoeducational groups, activity groups, task groups, and support groups are often led by registered nurses and provide significant treatment as part of the multidisciplinary treatment plan.
- Advanced practice registered nurses may lead psychotherapy groups based on various theoretical models.
- Challenging member behaviors such as silence, complaining, or demoralizing can be especially difficult. A variety of interventions are recommended to minimize the disruption to the group and maximize the benefit to the patient who is engaging in these behaviors.

CRITICAL THINKING

1. You are assigned to work with Mary, a 30-year-old who was admitted to the psychiatric unit with major depression and a suicide attempt. Her nurse has told her she needs to attend group therapy. While lying in bed and staring at the ceiling, Mary tells you that she is a private person and that listening to other people's problems won't help and will only make her more depressed.
   A. How would you describe the benefits of group therapy to Mary?

B. What intervention(s) might make it easier for Mary to attend group therapy?

2. Construct an outline for a medication teaching group that would cover information useful for your patients. If possible co-lead this group with a staff member with guidelines from your instructor.

3. Ms. Rodriguez is a 22-year-old Puerto Rican–born nursing student admitted to the psychiatric unit after a nearly lethal overdose of acetaminophen. She admits to drinking excessively for the past six months. She is at risk of failing school. She complains of depressed mood, a loss of interest in her studies, decreased concentration, and social isolation. In the dual-diagnosis group, she has been silent for the past two sessions and sits staring at the floor.
   A. What is your evaluation of Ms. Rodriguez's situation?
   B. What might Ms. Rodriguez's nonverbal behavior mean?
   C. What approach would you use to involve her more in the group?
   D. What criteria could you use to evaluate the effectiveness of your intervention?
   E. What cultural implications should you consider?

CHAPTER REVIEW

1. The nurse is caring for four patients. Which patient would not be appropriate to consider for group therapy? The patient who:
   1. has limited financial resources.
   2. is acutely manic.
   3. has few friends on the unit.
   4. does not speak up often, yet listens to others.

2. The nurse tells group members that they will be working on expressing conflicts during the current group session. Which phase of group development is represented?
   1. Formation phase
   2. Orientation phase
   3. Working phase
   4. Termination phase

3. Group members are having difficulty deciding what topic to cover in today's session. Which nurse leader response reflects autocratic leadership?
   1. "We are talking about fear of rejection today."
   2. "Let's go around the room and make suggestions for today's topic."
   3. "I will let you come to a conclusion together about what to talk about."
   4. "I'll work with you to find a suitable topic for today."

4. The nurse is planning care which will include a dual-diagnosis group. Which patient would be appropriate for this group? The patient with:
   1. depression and suicidal tendencies.
   2. anxiety and frequent migraine headaches.
   3. bipolar disorder and anorexia nervosa.
   4. schizophrenia and alcohol abuse.

5. A patient continues to dominate the group conversation despite having been asked to allow others to speak. What is the most appropriate nursing response?
   1. "You are monopolizing the conversation."
   2. "When you talk constantly, it makes everyone feel angry."
   3. "You are supposed to allow others to talk also."
   4. "When you speak out of turn, I feel concerned that others cannot participate equally."

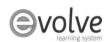

Visit the Evolve website for an **Audio Chapter Summary, Chapter Review Answers & Rationales, Critical Thinking Answer Guidelines,** and additional resources related to the content in this chapter: **http://evolve.elsevier.com/Varcarolis/foundations**

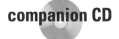

Use the Companion CD to prepare for tests and the NCLEX® Examination with **Test-Taking Strategies** for psychiatric mental health nursing and hundreds of **Review Questions.**

REFERENCES

American Psychiatric Nurses Association, International Society of Psychiatric-Mental Health Nurses, & American Nurses Association. (2007). *Psychiatric-mental health nursing: Scope and standards of practice.* Silver Spring, MD: NurseBooks.org.

Benne, K. D., & Sheats, P. (1948). Functional roles of group members. *Journal of Social Issues, 4*(2) 41–49.

Chadwick, P., Taylor, K. N., & Abba, N. (2005). Mindfulness groups for people with psychosis. *Behavioural and Cognitive Psychotherapy, 33,* 351–359.

Drake, R. E., Essock, S. M., Shaner, A., Carey, K. B., Minkoff, K., Kola, L., et al. (2001). Implementing dual-diagnosis services for clients with severe mental illness. *Psychiatric Services, 52,* 469–476.

Hayes, S. A., Hope, D. A., Terryberry-Spohr, L. S., Spaulding, W. D., Vandyke, M., Elting, D. T., et al. (2006).

Discriminating between cognitive and supportive group therapies for chronic mental illness. *The Journal of Nervous and Mental Disease, 194,* 603–609.

Sadock, B. J., & Sadock, V. A. (2008). *Kaplan & Sadock's concise textbook of clinical psychiatry* (3rd ed.). Philadelphia: Lippincott Williams & Wilkins.

Winship, G. (2007). A qualitative study into the experience of individuals involved in a mindfulness group within an acute inpatient mental health unit. *Journal of Psychiatric and Mental Health Nursing, 14,* 603-608.

Yalom, I. D. (2005). *The theory and practice of group psychotherapy* (5th ed.). New York: Basic Books.

CHAPTER **35**

Family Interventions

Sylvia Stevens and Verna Benner Carson

Key Terms and Concepts

behavioral family therapy, 754
boundaries, 750
clear boundaries, 750
diffuse or enmeshed boundaries, 750
family systems theory, 754
family triangle, 756
flexibility, 754

genogram, 758
insight-oriented family therapy, 754
multigenerational issues, 758
nuclear family, 757
psychoeducational family therapy, 763
rigid or disengaged boundaries, 750
sociocultural context, 758

Objectives

1. Discuss the characteristics of a healthy family using clinical examples.
2. Differentiate between functional and dysfunctional family patterns of behavior as they relate to the five family functions.
3. Compare and contrast insight-oriented family therapy and behavioral family therapy.
4. Identify five family theorists and their contributions to the family therapy movement.
5. Analyze the meaning and value of the family's sociocultural context when assessing and planning intervention strategies.

6. Construct a genogram using a three-generation approach.
7. Formulate seven outcome criteria that a counselor and family might develop together.
8. Identify some strategies for family intervention.
9. Distinguish between the nursing intervention strategies of a basic level nurse and those of an advanced practice nurse with regard to counseling and psychotherapy and psychobiological issues.
10. Explain the importance of the nurse's role in psychoeducational family therapy.

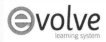 Visit the Evolve website for an **Audio Glossary & Flashcards**, **Concept Map Creator**, and additional resources related to the content in this chapter: **http://evolve.elsevier.com/Varcarolis/foundations**

In Western culture, the uniqueness of the individual and the search for autonomy is celebrated, yet we are defined and sustained by interlocking systems of human relationships, including the relationships we develop with our own family members (Nichols, 2004). Many of us struggle with these personal family relationships and wish they were better. When families are discussed, the tone ranges from a negative focus on differences and dissension to a positive focus on loyalty, tolerance, mutual aide, and assistance.

The individual learns a range of social and emotional responses through the family; it is the training ground for interacting in the greater community. Most people struggle to fully understand the forces that influence family functioning, even when they evaluate their family as "normal." When a family is plagued with depression, anxiety, and/or unhappy relationships, the individual may have similar interpersonal patterns and carry these same problems into adult life. Some families need psychotherapeutic intervention during the early years of a child's development to correct maladaptive patterns in order to limit the psychological impairment.

Family therapy is defined as a psychotherapeutic process that focuses on changing the interactions among the people who make up the family or marital unit (Sadock & Sadock, 2008). It also serves to improve the family itself, the subsystems within the family, and the individuals who make up the family. It focuses on evaluating these relationships and the communication patterns, structure, and rules that govern the nature of them.

FAMILY

What is a family? There are many different types of families, each defined by reciprocal relationships in which people are committed to one another. A family can consist of a married couple with children, two people of the same sex committed to each other and living together, a married couple without children, a remarriage in which a parent, stepparent, and children and/or stepchildren all live together, a single adult with an adopted child, a gay or lesbian couple raising biological, adopted, or stepchildren, a tri-generational group in which grandparent(s), parent(s), and child(ren) all live together as a cohesive unit.

The family is the primary system to which a person belongs, and in most cases, it is the most powerful system of which a person will ever be a member. Birth, puberty, marriage, and death can all be considered family experiences. The family can be the source of love or hate, pride or shame, security or insecurity. Although individual family members have roles and functions, the overriding value in families lies in the relationships among family members. It is these family relationships that provide the primary context of human development. "Family" comprises the entire system of at least three, and frequently four, generations. Many family theorists consider the intergenerational connectedness of the family to be one of our greatest human resources.

Family Functions

Healthy families provide members with tools that guide effective functioning in intimate relationships, the workplace, their culture, and society in general. These tools are acquired through the activities associated with family life, which can be divided into five functions: (1) management, (2) boundaries, (3) communication, (4) emotional-supportive, and (5) socialization (Nichols, 2004). Although family therapists may use various assessment strategies, these five areas are always included. Figure 35-1 presents an assessment tool developed by Roberts (1983) that the family counselor can use to evaluate these five areas of function.

Management

Every day in every family, decisions are made regarding issues of power, rule making, and provision of financial support. Other management issues include future planning and goods allocation (i.e., who gets what within the family). In healthy families, it is usually the adults in the family who agree as to how these functions are to be performed. In families with a single parent, these management functions may sometimes become overwhelming, and single parents can benefit from discussions with other adults. In more chaotic families, an inappropriate member, such as a teenager, may be the one who makes these decisions. Although children learn decision-making skills as they mature and increasingly make decisions and choices about their own lives, they should not be expected or forced to take on this responsibility for the family.

Boundaries

Boundaries maintain a distinction between individuals in the family. Boundaries may be clear, diffuse, rigid, or inconsistent. Most families are combinations of these boundary types (Goldenberg & Goldenberg, 2008). Clear boundaries are well understood by all members of the family and give family members a sense of "I-ness" and also "we-ness." They help define the roles of members within the family and allow members to function without unnecessary interference from other members. However, they are not so rigid as to restrict contact among family members. For example, a mother tells her 14-year-old daughter, "You don't need to worry whether your little brother eats his breakfast. Your father and I will handle that." This boundary may be redefined: "I want you to make sure that your little brother gets his homework done while your father and I are at the movies."

Diffuse or enmeshed boundaries refer to a blending together of the roles, thoughts, and feelings of the individual family members so that clear distinctions fail to emerge. The members of a family that operates with diffuse or enmeshed boundaries are more prone to psychological or psychosomatic symptoms. A common phenomenon within families with diffuse boundaries is that individuals expect other members of the family to know what they are thinking ("Why did you take that? You know I wanted it!") and believe they know what other family members are thinking ("I know exactly why you did that!").

Rigid or disengaged boundaries are those in which the rules and roles are consistently adhered to no matter what; thus rigid boundaries prevent family members from trying out new roles or, in some cases, from taking on more mature functions as time goes on. In families in which rigid boundaries predominate, isolation may be marked. Family members are often cut off from the community and outside influences, and even from each other.

FAMILY FUNCTION CHECKLIST

Client Family _____ Date of Assessment _____

Family Functions	Observed Behavior	Assessed Need Level (I-IV)	Suggested Nursing Responses
I. *Management function* A. Use of power for all family members B. Rule making clear, accepted C. Fiscal support adequate D. Successful negotiations with extrafamilial systems E. Future planning present			
II. *Boundary function* A. Clear individual boundaries B. Clear generational boundaries C. Clear family boundaries			
III. *Communication function* A. Straight messages B. No manipulation C. Safe expression of positive and negative feelings			
IV. *Emotional-supportive function* A. Mutual positive regard B. Deals with conflict C. Uses resources for all family members D. Allows growth for all family members			
V. *Socialization function* A. Children growing and developing in a healthy pattern B. Mutual negotiation of roles by age and ability C. Parents feeling good about parenting D. Spouses happy with each other's role behavior			

Figure 35-1 Family Function Checklist. (From Roberts, F. B. [1983]. An interaction model for family assessment. In I. W. Clements & F. B. Roberts [Eds.], *Family health: A theoretical approach to nursing care* [p. 202]. New York: Wiley. Copyright © 1983 John Wiley & Sons. Reprinted by permission of John Wiley & Sons, Inc.)

VIGNETTE

Kristina is a single parent living on public assistance; she has two preschool-aged children. A teenage mother, Kristina is studying for a general equivalency degree and working part time as a seamstress. Her mother, Sandra, helps to watch the children, and discipline of the children is an issue of contention between Kristina and Sandra. Kristina's mother thinks that the children are allowed to run wild under Kristina's care. ▪

When boundaries are functioning properly, family members work out arrangements in there is compromise based on understanding of appropriate roles. Each generation within the family are made aware of how decisions will be made and clearly understand who is in charge and when they are in charge. Blurred boundary function results in family members interfering with each other's goals, resulting in tension and anxiety between family members. Children in families such as this become confused, engage in manipulative and perhaps age-inappropriate behavior, and feel insecure.

Communication

Communication patterns are extremely important in family life. Healthy communication patterns are characterized by clear and comprehensible messages (e.g., "I would like to go now," or "I don't like it when you interrupt what I'm saying"). Healthy communication within the family encourages members to ask for what they want and express their feelings appropriately. Feelings of affection and conflict are both openly expressed. Family members are able to ask for what they want and get the attention they need without resorting to manipulation. When communication among family members is unclear, it cannot be used as a means to solve problems or to resolve conflict; therefore, the cardinal rule for effective and functional communication in families is: "Be clear and direct in saying what you want and need."

As simple as this may seem, it is one of the hardest skills to activate in a family system. To be direct, individuals must first have a sense that the self is respected and loved; they then feel entitled to take a stand and set boundaries with others. The consequences of being clear and direct may be unpleasant in a family system in which boundaries are enmeshed and confusion is the norm. To attempt to change a family pattern is to pit oneself against the status quo. Explicitly stating what one wants and needs is especially difficult when one believes that family members should already know—especially if the family member is a spouse, a parent, or a close sibling. No one is able to mind-read, but emotionally undifferentiated members may think that this is possible. The following vignette describes a spousal situation that shows how easily communication can be misunderstood when clear and direct messages are not sent, and Box 35-1 identifies some unhealthy communication patterns.

VIGNETTE

Liz would like to spend more time with her husband, Michael, on the weekends; however, Michael always seems to be busy doing projects around the house or talking with friends on the telephone. Liz feels that he does not notice her, or maybe is not interested in her, so she spends a lot of time working out or playing tennis. Michael figures that Liz is doing what she wants to do and that it makes her happy, so he contents himself with finding things to do alone. The result is that Liz and Michael spend little time together. Liz finally confronts Michael clearly and directly about his "disinterest" in her and tells him what she wants and needs—to spend more time together on the weekends. Michael replies that he had no idea she felt that way. He had thought she enjoyed the way things were, and he would like to have more time together too. ∎

Emotional Support

All families encounter conflicts, and no family is 100% "functional." However, in a healthy family, feelings of affection are generally uppermost, and anger and conflict do not dominate the family's pattern of interaction. Healthy families are concerned with each other's needs, and most of the family members' emotional and physical needs are met most of the time. When peoples' emotional needs are met, they feel support from those around them and are free to grow and explore new roles and facets of their personalities. A family that is dominated by conflict and anger alienates its members, leaving them isolated, fearful, and impaired emotionally.

Socialization

It is within families that each member learns socialization skills. People learn how to interact, negotiate, and plan; they adopt coping skills. This is most evident in the socialization of children. Children learn how to function effectively within the family, and then they apply those skills in society. Parents are socialized

---

BOX 35-1 Examples of Dysfunctional Communication

Manipulating

Instead of asking directly for what is wanted, family members manipulate others to get what they want. For example, a child starts a fight with a sibling to get attention. Another example is a family member's making requests with strings attached, so that the other person has a difficult time refusing the request: "If you do this for me, I won't tell Daddy you are getting poor grades in school."

Distracting

To avoid functional problem solving and resolve conflicts within the family, family members introduce irrelevant details into problematic issues.

Generalizing

When dealing with problematic family issues, members use global statements like "always" and "never" instead of dealing with specific problems and areas of conflict. Family members may say "Harry is always angry" instead of "Harry, what is upsetting you?"

Blaming

Family members blame others for failures, errors, or negative consequences of an action to keep the focus away from themselves. This is a response to fear of being blamed by others.

Placating

Family members pretend to be inadequate but well meaning to keep peace in the family at any price: "Don't yell at the children, dear. *I* put the shoes on the stairs."

---

into their family role by the demands of each child throughout the developmental stages of their children. The parents' role changes again when the children mature and leave home, and the partners may renegotiate the pattern of their lives together. As time goes on, the parents may need their adult children's help if they become less able to care for their own needs. Each phase brings new demands and requires new approaches to deal with changes as people become socialized into new roles. Families have difficulty negotiating role change, and changes often increase the stress within families for a time. In response to the family's developmental life cycle, healthy families are flexible in adapting to new roles.

Family Life Cycle

The life cycle of the individual takes place within the family life cycle, which is the primary context of human development. The family is a system that moves through time, and family stress is often the greatest at transition points or when an interruption or a dislocation occurs. Transition points include the birth of a child, employment changes, children leaving home, and retirement. Interruptions or dislocations could include a serious illness, death, or divorce. At these times, therapeutic efforts often need to be directed toward helping family members reorganize so that they can then proceed developmentally. If a family member feels there is no way to function within the system, the pressures can, in the extreme, lead to mental illness or suicide. The development of symptoms should be viewed not only as a response to an interruption or a dislocation in the family life cycle but also as a solution to a stressful situation. This model assumes a traditional family organization and must be modified for those are considered "less traditional."

In the traditional Northern European family type, there are six main phases of the family life cycle: (1) launching the single young adult, (2) joining families through couple formation, (3) becoming parents and caring for young children, (4) parenting adolescents, (5) launching children and moving on, and (6) experiencing later life. Not all families go through these phases. In the divorce and postdivorce family life cycle, there are four other phases, and in the remarried family life cycle there are two additional phases.

THEORY

The basic framework of family therapy took root in the 1960s and 1970s. In clinical settings, therapists were beginning to notice the effects of the social milieu on their patients, the therapeutic community became established as a treatment modality, and group therapy and psychodrama (see Chapter 34) were developed. All these changes were based on observations of patients and a belief that social systems played an integral role in psychological functioning and treatment. An **interactive** (interpersonal) rather than **indwelling** (intrapsychic Freudian) model of mental illness was becoming more widely accepted. These influences paved the way for an interest in the family system as it related to psychiatric disorders.

Virginia Satir (1972, 1983) and Jay Haley (1980, 1996), two leading theorists of the same era, moved the focus from the patient's symptoms to the patient's position and relationships within the family. Salvador Minuchin (1974, 1996), a structural therapist, established the legitimacy of family therapy within psychiatry. Bowen (1985, 1988) was a leading proponent of the family systems model. He underplayed problem resolution, focusing instead on the long-term differentiation process of individual family members.

The terms *strategic* and *structural* are used to identify the frameworks adopted by specific therapists. A **strategic model of family therapy** assumes that changing any single element in the family system will bring about change in the entire system. Briefly, the aim of strategic therapy is to change the patterns, rules, and meaning of family interactions.

VIGNETTE

Eight-year-old Tommy Gomez, who is hyperactive and disruptive at school and at home, is brought to the community mental health clinic to be evaluated for attention deficit hyperactivity disorder (ADHD). The nurse clinician performs an assessment and finds that a great deal of turmoil exists within the Gomez family. The family is composed of Tommy's married parents, their two other children, and a grandmother. Tommy's father has just lost his job, and his grandmother was recently diagnosed with bladder cancer. Tommy's mother is planning to file for separation because of constant, unresolved arguments with her husband. The nurse clinician who views this family from a strategic model would not focus solely on Tommy but would view Tommy's symptoms as a function of many difficult losses and transitions that are stressing the entire family's coping mechanisms.

The nurse identifies the multiple stressors in this family, believing that Tommy's symptoms of hyperactivity and acting out are related to the severe stresses in the family system. Once the issues within the family are addressed and plans are made to deal with these issues, perhaps Tommy's symptoms will subside. She refers the couple to a family therapist. In the meantime, she encourages the couple to focus more on their own issues and less on Tommy's behavior. An appointment is made to go to the clinic in 1 month, where Tommy will be reevaluated. ∎

The previous vignette is an example of a family in which a pattern of communication, partly cultural, excludes any discussion with the children. All decisions, whether or not they involve the children, are made without informing them. Consequently, the children in this family often feel powerless, and Tommy has begun to engage in destructive behavior at school, which has precipitated a visit to a family therapist. A family therapist who uses the strategic model might work with the family to change their rigid pattern of communication to allow the children to be informed earlier in the decision-making process. The children could comment and offer suggestions about how issues could be resolved. Tommy may be less anxious and less of a behavior problem because he has been given a sense of control over some aspects of his life. This intervention would result in a systemic change in the way the Gomez family communicates.

The **structural model of family therapy** explains family problems from the perspective of dysfunctional boundary and role structure. These problems become evident when the family is exposed to a stressor or a transition point and find they are unable to adapt to changing conditions (Goldenberg & Goldenberg, 2008). A therapist using the structural model with the Gomez family, rather than focusing on changing a specific pattern, would highlight the importance of boundaries between the parental and sibling (child) subsystems. At the same time, the therapist would emphasize the importance of flexibility in the family system that would allow for the changes inherent to normal growth and development.

The aims of family systems theory are to decrease emotional reactivity and encourage differentiation among individual family members (i.e., increase each member's sense of self). The parents or adults in the system would be encouraged to consider emotional patterns learned in their family of origin and attempt to utilize extended family resources to reengage in more mature patterns of interaction. Children who are identified as the "problem" receive counseling and behavior therapy but are not the focus of the therapy. Instead, the couple or parent is encouraged to consider

system factors that may contribute to the child's emotional and/or behavioral problems.

In family therapy, there is no single, accepted model for treating families. All the shapers of family theory have made substantial contributions to the field of family therapy. In addition, all techniques are not applicable to all problems, and the experienced clinician must be discerning. Most of the theoretical schools of or approaches to marital and family therapy fall into two broad classifications: insight-oriented family therapy or behavioral family therapy. Table 35-1 summarizes some of the types of therapy in each classification, describes their basic concepts and approaches, and lists the major theorists.

Working with the Family

Many concepts are widely used in working with families. The concepts of the identified patient, the family triangle, and the nuclear family emotional system are discussed here. Box 35-2 describes other concepts relevant to family work.

TABLE 35-1 Insight-Oriented and Behavioral Therapy

Type of Therapy	Concepts	Major Theorists
INSIGHT-ORIENTED FAMILY THERAPY		
Psychodynamic therapy	Problems arise from: • Developmental arrest • Current interactions • Projections • Current stresses Improvement through insight into problematic relationships originating in the past	Nathan Ackerman James Framo Ivan Boszormenyi-Nagy
Family-of-origin therapy	Family viewed as an emotional relationship system: • Goal is to foster differentiation and decrease emotional reactivity • Concept of triangulation • Emphasis on the family of origin	Murray Bowen
Experimental-existential therapy	Goal of therapy is to encourage the growth of family: • Symptoms express family pain • Family is responsible for its own solutions • Therapist uses nurturing and identifies dysfunctional communication patterns	Carl Whitaker Virginia Satir Leslie Greenberg Susan Johnson
BEHAVIORAL FAMILY THERAPY		
Structural therapy	Focus is on organizational patterns, boundaries, systems and subsystems, and use of scapegoating: • Restructures dysfunctional triangles • Clarifies boundaries • Looks at enmeshment and disengagement (excessive distance) issues	Salvador Minuchin

Continued

TABLE 35-1 Insight-Oriented and Behavioral Therapy—cont'd

Type of Therapy	Concepts	Major Theorists
BEHAVIORAL FAMILY THERAPY		
Strategic therapy	Goal is to change repetitive and maladaptive interaction patterns: • Identifies inequality of power, life-cycle perspectives, and use of double-bind messages • Uses paradox • Prescribes rituals	Jay Haley Chloe Madanes Milan group (Mara Palazzoli, Gianfranco Cecchin, Giuliana Prata)
Cognitive-behavioral therapy	Based on learning theory; focuses on changing cognition and behavior: • Problem solving and solutions focus on present situations • Skills training is emphasized	Gerald Patterson Richard Stuart Robert Liberman

---

BOX 35-2 Central Concepts of Family

Boundaries: Clear boundaries are those that maintain distinctions between individuals within the family and between the family and the outside world. Clear boundaries allow for balanced flow of energy between members. Roles of children and parent or parents are clearly defined. Diffuse or enmeshed boundaries are those in which there is a blending together of the roles, thoughts, and feelings of the individuals so that clear distinctions among family members fail to emerge. Rigid or disengaged boundaries are those in which the rules and roles are adhered to no matter what.

Triangulation: The tendency, when two-person relationships are stressful and unstable, to draw in a third person to stabilize the system through formation of a coalition in which the two join the third.

Scapegoating: A form of displacement in which a family member (usually the least powerful) is blamed for another's or another family member's distress. The purpose is to keep the focus off the painful issues and the problems of the blamers. In a family, the blamers are often the parents and the scapegoat a child.

Double bind: A situation in which a positive command (often verbal) is followed by a negative command (often nonverbal), which leaves the recipient confused, trapped, and immobilized because there is no appropriate way to act. A double bind is a "no-win" situation in which you are "darned if you do, darned if you don't."

Hierarchy: The function of power and its structures in families, differentiating parental and sibling roles and generational boundaries.

Family life cycle: The family's developmental process over time; refers to the family's past course, its present tasks, and its future course.

Differentiation: The ability to develop a strong identity and sense of self while at the same time maintaining an emotional connectedness with one's family of origin.

Sociocultural context: The framework for viewing the family in terms of the influence of gender, race, ethnicity, religion, economic class, and sexual orientation.

Multigenerational issues: The continuation and persistence from generation to generation of certain emotional interactive family patterns (e.g., reenactment of fairly predictable and almost ritual-like patterns; repetition of themes or toxic issues; and repetition of reciprocal patterns such as those of overfunctioner and underfunctioner).

The Family as a System

Every family can be viewed as a unique system. Each has its own structure, rules, and history of how it handles life problems and crises. Focusing on family patterns and interaction is basic to marital family therapy. The focus is *not* on an individual, as it is in traditional therapy, but rather on the interpersonal process of the family group (Nichols, 2004).

The Identified Patient

The **identified patient** is the individual in the family whom everyone regards as "the problem." A descriptive term for this person is also the "family symptom-bearer." This family member is generally the focus of most of the family system's anxiety. She or he may serve to divert the attention from other more serious and debilitating problems within the family, such as a crumbling marriage, substance abuse, or infidelity. Furthermore, the symptoms of the identified patient may serve as a stabilizing mechanism to bring about customary behavior in a distressed family (Goldenberg & Goldenberg, 2008). The identified patient may even be aware at some level of the role he serves in order to "save" the family. For example, adult children may sacrifice their autonomy by staying in the home to hold the parents together.

When a family comes for treatment, the presenting problem, which is usually related to one member of the family, must be addressed before the underlying systemic problem is dealt with. The family member who is the identified patient may or may *not* be the one who initially seeks help from inpatient or outpatient services.

When working with families, it is important to consider not only the family as a system in a particular stage of life-cycle development but also the individual developmental stage of each member. For example, a family may present with parents in Erikson's stage of generativity vs. stagnation, adolescent children dealing with identify vs. role confusion issues, a school-age child facing challenges of industry vs. inferiority, and grandparents dealing with ego integrity vs. despair. While no individual exactly fits Erikson's stages based on chronological age alone, most people are challenged by both their current life tasks and the tasks of their family. Thus, there is more than one perspective to be considered when looking at the identi-

fied patient in terms of the family system. The focus is on the family system's anxiety.

Family Triangles

Bowen (1985) described an important and common relationship process in families; it can be seen as a system of interlocking triangles. When tension in a family is low, the dyad or two-person system may interact comfortably, although some tension lies in the struggle between closeness and independence. When the tension in a close twosome builds, a third person (child, friend, parent) may be brought in to help lower the tension. The **family triangle** (Figure 35-2) then becomes the basic building block of interpersonal relationships. All triangles contain a close side, a distant side, and a side in which conflict or tension exists between two people (Nelson, 2003).

The intensity of the triangling process varies among families and within the same family over time because triangles create emotional instability. **Differentiation** refers to the ability of the individual to establish a unique identity while remaining emotionally connected to the family of origin. The lower the level of differentiation in a family, the higher the tension is, and the more important the role of triangling is to the lowering of tension and the preservation of emotional stability. As the family becomes stressed, for whatever reasons, the anxiety in the system is triggered, and the triangles become more active.

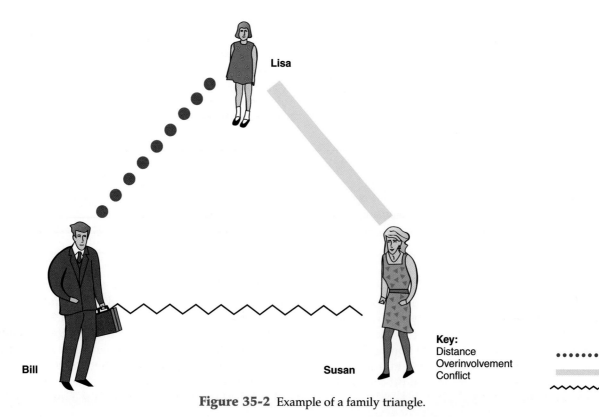

Figure 35-2 Example of a family triangle.

A common problem that occurs in families is the setting up of a triangle among two parents and a child; one parent is overinvolved with the child, and the other plays a more peripheral role. In this situation, the child eventually becomes the means by which the parents communicate with each other about issues they cannot deal with directly. In other words, spousal conflicts may be brought into the parental arena, where they clearly do not belong.

VIGNETTE

Six-year-old Hailey is having trouble making friends. Her mother, Megan, has been feeling anxious and helpless as she tries to find ways to engage Hailey with other youngsters. Megan develops an overprotectiveness that further inhibits Hailey from venturing out to make friends. Megan feels that her husband, Sean, is uncaring and disinterested because he thinks that she should be more relaxed about Hailey's social life and let things develop naturally. Sean's job requires that he travel most of the week, so he is not involved with Megan's daily experiences and struggles with Hailey.

In the spousal arena, Megan and Sean have been avoiding intimacy for almost a year. Megan is angry with Sean for spending so much time with his parents, which further casts him in a peripheral role in their nuclear family, and Sean is angry with Megan, sensing her rejection of him. Both are feeling isolated and alienated and are consequently angry with each other. Neither Sean nor Megan addresses this issue directly. Instead, they play out their anger in the parental arena as they battle over how to handle Hailey's social isolation. ■

The Nurse's Response to Triangulation. Although basic level nurses do not provide family therapy, they do interact with patients and families. Nurses should be aware that they carry their own family-of-origin issues, which may affect their responses. When this happens, the nurse may become "triangled" into the family's system. It is critical that the nurse's personal work on his or her own differentiation process continues while providing care for families. The nurse's continued self-assessment is necessary to maintain emotional stability in the face of a chaotic family situation, in which the nurse's own issues may be playing out.

For advanced practice nurses who engage in family therapy, holding family members accountable for themselves—making clear that the responsibility for change is theirs and not that of the nurse—is a way of remaining clear of their triangles. For example, the nurse therapist could become triangled into a family system in any number of ways: perhaps the nurse recently experienced the loss of a family member; the nurse may belong to an enmeshed family system, in which the children are regularly drawn into spousal arguments; or perhaps stubbornness is an unresolved issue for the nurse. Any of these possibilities could allow the nurse to become triangled into a family system, which makes good therapeutic intervention difficult, if not impossible. The likelihood is high that nurse clinicians will become triangled into others' family systems to engage in their own family battles.

Engaging in personal family-of-origin therapy and regular supervision are always recommended when nurse therapists work with individuals, couples, or families. Supervision can be conducted with peer professionals, in groups, or privately with a more experienced clinician. One indication that a nurse is being triangled is that his or her level of anxiety is greater than the situation warrants.

The Nuclear Family Emotional System

The term **nuclear family** refers to a parent or parents and the children under the parents' care. Bowen (1985) developed the concept of a *nuclear family emotional system*, which is defined as the flow of emotional processes within the nuclear family. In this concept, symptoms are viewed as belonging to the nuclear family emotional system rather than to any one individual. Within the system, a distinction is made between conventional medical (psychiatric) diagnosis and family diagnosis; rather than viewing a symptom as reflecting a disease that is confined to a patient, Bowen identified an emotional process that transcends the boundaries of a patient and encompasses the family relationship system. The earlier example of 8-year-old Tommy, who was believed by his family and others to have ADHD, is one in which Tommy's symptoms could be viewed as reflecting the family's conflicts and changes.

Refer to Box 35-2 for a summary of concepts central to family life.

APPLICATION OF THE NURSING PROCESS

ASSESSMENT

Assessment is typically intermixed with treatment, rather than constituting a distinct phase. Assessment should have multiple foci, including:
- The family system
- Family subsystems
- Individual members of the family

Essential information regarding sociocultural issues, past medical and mental illness, family interactions and communication styles, and areas of stress within the family needs to be obtained. Nichols (2004) identifies a number of issues that should be assessed in family therapy:
- Phases of the family life cycle
- Sociocultural context
- Multigenerational issues

Sociocultural Context

Rather than an isolated unit, the family is viewed in a sociocultural context, in which the issues of gender, race, ethnicity, class, sexual orientation, and religion are considered equally. Each of these contextual issues affects the family's specific values, norms, traditions, roles, and rules. For example, the way the family relates to a terminally ill family member may be decidedly different in a first-generation Italian American Catholic family than in a Japanese family or in an African American Baptist family. Therefore, the nurse clinician needs to ask how this family's cultural and religious beliefs affect the patient's presenting problem and what impact they have on the family's available options.

In regard to gender, the position of women in U.S. society needs to be understood in terms of job opportunities, earning power, and status, which for most women are secondary to those of men. Gender and culture must be viewed together, because the relative status of males and females differs according to culture. In particular, people from Asian and Latin cultures living in the United States have difficulty understanding gender roles in this country.

With regard to race and ethnicity, it is extremely important that nurses be aware of and understand the mores, practices, and beliefs of the many different cultures that exist in the United States (see Chapter 6). This cultural sensitivity prepares the nurse clinician to make effective interventions for families in times of crisis or psychiatric emergency. Because U.S. society does not overtly make class distinctions, viewing the family in the context of class may not come easily and indeed may be uncomfortable. In fact, class is often considered by most therapists to be the "last taboo." Although it is unspoken, most people in the United States do have a definite sense of the class to which they belong. It is most often defined in terms of money, education, and taste, and only with gentle questioning do these defining issues come to the fore.

Sexual orientation is another part of the context that often gets overlooked. When gathering family information, the nurse must ask questions regarding sexual orientation (e.g., in terms of long-term relationships). Finally, the context of religion figures prominently in a large percentage of the population, and this context includes many beliefs about why a person becomes ill and how that person should be treated. When the family is viewed in a sociocultural context, religion and spiritual values are important issues for consideration.

Multigenerational Issues

The influence of family is not restricted to the members of a household. Family is composed of the entire emotional system of at least three, and sometimes four, generations. This means that the family is affected by multigenerational issues. Through this intergenerational system, various patterns (e.g., involving geographical distance between members, suicide, divorce, addiction, affairs, grief, triangles, and loss) are passed down through the generations. The messages and legacies of the multigenerational family relate in some way to the patient's presenting problem. For example, in a family with adolescents in which the grandmother is terminally ill with cancer, if a pattern of addiction is already established in the family, the impending loss of an important family figure may exacerbate an addiction in one of the family members. An astute nurse may express concern to the family regarding this possibility, perhaps preventing the development of a serious problem.

This family may also have a preferred pattern of dealing with grief by using denial and by not allowing the outward expression of painful feelings. If this is the case, the nurse guides the family into learning about other, more acceptable and healthier ways of dealing with grief, because unexpressed feelings of grief may lead to further symptomatic behaviors in other family members. One way to identify multigenerational issues is by constructing a genogram.

Constructing a Genogram

The genogram is a format for efficiently providing a clinical summary of information and relationships across at least three generations of a family. It is an invaluable assessment tool that provides a graphic display of complex patterns and serves as a source of hypotheses as to how the presenting problem connects to the family context and the evolution of the family.

Bowen (1985) provided much of the conceptual framework for the analysis of genogram patterns. He proposed that the family is organized according to generation, age, sex, roles, functions, and interests, and suggested that where each individual fits into the family structure influences the family functioning, relational patterns, and type of family formed in the next generation. He further contended that sex and birth order shape sibling relationships and characteristics. Also, some issues tend to be played out from generation to generation through persisting interactive emotional patterns. A major concept is that of triangling, which was discussed earlier.

By creating a genogram, the nurses are able to map the family structure and record family information. This information should include demographic data such as location, occupation, and educational level. Functional information regarding medical, emotional, and behavioral status is also recorded. Finally, critical events must be noted (e.g., important transitions, moves, job changes, separations, illnesses, and deaths). Figure 35-3 provides an example of a genogram derived from the data from the family in the following vignette.

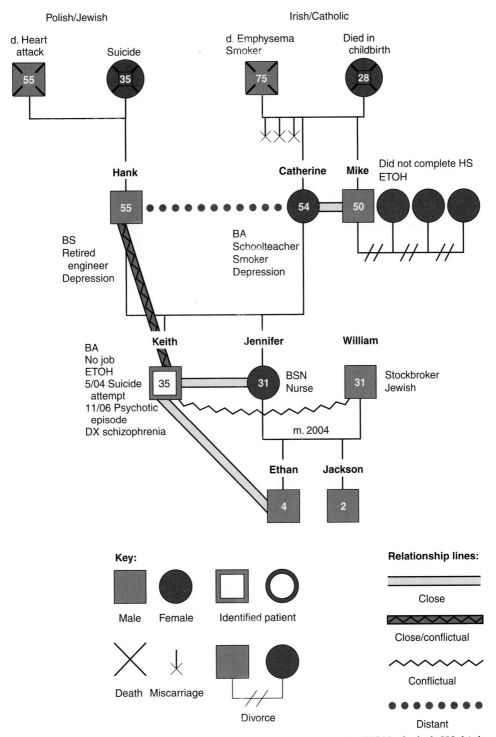

Figure 35-3 Genogram of the Schneider family. *DX,* Diagnosis; *ETOH,* alcohol; *HS,* high school; *m.,* married.

VIGNETTE

Hank and Catherine Schneider are both college educated, and each suffers from intermittent depression. Hank is an only child whose father died of a heart attack at age 55, Hank's present age. Hank's mother committed suicide at age 35. This is a toxic subject in Hank's family of origin. In Catherine's family of origin, she is the eldest, born after three miscarriages. Much pressure and many expectations were placed on her. Catherine's brother Mike was born 4 years after Catherine, and their mother died during Mike's birth. Mike never finished high school, has a serious alcohol addiction, and has had three marriages that ended in divorce. One can speculate about the level of guilt Mike may feel regarding the loss of his mother.

Hank and Catherine have two children, Keith and Jennifer. Keith, the identified patient, is 35 years old, has a college degree, and has not been able to hold down a job. He also has an addiction to alcohol. In 2004, Keith made a suicide attempt. In November 2006, Keith experienced a psychotic episode for which he was hospitalized, and he was diagnosed as having schizophrenia. His younger sister Jennifer has a college degree and works as a nurse. She married William in 2004, the year Keith attempted suicide. Jennifer and William have two young children, 4 and 2 years of age. ∎

Other Assessment Tools

Other tools are available to help the practitioner assess how the family functions as a unit and to identify individual members' perceptions of how the family communicates; how they deal with emotional issues such as anger, conflict, and affection; how they work together as a unit to plan and solve problems; how they make the important decisions for the family; and how they function generally. A focused interview, one in which the nurse can ask these questions directly, or an assessment tool can be used to obtain this information.

A careful family assessment can be a vital part of the treatment if the family has as one of its members a person with a severe mental illness. Finkelman (2000) emphasizes the need to form a partnership with the family to reintegrate the ill person into the family and home.

Self-Assessment

All nurses interact with families, whether in hospital acute care settings or in community-based settings. Most nurses come from a family, and because no family is perfect, all nurses are subject to forming triangles when anxious, to becoming defensive when personal family anxieties are aroused, or to experiencing role blurring or loosening of self-boundaries when sensitive personal issues and conflicts are triggered.

An advanced practice nurse educated at the master's level, with special training in family work, is usually best qualified to conduct family therapy. It is not uncommon for the nurse therapist to experience intense anxiety during the process of working with families. When this happens, it is important to be able to draw back emotionally and examine the source of the anxiety; it may be that the nurse is responding to her or his own personal family issues. When the nurse therapist's experience is one of getting drawn into the patient family dynamics rather than maintaining an objective stance, discussing these issues with a professional peer or supervisor is extremely important to maintain effectiveness. The nurse should identify

a time when he or she reacted intensely (positively or negatively) to either a patient or a patient's situation. How was this issue dealt with later in conference? Common issues with which health care workers may intensely identify are alcohol or drug use, family abuse, codependency, rescue fantasies, and lifestyles. These and many other issues that evoke strong feelings need to be addressed before the nurse can see clearly the patient and the patient's situation and needs. Self-assessment is a crucial component of effective nursing care, not only in psychiatric nursing but also in other nursing specialties.

DIAGNOSIS

Families have many needs at different times in their development. Family life often involves new members, deaths, mental and physical illnesses, economic challenges, developmental crises, and unanticipated changes or decline. Severe dysfunctional patterns (e.g., marked relational conflict, sexual misconduct, abuse, violence, and suicide) exist within many families that cause physical or mental anguish to the members.

Numerous nursing diagnoses are useful in working with families, and Box 35-3 identifies some of them. The *Diagnostic and Statistical Manual of Mental Disorders*, fourth edition, text revision *(DSM-IV-TR)* (American Psychiatric Association [APA], 2000) also identifies areas that can become targets of medical or psychiatric attention. These areas come under the heading of "other conditions that may be a focus of clinical attention."

BOX 35-3   Possible Nursing Diagnoses for Family Interventions

- Impaired parenting
- Sexual dysfunction
- Interrupted family processes
- Dysfunctional family processes
- Caregiver role strain
- Risk for caregiver role strain
- Spiritual distress
- Risk for compromised resilience
- Ineffective denial
- Ineffective family therapeutic regimen management
- Deficient knowledge
- Impaired verbal communication
- Defensive coping

Data from North American Nursing Diagnosis Association International (NANDA-I) (2009). *NANDA-I nursing diagnoses: Definitions and classification 2009-2011.* Oxford, United Kingdom: Author.

These *DSM-IV-TR* categories are as follows:

- Relational problems (related to a mental disorder or a generic medical condition, sibling relational problem or problems)
- Problems related to abuse or neglect (includes physical and sexual abuse and neglect of a child, and physical or sexual abuse of an adult)
- Bereavement (may cause considerable impairment and complications)
- Identity problems
- Religious or spiritual problems
- Age-related decline
- Acculturation problems

OUTCOMES IDENTIFICATION

Although different therapists may adhere to different theories and use a wide variety of methods, the goals of family therapy (Nichols, 2004) are basically the same:

- To reduce dysfunctional behavior of individual family members
- To resolve or reduce intrafamily relationship conflicts
- To mobilize family resources and encourage adaptive family problem-solving behaviors
- To improve family communication skills
- To heighten awareness and sensitivity to other family members' emotional needs and help family members meet their needs
- To strengthen the family's ability to cope with major life stressors and traumatic events, including chronic physical or psychiatric illness
- To improve integration of the family system into the societal system (e.g., school, medical facilities, workplace, and especially the extended family)
- To promote appropriate individual psychosocial development of each member of the family

Family psychoeducational treatment is often provided by nurses. Goals a nurse can use for psychoeducational teaching with a family include:

- Learning to accept the illness of a family member
- Learning to deal effectively with an ill member's symptoms, such as hallucinations, delusions, poor hygiene, physical limitations, paranoia, and aggression
- Understanding what medications can and cannot do and when the family should seek medical advice
- Learning what community resources are available and how to access them
- Feeling less anxiety and regaining or acquiring a sense of control and balance in family life

PLANNING

The immediate and long-term needs of the family should be determined. For example, is the family in crisis—that is, is one of the members homicidal, suicidal, abusive, or being abused? Do protective services need to be called? Is hospitalization necessary to protect a suicidal or self-mutilating member?

Is there a crisis at one of the family's developmental phases? What are the family's coping mechanisms at this time? What kinds of new skills can family members use at this time to help them facilitate resolution of normal life-cycle crises? Do family members need to be taught conflict management skills, problem-solving skills, parenting skills, limit-setting skills?

Is there a need for psychoeducational family interventions? Nurses are becoming adept at helping family members learn about the physical illness of an afflicted family member (e.g., severe mental illness, dementia), understand what medications can do (as well as side effects, etc.), and identify support groups and community resources to help the family cope with crisis and improve the quality of life for all of its members. How extensive is the family's knowledge deficit?

Where should a family be referred for optimal outcomes? Is there a problem with substance abuse, depression, unrealistic expectations of members, anger, or conduct disorder?

A careful analysis of the data from a sound assessment helps the nurse and other members of the health care team to identify the most appropriate family interventions for troubled families.

IMPLEMENTATION

Family therapy has been applied to virtually every type of disorder among children, adolescents, and adults and has demonstrated efficacy for each population studied (Liddle & Rowe, 2004; Pinsof & Wynne, 2000). Family-based interventions enhance the involvement of patients and other family members, and impressive retention rates have been demonstrated for such therapy. Family therapy appears to be particularly effective in the treatment of substance abuse disorders, child behavioral problems, and marital relationship distress, and as an element of the treatment plan for schizophrenia (Liddle & Rowe, 2004).

Counseling and Communication Techniques

The basic level nurse clinician may provide counseling through the use of a problem-solving approach to address an immediate family difficulty related to health or well-being. Developing and practicing good listening skills and viewing family members in a positive, nonjudgmental way are critically important qualities for nurses at all levels, regardless of the practice setting.

An important function of basic level nurses is to respond to cues from various family members that indicate the degree and amount of stress the family system is experiencing. These critical observations need to be readily reported so that appropriate interventions may be made in a timely manner. Some indicators of stress in a family system are the following:

- Inability of the family or a family member to understand and act on certain recommended treatment directives
- Various somatic complaints among family members
- High degree of anxiety
- Depression
- Problems in school
- Drug use

Promoting and monitoring a family's mental health can occur in virtually any setting and often requires making the most of an opportune moment. There does not have to be a formal meeting. Sometimes an informal conversation **(therapeutic encounter)** can have the greatest effect. Following a few general guidelines can help the nurse remain nonjudgmental in the information presented, as well as in the tone of voice and questions asked. For example, the question "Don't you think you should at least try to comply with your medical regimen?" would probably cause the patient to tune the nurse out, whereas the invitation "Tell me what your medical regimen is like" could open the door to understanding and problem solving in a collaborative rather than a hierarchical way.

A nonjudgmental manner promotes open and flexible communication among all professionals and family members in the caregiving system. If other family members are involved in the conversation, whether in the hospital unit or a family therapy session, the nurse should consider each member's view, for example, by asking how the individual member's medical regimen affects the way the family functions and what the individual members consider a possible solution to the problem.

Information should be imparted in a clear and understandable manner to all family members so they can decide what to do with the information. This is both a respectful and an empowering way to work with families, indicating to them that *they* are the ones who are accountable and responsible for how they choose to use the information.

The perspective of each family member must be elicited and heard. Often, some family members hear another member's view for the first time in this democratic forum, and many times they are surprised ("I didn't know you felt that way"). The more family input there is, the more options usually exist for alternative ways of managing problematic situations. This approach defines the family as the central psychosocial unit of care. The following vignette provides an example of maintaining neutrality and hearing from all members.

VIGNETTE

Ms. Conway, the head nurse on the adolescent psychiatric unit, is concerned about all the negative comments the staff members are making regarding the fact that none of Aaron's family has been in to visit him for over a week. In fact, she is concerned that Aaron is picking up the staff's feelings as well. After many attempts, Ms. Conway finally reaches Aaron's mother by telephone and begins to assess the situation. She discovers that Aaron's mom is divorced and is working double shifts to meet the family's expenses. There is a 2-year-old at home and a set of twins in the fourth grade.

Aaron's mother had been planning to visit on the weekend, but the babysitter called to say she was sick. Once Ms. Conway is able to see the situation from another perspective, that this is a family with young children that is struggling to make ends meet, she calls a staff meeting to address the situation. ■

Further interventions in this situation would be to problem-solve with Aaron and his mother concerning what is realistic for each of them regarding visiting. Perhaps an extended family member or a friend can visit when the mother cannot. Longer-range planning for supervision for Aaron when he is discharged should also be discussed as family supports are identified and assessed.

Unfortunately, negative comments about family members by staff occur all too often. This can present a difficult situation for the nursing student, who is entering the culture of the unit as an outsider and who realizes the negative effects this behavior has on family members. It is appropriate for the student to first seek supervision from the instructor so that the most effective approach can be planned out beforehand. One useful technique is for the student to ask questions of the supervising nurse and staff in such a manner that alternative ways of viewing the family in a broader perspective are embedded in the questions. An example of this is "Has anyone had a chance to contact Aaron's mother to see if there are any problems?" or "I wonder what it's like for Aaron's mother to have her son in a psychiatric unit."

Family Therapy

The advanced practice registered nurse (APRN) who has graduate or postgraduate training in family therapy may conduct private family therapy sessions. With regard to psychobiological interventions, the APRN may have prescriptive authority (depending on the state's nurse practice act and the nurse's qualifications).

Family therapy is viewed by professionals as appropriate for most situations, although it may be contraindicated in some circumstances (Nichols, 2004):

- When the therapeutic environment is not safe, and someone will be harmed by information, uncontrolled anxiety, or hostility
- When there is a lack of willingness to be honest
- When there is an unwillingness to maintain confidentiality
- When a parental conflict involves issues of sexuality which are not appropriate for the children

In most other situations, however, family therapy is useful, especially when it is combined with psychopharmacology in the treatment of families who have a member with a mental illness such as bipolar disorder, depression, or schizophrenia. Other families may choose psychoeducational family therapy and/or self-help groups, which are good options that may be less costly and time consuming. The following subsections introduce the student to (1) traditional family therapy intervention strategies, (2) psychoeducational groups, and (3) self-help groups that may benefit families and family members.

Traditional Family Therapy

Family therapists use a wide variety of theoretical philosophies and techniques to bring about change in dysfunctional patterns of behavior and interaction. Some therapists may focus on the here and now, whereas others may rely more heavily on the family's history and reports of what happened between sessions. As stated earlier, most family therapists use an eclectic approach, drawing on a variety of techniques to fit the particular personality and strengths of the family.

Multiple-family group therapy is often used with families who have a hospitalized family member in an inpatient setting. These groups can help family members identify and gain insight into their own problems as they are reflected in the problems of other families. Several families meet in one group with one or more therapists, usually once a week until their ill family member is discharged; these groups often continue for a specific period of time after the patient is discharged.

Psychoeducational Family Therapy

Psychoeducational family therapy has proven immensely effective, especially as a family treatment method combined with other modalities (e.g., psychopharmacology). One of the areas in which psychoeducational family training has been applied most successfully is in treatment of the patient with schizophrenia. Families are extremely valuable and positive resources for patients. Family work promotes and supports families in coping with a family member with a severe mental illness.

The primary goal of psychoeducational family therapy is the sharing of mental health care information. Family education groups help family members better understand their member's illness, prodromal symptoms (symptoms that may appear before a full relapse), medications needed to help reduce the symptoms, and more. Psychoeducational family meetings or multiple family meetings allow feelings to be shared and strategies for dealing with these feelings to be developed. Painful issues of anger or loss, feelings of stigmatization or sadness, and feelings of helplessness can be shared and put in a perspective that the family and individual members can deal with more satisfactorily. Psychoeducational family groups are extremely useful for people with all kinds of mental, as well as medical, disorders.

Psychoeducational groups have also proven helpful in parent management training such as teaching a parent to work with a child with a conduct disorder.

Self-Help Groups

Self-help groups can be divided into two types. One type is for groups of people who have a personal problem or social deprivation. The second is for families with a member who has a specific problem or condition. Self-help groups acknowledge the needs of family members. Some groups may focus on families with healthy members, whereas others offer assistance to families whose members may be experiencing a health disorder or crisis. Most health professionals are aware that for any developmental event, life crisis, or health disorder, a related mutual-aid group exists. These health professionals are in the best position to help patients and their families find additional support and information. For many people, self-help groups can be healing.

Case Management

The family's culture, ethnicity, socioeconomic status, and stage of family life cycle, as well as its unique patterns and beliefs about illness, all affect an individual's progress and response to case management. The family is the most powerful group to which an individual may ever belong, and it is vital that the nurse not discount or ignore the importance of the family's influence on its members when planning care. To a great extent, case management entails teaching, giving appropriate referrals, and offering emotional support.

VIGNETTE

David Gardiner, age 21 years, is leaving the hospital after experiencing his first psychotic episode while taking his final examinations before graduation from college. David is being discharged back to his family, which consists of his mother and father; his maternal grandfather, who has been recently bedridden; and a younger brother Todd, who is 17 years of age. David's diagnosis is paranoid schizophrenia.

The nurse takes a psychoeducational approach with the family. Issues and needs are addressed by the nurse during family meetings while David is still hospitalized and later in follow-up family therapy after discharge. Initial interventions involve imparting information about David's mental illness through reading materials and discussion. The nurse also gives the family information on and telephone numbers of psychosocial support groups and a local chapter of the National Alliance for the Mentally Ill (NAMI).

The nurse performs ongoing assessment of the family's strengths and weaknesses, including family supports and community support. She identifies some of the areas that may need to be addressed during the next few meetings. Some of these issues include reorganizing family roles to accommodate a family member with a newly diagnosed serious mental illness; managing the bedridden grandfather; attending to Todd's probable fears that he too may have this illness; dealing with potential parental guilt feelings from a genetic point of view; planning how to mobilize, should David experience another psychotic episode; managing medication and emphasizing the importance of adherence to the medication regimen; dealing with concerns about David's future and formulating realistic expectations; coping with feelings of loss for what was and what was hoped for; and finally, maintaining the integrity and functioning of the spousal subsystem.

The nurse discusses these and other issues with the family and identifies where and how these issues can best be addressed. For example, a visiting nurse is called in to evaluate the grandfather's situation and need for support in the home, and a multiple-family psychoeducation group is formed to increase the family's understanding of David's illness, help the family learn ways to cope with common problems that may arise, and provide a place for family members to share their feelings of loss and grief. ■

Pharmacological Interventions

The nurse is often the first to explain to the family the purpose of a prescribed medication, the desired effects, possible side effects, and adverse reactions. The following vignette describes a situation that occurred at the time of discharge.

VIGNETTE

Susan Harris, a 45-year-old account executive and mother of three teenagers, has been referred by her physician to the mental health center for treatment of acute depression. The psychiatrist there has prescribed an antidepressant. Routinely, new patients are seen by the nurse clinician for a review of medications as part of

the health teaching. Unfortunately, the nurse clinician is engaged with another patient in crisis at the time and misses meeting with Susan and her husband.

One week later, Susan makes an appointment with the clinical specialist, complaining of symptoms of insomnia and lack of sexual desire, which is a concern for both Susan and her husband. Susan fears that she is getting worse and "going crazy." During the appointment, the nurse clinician reviews with Susan the side effects and adverse reactions associated with antidepressants. She informs Susan that the medication she is taking might not reach its full effects for 3 weeks or longer. She also explains that sleeplessness and lowered sexual drive are common side effects of the group of medications known as selective serotonin reuptake inhibitors (SSRIs), which includes the drug Susan is taking. They discuss ways to combat these side effects (see Chapter 13). The nurse urges Susan to continue taking the medication; however, if the side effects continue, the medication can be changed. Susan is due to visit the clinic 2 weeks later for follow-up. The nurse urges Susan to discuss the side effects of the medication with her husband and encourage him to come with her to the clinic at her next appointment. ■

Certainly, the more information family members have at their disposal, the less anxiety will distort their observations and decision making after discharge. Because of untoward circumstances in this case, the nurse clinician on the unit did not review Susan's medication with her before she was discharged. The clinical specialist needs to closely monitor Susan to determine whether her symptoms represent an exacerbation of her depression or a reaction to the antidepressant medication. If Susan is having a reaction to the medication, the nurse may consult with a physician so that another medication can be tried.

EVALUATION

In the treatment of families, evaluation focuses on whether family members are more functional, conflicts are reduced or resolved, communication skills are improved, coping is strengthened, and the family is more integrated into the societal system.

KEY POINTS TO REMEMBER

- Family therapy is based on a variety of theoretical concepts.
- The aim of family therapy is to decrease emotional reactivity among family members and to encourage differentiation among individual family members.
- The primary characteristics essential to healthy family functioning are flexibility and clear boundaries.

- It is important to be aware of the phases in the changing family life cycle of a traditional family, a divorced family, and a remarried family.
- Family-oriented approaches that include helping a family gain insight and make behavioral changes are most successful.
- The genogram is an efficient clinical summary and format for providing information and defining relationships across at least three generations.
- The family's culture, ethnicity, socioeconomic status, and life-cycle phase, as well as its unique patterns and beliefs about illness, all affect the individual patient's progress and response to case management.
- Assessment of the family includes a focus on the phase of the family life cycle, multigenerational issues, the individual developmental stage of each member, and the family's sociocultural status.
- Nurses with basic training are frequently called upon to conduct psychoeducation with families.
- Nurses who have specialized training and are certified provide family therapy using a variety of theoretical approaches.

CRITICAL THINKING

1. Select a family with whom you've gotten to work during your clinical experience. Evaluate this family's status in terms of functionality/dysfunctionality with reference to the five family functions described in the text (i.e., management function, boundary function, communication function, emotional-supportive function, and socialization function).

2. Create your own personal genogram, including at least three generations. Be sure to include the following:
   A. Location, occupation, and educational level
   B. Critical events such as births, marriages, moves, job changes, separations, divorces, illnesses, deaths
   C. Relationship patterns, if possible, such as cutoffs, distancing, overinvolvement, and conflict

3. A family has just found out that their young son is going to die. The parents have been fighting and blaming each other for ignoring the child's ongoing symptom of leg pain, which was eventually diagnosed as advanced cancer. There are two other siblings in the family.
   A. How would you apply family concepts to help this family?
   B. What would be your outcome criterion?

CHAPTER REVIEW

1. Jeff is a single, noncustodial parent in the postdivorce phase. He will be hospitalized for several days following surgery. Which primary concern of Jeff's should the nurse anticipate during this time?
   1. Mourning the loss of his nuclear family
   2. Wondering how to deal with his spouse's extended family
   3. Attempting to restructure the relationship with his former spouse
   4. Finding ways to continue to effectively parent his child

2. While the nurse works with a family, the father—with a smirk on his face—states, "I love my wife, and she's a good woman who would do anything for her family" and rolls his eyes. Which behavior should the nurse recognize?
   1. Triangulation
   2. Scapegoating
   3. Double-binding
   4. Differentiation

3. The family member the nurse should refer to individual therapy rather than family therapy is the:
   1. mother who has anxiety controlled by medication.
   2. father who is questioning his sexuality.
   3. brother who is verbally angry with parents.
   4. sister who has consented to maintaining confidentiality.

4. The nurse is evaluating the family therapy experience. Which behavior would indicate to the nurse that further family therapy is indicated?
   1. Wife has set aside 15 minutes daily to connect with husband.
   2. Son's grades have risen from a "D" average to a "C" average.
   3. Daughter's headaches have subsided.
   4. Mother has stopped using illicit substances; father's use has decreased.

5. The nurse is conducting family therapy. Which nursing intervention would be appropriate for an advanced practice nurse?
   1. Mobilizing family resources and encouraging adaptive family problem-solving behaviors
   2. Improving family communication skills
   3. Explaining what medications can and cannot do
   4. Prescribing pharmaceutical treatment

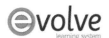
Visit the Evolve website for an **Audio Chapter Summary, Chapter Review Answers & Rationales, Critical Thinking Answer Guidelines**, and additional resources related to the content in this chapter: **http://evolve.elsevier.com/Varcarolis/foundations**

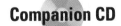 **Companion CD** Use the Companion CD to prepare for tests and the NCLEX® Examination with **Test-Taking Strategies** for psychiatric mental health nursing and hundreds of **Review Questions.**

References

American Psychiatric Association. (2000). *Diagnostic and statistical manual of mental disorders (DSM-IV-TR)* (4th ed., text rev.). Washington, DC: Author.

Bowen, M. (1985). *Family therapy in clinical practice*. New York: Jason Aronson.

Finkelman, A. W. (2000). Psychiatric patients and families: Moving from catastrophic event to long-term coping. *Home Care Provider, 5*(4), 142–147.

Goldenberg, H., & Goldenberg, I. (2008). *Family therapy: An overview* (7th ed.). Belmont, CA: Thomson.

Haley, J. (1980). *Leaving home*. New York: McGraw-Hill.

Haley, J. (1996). *Learning and teaching therapy*. New York: Guilford.

Liddle, H. A., & Rowe, C. L. (2004). Advances in family therapy research. In M. P. Nichols (Ed.), *Family therapy: Concepts and methods* (6th ed.). New York: Pearson Education.

Minuchin, S. (1974). *Families and family therapy*. Cambridge, MA: Harvard University Press.

Minuchin, S. (1996). *Mastering family therapy*. New York: John Wiley & Sons, Inc.

Nelson, T. S. (2003). Transgenerational family therapies. In L. L. Hecker & J. L. Wetchler (Eds.), *An introduction to marriage and family therapy*. New York: Haworth Clinical Practice Press.

Nichols, M. P. (2004). *Family therapy: Concepts and methods* (6th ed.). New York: Pearson Education.

North American Nursing Diagnosis Association International (NANDA-I). (2009). *NANDA-I nursing diagnoses: Definitions and classification 2009–2011*. Oxford, United Kingdom: Author.

Pinsof, W. M., & Wynne, L. C. (2000). Toward progress research: Closing the gap between family therapy practice and research. *Journal of Marital and Family Therapy, 26*(1), 1–8.

Roberts, F. B. (1983). An interaction model for family assessment. In I. W. Clements & F. B. Roberts (Eds.), *Family health: A theoretical approach to nursing care* (pp. 189–204). New York: Wiley.

Sadock, B. J., & Sadock, A. (2008). *Kaplan & Sadock's concise textbook of clinical psychiatry*. (3rd ed.). Philadelphia: Lippincott.

Satir, V. (1972). *Peoplemaking*. Palo Alto, CA: Science and Behavior Books.

Satir, V. (1983). *Conjoint family therapy*. Palo Alto, CA: Science and Behavior Books.

CHAPTER 36

Integrative Care

Rothlyn P. Zahourek and Charlotte Eliopoulos

Key Terms and Concepts

acupuncture, 772
aromatherapy, 777
chiropractic medicine, 777
complementary and alternative medicine (CAM), 767
conventional health care system, 767
healing touch, 780
herbal therapy, 776

holism, 771
homeopathy, 773
integrative care, 767
naturopathy, 773
Reiki, 780
therapeutic touch, 779

Objectives

1. Define the terms, *integrative care* and *complementary and alternative medicine*.
2. Identify trends in the use of nonconventional health treatments and practices.
3. Explore the category of alternative medical systems, along with the four domains of integrative care: mind-body approaches, biologically based interventions, manipulative approaches, and energy therapies.
4. Discuss the techniques used in major complementary therapies and potential applications to psychiatric mental health nursing practice.
5. Discuss how to educate the public in the safe use of integrative modalities and avoidance of false claims and fraud related to the use of alternative and complementary therapies.
6. Explore information resources available through literature and online sources.

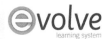 Visit the Evolve website for an **Audio Glossary & Flashcards**, **Concept Map Creator**, and additional resources related to the content in this chapter: **http://evolve.elsevier.com/Varcarolis/foundations**

This chapter considers *integrative medicine* within the broader concept of *integrative care* **as part** of a holistic nursing philosophy. This field is also referred to as **complementary and alternative medicine (CAM)**. Since these terms are widely accepted, they will be used interchangeably throughout this chapter. **Integrative care** places the patient at the center of care, focuses on prevention and wellness, and attends to the patient's physical, mental, and spiritual needs (Institute of Medicine, 2009). Many of the philosophical underpinnings for the approaches presented in this chapter are derived from non-Western cultural traditions or are based on newer concepts from quantum physics and studies in the nature of energy and reality. Integrative care is directed at healing and considers the whole person (mind, body, and spirit), along with the lifestyle of the person. The therapeutic relationship is considered part of the treatment, which includes both conventional and alternative therapies (Rakel, 2007). Integrative care may be used as a substitute for or combined with conventional therapies or treatments.

INTEGRATIVE CARE IN THE UNITED STATES

The **conventional health care system** (also referred to as *allopathic, mainstream,* or *orthodox medicine; regular medicine;* and *biomedicine*) in the United States is based largely on highly controlled, evidence-based scientific research. Rakel and Weil (2003) contrast conventional and integrative health care by noting that conventional medicine focuses on what is done to the patient, whereas integrative practices seek healing within the body-mind of an actively participating patient.

Because of growing interest in and use of CAM in the United States, the National Institutes of Health (NIH) established the National Center for Complementary and Alternative Medicine (NCCAM) in 1998. The NCCAM supports fair and scientific evaluation of integrative therapies and dissemination of information that allows health care providers to make good choices regarding the safety and appropriateness of CAM. To address the need for better research, Congress allocated $117 million toward alternative medicine research in 2004 (WNBC.com, 2004), and the World Health Organization (WHO) issued guidelines for ensuring the safety and efficacy of preparations in the multibillion-dollar herbal market (Hasselberger, 2004). Research centers continue to be established to treat and study such areas as pain and addictions management.

In May of 2008, the NCCAM and the National Center for Health Statistics (NCHS) released findings on the use of CAM in the United States. The data come from NCHS's *National Health Interview Survey,* for which 31,000 people were surveyed regarding their use of 26 complementary and alternative treatments (Barnes et al., 2008). Below is a summary of their findings:

- About 38% of adults (up from 36% in 2002) and almost 12% of children in the United States use some type of CAM.
- Use of CAM by adults is greater among women and those with higher levels of education and higher incomes.
- The most commonly used therapies are nonvitamin, nonmineral products such as fish oil/omega 3, glucosamine, echinacea, and flaxseed.
- Adults are most likely to use CAM for musculoskeletal problems such as back, neck, or joint pain.
- The use of CAM therapies for head or chest colds showed a substantial decrease from 2002 to 2007.

Since the previous survey taken in 2002, the use of CAM has held fairly steady. Several treatment methods increased from 2002 to 2007, including massage, acupuncture, and naturopathy. This increased use may be due to a greater availability of practitioners and facilities, along with more exposure through the media. Box 36-1 lists the types of CAM included in the 2007 *National Health Interview Survey,* and Figure 36-1 is a graph comparing the 10 most commonly used therapies among adults surveyed.

Children were not included in the 2002 NCHS survey, but the 2007 study revealed that the children of

---

BOX 36-1 CAM Therapies Included in the 2007 National Health Interview Survey

- Acupuncture*
- Ayurveda*
- Biofeedback*
- Chelation therapy*
- Chiropractic or osteopathic manipulation*
- Deep breathing exercises
- Diet-based therapies
  - Atkins diet
  - Macrobiotic diet
  - Ornish diet
  - Pritikin diet
  - South Beach diet
  - Vegetarian diet
  - Zone diet
- Energy healing therapy/Reiki*
- Guided imagery
- Homeopathic treatment
- Hypnosis*
- Massage*
- Meditation

- Movement therapies
  - Alexander technique
  - Feldenkreis
  - Pilates
  - Trager psychophysical integration
- Natural products (nonvitamin and nonmineral)
- Naturopathy*
- Progressive relaxation
- Qi gong
- Tai chi
- Traditional healers*
  - Botanica
  - Curandero
  - Espiritista
  - Hierbero or Yerbera
  - Native American healer/Medicine man
  - Shaman
  - Sobador
- Yoga

*Practitioner-based therapy.

Data from Barnes, P. M., Bloom, B., & Nahin, R. (2008). *Centers for Disease Control and Prevention National Health Statistics Report #12. Complementary and alternative medicine use among adults and children: United States, 2007.* <http://nccam.nih.gov/news/2008/nhsr12.pdf> Accessed 28.02.2009.

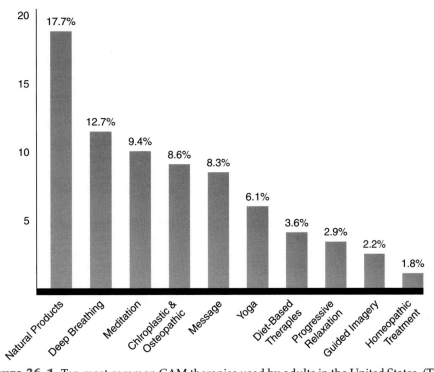

Figure 36-1 Ten most common CAM therapies used by adults in the United States. (The American Nurses Association and the American Holistic Nurses Association (2007) recognize holistic nursing as a specialty which they describe in *Holistic Nursing: Scope and Standards of Practice*.)

parents who use natural supplements, not surprisingly, were more likely to use them as well. The profile for a child who uses supplements is one who is white, non-Hispanic, adolescent, insured, lives in the western portion of the country, and has educated parents. Another factor that related to use of supplements was the presence of health conditions and frequent visits to the primary care provider.

Research

Although research on the efficacy of CAM is increasing, studies in the field are minimal when compared to those of conventional medicine. Several reasons for this include the (1) relatively recent use of some of these therapies in the United States, (2) lack of financial incentive to support the research, and (3) difficulties encountered when researching these modalities (Box 36-2). If a pharmaceutical company studies and patents a drug, it can reap considerable financial return; however, an herb cannot be patented and exclusively marketed, so there is little incentive to invest in researching its uses and effects. Governmental sources of funding such as the NCCAM and NIH, as well as nonprofit groups, are continuing to sponsor research that should contribute to further understanding of CAM. Nursing groups such as Healing Touch International and the American

Holistic Nurses Association (AHNA) are emphasizing research and are beginning to catalogue research on their websites.

BOX 36-2 CAM Research Challenges

- Individual, cultural, and environmental variables
- Lack of or limited funding sources
- Time as a variable to measure change
- Interpretation and meaning of an experience
- Impact of other intervening life experiences
- Effect and timing of a specific intervention or approach on a particular problem, specifically placebo and experimental effects
- Personality, belief systems, spiritual practices, and temperament of both the researcher and participants
- Difficulty trying to standardize modalities, variations in methods, approach and skill of the researcher
- Influence of studying a phenomenon or person within a naturalistic setting
- Interpretation of results
- The recognized value of both qualitative and quantitative results
- Acknowledging the importance of the relationship between the healer and the one being healed

Data from Zahourek, R. (2005). Intentionality: Evolutionary development in healing. *Journal of Holistic Nursing, 23*(1), 89–109.

CONSUMERS AND INTEGRATIVE CARE

Consumers are attracted to integrative care for a variety of reasons, including:

- A desire to be an active participant in one's health care and engage in holistic practices that can promote health and healing
- A desire to find therapeutic approaches that seem to carry lower risks than medications
- A desire to find less expensive alternatives to high-cost conventional care
- Positive experiences with holistic, integrative CAM practitioners, who tend to spend more time with and learn about their patients as a whole
- Dissatisfaction with the practice style of conventional medicine (e.g., rushed office visits, short hospital stays)
- A need to find modalities and remedies that provide comfort for chronic conditions for which no conventional medical cure exists, such as anxiety, chronic pain, and depression

The knowledgeable consumer, relying on health information available through public libraries, popular bookstores, and the Internet, may question conventional health care. It is essential that nurses maintain up-to-date knowledge of these modalities, continue to evaluate the evidence supporting the effectiveness and safety of CAM, and be able to guide patients in their safe use of these treatments. For example, consumers are using herbal remedies to treat a variety of psychiatric conditions. However, herbs used without the guidance of a knowledgeable practitioner can have serious side effects and interactions with other herbs and drugs.

Safety and Efficacy

People who use CAM therapies often do so without informing their conventional health care providers, which poses some risk. In the United States, there are no standards or regulations that guarantee the safety or efficacy of herbal products. Herbs and other food supplements do not have to undergo the same safety review as over-the-counter and prescription medications. Some consumers may believe that if they purchase a natural substance at a health food store, it must be safe and effective; however, "natural" does not mean "harmless." Herbal products and supplements may contain powerful active ingredients that can cause damage if taken inappropriately. Furthermore, the consumer cannot be sure that the amount of the herb or other active ingredient listed on the label is actually the amount in the product. Consumers may waste a great deal of money and risk their health on unproven, fraudulently marketed, useless, or harmful products and treatments (Box 36-3).

BOX 36-3   Warning Signs of Fraud

- The product is advertised as a quick and effective cure-all for a wide range of ailments.
- The promoters use words like "scientific break-through, miraculous cure, exclusive product, secret ingredient, or ancient remedy."
- The text is written using impressive terminology to disguise lack of good science.
- The promoter claims the government, the medical profession, or research scientists have conspired to suppress the product.
- The advertisement includes undocumented case histories claiming amazing results.
- The product is advertised as available from only one source, and payment is required in advance.
- The promoter promises a "no-risk, money-back guarantee."

Adapted from National Center for Complementary and Alternative Medicine. (2001). *FTC and FDA take action against internet scams and questionable health claims. NCCAM Newsletter 2001, Fall.* <http://nccam.nih.gov/news/newsletter/fall2001/3.htm>> Accessed 28.02.2009.

Another concern regarding CAM therapies is that diagnosis and treatment may be delayed while patients try alternative interventions, which is common with mental health symptoms such as major depression and anxiety. On the other hand, many CAM practitioners can recount stories of patients who have been injured by a noncaring conventional medical system or suffered terrible consequences from the use of conventional pharmaceuticals.

Cost

The growth in the use of CAM therapies is also linked to the rising cost of conventional medical care. There is mounting pressure to control health care spending in the United States and many other countries, and efforts are focused on the development of less expensive treatments. Before we can adopt alternative methods of treatment, however—even those that are less expensive—it is essential that we have reliable information about the clinical effectiveness of these treatment methods. Research on herbs such as St. John's wort, valerian, and ginkgo biloba and mind-body interventions such as yoga and meditation is extensive, and results are available on the NCCAM website. These supplements and approaches may prove effective and less costly than prescription drugs that produce similar results; however, it is imperative that data be available to identify the desired and adverse effects of these treatments.

Reimbursement

Payment for CAM services comes from a wide array of sources, although third-party coverage is still the exception rather than the rule. Research in the 1990s revealed that more money was being spent out of pocket on CAM than on primary care visits (Eisenberg, 1993), and out-of-pocket payments remain the principal source of spending on CAM. Some health insurance companies include coverage for certain modalities, particularly chiropractic medicine, nutritional care, massage, mind-body approaches, and acupuncture (Dumoff, 2004). The covered benefits are quite narrowly defined, however. For instance, acupuncture can be used in some plans only as an alternative to anesthesia.

Placebo Effect

Some people make the claim that integrative therapies work through a mechanism known as the *placebo effect*. This placebo effect refers to a treatment which actually does nothing, yet the condition for which it is used improves. The improvement comes about based on the power of suggestion and a belief that the treatment works. Research continues and is necessary to refute or support this claim. Yet, integrative care is based on optimism; a positive approach and the use of positive suggestions, no matter what treatment modality is being implemented, has a greater chance of success than if communication is negative or fosters a poor response. The placebo effect can be most powerful when the need is greatest and a trusting relationship has been established between patient and care giver. Saying "This will hurt" (more negative) may result in a *negative* placebo effect, whereas "This may cause some brief discomfort, but I know it can make you better" (more positive) may result in a *positive* placebo effect. A major report on the mechanism and value of the placebo as a mind-body response can be found in the *CAM at the NIH* newsletter (NCCAM, Summer, 2007b).

INTEGRATIVE NURSING CARE

The American Nurses Association (ANA) recognizes holistic nursing as a specialty, and they published *Holistic Nursing: Scope and Standards of Practice* in 2007. Holistic nursing is defined as "all nursing that has healing the whole person as its goal" (AHNA, 1998). Holism is described as involving (1) the identification of the interrelationships of the bio-psycho-social-spiritual dimensions of the person, recognizing that the whole is greater than the sum of its parts, and (2) understanding of the individual as a unitary whole in mutual process with the environment (AHNA, 2004).

Holistic nursing accepts both views and believes that the goals of nursing can be achieved within either framework.

Nurses in any setting should have a basic knowledge of treatments used in integrative care for several reasons. One is that they care for patients who increasingly are using a variety of unconventional modalities to meet their health needs. To fully understand the needs of patients, it is essential that nurses ask questions about the use of CAM as part of a holistic assessment. Currently this is encouraged by both NCCAM (2008e) and by newer standards of nursing practice. Nursing education programs are including basic integrative modalities such as relaxation and imagery in nursing curricula, and some may include energy-based approaches such as therapeutic touch.

Holistic assessments include the traditional areas of inquiry such as history, present illness, family medical history, history of surgeries, as well as medications taken and response to these medications. However, the holistic-integrative assessment also includes areas such as the quality of social relationships, the meaning of work, the impact of major stressors in the person's life, strategies used to cope with stress (including relaxation, meditation, deep breathing, etc.), and the importance of spirituality and religion and cultural values in the person's life. Patients also are asked what they really love, how this is manifested in their lives, what their strengths are, and to identify the personal gifts they bring to the world (Maizes et al., 2003).

Obtaining Credentials in Integrative Care

In 2004, almost 75% of U.S. medical schools had some type of curriculum offering in the area of integrative care (Lee et al., 2004). Presently there are five graduate programs in the United States that prepare nurses with a specialty in holistic nursing. Doctor of Nursing Practice (DNP) programs with an emphasis in holistic nursing are also now in development. Numerous post-masters certificate programs exist for advanced practice registered nurses (APRNs) and clinical nurse specialists (CNSs) from other specialty areas. The American Holistic Nursing Credentialing Center (AHNCC) offers two levels of certification: the holistic nurse–board certified (HN-BC) and the advanced holistic nurse–board certified (AHN-BC). Credentialing procedures are also in place for many of the non-nursing modalities, such as acupuncture, chiropractic medicine, naturopathy, and massage therapy. Efforts are being made to legitimize integrative care through credentialing of integrative physicians and nonphysician practitioners, including nurses.

CLASSIFICATION OF INTEGRATIVE CARE

NCCAM has developed a system of classification for CAM therapies. One classification, *alternative medical systems*, identifies entire systems of care and traditions that have evolved separately from conventional Western medicine. Integrative care is also classified according to a general approach to care and is separated into four domains: (1) mind-body approaches, (2) biologically based practices, (3) manipulative practices, and (4) energy therapies. An additional category, *alternative medical systems*, includes comprehensive systems that evolved separately from conventional modalities (e.g., traditional Chinese medicine and Ayurvedic medicine).

Alternative Medical Systems

Ayurvedic Medicine

Ayurvedic (pronounced "eye-yur-VEH-dik") medicine originated in India around 5000 BC and is one of the world's oldest and most complete medical systems. *Ayurveda* means "the science of life" and is a philosophy that emphasizes individual responsibility for health. It is holistic, promotes prevention, recognizes the uniqueness of the individual, and offers natural treatments (Pai et al., 2004).

Traditional Chinese Medicine

Traditional Chinese medicine (TCM) provides the basic theoretical framework for many CAM therapies, including acupuncture, acupressure, transcendental meditation, tai chi, and qi gong. TCM is derived from the philosophy of Taoism and emphasizes the need to promote harmony (health) or bring order out of chaos (illness). TCM is a vast medical system based on a constellation of concepts, theories, laws, and principles of energy movement within the body. Therapy is aimed at addressing the patient's illness in relation to the complex interaction of mind, body, and spirit.

Adherents of TCM say that it addresses not only symptoms but also what they call "cosmologic" events— events that relate to the dynamics of the universe. According to Taoists, the life force (qi, chi) is a two-part force (yin and yang); these parts are complementary and equally important. The goal of life is *transformation*— returning to and being reabsorbed into the qi, which circulates throughout the universe and in our bodies in precise channels called *meridians*. These meridians become significant in the practice of acupuncture, touch therapy, and the more recent energy-based therapies used to treat emotional symptoms and promote mental health.

Health is the balance between yin and yang, and illness emanates from imbalances. The TCM practitioner uses the history and physical examination to understand the imbalances of mind, body, and spirit that have caused the patient's illness. Diagnosis involves both questioning and observing body structure, skin color, breath, body odors, nail condition, voice, gestures, mood, and pulse. Eastern goals, perspectives, and stages of healing are useful in treating mental illnesses, many of which are long term. The goals of healing in Eastern medicine include:

- Being in harmony with one's environment and with all of creation in mind, body, and spirit
- Reawakening the spirit to its possibilities
- Reconnecting with life's meaning

Also, active participation in TCM treatment is essential as healing progresses through a series of stages (Box 36-4).

According to Jackonson and Keegan (2008) a *chakra* is the "specific center of consciousness in the human energy system that allows for the inflow and directing of energy from outside, as well as for outflow from the individual's energy field" (p. 347). There are seven major chakras that relate to the spine and many minor ones throughout the body.

Tai chi and yoga are modalities based on the principles of TCM. Both can be helpful to people experiencing anxiety and depression to increase a sense of well-being and reduce symptoms of stress and depression.

Acupuncture. Acupuncture has become an increasingly popular therapy in the United States. It is performed by a skilled practitioner and involves the placement of needles into the skin at meridian points

---

BOX 36-4 Stages of Healing in Traditional Chinese Medicine

- **Awakening**—represents a time, often triggered by crisis or illness, in which the person is said to sense a need for change, a feeling of diminution in the quality of life.
- **Intentionality and focus**—occurs when the person desires to change his or her consciousness from patterns of "disharmony" to patterns of healthy behaviors and seeks to ease the pain of spiritual discomfort and to obtain help.
- **Commitment**—occurs when the person forges healing relationships and establishes goals for change.
- **Transformation**—occurs when mutual, creative, active participation occurs between practitioner and patient directed toward ongoing change in mind, body, and spirit.
- **Attainment**—occurs when the patient incorporates new, healthy behaviors, has a sense of well-being, and accepts new challenges for growth; he or she has a willingness to evaluate and change to move toward greater levels of wholeness.
- **Empowerment**—occurs when the person feels a sense of stability and harmony.

to modulate the flow of qi. Sometimes acupuncture needles are inserted and removed immediately and at other times they are twirled, attached to electrodes for stimulation, or allowed to remain in place for a time. Sensations are described as rushing, warmth, or tingling and occasionally painful. Acupuncture is thought to stimulate physical responses such as changes in brain activity, blood chemistry, endocrine functions, blood pressure, heart rate, and immune-system response. Acupuncture can play a role in regulating blood cell counts, relieving pain by triggering endorphin production and controlling blood pressure.

Most people use acupuncture for pain relief (headache, back pain, osteoarthritis, or neck pain), but it also has been used to manage symptoms of withdrawal from substances and is useful in emotional disorders (Freeman & Lawlis, 2004). Researchers conducted a pilot study evaluating the use of acupuncture for patients with posttraumatic stress disorder (PTSD) (Hollifield et al., 2007). They analyzed anxiety, depression, and impairment in 73 people with PTSD. For a 12-week period, one group was treated with acupuncture, a second group with cognitive behavioral (CBT) group therapy, and a third group was placed on a waiting list. Both the CBT and the acupuncture group did better than the control group and maintained the improvement for 3 months after the treatment.

Homeopathy and Naturopathy

Homeopathy and naturopathy are examples of Western alternative medical systems. Homeopathy uses small doses (dilutions) of specially prepared plant extracts, herbs, minerals, and other materials to stimulate the body's defense mechanisms and healing processes. Infinitesimally small doses of diluted preparations that produce symptoms mimicking those of an illness are used to help the body heal itself. Homeopathy is based on the Law of Similars ("like cures like"), and dilutions are prescribed to match the patient's illness/symptom and personality profile. Healing occurs from the inside out, and symptoms disappear in the reverse order they appeared.

Homeopathy has been used in the treatment of short-term acute illnesses, migraine pain, allergies, chronic fatigue, otitis media, immune dysfunction, digestive disorders, and colic. It has also been used in the treatment of emotional disorders such as depression and anxiety. It is contraindicated as a treatment for advanced diseases, cancer, sexually transmitted diseases, conditions involving irreparable damage (e.g., defective heart valves), or brain damage due to stroke (Freeman & Lawlis, 2004).

Homeopathic remedies are available over the counter, but consumers should have a full evaluation by a homeopathic practitioner before using any treatments. Consumers who are given what is called a "constitutional remedy" to treat a specific symptom should be informed that occasionally the symptom will worsen before it gets better (e.g., a patient with anxiety should be warned not to fear a panic attack if anxiety worsens).

Naturopathy emphasizes health restoration rather than disease treatment and combines nutrition, homeopathy, herbal medicine, hydrotherapy, light therapy, therapeutic counseling, and other therapies. The underlying belief is that the individual assumes responsibility for his or her recovery. While psychiatric mental health nurses may not practice in these traditions, knowledge of the basic premises can be useful when assessing, treating, and referring patients. Such holistic concepts are also useful in considering the body-mind-spirit nature of mental health and illness.

Mind-Body Approaches

Mind-body (MB) approaches make use of the continuous interaction between mind and body. Most of these techniques emphasize facilitating the mind's capacity to affect bodily function and symptoms, but the reverse (bodily illness affects on mental health) is also part of the equation. These approaches are based on the recent research advances in psychoneuroimmunology and psychoneuroendocrinology.

The MB relationship is well accepted in conventional medicine and probably is the domain most familiar to psychiatric mental health nurses and nurses in general. Many of the MB interventions, such as cognitive-behavioral therapy, relaxation techniques, guided imagery, hypnosis, and support groups are now considered mainstream and have been the subject of considerable research (Anselmo, 2009; Schaub & Dossey, 2009). Research substantiates that these approaches dampen the parasympathetic responses in trauma that can lead to chronic health problems, PTSD, anxiety, and depression. Kwekkeboom and Grettarsdottir (2006) reviewed randomized trials of relaxation interventions for the treatment of pain in adults from 1996-2005. Many of the studies had weak methodology, but 8 of the 15 showed support of relaxation techniques (jaw relaxation and systematic relaxation) for arthritis and postoperative pain. Meditation, prayer, spiritual healing, and therapies using creative outlets such as dance, music, and art are less researched and continue to be categorized as CAM.

Guided Imagery

The use of **guided imagery** has been in the nursing literature for at least 3 decades. Different forms of imagery include (1) behavioral rehearsal imagery, (2) impromptu imagery, (3) biologically based imagery, and (4) symbolic and metaphoric imagery. Imagery is a holistic phenomenon as a "multidimensional mental representation of reality and fantasy that includes not only visual pictures, but also remembrance of situations and experiences such as sound, smell, touch, movement and taste" (Zahourek 2002, p. 113).

Imagery is used as a therapeutic tool for treating anxiety, pain, psychological trauma, and PTSD. Imagery may be combined with cognitive-behavioral therapy to help war veterans and people who have survived natural disasters. Imagery is used to enhance coping prior to childbirth or surgery, augment treatment, and minimize side effects of medications. It may help people cope with difficult times if they can imagine themselves as strong, coping, and eventually finding meaning in their experience.

Reed (2007) describes several uses of imagery in clinical practice, as well as a successful hospital program and pilot study to evaluate the impact of imagery on pain and patients' opioid use. The study group that received the imagery intervention had significantly more pain relief and required fewer pain medications.

Biofeedback

Biofeedback is the use of some form of external equipment or method of feedback (some as simple as a handheld thermometer) that informs a person about his or her psychophysiological processes and state of arousal (Anselmo, 2009). This process enables the person to begin to voluntarily control reactions that were previously outside conscious awareness. Biofeedback has been extensively practiced and researched since the 1960s, and many nurses now hold certification in this modality.

Hypnosis and Therapeutic Suggestion

Hypnosis is both a state of awareness (consciousness) and an intervention. As a state of consciousness, hypnosis is a natural focusing of attention that varies from mild to greater susceptibility to suggestion. In stress states, people are more susceptible to suggestion because their focus of attention is narrowed. People who dissociate in traumatic situations are in a trance-like state. When we use relaxation and imagery techniques, individuals frequently will enter a similarly altered state of awareness, or trance-like state.

Meditation

Several forms of **meditation** are available to people and have in recent years become popular self-help methods to reduce stress and promote wellness. Meditation practices include such simple behaviors as consciously breathing and focusing attention while walking. Other forms include transcendental meditation and mindfulness meditation developed by Benson and Kabat-Zinn. "Each practice cultivates a qualitative state of mind that can induce a deep experience of relaxation and calm" (Anselmo, 2009, p. 265).

Rhythmic Breathing

Kitko (2007) describes rhythmic breathing as an easy-to-learn-and-implement MB intervention for pain. The nurse helps the patient focus on an activity (purposeful breath) and in so doing, usually breathes with the patient. This enhances the relaxation response in both nurse and patient and has implications for nurses working with agitated psychiatric patients.

Prayer and Spirituality

Historically, there is a precedent for the inclusion of prayer and other spiritual practices as part of the care of the psychiatric patient. In England, a Quaker named William Tuke witnessed the failure of common practices of bleeding, purging, and ice baths that were used in the treatment of the mentally ill. He instituted compassionate psychological and spiritual treatments based on the idea that insanity was a disruption of both mind and spirit.

In the mid-1840s, the first form of psychiatric care in the United States was called "moral treatment." Religious superintendents ran the first mental institutions in Philadelphia, Hartford, and Worcester. A positive attitude toward prayer and spiritual practices continued in the United States until the influence of Sigmund Freud (1908 until 1939), who spoke and wrote about the emotionally destructive aspects of religion. These views subsequently influenced psychiatry's attitude toward religion for many years (Koenig, 2002).

Today there is increasing interest in the use of spiritual interventions; many psychiatric patients have significant spiritual needs. Some feel angry with God for allowing them to suffer with disorders that affect every aspect of their lives. Some need to address issues of forgiveness, for example, for friends and family who have rejected them or been judgmental because of the psychiatric illness. Other patients may wish to seek forgiveness because of hurt they have caused others. Many patients rely on God as their source of strength and maintain a deep, abiding faith despite the circumstances of their illnesses (Carson & Koenig, 2004).

O'Reilly (2004) emphasizes the value of psychiatric mental health nurses who use spiritual assessment tools and interventions to support a patient's move toward wholeness and healing. One challenge in meeting the spiritual needs of psychiatric patients is in maintaining appropriate boundaries. Patients may experience difficulty in knowing where their own beliefs stop and those of the health care professional begin. The patient is in a vulnerable position of perhaps being unfairly influenced by someone with strong beliefs. In meeting the spiritual needs of psychiatric patients, it is imperative that nurses be continually aware and respectful of boundary issues and never impose beliefs on the patient.

To support the spiritual needs of psychiatric patients, we first assess the patient's beliefs and practices. The assessment itself is a powerful intervention. When we ask a patient about the importance of spiritual issues in his or her life, we are not only encouraging discussion, we are also communicating that we are interested in and comfortable talking about an area of the patient's life. Asking about prayer, sources of hope and strength, and the patient's preferred spiritual practices allows us to know how we can provide spiritual support for the patient.

Biologically Based Therapies

Biologically based therapies include the use of dietary supplements such as vitamins, minerals, herbs or other botanicals; amino acids; and substances such as enzymes, organ tissues, and metabolites. Some supplements are expensive (e.g., SAM-E) and others are not well controlled when purchased over the counter (e.g., St. John's wort, kava kava, valerian, etc). Psychiatric mental health nurses need to be aware of therapies available and in common use, and they must also consult state board of nursing regulations.

With the proliferation of literature on herbal remedies and the accessibility of the products, increasing numbers of consumers are using these products to manage symptoms. Purchasing over-the-counter medications allows people to bypass a visit to a health care provider, thereby eliminating the cost and inconvenience of a visit, as well as the real or perceived stigma on the part of the health care provider and others of a psychiatric label.

Diet and Nutrition

Because psychiatric illness affects the whole person, it is not surprising that patients with mental illnesses frequently have nutritional disturbances. Often their diets are deficient in the proper nutrients, or they may eat too much or too little. Obesity and diabetes coexist at a greater than average rate in people with psychiatric disorders. Nutritional states may also cause psychiatric disturbances. Anemia, a common deficiency disease, is often accompanied by depression.

It is essential that nurses assess the patient's nutritional status and practices and address this area in health teaching. Assess for the use of nutrients such as vitamins, protein supplements, herbal preparations, enzymes, and hormones that are considered dietary supplements. These dietary supplements are sold without the premarketing safety evaluations required of new food ingredients. Dietary supplements can be labeled with certain health claims if they meet published requirements of the U.S. Food and Drug Administration (FDA) and may contain a disclaimer saying that the supplement has not been evaluated by the FDA and is not intended to diagnose, treat, cure, or prevent any disease.

Some nutritional supplements interact with medications. There are well-known interactions with vitamins (e.g., vitamin E and anticoagulants), but interactions with other supplements are not as easily recognized. Nurses should specifically ask about the use of supplements during the assessment and should not expect patients to share this information without being asked. Nurses can review the use of the supplements and the potential interactions with foods, drugs, and other supplements to reduce risks. An example of a serious hypertensive reaction can occur when a patient who is taking a monoamine oxidase inhibitor (MAOI) for depression ingests a food that contains tyramine, such as aged cheese, pickled or smoked fish, or wine.

Megavitamin therapy, also called *orthomolecular therapy*, is a nutritional therapy that involves taking large amounts of vitamins, minerals, and amino acids. The theory is that the inability to absorb nutrients from a proper diet alone may lead to the development of different illnesses. The earliest use of megavitamin therapy was for the treatment of schizophrenia, for which niacin was recommended. High-dose injections of vitamin C, also known as *ascorbate* or *ascorbic acid*, reduced tumor weight and growth rate by about 50 percent in mice with brain, ovarian, and pancreatic cancers. Researchers traced ascorbate's anti-cancer effect to the formation of hydrogen peroxide in the extracellular fluid surrounding the tumors (National Institutes of Health [NIH], 2008). Normal cells were unaffected.

Avoiding artificial food coloring became popular in the 1970s for treating children with attention deficit hyperactivity disorder (ADHD) and other developmental disorders. This therapy seems to move in and out of vogue and claims effectiveness in treating a variety of conditions, including acne, mild depression, arthritis, and Down's syndrome (O'Mathuna & Larimore, 2001).

Nutritional therapies are used to treat a variety of disorders, including depression, anxiety, ADHD, menopausal symptoms, dementia, and addictions. For instance, lower rates of anxiety and depression are reported among vegetarians than among nonvegetarians. An analysis of the vegetarian diet found a higher antioxidant level compared with the nonvegetarian diet, which suggests that antioxidants may play a role in the prevention of depression. Eating breakfast regularly improves mood, enhances memory, increases energy, and promotes feelings of calmness (Mehl-Madrona, 2004).

The efficacy of **Omega-3 fatty acids** continues to be studied in the treatment of depression and bipolar depression. In a meta-analysis of studies of omega-3 supplements, Eisenberg and colleagues (2006) concluded that they could recommend them as adjuncts to standard treatment for depression and bipolar disorder. Chiu et al., (2008) reviewed epidemiological evidence, preclinical trials, and case-controlled studies on the use of omega-3 fatty acids and recommends that patients with depression and bipolar depression follow the same guidelines as for the American Heart Association. These stipulate that adults eat fish at least twice a week. Patients with mood disorders, impulse-control disorders, and psychotic disorders should consume 1 gram of omega-3 fatty acids a day.

A supplement of 1 to 9 grams per day may be used, depending on dietary intake (Chiu et al., 2008).

Certain nutritional supplements, including S-adenosyl methionine (SAMe) and the B vitamins, especially vitamin B_6 and folic acid, also appear to improve depression (Mehl-Madrona, 2004). Currently, B vitamins and folic acid are also being seen more favorably for the management of bipolar illness and schizophrenia. According to Lake (2006), these vitamins often augment conventional care with antipsychotic, antidepressant, and antimanic medications. The researchers recommend that combining such approaches with exercise and meditative practices such as yoga is helpful. In a recent random controlled trail investigating vitamins B_{12} and B_6 and folic acid for the onset of depressive symptoms in older men (Ford et al., 2008), the vitamin supplements were found to be no more effective than placebo. Again, research results of such studies vary, and one may need to look carefully at the populations studied and the design of the study, as well as compare the results with other similar studies.

Herbal Therapy

A growing number of people in the United States are using herbal therapy for preventive and therapeutic purposes and report good results. However, since manufacturers are not required to submit proof of safety or efficacy to the FDA, providers should be vigilant about their patients' use of herbal therapies. Food products are also supplemented with herbs, which may result in untoward reactions. For example, ginseng has anticoagulant effects. Drinking ginseng tea may increase the effects of prescription anticoagulants, and the consequences could be a seriously delayed clotting time.

St. John's wort has been used for centuries to improve mood and to alleviate pain. In ancient times, herbalists wrote of its efficacy as a sedative, antimalarial agent, and balm for burns and wounds (NCCAM, 2008a). People may use St. John's wort instead of traditional antidepressants to avoid the side effects (dry mouth, nausea, headache, diarrhea, and impaired sexual function). St. John's wort may be less costly (depending on insurance coverage), has fewer side effects (dry mouth, dizziness, gastrointestinal symptoms, photosensitivity, and fatigue), and does not require a prescription.

St. Johns' wort has been extensively researched and was generally found to be as effective as antidepressants in the treatment of mild to moderate depression (Randlov et al., 2006), but now its usefulness in treating severe depression has been established (Linde et al., 2008). The most recent studies suggest that St. John's wort has similar efficacy to standard antidepressants and causes fewer side effects. Because St. John's wort is not regulated by the FDA, concentrations of the active ingredients may vary from preparation to preparation, which may account for some variation in research results.

Regulated preparations of St. John's wort are reasonably safe, but people should be cautioned not to take it if they are already taking an SSRI antidepressant. St. John's wort is mildly serotonergic and may cause serotonin syndrome. St John's wort also interacts negatively with other medications, including birth control pills, the antirejection transplant drug cyclosporine, Indivir and other anti-HIV medications, Irintocan and other cancer medications, and anticoagulants. Its safety has not been established for use during pregnancy or in children.

Ginkgo biloba has been used for the treatment of cerebral insufficiency, but this condition is broadly defined and ranges from memory loss to emotional instability. In a double-blind, random-controlled pilot study (Dodge et al., 2008) of 118 people over 85 years of age, participants took 80 mg of gingko extract three times a day. Those who were medication adherent did better on memory tests and had less decline than the placebo group and the ginkgo group who did not take the medication as directed.

According to NCCAM (2008f) other studies have failed to demonstrate that Ginkgo was effective in improving memory. Ginkgo tends to be well tolerated, with rare, nonspecific side effects of gastrointestinal distress, headache, and allergic skin reactions. Ginkgo has anticoagulant effects and can cause bleeding in individuals who are using anticoagulants and antiplatelet agents or who are anticipating an invasive or operative procedure (NCCAM, 2008f). Ginkgo should be used with caution by patients who consume alcohol or who have other risk factors for hemorrhagic stroke (Kligler & Lee, 2004).

Black cohosh is an extract from a root that was used for centuries by Native Americans to ease the pain of rheumatism, sore throats, and menstrual problems. It continues to be popular as a way of decreasing hot flashes and as an alternative to hormone replacement therapy for women in menopause. Other uses are for treatment of menstrual cramping and indigestion. Five clinical studies were conducted in Germany using a commercial black cohosh product called Remifemin, which is a standardized extract. These studies supported the effectiveness of black cohosh in relieving menopausal symptoms (O'Mathuna & Larimore, 2001). More recent reports from NCCAM (2008b) have not supported the efficacy.

Kava kava and **valerian** are both taken for anxiety. Kava is an herb from the South Pacific used in traditional ceremonial rites in Micronesian culture. Kava has also been used for analgesic and anesthetic properties. Kava was considered not only effective but safe until 2002, when at least 25 cases of liver toxicity, including hepatitis, cirrhosis, and liver failure, were linked to its use. The FDA issued a consumer advisory based on this potential risk, and

NCCAM discontinued its research (NCCAM, 2008c). According to Lake (2007), the cases of liver failure were associated with a processing error in the production of a **single** batch of Kava. This herbal medicine has been associated with dystonias (abnormal muscle movements), and scaly, yellow skin when taken long term.

Valerian is used as an antianxiety agent and has also been reported to have antidepressant and sedative properties (Mehl-Madrona, 2004). Valerian is a root that when brewed as a tea has sedative, tranquilizing, and sleep-inducing effects. Valerian can also be made into a variety of extracts and tinctures, which may also contain other ingredients (Mehl-Madrona, 2004). It is generally recognized as safe for the treatment of insomnia when taken at the recommended dosages. Mild side effects at recommended dosages include headache, dizziness, tiredness, and upset stomach (NCCAM, 2008d). The major drug interactions are with other sedative-hypnotic agents, and the sedative effect of valerian may potentiate the effects of other central nervous system depressants.

Herbal teas have long been used for their sedative-hypnotic effects. Common ingredients in these teas, in addition to valerian, are hops, lemon balm, chamomile, and passionflower. The most studied of these is chamomile, a tea widely used as a folk remedy. Chamomile extract has been found to bind with gamma-aminobutyric acid (GABA) receptors. These teas, along with improved sleep hygiene, may be part of a set of interventions for insomnia; they are generally safely recommended but should be used with awareness of their potential effects, side effects, and interactions.

Figure 36-2 shows a comparison of the most commonly used natural products as reported by adults in the 2002 (A) and 2007 (B) *National Health Interview Survey* conducted by the NCHS.

Aromatherapy

Aromatherapy, the use of essential oils for enhancing physical and mental well-being and healing, is a popular therapy in the mainstream market. Essential oils, often derived from herbs and plants, may be applied directly to the skin or an object such as cotton or diffused into the atmosphere through a diffuser. Essential oils are believed to stimulate the release of neurotransmitters in the brain. The sense of smell connects with the part of the brain that controls the autonomic (involuntary) nervous system. Depending on the essential oil used, the resulting affects are calming, pain reducing, stimulating, sedating, or euphoria producing.

Some nurses are trained in this art, and various oils have been introduced into hospitals, nursing homes, and hospice situations. Because these oils are believed

to have unique energetic characteristics that facilitate changes in the human energy field, these interventions may also be seen as energy therapies (Smith & Kyle, 2008). Research evidence exists that combining aromatherapy with massage reduces anxiety and fosters mood elevation and stress reduction (Maddocks-Jennings & Wilkinson, 2004).

There are anecdotal reports that aromatherapy is useful for pain relief, memory improvement, and wound healing. Smith and Kyle (2008, p. 7) provide a convenient chart on how various classifications of oils affect people:

- Rooty oils such as patchouli and valerian affect calming, grounding, and stabilizing.
- Floral oils such as ylang-ylang and jasmine create mood uplifting, relaxation, and sensuality.
- Green herbaceous oils such as lavender and chamomile create balance, regulation, and clarification.

Some individuals, particularly those with pulmonary disease, may be sensitive or allergic to essential oils when they come into contact with the skin or are inhaled. To prevent an allergic reaction, it is essential to dilute oils, administer a small amount, and perform a 24-hour skin patch test before massaging any essential oil into the skin.

Manipulative Practices

The next group of treatments is based on physically touching another person. (Therapeutic touch is included among the energy therapies since it technically does not involve physical touching of a patient.) The use of any physical touch in psychiatric mental health nursing practice continues to be controversial. Some believe it is not used enough, but most believe it should be used sparingly, with clear intent, recognizing that maintenance of therapeutic boundaries is extremely important, particularly with patients who have psychiatric disorders and might misinterpret touch.

Chiropractic Medicine

Chiropractic medicine is one of the most widely used integrative therapies. The term *chiropractic* comes from the Greek words *praxis* and *cheir*, meaning "practice" or "treatment by hand." Chiropractic medicine focuses on the relationship between structure and function and the way that relationship affects the preservation and restoration of health, using manipulative therapy as a treatment tool.

Daniel David Palmer, a grocery store owner, developed the method in the late 1800s in an effort to heal others without drugs. Palmer developed a series of manipulative procedures to bring health to muscles, nerves, and organs that had gotten out of alignment; he referred to these misalignments as *subluxations*. He believed that subluxations were metaphysical and

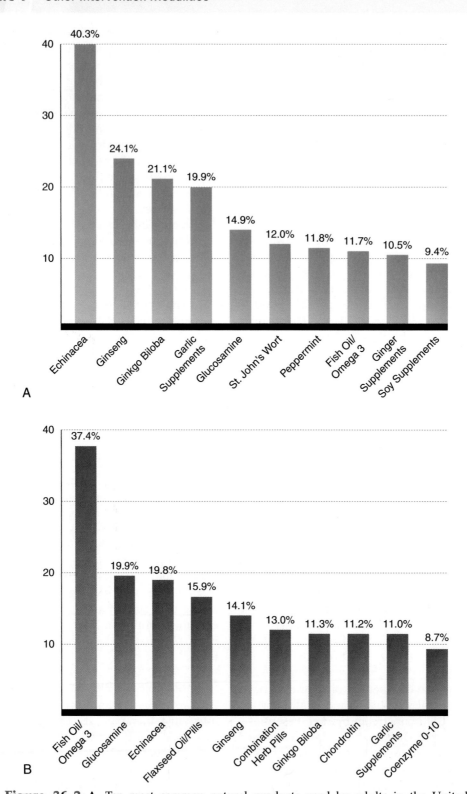

Figure 36-2 A, Ten most common natural products used by adults in the United States-2002. (From Barnes, P. M., Powel-Griner, E., McFann, K., & Nahin, R. [2004]. Centers for Disease Control and Prevention Advance Data Report #343. Complementary and alternative medicine use among adults: United States, 2002. Hyattsville, MD: National Center for Health Statistics.) **B,** Ten most common natural products used by adults in the United States-2007. (From Barnes, P. M., Bloom, B., & Nahin, R. [2008]. Centers for Disease Control and Prevention National Health Statistics Report #12. Complementary and alternative medicine use among adults and children: United States, 2007. Hyattsville, MD: National Center for Health Statistics.)

that they interfered with the flow through the body of "innate intelligence" (spirit or life energy).

Contemporary chiropractic medicine continues to be based on the theory that energy flows from the brain to all parts of the body through the spinal cord and spinal nerves. Manipulation of the spinal column, called *adjustment*, returns the vertebrae to their normal positions. Back pain is the most common reason people seek chiropractic treatment, but chiropractic manipulation is used to treat a variety of other conditions, including pain, allergies, and asthma (NCCAM, 2003). Manipulation is also helpful in reducing migraine, tension, or cervicogenic headache pain. Many chiropractors also treat patients with depression, anxiety, and chronic pain. Chiropractic treatment may be done in conjunction with herbs and supplements.

In randomized clinical trials investigating the treatment of tension headaches, one group of patients was treated with chiropractic manipulation, and another group received pain medication. Both groups experienced relief of pain, but there were fewer side effects from manipulation than from the use of medication (Freeman & Lawlis, 2004).

Massage Therapy

Massage therapy includes a broad group of medically valid therapies that involve rubbing or moving the skin. Massage therapists employ four basic techniques: effleurage (long, gliding strokes over the skin), pétrissage (kneading of the muscles to increase circulation), vibration and percussion (a series of fine or brisk movements that stimulate circulation and relaxation), and friction (which is decreased with the use of massage oils). Probably the best known massage technique in the United States is **Swedish massage**, which provides soothing relaxation and increases circulation. Japanese **Shiatsu massage** was strongly influenced by traditional Chinese medicine and developed from acupressure. It originated as a way to detect and treat problems in the flow of life energy (Japanese *ki*). The shiatsu practitioner uses fingers, thumbs, elbows, knees, or feet to apply pressure by massaging various parts of the body, known as *acupoints*.

Reflexology

Reflexology is yet another type of massage that focuses on the feet, hands, or ears. This approach is based on the belief that zones and points on these areas (most commonly the feet) correspond to other parts of the body. The purpose of treatments is to open blocked nerve pathways and improve circulation in the feet to treat problems that may exist elsewhere in the body (Riley et al., 2004). Research on this intervention is scarce at present. Morris (2006) completed a pilot study with peri- and postmenopausal women using hand, ear, and foot reflexology. Results indicated that

women were more relaxed and had more sleep after a 50-minute reflexology session once a week.

Energy Therapies

Energy therapy is a growing field that includes therapies originating from many parts of the world. It is based on the belief that nonphysical bioenergy forces pervade the universe and people. Explanations vary as to the nature of this energy, the form of the therapies, and the rationale for how healing is believed to occur. Some cultures believe the energy comes from God. Those who practice shamanic healing rituals believe the energy comes from various spirits through a priest or shaman.

In the 1970s when the United States opened diplomatic relations with China, the Western world was introduced to the use of acupuncture and other energy therapies common in TCM. The energy is referred to as *qi* in TCM, *prana* in Indian Ayurvedic medicine, *ki* in Japanese medicine, and by a variety of other names in other cultures. The NCCAM (2007a) coined the term *biofield energy*. This energy takes a particular form in each person called the *human energy field* or *aura*. This energy field is said to contain a number of layers, each with energy of different frequencies. Energy is transferred between layers and eventually into the physical body through *chakras*. Disturbances of the energy field are the cause of illness, and healing can occur only when the human energy field is balanced and energy is flowing freely.

More than 50 years ago, Russian researchers produced photographs of what they thought were human energy fields. The images captured by Kirlian photography show auras and streams of light emanating from people's hands and even from the leaves of plants. The conclusion was that the health of the person or organism could be evaluated by noting the intensity, shape, and color of these emanations. Unfortunately, the patterns on the Kirlian photographs have since been dismissed as explainable by variations in the techniques used in the photography.

Practitioners of energy medicine believe that they are able to increase their awareness of the human energy field and enhance healing through meditation and centering (finding the calm space within yourself) (Zahourek, 2005). Practitioners believe they can then detect problems in others' energy fields and adjust the quality or create balance. This is accomplished by placing one's hands in or through these fields to direct the energy through visualized or actual pressure and/or manipulation of the body.

Therapeutic touch, healing touch, and Reiki are the most common energy therapies practiced by nurses. The AHNA and Healing Touch International offer certificate courses in healing touch. Other examples of energy medicine include Thought field therapy and emotional freedom technique and their derivatives.

Therapeutic Touch

Therapeutic touch is a modality developed in the 1970s by Dolores Krieger, a nursing professor at New York University, and Dora Kunz, a Canadian healer. The premise for therapeutic touch is that healing is promoted by balancing the body's energies. In preparation for a treatment session, practitioners focus completely on the person receiving the treatment, without any other distraction. Practitioners then assess the energy field, clear and balance it through hand movements, and/or direct energy in a specific region of the body. The therapist does not physically touch the patient. After undergoing a session of therapeutic touch, patients report a sense of deep relaxation.

Practitioners of therapeutic touch believe that the therapy is useful in relieving premenstrual syndrome, depression, complications in premature babies, and secondary infections associated with human immunodeficiency virus (HIV) infection; lowering blood pressure; decreasing edema; easing abdominal cramps and nausea; resolving fevers; and accelerating the healing of fractures, wounds, and infections.

Therapeutic touch has uncertain research support. Two meta-analyses studies that reviewed the research literature (Peters, 1999; Winstead-Fry & Kijek, 1999) found that therapeutic touch reduced anxiety and pain and promoted comfort for people in various conditions of illness and recovery. However, in five studies on wound healing, two showed faster wound healing with therapeutic touch, two showed slower wound healing with therapeutic touch, and one showed no difference. A review of research involving therapeutic touch reveals similar patterns (Aetna Intelihealth, 2003; CAMline, 2003; Eisenberg et al., 2001).

Engebretson and Wardell (2007) explain that biomedical research on energy therapies presents several challenges. First, examining energy therapies is not like trying to investigate a disease or symptom. Determining a method to measure the success of touch therapies is difficult, since their success is based on restoring balance and total healing, which are not easily quantified. Further, establishing the appropriate time for an intervention to take effect and the dosage of an energy therapy is currently impossible. Finally, establishing control groups and dealing with personality variables with individual healers and patients confounds results.

Healing Touch

Healing touch is a derivative of therapeutic touch developed by a registered nurse, Janet Mentgen, in the early 1980s. Healing touch combines several energy therapies and is based on the belief that the body is a complex energy system that can be influenced by another through that person's intention for healing and well-being. Healing touch is related to therapeutic touch in the belief that working energetically with people to achieve their highest level of well-being, and not necessarily relieving a specific symptom, is the goal.

A unified international program of study has evolved that teaches and certifies practitioners of healing touch. Healing touch involves gentle laying on of hands on a clothed body or moving over the body in the energy field. The practitioner may focus on a specific problem area or the full body. In a review of over 30 studies on healing touch, Wardel and Weymouth (2004) found that although the studies reported positive results in reducing stress, anxiety, and pain and enhancing healing time and quality of life, the quality of the research was such that results could not be generalized to other settings and therapists.

Reiki

The Japanese spiritual practice of Reiki has become an increasingly popular modality for nurses to learn and practice. Reiki is an energy-based therapy in which the practitioner's energy is connected to a universal source (chi, qi, prana) and is transferred to a recipient for physical or spiritual healing (Miles & True, 2003). Numerous hospitals, hospices, cancer support groups, and clinics are now offering Reiki in complementary programs. Nursing research has been conducted on such topics as reducing anxiety and pain following abdominal hysterectomy, self-care for nurses, and orthopedic pain (Vitale & O'Conner, 2007; Brathovde, 2006; DiNucci, 2005). LaTorre (2005) describes its use as an adjunct in psychotherapy. People may be hesitant about using Reiki because (1) there is little scientific support for Reiki, and acceptance of its teaching about ki is a matter of faith; (2) the possibility exists that effects are due to a placebo effect; (3) it is incompatible with their religious beliefs; and (4) government regulation and licensing is controversial.

Thought Field Therapy and Emotional Freedom Technique

Thought field therapy (TFT) was first developed by Roger Callahan in the 1980s and then modified in the 1990s by Gary Craig, who called his version the *emotional freedom technique* (EFT) (Borgatti, 2008). The basis for these interventions is the idea that negative emotions are the result of energy imbalances and blocks in the body. The goal is to release these blocks and view the problem with less distress by tapping specific acupuncture points and meridians and repeating a positive mantra. EFT is relatively easy to integrate into a psychotherapy or psychopharmacology practice and has some beginning research to support its practice (Wells et al., 2003).

Bioelectromagnetic-Based Therapies

In contrast, bioelectromagnetic-based therapies involve the unconventional use of electromagnetic fields, such as pulsed fields, magnetic fields, or alternating-current or direct-current fields. Transcranial magnetic therapy

(TMS) and vagus nerve stimulus (VNS) treatments for depression are in this category. In TMS, pulsating magnetic fields are sent through a metal coil attached to the person's scalp (see Chapter 13, Figure 13-4). High-frequency pulses stimulate, and low-frequency pulses dampen neural impulses. A recent study indicates that when low-frequency TMS is used to "stun" parts of the brain of a person with schizophrenia, it tends to decrease auditory hallucinations (Aleman et al., 2007). TMS has been approved by the FDA for the treatment of depression (see Chapter 13).

Vagus nerve stimulation (VNS) was originally developed for epilepsy and showed some promise in treating medication-resistant depression. It is an extremely expensive surgical procedure (see Chapter 13, Figure 13-5), and after reviewing the data on this intervention, Medicare determined that it was not sufficiently effective to reimburse (Block, 2008).

The websites of both the NCCAM (http://nccam.nih.gov) and the NIH (http://nih.gov) provide detailed information and reviews about other complementary and alternative therapies. Table 36-1 summarizes integrative approaches to psychiatric disorders.

KEY POINTS TO REMEMBER

- A philosophy of holism and promoting a therapeutic relationship are at the heart of psychiatric mental health nursing and are important no matter what modality is used, conventional or integrative.
- Complementary, alternative, and integrative therapies are in demand as consumers seek a broader range of therapies than those offered by traditional medicine.
- With the availability of information on the Internet, consumers are more likely to have researched their symptoms or condition and identified potential CAM treatments.
- Nurses are in an ideal position to guide patients to reliable resources, such as the NCCAM, that provide up-to-date information for health care practitioners and consumers.
- Nurses need to keep abreast of current research about major CAM therapies so that they can promote holistic integrative care by informing patients and members of the health care team of CAM therapies that could be beneficial, affordable, and safe; help patients avoid wasting money on useless therapies; guide patients in discerning which therapies could be harmful for them; and help patients to maximize the benefits of CAM therapies.

CRITICAL THINKING

1. As a nurse, you may have patients who use integrative therapies in conjunction with the conventional therapies prescribed by the health care provider. Identify issues that are important to assess, and discuss how you would ask about the use of these nonconventional practices.

2. Discuss how herbal products sold in the United States can vary in quality. How does a patient determine the efficacy of the herb?

3. What can a patient do to guarantee the quality and dosage of an herbal product? What are resources for the patient and nurse to learn about the efficacy and safety of herbs and supplements?

4. By visiting their websites, determine how the NCCAM and other informational resources, such as the AHNA, provide information for the consumer and professionals.

CHAPTER REVIEW

1. A patient has questioned the nurse about safety of an herbal supplement. Which nursing response is most appropriate?
   1. "Herbal supplements are regulated by the FDA."
   2. "Natural ingredients in herbal supplements are harmless."
   3. "Your primary care provider should be aware of any supplements you take."
   4. "Marketing for herbal supplements demonstrates that all supplements are safe."

2. Which patient should the nurse identify that might benefit from biofeedback? The one who:
   1. is afraid of flying.
   2. is about to give birth.
   3. wants to quit smoking.
   4. wants to relax and promote well-being.

3. The nurse is teaching a patient taking a monoamine oxidase inhibitor (MAOI) for depression. Which food should the nurse encourage the patient to eat?
   1. Smoked fish
   2. Fresh vegetables
   3. Red wine
   4. Cheese

4. A patient with menstrual problems asks the nurse which supplement might be helpful to her. Which supplement should the nurse suggest for the patient to discuss with her primary care provider?
   1. Black cohosh
   2. St. John's Wort
   3. Kava kava
   4. Ginkgo biloba

5. Which nursing question(s) should be included in a holistic assessment? *Select all that apply.*
   1. "Are your parents still living?"
   2. "Have you undergone any surgeries in the past?"
   3. "What gives you a sense of meaning and purpose in life?"
   4. "What methods do you use to cope with stress?"
   5. "Do you feel safe in your relationships?"

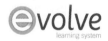

Visit the Evolve website for an **Audio Chapter Summary, Chapter Review Answers & Rationales, Critical Thinking Answer Guidelines,** and additional resources related to the content in this chapter: **http://evolve.elsevier.com/Varcarolis/foundations**

Companion CD   Use the Companion CD to prepare for tests and the NCLEX® Examination with **Test-Taking Strategies** for psychiatric mental health nursing and hundreds of **Review Questions.**

References

Aetna Intelihealth. (2003). *Therapeutic touch.* Retrieved April 17, 2005, from http://www.Intelihealth.com/IH/ihtIH/WSIHW000/8513/34968/358873.html?d=dmtContent

Aleman, A., Summer, L., & Kahn, R. (2007). Efficacy of slow repetitive magnetic stimulation on auditory hallucinations. *Journal of Clinical Psychiatry, 68,* 416–421.

American Holistic Nurses Association. (1998). *Description of Holistic Nursing.* Flagstaff, AZ: AHNA.

American Holistic Nurses Association. (2004). *What is Holistic Nursing.* Retrieved November 26, 2006. www.ahna.org

American Nurses Association & American Holistic Nurses Association. (2007). *Holistic nursing: Scope and standards of practice.* Silver Spring, MD: Author.

Anselmo, J. (2009). Relaxation. In B. Dossey & L. Keegan (Eds.), *Holistic nursing: A handbook for practice* (5th ed.). Sudbury, MA: Jones and Bartlett.

Barnes, P. M., Bloom, B., & Nahin, R. (2008). Center for Disease Control National Health Statistics Report #12. Complementary and alternative medicine use among adults and children: United States, 2007. Retrieved February 28, 2009 from http://nccam.nih.gov/news/2008/nhsr12.pdf

Block, D. R. (2008). Brain stimulation therapies for treatment-resistant depression: Evidence for the use of neurostimulating techniques. *Psychiatric Times, 25*(1), 37–38.

Borgatti, J. C. (2008). Tap your way to fast relief. *American Nurse Today, 3*(1), 32–33.

Brathovde, A. (2006). A pilot study of Reiki for self-care of nurses and healthcare providers. *Holistic Nursing Practice, 20*(2), 95–100.

Mline, C. A. (2003). *CAM therapies and practitioners: Therapeutic touch.* Retrieved December 17, 2004, from http://www.camline.org/therapiesPractitioners/therapeutic_touch/description.html

Carson, B., & Koenig, H. G. (2004). *Spiritual caregiving: Healthcare as a ministry.* Philadelphia: Templeton Foundation Press.

Chiu, C. C., Liu, J. P., & Su, K. P. (2008). The use of omega-3 fatty acids in the treatment of depression: The lights and shadows. *Psychiatric Times, 25*(9), 76–80.

DiNucci, E. M. (2005). Energy healing: A complementary treatment for orthopedic and other conditions. *Orthopedic Nursing, 24,* 259–269.

Dodge, H. H., Zitzelberger, T., Oken, B. S., Howieson, D., & Kaye, J. (2008). A randomized placebo controlled trial of gingko biloba for prevention of cognitive decline. *Neurology, 70*(19 Pt 2), 1809–1817.

Dumoff, A. (2004). Legal and ethical issues in integrative medicine. In B. Kligler & R. Lee (Eds.), *Integrative medicine: Principles for practice* (pp. 845–874). New York: McGraw-Hill.

Eisenberg, D. M. (1993). Unconventional medicine in the United States: Prevalence, costs, and patterns of use. *New England Journal of Medicine, 328,* 246–252.

Eisenberg, D. M., Davis, R. B., Waletzky, J., Yager, A., Landsberg, L., Aronson, M., et al. (2001). Inability of an "energy transfer diagnostician" to distinguish between fertile and infertile women. *Medscape General Medicine, 3*(1). Retrieved March 1, 2009 from http://www.medscape.com/viewarticle/408093

Eisenberg, D. M., Kessler, R. C., Van Rompay, M. I., Kaptchuk, T. J., Wilkey, S. A., Apple, S., et al. (2006). Perceptions about complementary therapies relative to conventional therapies among adults who use both: Results from a national survey. *Annals of Internal Medicine, 135,* 344–351.

Engebretson, J., & Wardell, D. W. (2007). Energy-based modalities. *Nursing Clinics of North America, 42,* 243–260.

Ford, A. H., Flicker, L., Thomas, J., Norman, P., Jamrozik, K., & Almedia, O. P. (2008). Vitamins B_{12}, B_6, and folic acid for onset of depressive symptoms in older men: Results from a 2-year placebo-controlled trial. *Journal Clinical Psychiatry, 69,* 1203–1209.

Freeman, L. W., & Lawlis, G. F. (Eds.). (2004). *Mosby's complementary and alternative medicine: A research based approach.* St Louis: Mosby.

Hasselberger, S. (2004). *WHO issues guidelines for herbal medicine: Press exaggerates warnings.* Retrieved May 22, 2005, from http://www.newmediaexplorer.org/Sepp/2004/06/30/who_issues_guidelines_for_herbal_medicine_press_exaggerates_warnings.htm#

Hollifield, M., Sinclair-Lian, N., Warner, T. D., & Hammerschlag, R. (2007). Acupuncture for posttraumatic stress disorder: A randomized controlled pilot trial. *Journal Nervous Mental Disorder, 195,* 504–513.

Institute of Medicine. (2009, February). Summit on integrative medicine and the health of the public. Retrieved March 1, 2009 from http://sev.prnewswire.com/health-care-hospitals/20090227/DC7670827022009-1.html#

Jackonson, C., & Keegan, L. (2008). Touch. In B. M. Dossey & L. Keegan (Eds.), *Holistic nursing: A handbook for practice* (5th ed., pp. 171–194. Sudbury, MA: Jones & Bartlett.

Kitko, J. (2007). Rhythmic breathing as a nursing intervention. *Holistic Nursing Practice, 21,* 2.

Kligler, B., & Lee, R. (2004). *Integrative medicine: Principles for practice.* New York: McGraw-Hill.

Koenig, H. G. (2002). *Spirituality in patient care: Why, how, when and what.* Philadelphia: Templeton Foundation Press.

Kwekkeboom, K. L., & Grettarsdottir, L. (2006). A systematic review of relaxation interventions for pain. *Journal of Nursing Scholarship, 38,* 269–277.

Lake, J. (2006). *Textbook of integrative mental health care.* New York: Thieme.

Lake, J. (2007). Integrative management of anxiety. *Psychiatric Times, 24*(12), 13–17.

LaTorre, M. A. (2005). The use of Reiki in psychotherapy. *Perspectives in Psychiatric Care, 41*(4), 184–187.

Lee, R., Kligler, B., & Shiflett, S. (2004). Integrative medicine: Basic principles. In B. Kligler & R. Lee (Eds.), *Integrative medicine: Principles for practice* (pp. 3–24). New York: McGraw-Hill.

Linde, K., Berner, M., Kriston, L. (2008). St John's wort for major depression. *Cochrane Database of Systematic Reviews,* Issue 4. Art No.: CD000448. DOI:10.1002/14561858. CD000448.pub3.

Maddocks-Jennings, W., & Wilkinson, J. M. (2004). Aromatherapy practice in nursing: Literature review. *Journal of Advanced Nursing, 48*, 933–103.

Maizes, V., Koffler, K., & Fleishman, S. (2003). The integrative assessment. In D. Rakel (Ed.), *Integrative medicine* (pp. 11–16). Philadelphia: Saunders.

Mehl-Madrona, L. (2004). Integrative approach to psychiatry. In B. Kligler & R. Lee (Eds.), *Integrative medicine: Principles for practice* (pp. 623–666). New York: McGraw-Hill.

Miles, P., & True, G. (2003). Reiki: Review of biofield therapy history, theory, practice, and research. *Alternative Therapies in Health and Medicine, 9*(2), 62–72.

Morris, D. (2006). Pilot study using reflexology. *Beginnings, 26*(5), 28–29.

National Center for Complementary and Alternative Medicine. (2003, November). *Research report: About chiropractic and its use in treating low-back pain.* Retrieved April 17, 2005, from http://nccam.nih.gov/health/chiropractic/

National Center for Complementary and Alternative Medicine. (2007a, March). *Energy Medicine: An overview.* Retrieved September 10, 2008, from http://nccam.nih.gov/health/backgrounds/energymed.htm

National Center for Complementary and Alternative Medicine. (2007b, Summer). Placebo: sugar, shams, therapies or all of the above. *CAM at the NIH, 14*(3), 1–2, 4–5.

National Center for Complementary and Alternative Medicine. (2008a, March). *Herbs at a glance: St John's wort.* Retrieved August 8, 2008, from http://nccam.nih.gov/health/stjohnswort

National Center for Complementary and Alternative Medicine. (2008b, March). *Herbs at a glance: Black Cohosh.* Retrieved September 10, 2008, from http://nccam.nih.gov/health/blackcohosh

National Center for Complementary and Alternative Medicine. (2008c, June). *Herbs at a glance: Kava.* Retrieved Aug 17, 2008, from http://nccam.nih.gov/health/kava

Natinal Center for Complementary and Alternative Medicine. (2008d, June). *Herbs at a glance: Valerian.* Retrieved Aug 17, 2008, from http://nccam.nih.gov/health/valerian

National Center for Complementary and Alternative Medicine. (2008e, July). New campaign encourages open communication about CAM. *CAM at the NIH, 15*(2), 1–2.

National Center for Complementary and Alternative Medicine. (2008f, November). *Herbs at a glance: Gingko.* Retrieved July 1, 2009 from http://nccam.nih.gov.health/ginkgo

National Institutes of Health. (2008). Vitamin C injections slow tumor growth in mice. Retrieved May 7, 2009, from http://www.nih.gov/news/health/aug2008/niddk-04.htm

O'Mathuna, D., & Larimore, W. (2001). *Alternative medicine: The Christian handbook.* Grand Rapids, MI: Zondervan.

O'Reilly. (2004). Spirituality and mental health clients. *Journal of Psychosocial Nursing and Mental Health Services, 42*(7), 44–53.

Pai, S., Shanbhag, V., & Archarya, S. (2004). Ayurvedic medicine. In B. Kligler & R. Lee (Eds.), *Integrative medicine: Principles for practice* (pp. 219–240). New York: McGraw-Hill.

Peters, R. M. (1999). The effectiveness of therapeutic touch: A meta-analytic review. *Nursing Science Quarterly, 12*(1), 52–61.

Rakel, D., & Weil, A. (2003). Philosophy of integrative medicine. In D. Rakel (Ed.), *Integrative medicine* (p. 7). Philadelphia: Saunders.

Rakel, R. (2007). *Integrative medicine.* Philadelphia: Saunders.

Randlov, C., Mehlsen, J., Thomsen, C. F., Hedman, C., Von Fircks, H., & Winther, K. (2006). The efficacy of St. John's Wort in patients with minor depressive symptoms or dysthymia—a double-blind placebo-controlled study. *Phytomedicine, 13*(4), 215–221.

Reed, T. (2007). Imagery in the clinical setting: A tool for healing. *Nursing Clinics of North America, 42*(2), 261–277.

Riley, D., Ehling, D., & Saucier, K. (2004). Movement and body-centered therapies. In B. Kligler & R. Lee (Eds.), *Integrative medicine: Principles for practice* (pp. 241–254). New York: McGraw-Hill.

Schaub, B. G., & Dossey, B. M. (2009). Imagery. In B. M. Dossey, & L. Kegan (Eds.), *Holistic Nursing: A Handbook for Practice* (5th ed.). Sudbury, MA: Jones & Bartlett.

Smith, M. C., & Kyle, L. (2008). Holistic foundations of aromatherapy for nursing. *Holistic Nursing Practice, 22*(1), 3–9.

Transcranial Magnetic Stimulation: The saga continues. (2008). *The Carlat Report, 6*(1), 1,3.

Vitale, A., & O'Conner, P. (2007). An integrative review of Reiki touch therapy research. *Holistic Nursing Practice, 21*(4), 167–179.

Wells, S., Polglase, K., Andrews, H. B., Carrington, P., & Baker, A. H. (2003). Evaluation of meridian based intervention: Emotional freedom technique (EFT) for reducing specific phobias for small animals. *Journal of Clinical Psychology, 59*, 943–966.

Winstead-Fry, P., & Kijek, J. (1999). An integrative review and meta-analysis of Therapeutic Touch literature. *Alternative Therapies in Health and Medicine, 5*(6), 58–67.

WNBC.com. (2004, February 10). Complementary and alternative medicine undergoes new scrutiny: Americans spend $30 billion on alternative therapies. Retrieved April 6, 2005, from http://www.wnbc.com/print/2815485/detail.html

Zahourek, R. P. (2002). *Imagery in holistic health and healing.* Philadelphia: F.A. Davis Co.

Zahourek, R. (2005). Intentionality: evolutionary development in healing. *Journal of Holistic Nursing, 23*(1), 89–109.

APPENDIX A

DSM-IV-TR Classification*

NOS, Not Otherwise Specified.

An *x* appearing in a diagnostic code indicates that a specific code number is required.

An ellipsis (…) is used in the names of certain disorders to indicate that the name of a specific mental disorder or general medical condition should be inserted when recording the name (e.g., 293.0 Delirium Due to Hypothyroidism).

If criteria are currently met, one of the following severity specifiers may be noted after the diagnosis:
- Mild
- Moderate
- Severe

If criteria are no longer met, one of the following specifiers may be noted:
- In Partial Remission
- In Full Remission
- Prior History

DISORDERS USUALLY FIRST DIAGNOSED IN INFANCY, CHILDHOOD, OR ADOLESCENCE

Mental Retardation

NOTE: These are coded on Axis II.
317   Mild Mental Retardation
318.0 Moderate Mental Retardation
318.1 Severe Mental Retardation
318.2 Profound Mental Retardation
319   Mental Retardation, Severity Unspecified

Learning Disorders

315.00 Reading Disorder
315.1   Mathematics Disorder
315.2   Disorder of Written Expression
315.9   Learning Disorder NOS

Motor Skills Disorder

315.4   Developmental Coordination Disorder

*From American Psychiatric Association. (2000). *Diagnostic and statistical manual of mental disorders* (4th ed., text rev.) *(DSM-IV-TR)*. Washington, DC: Author.

Communication Disorders

315.31 Expressive Language Disorder
315.32 Mixed Receptive-Expressive Language Disorder
315.39 Phonologic Disorder
307.0   Stuttering
307.9   Communication Disorder NOS

Pervasive Developmental Disorders

299.00 Autistic Disorder
299.80 Rett's Disorder
299.10 Childhood Disintegrative Disorder
299.80 Asperger's Disorder
299.80 Pervasive Developmental Disorder NOS

Attention-Deficit and Disruptive Behavior Disorders

314.xx Attention-Deficit/Hyperactivity Disorder
  .01   Combined Type
  .00   Predominantly Inattentive Type
  .01   Predominantly Hyperactive-Impulsive Type
314.9   Attention-Deficit/Hyperactivity Disorder NOS
312.xx Conduct Disorder
  .81   Childhood-Onset Type
  .82   Adolescent-Onset Type
  .89   Unspecified Onset
313.81 Oppositional Defiant Disorder
312.9   Disruptive Behavior Disorder NOS

Feeding and Eating Disorders of Infancy or Early Childhood

307.52 Pica
307.53 Rumination Disorder
307.59 Feeding Disorder of Infancy or Early Childhood

Tic Disorders

307.23 Tourette's Disorder
307.22 Chronic Motor or Vocal Tic Disorder
307.21 Transient Tic Disorder
       Specify if: Single Episode/Recurrent
307.20 Tic Disorder NOS

Elimination Disorders

___.___ Encopresis
787.6 With Constipation and Overflow Incontinence
307.7 Without Constipation and Overflow Incontinence
307.6 Enuresis (Not Due to a General Medical Condition)
Specify type: Nocturnal Only/Diurnal Only/ Nocturnal and Diurnal

Other Disorders of Infancy, Childhood, or Adolescence

309.21 Separation Anxiety Disorder
Specify if: Early Onset
313.23 Selective Mutism
313.89 Reactive Attachment Disorder of Infancy or Early Childhood
Specify type: Inhibited Type/Disinhibited Type
307.3 Stereotypic Movement Disorder
Specify if: With Self-Injurious Behavior
313.9 Disorder of Infancy, Childhood, or Adolescence NOS

DELIRIUM, DEMENTIA, AND AMNESTIC AND OTHER COGNITIVE DISORDERS

Delirium

293.0 Delirium Due to ... *[Indicate the General Medical Condition]*
___.___ Substance Intoxication Delirium *(refer to Substance-Related Disorders for substance-specific codes)*
___.___ Substance Withdrawal Delirium *(refer to Substance-Related Disorders for substance-specific codes)*
___.___ Delirium Due to Multiple Etiologies *(code each of the specific etiologies)*
780.09 Delirium NOS

Dementia

294.xx Dementia of the Alzheimer's Type, With Early Onset *(also code 331.0 Alzheimer's disease on Axis III)*
.10 Without Behavioral Disturbance
.11 With Behavioral Disturbance
294.xx Dementia of the Alzheimer's Type, With Late Onset *(also code 331.0 Alzheimer's disease on Axis III)*
.10 Without Behavioral Disturbance
.11 With Behavioral Disturbance
290.xx Vascular Dementia
.40 Uncomplicated
.41 With Delirium
.42 With Delusions
.43 With Depressed Mood
Specify if: With Behavioral Disturbance

Code presence or absence of a behavioral disturbance in the fifth digit for Dementia Due to a General Medical Condition:
0 = Without Behavioral Disturbance
1 = With Behavioral Disturbance
294.1x Dementia Due to HIV Disease *(also code 042 HIV on Axis III)*
294.1x Dementia Due to Head Trauma *(also code 854.00 head injury on Axis III)*
294.1x Dementia Due to Parkinson's Disease *(also code 332.0 Parkinson's disease on Axis III)*
294.1x Dementia Due to Huntington's Disease *(also code 333.4 Huntington's disease on Axis III)*
294.1x Dementia Due to Pick's Disease *(also code 331.1 Pick's disease on Axis III)*
294.1x Dementia Due to Creutzfeldt-Jakob Disease *(also code 046.1 Creutzfeldt-Jakob disease on Axis III)*
294.1x Dementia Due to ... *[Indicate the General Medical Condition not listed above] (also code the general medical condition on Axis III)*
___.___ Substance-Induced Persisting Dementia *(refer to Substance-Related Disorders for substance-specific codes)*
___.___ Dementia Due to Multiple Etiologies *(code each of the specific etiologies)*
294.8 Dementia NOS

Amnestic Disorders

294.0 Amnestic Disorder Due to ... *[Indicate the General Medical Condition]*
Specify if: Transient/Chronic
___.___ Substance-Induced Persisting Amnestic Disorder (refer to Substance-Related Disorders for substance-specific codes)
294.8 Amnestic Disorder NOS

Other Cognitive Disorders

294.9 Cognitive Disorder NOS

MENTAL DISORDERS DUE TO A GENERAL MEDICAL CONDITION NOT ELSEWHERE CLASSIFIED

293.89 Catatonic Disorder Due to ... *[Indicate the General Medical Condition]*
310.1 Personality Change Due to ... *[Indicate the General Medical Condition]*
Specify type: Labile Type/Disinhibited Type/ Aggressive Type/Apathetic Type/Paranoid Type/ Other Type/Combined Type/Unspecified Type
293.9 Mental Disorder NOS Due to ... *[Indicate the General Medical Condition]*

SUBSTANCE-RELATED DISORDERS

The following specifiers may be applied to Substance Dependence as noted:
[a]With Physiologic Dependence/Without Physiologic Dependence

[b]Early Full Remission/Early Partial Remission/Sustained Full Remission/Sustained Partial Remission
[c]In a Controlled Environment
[d]On Agonist Therapy
The following specifiers apply to Substance-Induced Disorders as noted:
[I]With Onset During Intoxication/[W]With Onset During Withdrawal

Alcohol-Related Disorders

Alcohol Use Disorders

303.90 Alcohol Dependence[a,b,c]
305.00 Alcohol Abuse

Alcohol-Induced Disorders

303.00 Alcohol Intoxication
291.81 Alcohol Withdrawal
     Specify if: With Perceptual Disturbances
291.0 Alcohol Intoxication Delirium
291.0 Alcohol Withdrawal Delirium
291.2 Alcohol-Induced Persisting Dementia
291.1 Alcohol-Induced Persisting Amnestic Disorder
291.x Alcohol-Induced Psychotic Disorder
     .5 With Delusions[I,W]
     .3 With Hallucinations[I,W]
291.89 Alcohol-Induced Mood Disorder[I,W]
291.89 Alcohol-Induced Anxiety Disorder[I,W]
291.89 Alcohol-Induced Sexual Dysfunction[I]
291.89 Alcohol-Induced Sleep Disorder[I,W]
291.9 Alcohol-Related Disorder NOS

Amphetamine (or Amphetamine-Like)–Related Disorders

Amphetamine Use Disorders

304.40 Amphetamine Dependence[a,b,c]
305.70 Amphetamine Abuse

Amphetamine-Induced Disorders

292.89 Amphetamine Intoxication
     Specify if: With Perceptual Disturbances
292.0 Amphetamine Withdrawal
292.81 Amphetamine Intoxication Delirium
292.xx Amphetamine-Induced Psychotic Disorder
     .11 With Delusions[I]
     .12 With Hallucinations[I]
292.84 Amphetamine-Induced Mood Disorder[I,W]
292.89 Amphetamine-Induced Anxiety Disorder[I]
292.89 Amphetamine-Induced Sexual Dysfunction[I]
292.89 Amphetamine-Induced Sleep Disorder[I,W]
292.9 Amphetamine-Related Disorder NOS

Caffeine-Related Disorders

Caffeine-Induced Disorders

305.90 Caffeine Intoxication

292.89 Caffeine-Induced Anxiety Disorder[I]
292.89 Caffeine-Induced Sleep Disorder[I]
292.9 Caffeine-Related Disorder NOS

Cannabis-Related Disorders

Cannabis Use Disorders

304.30 Cannabis Dependence[a,b,c]
305.20 Cannabis Abuse

Cannabis-Induced Disorders

292.89 Cannabis Intoxication
     Specify if: With Perceptual Disturbances
292.81 Cannabis Intoxication Delirium
292.xx Cannabis-Induced Psychotic Disorder
     .11 With Delusions[I]
     .12 With Hallucinations[I]
292.89 Cannabis-Induced Anxiety Disorder[I]
292.9 Cannabis-Related Disorder NOS

Cocaine-Related Disorders

Cocaine Use Disorders

304.20 Cocaine Dependence[a,b,c]
305.60 Cocaine Abuse

Cocaine-Induced Disorders

292.89 Cocaine Intoxication
     Specify if: With Perceptual Disturbances
292.0 Cocaine Withdrawal
292.81 Cocaine Intoxication Delirium
292.xx Cocaine-Induced Psychotic Disorder
     .11 With Delusions[I]
     .12 With Hallucinations[I]
292.84 Cocaine-Induced Mood Disorder[I,W]
292.89 Cocaine-Induced Anxiety Disorder[I,W]
292.89 Cocaine-Induced Sexual Dysfunction[I]
292.89 Cocaine-Induced Sleep Disorder[I,W]
292.9 Cocaine-Related Disorder NOS

Hallucinogen-Related Disorders

Hallucinogen Use Disorders

304.50 Hallucinogen Dependence[b,c]
305.30 Hallucinogen Abuse

Hallucinogen-Induced Disorders

292.89 Hallucinogen Intoxication
292.89 Hallucinogen Persisting Perception Disorder (Flashbacks)
292.81 Hallucinogen Intoxication Delirium
292.xx Hallucinogen-Induced Psychotic Disorder
     .11 With Delusions[I]
     .12 With Hallucinations[I]
292.84 Hallucinogen-Induced Mood Disorder[I]
292.89 Hallucinogen-Induced Anxiety Disorder[I]
292.9 Hallucinogen-Related Disorder NOS

Inhalant-Related Disorders

Inhalant Use Disorders

304.60 Inhalant Dependence[b,c]
305.90 Inhalant Abuse

Inhalant-Induced Disorders

292.89 Inhalant Intoxication
292.81 Inhalant Intoxication Delirium
292.82 Inhalant-Induced Persisting Dementia
292.xx Inhalant-Induced Psychotic Disorder
  .11 With Delusions[I]
  .12 With Hallucinations[I]
292.84 Inhalant-Induced Mood Disorder[I]
292.89 Inhalant-Induced Anxiety Disorder[I]
292.9 Inhalant-Related Disorder NOS

Nicotine-Related Disorders

Nicotine Use Disorder

305.1 Nicotine Dependence[a,b]

Nicotine-Induced Disorder

292.0 Nicotine Withdrawal
292.9 Nicotine-Related Disorder NOS

Opioid-Related Disorders

Opioid Use Disorders

304.00 Opioid Dependence[a,b,c,d]
305.50 Opioid Abuse

Opioid-Induced Disorders

292.89 Opioid Intoxication
  Specify if: With Perceptual Disturbances
292.0 Opioid Withdrawal
292.81 Opioid Intoxication Delirium
292.xx Opioid-Induced Psychotic Disorder
  .11 With Delusions[I]
  .12 With Hallucinations[I]
292.84 Opioid-Induced Mood Disorder[I]
292.89 Opioid-Induced Sexual Dysfunction[I]
292.89 Opioid-Induced Sleep Disorder[I,W]
292.9 Opioid-Related Disorder NOS

Phencyclidine (or Phencyclidine-Like)– Related Disorders

Phencyclidine Use Disorders

304.60 Phencyclidine Dependence[b,c]
305.90 Phencyclidine Abuse

Phencyclidine-Induced Disorders

292.89 Phencyclidine Intoxication
  Specify if: With Perceptual Disturbances
292.81 Phencyclidine Intoxication Delirium
292.xx Phencyclidine-Induced Psychotic Disorder

  .11 With Delusions[I]
  .12 With Hallucinations[I]
292.84 Phencyclidine-Induced Mood Disorder[I]
292.89 Phencyclidine-Induced Anxiety Disorder[I]
292.9 Phencyclidine-Related Disorder NOS

Sedative-, Hypnotic-, or Anxiolytic-Related Disorders

Sedative, Hypnotic, or Anxiolytic Use Disorders

304.10 Sedative, Hypnotic, or Anxiolytic Dependence[a,b,c]
305.40 Sedative, Hypnotic, or Anxiolytic Abuse

Sedative-, Hypnotic-, or Anxiolytic-Induced Disorders

292.89 Sedative, Hypnotic, or Anxiolytic Intoxication
292.0 Sedative, Hypnotic, or Anxiolytic Withdrawal
  Specify if: With Perceptual Disturbances
292.81 Sedative, Hypnotic, or Anxiolytic Intoxication Delirium
292.81 Sedative, Hypnotic, or Anxiolytic Withdrawal Delirium
292.82 Sedative-, Hypnotic-, or Anxiolytic-Induced Persisting Dementia
292.83 Sedative-, Hypnotic-, or Anxiolytic-Induced Persisting Amnestic Disorder
292.xx Sedative-, Hypnotic-, or Anxiolytic-Induced Psychotic Disorder
  .11 With Delusions[I,W]
  .12 With Hallucinations[I,W]
292.84 Sedative-, Hypnotic-, or Anxiolytic-Induced Mood Disorder[I,W]
292.89 Sedative-, Hypnotic-, or Anxiolytic-Induced Anxiety Disorder[W]
292.89 Sedative-, Hypnotic-, or Anxiolytic-Induced Sexual Dysfunction[I]
292.89 Sedative-, Hypnotic-, or Anxiolytic-Induced Sleep Disorder[I,W]
292.9 Sedative-, Hypnotic-, or Anxiolytic-Related Disorder NOS

Polysubstance-Related Disorder

304.80 Polysubstance Dependence[a,b,c,d]

Other (or Unknown) Substance-Related Disorders

Other (or Unknown) Substance Use Disorders

304.90 Other (or Unknown) Substance Dependence[a,b,c,d]
305.90 Other (or Unknown) Substance Abuse

Other (or Unknown) Substance-Induced Disorders

292.89 Other (or Unknown) Substance Intoxication
  Specify if: With Perceptual Disturbances

292.0 Other (or Unknown) Substance Withdrawal
Specify if: With Perceptual Disturbances

292.81 Other (or Unknown) Substance-Induced Delirium

292.82 Other (or Unknown) Substance-Induced Persisting Dementia

292.83 Other (or Unknown) Substance-Induced Persisting Amnestic Disorder

292.xx Other (or Unknown) Substance-Induced Psychotic Disorder
   .11 With Delusions[I,W]
   .12 With Hallucinations[I,W]

292.84 Other (or Unknown) Substance-Induced Mood Disorder[I,W]

292.89 Other (or Unknown) Substance-Induced Anxiety Disorder[I,W]

292.89 Other (or Unknown) Substance-Induced Sexual Dysfunction[I]

292.89 Other (or Unknown) Substance-Induced Sleep Disorder[I,W]

292.9 Other (or Unknown) Substance-Related Disorder NOS

SCHIZOPHRENIA AND OTHER PSYCHOTIC DISORDERS

295.xx Schizophrenia
The following Classification of Longitudinal Course applies to all subtypes of Schizophrenia:
  Episodic With Interepisode Residual Symptoms (*specify if:* With Prominent Negative Symptoms)/Episodic With No Interepisode Residual Symptoms
  Continuous (*specify if:* With Prominent Negative Symptoms)
  Single Episode in Partial Remission (*specify if:* With Prominent Negative Symptoms)/Single Episode In Full Remission
  Other or Unspecified Pattern
   .30 Paranoid Type
   .10 Disorganized Type
   .20 Catatonic Type
   .90 Undifferentiated Type
   .60 Residual Type

295.40 Schizophreniform Disorder
Specify if: Without Good Prognostic Features/With Good Prognostic Features

295.70 Schizoaffective Disorder
Specify type: Bipolar Type/Depressive Type

297.1 Delusional Disorder
Specify type: Erotomanic Type/Grandiose Type/Jealous Type/Persecutory Type/Somatic Type/Mixed Type/Unspecified Type

298.8 Brief Psychotic Disorder
Specify if: With Marked Stressor(s)/Without Marked Stressor(s)/With Postpartum Onset

297.3 Shared Psychotic Disorder

293.xx Psychotic Disorder Due to … *[Indicate the General Medical Condition]*

   .81 With Delusions
   .82 With Hallucinations

____.___ Substance-Induced Psychotic Disorder (*refer to Substance-Related Disorders for substance-specific codes*)
Specify if: With Onset During Intoxication/With Onset During Withdrawal

298.9 Psychotic Disorder NOS

MOOD DISORDERS

Code current state of Major Depressive Disorder or Bipolar I Disorder in fifth digit:
  1 = Mild
  2 = Moderate
  3 = Severe Without Psychotic Features
  4 = Severe With Psychotic Features
  Specify: Mood-Congruent Psychotic Features/Mood-Incongruent Psychotic Features
  5 = In Partial Remission
  6 = In Full Remission
  0 = Unspecified
The following specifiers apply (for current or most recent episode) to Mood Disorders as noted:
  [a]Severity/Psychotic/Remission Specifiers
  [b]Chronic
  [c]With Catatonic Features
  [d]With Melancholic Features
  [e]With Atypical Features
  [f]With Postpartum Onset
The following specifiers apply to Mood Disorders as noted:
  [g]With or Without Full Interepisode Recovery
  [h]With Seasonal Pattern
  [i]With Rapid Cycling

Depressive Disorders

296.xx Major Depressive Disorder
   .2x Single Episode[a,b,c,d,e,f]
   .3x Recurrent[a,b,c,d,e,f,g,h]

300.4 Dysthymic Disorder
Specify if: Early Onset/Late Onset
Specify: With Atypical Features

311 Depressive Disorder NOS

Bipolar Disorders

296.xx Bipolar I Disorder
   .0x Single Manic Episode[a,c,f]
   Specify if: Mixed
   .40 Most Recent Episode Hypomanic[g,h,i]
   .4x Most Recent Episode Manic[a,c,f,g,h,i]
   .6x Most Recent Episode Mixed[a,c,f,g,h,i]
   .5x Most Recent Episode Depressed[a,b,c,d,e,f,g,h,i]
   .7 Most Recent Episode Unspecified[g,h,i]

296.89 Bipolar II Disorder[a,b,c,d,e,f,g,h,i]
Specify (current or most recent episode):
Hypomanic/Depressed

301.13 Cyclothymic Disorder

296.80 Bipolar Disorder NOS
293.83 Mood Disorder Due to... *[Indicate the General Medical Condition]*
  Specify type: With Depressive Features/With Major Depressive-Like Episode/With Manic Features/With Mixed Features
___.__ Substance-Induced Mood Disorder *(refer to Substance-Related Disorders for substance-specific codes)*
  Specify type: With Depressive Features/With Manic Features/With Mixed Features
  Specify if: With Onset During Intoxication/ With Onset During Withdrawal
296.90 Mood Disorder NOS

ANXIETY DISORDERS

300.01 Panic Disorder Without Agoraphobia
300.21 Panic Disorder With Agoraphobia
300.22 Agoraphobia Without History of Panic Disorder
300.29 Specific Phobia
  Specify type: Animal Type/Natural Environment Type/Blood-Injection-Injury Type/Situational Type/Other Type
300.23 Social Phobia
  Specify if: Generalized
300.3 Obsessive-Compulsive Disorder
  Specify if: With Poor Insight
309.81 Posttraumatic Stress Disorder
  Specify if: Acute/Chronic
  Specify if: With Delayed Onset
308.3 Acute Stress Disorder
300.02 Generalized Anxiety Disorder
293.84 Anxiety Disorder Due to... *[Indicate the General Medical Condition]*
  Specify if: With Generalized Anxiety/With Panic Attacks/With Obsessive-Compulsive Symptoms
___.__ Substance-Induced Anxiety Disorder *(refer to Substance-Related Disorders for substance-specific codes)*
  Specify if: With Generalized Anxiety/With Panic Attacks/With Obsessive-Compulsive Symptoms/With Phobic Symptoms
  Specify if: With Onset During Intoxication/ With Onset During Withdrawal
300.00 Anxiety Disorder NOS

SOMATOFORM DISORDERS

300.81 Somatization Disorder
300.82 Undifferentiated Somatoform Disorder
300.11 Conversion Disorder
  Specify type: With Motor Symptom or Deficit/ With Sensory Symptom or Deficit/With Seizures or Convulsions/With Mixed Presentation
307.xx Pain Disorder
  .80 Associated With Psychologic Factors
  .89 Associated With Both Psychologic Factors and a General Medical Condition
    Specify if: Acute/Chronic
300.7 Hypochondriasis
  Specify if: With Poor Insight
300.7 Body Dysmorphic Disorder
300.82 Somatoform Disorder NOS

FACTITIOUS DISORDERS

300.xx Factitious Disorder
  .16 With Predominantly Psychologic Signs and Symptoms
  .19 With Predominantly Physical Signs and Symptoms
  .19 With Combined Psychologic and Physical Signs and Symptoms
300.19 Factitious Disorder NOS

DISSOCIATIVE DISORDERS

300.12 Dissociative Amnesia
300.13 Dissociative Fugue
300.14 Dissociative Identity Disorder
300.6 Depersonalization Disorder
300.15 Dissociative Disorder NOS

SEXUAL AND GENDER IDENTITY DISORDERS

Sexual Dysfunctions

The following specifiers apply to all primary Sexual Dysfunctions:
  Lifelong Type/Acquired Type
  Generalized Type/Situational Type
  Due to Psychologic Factors/Due to Combined Factors

Sexual Desire Disorders

302.71 Hypoactive Sexual Desire Disorder
302.79 Sexual Aversion Disorder

Sexual Arousal Disorders

302.72 Female Sexual Arousal Disorder
302.72 Male Erectile Disorder

Orgasmic Disorders

302.73 Female Orgasmic Disorder
302.74 Male Orgasmic Disorder
302.75 Premature Ejaculation

Sexual Pain Disorders

302.76 Dyspareunia (Not Due to a General Medical Condition)
306.51 Vaginismus (Not Due to a General Medical Condition)

Sexual Dysfunction Due to a General Medical Condition

625.8   Female Hypoactive Sexual Desire Disorder Due to…*[Indicate the General Medical Condition]*
608.89 Male Hypoactive Sexual Desire Disorder Due to…*[Indicate the General Medical Condition]*
607.84 Male Erectile Disorder Due to…*[Indicate the General Medical Condition]*
625.0   Female Dyspareunia Due to…*[Indicate the General Medical Condition]*
608.89 Male Dyspareunia Due to…*[Indicate the General Medical Condition]*
625.8   Other Female Sexual Dysfunction Due to…*[Indicate the General Medical Condition]*
608.89 Other Male Sexual Dysfunction Due to…*[Indicate the General Medical Condition]*
____.__ Substance-Induced Sexual Dysfunction *(refer to Substance-Related Disorders for substance-specific codes)*
        Specify if: With Impaired Desire/With Impaired Arousal/With Impaired Orgasm/With Sexual Pain
        Specify if: With Onset During Intoxication
302.70 Sexual Dysfunction NOS

Paraphilias

302.4   Exhibitionism
302.81 Fetishism
302.89 Frotteurism
302.2   Pedophilia
        Specify if: Sexually Attracted to Males/Sexually Attracted to Females/Sexually Attracted to Both
        Specify if: Limited to Incest
        Specify type: Exclusive Type/Nonexclusive Type
302.83 Sexual Masochism
302.84 Sexual Sadism
302.3   Transvestic Fetishism
        Specify if: With Gender Dysphoria
302.82 Voyeurism
302.9   Paraphilia NOS

Gender Identity Disorders

302.xx Gender Identity Disorder
  .6   In Children
  .85   In Adolescents or Adults
        Specify if: Sexually Attracted to Males/Sexually Attracted to Females/Sexually Attracted to Both/Sexually Attracted to Neither
302.6   Gender Identity Disorder NOS
302.9   Sexual Disorder NOS

EATING DISORDERS

307.1   Anorexia Nervosa
        Specify type: Restricting Type; Binge-Eating/Purging Type
307.51 Bulimia Nervosa
        Specify type: Purging Type/Nonpurging Type
307.50 Eating Disorder NOS

SLEEP DISORDERS
Primary Sleep Disorders

Dyssomnias

307.42 Primary Insomnia
307.44 Primary Hypersomnia
        Specify if: Recurrent
347   Narcolepsy
780.59 Breathing-Related Sleep Disorder
307.45 Circadian Rhythm Sleep Disorder
        Specify type: Delayed Sleep Phase Type/Jet Lag Type/Shift Work Type/Unspecified Type
307.47 Dyssomnia NOS

Parasomnias

307.47 Nightmare Disorder
307.46 Sleep Terror Disorder
307.46 Sleepwalking Disorder
307.47 Parasomnia NOS

Sleep Disorders Related to Another Mental Disorder

307.42 Insomnia Related to…*[Indicate the Axis I or Axis II Disorder]*
307.44 Hypersomnia Related to…*[Indicate the Axis I or Axis II Disorder]*

Other Sleep Disorders

780.xx Sleep Disorder Due to…*[Indicate the General Medical Condition]*
  .52   Insomnia Type
  .54   Hypersomnia Type
  .59   Parasomnia Type
  .59   Mixed Type
____.__ Substance-Induced Sleep Disorder *(refer to Substance-Related Disorders for substance-specific codes)*
        Specify type: Insomnia Type/Hypersomnia Type/Parasomnia Type/Mixed Type
        Specify if: With Onset During Intoxication/With Onset During Withdrawal

IMPULSE-CONTROL DISORDERS NOT ELSEWHERE CLASSIFIED

312.34 Intermittent Explosive Disorder
312.32 Kleptomania
312.33 Pyromania
312.31 Pathologic Gambling
312.39 Trichotillomania
312.30 Impulse-Control Disorder NOS

ADJUSTMENT DISORDERS

309.xx Adjustment Disorder
.0 With Depressed Mood
.24 With Anxiety
.28 With Mixed Anxiety and Depressed Mood
.3 With Disturbance of Conduct
.4 With Mixed Disturbance of Emotions and Conduct
.9 Unspecified
Specify if: Acute/Chronic

PERSONALITY DISORDERS

NOTE: These are coded on Axis II.
301.0 Paranoid Personality Disorder
301.20 Schizoid Personality Disorder
301.22 Schizotypal Personality Disorder
301.7 Antisocial Personality Disorder
301.83 Borderline Personality Disorder
301.50 Histrionic Personality Disorder
301.81 Narcissistic Personality Disorder
301.82 Avoidant Personality Disorder
301.6 Dependent Personality Disorder
301.4 Obsessive-Compulsive Personality Disorder
301.9 Personality Disorder NOS

OTHER CONDITIONS THAT MAY BE A FOCUS OF CLINICAL ATTENTION

Psychologic Factors Affecting Medical Condition

316 ...*[Specified Psychologic Factor] Affecting...[Indicate the General Medical Condition]*
Choose name based on nature of factors:
  Mental Disorder Affecting Medical Condition
  Psychological Symptoms Affecting Medical Condition
  Personality Traits or Coping Style Affecting Medical Condition
  Maladaptive Health Behaviors Affecting Medical Condition
  Stress-Related Physiological Response Affecting Medical Condition
  Other or Unspecified Psychological Factors Affecting Medical Condition

Medication-Induced Movement Disorders

332.1 Neuroleptic-Induced Parkinsonism
333.92 Neuroleptic Malignant Syndrome
333.7 Neuroleptic-Induced Acute Dystonia
333.99 Neuroleptic-Induced Acute Akathisia
333.82 Neuroleptic-Induced Tardive Dyskinesia

333.1 Medication-Induced Postural Tremor
333.90 Medication-Induced Movement Disorder NOS

Other Medication-Induced Disorder

995.2 Adverse Effects of Medication NOS

Relational Problems

V61.9 Relational Problem Related to a Mental Disorder or General Medical Condition
V61.20 Parent-Child Relational Problem
V61.10 Partner Relational Problem
V61.8 Sibling Relational Problem
V62.81 Relational Problem NOS

Problems Related to Abuse or Neglect

V61.21 Physical Abuse of Child *(code 995.5 if focus of attention is on victim)*
V61.21 Sexual Abuse of Child *(code 995.5 if focus of attention is on victim)*
V61.21 Neglect of Child *(code 995.5 if focus of attention is on victim)*
___.__ Physical Abuse of Adult
V61.12 (if by partner)
V62.83 (if by person other than partner) *(code 995.81 if focus of attention is on victim)*
___.__ Sexual Abuse of Adult
V61.12 (if by partner)
V62.83 (if by person other than partner) *(code 995.83 if focus of attention is on victim)*

Additional Conditions That May Be a Focus of Clinical Attention

V15.81 Noncompliance With Treatment
V65.2 Malingering
V71.01 Adult Antisocial Behavior
V71.02 Child or Adolescent Antisocial Behavior
V62.89 Borderline Intellectual Functioning
    NOTE: *This is coded on Axis II.*
780.9 Age-Related Cognitive Decline
V62.82 Bereavement
V62.3 Academic Problem
V62.2 Occupational Problem
313.82 Identity Problem
V62.89 Religious or Spiritual Problem
V62.4 Acculturation Problem
V62.89 Phase of Life Problem

ADDITIONAL CODES

300.9 Unspecified Mental Disorder (nonpsychotic)
V71.09 No Diagnosis or Condition on Axis I
799.9 Diagnosis or Condition Deferred on Axis I
V71.09 No Diagnosis on Axis II
799.9 Diagnosis Deferred on Axis II

APPENDIX B

Historical Synopsis of Psychiatric Mental Health Nursing

Pre-1860

Nursing care for young, ill, and vulnerable people has existed as long as the human race. Care was given by family members, other relatives, servants, neighbors, members of religious orders or humanitarian societies, or by convalescing patients or prisoners.

1860

Florence Nightingale. Established Nightingale School at St. Thomas's Hospital in London after the Crimean War and worked with untrained women caring for soldiers. *Founder of modern-day nursing.*

1860-1880

Nightingale emphasized the maintenance of a healthful environment, personal hygiene, cleanliness, and healthful living habits, such as adequate nutrition, exercise, and sleep, so that nature could heal. Emphasized kindness toward patients along with custodial care.

Linda Richards. First graduate nurse and first psychiatric nurse in the United States. After study under Florence Nightingale, organized nursing services and educational programs in Boston City Hospital and in several state mental hospitals in Illinois.

Dorothea Dix. Worked to reform psychiatric care in mental hospitals and to correct overcrowding and the insufficient number of physicians and attendants.

1882

First school to prepare nurses to care for patients with acute and chronic mental illness opened at McLean Hospital, Waverly, Massachusetts, through collaboration of Linda Richards and Dr. Edward Cowles.

1890-1930

Nurses with special preparation recognized by some administrative psychiatrists in state and private hospitals for their preparation. Nurses relieved of menial housekeeping chores to engage in physical custodial care of patients. Role primarily to assist physician or carry out procedures for physical care. Few psychological nursing skills. Psychologically concerned with maintaining kind, tolerant attitude and humane treatment.

1920

Harriet Bailey. *First nurse educator to write a psychiatric nursing text,* Nursing Mental Disease, *1920.* She wrote of the importance of a nurse's knowing mental illness and of teaching mental health nursing, and she worked for provision of student experiences in psychiatry. She argued for more holistic care of patients.

1926

Euphemia "Effie" Jane Taylor. Became the first psychiatric nurse to be appointed Professor of Nursing at Yale University School of Nursing.

1937

National League for Nursing recommended that psychiatric nursing be included in the basic nursing curriculum.

1940

Publication of *Psychiatry for Nurses* by Louis Karnosh, a psychiatrist, and Edith Gage, a registered nurse.

1946

National Mental Health Act authorizes the establishment of the National Institute of Mental Health, with funds and programs to train professional psychiatric personnel, conduct psychiatric research, and aid in the development of mental health programs at the state level. Provided impetus for psychiatric nursing as a specialty.

1950-1960

Nurse's role included physical care, administration of medications, and maintenance of therapeutic milieu. Less emphasis on physical restraints.

Ruth Matheney and Mary Topalis. Emphasized importance of milieu therapy and the nurse's use of this intervention.

1952

Hildegard E. Peplau. Formulated first systematic theoretical framework in psychiatric nursing, presented in *Interpersonal Relations in Nursing*, 1952. Emphasized nursing as an interpersonal process and that psychological techniques and theoretical concepts are essential to nursing practice. Defined steps in nurse-patient relationship:

1. Nurse helps patient examine situational factors through observation of behavior.
2. Nurse helps patient describe and analyze behavior.
3. Nurse formulates with patient connections between feelings and behavior.
4. Nurse encourages patient to improve interpersonal competence through testing new behavior.
5. Nurse validates with patient when new behavior is integrated into personality structure.

1953

The Therapeutic Community by Maxwell Jones, in Great Britain, laid basis for movement in United States toward milieu therapy and for nurse's role in this therapy.

1954

Advent of the use of the antipsychotic medication, chlorpromazine (Thorazine), in the United States; synthesized in France in 1950.

1956

National Conference on Graduate Education in Psychiatric Nursing introduced concept of psychiatric clinical nurse specialist. Theorists begin to differentiate functions based on master's level of preparation in nursing.

1957

June Mellow. Introduced second theoretical approach to psychiatric nursing, called "nursing therapy," which applied psychoanalytical theory in one-to-one interactions with patients who had schizophrenia. Emphasized the provision of corrective emotional experiences rather than investigating pathological processes.

1958

American Nurses Association established Conference Group on Psychiatric Nursing.

1959

Accredited schools of nursing had to have own psychiatric nursing curriculum and instructor, per National League for Nursing. They could no longer buy services of hospitals to supply education.

1960-1970

Hildegard E. Peplau, Gertrude Ujhely, Joyce Travelbee, Shirley Burd, Loretta Bermosk, Joyce Hays, Catherine Norris, Gertrude Stokes, Anne Hargreaves, Dorothy Gregg, and Sheila Rouslin. Nursing leaders emphasized importance of self-awareness and use of self, nurse-patient relationship therapy, therapeutic communication, and psychosocial aspects of general nursing. Peplau identified the manifestations of anxiety and formulated steps in anxiety intervention now used by all health care professions. All of these nursing leaders converted various psychological concepts into operational definitions for use in nursing.

1960-1965

Sheila Rouslin and Suzanne Lego. Opened private practices in psychotherapy.

1961

Anne Burgess and Donna Aguilera. Engaged in crisis work and short-term therapy as well as long-term therapy. Applied crisis theory to psychiatric nursing.

Ida Orlando. Initiated term *nursing process* and began to delineate its components. Presented general theoretical framework for all nurse-patient relationships that focused on the patient identifying the meaning of behavior and what the nurse could do to help. She wrote the classic book, *The Dynamic Nurse-Patient Relationship*.

Hildegard E. Peplau. Promoted primary role of nurse as psychotherapist or counselor rather than as mother surrogate, socializer, or manager.

1963

The Comprehensive Community Mental Health Act was passed, providing an impetus for nurses to move from hospitals to community settings.

1967

American Nurses Association presented "Position Paper on Psychiatric Nursing," which endorsed the role of clinical specialist as therapist in individual, group, family, and milieu therapies.

American Nurses Association, Division on Psychiatric and Mental Health Nursing Practice, published first *Statement on Psychiatric and Mental Health Nursing Practice.*

1970-1980

Sheila Rouslin. Because of her leadership, certification of clinical specialists in psychiatric nursing begun by Division of Psychiatric Mental Health Nursing, New Jersey State Nurses Association. Later, certification developed by American Nurses Association.

Shirley Smoyak. Defined the patient as individual, group, family, or community; defined the nurse as family therapist; defined the expanded role of nurse.

Gwen Marram and Irene Burnside. Emphasized that nurses with graduate-level preparation could conduct group and family psychotherapy.

Carolyn Clark. Emphasized the usefulness of a systems framework for psychiatric nurses. Also emphasized the importance of nurses acting as change agents and researchers.

Bonnie Bullough. Emphasized legal and ethical aspects of psychiatric care.

Madeleine Leininger. Reemphasized care of whole person. Introduced implications of cultural diversity for mental health services and psychiatric treatment.

1973

The American Nurses Association (ANA) published *Standards of Psychiatric-Mental Health Nursing*. Certification of Psychiatric-Mental Health Nurse Generalists was established by the ANA.

1976

American Nurses Association, Division on Psychiatric and Mental Health Nursing Practice published revised *Statement on Psychiatric and Mental Health Nursing Practice*.

1978

Report of The President's Commission on Mental Health concluded that deinstitutionalization and discharge of patients to community facilities had not worked as expected and that improved financial, social, medical, and nursing resources, research, and coordination of services were needed.

1979

ANA established certification of Psychiatric-Mental Health Nurse Specialists.

1980-1990

Anne Burgess. Formulated a theory of victimology based on extensive studies of adult and child victims of rape and abuse, child victims of neglect, and family violence of incest and battering. Described rape-trauma syndrome, silent rape trauma, and compound reactions to rape.

Lee Ann Hoff. Expanded crisis theory to be used in nursing practice. Contributed to theory of suicidology. Described battering syndrome after performing research on battered women and battered elderly.

1982

American Nurses Association Executive Committee and Standards Committee, Division on Psychiatric and Mental Health Nursing Practice, published *Standards of Psychiatric and Mental Health Nursing Practice*.
Century Celebration of Psychiatric Nursing, Washington, DC.

1987

Maxine E. Loomis, Anita O'Toole, Marie Scott Brown, Patricia Pothier, Patricia West, and Holly S. Wilson. Began the development of a classification system for psychiatric and mental health nursing, first published in the newly established journal *Archives of Psychiatric Nursing*, 1(1), 16-24, 1987.

1988

National Institute of Mental Health Epidemiological Catchment Area Study published.

1990

Suzanne Lego. Opened the first psychoanalytic training program for nurses at Columbia University School of Nursing.

Americans with Disabilities Act passed by U.S. Congress. President George H.W. Bush declared the 1990s as the "Decade of the Brain."

1994

Carolyn V. Billings, Jean Blackburn, Mickie Ceimone, Carol Dashiff, Kathleen Scharer, Anita O'Toole, and Carole A. Shea. Composed a task force to:
- Revise *Statement on Psychiatric and Mental Health Nursing Practice*, updating the scope and functions for nurses certified at the basic level and those certified at the advanced practice level.
- Revise *Standards of Psychiatric and Mental Health Nursing Practice*, describing professional nursing activities that are demonstrated by the nurse throughout the nursing process for both the basic level certified psychiatric nurse and the advanced practice psychiatric nurse, and standards of professional performance.

Essentials of Psychiatric Nursing, 14th edition, by Cecelia Taylor (originally published as *Psychiatry for Nurses* in 1940) was published.

1995

The *Journal of the American Psychiatric Nurses Association* began publication.

2000

Grayce Sills, Karen A. Ballard, Carolyn V. Billings, and others. Composed a task force to revise *Scope and Standards of Psychiatric Mental Health Nursing*.

2003

Twenty-five years after the last presidential commission, The President's New Freedom Commission released it's report emphasizing the importance of mental health to overall health. Recommendations included the reduction of disparities and stigma, the promotion of recovery, resilience, and early mental health interventions, and expanding research and technology for mental health care.

2007

A revised *Psychiatric-Mental Health Nursing: Scope and Standards of Practice* was developed jointly by the American Psychiatric Nurses Association, the International Society of Psychiatric-Mental Health Nurses, and the American Nurses Association.

Adapted from Murray, R.B. (1991). The nursing process and emotional care. In R.B. Murray and M.M.W. Huelskoetter (Eds.), *Psychiatric mental health nursing—giving emotional care* (3rd ed., pp. 94–97). Norwalk, CT: Appleton & Lange.

Glossary

A

abstract thinking The ability to conceptualize ideas (e.g., finding meaning in proverbs).

abuse An act of misuse, deceit, or exploitation; wrong or improper use of or action toward another, resulting in injury, damage, maltreatment, or corruption.

accommodation The ability to change one's way of thinking to introduce new ideas, objects, or experiences.

acculturation Adapting to the beliefs, values, and practices of a new cultural setting.

acquaintance (or date) rape A rape in which the perpetrator is known to, and presumably trusted by, the person raped.

acrophobia Fear of high places.

acting-out behaviors Behaviors that originate on an unconscious level to reduce anxiety and tension. Anxiety is displaced from one situation to another in the form of observable responses (e.g., anger, crying, or violence).

active listening Being aware of the patient's verbal and nonverbal communications while monitoring personal verbal and nonverbal communications.

activities of daily living The activities such as eating, attending to hygiene, eating, and toileting that are necessary to live independently as an adult.

acupuncture An aspect of traditional Chinese medicine that involves the placement of needles into the skin at meridian points to modulate the flow of *qi*.

acute anxiety Anxiety that is precipitated by an imminent loss or a change that threatens an individual's sense of security.

acute dystonia Acute, often painful, sustained contraction of muscles, usually of the head and neck, which typically occur from 2 to 5 days after the introduction of antipsychotic medications.

acute stress disorder Severe fear, helplessness, or horror that occurs within 1 month of exposure to extreme stress.

addiction Obsession, compulsion, or loss of control with respect to use of a drug (e.g., alcohol), with genetic, psychosocial, and environmental factors that influence its development. Use of the drug continues despite the presence of related problems and a tendency to relapse after stopping use.

adjustment disorder A psychological response to identifiable stressor(s), with symptoms developing within 3 months of the stressor(s).

admission criteria Criteria for admitting an individual to an inpatient psychiatric unit. Criteria begin with the premise that the person is suffering from a mental illness, and there is evidence of one or more of the following: (1) imminent danger of harming self, (2) imminent danger of harming others, or (3) unable to care for basic needs, placing individual at imminent risk of harming self.

Adult Children of Alcoholics (ACOA) A support group for adult children of alcoholics, who often experience similar difficulties and problems in their adult lives as a result of having an alcoholic parent or parents.

adult day care A nonresidential facility that provides services and activities to elderly or handicapped individuals.

advance directive Directions provided by a patient for clinicians to follow in the event of a serious illness.

advanced practice forensic nurse A nurse who has completed graduate education with a broad focus in forensic nursing and obtained credentials as a clinical nurse specialist, certified nurse-midwife, or nurse practitioner.

advanced practice registered nurse–psychiatric mental health (APRN-PMH) A nurse generalist who has obtained additional training to provide care as a clinical nurse specialist with advanced nursing expertise or as a nurse practitioner who diagnoses, prescribes, and treats psychiatric disorders.

adventitious crisis A crisis that is not part of everyday life but involves an event that is unplanned and accidental. Adventitious crises include natural disasters and crimes of violence such as rapes or muggings.

affect The external manifestation of feeling or emotion which is manifested in facial expression, tone of voice, and body language. For example, a patient may be said to have a *flat affect*, meaning that there is an absence or a near absence of facial expression. The term may be used loosely to describe a feeling, emotion, or mood.

affective symptoms Symptoms involving emotions and their expression.

ageism A system of destructive, erroneous beliefs about the elderly; a bias against older people based solely on their age.

aggression Any verbal or nonverbal (actual or attempted, conscious or unconscious) forceful means of harm or abuse of another person or object.

agnosia Loss of the ability to recognize familiar objects. For example, a person may be unable to identify familiar sounds, such as the ringing of a doorbell (auditory agnosia), or familiar objects, such as a toothbrush or keys (visual agnosia).

agoraphobia An anxiety disorder characterized by fear of being in places or situations in which escape might be difficult or embarrassing or in which help may not be available should an anxiety attack occur.

agraphia   Loss of a previous ability to write, resulting from brain injury or brain disease.

akathisia   Regular rhythmic movements, usually of the lower limbs; constant pacing may also be seen; often noticed in people taking antipsychotic medication.

akinesia   Absence or diminution of voluntary motion. Akinesia is usually accompanied by a parallel reduction in mental activity.

Al-Anon   A support group for spouses and friends of alcoholics.

Alateen   A nationwide network for children older than 10 years of age who have alcoholic parents.

alcohol withdrawal delirium   An organic mental disorder that occurs 40 to 48 hours after cessation or reduction of long-term heavy alcohol intake and that is considered a medical emergency; often referred to by the older term *delirium tremens* (DTs).

alcoholic hallucinations   Visual and tactile hallucinations reported to occur in alcohol-dependent patients suffering from alcohol withdrawal delirium.

Alcoholics Anonymous (AA)   A self-help group for recovering alcoholics that provides support and encouragement to those involved in continuing recovery.

alcoholism   The end stage of the continuum that includes addiction to and dependence on alcohol.

alternate personality (alter) or subpersonality   A distinct personality state that recurrently takes control of a behavior of a person with dissociative identity disorder.

Alzheimer's disease (AD)   A primary cognitive impairment disorder characterized by progressive deterioration of cognitive functioning, with the end result that the person may not recognize once-familiar people, places, and things. The ability to walk and talk is absent in the final stages.

ambivalence   The holding, at the same time, of two opposing emotions, attitudes, ideas, or wishes toward the same person, situation, or object.

amnesia   Loss of memory for events within a specific period of time; may be temporary or permanent.

anergia   Lack of energy; passivity.

anger   An emotional response to the perception of frustration of desires or threat to one's needs.

anhedonia   The inability to experience pleasure.

anorexia nervosa   A medical term that signifies a loss of appetite. A person with anorexia nervosa, however, may not have any loss of appetite and often is preoccupied with food and eating. A person with this disorder may suppress the desire for food in order to control his or her eating.

anosognosia   A patient's inability to realize that he or she is ill; caused by the illness itself.

antagonists   Drugs that block or depress the normal response of a specific receptor by only partly fitting the receptor site.

antianxiety drugs   Drugs prescribed, usually on a short-term basis, to reduce anxiety. May be referred to as *anxiolytics*.

anticholinergic side effects   Side effects of some medications (e.g., neuroleptics and tricyclic antidepressants) that include dry mouth, constipation, urinary retention, blurred vision, and dry mucous membranes.

anticholinesterase drugs   Drugs that prevent the destruction of acetylcholine within the parasympathetic nervous system. Increasing acetylcholine slows heart action, lowers blood pressure, increases secretion, and increases contraction of smooth muscles.

anticipatory grief   Grief that occurs before an actual loss. During this time, painful feelings may be partially resolved.

anticonvulsant drugs   Drugs commonly used to treat epilepsy; suppress the rapid and excessive firing of neurons and are used as mood stabilizers.

antidepressants   Drugs predominantly used to elevate mood in people who are depressed.

antimanic drugs   Drugs used in the treatment of a manic state to lower an elevated and unstable mood and to reduce irritability and aggressiveness.

antipsychotic drugs   Drugs used to decrease hallucinations, delusions, and disorganized thinking. Conventional antipsychotics target the neurotransmitter, dopamine. Atypical antipsychotics target dopamine and other neurotransmitters, including serotonin; drugs in this classification not only reduce psychotic symptoms but also increase mood and motivation.

antisocial personality disorder   A syndrome in which a person lacks the capacity to relate to others, does not experience discomfort in inflicting or observing pain in others, and may manipulate others for personal gain. Common characteristics and behaviors include crimes against society, aggressiveness, inability to feel remorse, untruthfulness and insincerity, unreliability, and failure to follow any life plan.

anxiety   A state of feeling apprehension, uneasiness, uncertainty, or dread; results from a real or perceived threat whose actual source is unknown or unrecognized.

apathy   A state of indifference.

aphasia   Difficulty in the formulation of words; loss of language ability. In extreme cases, a person may be limited to a few words, may babble, or may become mute.

apraxia   Loss of ability to perform purposeful movements. For example, a person may be unable to shave, to dress, or to perform other once-familiar and purposeful tasks.

aromatherapy   The use of essential oils for enhancing physical and mental well-being and healing.

assault   An intentional threat designed to make the victim fearful; produces reasonable apprehension of harm.

assertive community treatment (ACT)   An intensive type of case management developed in response to community-living needs of people with serious, persistent psychiatric symptoms and patterns of repeated hospitalization for services such as emergency room and inpatient care.

assertiveness Asking for what one wants or acting to get what one wants in a way that respects the rights and feelings of other people.

assertiveness training Instruction in communication skills that help people ask directly in appropriate (nondemanding, nonthreatening, nondemeaning) ways for what they want.

assimilation The incorporation of new ideas, objects, and experiences into the framework of one's thoughts.

associative looseness A disturbance of thinking in which ideas shift from one subject to another in an oblique or unrelated manner.

attempted rape Physical attempts and verbal threats of rape.

attention deficit hyperactivity disorder (ADHD) A behavioral disorder usually manifested before the age of 7 years that includes overactivity, chronic inattention, and difficulty dealing with multiple stimuli.

atypical antipsychotics A classification of antipsychotic medications, also known as *second-generation antipsychotics*, which commonly interact with serotonin as well as dopamine receptors. They are considered the first line of treatment for psychosis and have a low profile for extrapyramidal side effects.

autism A state in which thinking is not bound to reality but reflects the private perceptual world of the individual.

autistic thinking Thoughts, ideas, or desires derived from internal private stimuli or perceptions that often are incongruent with reality. Hallucinations, delusions, and neologisms are examples of autistic thinking.

automatic obedience The performance of all simple commands in a robotlike fashion; may be present in catatonia.

automatic thoughts Rapid, unthinking responses based on unique assumptions about ourselves and the world. These assumptions may be realistic or distorted. Common distortions include focusing on negative details and catastrophizing, which is assuming the worst possible outcome.

aversion therapy A behavioral technique that uses negative reinforcement or conditioning to alter or eliminate an unwanted or negative behavior.

avoidant personality disorder A personality disorder in which the central characteristics are an extreme sensitivity to rejection and robust avoidance of interpersonal situations.

avolition Lack of motivation.

axon The part of the neuron that conveys electrical impulses away from the cell body.

B

basal ganglia Pockets of integrating gray matter deep within the cerebrum; involved in the regulation of movement, emotions, and basic drives.

basic level registered nurse Any nurse with basic training (diploma, associate degree, baccalaureate degree) in nursing.

battering Physical attack such as hitting, kicking, biting, throwing, and burning.

battery The harmful or offensive touching of another person.

behavior modification A treatment modality that focuses on modifying and changing specific observable dysfunctional patterns of behavior by means of stimulus-and-response conditioning. Examples of behavioral therapy techniques include operant conditioning, token economy, systematic desensitization, aversion therapy, and flooding.

behavioral family therapy A treatment in which family members identify undesirable behaviors, how they can unlearn these behaviors, and how they can learn more desirable behaviors. This type of therapy is a method of direct treatment in which goals are immediately established and an action plan is developed and monitored.

behavioral therapy A treatment method that is concerned with patterns of behavior rather than inner motivations. Maladaptive responses are replaced with adaptive responses.

Benson's relaxation techniques Techniques that allow a patient to switch from the sympathetic mode of the autonomic nervous system to a state of relaxation by focusing on a pleasant mental image in a calm and peaceful environment.

bereavement The period of grieving following a death; derived from the Old English word *berafian*, meaning "to rob."

bibliotherapy The use of literature to assists the individual to express feelings, gain insight into feelings and behavior, and learn new ways to cope with difficult situations.

binge eating disorder An eating disorder in which individuals engage in repeated episodes of binge eating, after which they experience significant distress.

binge-purge cycle An episodic, uncontrolled, rapid ingestion of large quantities of food over a short period of time, followed by purging (vomiting; overexercising; misusing laxatives, diuretics, or other medications); seen in people with bulimia nervosa.

bioethics The study of specific ethical questions that arise in health care.

biofeedback A technique for gaining conscious control over unconscious body functions, such as blood pressure and heartbeat, to achieve relaxation or the relief of stress-related physical symptoms; involves the use of self-monitoring equipment.

biologically based mental illnesses Mental health disorders listed in the *DSM-IV-TR.*

biofeedback Feedback obtained by sensitive instruments that provide immediate and exact information regarding muscle activity, brain waves, skin temperature, and other bodily functions.

bipolar disorders Mood disorders that include one or more manic episodes and usually one or more depressive episodes.

bipolar I disorder A form of bipolar disorder in which at least one episode of mania alternates with major depression.

bipolar II disorder A form of bipolar disorder in which hypomanic episodes alternate with major depression.

bisexuality Sexual attraction toward both males and females, which may be acted on by engaging in both heterosexual and homosexual activities.

blocking A sudden obstruction or interruption in the spontaneous flow of thinking or speaking that is perceived as an absence or deprivation of thought.

blood alcohol level (BAL) The concentration of alcohol in a person's blood.

body dysmorphic disorder A somatoform disorder that involves preoccupation with an imagined defective body part, resulting in obsessional thinking and compulsive behavior.

body image One's internalized sense of the physical self.

borderline personality disorder A disorder characterized by disordered images of self, impulsive and unpredictable behavior, marked shifts in mood, and instability in relationships with others.

boundaries Those functions that maintain a clear distinction among individuals within a family or group and between family members and the outside world. Boundaries may be clear, diffuse, rigid, or inconsistent.

bulimia nervosa Episodes of excessive and uncontrollable intake of large amounts of food (binges), usually alternating with compensatory activities such as self-induced vomiting, use of cathartics and/or diuretics, and self-starvation. These alternating behaviors characterize the eating disorder bulimia nervosa.

C

caring presence Refers to the therapeutic benefit of simply being available and present for patients.

case management Duties of a health care worker (e.g., a nurse) that involve assuming responsibility for a patient or group of patients—arranging assessments of need, formulating a comprehensive plan of care, arranging for delivery of services to address individual patient needs, and assessing and monitoring the services delivered.

catatonia A state of psychologically induced immobilization, at times interrupted by episodes of extreme agitation.

catecholamines A group of biogenic amines that are derived from phenylalanine and contain catechol as the aromatic portion. Certain of these amines, such as epinephrine, norepinephrine, and dopamine, are neurotransmitters and exert an important influence on peripheral and central nervous system activity.

cathexis A psychoanalytical term used to describe the emotional attachment or bond to an idea, an object, or, most commonly, a person.

character The sum of a person's relatively fixed personality traits and habitual modes of response.

chemical restraint A drug given for the specific purpose of inhibiting a certain behavior or movement.

child abuse—battering Physical assault of a child, such as hitting, kicking, biting, throwing, and burning.

child abuse—neglect A type of child abuse that can be physical (e.g., failure to provide medical care), developmental (e.g., failure to provide emotional nurturing and cognitive stimulation), educational (failure to provide educational opportunities to the child in accordance with the state's education laws), or a combination of these.

child abuse—physical endangerment Reckless behaviors toward a child that could lead to the child's serious physical injury, such as leaving a young child alone or placing the child in a hazardous environment.

child abuse—sexual Sexual maltreatment of a child, which can take many forms. Essentially it is those acts designed to stimulate the child sexually or to use a child for sexual stimulation, either for the perpetrator or for another person.

chiropractic medicine Focuses on the relationship between structure and function and the way relationship affects the preservation and restoration of health, using manipulative therapy as a treatment tool.

chronic anxiety Anxiety a person has lived with for a long time. Chronic anxiety may take the form of chronic fatigue, insomnia, discomfort in daily activities, or discomfort in personal relationships.

chronic illness An illness that has persisted over a long period of time and generally involves progressive deterioration, with a resulting increase in functional impairment, symptoms, and disability.

chronic pain Pain that a patient has had for longer than 6 months.

circadian rhythm A 24-hour biological rhythm that influences specific regulatory functions such as the sleep/wake cycle, body temperature, and hormonal and neurotransmitter secretions. The 24-hour biological rhythm is controlled by a "pacemaker" in the brain that sends messages to various systems in the body such as those mentioned.

circumstantial speech A pattern of speech characterized by indirectness and delay before the person gets to the point or answers a question; the person gets caught up in countless details and explanations.

civil rights The rights of personal liberty guaranteed under two U.S. constitutional amendments.

clang association The meaningless rhyming of words, often in a forceful manner.

classical conditioning Bringing about involuntary behavior or reflexes through conditioned responses to stimuli.

clear boundaries Boundaries that are understood by all members of the family and give family members a sense of "I-ness" and also "we-ness."

clinical epidemiology A broad field that addresses what happens after people with illnesses are seen by providers of clinical care.

clinical pathway A written plan or "map" identifying predetermined times that specific nursing and medical interventions (e.g., diagnostic studies, treatments, activities, medications, teaching, discharge teaching) will be implemented (e.g., day 1 or day 2 for hospital settings, or week 1 or month 2 for community-based settings).

clinical supervision A mentoring relationship which is characterized by evaluation and feedback and a gradual increase in autonomy and responsibility.

closed-ended questions Questions that elicit a "yes" or "no" response. They are useful for getting information efficiently, as in an assessment, but do little to encourage the sharing of feelings.

codependence A term used to describe coping behaviors that prevent individuals from taking care of their own needs and have as their core a preoccupation with the thoughts and feelings of another or others. It usually refers to the dependence of one person on another person who is addicted in one form or another.

codes Psychiatric emergencies.

cognition The act, process, or result of knowing, learning, or understanding.

cognitive disorders Psychiatric disorders that are manifested in deficits in memory, perception, and problem-solving.

cognitive distortions Inaccurate and irrational automatic thoughts or ideas that lead to false assumptions and misinterpretations.

cognitive impairment syndrome/disorder A disturbance in orientation, memory, intellect, judgment, and affect due to physiological changes in the brain. Delirium and dementia are two examples of cognitive impairment syndromes. An older term is *chronic mental disorder*.

cognitive reframing A process of changing the individual's perceptions of stress by reassessing a situation and replacing irrational beliefs.

cognitive rehearsal A technique in which a patient imagines each successive step in the sequence leading to completion of a task, identifying potential "roadblocks" (cognitive, behavioral, or environmental), and planning strategies to deal with them before they produce an unwanted failure experience.

cognitive symptoms Abnormalities in how a person thinks.

cognitive therapy A treatment method (particularly useful for depressive disorders) that emphasizes the revision of a person's maladaptive thought processes, perceptions, and attitudes.

cognitive-behavioral therapy (CBT) An effective therapeutic modality that seeks to identify negative and irrational patterns of thought and challenge them based on rational evidence and thoughts.

command hallucinations "Voices" that direct the person to take action.

community nursing center (CNC) A nurse-managed center that provides direct access to professional nurses who offer holistic, patient-centered health services for reimbursement.

comorbid condition A condition that occurs along with another disorder.

compensation Making up for deficits in one area by excelling in another area in order to raise or maintain self-esteem.

competency The capacity to understand the consequences of one's decisions.

competency evaluator A forensic nurse who assesses mental health or illness, conducts forensic interviews, provides documentation, completes a formal report to the court, and testifies as an expert witness regarding the competency of the defendant.

complementary and alternative medicine (CAM) A group of diverse medical and health care systems, practices, and products that are not generally considered part of conventional medicine.

completed suicide A suicide attempt that results in death.

compulsion Repetitive, seemingly purposeless behaviors performed according to certain rules known to the patient to temporarily reduce escalating anxiety.

concrete thinking Thinking grounded in immediate experience rather than abstraction. There is an overemphasis on specific detail as opposed to general and abstract concepts.

conditional release A release from an inpatient psychiatric facility that is contingent upon outpatient commitment.

conduct disorder A psychiatric disorder characterized by a persistent pattern of behavior in which the rights of others are violated and age-appropriate societal norms or rules are disregarded.

confabulation The filling in of a memory gap with a detailed fantasy believed by the teller. The purpose is to maintain self-esteem. It is seen in organic conditions such as Korsakoff's psychosis.

confidentiality The ethical responsibility of a health care professional that prohibits the disclosure of privileged information without the patient's informed consent.

conflict A disagreement between two or more people or groups.

conscious   Denoting experiences that are within a person's awareness.

consensual validation   The reality checking of thoughts, feelings, and actions with others. If a child grows up in an environment in which the chance to validate thoughts, feelings, and behaviors is decreased, the child's ability to perceive reality is greatly impaired.

consultant   An expert who gives advice.

contract   A written or stated agreement between patient and caregiver that contains the place, time, date, and duration of meetings.

controlled style of coping   A coping style characterized by a high degree of objectivity and intellectualization which tends toward focusing on understanding what is happening.

conventional antipsychotics   The original classification of antipsychotic medications, also known as *typical antipsychotics* and *first-generation antipsychotics*, which work by D_2 receptor antagonism. They are accompanied by a variety of side effects, including extrapyramidal symptoms. Effective in the treatment of positive symptoms (e.g., delusions, hallucinations, disorganized thought) but not negative symptoms (e.g., depression, avolition, anhedonia).

conventional health care system   Also known as *allopathic, mainstream,* or *orthodox* medicine; *regular medicine; and biomedicine;* based largely on highly controlled, evidence-based scientific research.

conversion   An unconscious defense mechanism in which anxiety is expressed as a physical symptom that has no organic cause.

conversion disorder   A somatoform disorder characterized by the presence of deficits in voluntary motor or sensory functions, including blindness, paralysis, movement disorder, gait disorder, numbness, paresthesia, loss of vision or hearing, or episodes resembling epilepsy.

co-occuring disorders   Disorders that occur at the same time as the psychiatric disorder and may be associated with the disorder.

coping mechanism   A way of adjusting to environmental stress without altering one's goals or purposes. A coping mechanism may be either conscious or unconscious.

coping skills   Skills that enable a patient to develop healthier ways of looking at and dealing with illness.

coping styles   Discrete personal attributes that people have and can develop to help manage stress.

copycat suicide   A suicide that follows a highly publicized suicide of a public figure, idol, or peer in the community.

correctional nursing   Nursing that occurs in correctional facilities and is defined by the location of the work or the legal status of the patient, rather than by the role functions performed.

cotherapist   A therapist who shares responsibility for therapeutic work, usually work done with groups or with families.

countertransference   The tendency of the nurse (therapist, social worker) to displace onto the patient feelings that are a response to people in the nurse's past. Strong positive or strong negative reactions to a patient may indicate countertransference.

criminal profiler   A person who attempts to provide law enforcement officials with specific information about the type of individual who may have committed a certain crime.

crisis   A temporary state of disequilibrium (high anxiety) in which a person's usual coping mechanisms or problem-solving methods fail. Crisis can result in personality growth or disorganization.

crisis intervention   A brief, active, and collaborative therapy that draws on an individual's personal coping abilities and resources within the family, health care setting, or community.

critical incident stress debriefing (CISD)   A seven-phase group meeting that offers individuals who have experienced a crisis the opportunity to share their thoughts and feelings in a safe and controlled environment.

cultural competence   The nurse's act of adjusting his or her practices to meet the patient's cultural beliefs, practices, needs, and preferences.

cultural filters   Filters through which each of us interprets ourselves, others, and the world around us.

culture   The total lifestyle of a given people, the social legacy the individual acquires from his or her group, or the environment that is the creation of humankind.

culture-bound syndromes   Sets of signs and symptoms common in a limited number of cultures but virtually nonexistent in most other cultural groups.

cunnilingus   Oral sexual contact with the female sex organs.

cyclothymia   A chronic mood disturbance (of a least 2 years' duration) involving both hypomanic and dysthymic mood swings. Delusions are never present, and these mood swings usually do not warrant hospitalization or grossly impair a person's social, occupational, or interpersonal functioning.

D

decode   Interpret the meaning of autistic communications, such as those characterized by looseness of associations.

decompensation   Deterioration of mental health and loss of control due to inability to compensate for mental illness due to stress.

de-escalation techniques   Intentional techniques used for reduction of the intensity of a conflict.

defense mechanisms   Unconscious intrapsychic processes used to ward off anxiety by preventing conscious awareness of threatening feelings. Defense mechanisms can be used in a healthy or a not-so-healthy manner. Examples are repression, projection, sublimation, denial, and regression.

deinstitutionalization   Shifting of psychiatric patients from state hospitals to the community.

delayed grief A dysfunctional reaction to grief in which a person may not experience the pain of loss; however, the pain is manifested as chronic depression, intense preoccupation with body functioning (hypochondriasis), phobic reactions, or acute insomnia.

delirium An acute, usually reversible alteration in consciousness typically accompanied by disturbances in thinking, memory, attention, and perception; the syndrome has multiple causes.

delirium tremens (DTs) See *alcohol withdrawal delirium.*

delusion A false belief held to be true even with evidence to the contrary (e.g., the false belief that one is being singled out for harm by others).

dementia A progressive and usually irreversible deterioration of cognitive and intellectual functions and memory without impairment in consciousness.

dendrite The part of the neuron that conveys electrical impulses toward the cell body.

denial Escaping unpleasant realities by ignoring their existence.

dependent personality disorder A personality disorder in which a person has a pattern of establishing relationships in which he or she is submissive, passive, self-doubting, and avoidant of responsibility.

depersonalization A phenomenon whereby a person experiences a sense of unreality of or estrangement from the self. For example, one may feel that limbs or extremities have changed, that one is seeing self and events from a distance, or that one is in a dream.

depersonalization disorder A dissociative disorder in which there is a persistent or recurrent alteration in the perception of the self while reality testing remains intact.

depressive mood syndrome A depressed mood or loss of interest that lasts at least 2 weeks and is accompanied by symptoms such as weight loss and difficulty concentrating.

derealization The false perception by a person that his or her environment has changed. For example, everything seems bigger or smaller, or familiar objects appear strange and unfamiliar.

desensitization The reduction of intense reactions to a stimulus (as in a phobia) by repeated exposure to the stimulus in a weaker or milder form.

detachment An interpersonal and intrapersonal dissociation from affective expression. Therefore, the individual appears cold, aloof, and distant. This behavior is thought to be learned and is viewed as defensive.

***Diagnostic and Statistical Manual of Mental Disorders*, 4th edition, text revision (*DSM-IV-TR*)** A classification of mental disorders that includes descriptions of diagnostic categories. The *DSM-IV-TR* is the most widely accepted system of classifying abnormal behaviors used in the United States today.

diathesis-stress model A general theory that explains psychopathology using a multi-causational systems approach.

diffuse or enmeshed boundaries A blending together of roles, thoughts, and feelings of individuals so that clear distinctions among family members (or others) fail to emerge.

disenfranchised grief Grief that cannot be publicly acknowledged because the loss is not congruent with a socially recognized and sanctioned relationship.

disorientation Confusion and impaired ability to identify time, place, and person.

displacement Transfer of emotions associated with a particular person, object, or situation to another person, object, or situation that is nonthreatening.

dissociation An unconscious defense mechanism that allows blocking of overwhelming anxiety stemming from disintegration of functions of consciousness, memory, identity, or perception of environment.

dissociative amnesia A dissociative disorder marked by the inability to recall important personal information, often of a traumatic or stressful nature.

dissociative disorders Disorders reflecting a disturbance in the normally well-integrated continuum of consciousness, memory, identity, and perception.

dissociative fugue A dissociative disorder characterized by sudden, unexpected travel away from the customary locale and inability to recall one's identity and information about some or all of the past.

dissociative identity disorder (DID) A dissociative disorder in which two or more distinct personality states recurrently take control of behavior.

distractibility Inability to maintain attention; tendency to shift from one area or topic to another with minimal provocation.

distress A negative, draining energy that results in anxiety, depression, confusion, helplessness, hopelessness, and fatigue.

double messages Conflicting messages (also known as *mixed messages*).

double-bind messages Communication that contains two contradictory messages given by the same person at the same time, to which the receiver is expected to respond. Constant double-bind situations result in feelings of helplessness, fear, and anxiety in the recipient of such messages.

drug abuse Defined by the American Psychiatric Association as the maladaptive and consistent use of a drug despite the presence of social, occupational, psychological, or physical problems exacerbated by such drug use; or recurrent use in situations that are physically hazardous, such as driving while intoxicated.

drug dependence Impaired control of drug use despite adverse consequences, the development of tolerance to the drug, and the occurrence of withdrawal symptoms when drug intake is reduced or stopped.

drug interaction The reciprocal action between two or more drugs taken simultaneously, which produces an effect different from the usual effects of either drug taken alone. The interacting drugs may be potentiating or inhibitory, and serious side effects may result.

drug tolerance   A need for higher and higher dosages of a drug to achieve intoxication or the desired effect.

dual diagnosis   The coexistence of a psychiatric disease with substance abuse. A person with a dual diagnosis is chronically dependent on a drug or alcohol and also has another psychiatric disorder such as a depressive or personality disorder.

duty to protect   Ethical and legal obligations of health care workers to protect patients from physically harming themselves or others.

duty to warn   An obligation that may result in the breach of confidentiality on the part of the health care worker to warn third parties when they may be in danger from a patient.

dyskinesia   Involuntary muscular activity, such as tic, spasm, or myoclonus.

dyspareunia   Persistent genital pain in either a male or a female before, during, or after sex.

dyssomnias   Sleep disturbances associated with the initiation and maintenance of sleep or of excessive sleepiness.

dysthymic disorder (DD)   A mild to moderate mood disturbance characterized by a chronic depressive syndrome that is usually present for many years. The depressive mood disturbance is hard to distinguish from the person's usual pattern of functioning, and the person has minimal social or occupational impairment.

dystonia   Abnormal muscle tonicity resulting in impaired voluntary movement. May occur as an acute side effect of neuroleptic (antipsychotic) medication, in which it manifests as muscle spasms of the face, head, neck, and back.

E

echolalia   Repeating of the last words spoken by another; mimicry or imitation of the speech of another person.

echopraxia   Mimicry or imitation of the movements of another person.

economic abuse   The withholding of financial support or the illegal or improper exploitation of funds or other resources for one's personal gain.

ego   One of three psychological processes that make up the Freudian system of personality (id, ego, superego). The ego is one's sense of self and provides such functions as problem solving, mobilization of defense mechanisms, reality testing, and the capability of functioning independently. The ego is said to be the mediator between one's primitive drives (the id) and internalized parental and social prohibitions (the superego).

ego boundaries   The individual's perception of the boundaries between himself or herself and the external environment.

ego-alien/ego-dystonic   Synonymous terms used to describe symptoms that are unacceptable to the person who has them and are incompatible with the person's view of himself or herself (e.g., fear of cats).

ego-syntonic   A term used to describe symptomatic behaviors or beliefs that do not seem to bother the person or that seem right to the person. For example, a very paranoid person who wrongly believes that the government is out to get him or her truly believes this thought, and it is consistent with the way this person experiences life.

egocentric   Self-centered.

electroconvulsive therapy (ECT)   An effective treatment for depression in which a grand mal seizure is induced by passing an electrical current through electrodes that are applied to the temples. The administration of a muscle relaxant minimizes seizure activity and prevents damage to long bones and cervical vertebrae.

electronic health care   The provision of health care through methods which are not face-to-face but rather through an electronic medium.

elopement   Escape or leaving a psychiatric treatment facility without medical authorization or recommendation.

emotional abuse   Depriving an individual of a nurturing atmosphere in which he or she can thrive, learn, and develop. Emotional abuse takes many forms (e.g., terrorizing, demeaning, consistently belittling, withholding warmth).

empathy   The ability of one person to get inside another's world and see things from the other person's perspective and to communicate this understanding to the other person.

enabling   Helping a chemically dependent individual avoid experiencing the consequences of his or her drinking or drug use. It is one behavioral component of a codependency role.

enculturation   The process in which a culture's worldview, beliefs, values, and practices are transmitted to its members.

endorphins   Naturally produced chemicals (peptides) with morphinelike action. They are usually found in the brain and are associated with reduction of pain and feelings of well-being.

enmeshed boundaries   See *blurred or diffuse boundaries.*

enuresis   Nocturnal and/or daytime involuntary discharge of urine.

epidemiology   The quantitative study of the distribution of mental disorders in human populations.

epinephrine (adrenaline)   A catecholamine secreted by the adrenal gland and by fibers of the sympathetic nervous system. It is responsible for many of the physical manifestations of fear and anxiety.

ethical dilemma   A situation in which there is a conflict between two or more courses of action, each carrying favorable and unfavorable consequences.

ethics   The discipline concerned with standards of values, behaviors, or beliefs adhered to by individuals or groups.

ethnicity   The common heritage and history shared by a specific ethnic group.

ethnocentrism   The universal tendency of humans to think their way of thinking and behaving is the only correct and natural way.

ethnopharmacology A relatively new field of medicine that investigates the genetic and ethnic variations in drug pharmacokinetics.

eustress A positive type of stress that reflects a person's confidence in the ability to successfully master given demands or tasks.

euthymia A normal, moderate mood state, neither depressed or manic.

evidence-based practice A method of care that integrates the latest and best available research.

excessive sleepiness (ES) A subjective report of difficulty staying awake that is serious enough to impact social and vocational functioning and increase the risk for accident or injury.

exhibitionism An illegal activity that involves the intentional display of the genitals in a public place.

expert witness A witness recognized by the court as having a certain level of skill or expertise in a designated area and possesses superior knowledge because of education or specialized experience.

expressed style of coping Overt behaviors such as crying, withdrawing, smoking, abusing alcohol and drugs, wanting to talk, acting confused or disoriented, and even laughing and joking as a way of getting through difficult times.

extinction In operant conditioning, extinction occurs when reinforcement no longer results in a given behavior or response; in classical conditioning, extinction occurs when the stimulus no longer produces a response.

extrapyramidal side effects (EPSs) A variety of signs and symptoms that are often side effects of the use of certain psychotropic drugs, particularly the phenothiazines. Three reversible extrapyramidal side effects are acute dystonia, akathisia, and pseudoparkinsonism. A fourth, tardive dyskinesia, is the most serious and is not reversible.

F

fact witness A witness who testifies in court regarding what was *personally* seen, heard, performed, or documented regarding a patient's care and testifies first-hand experience only.

factitious disorders Psychiatric disorders in which people consciously pretend to be ill to get emotional needs met and attain the status of "patient."

factitious disorder by proxy Also known as *Munchausen syndrome by proxy*, a factitious disorder in which a caregiver deliberately feigns illness in a vulnerable dependent, usually a child, for the purpose of the attention, excitement, and treatment by health care providers of that dependent.

false imprisonment May be a misdemeanor or tort brought against health care workers who illegally hold people in confinement. Confinement includes restraint within a limited area and restraint within an institution.

family system Those individuals who make up the family unit and contribute to the functional state of the family as a unit.

family systems theory A theory of human behavior that views the family as an emotionally connected unit and describes their interactions through a systems perspective.

family therapy A treatment modality that focuses on the relationships within the family system.

family triangle A dysfunctional phenomenon in which a third person is brought into a two-person relationship to help relieve anxiety or stress between two family members. Triangles are dysfunctional because the lowering of anxiety comes from diversion from the conflict rather than from resolution of the conflict between the two members.

family violence The intentional intimidation, abuse, or neglect of children, adults, or elders by a family member, intimate partner, or caretaker in order to gain power and control over the victim.

fantasy Mental imagery that is unrestrained by reality and represents an attempt to solve problems in a private world. One difference between a healthy person and a schizophrenic, for example, is that a schizophrenic may not know where fantasy ends and reality begins.

fear A reaction to a specific danger.

feedback Communication of one person's impressions of and reactions to another person's actions or verbalizations.

fellatio Oral sexual contact with the penis.

fetish An object or part of the body to which sexual significance or meaning is attached.

fetishism A sexual disorder characterized by a sexual focus on objects that are intimately associated with the human body.

fight-or-flight response The body's physiological response to fear or rage that triggers the sympathetic branch of the autonomic nervous system as well as the endocrine system. This response is useful in emergencies; however, a sustained response can result in pathophysiological changes such as high blood pressure, ulcers, and cardiac problems.

flashbacks Transitory recurrences of perceptual disturbance caused by a person's earlier hallucinogenic drug use when he or she is in a drug-free state.

flight of ideas A continuous flow of speech in which the person jumps rapidly from one topic to another. Sometimes the listener can keep up with the changes; at other times, it is necessary to listen for themes in the incessant talking. Themes often include grandiose and fantasized evaluation of personal sexual prowess, business ability, artistic talents, and so forth.

forensic nurse examiner A forensic psychiatric nurse who conducts court-ordered evaluations regarding legal sanity or competency to proceed, responds to specific medicolegal questions as requested by the court, and renders an expert opinion in a written report or courtroom testimony.

forensic nurse generalist A nurse with a baccalaureate or associate degree or diploma who has acquired additional knowledge and skills by completing a certificate program in forensic nursing.

forensic nursing The application of nursing science and care to public or legal proceedings or the application of forensic aspects of health care combined with the biopsychosocial education of the registered nurse.

forensic psychiatric nurse A psychiatric nurse prepared at the generalist or advanced practice level who cares for patients and/or victims involved with the forensic system.

formication A tactile hallucination or illusion involving the sensation of insects crawling on the body or under the skin.

Four Gifts of Resolving Relationships A means of opening conversations about a coming separation; the four gifts include forgiveness, love, gratitude, and farewell.

frotteurism A sexual disorder characterized by rubbing or touching a nonconsenting person.

frustration The curtailment of personal goals, satisfaction, or security by conditions of external reality or by internal controls.

fugue An altered state of consciousness involving both memory loss (as in psychogenic amnesia) and travel away from home or from one's usual work locale; that is, fugue involves flight as well as forgetfulness. Often called *psychogenic* or *dissociative fugue.*

G

gamma-aminobutyric acid (GABA) The major inhibitory neurotransmitter in the central nervous system; targeted by drugs that reduce anxiety.

gender dysphoria A person's feelings of unease about his maleness or her femaleness.

gender identity The sense of maleness or femaleness.

gender identity disorder A sexual disorder defined as a strong and persistent cross-gender identification.

general adaptation syndrome (GAS) The body's organized response to stress, as elucidated by Hans Selye. It progresses through three stages: (1) the stage of alarm, (2) the stage of resistance, and (3) the stage of exhaustion.

generalized anxiety disorder (GAD) Anxiety disorder characterized by excessive anxiety or worry about numerous things, lasting for 6 months or longer.

genogram A systematic diagram of the three-generational relationships within a family system.

genuineness Self-awareness of one's feelings as they arise within the nurse-patient relationship and the ability to communicate them when appropriate.

grandiosity Exaggerated belief in or claims about one's importance or identity.

grief The subjective feelings and affect that are precipitated by a loss.

group Two or more individuals who have a relationship with one another, are interdependent, and may share some norms.

group content All that is said in a group.

group dynamics The interactions and interrelations among members of a therapy group and between members and the therapist. The effective use of group dynamics is essential in group treatment.

group norms Expectations for behavior in the group that develop over time and provide structure for members.

group process The interaction continually taking place among members of a group.

group psychotherapy Psychotherapy based on the examination of group interaction with a view toward understanding and eventually changing the ways in which patients interact with others.

group themes Members' expressed ideas or feelings that recur and have a common thread.

group work A method whereby individuals with common purpose come together and benefit by both giving and receiving feedback within the dynamic and unique context of group life.

guided imagery A process whereby a person is led to envision images that are both calming and health enhancing.

H

hallucination A sense perception (seeing, hearing, tasting, smelling, or touching) for which no external stimulus exists (e.g., hearing voices when none are present).

healing touch A derivative of therapeutic touch that combines several energy therapies and is based on the belief that the body is a complex energy system that can be influenced by another through that person's intention for healing and well-being.

Health Insurance Portability and Accountability Act (HIPAA) A bill enacted in 1996 that established national standards for the protection of electronic medical records.

health maintenance organization (HMO) An organization that contracts with a group or individuals to offer designated health care services to plan members for a fixed, prepaid premium (an example of a managed care program).

health teaching Identification of the health education needs of the patient and teaching of basic physical and mental health principles.

herbal therapy The use of plants or plant products to improve health, prevent illness, and/or treat illness.

histrionic personality disorder A personality disorder in which there is a dramatic presentation of oneself with pervasive and excessive emotionality in order to seek attention, love, and admiration.

holism Involves (1) the identification of the interrelationships of the bio-psycho-social-spiritual dimensions of the person, recognizing that the whole is greater than the sum of its parts and (2) understanding of the individual as a unitary whole in mutual process with the environment.

homelessness—chronic Long-term lack of a home or permanent residence. It represents the final stage in a lifelong series of crises and missed opportunities and is the culmination of a gradual disengagement from supportive relationships and institutions.

homeopathy A Western alternative medical system in which small doses (dilutions) of specially prepared plant extracts, herbs, minerals, and other materials are used to stimulate the body's defense mechanisms and healing processes.

homosexuality Sexual attraction to or preference for persons of the same sex.

hopelessness The belief of a person that no one can help him or her; extreme pessimism about the future.

hospice Physician services, nursing visits, medical equipment, medications, some supplies related to the terminal illness, social work, counseling services, spiritual care, volunteer services, bereavement services, and physical, dietary, speech, and occupational therapy offered to patients with terminal illnesses and their families as support at the end of life.

hospice philosophy A philosophy characterized by the acceptance of death as a natural conclusion to life and the belief that patients rather than health care providers should make the end-of-life decisions about how they want to live and die.

hostage negotiator A consultant who addresses the mental state of the perpetrator and recommends appropriate negotiation strategies.

hostility Anger that is destructive in nature and purpose.

hotline A telephone crisis counseling service often used in crisis intervention centers to provide immediate contact between a person in crisis and a counselor.

human rights abuses Those actions that violate the basic rights of human beings.

hypermetamorphosis The desire to touch everything in sight.

hyperorality The desire to taste everything, chew everything, and put everything into one's mouth.

hypersomnia The spending of increased time in sleep, possibly to escape from painful feelings; however, the increased sleep is not experienced as restful or refreshing.

hypervigilance A state of extraordinary alertness.

hypnotic A classification of drugs used to promote sleep.

hypoactive sexual desire A sexual desire disorder characterized by a deficiency or absence of sexual fantasies or desire for sexual activity.

hypochondriasis Excessive preoccupation with one's physical health in the absence of any organic pathology.

hypomania An elevated mood with symptoms less severe than those of mania. A person in hypomania does not experience impairment in reality testing, nor do the symptoms markedly impair the person's social, occupational, or interpersonal functions.

hysterical personality disorder A disorder characterized by dramatic, emotionally intense, unstable behavior.

I

id One of three psychological processes that make up the Freudian system of personality (id, ego, and superego). The id is the source of all primitive drives and instincts and is considered to be the reservoir of all psychic energy.

idea of reference The false impression that outside events have special meaning for oneself.

identification Unconscious assumption of the thoughts, mannerisms, or behaviors of a person or group in order to decrease anxiety.

identity Sense of self based on experience, memories, perceptions, and emotions.

illusion An error in the perception of a sensory stimulus. For example, a person may mistake polka dots on a pillow for hairy spiders.

implied consent A form of consent that is not expressly given but implied from circumstances of a person's particular situation or a person's actions, especially in life-threatening or serious situations.

impotence The inability to achieve or maintain a penile erection of sufficient quality to engage in successful sexual intercourse.

impulsiveness The tendency to engage in actions that are abrupt, unplanned, and directed toward immediate gratification.

incest A sexual relationship between persons who are close biological relatives.

incidence Refers to the number of new cases of mental disorders in a healthy population within a given period of time.

indigenous culture The people and culture that have inhabited a country for thousands of years (e.g., Maoris of New Zealand, Australian aborigines, native Hawaiians, and natives of North and South America).

informal admission One type of voluntary admission in which there is no formal or written application.

informed consent A legal term that indicates that a person has been provided with a basic understanding of risks, benefits, and alternatives and is receiving treatment voluntarily.

insight Understanding and awareness of the reasons for and meaning behind one's motives and behavior.

insight-oriented family therapy A traditional therapeutic modality that emphasizes understanding the origins of problems in order to address them.

insomnia Inability to fall asleep or to stay asleep, early morning awakening, or both.

institutionalization The provision of psychiatric care in a custodial setting, typically viewed as a restrictive environment. When overused or used inappropriately, institutionalization can result in apathy, dependency, and stagnation and impede a person's ability to function normally outside the institution.

integrative care   Care that places the patient at the center of care, focuses on prevention and wellness, and attends to the patient's physical, mental, and spiritual needs.

intellectualization   The excessive use of reasoning, logic, or words to avoid confronting undesirable impulses, emotions, and interpersonal situations.

interpersonal psychotherapy   A therapeutic modality that emphasizes what goes on between people. The basis of the therapy is on building interpersonal skills and correcting faulty processes of interacting.

intentional torts   Willful and intentional acts that violate another person's rights or property.

intimacy   Emotional closeness.

intoxication   Maladaptive behavioral or psychological changes caused by excessive use of a drug or alcohol.

intrapsychic   Internal psychological processes.

introjection   The process by which a person incorporates or takes into his or her own personality qualities or values of another person or group with whom intense emotional ties exist.

intuition   Knowledge or insight gained without conscious rational thinking.

isolation   The separation of thought, ideas, or actions from their emotional aspects.

involuntary admission   Admission to a psychiatric facility without the patient's consent.

involuntary outpatient admission   Court mandates for medication and other treatments as a condition for remaining in the community rather than in the hospital. These mandates are controversial and not used in all communities in the United States.

J

journaling   Keeping a diary which may be informal or part of a treatment plan of daily events, activities, and feelings.

judgment   The ability to make logical, rational decisions.

L

la belle indifférence   An affect or attitude of inappropriate unconcern about a symptom that is seen when the symptom is unconsciously used to lower anxiety.

labile   Characterized by rapid shifts in mood which may be as dramatic as laughing one minute and crying the next; unstable.

late-life mental illness   Psychiatric disorders not discovered earlier in life but evident in older years.

least restrictive alternative doctrine   Mandates that the least restrictive and least disruptive means be used to achieve a specific purpose.

legal sanity   An individual's ability to distinguish right from wrong with reference to the act charged, capacity to understand the nature and quality of the act charged, and capacity to form the intent to commit the crime.

lesbian   A homosexual who is female.

lethality   The relative deadliness of a chosen suicide method. For example, a shotgun has a high degree of lethality.

libido   Sexual desire, drive, and pleasure.

light therapy   A first-line treatment of seasonal affective disorder (SAD) in which the patient is exposed to 30 to 45 minutes of exposure daily to a 10,000-lux light source.

limbic system   The part of the brain that is related to emotions and is referred to by some as the "emotional brain." It is involved in the mediation of fear and anxiety; anger and aggression; love, joy, and hope; and sexuality and social behavior.

limit setting   The reasonable and rational setting of parameters for patient behavior that provide control and safety.

lithium carbonate   Known as an antimanic drug because it can stabilize the manic phase of a bipolar disorder. When effective, it can modify future manic episodes and protect against future depressive episodes.

living will   An expression by a person, while competent, of his or her preference that life-sustaining treatment be continued, withheld, or withdrawn if he or she becomes terminally ill and is no longer able to make health care decisions.

long-term involuntary admission   Used for extended care and treatment of those with mental illness. Commitments are obtained through medical certification, judicial hearings, or administrative action.

looseness of association   A pattern of thinking that is haphazard, illogical, and confused and in which connections in thought are interrupted; it is seen primarily in schizophrenic disorders.

M

magical thinking   The belief that simply thinking something can make it happen; it is seen in children and psychotic patients.

major depressive disorder (MDD)   A mood disorder in which the patient presents with a history of one or more major depressive episodes and no history of manic or hypomanic episodes.

malingering   A conscious effort to deceive others, often for financial gain, by pretending to have physical symptoms.

malpractice   An act or omission to act that breaches the duty of due care and results in or is responsible for a person's injuries.

managed behavioral health care organizations (MBHOs)   Managed care plans that developed separately from medical services to provide mental health and substance-abuse treatment.

managed care   A term referring to an organized system that integrates cost management and provision of health care. Health maintenance organizations (HMOs), preferred provider organizations (PPOs), and managed care options offered by government and private indemnity health insurance plans are the basic types of managed care organization.

managed care plans Care plans that provide members with a list of health care providers they may visit and then either cover the entire cost or collect co-pays from members.

mania An unstable elevated mood in which delusion, poor judgment, and other signs of impaired reality testing are evident. During a manic episode, patients have marked impairment of social, occupational, and interpersonal functioning.

manipulation Purposeful behavior directed at getting one's needs met, sometimes without regard for the needs, goals, and feelings of others.

masochism The deriving of unconscious or conscious gratification from the experience of mental or physical pain; often used to refer to deviant sexual behaviors.

maturational crisis A normal state in growth and development in which a specific maturational task must be learned, but old coping mechanisms are no longer adequate or acceptable.

meditation A discipline for training the mind to develop greater calm and then using that calm to bring penetrative insight into one's experience.

mental health A state of well-being in which each individual is able to realize his or her own potential, cope with the normal stresses of life, work productively and fruitfully, and make a contribution to the community.

mental health continuum A conceptual line used to represent levels of mental health and mental illness that vary from person to person and vary for a particular person over time.

mental health parity Recognition by health insurance companies that mental illnesses are as debilitating and in need of proper treatment as physical illnesses.

mental illness A clinically significant behavioral or psychological syndrome marked by the patient's distress, disability, or the risk of suffering disability or loss of freedom.

mental status examination A formal assessment of cognitive functions such as intelligence, thought processes, and capacity for insight.

metabolic syndrome Weight gain, dyslipidemia, and altered glucose metabolism caused by atypical antipsychotic drugs.

mild anxiety Occurs in the normal experience of everyday living.

milieu The physical and social environment of an individual.

milieu therapy A general term for any therapeutic setting that focuses on control of the environment (both physical and social) to effect positive change.

mindfulness A centuries-old form of meditation that emphasizes awareness of ourselves and our mental activity from moment to moment.

mnemonic disturbance Loss of memory.

modeling A technique in which desired behaviors are demonstrated. The patient learns to imitate these behaviors in appropriate situations.

moderate anxiety The second level on a four-tiered anxiety continuum, moderate anxiety results in selective inattention and some diminished thinking, although learning and problem solving can still occur. Symptoms include tension, pounding heart, increased pulse and respiration rate, perspiration, gastric discomfort, headache, urinary urgency, voice tremors, and shaking.

monoamine oxidase inhibitors (MAOIs) A classification of antidepressants that inhibit monoamine oxidase, an enzyme that breaks down amines such as serotonin and norepinephrine. The use of an MAOI necessitates the adoption of a tyramine-free diet because of potentially fatal interactions.

mood A pervasive and sustained emotion that, when extreme, can markedly color the way the individual perceives the world.

mood disorders A category of disorders characterized by disturbances of mood that range from elation to depression and interfere with normal functioning.

mood stabilizers Classes of drugs used to treat mood disorders; include lithium and anticonvulsants.

mourning The process by which grief is resolved.

multidisciplinary treatment plan A plan developed with input from a diverse group of health care professionals (e.g., nurses, social workers, psychologists, physicians).

multigenerational issues Various family patterns passed down through the generations.

multiple personality disorder A severe dissociative disorder in which one or more distinct subpersonalities exist within an individual, each of which may be dominant at different times. Each subpersonality is a complex unit with its own memories, behavioral patterns, and social relationships, which may be very different from those of the primary personality.

Munchausen syndrome A psychiatric syndrome in which a person, usually one knowledgeable of medical treatment, purposefully produces symptoms of a disease, illness, or trauma in order to elicit help, care, and treatment from medical personnel.

N

narcissism Self-preoccupation and lack of empathy for others; the narcissistic person is very self-centered, self-involved, and self-important; narcissism is normal in children but pathological when it occurs in adults to the same degree.

narcissistic personality disorder A disorder characterized by a pervasive pattern of grandiosity, need for admiration, and lack of empathy for others.

National Alliance on Mental Illness (NAMI) A national support group for families of the mental ill, with many local and state affiliates; provides educational programs and political action.

naturopathy A Western alternative medical system that emphasizes health restoration rather than disease treatment and combines nutrition, homeopathy, herbal medicine, hydrotherapy, light therapy, therapeutic counseling, and other therapies.

negative reinforcement Increasing the probability of a behavior by removing unpleasant consequences; it is not punishment. This concept is related to positive reinforcement, which rewards or gives in to a specific behavior. A mouse that learns to press a lever to stop a shock has undergone negative reinforcement.

negative symptoms The absence of something that should be present (e.g., apathy, lack of motivation, anhedonia, poor thought processes).

negativism Opposition or resistance, either covert or overt, to outside suggestions or advice.

neglect A form of abuse that involves failure to provide for or attend to basic physical, emotional, educational, or medical needs of another.

negligence An act, or failure to act, that breaches the duty of due care and results in or is responsible for another person's injuries.

neologism A word a person makes up that has meaning only for that person; often part of a delusional system.

neuroleptic malignant syndrome (NMS) A rare and sometimes fatal reaction to high-potency neuroleptic drugs. Symptoms include muscle rigidity, fever, and elevated white blood cell count. It is thought to result from dopamine blockage at the basal ganglia and hypothalamus.

neurons Specialized cells in the central nervous system. Each neuron has a cell body, an axon, and dendrites.

neurotransmitter A chemical substance that functions as a neural messenger. Neurotransmitters are released from the axon terminal of the presynaptic neuron when stimulated by an electrical impulse.

nihilism A delusion that the self or part of the self does not exist.

no-suicide contract A contract made between a nurse or counselor and a patient, outlined in clear and simple language, in which the patient states that he or she will not attempt self-harm and in which specific alternatives are given for the person instead.

nontherapeutic communication Any method of communication that detracts from the therapeutic relationship.

nonverbal communication Communication without words, such as body language, eye contact, facial expressions, or gestures.

nuclear family A family that includes a parent or parents and the children under the parents' care.

nurse coroner/death investigator A nurse who makes expert judgments of the circumstances of death based on observations of history, symptomatology, autopsy results, toxicology, other diagnostic studies, and evidence revealed in other areas of the case.

nursing The diagnosis and treatment of human responses to actual or potential health problems.

Nursing Interventions Classification (NIC) A listing of research-based nursing intervention labels that provide standardization of expected nursing interventions.

Nursing Outcomes Classification (NOC) A classification system which defines and describes patient outcomes to nursing interventions.

O

obesity A condition characterized by a body weight that is at least 20% higher than the acceptable standard or ideal weight.

obsession An idea, impulse, or emotion that cannot be put out of consciousness; the condition can be mild or severe.

obsessive-compulsive personality disorder A personality disorder in which the key characteristic is perfectionism with a focus on orderliness and control.

Omnibus Budget Reconciliation Act (OBRA) The 1990 act that declared that nursing home residents have the right to be free from unnecessary drugs and physical restraints.

open-ended questions Questions that encourage lengthy responses and information about experiences, perceptions, or responses to a situation and cannot be answered by a simple "yes" or "no" response.

operant conditioning A type of behavior modification in which voluntary behaviors are increased or decreased through reinforcement or punishment.

oppositional defiant disorder A psychiatric disorder characterized by a recurrent pattern of negativistic, disobedient, hostile, defiant behavior toward authority figures, without going so far as to seriously violate the basic rights of others.

organic mental disorder A specific brain syndrome for which a cause is known; for example, alcohol withdrawal delirium or Alzheimer's disease.

orientation The ability to identify the correct time, place, and person.

orientation phase The phase of the nurse-patient relationship in which the nurse and patient meet, and the nurse conducts the initial interview.

outcome criteria Hoped-for outcomes that reflect the maximal level of patient health that can realistically be achieved through nursing interventions.

outpatient commitment Provides mandatory treatment in a less restrictive setting.

overt anxiety Anxiety in which the attendant physical, physiological, and cognitive symptoms are evident and may be assessed.

P

pain disorder   A somatoform disorder in which testing rules out any organic cause of the patient's pain; the pain leads to significant impairment.

palliative care   See *hospice*.

panic   Sudden, overwhelming anxiety of such intensity that it produces disorganization of the personality, loss of rational thought, and inability to communicate, along with specific physiological changes.

panic disorder (PD)   An anxiety disorder in which panic attacks are the key feature.

paranoia   A state characterized by the presence of intense and strongly defended irrational suspicions. These ideas cannot be corrected by experience and cannot be modified by facts or reality.

paranoid personality disorder   A personality disorder in which the key characteristics are distrust and suspiciousness toward others based on the belief (unsupported by evidence) that others want to exploit, harm, or deceive.

paraphilias   Also known as *sexual impulse disorders*, these sexual disorders are characterized by acts or sexual stimuli that are outside of what society considers normal but necessary for some individuals to experience desire, arousal, and orgasm.

parasomnias   Sleep disorders characterized by unusual or undesirable behaviors or events that occur during sleep/wake transitions, certain stages of sleep, or during arousal from sleep.

parasuicide   Self-injury with clear intent to cause bodily harm or death.

passive-aggressive behavior   Behavior that represents an indirect expression of anger or aggressive feelings. Behavior may seem passive but is motivated by unconscious anger and often triggers anger and frustration in others. Examples of passive-aggressive behavior are being late, forgetting, making "mistakes," and acting obtuse.

Patient Self-Determination Act (PSDA)   The 1990 act that requires health care facilities to provide clear written information for every patient regarding his or her legal right to make health care decisions, including the right to accept or refuse treatment.

pedophilia   A sexual disorder that involves sexual activity with a prepubescent child.

peer review   Review of clinical practice with peers, supervisors, or consultants.

perception   The mental process by which intellectual, sensory, and emotional data are organized logically or meaningfully.

perpetrators   Those who initiate violence.

perseveration   The involuntary repetition of the same thought, phrase, or motor response (e.g., brushing teeth, walking); it is associated with brain damage.

personality   Deeply ingrained personal patterns of behavior, traits, and thoughts that evolve, both consciously and unconsciously, as a person's style and way of adapting to the environment.

personality disorder   An enduring pattern of experience and behavior that deviates significantly from the expectations within the individual's culture.

pervasive developmental disorder (PDD)   A psychiatric disorder characterized by severe and pervasive impairment in reciprocal social interaction and communication skills, usually accompanied by stereotypical behavior, interests, and activities.

pharmacodynamics   The physiological actions and effects of drugs in the body; this includes receptor binding, postreceptor effects, and chemical interactions.

pharmacokinetics   The physiological actions, effects, and responses of the body to drugs; this includes absorption, distribution, excretion, onset of action, duration of effect, and the influence of substances such as enzymes.

phenomena of concern   The central interests of a particular discipline. In nursing they are commonly considered to be person, health, environment, and nursing.

phobia   An intense irrational fear of an object, situation, or place. The fear persists even though the object of the fear is harmless and the person is aware of the irrationality.

physical abuse   The infliction of physical pain or bodily harm.

physical restraint   Any manual method or mechanical device, material, or equipment that inhibits free movement.

physical stressors   Environmental and physical conditions that elicit the stress response.

play therapy   An intervention that allows a child to symbolically express feelings such as aggression, self-doubt, anxiety, and sadness through the medium of play.

pleasure principle   A tendency to seek immediate gratification of impulses and tension reduction; the id operates according to the pleasure principle.

polydrug abuse   The pathological use of more than one drug.

polypharmacy   The taking of more than one drug at any given time.

positive reinforcement   The presentation of a reward immediately following a behavior, making the behavior more likely to occur in the future.

positive symptoms   The presence of something that is not normally present (e.g., hallucinations, delusions, bizarre behavior, paranoia).

posttraumatic stress disorder (PTSD)   An anxiety disorder characterized by persistent reexperiencing of a highly traumatic event that involved actual or threatened death or serious injury to self or others, to which the individual responded with intense fear, helplessness, or horror.

postvention   Therapeutic interventions with the significant others of an individual who has committed suicide.

poverty of speech   A speech pattern characterized by brevity and uncommunicativeness.

preconscious Unconscious thoughts (including memory) that are available for retrieval to the conscious at any time.

premature ejaculation A sexual dysfunction in which a man persistently or recurrently achieves orgasm and ejaculation before he wishes to.

pressure of speech A speech pattern characterized by forceful energy manifested in frantic, jumbled speech, as when an individual with mania struggles to keep pace with racing thoughts.

prevalence Refers to the total number of cases of a disease within a population at a given time.

primary anxiety Anxiety that is due to intrapersonal or intrapsychic causes, such as a phobia.

primary care Care that promotes mental health and reduces mental illness to decrease the incidence of crisis.

primary dementia Dementia that is irreversible, progressive, and not secondary to any other disorder.

primary depression A depressive mood episode that is not due to known organic factors and is not part of another psychotic disorder such as schizophrenia.

primary gain The anxiety relief resulting from the use of defense mechanisms or symptom formation such as somatization (e.g., getting a headache instead of feeling angry).

primary intervention Intervention that includes activities to provide support, information, and education to prevent suicide.

primary prevention Activities that provide support, information, and education, with the goal of prevention.

primary process In psychoanalytic theory, a primitive and unconscious psychological activity in which the id attempts to reduce tension by forming an image of or hallucinating the object that would satisfy its need.

progressive muscle relaxation (PMR) A method of decreasing anxiety in which the individual tenses groups of muscles as tightly as possible for 8 seconds and then suddenly releases them.

projection The unconscious attributing of one's own intolerable wishes, emotions, or motivations to another person.

projective identification A primitive form of projection used to externalize aggressive feelings. Once projection has occurred, fear of the person who is the object of the projection is coupled with a desire to control the person.

prolonged grief A dysfunctional grief reaction in which the bereaved remains intensely preoccupied with memories of the deceased many years after the person has died.

pseudodementia A disorder that mimics dementia.

pseudoparkinsonism A medication-induced temporary constellation of symptoms associated with Parkinson's disease: tremor, reduced accessory movements, impaired gait, and stiffening of muscles.

psychiatric case management A program that coordinates services for individual patient care.

psychiatric liaison nurse A nurse with a master's degree and a background in psychiatric and medical-surgical nursing. The liaison nurse functions as a nursing consultant in addressing psychosocial concerns and as a clinician in helping the patient deal more effectively with physical and emotional problems.

psychiatric mental health nursing This specialty area in nursing and core mental health profession promotes mental health through the nursing process in the treatment of mental health problems and psychiatric disorders.

psychiatry The science of treating disorders of the psyche. It is the medical specialty involved in the study, diagnosis, treatment, and prevention of mental disorders.

psychiatry's definition of mental health A definition of mental health that evolves over time and is shaped by the prevailing culture and societal values. It reflects changes in cultural norms, society's expectations, political climates, and even reimbursement criteria by third-party payers.

psychodynamic therapy A therapeutic modality based on classical psychoanalysis, but with less focus on the early development of pathology. It uses free association, dream analysis, transference, and countertransference. The therapist is actively involved and interacts with the client in the here and now.

psychoeducation A strategy of teaching patients and their families about disorders, treatments, coping techniques, and resources. Helps empower patients and families by having them become more involved and prepares them to participate in their own care once they have the requisite knowledge.

psychoeducational group A group set up to increase knowledge or skills about a specific somatic or psychological subject and allow members to communicate emotional concerns.

psychogenic Denoting a physical condition caused by psychological factors.

psychogenic amnesia The loss of memory for an event or period of time that is associated with overwhelming anxiety and pain. The loss of memory is related to psychological stress.

psychological autopsy Retrospective review of the deceased person's life within several months of the death to establish likely diagnoses at the time of death.

psychomotor agitation Constant involvement in some tension-relieving activity, such as constantly pacing, biting one's nails, smoking, or tapping one's fingers on a tabletop.

psychomotor retardation Extreme slowness of and difficulty in movements that in the extreme can entail complete inactivity and incontinence.

psychoneuroimmunology Study of the links among stress, the immune system, and disease.

psychosexual development Emotional and sexual growth from birth to adulthood.

psychosis An extreme response to psychological or physical stressors that leads to pronounced distortion or disorganization of affective response, psychomotor function, and behavior. Reality testing is impaired, as evidenced by hallucinations or delusions.

psychosocial rehabilitation The development of the skills necessary for a person with chronic mental illness to live independently.

psychosomatic An older term describing the interaction of the mind (*psyche*) and the body (*soma*).

psychotherapy A treatment modality based on the development of a trusting relationship between the patient and therapist for the purpose of exploring and modifying the patient's behavior in a positive direction.

psychotropic drugs Drugs that have an effect on psychic function, behavior, or experience.

Q

quality of life The degree of enjoyment or satisfaction a person experiences with normal life activities.

R

race A group of humans within the population that share common heritable characteristics such as color of skin, eyes, and hair.

racism A belief that inherent differences between races determine people's achievement and that one's own race is superior.

rape See *sexual assault/rape.*

rape-trauma syndrome A syndrome characterized by an acute phase and a long-term reorganization process that occurs after an actual or attempted sexual assault. Each phase has separate symptoms.

rapid cycling Experiencing four or more mood episodes in a 12-month period.

rapport A relationship characterized by trust, support, and understanding.

rationalization Justification of illogical or unreasonable ideas, actions, or feelings by the development of acceptable explanations that satisfy the teller as well as the listener.

reaction-formation (overcompensation) The process of keeping unacceptable feelings or behaviors out of awareness by developing the opposite emotion or behavior.

reality principle The ability to delay immediate gratification and modify desires in accordance with the demands of society and external reality. The ego operates according to the reality principle.

reality testing A process by which a person is objectively able to evaluate the external world and adequately distinguish it from the internal world (the self).

receptors Protein molecules located within or on the outer membrane of cells of various tissues, such as neurons, muscle, and blood vessels. A receptor receives chemical stimulation that causes a chemical reaction resulting in either stimulation or inhibition of the activity of the cell.

recovery model Conceptual model of psychiatric illness that stresses hope, living a full and productive life, and eventual recovery.

reframing A technique of changing the viewpoint of a situation and replacing it with another viewpoint that fits the facts equally well but alters the entire meaning.

refugee An immigrant who has left his or her native country to escape intolerable conditions and would have preferred to stay in the original culture.

regression In the face of overwhelming anxiety, the return to an earlier, more comforting (although less mature) way of behaving.

rehabilitation A concept focused on managing patients' deficits and helping them learn to live with their illnesses. Criticized by the consumer movement as being paternalistic and focused on living with disability rather than on quality of life and eventual cure.

Reiki An energy-based therapy in which the practitioner's energy is connected to a universal source (*chi, qi, prana*) and is transferred to a recipient for physical or spiritual healing.

relapse A recurrence of the manifestations of a disease after a period of improvement; in a substance use disorder, the process of becoming dysfunctional in sobriety that ends in a return to chemical use.

relapse prevention Identifying and preventing risky situations that may result in psychological deterioration or substance abuse.

relaxation response A set of physiological changes that result in decreased activity of the sympathetic part of the autonomic nervous system and a shift to the parasympathetic mode, which induces a state of relaxation. It is the opposite of the fight-or-flight response and has a stabilizing effect on the nervous system.

repression The exclusion of unpleasant or unwanted experiences, emotions, or ideas from conscious awareness; considered the first line of psychological defense.

resilience The ability to adapt and cope which helps people to face tragedies, loss, trauma, and severe stress.

respite care Temporary supervision and care of a patient who lives with his or her family. The purpose of respite care is to provide the family with some relief from the demands of the patient's need for continuous care.

restraint See *physical restraint* and *chemical restraint.*

reticular activating system (RAS) The part of the brain stem that mediates alertness, arousal, and motivation; serves to filter out repetitive stimuli to prevent overload.

reuptake The return of neurotransmitters to the presynaptic cell after communication with receptors on the postsynaptic cell.

right to privacy The legal expectation of privacy concerning the sharing medical information.

right to refuse treatment The right to reject forced treatment. This right takes into consideration the person's right for choice, or autonomy, and beneficence, actions which benefit others.

right to treatment The right to expect appropriate and adequate treatment.

rigid or disengaged boundaries Adherence to the "rules and roles" within a family, no matter what the situation. Rigid boundaries prevent family members from trying out new roles or taking on more mature functions.

ritual A repetitive action that a person must execute over and over until he or she is exhausted or anxiety is decreased; it is often performed to lessen the anxiety triggered by an obsession.

role-playing A technique used in individual, group, or family therapy in which the therapist or a group member acts out the behavior of another member to increase that individual's ability to see a situation from another point of view. This technique helps people practice skills in a safe environment before they try them in real-life situations.

S

SAD PERSONS scale A simple and practical assessment tool to evaluate potentially suicidal patients.

sadism The deriving of sexual pleasure and erotic gratification from the infliction of pain, abuse, or humiliation on another.

safety plan A plan for rapid escape when abuse recurs.

scapegoat A member of a group or family who becomes the target of others' aggression but who may not be the actual cause of their hostility or frustration.

schizoaffective disorder A disorder that includes a mixture of schizophrenic and affective symptoms (i.e., alterations in mood as well as disturbances in thought); it is considered by some to be a severe form of bipolar disorder.

schizoid personality disorder A personality disorder in which there is a serious defect in interpersonal relationships. Characteristics include lack of warmth, aloofness, and indifference to the feelings of others.

schizotypal personality disorder A personality disorder in which strikingly odd characteristics (e.g., magical thinking, derealization, perceptual distortions, rigid ideas) are expressed.

schizophrenia A group of mental disorders characterized by severe disturbance of thought and associative looseness, impaired reality testing (hallucinations, delusions), and limited socialization.

seasonal affective disorder (SAD) A recently studied syndrome that appears to affect mostly women and is characterized by hypersomnia, fatigue, weight gain, irritability, and interpersonal difficulties during the winter months. It has been successfully managed with daily treatments of 2 to 3 hours of bright light.

seclusion The last step in a process to maximize the safety of a patient and others, in which the patient is placed alone in a specially designed room for protection and close observation.

seclusion protocol Proper reporting procedure through the chain of command when a patient is to be secluded.

secondary anxiety Anxiety that is due to physiological abnormalities such as certain medical disorders (e.g., neurological, endocrine, or circulatory) or is secondary to a pervasive psychiatric disorder such as depression.

secondary care Care that establishes intervention during an acute crisis to prevent prolonged anxiety from diminishing personal effectiveness and personality organization.

secondary dementia Dementia that is due to an underlying disease process, such as a metabolic, nutritional, or neurological disorder. Dementia related to acquired immunodeficiency syndrome is an example.

secondary depression A depressive mood syndrome that is caused by a physical illness or another psychiatric disorder or is part of an organic mental disorder; essentially, it is depression secondary to other causes.

secondary gain Those advantages a person realizes from whatever symptoms or relief behaviors he or she employs. These advantages include increased attention from others, avoidance of expected responsibilities, financial gain, and the ability to manipulate others in the environment.

secondary intervention Treatment of an actual suicidal crisis.

secondary prevention Involves early intervention in abusive situations to minimize their disabling or long-term effects.

secondary process In psychoanalytic theory, a process consistent with the reality principle; that is, realistic thinking.

selective inattention The failure to notice or attend to an almost infinite number of more-or-less meaningful details of one's own living that might cause anxiety. A concept articulated by H.S. Sullivan.

selective serotonin reuptake inhibitors (SSRIs) First-line antidepressants that block the reuptake of serotonin, permitting serotonin to act for an extended period at the synaptic binding sites in the brain.

self-care activities See *activities of daily living.*

self-concept A person's image of the self.

self-esteem The individual's feeling that he or she has worth or value.

self-help group   A group of people with similar problems or concerns who meet to receive peer support and encouragement and work together using their strengths to gain control over their lives.

self-mutilation   The act of self-induced pain or injury without the intent to kill oneself.

serious mental illness (SMI)   Mental disorders that interfere with some area of social functioning.

sex reassignment surgery   A surgical procedure that reshapes sexual organs from one gender to another.

sexual abuse   Any form of sexual contact or exposure without consent or in circumstances in which the victim is incapable of giving consent.

sexual assault/rape   Forced and violent vaginal, anal, or oral penetration against an adult victim's will and without the victim's consent. Legal definitions vary from state to state.

sexual assault nurse examiner (SANE)   The first specialized forensic role for nurses, SANEs are forensic nurse generalists who receive training in the care of adult and pediatric victims of sexual assault.

sexual disorders   Psychiatric disorders in which sexual problems are considered to be socially atypical, have the potential to disrupt meaningful relationships, and may result in insult or even significant injury to other people.

sexual dysfunction   A disturbance in the desire, excitement, or orgasm phases of the sexual response cycle or pain during sexual intercourse.

shelters or safe houses   Temporary residences that serve as refuges for abused spouses.

situational crisis   A crisis arising from an external as opposed to an internal source. Most people experience situational crises to some extent during the course of their lives (e.g., the death of a loved one, marriage, divorce, or a change in health status).

sleep architecture   The structural organization of NREM and REM sleep.

sleep continuity   The distribution of sleep and wakefulness across the sleep period.

sleep deprivation   A state that occurs from a discrepancy between hours of sleep obtained and hours of sleep required for optimal functioning.

sleep efficiency   Ratio of sleep duration to time spent in bed.

sleep fragmentation   Disruption of sleep stages as indicated by excessive amounts of stage 1 sleep, multiple brief arousals, and frequent shifts in sleep staging.

sleep hygiene   Conditions and practices that promote continuous and effective sleep.

sleep latency   The time it takes to go to sleep.

sleep restriction   Limiting the total sleep time, which creates a temporary, mild state of sleep deprivation and strengthens the sleep homeostatic drive.

social phobia   A phobia of an interpersonal nature, such as fear of public speaking, fear of eating in front of others, or fear of writing or performing in public.

social relationship   A relationship that is primarily initiated for the purpose of friendship, socialization, enjoyment, or accomplishment of a task.

social skills training   Training that uses the principles of guidance, demonstration, practice, and feedback to enhance a patient's skills in community living. Training focuses on skills such as introducing oneself, starting and ending a conversation, asking for assistance, and other simple yet essential social interactions; it is often helpful in combating the negative symptoms of schizophrenia.

sociocultural context   The culture that a person lives in, which includes the people and environment with whom the person interacts.

somatic therapy   Treatment that involves the body, such as the use of medications or electroconvulsive therapy.

somatization   The expression of psychological stress through physical symptoms.

somatization disorder   A psychiatric problem in which a person chronically and persistently complains of multiple physical problems that have no physical origin and interfere with day-to-day functioning.

somatoform disorders   Psychiatric disorders in which the patient's physical symptoms suggest a physical disorder for which there is no demonstrable cause and a strong presumption that the symptoms are linked to psychobiological factors exists.

specific phobias   Fear and avoidance of a single object, situation, or activity; very common in the general population.

spirituality   The devotion or receptiveness to religious or moral values. Spirituality includes a search for meaning and purpose; a relationship with a higher being; and adherence to transcendent values such as hope, love, forgiveness. It is frequently experienced through a formal faith tradition.

splitting   A primitive defense mechanism in which the person sees self or others as all good or all bad, failing to integrate the positive and negative qualities of the self and others into a cohesive whole.

spousal (or marital) rape   A rape in which the perpetrator (nearly always the male) is married to the person raped.

stereotyping   The assumption that all people in a similar cultural, racial, or ethnic group think and act alike.

stereotyped behavior   A motor pattern that originally had meaning to the person (e.g., sweeping the floor or washing windows) but has become mechanical and lacks purpose.

stigma   Negative attitudes or behaviors toward a person or group, based on a belief that they possess negative traits.

stimulus control   Adherence to five basic principles that decrease the negative associations between the bed and bedroom and strengthen the stimulus for sleep.

stress   A physical, emotional, or psychological demand that can lead to growth or overwhelm the ability to cope and lead health problems.

stressors Psychological or physical stimuli that are incompatible with current functioning and require adaptation.

stupor A state in which a person is dazed and awareness of his or her environment appears deadened. For example, a person may sit motionless for long periods of time and in extreme cases may appear to be in a coma.

subconscious Experiences, thoughts, feelings, and desires that are not in immediate awareness but can be recalled to consciousness; often called the *preconscious*. The subconscious mind helps repress unpleasant thoughts or feelings.

sublimation The unconscious process of substituting constructive and socially acceptable activities for strong impulses that are not acceptable in their original form, such as strong aggressive or sexual drives.

substance-abuse intervention A meeting in which the significant others of a person with an addiction point out current problems and offer treatment alternatives.

suicidal ideation Thoughts a person has regarding killing himself or herself.

suicide The ultimate act of self-destruction in which a person purposefully ends his or her own life.

suicide attempt Any willful, self-inflicted, life-threatening attempt at suicide that did not lead to death.

suicide gesture A suicide attempt that is planned to be discovered and is made for the purpose of influencing or manipulating others.

sundowning Increasing destabilization of cognitive abilities (e.g., confusion) and lability of mood during the late afternoon, early evening, or night. Seen in people with cognitive disorders.

superego One of three psychological processes that make up the Freudian system of personality (id, ego, and superego). The superego is the internal representative of the values, ideals, and moral standards of society. The superego is said to be the moral arm of the personality.

support group A group that uses a variety of modalities to help people cope with overwhelming situations or alter unwanted behaviors during stressful periods.

supported employment Work and training in supportive settings for people with disabilities that helps them to become active workforce members.

supportive psychotherapy Psychotherapy that focuses on supporting the patient at the current stage of illness rather than confronting possible problems and pushing the patient towards change.

suppression The conscious removal from awareness of disturbing situations or feelings; the only defense mechanism that operates on a conscious level.

survivor A term often used instead of *victim* because of its positive and assertive associations with recovery and healing.

symbolization The process by which one object or idea comes to represent another. For example, the nurse's keys on a locked unit may represent power and autonomy, or a fancy house may represent prestige and power.

synapse The gap between the membrane of one neuron and the membrane of another neuron. The synapse is the point at which the transmission of the nerve impulse occurs.

synesthesia A condition in which the stimulation of one sense also gives rise to a subjective sensation in another sense, such as hearing colors or seeing sounds; the phenomenon may be experienced by people taking hallucinogenic drugs.

T

tangentiality A disturbance in associative thinking in which the speaker goes off the topic. When it happens frequently and the speaker does not return to the topic, interpersonal communication is destroyed.

Tarasoff **decision** A California court decision that imposes a duty on the therapist to warn the appropriate person or persons when the therapist becomes aware that a patient presents a risk of harm to a specific person or persons.

tardive dyskinesia A serious and irreversible side effect of the phenothiazines and related drugs; consists of involuntary tonic muscle spasms typically involving the tongue, fingers, toes, neck, trunk, or pelvis.

temperament The style of behavior a child habitually uses to cope with the demands and expectations of the environment.

temporary admission Admitting patients with acute psychiatric symptoms on an emergency basis upon written order of a primary care provider for a limited amount of time.

termination phase The final, integral phase of the nurse-patient relationship.

tertiary care Care that provides support for those who have experienced a severe crisis and are now recovering from a disabling mental state.

tertiary intervention Also known as *postvention*, interventions with the family and friends of a person who has committed suicide.

tertiary prevention Involves nurses facilitating the healing and rehabilitative process by counseling individuals and families, providing support for groups of survivors, and assisting survivors of violence to achieve their optimal level of safety, health, and well-being.

therapeutic communication techniques Responses that maximize nurse-patient interactions.

therapeutic communities A group approach to treatment where patients and therapists live together in an environment based on the concepts of therapeutic milieus.

therapeutic encounter A brief, informal meeting between nurse and patient in which the relationship is useful and important for the patient.

therapeutic factors Aspects of the group experience that leaders and members have identified as facilitating therapeutic change.

therapeutic games Games the nurse can play with a child to facilitate the development of a therapeutic relationship and provide opportunity for conversation.

therapeutic index The ratio of the therapeutic dose of a drug and the toxic dose of a drug.

therapeutic relationship A relationship requiring that the nurse maximize his or her communication skills, understanding of human behaviors, and personal strengths in order to enhance personal growth in the patient. This relationship occurs in all clinical settings, not just those on a psychiatric unit.

therapeutic touch An energy therapy in which the practitioner focuses completely on the person receiving the treatment, assesses the energy field, clears and balances the energy field through hand movements, and/or directs energy in a specific region of the body.

therapeutic use of self Creative use of unique personality traits and talents to form positive bonds with others.

time-out The removal or disengagement of an individual (especially a child) from a situation so that the person can regain self-control.

token economy A behavioral approach to eliciting desired behaviors that involves application of the principles and procedures of operant conditioning; it is generally used in the management of a social setting such as a ward, classroom, or halfway house. Targeted behaviors are awarded tokens that can be exchanged for desired goods or privileges.

tolerance The physiological decrease in reaction to a drug with repeated administrations of the same dose.

tort A civil wrong for which money damages (or other relief) may be obtained by the injured party (plaintiff) from the wrongdoer (defendant).

transcranial magnetic stimulation (TMS) A noninvasive treatment modality that uses MRI-strength magnetic pulses to stimulate focal areas of the cerebral cortex.

transference The experiencing of thoughts and feelings toward a person (often the therapist) that were originally held toward a significant person in one's past. Transference is a valuable tool used by therapists in psychoanalytical psychotherapy.

transinstitutionalization The shifting of a person or population from one form of institution to another, such as from state hospitals to jails, prisons, nursing homes, or shelters.

transsexual A person who has an early and persistent feeling that he or she is trapped in a body with the wrong genitals. The individual believes that he or she is, and was always meant to be, of the opposite sex.

transsexualism The most extreme form of gender dysphoria, in which a person wishes to change his or her anatomical sexual characteristics to those of the opposite sex.

trauma-informed care An older, recently reintroduced concept of providing care based on the notion that disruptive psychiatric patients often have histories that include violence and victimization.

triangle See *family triangle.*

tricyclic antidepressants Drugs that inhibit the reuptake of norepinephrine and serotonin by the presynaptic neurons in the CNS, increasing the amount of time norepinephrine and serotonin are available to the postsynaptic receptors.

U

unconditional release Termination of a patient-institutional relationship.

unconscious The repressed memories, feelings, thoughts, or wishes that are not available to the conscious mind. Usually, these unconscious memories, feelings, thoughts, or wishes are associated with intense anxiety and can greatly affect an individual's behavior.

undoing An act or behavior unconsciously designed to make up for or negate a previous act or behavior (e.g., bringing the boss a present after talking about the boss unfavorably to co-workers).

unintentional torts Unintended acts against another person that produce injury or harm.

V

vaginismus Spasm of the vagina which leads to pain, burning, discomfort, and the inability to engage in sexual intercourse.

vagus nerve stimulation Originally used as a treatment for epilepsy, a pacemaker-like device is implanted surgically into the left chest wall from which a thin, flexible wire is threaded up and wrapped around the vagus nerve on the left side of the neck. Electrical stimulation of the vagus nerve is thought to boost the level of neurotransmitters, improving mood and the action of antidepressants.

validate See *consensual validation.*

validation therapy A therapeutic modality that is typically used for older adults and focuses on emotional themes rather than content.

values Abstract standards that represent an ideal, either positive or negative.

values clarification A process of self-discovery in which a person explores and determines his or her personal values and identifies what priority these values hold in personal decision making. This process can lead to increased awareness of why the person behaves in certain ways.

vegetative signs of depression Significant changes from normal functioning in those activities necessary to support physical life and growth, such as eating, sleeping, elimination, and sex, during a depressive episode.

verbal communication All of the words a person speaks.

violence An objectionable act that involves intentional use of force that results in, or has the potential to result in, injury to another person.

vocational rehabilitation State agencies that emphasized extensive prevocational training and employment in sheltered workshops before placement in competitive jobs; success of this type of program was low.

voluntary admission Inpatient care sought by the patient or the patient's guardian through a written application to the facility.

voyeurism An illegal activity that involves seeking sexual arousal through viewing, usually secretly, other people in intimate situations.

vulnerable person The family member upon whom abuse is perpetrated.

W

waxy flexibility Excessive maintenance of posture; for example, after the arms or legs are placed in a certain position, the individual holds that same position for hours.

withdrawal The negative physiological and psychological reactions that occur when a drug taken for a long period of time is reduced in dosage or no longer taken.

word salad A mixture of words meaningless to the listener and to the speaker as well.

working phase The phase of the nurse-patient relationship during which the nurse and patient identify and explore areas that are causing problems in the patient's life.

worldview A system for thinking about how the world works and how people should behave in it and in relationships with one another.

writ of habeas corpus A "formal written order" to "free the person."

Index

A

Abandonment, 132
Abilify. See Aripiprazole (Abilify).
Abnormal Involuntary Movement Scale (AIMS), 68, 331, 332*f*
Abnormal movements
  medication-induced, 328–331, 329*t*, 791
  rating scales for, 146*t*
Abuse, 584. See also Child abuse; Sexual assault.
  abuse protection support for, 600*b*
  advanced practice interventions for, 602–603
  assessment of, 589–596
    general, 589–591
    guidelines for, 595*b*
    during home visit, 594*b*
    interview guidelines for, 590–591, 590*b*
    key areas for, 590, 590*b*, 591–595
    older adults and, 667–668
    presenting problems in, 592*b*
    records for, 595
    screening tool for, 591*f*
    self-, 595–596, 596*t*
  case management for, 600–601
  case study and nursing care plan for, 604*b*
  comorbidity with, 587
  counseling for, 598–600
  cycle of violence in, 585, 586*f*
  epidemiology of, 585–587, 586*t*, 587*t*
  etiology of, 587–589
  evaluation of, 603–606
  group psychotherapy for, 603
  health teaching and promotion for, 601
  human rights, 702–703
  implementation for, 597–603
  milieu management for, 601
  myth vs. fact about, 593*t*
  nursing diagnosis for, 596–597, 596*t*
  outcomes identification for, 597, 597*t*
  personalized safety guide for, 599*b*
  planning for, 597
  prevention of, 601–602
  problems related to, 791
  reporting, 127–128, 127*b*, 131, 597–598, 598*b*
  self-care activities for, 601
  types of, 584–585
  verbal, 578, 579*b*
Abuse protection support, 600–601, 600*b*
Acamprosate (Campral), 425
Acceptance of dying, 708, 716
Accepting statement, 181*t*
Accountability, 158
Acculturation, 111
Acetaminophen, 661
Acetylcholine (ACh), 50*t*, 51, 52*b*
  antidepressant drugs and, 63*f*, 64
  antipsychotic drugs and, 68–69
  depression and, 251
Acetylcholinesterase, 51, 52*b*
Acquaintance (or date) rape, 611, 611*t*
Actigraphy, 465
Active listening, 179–180, 720
Active participation, 169
Activity theory of aging, 665
Acupoints, 779
Acupuncture, 772–773, 779

Acute care, 76–77
  anger or aggression in, 577–579, 577*b*, 579*b*
  for child/adolescent disorders, 630–631
  community vs., 90, 91*t*
  for eating disorders, 352, 356–357
  entry to, 78
  funding for, 77–78
  multidisciplinary team in, 79–80, 79*b*, 80*b*
  nursing care in, 80–85
  nursing diagnoses, outcomes, and interventions for, 81*t*
  for older adults, 668–669
  patient rights for, 78–79, 79*b*
Acute dystonia, 328, 329*t*
Acute phase
  of bipolar disorder, 288, 289, 290, 291*t*
  of depression, 259
  of rape-trauma syndrome, 612–613, 612*b*
  of schizophrenia, 311–312, 320, 321–322, 321*t*
Acute stress disorder, 223–224, 223*b*, 223*f*
Adapin. See Doxepin (Adapin, Sinequan).
Adderall, 71, 644*t*
Addiction, 407
  relapse and, 409–410
  theories of, 407–408
Adherence to treatment
  in acute care, 83
  bipolar disorder and, 290, 299
  in community, 92
  depression and, 696–698
  interventions to improve, 681*b*
  serious mental illness and, 681–682, 689
Adjustment disorders, 649, 791
Administration, nursing role in, 90*t*
Administration on Aging, 673
Admission, 120–122
  involuntary, 78, 78*b*, 120, 124, 689
  nursing diagnoses, outcomes, and interventions during, 81*t*
  procedures for, 78–79
Admission assessment, 80–81, 663
Admission criteria, 76–77, 78
Adolescent-onset conduct disorder, 642
Adolescents. See also Children.
  abuse of, 587, 588, 589
  antidepressant drugs and, 268–269, 554
  assessment of, 140–141, 141*b*
  brain development in, 628–629
  depression in, 249, 255
  disorders of, 626–627, 784
    epidemiology of, 627
    etiology of, 628–630
    nursing care for, 630–637
  hostility toward gay, lesbian, and bisexual, 631*b*
  mentally healthy, 631, 632*b*
  pregnancy and birth trauma in, 226*b*
  psychosocial crises of, 29*t*
  suicide risk among, 549, 551, 551*b*
  violence among, 628, 629*b*
  yoga for, 648*b*
Adrenal glands, 47
Adrenalin, 197
Adult day care, 673

Adults. See also Older adults.
  abuse of dependent or disabled, 127–128
  psychosocial crises of, 29*t*
  serious mental illness in, 678–679, 678*b*
Advance directives, 663–665, 663*b*
  for dying patient, 707–708
  nursing role for, 663*b*, 664–665
  rights regarding, 124
  for serious mental illness, 687
Advanced practice forensic nurse, 726–727, 728
Advanced practice interventions, 18*t*, 139*f*
  for abuse, 602–603
  for anorexia nervosa, 353–354, 354*b*
  for anxiety disorders, 238–239
  for bipolar disorder, 299
  for bulimia nervosa, 357, 357*b*
  in community settings, 90*t*
  for depression, 260–269
  for dissociative disorders, 521–523
  for family therapy, 762–763
  for older adults, 669–670
  for personality disorders, 455, 455*f*
  for schizophrenia, 336–337
  for sexual assault, 618–619
  for sexual disorders, 498–499
  for sexual dysfunction, 490*t*, 491–492, 492*b*
  for sleep disorders, 476–477
  for somatoform disorders, 512, 513*t*
  standards for, 151
  for substance abuse, 427
  for suicidal patient, 559
Advanced practice registered nurse–psychiatric mental health (APRN-PMH), 19, 80
  child/adolescent care by, 631
  forensic, 726–727, 728
  group leadership by, 741–742, 743–746
Adventitious crisis, 532
Advice, giving, 184*t*, 186
Advocacy, patient, 20–21
Affect
  depression and, 254
  schizophrenia and, 307, 314, 317, 317*t*
Affection, additional, 646
Affective symptoms of schizophrenia, 312, 313*f*, 318
African Americans
  depression and, 654*b*
  preventing violence among, 629*b*
  suicide among, 551–552
Age
  assessment and, 140–141
  suicide risk and, 548, 549, 655*f*
Ageism, 662–663, 665
Aggression, 565. See also Violence.
  assessment of, 568–570, 568*b*, 569*b*
  case management for, 572–573
  clinical picture of, 565–566
  cognitive deficits and, 579–580, 580*b*
  comorbidity with, 566
  conduct disorder and, 642
  de-escalation techniques for, 572, 572*b*
  epidemiology of, 566
  etiology of, 566–568

Note: Page numbers followed by *f* indicate figures; *t*, tables; and *b*, boxes.

ANSWERS TO CHAPTER REVIEW QUESTIONS

Visit the Evolve website at **http://evolve.elsevier.com/Varcarolis/foundations** for the rationale, relevant step of the nursing process, NCLEX® Client Needs category, cognitive level, and text page reference(s) for each question.

Chapter 1
3
4
1, 2, 5
1
3, 4, 5

Chapter 2
1
4
2
3
4

Chapter 3
1
3
3
2
1

Chapter 4
2
2, 3, 5, 6
1, 2, 3, 5, 6
3
4

Chapter 5
1, 4, 5, 6
4
2
2
1

Chapter 6
3
2
1, 3, 4
1
4

Chapter 7
4
2, 4, 5
2
4
1, 2, 3, 5

Chapter 8
1, 2, 3, 4
1, 2, 5
2
4
1

Chapter 9
3
2
4
1, 2, 5, 6
1

Chapter 10
1
2
3
3, 5
3

Chapter 11
2
3
3
1
4

Chapter 12
3
1, 3, 5
3
1
1, 2, 3, 4, 5, 6

Chapter 13
4
3
2
2
2

Chapter 14
4
1
1
3
1, 3, 5

Chapter 15
2
4, 5
1, 2, 3, 6, 7
2
1, 2

Chapter 16
3
4
1
2
1, 2, 4, 5

Chapter 17
2
2, 3, 5, 6, 7
4
1
4, 5, 6, 7

Chapter 18
2
2
3
3
1

Chapter 19
2
2
4
1, 2, 5
4, 6, 7

Chapter 20
3
2
4
1
3

Chapter 21
2
1
3
1, 2, 3, 4, 6
4

Chapter 22
2
1
3
4
3, 4

Chapter 23
1
4
1
2
4

Chapter 24
1, 2, 3, 4, 5, 6
3
2, 4, 5, 6
1, 3, 4, 6
2, 3, 5

Chapter 25
2
1, 2, 3, 4, 5
1, 3, 4
1
1

Chapter 26
3
1, 3, 6
4
1, 5, 6
2, 3, 5, 6

Chapter 27
1
3
1
2
1, 3, 5

Chapter 28
3
4
1
4
2

Chapter 29
3
2
2
4
3

Chapter 30
3
1, 3, 5
2
4
2, 3, 4, 5, 6

Chapter 31
4
3
2
1
1, 3, 4, 5

Chapter 32
4
2
1
4
1

Chapter 33
3
2
1
3
2

Chapter 34
2
3
1
4
4

Chapter 35
4
3
2
4
4

Chapter 36
3
1
2
1
1, 2, 3, 4, 5

NANDA INTERNATIONAL-APPROVED NURSING DIAGNOSES

Activity intolerance
Activity intolerance, Risk for
Activity planning, Ineffective
Airway clearance, Ineffective
Allergy response, Latex
Allergy response, Risk for latex
Anxiety
Anxiety, Death
Aspiration, Risk for
Attachment, Risk for impaired parent/
  infant/child
Autonomic dysreflexia
Autonomic dysreflexia, Risk for

Behavior, Risk-prone health
Bleeding, Risk for
Body image, Disturbed
Body temperature, Risk for imbalanced
Bowel incontinence
Breastfeeding, Effective
Breastfeeding, Ineffective
Breastfeeding, Interrupted
Breathing pattern, Ineffective

Cardiac output, Decreased
Cardiac perfusion, Risk for decreased
Cardiac tissue perfusion, Risk for
  ineffective
Caregiver role strain
Caregiver role strain, Risk for
Cerebral tissue perfusion, Risk for
  ineffective
Childbearing process, Readiness for
  enhanced
Comfort, Readiness for enhanced
Comfort, Impaired
Communication, Impaired verbal
Communication, Readiness for
  enhanced
Conflict, Decisional
Conflict, Parental role
Confusion, Acute
Confusion, Chronic
Confusion, Risk for acute
Constipation
Constipation, Perceived
Constipation, Risk for
Contamination
Contamination, Risk for
Coping, Compromised family
Coping, Defensive
Coping, Disabled family
Coping, Ineffective
Coping, Ineffective community
Coping, Readiness for enhanced
Coping, Readiness for enhanced
  community
Coping, Readiness for enhanced family

Death syndrome, Risk for sudden infant
Decision making, Readiness for enhanced
Denial, Ineffective
Dentition, Impaired
Development, Risk for delayed
Diarrhea

Dignity, Risk for compromised human
Distress, Moral
Disuse syndrome, Risk for
Diversional activity, Deficient

Electrolyte imbalance, Risk for
Energy field, Disturbed
Environmental interpretation
  syndrome, Impaired

Failure to thrive, Adult
Falls, Risk for
Family processes: alcoholism,
  Dysfunctional
Family processes, Interrupted
Family processes, Readiness for
  enhanced
Fatigue
Fear
Fluid balance, Readiness for
  enhanced
Fluid volume, Deficient
Fluid volume, Excess
Fluid volume, Risk for deficient
Fluid volume, Risk for imbalanced

Gas exchange, Impaired
Gastrointestinal motility, Dysfunctional
Gastrointestinal motility, Risk for
  dysfunctional
Gastrointestinal tissue perfusion, Risk
  for ineffective
Glucose level, Risk for unstable
Grieving
Grieving, Complicated
Grieving, Risk for complicated
Growth and development, Delayed

Health maintenance, Ineffective
Health management, Ineffective self
Health management, Readiness for
  enhanced self
Health-seeking behaviors
Home maintenance, Impaired
Hope, Readiness for enhanced
Hopelessness
Hyperthermia
Hypothermia

Identity, Disturbed personal
Immunization status, Readiness for
  enhanced
Incontinence, Functional urinary
Incontinence, Overflow urinary
Incontinence, Reflex urinary
Incontinence, Stress urinary
Incontinence, Total urinary*
Incontinence, Urge urinary
Incontinence, Risk for urge urinary
Infant behavior, Disorganized
Infant behavior, Risk for disorganized
Infant behavior, Readiness for
  enhanced organized
Infant feeding pattern, Ineffective
Infection, Risk for

Injury, Risk for
Injury, Risk for perioperative-positioning
Insomnia
Intracranial adaptive capacity, Decreased

Jaundice, Neonatal

Knowledge, Deficient
Knowledge, Readiness for enhanced

Lifestyle, Sedentary
Liver function, Risk for impaired
Loneliness, Risk for

Maternal/Fetal dyad, Risk for
  disturbed
Memory, Impaired
Mobility, Impaired bed
Mobility, Impaired physical
Mobility, Impaired wheelchair

Nausea
Neglect, Self
Neglect, Unilateral
Noncompliance
Nutrition: less than body
  requirements, Imbalanced
Nutrition: more than body
  requirements, Imbalanced
Nutrition, Readiness for enhanced
Nutrition: more than body
  requirements, Risk for imbalanced

Oral mucous membrane, Impaired

Pain, Acute
Pain, Chronic
Parenting, Readiness for enhanced
Parenting, Impaired
Parenting, Risk for impaired
Peripheral neurovascular dysfunction,
  Risk for
Peripheral tissue perfusion,
  Ineffective
Poisoning, Risk for
Post-trauma syndrome
Post-trauma syndrome, Risk for
Power, Readiness for enhanced
Powerlessness
Powerlessness, Risk for
Protection, Ineffective

Rape-trauma syndrome
Rape-trauma syndrome: compound
  reaction*
Rape-trauma syndrome: silent
  reaction*
Relationship, Readiness for enhanced
Religiosity, Impaired
Religiosity, Readiness for enhanced
Religiosity, Risk for impaired
Relocation stress syndrome
Relocation stress syndrome, Risk for
Renal perfusion, Risk for ineffective
Resilience, Impaired individual

Resilience, Readiness for enhanced
Resilience, Risk for compromised
Role performance, Ineffective

Self-care, Readiness for enhanced
Self-care deficit, Bathing/hygiene
Self-care deficit, Dressing/grooming
Self-care deficit, Feeding
Self-care deficit, Toileting
Self-concept, Readiness for enhanced
Self-esteem, Chronic low
Self-esteem, Situational low
Self-esteem, Risk for situational low
Self-mutilation
Self-mutilation, Risk for
Sensory perception, Disturbed
Sexual dysfunction
Sexuality pattern, Ineffective
Shock, Risk for
Skin integrity, Impaired
Skin integrity, Risk for impaired
Sleep deprivation
Sleep, Readiness for enhanced
Sleep pattern, Disturbed
Social isolation
Social interaction, Impaired
Sorrow, Chronic
Spiritual distress
Spiritual distress, Risk for
Spiritual well-being, Readiness for
  enhanced
Stress overload
Suffocation, Risk for
Suicide, Risk for
Surgical recovery, Delayed
Swallowing, Impaired

Therapeutic regimen management,
  Effective*
Therapeutic regimen management,
  Ineffective community*
Therapeutic regimen management,
  Ineffective family
Thermoregulation, Ineffective
Thermoregulation, Ineffective
Thought processes, Disturbed*
Tissue integrity, Impaired
Tissue perfusion, Ineffective
Transfer ability, Impaired
Trauma, Risk for

Urinary elimination, Impaired
Urinary elimination, Readiness for
  enhanced
Urinary retention

Vascular trauma, Risk for
Ventilation, Impaired spontaneous
Ventilatory weaning response,
  Dysfunctional
Violence, Risk for other-directed
Violence, Risk for self-directed

Walking, Impaired
Wandering